Jane Kitchen

WHAT THE EXPERTS ARE SAYING ABOUT
THE PDR® POCKET GUIDE
TO PRESCRIPTION DRUGS™

"The premier professional drug reference now gives
consumers their best guide to medical problems and
the medications prescribed for them. . . . Clear,
readable, comprehensive."

> —Barrie R. Cassileth, Ph.D., adjunct professor,
> University of North Carolina and
> Duke University Medical Center

"A must for every household where there are concerns about the safe use of medications. It is an
ideal way to clarify and supplement the information provided by your health care provider."

> —Jack M. Rosenberg, Pharm.D., Ph.D.,
> professor of clinical pharmacy and pharmacology and
> director of the Division of Pharmacy Practice,
> Arnold & Marie Schwartz College Pharmacy
> and Health Sciences, Long Island University

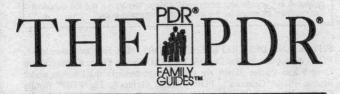

THE PDR PDR FAMILY GUIDES™

POCKET GUIDE

TO PRESCRIPTION DRUGS™

FOURTH EDITION
REVISED AND UPDATED

Based on Physicians' Desk Reference®,
the Nation's Leading Professional Drug Handbook

POCKET BOOKS
New York   London   Toronto   Sydney   Singapore

PHYSICIANS' DESK REFERENCE®, PDR®, PDR For Ophthalmology®, PDR For Nonprescription Drugs®, The PDR® Family Guide to Prescription Drugs® and Pocket PDR® are registered trademarks used herein under license. PDR® Generics™, PDR® Family Guides™, The PDR® Family Guide to Women's Health and Prescription Drugs™, The PDR® Family Guide to Nutrition and Health™, The PDR® Family Guide to Over-The-Counter Drugs™, The PDR® Family Guide Encyclopedia of Medical Care™, PDR Companion Guide™, PDR® Medical Dictionary™, PDR® Nurse's Dictionary™, PDR® Nurse's Handbook™, PDR® Electronic Library™, and PDR® Drug Interactions, Side Effects, Indications, Contraindications System™ are trademarks used herein under license.

Officers of Medical Economics Company: *President and Chief Executive Officer:* Curtis B. Allen; *Vice President, New Media:* L. Suzanne BeDell; *Vice President, Corporate Human Resources:* Pamela M. Bilash; *Vice President and Chief Information Officer:* Steven M. Bressler; *Chief Financial Officer:* Christopher Caridi; *Vice President, Finance:* Claudia Flowers; *Vice President and Controller:* Barry Gray; *Vice President, New Business Planning:* Linda G. Hope; *Vice President, Business Integration:* David A. Pitler; *Vice President, Healthcare Publishing Business Management:* Donna Santarpia; *Senior Vice President, Directory Services:* Paul Walsh; *Senior Vice President, Operations:* John R. Ware; *Senior Vice President, Internet Strategies:* Raymond Zoeller

POCKET BOOKS, a division of Simon & Schuster Inc.
1230 Avenue of the Americas, New York, NY 10020

ISBN: 0-671-78643-1

First Pocket Books printing of this revised fourth edition May 2000

10 9 8 7 6 5 4 3 2 1

POCKET and colophon are registered trademarks of Simon & Schuster Inc.

Front cover photograph by Jeffrey Sylvester/FPG International

Printed in the U.S.A.

Publisher's Note

The drug information contained in this book is based on product labeling published in the 1999 edition of *Physicians' Desk Reference®*, supplemented with facts from other sources the publisher believes reliable. While diligent efforts have been made to assure the accuracy of this information, the book does not list every possible action, adverse reaction, interaction, and precaution; and all information is presented without guarantees by the authors, consultants, and publisher, who disclaim all liability in connection with its use.

This book is intended only as a reference for use in an ongoing partnership between doctor and patient in the vigilant management of the patient's health. It is not a substitute for a doctor's professional judgment, and serves only as a reminder of concerns that may need discussion. All readers are urged to consult with a physician before beginning or discontinuing use of any prescription drug or undertaking any form of self-treatment.

Brand names listed in this book are intended to represent only the more commonly used products. Inclusion of a brand name does not signify endorsement of the product; absence of a name does not imply a criticism or rejection of the product. The publisher is not advocating the use of any product described in this book, does not warrant or guarantee any of these products, and has not performed any independent analysis in connection with the product information contained herein.

Contents

Contents

The PDR® Pocket Guide to Prescription Drugs based on the seventh edition of The PDR® Family Guide to Prescription Drugs®

Contributors and Consultants

Editor-in-Chief: David W. Sifton
Director of New Business Development and Professional Services: Mukesh Mehta, R Ph
Art Director: Robert Hartman

Managing Pharmaceutical Editor: Maria Deutsch, MS, R Ph, CDE

Writers: Nancy K. Bannon; Kathleen Rodgers, R Ph

Assistant Editors: Paula Benus; Gwynned L. Kelly; Ann Marevis

Illustrations: Christopher Wikoff, MAMS

Editorial Production: *Director of Production:* Carrie Williams; *Manager of Production:* Kimberly H. Vivas; *Senior Production Coordinator:* Amy B. Brooks; *Senior Digital Imaging Coordinator:* Shawn W. Cahill; *Digital Imaging Coordinator:* Frank J. McElroy, III; *Electronic Publishing Designer:* Robert K. Grossman

Medical Economics Company

Senior Vice President, Directory Services: Paul Walsh

Director of Product Management: Mark A. Friedman

Associate Product Manager: Bill Shaughnessy

Director of Sales: Dikran N. Barsamian

National Sales Manager, Medical Economics Trade Sales: Bill Gaffney

Promotion Manager: Donna L. Doyle

Board of Medical Consultants

Gary D. Koenig, MD
Florissant, MO

Mitchell R. Lester, MD
James F. Murray Fellow, Pediatric Allergy and
Immunology
National Jewish Center for Immunology and Respiratory
Medicine, Denver, CO

Younghee Limb, MD
Assistant Professor of Internal Medicine
State University of New York, Stony Brook, NY

Gardiner Morse, MS
Executive Editor, AIDS Clinical Care, Waltham, MA

Louis V. Napolitano, MD
Senior Attending Physician
Hackensack Medical Center, Hackensack, NJ

Mark D. Ravenscraft, MD
Medical Director, Renal Transplantation
St. John's Mercy Medical Center, St. Louis, MO

Martin I. Resnick, MD
Professor and Chairman, Department of Urology
Case Western Reserve University, Cleveland, OH

Frank Simo, MD
Assistant Clinical Professor, Department of
Otolaryngology
St. Louis University, St. Louis, MO

Karl Singer, MD
Exeter Family Medicine Associates, Exeter, NH

Eugene W. Sweeney, MD
Assistant Clinical Professor of Dermatology
Columbia College of Physicians and Surgeons,
New York, NY

Guy D. Eslick, MD,
Princeton, NJ

Mitchell R. Lester, MD
Fellow in Allergy and
Immunology
National Jewish Center for Immunology and Respiratory
Medicine, Denver, CO

Gregory Lamb, MD
Assistant Professor of Internal Medicine
State University of New York, Stony Brook, NY

Carolyn Nurse, MS
Executive Editor, AIDS Clinical Care, Waltham, MA

Louis V. Napolitano, MD
Senior Attending Physician
Hackensack Medical Center, Hackensack, NJ

Mary D. Rheeseman, MD
Medical Director, Renal Transplantation
St. John's Mercy Medical Center, St. Louis, MO

Marshall Remtel, MD
Professor and Chairman, Department of Urology
Case Western Reserve University, Cleveland, OH

Frank Simon, MD
Assistant Clinical Professor, Department of
Otolaryngology
St. Louis University, St. Louis, MO

Kim Siegel, MD
Exeter Family Medicine Associates, Exeter, NH

Duncan W. Sweeney, MD
Assistant Clinical Professor of Dermatology
Columbia College of Physicians and Surgeons
New York, NY

Foreword

Like its predecessors, this new edition of *The PDR Pocket Guide to Prescription Drugs* strives to make the many benefits of modern pharmaceuticals—as well as their undeniable risks—as clear and simple as can be. Unlike other books in the field, *The PDR Pocket Guide* discloses all important side effects specifically attributed to the drug by the manufacturer, no matter how rare. As a safeguard against error, it also provides you with full information on standard dosage recommendations. It tells exactly what to do when you miss a dose of your medication, while alerting you to the warning signs of an overdose. And to help you find all these facts as quickly as possible, it lists each medication under its familiar brand name—with a cross-reference in case the drug is dispensed generically.

Still, despite the depth and detail of the information you'll find here, *The PDR Pocket Guide* is not a replacement for your doctor's advice. Instead, it serves as a reminder of the basic instructions and caveats that all too often are forgotten by the time a patient leaves the doctor's office, as well as providing you with a checklist of the problems and conditions that you must be certain the doctor knows about—facts that might call for a change in your prescription.

In this way, the book is designed to serve as an aid in an ongoing dialogue between you and your doctor—a collaboration that's necessary for any treatment to work. Just as the doctor must tell you how and why to use a particular drug, you must tell the doctor how it affects you, reporting any reactions or drug interactions you suspect you may have. And while it's up to the doctor to devise your treatment strategy, it's up to you to make sure that the right doses are administered at the right times, and that the prescribed course of therapy is completed as planned.

Physicians' Desk Reference has been providing doctors with the information needed for safe, effective drug therapy for over 50 years. Designed especially for healthcare professionals, it presents the facts in a detailed, technical format approved by the Food and Drug Administration. Now, to make the key facts buried in this wealth of data accessible to everyone, *The PDR Pocket Guide* has stripped away the medical shorthand and technical terminology, and presented the core of this information in a simple, standard format designed for maximum convenience and ease of use by the consumer.

Almost all the information you'll find in *The PDR Pocket Guide*'s consumer drug profiles has been extracted from PDR itself. When necessary, however, selected facts have been added from other sources—in particular, the databases maintained by PDR's sister company, MICROMEDEX, INC. Generally, this extra information describes uses for a drug that are still awaiting formal FDA approval, or supplies instructions meant specifically for the patient, such as how to make up a missed dose.

Modern drug therapy is a vast and complicated field—so complicated that, for many questions about medicines, the answer varies with each patient. *The PDR Pocket Guide to Prescription Drugs* gives you general guidelines for safe drug use; but only your doctor, evaluating the unique details of your case, can give you the exact instructions best suited for you. The goal of this book is simply to alert you to the most pertinent questions to ask, and to help clarify your doctor's answers—in short, to give you the tools you need to supervise your own medical care as effectively as possible. We wish you good health.

Robert W. Hogan, MD
Chair, Board of Medical Consultants

How to Use This Book

Modern medicines spare us all an incredible amount of suffering. If you doubt it, imagine a world without antibiotics to cure infections, analgesics to alleviate pain, or any of the many drugs we use to ease stiff joints and help weakened hearts.

But today's potent medicines are not without their risks. For certain people, at certain times, some drugs can cause problems. And for all people, misusing a medication is an invitation to trouble. The purpose of this book is to alert you to those times and those conditions which should make you wary, and to help you use all of your medications safely and effectively.

This book is not a substitute for a visit to the doctor. Only a doctor can weigh all the diverse aspects of your condition and choose the treatment most likely to meet your needs. What we hope this book can do, however, is help you sort out the facts and questions that deserve further discussion. Your doctor, after all, can respond only to the problems and concerns you mention. And a seemingly unimportant question could ultimately reveal a crucial aspect of your particular case.

The Drug Profiles

The drug profiles are designed to give you detailed information on the nation's most frequently prescribed prescription drugs, plus a few widely used over-the-counter medications. Though the section covers more than 1,000 products, it is not all-inclusive. If you do not find a profile for a particular prescription you've received, you shouldn't be concerned. There are a number of specialized, yet valuable drugs in current use that have been omitted here due to lack of space.

Most prescription products have two names—a generic chemical name and a manufacturer's brand name. Both are listed alphabetically in this book, with a profile of the drug appearing under the more familiar of the two. In most instances, that means the brand name. In a few cases—such as insulin, for example—the generic name heads the profile. In either case, the drug's other name gives you a cross-reference to the profile.

If there is more than one brand of a drug, you'll usually find the profile under the name that's most frequently prescribed. For example, information on amoxicillin can be found in the profile of Amoxil, the nation's leading brand. Other brands of amoxicillin, such as Trimox and Wymox, are cross-referenced to the Amoxil entry.

The drug profiles begin with correct pronunciation of the name, followed by the other brand and generic names for the drug. The information that follows these names is divided into 10 sections. Here's what you'll find in each.

Why is this drug prescribed?
This section provides an overview of the major diseases and disorders for which the drug is generally given. It names each basic problem, but does not go into technical details. For instance, the information here will confirm that a particular antibiotic is used to fight, say, upper respiratory tract infections. The section does not, however, attempt to list all the specific germs that the antibiotic is capable of eliminating.

Most important fact about this drug
Highlighted here is one key point—out of the dozens found in a typical profile—that is especially worthwhile to remember. We've placed it here for the sake of emphasis. Never regard this section as a definitive summary of the drug.

How should you take this medication?
Some drugs should never be taken with meals. Others must be. This section details such special instructions, including how and when to take the medication, and any dietary restrictions that may apply. Also found here is advice on what to do when you forget a dose, and any special storage requirements that apply.

What side effects may occur?
Shown here are the potential side effects that the manufacturer has listed in the drug's FDA-approved product labeling. Virtually any drug will occasionally cause an unwanted reaction. However, even the most common of these reactions is generally seen in only a small minority of patients. For that reason, presence of a long list of possible side effects does not mean that the drug is unusually dangerous

or trouble-prone. In fact, your odds of experiencing even one of these effects are typically very low. Not listed are the side effects that can be detected only by a physician or analysis in a laboratory.

Why should this drug not be prescribed?

A few drugs are known to be harmful under certain specific conditions, which are detailed here—the most common being hypersensitivity to the drug itself. If you think one of these restrictions applies to you, you should alert your doctor immediately. If you're correct, he or she may decide to use an alternative treatment.

Special warnings about this medication

This cautionary information is presented as a double check. If it includes any problems or conditions that your doctor may be unaware of, be sure to bring them to his or her attention. Chances are that no change in treatment will be called for; but it's worth making sure. In any event, do not take this information as a signal to change your dosage or discontinue the drug without consulting your doctor. Such a change might well do more harm than good.

Possible food and drug interactions
when taking this medication

In this section you'll find a list of specific drugs—and types of drugs—that have been known to interact with the medicine being profiled. Generally, the list includes a few examples of each type. However, it is far from inclusive. If you're not certain whether a medication you're taking falls into one of these categories, be sure to check with your doctor or pharmacist.

Remember, too, that the chances of an interaction—and its intensity if one occurs—vary from person to person. In many cases, the benefits of the two medicines may outweigh the results of an interaction. Don't stop taking either drug without first consulting your doctor.

Special information
if you are pregnant or breastfeeding

Very few medicines have been definitively proved safe for use during pregnancy. On the other hand, only a handful are known to be inevitably harmful. Most drugs fall in-between, in a gray area where no harm has been reported, but neither has safety been conclusively proved. With many of these drugs, the small theoretical risk they pose may be overshadowed by your need for treatment. This section will tell you whether a drug has been confirmed safe, is known to be dangerous, or is part of that large group about which scientists are not really sure.

Recommended dosage

Shown here are excerpts of the dosage guidelines your doctor uses. They generally present a range of doses recommended for typical cases, and sometimes include a recommended maximum. The information is presented as a convenient double check in case you suspect a misunderstanding or a typographical error on your prescription label. It is not useful for determining an exact dosage yourself. The dose that's best for you depends on numerous factors—such as your age, weight, physical condition, and response to the drug—that can be properly evaluated only by your doctor.

Overdosage

As another safety measure, this section lists, when available, the signs of an overdose. If the symptoms listed in this section lead you to suspect an overdose, your best response is to seek emergency medical attention immediately.

Other Features

The book includes several other sections that you'll find useful when faced with certain specific problems.

The Disease and Disorder Index enables you to quickly identify drugs available for a particular medical condition. Arranged alphabetically by ailment, it lists all the medications profiled in the book.

You'll also find the following special sections.

Product Identification Guide

It's wise to keep all your prescription medications in their original bottles or vials. However, if they do somehow get mixed up, you may find this section helpful for sorting them out. It includes actual-size photographs of the leading products discussed in the book, arranged alphabetically by brand name. Manufacturers occasionally change the color and shape of a product, so if a prescription does not match the photo shown here, check with your pharmacist before assuming there's been a mistake.

The Appendices

This section provides you with two important safeguards that every home should always have handy. One is a brief guide to safe medication use. The other—for ready reference in an emergency—is a directory of poison control centers.

The Doctor-Patient Partnership

Although doctors today can often work miracles with advanced technology and sophisticated medicines, they still need the help of the patient to make most treatments work. No matter how potent the medication, it can still prove worthless if you fail to take it properly. Likewise, if you react badly to a drug, or have a condition that makes it dangerous, there is nothing any doctor can do about it unless you report the problem.

This book is offered as an aid in this cooperative effort with your doctor. We hope it suggests the right questions to ask, while allaying any unwarranted concerns you might have. Most of all, we hope it helps in some small way to make all of your treatments as effective as they can possibly be.

and share of a product, so if a prescription does not match the photo above it here, check with your pharmacist before assuming there's been a mistake.

The Appendices

This section provides you with two important appendices that every home should always have handy. One is a brief guide to safe medication use. The other — for ready reference in an emergency — is a directory of poison control centers.

The Doctor-Patient Partnership

Although doctors today can often work miracles with advanced technology and sophisticated medicines, they still need the help of the patient to make most treatments work. No matter how potent the medication, it won't prove worthwhile if you fail to take it properly. Likewise, if you react badly to a drug, or have a condition that makes it dangerous, there is nothing any doctor can do about it unless you report the problem.

This book is offered as an aid in this cooperative effort with your doctor. We hope it reveals the right questions to ask, while allaying any unwarranted concerns you might have. Most of all, we hope it helps us and shall way to make all your treatments as effective as they can possibly be.

Drug Profiles

Generic name:

ACARBOSE

See Precose, page 1029.

Brand name:

ACCOLATE

Pronounced: ACK-o-late
Generic name: Zafirlukast

Why is this drug prescribed?
Accolate helps prevent asthma attacks. It is prescribed for long-term treatment.

Most important fact about this drug
Accolate will not stop an asthma attack once it starts. You will still need to use an airway-opening medication when an attack occurs.

How should you take this medication?
Accolate should be taken twice every day, whether or not you have had any recent asthma attacks. Do not take the medication with food. Allow at least 1 hour to pass before eating, or wait for 2 hours after a meal. You can continue to take Accolate while using another medication to stop an attack.

- *If you miss a dose...*
  Take it as soon as you remember. If it is almost time for your next dose, skip the one you missed and go back to your regular schedule. Do not take 2 doses at once.

- *Storage instructions...*
  Store at room temperature in a dark, dry place.

What side effects may occur?
Side effects cannot be anticipated. If any develop or change in intensity, inform your doctor as soon as possible. Only your doctor can determine if it is safe for you to continue taking Accolate.

- *More common side effects may include:*
  Headache, infection, nausea

- *Less common side effects may include:*
  Accidental injury, abdominal pain, allergic reactions (hives; swelling of the lips, tongue, face, arms, and legs; rash), back pain, diarrhea, dizziness, fever, generalized pain, indigestion, muscle aches, vomiting, weakness

Why should this drug not be prescribed?
If you have had an allergic reaction to Accolate or to any of its ingredients, avoid this drug.

Special warnings about this medication
While taking Accolate, you should not stop—or even cut down on—any other asthma medication you are using unless your doctor recommends it. Remember that Accolate is not an airway-opening medication. You will still need an inhaler to stop an attack.

If you have been taking an oral steroid drug and your doctor does decide to cut back the dosage, there is a remote chance that complications will follow. Inform your doctor of any new symptoms.

Also call your doctor if you develop any of the following: pain in the upper right abdomen, nausea, fatigue, lethargy, itching, flu-like symptoms, or jaundice (yellowing of the skin and eyes). These are signs of a liver problem—a rare side effect of Accolate. If tests show the problem to be serious, you may have to stop using the drug. The symptoms will disappear after you stop taking the drug.

Possible food and drug interactions
when taking this medication
A full stomach can reduce Accolate's effectiveness. Do not take with meals.

If Accolate is taken with certain other drugs, the effects of either could be increased, decreased, or altered. It is especially important to check with your doctor before combining Accolate with the following:

Aspirin (Ecotrin, Genuine Bayer, others)
Astemizole (Hismanal)
Blood-thinning drugs such as Coumadin
Carbamazepine (Tegretol)
Cisapride (Propulsid)
Cyclosporine (Sandimmune, Neoral)
Erythromycin (E.E.S., E-Mycin, others)

Heart and blood pressure medications called calcium channel blockers,
   including Calan, Cardizem, and Procardia
Phenytoin (Dilantin)
Terfenadine (Seldane)
Theophylline (Theo-Dur, others)
Tolbutamide (Orinase)

Special information
if you are pregnant or breastfeeding

Accolate should be taken during pregnancy only if clearly needed. If you are
pregnant or plan to become pregnant, inform your doctor immediately.

Accolate does find its way into breast milk and should not be taken by
nursing mothers.

Recommended dosage

ADULTS AND CHILDREN 12 AND OVER

The usual dose is 1 tablet twice a day.

CHILDREN UNDER 12

Safety and effectiveness have not been studied in this age group.

Overdosage

No overdoses of Accolate have been reported. However, any medication
taken in excess can have serious consequences. If you suspect an overdose,
seek medical attention immediately.

Brand name:

ACCUPRIL

Pronounced: AK-you-prill
Generic name: Quinapril hydrochloride

Why is this drug prescribed?

Accupril is used in the treatment of high blood pressure. It can be taken
alone or in combination with a thiazide type of water pill such as
HydroDIURIL. Accupril is in a family of drugs known as "ACE inhibitors." It
works by preventing a chemical in your blood called angiotensin I from
converting into a more potent form that increases salt and water retention in
your body. Accupril also enhances blood flow throughout your blood vessels.

Along with other drugs, Accupril is also prescribed in the treatment of congestive heart failure.

Most important fact about this drug
You must take Accupril regularly for it to be effective. Since blood pressure declines gradually, it may be several weeks before you get the full benefit of Accupril; and you must continue taking it even if you are feeling well. Accupril does not cure high blood pressure; it merely keeps it under control.

How should you take this medication?
You can take Accupril with or without meals.

Alcohol may increase the effect of Accupril, and could cause dizziness or fainting. Avoid alcoholic beverages until you have checked with your doctor.

Take Accupril exactly as prescribed, and see your doctor regularly to make sure the drug is working properly without unwanted side effects. Do not stop taking this drug without first consulting your doctor.

- *If you miss a dose...*
  Take the forgotten dose as soon as you remember. However, if it is almost time for your next dose, skip the one you missed and go back to your regular schedule. Never try to "catch up" by doubling the dose.

- *Storage instructions...*
  Accupril can be stored at room temperature. Protect from light.

What side effects may occur?
Side effects cannot be anticipated. If any develop or change in intensity, inform your doctor as soon as possible. Only your doctor can determine if it is safe for you to continue taking Accupril.

- *More common side effects may include:*
  Dizziness, headache

- *Less common side effects may include:*
  Abdominal pain, coughing, fatigue, nausea, vomiting

- *Rare side effects may include:*
  Angina (severe chest pain), back pain, bleeding in the stomach or intestines, bronchitis, changes in heart rhythm, constipation, depression, dimmed vision, dizziness when first standing up, dry mouth or throat,

extremely high blood pressure, fainting, hair loss, heart attack, heart failure, hepatitis, high potassium, impotence, increased blood pressure, increased sweating, inflammation of the pancreas, inflammation of the sinuses, insomnia, itching, kidney failure, nervousness, numbness/tingling, palpitations, rapid heartbeat, sensitivity to light, severe allergic reactions, skin peeling, sleepiness, sore throat, stroke, swelling of the mouth and throat, vague feeling of illness, vertigo

Why should this drug not be prescribed?

If you are sensitive to or have ever had an allergic reaction to Accupril or similar drugs, such as Capoten and Vasotec, you should not take this medication. Make sure your doctor is aware of any drug reactions you have experienced.

Special warnings about this medication

If you develop swelling of the face, lips, tongue, or throat, or of your arms and legs, or have difficulty swallowing or breathing, you should contact your doctor immediately. You may need emergency treatment.

You may feel light-headed, especially during the first few days of Accupril therapy. If this occurs, notify your doctor. If you actually faint, stop taking the medication until you have consulted with your doctor.

Vomiting, diarrhea, and heavy perspiration can all deplete your body fluid; and dehydration can cause your blood pressure to drop. If this leads to light-headedness or fainting, you should check with your doctor.

Inform your doctor or dentist that you are taking Accupril before undergoing surgery or anesthesia.

Do not use potassium supplements or salt substitutes containing potassium without consulting your doctor.

If you develop a sore throat or fever, contact your doctor immediately. It could indicate a more serious illness.

If you are taking Accupril, your doctor will do a complete assessment of your kidney function and will watch it closely as long as you are taking this drug.

If you notice a yellow tinge to your skin and the whites of your eyes, stop taking the drug and notify your doctor immediately. This could be a sign of liver damage.

The safety and effectiveness of Accupril in children have not been established.

Possible food and drug interactions
when taking this medication

If Accupril is taken with certain other drugs, the effects of either could be increased, decreased, or altered. It is especially important to check with your doctor before combining Accupril with the following:

Diuretics such as Lasix
Lithium (Eskalith, Lithobid)
Potassium-sparing diuretics such as Aldactone, Dyazide, and Moduretic
Potassium supplements such as Slow-K and K-Dur
Salt substitutes containing potassium
Tetracycline (Sumycin)

Special information
if you are pregnant or breastfeeding

ACE inhibitors such as Accupril have been shown to cause injury and even death to the unborn child when used in pregnancy during the second and third trimesters. If you are pregnant, your doctor should discontinue Accupril as soon as possible. If you plan to become pregnant, make sure your doctor knows you are taking this medication. Accupril appears in breast milk and could affect a nursing infant. If this medication is essential to your health, your doctor may advise you to discontinue breastfeeding until your treatment is finished.

Recommended dosage

HIGH BLOOD PRESSURE

The usual starting dose is 10 or 20 milligrams taken once a day. If you have any problems with your kidneys or if you are also taking a diuretic, your starting dose may be lower. Depending on how your blood pressure responds, your doctor may increase your dose up to a total of 80 milligrams a day taken once a day or divided into two doses.

CONGESTIVE HEART FAILURE

The usual starting dose is 5 milligrams taken twice a day. Your doctor may increase the dose from week to week, up to as much as 20 to 40 milligrams daily, divided into 2 equal doses. If you have kidney problems, the dosage will be lower.

Overdosage

Any medication taken in excess can have serious consequences. If you suspect an overdose, seek medical attention immediately.

A severe drop in blood pressure is the primary sign of an Accupril overdose.

Brand name:

ACCUTANE

Pronounced: ACC-u-tane
Generic name: Isotretinoin

Why is this drug prescribed?

Accutane, a chemical cousin of vitamin A, is prescribed for the treatment of severe, disfiguring cystic acne that has not cleared up in response to milder medications such as antibiotics. It works on the oil glands within the skin, shrinking them and diminishing their output. You take Accutane by mouth every day for several months, then stop. The antiacne effect can last even after you have finished your course of medication.

Most important fact about this drug

Because Accutane can cause severe birth defects, including mental retardation and physical malformations, a woman *must not* become pregnant while taking it. If you are a woman of childbearing age, your doctor will ask you to sign a detailed consent form before you start taking Accutane. If you accidentally become pregnant while taking the medication, you should immediately consult your doctor.

How should you take this medication?

Take Accutane with food. Follow your doctor's instructions carefully.

Depending on your reaction to Accutane, your doctor may need to adjust the dosage upward or downward. If you respond quickly and very well, your doctor may take you off Accutane even before the 15 or 20 weeks are up.

After you finish taking Accutane, there should be at least a 2-month "rest period" during which you are off the drug. This is because your acne may continue to get better even though you are no longer taking the medication. Once the 2 months are up, if your acne is still severe, your doctor may want to give you a second course of Accutane.

Avoid consumption of alcoholic beverages.

Read the patient information leaflet available with the product.

Do not crush the capsules.

■ *If you miss a dose...*
  Take the forgotten dose as soon as you remember. If it is almost time for your next dose, skip the one you missed and go back to your regular schedule. Do not take 2 doses at the same time.

- *Storage instructions...*
  Store at room temperature, away from light.

What side effects may occur?

Side effects cannot be anticipated. If any develop or change in intensity, inform your doctor as soon as possible. Only your doctor can determine if it is safe for you to continue taking Accutane.

- *More common side effects may include:*
  Conjunctivitis ("pinkeye"), dry or fragile skin, dry or cracked lips, dry mouth, dry nose, itching, joint pains, nosebleed

- *Less common side effects may include:*
  Bowel inflammation and pain, chest pain, decreased night vision, decreased tolerance to contact lenses, delay in wound healing, depression, fatigue, headache, nausea, peeling palms or soles, rash, skin infections, stomach and intestinal discomfort, sunburn-sensitive skin, thinning hair, urinary discomfort, vision problems, vomiting

Why should this drug not be prescribed?

You should not take Accutane if you are sensitive to or have ever had an allergic reaction to parabens, the preservative used in the capsules.

If you are a woman of childbearing age, you should not take Accutane if you are pregnant, if you think there is a possibility you might get pregnant during the treatment, or if you are unable to keep coming back to the doctor for monthly checkups, including pregnancy testing.

Special warnings about this medication

When you first start taking Accutane, it is possible that your acne will get worse before it starts to get better.

If you are a woman of childbearing age and you are considering taking Accutane, you will be given both spoken and written warnings about the importance of avoiding pregnancy during the treatment. You will be asked to sign a consent form noting that:

- Accutane is a powerful, "last resort" medication for severe acne;
- You must not take Accutane if you are pregnant or may become pregnant during treatment;
- If you get pregnant while taking Accutane, your baby will be at high risk for birth defects;
- If you take Accutane, you must use 2 effective forms of birth control from 1 month before the start of treatment through 1 month after the end of treatment;

- You must test negative for pregnancy within 1 week before starting Accutane, and you must start Accutane on the second or third day of your menstrual period;
- You may participate in a program that includes an initial free pregnancy test and birth control counseling session;
- If you become pregnant, you must immediately stop taking Accutane and see your doctor;
- You have read and understood the Accutane patient brochure and asked your doctor any questions you had;
- You are not currently pregnant and do not plan to become pregnant for at least 30 days after you finish taking Accutane;
- You have been invited to participate in a survey of women being treated with Accutane.

Accutane may cause depression or other mental problems. In rare cases, it has prompted thoughts of suicide. If you begin to feel depressed or become troubled by suicidal thoughts, contact your doctor immediately.

Some people taking Accutane, including some who simultaneously took tetracycline, have experienced headache, nausea, and visual disturbances caused by increased pressure within the skull. See a doctor immediately if you have these symptoms; if the doctor finds swelling of the optic nerve at the back of your eye, you must stop taking Accutane at once and see a neurologist for further care.

Be careful driving at night. Some people have experienced a sudden decrease in night vision.

Some people taking Accutane have had problems regulating their blood sugar level.

You may not be able to tolerate your contact lenses during and after your therapy with Accutane.

You should stop taking Accutane immediately if you have abdominal pain, bleeding from the rectum, or severe diarrhea. You may have an inflammatory disease of the bowel.

You should not donate blood during your therapy with Accutane and for a month after you stop taking it.

Possible food and drug interactions
when taking this medication

While taking Accutane, do not take vitamin supplements containing vitamin A. Accutane and vitamin A are chemically related; taking them together is like taking an overdose of vitamin A.

Special information
if you are pregnant or breastfeeding

Accutane causes birth defects; do not use it while pregnant. Nursing mothers should not take Accutane because of the possibility of passing the drug on to the baby via breast milk.

Recommended dosage

The recommended dosage range for Accutane is 0.5 to 2 milligrams per 2.2 pounds of body weight, divided into 2 doses daily, for 15 to 20 weeks. The usual starting dose is 0.5 to 1 milligram per 2.2 pounds per day.

People whose disease is very severe or is primarily on the body may have to take up to the maximum recommended dose.

If after a period of 2 months or more off therapy, severe cystic acne persists, your doctor may prescribe a second course of therapy.

Overdosage

Any medication taken in excess can have serious consequences. If you suspect an overdose of Accutane, seek medical attention immediately.

- *Overdosage of Accutane, like overdosage of vitamin A, can cause:*
  Abdominal pain, dizziness, dry or cracked lips, facial flushing, incoordination and clumsiness, headache, vomiting

Generic name:

ACEBUTOLOL

See Sectral, page 1170.

Generic name:

ACETAMINOPHEN

See Tylenol, page 1362.

Generic name:

ACETAMINOPHEN WITH CODEINE

See Tylenol with Codeine, page 1365.

Generic name:

ACETAMINOPHEN WITH OXYCODONE

See Percocet, page 979.

Generic name:

ACETAZOLAMIDE

See Diamox, page 389.

Brand name:

ACHROMYCIN V

See Tetracycline, page 1289.

Brand name:

ACLOVATE

Pronounced: AK-low-vait
Generic name: Alclometasone dipropionate

Why is this drug prescribed?

Aclovate, a synthetic steroid medication of the cortisone family, is spread on the skin to relieve certain types of itchy rashes, including psoriasis.

Most important fact about this drug

When you use Aclovate, you inevitably absorb some of the medication through your skin and into the bloodstream. Too much absorption can lead to unwanted side effects elsewhere in the body. To keep this problem to a minimum, avoid using large amounts of Aclovate over large areas, and do not cover it with airtight dressings such as plastic wrap or adhesive bandages unless specifically told to by your doctor.

How should you use this medication?

Use Aclovate exactly as prescribed by your doctor and only to treat the condition for which your doctor prescribed it. The usual procedure is to spread a thin film of Aclovate cream or ointment over the rash and massage gently until the medication disappears. Do this 2 or 3 times a day.

For areas of deep-seated, persistent rash, your doctor may recommend a thick layer of Aclovate cream or ointment topped with waterproof bandaging, to be left in place for 1 to 4 days. If necessary, this procedure may be repeated 3 or 4 times. Do not use bandaging at all, however, unless your doctor so advises.

Aclovate is for use only on the skin. Be careful to keep it out of your eyes.

■ *If you miss a dose...*
Apply it as soon as you remember. If it is almost time for the next dose, skip the one you missed and go back to your regular schedule.

■ *Storage instructions...*
Store at room temperature.

What side effects may occur?
Side effects cannot be anticipated. If any develop or change in intensity, inform your doctor as soon as possible. Only your doctor can determine if it is safe for you to continue taking Aclovate.

■ *Side effects may include:*
Acne-like pimples, allergic rash/inflammation, burning, dryness, infection, irritation, itching, pale spots, prickly heat, rash, redness, stretch marks on skin

Why should this drug not be prescribed?
Do not use Aclovate if it has ever given you an allergic reaction.

Special warnings about this medication
Aclovate is for external use only. Do not let the cream or ointment get into your eyes. Avoid using the product on your face, underarms, or groin, unless the doctor tells you to.

Do not use Aclovate to treat diaper rash or apply it in the diaper area; waterproof diapers or plastic pants can increase unwanted absorption of Aclovate.

If your skin is inflamed or you have some other skin condition, tell your doctor. You may absorb more drug than usual.

If you use Aclovate over large areas of skin for prolonged periods of time, the amount of hormone absorbed into your bloodstream may eventually lead to

Cushing's syndrome: a moon-faced appearance, fattened neck and trunk, and purplish streaks on the skin. Children, because of their relatively larger ratio of skin surface to body weight, are particularly susceptible to overabsorption of hormone from Aclovate. The drug should not be used on children under 1 year of age or for more than 3 weeks in children older than 1 year.

Possible food and drug interactions
when taking this medication

Check with your doctor before combining Aclovate with other more potent steroids, since this could lead to undesirably large amounts of hormone circulating in your bloodstream.

Special information
if you are pregnant or breastfeeding

Drug absorbed from Aclovate cream or ointment into the bloodstream may find its way into an unborn child's blood, or may seep into breast milk. To avoid any possible harm to your child, use Aclovate very sparingly—and only with your doctor's permission—if you are pregnant or nursing a baby.

Recommended dosage

Apply a thin film of Aclovate cream or ointment to the affected skin areas 2 or 3 times daily; massage gently until the medication disappears.

Bandages that block out air may be used to control psoriasis and other severe skin rashes, if your doctor recommends them. Apply as follows:

1. Cover the affected area with a thick layer of Aclovate cream or ointment and a light gauze dressing, then cover the area with a pliable plastic film.
2. Seal the edges to the normal skin by adhesive tape or other means.
3. Leave the dressing in place 1 to 4 days and repeat the procedure 3 or 4 times as needed.

With this method of treatment, marked improvement is often seen in a few days. If an infection develops, the use of airtight bandages should be discontinued. Your doctor will recommend an alternative treatment.

Once your condition is under control, you should stop using Aclovate. If you don't see any improvement within 2 weeks, check with your doctor.

Overdosage

Any medication taken in excess can have serious consequences. If you suspect an overdose, seek medical attention immediately.

In a child, an overdose of Aclovate may cause increased pressure within the skull leading to bulging soft spots (in an infant's head) or headache. If this happens, see a doctor without delay.

Over the long term, overuse of Aclovate can interfere with a child's normal growth and development.

Generic name:

ACRIVASTINE WITH PSEUDOEPHEDRINE

See Semprex-D, page 1173.

Brand name:

ACTIGALL

Pronounced: AK-ti-gawl
Generic name: Ursodiol

Why is this drug prescribed?
Actigall is used to help dissolve certain kinds of gallstones. If you suffer from gallstones but do not want to undergo surgery to remove them, or if age, infirmity, or a poor reaction to anesthesia makes you a poor candidate for surgery, Actigall treatment may be a good alternative.

Actigall is also used to prevent gallstones in people on rapid-weight-loss diets.

Most important fact about this drug
Actigall is not a quick remedy. It takes months of Actigall therapy to dissolve gallstones; and there is a possibility of incomplete dissolution and recurrence of stones. Your doctor will weigh Actigall against alternative treatments and recommend the best one for you.

Actigall is most effective if your gallstones are small or "floatable" (high in cholesterol). In addition, your gallbladder must still be functioning properly.

How should you take this medication?
Take Actigall exactly as prescribed; otherwise the gallstones may dissolve too slowly or not dissolve at all. During treatment, your doctor will do periodic ultrasound exams to see if your stones are dissolving.

■ *If you miss a dose...*
Take it as soon as you remember, or at the same time as the next dose.

■ *Storage instructions...*
Store at room temperature in a tightly closed container.

What side effects may occur?
Side effects cannot be anticipated. If any develop or change in intensity, inform your doctor as soon as possible. Only your doctor can determine if it is safe for you to continue taking Actigall.

■ *Side effects may include:*
Abdominal pain, allergy, arthritis, back pain, bronchitis, chest pain, constipation, cough, diarrhea, dizziness, fatigue, flu-like symptoms, gas, hair loss, headache, indigestion, insomnia, joint pain, menstrual pain, muscle and bone pain, nasal inflammation, nausea, sinus inflammation, sore throat, stomach or intestinal disorder, upper respiratory tract infection, urinary tract infection, viral infection, vomiting

Why should this drug not be prescribed?
Do not take this medication if you are sensitive to or have ever had an allergic reaction to ursodiol or to other bile acids.

Actigall will not dissolve certain types of gallstones. If your doctor tells you that your gallstones are calcified cholesterol stones, radio-opaque stones, or radiolucent bile pigment stones, you are not a candidate for treatment with Actigall.

Also, if you have biliary tract (liver, gallbladder, bile duct) problems or certain liver and pancreas diseases, your doctor may not be able to prescribe Actigall for you.

Special warnings about this medication
Although Actigall is not known to cause liver damage, it is theoretically possible in some people. Your doctor may run blood tests for liver function before you start to take Actigall and again while you are taking it.

Possible food and drug interactions
when taking this medication
If Actigall is taken with certain other drugs, the effects of either could be increased, decreased, or altered. It is especially important to check with your doctor before combining Actigall with the following:

Aluminum-based antacid medications (Alu-Cap, Alu-Tab, Rolaids, others)

Cholesterol-lowering medications, such as Lopid, Mevacor, Questran, and Colestid

Estrogens such as Premarin

Oral contraceptives

Special information
if you are pregnant or breastfeeding

If you are pregnant or plan to become pregnant, inform your doctor immediately. So far, there is no evidence that Actigall can harm an unborn baby; but to be safe, the medication is not recommended during pregnancy. Caution is needed during breastfeeding; it is not known whether Actigall taken by a nursing mother passes into her breast milk.

Recommended dosage

DISSOLVING GALLSTONES

The recommended daily dosage is 8 to 10 milligrams per 2.2 pounds of body weight, divided into 2 or 3 doses.

PREVENTING GALLSTONES

The usual dose in people losing weight rapidly is 300 milligrams twice a day.

Overdosage

Although there have been no reports of overdose with Actigall, the most likely symptom of severe overdose would be diarrhea. Since any medication taken in excess can have serious consequences, you should seek medical attention immediately if you suspect an Actigall overdose.

Brand name:

ACTRON

See Orudis, page 937.

Generic name:

ACYCLOVIR

See Zovirax, page 1477.

Brand name:

ADALAT

See Procardia, page 1055.

Generic name:

ADAPALENE

See Differin, page 393.

Brand name:

ADDERALL

Pronounced: ADD-ur-all
Generic ingredients: Amphetamines

Why is this drug prescribed?
Adderall is prescribed in the treatment of attention-deficit disorder with hyperactivity, the condition in which a child exhibits a short attention span and becomes easily distracted, overly emotional, excessively active, and highly impulsive. It should be used as part of a broader treatment plan that includes psychological, educational, and social measures.

Adderall is also prescribed for narcolepsy (uncontrollable attacks of sleep).

Most important fact about this drug
Adderall, like all amphetamines, has a high potential for abuse. If used in large doses over long periods of time, it can cause dependence and addiction. Be careful to take Adderall only as prescribed.

How should you take this medication?
Never take more Adderall than your doctor has prescribed. Do not take it for a longer time or for any other purpose than prescribed.

Take the first dose upon awakening. If additional doses are prescribed, take them at intervals of 4 to 6 hours. Avoid late evening doses, which can interfere with sleep.

■ *If you miss a dose...*
 If you are taking 1 dose a day, and at least 6 hours remain before bedtime, take the dose as soon as you remember. If you don't remember until the

next day, skip the dose and go back to your regular schedule. Do not take a double dose.

If you are taking more than 1 dose a day, and you remember within an hour or so of the scheduled time, take the missed dose immediately. Otherwise, skip the dose and go back to your regular schedule. Never take 2 doses at once.

■ *Storage instructions...*
Store at room temperature in a tight, light-resistant container.

What side effects may occur?
Side effects cannot be anticipated. If any develop or change in intensity, tell your doctor as soon as possible. Only your doctor can determine if it is safe for you or your child to continue taking Adderall.

■ *Side effects may include:*
Changes in sex drive, constipation, depression, diarrhea, dizziness, dry mouth, exaggerated feelings of well-being, headache, high blood pressure, hives, impotence, insomnia, loss of appetite, mental disturbances, overstimulation, rapid or pounding heartbeat, restlessness, stomach and intestinal disturbances, tremor, twitches, unpleasant taste, weakened heart, weight loss, worsening of tics (including Tourette's syndrome)

Why should this drug not be prescribed?
Do not use Adderall if you have any of the following conditions:

Heart disease
Hardening of the arteries
High blood pressure
High pressure in the eye (glaucoma)
Overactive thyroid gland

Never take Adderall within 14 days of taking an antidepressant classified as an MAO inhibitor, including Nardil and Parnate. A potentially life-threatening spike in blood pressure could result.

Your doctor will not prescribe Adderall if you have ever had a reaction to similar stimulant drugs. The doctor will also avoid prescribing Adderall if you appear agitated or are prone to substance abuse.

Special warnings about this medication
If you have even a mild case of high blood pressure, take Adderall with caution. Be careful, too, about driving or operating machinery until you know how this drug affects you. It may impair judgment and coordination.

Adderall can make tics and twitches worse. If you or a family member has this problem (or the condition called Tourette's syndrome), make sure the doctor is aware of it.

If the problem is attention-deficit disorder, the doctor will do a complete history and evaluation before prescribing Adderall, taking particular account of the severity of the symptoms and the age of your child. If the problem is a temporary reaction to a stressful situation, Adderall is probably not called for.

At present, there has been no experience with long-term Adderall therapy in children. However, other amphetamine-based medications have been known to stunt growth, so your doctor will need to watch the child carefully.

Possible food and drug interactions
when taking this medication

If Adderall is taken with certain other drugs, the effects of either could be increased, decreased, or altered. It is especially important to check with your doctor before combining Adderall with the following:

Acetazolamide (Diamox)
Antihistamines such as Benadryl and Chlor-Trimeton
Drugs classified as MAO inhibitors, including the antidepressants Nardil and Parnate
Drugs that make the urine more acid, such as Uroquid-Acid No. 2
Fruit juices and vitamin C
Glutamic acid (an amino acid related to MSG)
High blood pressure medications such as Calan, Esimil, HydroDIURIL, Hytrin, Procardia, and Serpasil
Lithium (Lithonate)
Major tranquilizers such as Haldol and Thorazine
Meperidine (Demerol)
Methenamine (Urised)
Norepinephrine (Levophed)
Propoxyphene (Darvon)
Seizure medications such as Dilantin, phenobarbital, and Zarontin
"Tricyclic" antidepressants such as Norpramin, Tofranil, and Vivactil

Special information
if you are pregnant or breastfeeding

Heavy use of amphetamines during pregnancy can lead to premature birth or low birth weight. Avoid taking Adderall unless absolutely necessary. Amphetamines do find their way into breast milk, so you should not take Adderall while breastfeeding.

Recommended dosage
Whether the problem is attention-deficit disorder or narcolepsy, the doctor will keep the dosage as low as possible.

ATTENTION-DEFICIT DISORDER WITH HYPERACTIVITY

Children 3 to 5 years of age
The usual starting dose is 2.5 milligrams daily. Each week, the doctor will raise the daily dosage by 2.5 milligrams until the condition is under control.

Children 6 years of age and older
The usual starting dose is 5 milligrams once or twice a day. Each week, the daily dosage may be increased by 5 milligrams. Only in rare cases will a child need more than 40 milligrams per day.

The doctor may interrupt therapy occasionally to see if the drug is still needed.

NARCOLEPSY

Adults
The usual total daily dose ranges from 5 to 60 milligrams, taken as 2 or more smaller doses.

Children under 12 years of age
The usual starting dose is 5 milligrams daily. Each week, the doctor will raise the daily dose by 5 milligrams until the condition is under control.

Children 12 years of age and older
The usual starting dose is 10 milligrams daily, with weekly increases of 10 milligrams daily until the drug takes effect.

Overdosage
A large overdose of Adderall can be fatal. Warning signs of a massive overdose include convulsions and coma.

■ *Symptoms of Adderall overdose may include:*
 Abdominal cramps, assaultiveness, changes in blood pressure, confusion, diarrhea, hallucinations, heightened reflexes, high fever, irregular heartbeat, nausea, panic, rapid breathing, restlessness, tremor, vomiting

If you suspect an overdose, seek emergency treatment immediately.

Brand name:

ADIPEX-P

See Fastin, page 506.

Brand name:

ADVIL

See Motrin, page 830.

Brand name:

AEROBID

Pronounced: AIR-oh-bid
Generic name: Flunisolide
Other brand names: AeroBid-M, Nasalide

Why is this drug prescribed?

AeroBid is prescribed for people who need long-term treatment to control and prevent the symptoms of asthma. It contains an anti-inflammatory steroid type of medication and may reduce or eliminate your need for other corticosteroids. A nasal-spray form of the drug (Nasalide) is available for relief of hay fever.

Most important fact about this drug

AeroBid helps to reduce the likelihood of an asthma attack, but will not relieve one that has already started. To be effective as a preventive measure, it must be taken every day at regularly spaced intervals. It may be several weeks before you receive its full benefit.

How should you take this medication?

Take this medication at regular intervals, exactly as prescribed by your doctor.

Administration technique:
1. Place the metal cartridge inside the plastic container.
2. Remove the cap; inspect the mouthpiece for foreign objects.
3. Shake the inhaler thoroughly.
4. Tilt your head slightly and breathe out as completely as possible.

5. Hold the inhaler upright and put the plastic mouthpiece in your mouth; close your lips tightly around it.

6. Press down on the metal cartridge. At the same time, take a slow, deep breath through your mouth.

7. Hold your breath as long as you can. While holding your breath, stop pressing down on the cartridge and remove the mouthpiece from your mouth.

8. Allow at least 1 minute between inhalations.

To help reduce hoarseness, throat irritation, and mouth infection, rinse out with water after each use. If your mouth is sore or has a rash, tell your doctor.

Illustrated instructions for use are available with the product.

■ *If you miss a dose...*
Use it as soon as you remember. If it is almost time for your next dose, skip the one you missed and go back to your regular schedule. Do not take 2 doses at the same time.

■ *Storage instructions...*
Store away from heat or cold and light. Keep away from open flames.

What side effects may occur?
Side effects cannot be anticipated. If any develop or change in intensity, inform your doctor as soon as possible. Only your doctor can determine if it is safe for you to continue taking AeroBid.

■ *More common side effects may include:*
Cold symptoms, diarrhea, flu, headache, infection of the upper respiratory tract, nasal congestion, nausea, sore throat, unpleasant taste, upset stomach, vomiting

■ *Less common side effects may include:*
Abdominal pain, chest congestion, chest pain, cough, decreased appetite, dizziness, ear infection, eczema (inflamed skin with sores and crusting), fever, heartburn, hoarseness, inflamed lining of the nose, irritability, itching, loss of smell or taste, menstrual disturbances, nervousness, phlegm, rapid, fluttering heartbeat, rash, runny nose, shakiness, sinus congestion, sinus drainage, sinus infection, sinus inflammation, sneezing, swelling due to fluid retention, wheezing, yeastlike fungal infection of the mouth and throat

■ *Rare side effects may include:*
Acne, anxiety, blurred vision, bronchitis, chest tightness, chills, constipation, depression, difficult or labored breathing, dry throat, earache, excessive restlessness, eye discomfort, eye infection, faintness, fatigue, gas, general feeling of illness, head stuffiness, high blood pressure, hives, inability to fall or stay asleep, increased appetite, indigestion, inflammation of the tongue, laryngitis, moodiness, mouth irritation, nasal irritation, nosebleed, numbness, pneumonia, rapid heart rate, sinus discomfort, sluggishness, sweating, swelling of the arms and legs, throat irritation, vertigo, weakness, weight gain

Why should this drug not be prescribed?
This medication is not for treatment of prolonged, severe asthma attacks where more intensive measures are required.

If you are allergic or sensitive to AeroBid or other steroid drugs, advise your doctor. This medication may not be right for you.

Special warnings about this medication
Your asthma should be reasonably stable before treatment with AeroBid Inhaler is started. AeroBid should be started in combination with your usual dose of an oral steroid medication. After approximately 1 week, your doctor will start to withdraw gradually the oral steroid by reducing the daily or alternate daily dose. A slow rate of reduction is very important, as some people have experienced withdrawal symptoms such as joint and/or muscular pain, fatigue, and depression. Tell your doctor if you lose weight or feel light-headed. You may need to take more oral corticosteroid temporarily.

This medication is not useful when you need rapid relief of asthma symptoms.

Transferring from steroid tablet therapy to AeroBid Inhaler may produce allergic conditions that were previously controlled by the steroid tablet therapy. These include rhinitis (inflammation of the mucous membrane of the nose), conjunctivitis (pinkeye), and eczema.

Contact your doctor immediately if you have an asthma attack that isn't controlled by a bronchodilator while you are being treated with AeroBid. You may need an oral steroid drug.

While you are being treated with AeroBid, particularly at higher doses, your doctor will carefully observe you for any evidence of side effects such as the suppression of glandular function and diminished bone growth in children. If you have just had surgery or are under extreme stress, your doctor will also closely monitor you.

The use of AeroBid may cause a yeastlike fungal infection of the mouth, pharynx (throat), or larynx (voice box). If you suspect a fungal infection, notify your doctor. Treatment with antifungal medication may be necessary.

Since the contents of this inhalant are under pressure, do not puncture the container and do not use or store the medication near heat or an open flame. Exposure to temperatures above 120 degrees may cause the container to explode.

People taking drugs such as AeroBid that suppress the immune system are more open to infection. Take extra care to avoid exposure to measles and chickenpox if you've never had them or never had shots. Such diseases can be serious or even fatal when your immune system is below par. If you are exposed, tell your doctor immediately.

Also, if you have tuberculosis, a herpes infection of the eye, or any other kind of infection, make sure the doctor knows about it. You probably should not use AeroBid.

**Possible food and drug interactions
when taking this medication**
No interactions have been reported.

**Special information
if you are pregnant or breastfeeding**
The effects of AeroBid during pregnancy have not been adequately studied. If you are pregnant or plan to become pregnant, inform your doctor immediately. It is not known whether AeroBid appears in breast milk. If this medication is essential to your health, your doctor may advise you to discontinue breastfeeding your baby until your treatment with this medication is finished.

Recommended dosage
The AeroBid Inhaler system is for oral inhalation only.

ADULTS

The recommended starting dose is 2 inhalations twice daily, in the morning and evening, for a total daily dose of 1 milligram. The daily dose should not exceed 4 inhalations twice a day, for a total daily dose of 2 milligrams.

CHILDREN

For children 6 to 15 years of age, 2 inhalations may be used twice daily, for a total daily dose of 1 milligram.

The safety and effectiveness of this drug have not been established in children under 6 years of age.

Overdosage
Any medication taken in excess can have serious consequences. If you suspect an overdose, seek emergency medical treatment immediately.

Brand name:

AKTOB

See Tobrex, page 1312.

Generic name:

ALBUTEROL

See Proventil, page 1073.

Generic name:

ALCLOMETASONE

See Aclovate, page 11.

Brand name:

ALDACTAZIDE

Pronounced: al-DAK-tah-zide
Generic ingredients: Spironolactone, Hydrochlorothiazide

Why is this drug prescribed?
Aldactazide is used in the treatment of high blood pressure and other conditions that require the elimination of excess fluid from the body. These conditions include congestive heart failure, cirrhosis of the liver, and kidney disease. Aldactazide combines two diuretic drugs that help your body produce and eliminate more urine. Spironolactone, one of the ingredients, helps to minimize the potassium loss that can be caused by the hydrochloro-thiazide component.

Most important fact about this drug
If you have high blood pressure, you must take Aldactazide regularly for it to be effective. Since blood pressure declines gradually, it may be several weeks

before you get the full benefit of Aldactazide; and you must continue taking it even if you are feeling well. Aldactazide does not cure high blood pressure; it merely keeps it under control.

How should you take this medication?
Take Aldactazide exactly as prescribed. Stopping Aldactazide suddenly could cause your condition to worsen.

■ *If you miss a dose...*
Take it as soon as you remember. If it is almost time for your next dose, skip the one you missed and go back to your regular schedule. Never take 2 doses at the same time.

■ *Storage instructions...*
Store at room temperature.

What side effects may occur?
Side effects cannot be anticipated. If any develop or change in intensity, inform your doctor as soon as possible. Only your doctor can determine if it is safe for you to continue taking Aldactazide.

■ *Side effects may include:*
Abdominal cramps, breast development in males, change in potassium levels (leading to such symptoms as dry mouth, excessive thirst, weak or irregular heartbeat, and muscle pain or cramps), deepening of the voice, diarrhea, dizziness, dizziness on rising, drowsiness, excessive hairiness, fever, headache, hives, inflammation of blood vessels or lymph vessels, inflammation of the pancreas, irregular menstruation, lack of coordination, liver problems, loss of appetite, mental confusion, muscle spasms, nausea, postmenopausal bleeding, rash, red or purple spots on skin, restlessness, sensitivity to light, severe allergic reaction, sexual dysfunction, sluggishness, stomach bleeding, stomach inflammation, stomach ulcers, tingling or pins and needles, vertigo, vomiting, weakness, yellow eyes and skin, yellow vision

Why should this drug not be prescribed?
Aldactazide should not be used if you have acute kidney disease or liver failure, have difficulty urinating or are unable to urinate, or have high potassium levels in your blood.

If you are sensitive to or have ever had an allergic reaction to spironolactone, hydrochlorothiazide, or similar drugs, or if you are sensitive to sulfa drugs, you should not take this medication. Make sure your doctor is aware of any drug reactions you may have experienced.

Special warnings about this medication

This medication should be used only if your doctor has determined that the precise amount of each ingredient in Aldactazide meets your specific needs.

Potassium supplements (including salt substitutes) or diuretics that leave high levels of potassium in your body should not be used while taking Aldactazide, unless specifically recommended by your doctor.

If you are taking an ACE-inhibitor type of blood pressure medication such as Vasotec, this drug should be used with extreme caution.

If you have liver disease or lupus erythematosus (a disease that causes skin eruptions), Aldactazide should be used with caution.

Excessive sweating, dehydration, severe diarrhea, or vomiting could cause you to lose too much water and cause your blood pressure to become too low. Be careful when exercising and in hot weather.

Notify your doctor or dentist that you are taking Aldactazide if you have a medical emergency, and before you have surgery or dental treatment.

Possible food and drug interactions
when taking this medication

If Aldactazide is taken with certain other drugs, the effects of either could be increased, decreased, or altered. It is especially important to check with your doctor before combining Aldactazide with the following:

ACE-inhibitor blood pressure drugs such as Vasotec
Antigout medications such as Zyloprim
Digoxin (Lanoxin)
Diuretics such as Lasix and Midamor
Indomethacin (Indocin)
Insulin or oral antidiabetic drugs such as Micronase
Lithium (Lithonate)
Norepinephrine (Levophed)
Potassium supplements such as Slow-K
Steroids such as prednisone

Special information
if you are pregnant or breastfeeding

The effects of Aldactazide during pregnancy have not been adequately studied. If you are pregnant or plan to become pregnant, inform your doctor immediately. Aldactazide appears in breast milk and could affect a nursing infant. If this medication is essential to your health, your doctor may advise you to discontinue breastfeeding until your treatment is finished.

Recommended dosage

ADULTS

Congestive Heart Failure, Cirrhosis, Nephrotic Syndrome (kidney disorder)
The usual dosage is 100 milligrams each of spironolactone and hydrochlorothiazide daily, taken as a single dose or in divided doses. Dosage may range from 25 milligrams to 200 milligrams of each ingredient daily, depending on your individual needs.

High Blood Pressure
The usual dose is 50 milligrams to 100 milligrams each of spironolactone and hydrochlorothiazide daily, in a single dose or divided into smaller doses.

CHILDREN

The usual dose of Aldactazide should provide 0.75 milligram to 1.5 milligrams of spironolactone per pound of body weight.

Overdosage

Although there is no information on specific signs of Aldactazide overdose, any medication taken in excess can have serious consequences. If you suspect an overdose, seek medical attention immediately.

Brand name:

ALDACTONE

Pronounced: al-DAK-tone
Generic name: Spironolactone

Why is this drug prescribed?

Aldactone flushes excess salt and water from the body and controls high blood pressure. It is used in the diagnosis and treatment of hyperaldosteronism, a condition in which the adrenal gland secretes too much aldosterone (a hormone that regulates the body's salt and potassium levels). It is also used in treating other conditions that require the elimination of excess fluid from the body. These conditions include congestive heart failure, high blood pressure, cirrhosis of the liver, kidney disease, and unusually low potassium levels in the blood. When used for high blood pressure, Aldactone can be taken alone or with other high blood pressure medications.

Most important fact about this drug

If you have high blood pressure, you must take Aldactone regularly for it to be effective. Since blood pressure declines gradually, it may be several weeks before you get the full benefit of Aldactone; and you must continue taking it even if you are feeling well. Aldactone does not cure high blood pressure; it merely keeps it under control.

How should you take this medication?

Take Aldactone exactly as prescribed by your doctor. Stopping Aldactone suddenly could cause your condition to worsen.

■ *If you miss a dose...*
Take it as soon as you remember. If it is almost time for your next dose, skip the one you missed and go back to your regular schedule. Never take 2 doses at the same time.

■ *Storage instructions...*
Store at room temperature.

What side effects may occur?

Side effects cannot be anticipated. If any develop or change in intensity, inform your doctor as soon as possible. Only your doctor can determine if it is safe for you to continue taking Aldactone.

■ *Side effects may include:*
Abdominal cramps, breast development in males, change in potassium levels (leading to such symptoms as dry mouth, excessive thirst, weak or irregular heartbeat, and muscle pain or cramps), deepening of voice, diarrhea, drowsiness, excessive hairiness, fever, headache, hives, irregular menstruation, lack of coordination, lethargy, liver problems, mental confusion, postmenopausal bleeding, severe allergic reaction, sexual dysfunction, skin eruptions, stomach bleeding, stomach inflammation, ulcers, vomiting

Why should this drug not be prescribed?

You should not take Aldactone if you have kidney disease, an inability to urinate, difficulty urinating, or high potassium levels in your blood.

Special warnings about this medication

Potassium supplements or other diuretics that leave your potassium levels high, such as Maxzide, should not be used while taking Aldactone, unless specifically indicated by your doctor.

ACE inhibitors (Vasotec, Capoten), used for blood pressure and heart failure, should not be taken while using Aldactone.

If you are taking Aldactone, your kidney function should be given a complete assessment and should continue to be monitored.

If you have liver disease, your doctor will be cautious about using this medication.

Excessive sweating, dehydration, severe diarrhea, or vomiting could cause you to lose too much water and cause your blood pressure to become too low. Be careful when exercising and in hot weather.

Notify your doctor or dentist that you are taking Aldactone if you have a medical emergency, and before you have surgery or dental treatment.

Possible food and drug interactions
when taking this medication

If Aldactone is taken with certain other drugs, the effects of either could be increased, decreased, or altered. It is especially important to check with your doctor before combining Aldactone with the following:

  ACE inhibitors such as Vasotec and Capoten
  Digoxin (Lanoxin)
  Indomethacin (Indocin)
  Norepinephrine (Levophed)
  Other water pills such as Lasix and HydroDIURIL
  Other high blood pressure medications such as Aldomet and
    Procardia XL

Special information
if you are pregnant or breastfeeding

The effects of Aldactone during pregnancy have not been adequately studied. If you are pregnant or plan to become pregnant, inform your doctor immediately. Aldactone appears in breast milk and could affect a nursing infant. If this medication is essential to your health, your doctor may advise you to discontinue breastfeeding until your treatment with this medication is finished.

Recommended dosage

ADULTS

Primary Hyperaldosteronism

Initial dosages of this medication are used to determine the presence of primary hyperaldosteronism (too much secretion of the adrenal hormone aldosterone). People can be tested with this medication over either a long or a short period of time.

In the long test, you take 400 milligrams per day for 3 to 4 weeks. If your potassium levels and blood pressure are corrected with this dosage in this time period, your physician may assume you have this condition.

In the short test, you receive 400 milligrams per day for 4 days. A laboratory test compares potassium levels while you are on Aldactone and after the medication is stopped. Your doctor may then make a diagnosis.

After the diagnosis of primary hyperaldosteronism is made and confirmed by more tests, the usual dose is 100 to 400 milligrams per day, prior to surgery. In those who are not good candidates for surgery, this drug is given over the long term at the lowest effective dose.

Adult Edema (Congestive Heart Failure, Cirrhosis of the Liver, or Kidney Disorders)

The usual starting dosage is 100 milligrams daily either in a single dose or divided into smaller doses. However, your doctor may have you take daily doses as low as 25 milligrams or as high as 200 milligrams.

Your doctor may choose to adjust your dosage after an initial 5-day trial period or add another diuretic medication to this one.

Essential Hypertension (High Blood Pressure)

The usual starting dosage is 50 to 100 milligrams daily in a single dose or divided into smaller doses. This medication may be given with another diuretic or with other high blood pressure medications.

It may be up to 2 weeks before the full effect of this medication is seen. Your doctor can then adjust the dosage according to your response.

Hypokalemia (Potassium Loss)

Your doctor may have you take daily dosages of 25 milligrams to 100 milligrams when potassium loss caused by the effects of a diuretic cannot be treated by a potassium supplement.

CHILDREN

Edema (Swelling Due to Water Retention)
The usual starting dosage is 1.5 milligrams per pound of body weight daily in a single dose or divided into smaller doses.

Overdosage
Although no specific information on signs of Aldactone overdose is available, any medication taken in excess can have serious consequences. If you suspect an overdose, seek medical attention immediately.

Brand name:

ALDOMET

Pronounced: AL-doe-met
Generic name: Methyldopa

Why is this drug prescribed?
Aldomet is used to treat high blood pressure. It is effective when used alone or with other high blood pressure medications.

Most important fact about this drug
You must take Aldomet regularly for it to be effective. Since blood pressure declines gradually, it may be several weeks before you get the full benefit of Aldomet; and you must continue taking it even if you are feeling well. Aldomet does not cure high blood pressure; it merely keeps it under control.

How should you take this medication?
Take this medication exactly as prescribed. Try not to miss any doses. Do not stop taking the drug without your doctor's knowledge.

Drowsiness may occur when dosage is increased. If your doctor increases the amount of Aldomet you take, start the new dosage in the evening.

- *If you miss a dose...*
  Take it as soon as you remember. If it is almost time for your next dose, skip the one you missed and go back to your regular schedule. Never take 2 doses at the same time.

- *Storage instructions...*
  Keep Aldomet in the container it came in, tightly closed. Store Aldomet tablets at room temperature. Keep oral suspension in the refrigerator. Protect from light.

What side effects may occur?
Side effects cannot be anticipated. If any develop or change in intensity, inform your doctor as soon as possible. Only your doctor can determine if it is safe for you to continue taking Aldomet.

■ *More common side effects may include:*
Drowsiness during the first few weeks of therapy, fluid retention or weight gain, headache, weakness

■ *Less common or rare side effects may include:*
Anemia, Bell's palsy (paralysis of the face, making it look distorted), bloating, blood disorders, breast development in males, breast enlargement, changes in menstruation, chest pain, congestive heart failure, constipation, decreased mental ability, decreased sex drive, depression, diarrhea, dizziness when standing up, dry mouth, fever, gas, hepatitis, impotence, inflammation of the large intestine, inflammation of the pancreas, inflammation of the salivary glands, involuntary movements, joint pain, light-headedness, liver disorders, milk production, muscle pain, nasal stuffiness, nausea, nightmares, parkinsonism (tremors, shuffling walk, stooped posture, muscle weakness), rash, slow heartbeat, sore or "black" tongue, tingling or pins and needles, vomiting, yellow eyes and skin

Why should this drug not be prescribed?
If you have liver disease or cirrhosis, or if you have taken Aldomet before and developed liver disease, do not take this medication.

If you are sensitive to or have ever had an allergic reaction to Aldomet, or if you have been prescribed the oral suspension form of Aldomet and have ever had an allergic reaction to sulfites, you should not take this medication.

If you are taking drugs known as monoamine oxidase (MAO) inhibitors, you should not take Aldomet.

Special warnings about this medication
Before you begin taking Aldomet, your doctor should perform a complete study of your liver function, and it should be monitored periodically thereafter.

Aldomet can cause liver disorders. You may develop a fever, jaundice (yellow eyes and skin), or both, usually within the first 2 to 3 months of therapy. If either of these symptoms occurs, stop taking Aldomet and contact your doctor immediately. If the fever and/or jaundice were caused by the medication, your liver function should gradually return to normal.

If you have a history of liver disease, this medication should be used with caution.

Hemolytic anemia, a blood disorder in which red blood cells are destroyed, can develop with long-term use of Aldomet; your doctor will do periodic blood counts to check for this problem.

Aldomet can cause water retention or weight gain in some people. A diuretic will usually relieve these symptoms.

If you have asthma and are taking the liquid form of Aldomet, you could have an allergic reaction to the sulfite component of the liquid.

If you are on dialysis and are taking Aldomet for high blood pressure, your blood pressure may rise after your dialysis treatments.

Aldomet can cause you to become drowsy or less alert, especially during the first few weeks of therapy or when dosage levels are increased. If it affects you this way, driving or operating heavy machinery or participating in any hazardous activity that requires full mental alertness is not recommended.

Notify your doctor or dentist that you are taking Aldomet if you have a medical emergency and before you have surgery or dental treatment.

Possible food and drug interactions
when taking this medication

If Aldomet is taken with certain other drugs, the effects of either could be increased, decreased, or altered. It is especially important to check with your doctor before combining Aldomet with the following:

Antidepressants known as MAO inhibitors, including Nardil and Parnate
Dextroamphetamine (Dexedrine)
Imipramine (Tofranil)
Iron-containing products such as Feosol
Lithium (Lithonate)
Other blood pressure medications such as Catapres and Calan
Phenylpropanolamine (a decongestant used in common cold remedies
    such as Dimetapp, Entex LA, and others)
Propranolol (Inderal)
Tolbutamide (Orinase)

Special information
if you are pregnant or breastfeeding

The use of Aldomet during pregnancy appears to be relatively safe. However, if you are pregnant or plan to become pregnant, inform your doctor immediately. Aldomet appears in breast milk and could affect a nursing infant. If this medication is essential to your health, your doctor may advise you to discontinue breastfeeding until your treatment is finished.

Recommended dosage

ADULTS

The usual starting dose is 250 milligrams, 2 or 3 times per day in the first 48 hours of treatment. Your doctor may increase or decrease your dose over the next few days to achieve the correct blood pressure.

To reduce the effect of any sedation the medication may cause, dosage increases will usually be given in the evening.

The usual maintenance dosage is 500 milligrams to 2 grams per day divided into 2 to 4 doses. The maximum dose is usually 3 grams.

Your doctor will also adjust your dosage of Aldomet when it is taken in combination with certain other high blood pressure drugs.

If you take Aldomet with a non-thiazide high blood pressure medicine, your doctor will limit the initial dosage to 500 milligrams daily divided into small doses.

Dosages will be adjusted, and other high blood pressure drugs may be added, during the first few months of treatment with Aldomet. Those with reduced kidney function may require smaller doses. Older people who are prone to fainting spells due to arterial disease may also require smaller doses.

CHILDREN

The usual starting dose is 10 milligrams per 2.2 pounds of body weight daily, divided into 2 to 4 doses. Doses will be adjusted until blood pressure is normal. The maximum daily dose is usually 65 milligrams per 2.2 pounds of body weight or 3 grams, whichever is less.

OLDER ADULTS

Dosages of this drug are adjusted to each individual's needs. Lower doses may be prescribed by your doctor.

Overdosage

Any medication taken in excess can have serious consequences. If you suspect an overdose, seek medical attention immediately.

■ *Symptoms of Aldomet overdose may include:*
Bloating, constipation, diarrhea, dizziness, extreme drowsiness, gas, light-headedness, nausea, severely low blood pressure, slow heartbeat, vomiting, weakness

Generic name:

ALENDRONATE

See Fosamax, page 553.

Brand name:

ALEVE

See Anaprox, page 66.

Brand name:

ALLEGRA

Pronounced: ah-LEG-rah
Generic name: Fexofenadine hydrochloride
Other brand name: Allegra-D

Why is this drug prescribed?
Allegra relieves the itchy, runny nose, sneezing, and itchy, red, watery eyes that come with hay fever. Its effect begins in 1 hour and lasts 12 hours, peaking around the second or third hour. Allegra is one of the new type of antihistamines that rarely cause drowsiness.

In addition, to the antihistamine in Allegra, Allegra-D also contains the nasal decongestant pseudoephedrine.

Most important fact about this drug
Seldane, an antihistamine related to Allegra, has been implicated in dangerous interactions with the common antibiotic erythromycin, the antifungal medication ketoconazole (Nizoral), and several similar drugs. Allegra poses no such risks. It is also safe for people with liver disease.

How should you take this medication?
Take Allegra and Allegra-D only as prescribed.

■ *If you miss a dose...*
Take it as soon as you remember. If it is almost time for your next dose, skip the one you missed and go back to your regular schedule. Do not take 2 doses at once.

■ *Storage instructions...*
Store at room temperature. Protect blister packs from moisture.

What side effects may occur?
Side effects cannot be anticipated. If any develop or change in intensity, tell your doctor as soon as possible. Only your doctor can determine if it is safe for you to continue taking Allegra.

■ *Side effects of Allegra may include:*
Colds or flu, drowsiness, fatigue, indigestion, menstrual problems, nausea

■ *Side effects of Allegra-D may include:*
Abdominal pain, agitation, anxiety, back pain, dizziness, dry mouth, headache, heart palpitations, indigestion, insomnia, nausea, nervousness, respiratory tract infection, throat irritation

Why should this drug not be prescribed?
If Allegra or Allegra-D gives you an allergic reaction, avoid it in the future. Do not give either product to children under 12.

Do not take Allegra-D if you have glaucoma, urination problems, or severe high blood pressure or heart disease. Also avoid taking Allegra-D within 2 weeks of using an MAO-inhibitor drug such as Marplan, Nardil, or Parnate.

Special warnings about this medication
Use Allegra-D with caution if you have high blood pressure, diabetes, heart disease, increased pressure in the eyes, prostate problems, or hyperthyroidism. Stop using it and check with your doctor if it causes nervousness, dizziness, or sleeplessness.

**Possible food and drug interactions
when taking this medication**
No interactions with Allegra have been reported. Allegra-D, however, is known to interact with several prescription drugs. Avoid taking it within 2

weeks of using an MAO-inhibitor drug such as the antidepressants Marplan, Nardil, and Parnate, and check with your doctor before combining it with the following:

Mecamylamine (Inversine)
Methyldopa (Aldomet)
Reserpine (Diupress, Hydropres)

You should also avoid Allegra-D if you have a pacemaker and take digoxin (Lanoxin). And you should not combine it with over-the-counter antihistamines and decongestants.

Special information
if you are pregnant or breastfeeding
The effects of this drug during pregnancy have not been adequately studied. If you are pregnant or plan to become pregnant, inform your doctor immediately. It is not known whether Allegra appears in breast milk. If the drug is essential to your health, your doctor may advise you to stop nursing until your treatment is finished.

Recommended dosage

ALLEGRA

The usual dosage is 1 capsule (60 milligrams) twice a day. People with kidney problems should take only 1 dose a day.

ALLEGRA-D

Take 1 tablet twice a day. People with kidney problems should take only 1 tablet daily.

Overdosage
An overdose is unlikely to produce serious symptoms. Nevertheless, an excessive dose of any medicine can have serious consequences, so you should seek medical attention whenever an overdose is suspected.

Generic name:

ALLOPURINOL

See Zyloprim, page 1487.

Brand name:

ALORA

See Estraderm, page 490.

Generic name:

ALPRAZOLAM

See Xanax, page 1436.

Generic name:

ALPROSTADIL

See Caverject, page 217.

Brand name:

ALTACE

Pronounced: AL-tayce
Generic name: Ramipril

Why is this drug prescribed?

Altace is used in the treatment of high blood pressure. It is effective when used alone or in combination with other high blood pressure medications, especially thiazide-type water pills (diuretics). Altace works by preventing the conversion of a chemical in your blood called angiotensin I into a more potent substance that increases salt and water retention in your body. It also enhances blood flow in your circulatory system. It is a member of the group of drugs called ACE inhibitors.

Altace is also prescribed for people who show signs of congestive heart failure after a heart attack. It helps prevent the condition from getting worse.

Most important fact about this drug

If you are taking Altace for high blood pressure, you must take the drug regularly for it to be effective. Since blood pressure declines gradually, it may be several weeks before you get the full benefit of Altace; and you must continue taking it even if you are feeling well. Altace does not cure high blood pressure; it merely keeps it under control.

How should you take this medication?
Take this medication exactly as prescribed by your doctor. If you have difficulty swallowing the capsule, you can sprinkle the contents on a small amount (about 4 ounces) of applesauce, or mix the contents with 4 ounces of water or apple juice. Be sure to eat or drink the entire mixture so that you get the full dose of the drug. You can prepare the mixture ahead of time; it will keep for 24 hours at room temperature or 48 hours in the refrigerator.

■ *If you miss a dose...*
If you forget to take a dose, take it as soon as you remember. If it is almost time for your next dose, skip the one you missed and go back to your regular schedule. Never take 2 doses at the same time.

■ *Storage instructions...*
Store Altace at room temperature in a tightly closed container.

What side effects may occur?
Side effects cannot be anticipated. If any develop or change in intensity, inform your doctor as soon as possible. Only your doctor can determine if it is safe for you to continue taking Altace.

■ *More common side effects may include:*
Cough, headache (in people with high blood pressure); cough, dizziness, low blood pressure (in people with congestive heart failure)

■ *Less common or rare side effects may include:*
Abdominal pain, anemia, angina pectoris (chest pain), anxiety, arthritis, bruises, change in taste, constipation, convulsions, depression, diarrhea, difficulty swallowing, dizziness, dry mouth, fainting, fatigue, feeling of general discomfort, fever, fluid retention, heart failure, hearing loss, heart attack, impotence, inability to sleep, increased salivation, indigestion, inflammation of the stomach and intestines, irregular heartbeat, itching, joint pain or inflammation, labored breathing, light-headedness, loss of appetite, low blood pressure, memory loss, muscle pain, nausea, nerve pain, nervousness, nosebleed, rash, ringing in ears, skin reddening, skin sensitivity to light, sleepiness, sudden loss of strength, sweating, tingling or pins and needles, tremors, vertigo, very rapid heartbeat, vision changes, vomiting, weakness, weight gain

People prescribed the drug after a heart attack may also experience light-headedness when standing; more severe heart failure is also a possibility.

Why should this drug not be prescribed?
If you are sensitive to or have ever had an allergic reaction to Altace, or if you have a history of swelling of the face, tongue, or throat while taking similar drugs such as Capoten, Vasotec, and Zestril, you should not take this medication. Make sure that your doctor is aware of any drug reactions that you have experienced.

Special warnings about this medication
If you develop swelling of the face around your lips, tongue, or throat or difficulty swallowing, difficulty breathing, swelling of arms and legs, or infection, sore throat, and fever, you should contact your doctor immediately. You may have a serious side effect of the drug and need emergency treatment.

If you are taking Altace, your kidney function should be given a complete assessment and should continue to be monitored.

If you notice your skin or the whites of your eyes turning yellow, notify your doctor. Your liver may be affected, and you may have to stop taking Altace. Your doctor should routinely test your liver function while you are on this drug.

Altace should be used with caution if you have impaired liver or kidney function, or a disease of the connective tissue such as lupus erythematosus or scleroderma.

If you are taking diuretics and Altace, or have congestive heart failure, you may develop excessively low blood pressure.

Do not use salt substitutes containing potassium without consulting your doctor. Altace can cause increased potassium levels in your blood, especially if you have diabetes and kidney problems.

Light-headedness can occur when taking Altace, especially during the first days of therapy, and should be reported to your doctor. If fainting occurs, stop taking the medication and notify your doctor immediately.

Dehydration, excessive sweating, severe diarrhea, or vomiting could deplete your body's fluids, causing your blood pressure to drop dangerously.

ACE inhibitors such as Altace have been known to cause severe allergic reactions in people undergoing desensitization therapy with bee or wasp venom. These drugs have also caused severe reactions in kidney dialysis patients.

Possible food and drug interactions
when taking this medication

If Altace is taken with certain other drugs, the effects of either could be increased, decreased, or altered. It is especially important to check with your doctor before combining Altace with the following:

Alcohol
Diuretics such as hydrochlorothiazide (found in many blood pressure medicines)
Diuretics that don't wash out potassium, such as spironolactone (Aldactone) and the diuretic component in Dyazide, Maxzide, Moduretic, and others
Lithium (Lithonate, Eskalith)
Potassium supplements such as K-lyte and K-Tab
Potassium-containing salt substitutes

Special information
if you are pregnant or breastfeeding

When used during the second and third trimesters, Altace can lead to birth defects, prematurity, and death in developing and newborn babies. If you are pregnant or plan to become pregnant and are taking Altace, Altace should be discontinued as soon as possible. Contact your doctor immediately. Altace may appear in breast milk and could affect a nursing infant. If this medication is essential to your health, your doctor may advise you to avoid breastfeeding.

Recommended dosage

ADULTS

As a precaution, your doctor may have you take the first dose of Altace in his office. To reduce the risk of a severe drop in blood pressure, the dosage of any diuretic you're taking should be reduced or, if possible, eliminated.

High blood pressure

For patients not on diuretics, the usual starting dose is 2.5 milligrams, taken once daily. After blood pressure is under control, the dosage will range from 2.5 to 20 milligrams a day in a single dose or divided into 2 equal doses. If Altace proves insufficient, the doctor may then add a diuretic.

Heart failure after a heart attack

The usual starting dose is 2.5 milligrams taken twice a day. If your blood pressure drops severely, your doctor will reduce the dose to 1.25 milligrams, then slowly increase it back to the starting dose, aiming for a maintenance dose of 5 milligrams twice a day.

If you have kidney problems, your doctor may prescribe a lower than normal dose.

CHILDREN

The safety and effectiveness of Altace in children have not been established.

Overdosage

Any medication taken in excess can have serious consequences. If you suspect an overdose, seek medical attention immediately.

Symptoms of low blood pressure are likely to be the primary warning of an Altace overdose.

Brand name:

ALUPENT

Pronounced: AL-yew-pent
Generic name: Metaproterenol sulfate
Other brand name: Metaprel

Why is this drug prescribed?

Alupent is a bronchodilator prescribed for the prevention and relief of bronchial asthma and bronchial spasms (wheezing) associated with bronchitis and emphysema. Alupent Inhalation Solution is also used to treat acute asthmatic attacks in children 6 years of age and older.

Most important fact about this drug

Alupent's effects last up to 6 hours. It should not be used more frequently than your doctor recommends.

Increasing the number of doses can be dangerous and may actually make symptoms of asthma worse. Fatalities have occurred with excessive use of this medication.

If the dose your doctor recommends does not provide relief of your symptoms, if your symptoms become worse, or if side effects occur, seek medical attention immediately.

How should you take this medication?

Take this medication exactly as prescribed by your doctor.

■ *If you miss a dose...*
Take the dose as soon as you remember. Take any remaining doses for the day at equal intervals thereafter. Do not increase the total for the day or take 2 doses at the same time.

■ *Storage instructions...*
Store at room temperature. Protect from light and excessive humidity. Keep out of reach of children.

What side effects may occur?
Side effects cannot be anticipated. If any develop or change in intensity, inform your doctor as soon as possible. Only your doctor can determine if it is safe for you to continue taking Alupent.

■ *Side effects may include:*
Bad taste in mouth, cough, diarrhea, dizziness, fatigue, headache, high blood pressure, insomnia, nausea, nervousness, rapid or throbbing heartbeat, stomach and intestinal upset, throat irritation, tremors, vomiting, worsening or aggravation of asthma

Side effects can occur when a new aerosol container is used, even though you have had no trouble with the medication in the past. Replacing the container may solve the problem.

Why should this drug not be prescribed?
If you are sensitive to or have ever had an allergic reaction to Alupent or similar drugs, such as Proventil, you should not take this medication. Make sure your doctor is aware of any drug reactions you have experienced.

Unless you are directed to do so by your doctor, do not take this medication if you have an irregular, rapid heart rate.

Special warnings about this medication
When taking Alupent, you should not use other inhaled medications (called sympathomimetics) before checking with your doctor. Only your doctor can determine the sufficient amount of time between inhaled medications.

A single dose of nebulized Alupent used to treat an acute attack of asthma may temporarily relieve symptoms but not completely stop the attack.

Consult your doctor before using this medication if you have a heart condition or convulsive disorder (e.g., epilepsy), high blood pressure, hyperthyroidism, or diabetes mellitus. Alupent can cause significant changes in blood pressure.

Possible food and drug interactions
when taking this medication

If Alupent is taken with certain other drugs, the effects of either could be increased, decreased, or altered. It is especially important to check with your doctor before combining Alupent with the following:

MAO inhibitors (antidepressant drugs such as Nardil and Parnate)
Bronchodilators such as Ventolin and Proventil inhalers
Tricyclic antidepressants such as Elavil and Tofranil

Special information
if you are pregnant or breastfeeding

The effects of Alupent during pregnancy have not been adequately studied. If you are pregnant or plan to become pregnant, inform your doctor immediately. It is not known whether Alupent appears in breast milk. If this medication is essential to your health, your doctor may advise you to stop nursing your baby until your treatment is finished.

Recommended dosage

ADULTS

Inhalation Aerosol

The usual single dose is 2 to 3 inhalations. Inhalation should usually not be repeated more often than about every 3 to 4 hours. Total dosage per day should not exceed 12 inhalations.

Inhalation Solution 5%

Treatment usually need not be repeated more often than every 4 hours to relieve acute attacks of bronchospasm.

As part of a total treatment program for chronic breathing disorders, the inhalation solution may be taken 3 to 4 times per day, as determined by your doctor.

Inhalation solution is given by oral inhalation with the aid of a nebulizer or an intermittent positive pressure breathing (IPPB) apparatus.

The usual single dose with the nebulizer is 10 inhalations. However, a single dose of 5 to 15 inhalations can be taken, as determined by your doctor. The usual single daily dose with the IPPB is 0.3 milliliter diluted in approximately 2.5 milliliters of saline solution. The dosage range is 0.2 to 0.3 milliliter, as determined by your doctor.

Inhalation Solution 0.4% and 0.6% Unit-Dose Vials
The inhalation solution unit-dose vial is administered by oral inhalation using an intermittent positive pressure breathing (IPPB) apparatus. The usual adult dose is 1 vial per treatment. You usually should not need to repeat the treatment more often than every 4 hours for severe attacks of wheezing. You can use the unit-dose vials 3 to 4 times a day.

Syrup
The usual dose is 2 teaspoonfuls, 3 or 4 times a day.

Tablets
The usual dose is 20 milligrams, 3 or 4 times per day.

CHILDREN

Inhalation Aerosol
Alupent Inhalation Aerosol is not recommended for use in children under 12 years of age.

Inhalation Solution 5%
For children aged 6 to 12 years, the usual single dose is 0.1 milliliter, given by oral inhalation with a nebulizer. Dosage can be increased to 0.2 milliliter 3 to 4 times a day.

The unit-dose vial is not recommended for children under 12 years of age.

Syrup
The usual dose for children 6 to 9 years of age or weighing under 60 pounds is 1 teaspoonful, 3 or 4 times a day.

The usual dose for children over 9 years of age or weighing over 60 pounds is 2 teaspoonfuls, 3 or 4 times a day.

Tablets
The usual dose for children 6 to 9 years of age or weighing under 60 pounds is 10 milligrams, 3 or 4 times a day.

The usual dose for children over 9 years of age or weighing over 60 pounds is 20 milligrams, 3 or 4 times a day.

Tablets are not recommended for use in children under 6 years of age.

Overdosage
Any medication taken in excess can have serious consequences.

If you suspect an overdose, seek medical attention immediately.

■ *Symptoms of Alupent overdose may include:*
Dizziness, dry mouth, fatigue, general feeling of bodily discomfort,
headache, high or low blood pressure, inability to fall or stay asleep,
irregular heartbeat, nausea, nervousness, rapid, fluttery heartbeat, severe,
suffocating chest pain, tremors

Brand name:

AMARYL

Pronounced: AM-a-ril
Generic name: Glimepiride

Why is this drug prescribed?
Amaryl is an oral medication used to treat Type II (non-insulin-dependent)
diabetes when diet and exercise alone fail to control abnormally high levels
of blood sugar. Like other diabetes drugs classified as sulfonylureas, Amaryl
lowers blood sugar by stimulating the pancreas to produce more insulin.
Amaryl may also be used along with insulin and other diabetes drugs.

Most important fact about this drug
Always remember that Amaryl is an aid to, not a substitute for, good diet
and exercise. Failure to follow a sound diet and exercise plan may diminish
the results of Amaryl and can lead to serious complications such as
dangerously high or low blood sugar levels. Remember, too, that Amaryl is
not an oral form of insulin, and cannot be used in place of insulin.

How should you take this medication?
Do not take more or less of this medication than directed by your doctor.
Amaryl should be taken with breakfast or the first main meal.

■ *If you miss a dose...*
Take it as soon as you remember. If it is almost time for the next dose,
skip the one you missed and go back to your regular schedule. Do not take
2 doses at the same time.

■ *Storage instructions...*
Amaryl should be stored at room temperature in a well-closed container.

What side effects may occur?
Side effects cannot be anticipated. If any develop or change in intensity, tell
your doctor as soon as possible. Only your doctor can determine if it is safe
for you to continue taking Amaryl.

■ *Less common or rare side effects may include:*
Anemia and other blood disorders, blurred vision, diarrhea, dizziness, headache, itching, muscle weakness, nausea, sensitivity to light, skin rash and eruptions, stomach and intestinal pain, vomiting, yellow eyes and skin

Amaryl, like all oral antidiabetics, can result in hypoglycemia (low blood sugar). The risk of hypoglycemia can be increased by missed meals, alcohol, other medications, fever, injury, infection, surgery, and excessive exercise. To avoid hypoglycemia, closely follow the dietary and exercise regimen suggested by your doctor.

■ *Symptoms of mild low blood sugar may include:*
Blurred vision, cold sweats, dizziness, fast heartbeat, fatigue, headache, hunger, light-headedness, nausea, nervousness

■ *Symptoms of more severe low blood sugar may include:*
Coma, disorientation, pale skin, seizures, shallow breathing

Ask your doctor what steps you should take if you experience mild hypoglycemia. If symptoms of severe low blood sugar occur, contact your doctor immediately; severe hypoglycemia is a medical emergency.

Why should this drug not be prescribed?
Avoid Amaryl if you have ever had an allergic reaction to it.

Do not take Amaryl to correct diabetic ketoacidosis (a life-threatening medical emergency caused by insufficient insulin and marked by excessive thirst, nausea, fatigue, and fruity breath). This condition should be treated with insulin.

Special warnings about this medication
It's possible that drugs such as Amaryl may lead to more heart problems than diet treatment alone, or treatment with diet and insulin. If you have a heart condition, you may want to discuss this with your doctor.

When taking Amaryl, you should check your blood and urine regularly for abnormally high sugar (glucose) levels. The effectiveness of any oral antidiabetic, including Amaryl, may decrease with time. This may occur because of either a diminished responsiveness to the medication or a worsening of the diabetes.

Even people with well-controlled diabetes may find that stress such as injury, infection, surgery, or fever triggers a loss of control. If this happens, your doctor may recommend that you add insulin to your treatment with Amaryl or that you temporarily stop taking Amaryl and use insulin instead.

Possible food and drug interactions
when taking this medication

If Amaryl is taken with certain other drugs, the effects of either could be increased, decreased, or altered. It is especially important to check with your doctor before combining Amaryl with the following:

Airway-opening drugs such as Proventil and Ventolin
Aspirin and other salicylate medications
Chloramphenicol (Chloromycetin)
Corticosteroids such as prednisone (Deltasone)
Diuretics such as hydrochlorothiazide (HydroDIURIL) and chlorothiazide (Diuril)
Estrogens such as Premarin
Heart and blood pressure medications called beta blockers, including Tenormin, Inderal, and Lopressor
Isoniazid (Nydrazid)
Major tranquilizers such as Mellaril and Thorazine
MAO inhibitors (antidepressants such as Nardil and Parnate)
Miconazole (Monistat)
Nicotinic acid (Nicobid)
Nonsteroidal anti-inflammatory drugs such as Advil, Motrin, Naprosyn, Nuprin, Ponstel, and Voltaren
Oral contraceptives
Phenytoin (Dilantin)
Probenecid (Benemid)
Sulfa drugs such as Bactrim DS, Septra DS
Thyroid medications such as Synthroid
Warfarin (Coumadin)

Use alcohol with care; excessive alcohol intake can cause low blood sugar.

Special information
if you are pregnant or breastfeeding

Do not take Amaryl while pregnant. Since studies suggest the importance of maintaining normal blood sugar levels during pregnancy, your doctor may prescribe injected insulin instead. Drugs similar to Amaryl do appear in breast milk and may cause low blood sugar in nursing infants. You should not take Amaryl while nursing. If diet alone does not control your sugar levels, your doctor may prescribe injected insulin.

Recommended dosage

ADULTS

The usual starting dose is 1 to 2 milligrams taken once daily with breakfast or the first main meal. The maximum starting dose is 2 milligrams.

If necessary, your doctor will gradually increase the dose 1 or 2 milligrams at a time every 1 or 2 weeks. Your diabetes will probably be controlled on 1 to 4 milligrams a day; the most you should take in a day is 8 milligrams.

Weakened or malnourished people and those with adrenal, pituitary, kidney, or liver disorders are particularly sensitive to hypoglycemic drugs such as Amaryl and should start at 1 milligram once daily. Your doctor will increase your medication based on your response to the drug.

CHILDREN

Safety and effectiveness in children have not been established.

Overdosage
An overdose of Amaryl can cause low blood sugar (see "What side effects may occur?" for symptoms).

Eating sugar or a sugar-based product will often correct mild hypoglycemia. For severe hypoglycemia, seek medical attention immediately.

Brand name:

AMBIEN

Pronounced: AM-bee-en
Generic name: Zolpidem tartrate

Why is this drug prescribed?
Ambien is used for short-term treatment of insomnia (difficulty falling asleep or staying asleep, or early awakening). A relatively new drug, it is chemically different from other common sleep medications such as Halcion and Dalmane.

Most important fact about this drug
Sleep problems are usually temporary and require medication for a week or two at most. Insomnia that lasts longer could be a sign of another medical problem. If you find that you need this medicine for more than 7 to 10 days, be sure to check with your doctor.

How should you take this medication?
Ambien works very quickly. Take it just before going to bed. Take only the prescribed dose, exactly as instructed by your doctor.

■ *If you miss a dose...*
   Take Ambien only as needed. Never double the dose.

■ *Storage instructions...*
Store at room temperature. Protect from extreme heat.

What side effects may occur?
Side effects cannot be anticipated. If any develop or change in intensity, tell your doctor immediately. Only your doctor can determine whether it is safe to continue taking Ambien.

■ *More common side effects may include:*
Allergy, daytime drowsiness, dizziness, drugged feeling, headache, indigestion, nausea

■ *Less common side effects may include:*
Abdominal pain, abnormal dreams, abnormal vision, agitation, amnesia, anxiety, arthritis, back pain, bronchitis, burning sensation, chest pain, confusion, constipation, coughing, daytime sleeping, decreased mental alertness, depression, diarrhea, difficulty breathing, difficulty concentrating, difficulty swallowing, diminished sensitivity to touch, dizziness on standing, double vision, dry mouth, emotional instability, exaggerated feeling of well-being, eye irritation, falling, fatigue, fever, flu-like symptoms, gas, general discomfort, hallucination, hiccup, high blood pressure, high blood sugar, increased sweating, infection, insomnia, itching, joint pain, lack of bladder control, lack of coordination, lethargy, lightheadedness, loss of appetite, menstrual disorder, migraine, muscle pain, nasal inflammation, nervousness, numbness, paleness, prickling or tingling sensation, rapid heartbeat, rash, ringing in the ears, sinus inflammation, sleep disorder, speech difficulties, swelling due to fluid retention, taste abnormalities, throat inflammation, throbbing heartbeat, tremor, unconsciousness, upper respiratory infection, urinary tract infection, vertigo, vomiting, weakness

■ *Rare side effects may include:*
Abnormal tears or tearing, abscess, acne, aggravation of allergies, aggravation of high blood pressure, aggression, allergic reaction, altered production of saliva, anemia, belching, blisters, blood clot in lung, boils, breast pain, breast problems, breast tumors, bruising, chill with high temperature followed by heat and perspiration, decreased sex drive, delusion, difficulty urinating, excessive urine production, eye pain, facial swelling due to fluid retention, fainting, false perceptions, feeling intoxicated, feeling strange, flushing, frequent urination, glaucoma, gout, heart attack, hemorrhoids, herpes infection, high cholesterol, hives, hot flashes, impotence, inability to urinate, increased appetite, increased

tolerance to the drug, intestinal blockage, irregular heartbeat, joint degeneration, kidney failure, kidney pain, laryngitis, leg cramps, loss of reality, low blood pressure, mental deterioration, muscle spasms in arms and legs, muscle weakness, nosebleed, pain, painful urination, panic attacks, paralysis, pneumonia, poor circulation, rectal bleeding, rigidity, sciatica (lower back pain), sensation of seeing flashes of lights or sparks, sensitivity to light, sleepwalking, speech difficulties, swelling of the eye, thinking abnormalities, thirst, tooth decay, uncontrolled leg movements, urge to go to the bathroom, varicose veins, weight loss, yawning

Why should this drug not be prescribed?
There are no known situations in which Ambien cannot be used.

Special warnings about this medication
When sleep medications are used every night for more than a few weeks, some may lose their effectiveness. Remember, too, that you can become dependent on some sleep medications if you use them for a long time or at high doses.

Some people using Ambien have experienced unusual changes in their thinking and/or behavior. Alert your doctor if you notice a change.

Ambien and other sleep medicines can cause a special type of memory loss. It should not be taken on an overnight airplane flight of less than 7 to 8 hours, since "traveler's amnesia" may occur.

When you first start taking Ambien, until you know whether the medication will have any "carry over" effect the next day, use extreme care while doing anything that requires complete alertness, such as driving a car or operating machinery. Older adults, in particular, should be aware that they may be more apt to fall.

Use Ambien cautiously if you have liver problems. It will take longer for its effects to wear off.

If you take Ambien for more than 1 or 2 weeks, consult your doctor before stopping. Sudden discontinuation of a sleep medicine can bring on withdrawal symptoms ranging from unpleasant feelings to vomiting and cramps.

When taking Ambien, do *not* drink alcohol. It can increase the drug's side effects.

If you have breathing problems, they may become worse when you use Ambien.

Possible food and drug interactions
when taking this medication

If Ambien is used with certain other drugs, the effects of either drug could be increased, decreased, or altered. It is especially important to check with your doctor before combining Ambien with the following:

The major tranquilizer, chlorpromazine (Thorazine)
The antidepressant drug, imipramine (Tofranil)
Other drugs that depress the central nervous system, including Valium, Percocet, and Benadryl

Special information
if you are pregnant or breastfeeding

If you are pregnant or plan to become pregnant, inform your doctor immediately. Babies whose mothers take some sedative/hypnotic drugs may have withdrawal symptoms after birth and may seem limp and flaccid. Ambien is not recommended for use by nursing mothers.

Recommended dosage

ADULTS

The recommended dosage for adults is 10 milligrams right before bedtime. Your doctor will prescribe a smaller dose if you are likely to be sensitive to the drug or have a liver problem. Never take more than 10 milligrams of Ambien per day.

CHILDREN

Safety and effectiveness have not been established in children below the age of 18.

OLDER ADULTS

Because older people and those in a weakened condition may be more sensitive to Ambien's effects, the recommended starting dosage is 5 milligrams just before bedtime.

Overdosage

People who take too much Ambien may become excessively sleepy or even go into a light coma. The symptoms of overdose are more severe if the person is also taking other drugs that depress the central nervous system. Some cases of multiple overdose have been fatal.

If you suspect an overdose, seek medical attention immediately.

Generic name:

AMCINONIDE

See Cyclocort, page 317.

Brand name:

AMERGE

Pronounced: ah-MERJ
Generic name: Naratriptan hydrochloride

Why is this drug prescribed?
Amerge is used for relief of classic migraine headaches. It's helpful whether or not the headache is preceded by an aura (visual disturbances, usually sensations of halos or flickering lights). The drug works only during an actual attack. It will not reduce the number of headaches that develop.

Most important fact about this drug
Amerge should be used only for acute, classic migraine attacks. It should not be taken for other types of headache, including cluster headache and certain unusual types of migraine.

How should you take this medication?
Amerge may be taken any time after the headache starts. Swallow the tablet whole, with liquid. If you have no response, a partial response, or return of your headache after the first tablet, consult your doctor. You may take a second tablet, but should wait at least 4 hours after the first dose. Do not take more than 2 doses within 24 hours.

- *If you miss a dose...*
  Amerge is not for regular use. Take it only during an attack.

- *Storage instructions...*
  Store Amerge tablets at room temperature, away from heat and light. If your medication has expired (the expiration date is printed on the treatment pack), throw it away. If your doctor decides to stop your treatment, do not keep any leftover medicine unless your doctor recommends it.

What side effects may occur?
Side effects cannot be anticipated. If any develop or change in intensity,

inform your doctor as soon as possible. Only your doctor can determine if it is safe for you to continue taking Amerge.

■ *More common side effects may include:*
Nausea, sensation of pain and pressure, strange sensations

■ *Less common side effects may include:*
Decreased salivation, dizziness, drowsiness, fatigue, flu-like symptoms, ear/nose/throat infections, sensation of pain and pressure in the neck and throat, sensation of warmth or cold, sensitivity to light, tingling and stinging of the skin, vertigo, vomiting

■ *Rare side effects may include:*
Acid indigestion, allergic reactions, anxiety, blurred vision, constipation, chills and fever, cough, depression, diarrhea, fainting, increased blood pressure, increased thirst, increased urination, itching, joint and muscle stiffness, joint pain, loss of body fluids, muscle cramps and spasms, pneumonia, rapid heartbeat, ringing in the ears, sensitivity to sound, sinus and upper respiratory inflammation, skin rash, sleep disturbances, sweating, swelling, swollen and itchy patches of skin, taste and smell disturbances, thinking disturbances, tremors

Why should this drug not be prescribed?
You should avoid Amerge if you are prone to any type of impaired circulation, including angina (crushing chest pain), heart attack, stroke, or ischemic bowel disease. Also avoid Amerge if you have severe kidney or liver disease, or suffer from uncontrolled high blood pressure.

Do not use Amerge within 24 hours of another medication in the same drug class, such as Imitrex or Zomig, or an ergotamine-based medication such as Cafergot, D.H.E. 45 Injection, Migranol Nasal Spray, or Sansert.

If Amerge gives you an allergic reaction, stop using it and notify your doctor.

Special warnings about this medication
Amerge sometimes causes serious problems in people with heart disease. If you have heart disease, or know of any factors that make undetected heart disease a possibility, be sure to tell the doctor. Risk factors include high blood pressure, high cholesterol, diabetes, excess weight, smoking, a history of heart disease in your family, and menopause.

If there's any chance of a heart problem, your doctor may administer the first dose of Amerge in the office and monitor your response. After later doses, call your doctor immediately if you experience chest discomfort (including pain, heaviness, tightness), sudden or severe stomach pain, numbness or tingling, heat sensations, or facial flushing after taking Amerge.

Amerge is only for classic migraine headache. If the first dose fails to relieve your symptoms, your doctor should reevaluate you. Your problem may not be migraine.

If a headache feels different from any you've had previously, check with your doctor. It could be a warning of a problem unrelated to migraine.

If you have kidney or liver problems, or if you have any trouble with your eyes, inform your doctor.

Although very rare, severe and even fatal allergic reactions have occurred in people taking Amerge. Call your doctor immediately if you have shortness of breath; wheezing; palpitations; swelling of the eyelids, face, or lips; or a skin rash, lumps, or hives. Such reactions are more likely in people who have multiple allergies.

Amerge has not been tested in children or adults over age 65.

Possible food and drug interactions
when taking this medication
If Amerge is taken with certain other drugs, the effects of either may be increased, decreased, or altered. Do not combine Amerge with the following:

Ergot-containing drugs such as Cafergot and Ergostat
Sumatriptan (Imitrex)
Zolmitriptan (Zomig)
Antidepressants that boost serotonin levels, including Luvox, Paxil,
    Prozac, and Zoloft

Special information
if you are pregnant or breastfeeding
The effects of Amerge during pregnancy have not been adequately studied. If you are pregnant or plan to become pregnant, inform your doctor immediately. Amerge may appear in breast milk and could affect a nursing infant. If this medication is essential to your health, your doctor may advise you to discontinue breastfeeding while using Amerge.

Recommended dosage

ADULTS

Amerge comes in 1- and 2.5-milligram tablets. The most you should take at one time is 2.5 milligrams, and the maximum for each 24 hours is 5 milligrams. Doses should be spaced at least 4 hours apart.

If you have kidney or liver problems, the recommended dose is 1 milligram, with a 24-hour maximum of 2.5 milligrams.

Overdosage
Any medication taken in excess can have serious consequences. If you suspect an overdose, seek medical attention immediately.

- *Symptoms of Amerge overdose may include:*
  Light-headedness, loss of coordination, tension in the neck, tiredness

Generic name:

AMILORIDE WITH HYDROCHLOROTHIAZIDE

See Moduretic, page 817.

Generic name:

AMITRIPTYLINE

See Elavil, page 460.

Generic name:

AMITRIPTYLINE WITH PERPHENAZINE

See Triavil, page 1339.

Generic name:

AMLODIPINE

See Norvasc, page 910.

Generic name:

AMLODIPINE AND BENAZEPRIL

See Lotrel, page 732.

Generic name:

AMOXICILLIN

See Amoxil, page 58.

Generic name:

AMOXICILLIN, CLARITHROMYCIN, AND LANSOPRAZOLE

See Prevpac, page 1045.

Generic name:

AMOXICILLIN WITH CLAVULANATE

See Augmentin, page 113.

Brand name:

AMOXIL

Pronounced: a-MOX-il
Generic name: Amoxicillin
Other brand names: Trimox, Wymox

Why is this drug prescribed?

Amoxil, an antibiotic, is used to treat a wide variety of infections, including: gonorrhea, middle ear infections, skin infections, upper and lower respiratory tract infections, and infections of genital and urinary tract. In combination with other drugs such as Prevacid and Biaxin, it is also used to treat duodenal ulcers caused by *H. pylori* bacteria (ulcers in the wall of the small intestine near the exit from the stomach).

Most important fact about this drug

If you are allergic to either penicillin or cephalosporin antibiotics in any form, consult your doctor before taking Amoxil. There is a possibility that you are allergic to both types of medication; and if a reaction occurs, it could be extremely severe. If you take the drug and feel signs of a reaction, seek medical attention immediately.

How should you take this medication?

Amoxil can be taken with or without food. If you are using Amoxil suspension, shake it well before using.

■ *If you miss a dose...*
Take it as soon as you remember. If it is almost time for the next dose, and you take 2 doses a day, take the one you missed and the next dose 5 to 6 hours later. If you take 3 or more doses a day, take the one you missed and the next dose 2 to 4 hours later. Then go back to your regular schedule.

■ *Storage instructions...*
Amoxil suspension and pediatric drops should be stored in a tightly closed bottle. Discard any unused medication after 14 days. Refrigeration is preferable.

What side effects may occur?
Side effects cannot be anticipated. If any develop or change in intensity, inform your doctor as soon as possible. Only your doctor can determine if it is safe for you to continue taking Amoxil.

■ *Side effects may include:*
Agitation, anemia, anxiety, changes in behavior, confusion, diarrhea, dizziness, hives; hyperactivity, insomnia, nausea, rash, vomiting.

When used in combination with Prevacid and/or Biaxin for the treatment of ulcers, the most common side effects are changes in taste sensation, diarrhea, and headache.

Why should this drug not be prescribed?
You should not use Amoxil if you are allergic to penicillin or cephalosporin antibiotics (for example, Ceclor).

Special warnings about this medication
If you have ever had asthma, hives, hay fever, or other allergies, consult with your doctor before taking Amoxil.

You should stop using Amoxil if you experience reactions such as bruising, fever, skin rash, itching, joint pain, swollen lymph nodes, and/or sores on the genitals. If these reactions occur, stop taking Amoxil unless your doctor advises you to continue.

For infections such as strep throat, it is important to take Amoxil for the entire amount of time your doctor has prescribed. Even if you feel better, you need to continue taking Amoxil. If you stop taking Amoxil before your treatment time is complete, you may get other infections, such as glomerulonephritis (a kidney infection) or rheumatic fever.

If you are diabetic, be aware that Amoxil may cause a *false positive* Clinitest (urine glucose test) result to occur. You should consult with your doctor about using different tests while taking Amoxil.

Before taking Amoxil, tell your doctor if you have ever had asthma, colitis (inflammatory bowel disease), diabetes, or kidney or liver disease.

Possible food and drug interactions
when taking this medication

If Amoxil is taken with certain other drugs, the effects of either could be increased, decreased, or altered. It is especially important to check with your doctor before combining Amoxil with the following:

Chloramphenicol (Chloromycetin)
Erythromycin (E.E.S., PCE, others)
Oral contraceptives
Probenecid (Benemid)
Tetracycline (Achromycin V, others)

Special information
if you are pregnant or breastfeeding

Amoxil should be used during pregnancy only when clearly needed. If you are pregnant or plan to become pregnant, inform your doctor immediately. Since Amoxil may appear in breast milk, you should consult your doctor if you plan to breastfeed your baby.

Recommended dosage

Dosages will be determined by the type of infection being treated.

ADULTS

Ear, Nose, Throat, Skin, Genital, and Urinary Tract Infections

The usual dosage is 250 milligrams, taken every 8 hours.

Infections of the Lower Respiratory Tract

The usual dosage is 500 milligrams, taken every 8 hours.

Gonorrhea

The usual dosage is 3 grams in a single oral dose.

Gonococcal Infections Such as Acute, Uncomplicated Anogenital and Urethral Infections

3 grams as a single oral dose.

Ulcers

1 gram of Amoxil in combination with 500 milligrams of Biaxin and 30 milligrams of Prevacid taken every 12 hours for 14 days.

Alternatively, 1 gram of Amoxil can be taken with 30 milligrams of Prevacid every 8 hours for 14 days.

CHILDREN

Children weighing 44 pounds and over should follow the recommended adult dose schedule.

Children weighing under 44 pounds will have their dosage determined by their weight.

Dosage of Pediatric Drops:
Use the dropper provided with the medication to measure all doses.

All Infections Except Those of the Lower Respiratory Tract
Under 13 pounds:
  0.75 milliliter every 8 hours.
13 to 15 pounds:
  1 milliliter every 8 hours.
16 to 18 pounds:
  1.25 milliliters every 8 hours.

Infections of the Lower Respiratory Tract
Under 13 pounds:
  1.25 milliliters every 8 hours.
13 to 15 pounds:
  1.75 milliliters every 8 hours.
16 to 18 pounds:
  2.25 milliliters every 8 hours.

Children weighing more than 18 pounds should take the oral liquid. The required amount of suspension should be placed directly on the child's tongue for swallowing. It can also be added to formula, milk, fruit juice, water, ginger ale, or cold drinks. The preparation should be taken immediately. To be certain the child is getting the full dose of medication, make sure he or she drinks the entire preparation.

Overdosage

Any medication taken in excess can have serious consequences. If you suspect an overdose, seek medical attention immediately.

■ *Symptoms of Amoxil overdose may include:*
  Diarrhea, nausea, stomach cramps, vomiting

Generic name:

AMPHETAMINES

See Adderall, page 17.

Generic name:

AMPICILLIN

See Omnipen, page 922.

Brand name:

ANAFRANIL

Pronounced: an-AF-ran-il
Generic name: Clomipramine hydrochloride

Why is this drug prescribed?

Anafranil, a chemical cousin of tricyclic antidepressant medications such as Tofranil and Elavil, is used to treat people who suffer from obsessions and compulsions.

An obsession is a persistent, disturbing idea, image, or urge that keeps coming to mind despite the person's efforts to ignore or forget it—for example, a preoccupation with avoiding contamination.

A compulsion is an irrational action that the person knows is senseless but feels driven to repeat again and again—for example, hand-washing perhaps dozens or even scores of times throughout the day.

Most important fact about this drug

Serious, even fatal, reactions have been known to occur when drugs such as Anafranil are taken along with drugs known as MAO inhibitors. Drugs in this category include the antidepressants Nardil and Parnate. Never take Anafranil with one of these drugs.

How should you take this medication?

Take Anafranil with meals, at first, to avoid stomach upset. After your regular dosage has been established, you can take 1 dose at bedtime to avoid sleepiness during the day. Always take it exactly as prescribed.

This medicine may cause dry mouth. Hard candy, chewing gum, or bits of ice may relieve this problem.

■ *If you miss a dose...*
  If you take 1 dose at bedtime, consult your doctor. Do not take the missed dose in the morning. If you take 2 or more doses a day, take the missed dose as soon as you remember. If it is almost time for your next dose, skip

the one you missed and go back to your regular schedule. Do not take 2 doses at the same time.

■ *Storage instructions...*
Store at room temperature in a tightly closed container, away from moisture.

What side effects may occur?

Side effects cannot be anticipated. If any develop or change in intensity, inform your doctor as soon as possible. Only your doctor can determine if it is safe for you to continue taking Anafranil.

The most significant risk is that of seizures (convulsions). Headache, fatigue, and nausea can be a problem. Men are likely to experience problems with sexual function. Unwanted weight gain is a potential problem for many people who take Anafranil, although a small number actually lose weight.

■ *More common side effects may include:*
Abdominal pain, abnormal dreaming, abnormal tearing, abnormal milk secretion, agitation, allergy, anxiety, appetite loss, back pain, chest pain, confusion, constipation, coughing, depression, diarrhea, dizziness, dry mouth, extreme sleepiness, failure to ejaculate, fast heartbeat, fatigue, fever, flushing, fluttery heartbeat, frequent urination, gas, headache, hot flushes, impotence, inability to concentrate, increased appetite, increased sweating, indigestion, inflamed lining of nose or sinuses, itching, joint pain, light-headedness on standing up, memory problems, menstrual pain and disorders, middle ear infection (children), migraine, muscle pain or tension, nausea, nervousness, pain, rash, red or purple areas on the skin, ringing in the ears, sex-drive changes, sleeplessness, sleep disturbances, sore throat, speech disturbances, taste changes, tingling or pins and needles, tooth disorder, tremor, twitching, urinary problems, urinary tract infection, vision problems, vomiting, weight gain, weight loss (children), yawning

■ *Less common side effects may include:*
Abnormal skin odor (children), acne, aggression (children), eye allergy (children), anemia (children), bad breath (children), belching (children), breast enlargement, breast pain, chills, conjunctivitis (pinkeye), difficult or labored breathing (children), difficulty swallowing, difficulty or pain in urinating, dilated pupils, dry skin, emotional instability, eye twitching (children), fainting (children), hearing disorder (children), hives, irritability, lack of menstruation, loss of sense of identity, mouth inflammation

(children), muscle weakness, nosebleed, panic, paralysis (children), skin inflammation, sore throat (children), stomach and intestinal problems, swelling due to fluid retention, thirst, unequal size of pupils of the eye (children), vaginal inflammation, weakness (children), wheezing, white or yellow vaginal discharge

Why should this drug not be prescribed?

Do not take this medication if you are sensitive to or have ever had an allergic reaction to a tricyclic antidepressant such as Tofranil, Elavil, or Tegretol.

Be sure to avoid Anafranil if you are taking, or have taken within the past 14 days, an MAO inhibitor such as the antidepressants Parnate or Nardil. Combining Anafranil with one of these medications could lead to fever, seizures, coma, and even death.

Do not take Anafranil if you have recently had a heart attack.

Special warnings about this medication

If you have narrow-angle glaucoma (increased pressure in the eye) or are having difficulty urinating, Anafranil could make these conditions worse. Use Anafranil with caution if your kidney function is not normal.

If you have a tumor of the adrenal gland, this medication could cause your blood pressure to rise suddenly and dangerously.

Because Anafranil poses a possible risk of seizures, and because it may impair mental or physical ability to perform complicated tasks, your doctor will probably warn you to take special precautions if you need to drive a car, operate complicated machinery, or take part in activities such as swimming or climbing, in which suddenly losing consciousness could be dangerous. Note that your risk of seizures is increased:

- If you have ever had a seizure
- If you have a history of brain damage or alcoholism
- If you are taking another medication that might predispose you to seizures

As with Tofranil, Elavil, and other tricyclic antidepressants, an overdose of Anafranil can be fatal. Do not be surprised if your doctor prescribes only a small quantity of Anafranil at a time. This is standard procedure to minimize the risk of overdose.

Anafranil may cause your skin to become more sensitive to sunlight. Avoid prolonged exposure to sunlight.

Before having any kind of surgery involving the use of general anesthesia, tell your doctor or dentist that you are taking Anafranil. You may be advised to discontinue the drug temporarily.

When it is time to stop taking Anafranil, do not stop abruptly. Your doctor will have you taper off gradually to avoid withdrawal symptoms such as dizziness, fever, general feeling of illness, headache, high fever, irritability or worsening emotional or mental problems, nausea, sleep problems, vomiting.

Possible food and drug interactions when taking this medication

Avoid alcoholic beverages while taking Anafranil.

If Anafranil is taken with certain other drugs, the effects of either could be increased, decreased, or altered. It is especially important to check with your doctor before combining Anafranil with the following:

Barbiturates such as phenobarbital
Certain blood pressure drugs such as Ismelin and Catapres-TTS
Cimetidine (Tagamet)
Digoxin (Lanoxin)
Drugs that ease spasms, such as Donnatal, Cogentin, and Bentyl
Flecainide (Tambocor)
Fluoxetine (Prozac)
Haloperidol (Haldol)
Methylphenidate (Ritalin)
Major tranquilizers such as Thorazine
MAO inhibitors such as Nardil and Parnate
Paroxetine (Paxil)
Phenytoin (Dilantin)
Propafenone (Rythmol)
Quinidine (Quinidex)
Sertraline (Zoloft)
Thyroid medications such as Synthroid
Tranquilizers such as Xanax and Valium
Warfarin (Coumadin)

Special information if you are pregnant or breastfeeding

If you are pregnant or plan to become pregnant, inform your doctor immediately. Anafranil should not be used during pregnancy unless absolutely necessary; some babies born to women who took Anafranil have had withdrawal symptoms such as jitteriness, tremors, and seizures. Anafranil appears in breast milk. Your doctor may advise you to stop breastfeeding while you are taking Anafranil.

Recommended dosage

ADULTS

The usual recommended initial dose is 25 milligrams daily. Your doctor may gradually increase this dosage to 100 milligrams during the first 2 weeks. During this period you will be asked to take this drug, divided into smaller doses, with meals. The maximum daily dosage is 250 milligrams. After the dose has been determined, your doctor may direct you to take a single dose at bedtime, to avoid sleepiness during the day.

CHILDREN

The usual recommended initial dose is 25 milligrams daily, divided into smaller doses and taken with meals. Your doctor may gradually increase the dose to a maximum of 100 milligrams or 3 milligrams per 2.2 pounds of body weight per day, whichever is smaller. The maximum dose is 200 milligrams or 3 milligrams per 2.2 pounds of body weight, whichever is smaller. Once the dose has been determined, the child can take it in a single dose at bedtime.

Overdosage

An overdose of Anafranil can be fatal. If you suspect an overdose, seek medical attention immediately.

■ *Critical signs and symptoms of Anafranil overdose may include:*
Impaired brain activity (including coma), irregular heartbeat, seizures, severely low blood pressure

■ *Other signs and symptoms of overdosage may include:*
Agitation, bluish skin color, breathing difficulty, delirium, dilated pupils, drowsiness, high fever, incoordination, little or no urine output, muscle rigidity, overactive reflexes, rapid heartbeat, restlessness, severe perspiration, shock, stupor, twitching or twisting movements, vomiting

There is a danger of heart malfunction and even, in rare cases, cardiac arrest.

Brand name:

ANAPROX

Pronounced: AN-uh-procks
Generic name: Naproxen sodium
Other brand names: Aleve, Naprelan

Why is this drug prescribed?
Anaprox and Naprelan are nonsteroidal anti-inflammatory drugs used to relieve mild to moderate pain and menstrual cramps. They are also prescribed for relief of the inflammation, swelling, stiffness, and joint pain associated with rheumatoid arthritis and osteoarthritis (the most common form of arthritis), and for ankylosing spondylitis (spinal arthritis), tendinitis, bursitis, acute gout, and other conditions. Anaprox also may be prescribed for juvenile arthritis.

The over-the-counter form of naproxen sodium, Aleve, is used for temporary relief of minor aches and pains, and to reduce fever.

Most important fact about this drug
You should have frequent checkups with your doctor if you take Anaprox regularly. Ulcers or internal bleeding can occur without warning.

How should you take this medication?
Your doctor may ask you to take Anaprox with food or an antacid to avoid stomach upset. Take Aleve with a full glass of water.

Take this medication exactly as prescribed by your doctor.

If you are using Anaprox for arthritis, it should be taken regularly.

■ *If you miss a dose...*
Anaprox: Take the forgotten dose as soon as you remember. If it is almost time for your next dose, skip the one you missed and go back to your regular schedule. Never take 2 doses at the same time.

Naprelan: Take the forgotten dose only if you remember within 2 hours after the appointed time. Otherwise, skip the dose and go back to your regular schedule.

■ *Storage instructions...*
Store at room temperature in a tightly closed container.

What side effects may occur?
Side effects cannot be anticipated. If any develop or change in intensity, inform your doctor as soon as possible. Only your doctor can determine if it is safe for you to continue taking Anaprox.

■ *More common side effects of Anaprox may include:*
Abdominal pain, bruising, constipation, diarrhea, difficult or labored breathing, dizziness, drowsiness, headache, hearing disturbances, heartburn, indigestion, inflammation of the mouth, itching, light-headedness,

nausea, rapid, fluttery heartbeat, red or purple spots on the skin, ringing in the ears, skin eruptions, sweating, swelling due to fluid retention, thirst, vertigo, vision changes

■ *Less common or rare side effects of Anaprox may include:*
Abdominal bleeding, black stools, blood in the urine, change in dream patterns, chills and fever, colitis (inflammation of the large intestine), congestive heart failure, depression, general feeling of illness, hair loss, inability to concentrate, inability to sleep, inflammation of the lungs, kidney disease or failure, menstrual problems, muscle weakness and/or pain, peptic ulcer, severe allergic reactions, skin inflammation due to sensitivity to light, skin rashes, vomiting, vomiting blood, yellow skin and eyes

Naprelan shares some of the above side effects, but also has some of its own:

■ *More common side effects of Naprelan may include:*
Back pain, flu symptoms, infection, nasal inflammation, sinus inflammation, sore throat, urinary infection

■ *Less common side effects of Naprelan may include:*
Accidental injury, anemia, bronchitis, chest pain, cough increased, difficulty swallowing, fever, gas, high blood pressure, high blood sugar, joint pain, joint/tendon problems, leg cramps, "pins and needles" or tingling, stomach inflammation, weakness

■ *Rare side effects of Naprelan may include:*
Abscesses, amnesia, angina pectoris (severe chest pain), anxiety, belching, blood disorders, bone disorders, bursitis, certain cancers, confusion, digestive tract inflammation, emotional changeability, enlarged abdomen, eye or ear problems, fainting, gallstones, heart and blood vessel disorders, kidney stones, loss of appetite, migraine, nail disorders, neck pain or rigidity, nerve problems, nervousness, nosebleed, paralysis, pelvic pain, prostate problems, respiration and/or lung problems, skin disorders, stomach/intestinal/rectal hemorrhage or other disorders, tooth problems, ulcers, urinary problems, vaginal inflammation, vertigo, weight loss

Why should this drug not be prescribed?
If you are sensitive to or have ever had an allergic reaction to Anaprox, aspirin, or similar drugs such as Motrin, if you have had asthma attacks caused by aspirin or other drugs of this type, or if you have ever retained fluid

or had hives or nasal tumors, you should not take this medication. Make sure your doctor is aware of any drug reactions you have experienced.

Special warnings about this medication

Remember that peptic ulcers and bleeding can occur without warning.

This drug should be used with caution if you have kidney or liver disease. It can cause liver inflammation in some people.

Do not take aspirin or any other anti-inflammatory medications while taking Anaprox, unless your doctor tells you to do so.

Anaprox and Naprelan contain sodium. If you are on a low sodium diet, discuss this with your doctor.

Use with caution if you have heart disease or high blood pressure. This drug can increase water retention. It also may cause vision problems. If you experience any changes in your vision, inform your doctor.

This drug makes some people drowsy or less alert. Avoid driving, operating dangerous machinery, or participating in any hazardous activity that requires full mental alertness if you find that the drug has this effect on you.

Do not take Aleve for more than 10 days for pain or 3 days for fever. Contact your doctor if pain or fever persists or gets worse, if the painful area becomes red or swollen, or if you develop more than a mild digestive upset.

Possible food and drug interactions
when taking this medication

If Anaprox is taken with certain other drugs, the effects of either could be increased, decreased, or altered. It is especially important to check with your doctor before combining Anaprox with the following:

ACE inhibitors such as the blood pressure medication Capoten
Antiseizure drugs such as Dilantin
Aspirin
Beta blockers, including blood pressure drugs such as Inderal
Blood thinners such as Coumadin
Certain water pills (diuretics) such as Lasix
Lithium (Lithonate)
Methotrexate
Naproxen in other forms, such as Naprosyn
Oral diabetes drugs such as Micronase
Other pain relievers such as aspirin, acetaminophen (Tylenol), and
    ibuprofen (Motrin)
Probenecid (Benemid)

If you have more than 3 alcoholic drinks per day, check with your doctor before using painkillers.

Special information
if you are pregnant or breastfeeding
The effects of Anaprox during pregnancy have not been adequately studied. If you are pregnant or plan to become pregnant, inform your doctor immediately. Avoid Anaprox, Naprelan, and Aleve during the last 3 months of pregnancy. Anaprox appears in breast milk and could affect a nursing infant. If this medication is essential to your health, your doctor may advise you to discontinue breastfeeding until your treatment with this medication is finished.

Recommended dosage

ANAPROX: ADULTS

Mild to Moderate Pain, Menstrual Cramps, Acute Tendinitis and Bursitis
The starting dose is 550 milligrams, followed by 275 milligrams every 6 to 8 hours or 550 milligrams every 12 hours. You should not take more than 1,375 milligrams a day to start, or 1,100 milligrams a day thereafter.

Rheumatoid Arthritis, Osteoarthritis, and Ankylosing Spondylitis
The starting dose is 275 milligrams or 550 milligrams 2 times a day (morning and evening). Your physician can adjust the doses for maximum benefit. Symptoms should improve within 2 to 4 weeks.

Acute Gout
The starting dose is 825 milligrams, followed by 275 milligrams every 8 hours, until symptoms subside.

ANAPROX: CHILDREN

Juvenile Arthritis
The usual daily dosage is a total of 10 milligrams per 2.2 pounds of body weight, divided into 2 doses. Dosage should not exceed 15 milligrams per 2.2 pounds per day.

The safety and effectiveness of Anaprox have not been established in children under 2 years of age.

ANAPROX: OLDER ADULTS

Your doctor will determine the dosage based on your particular needs. Adjustments in the normal adult dosage may be needed.

NAPRELAN

Rheumatoid Arthritis, Osteoarthritis, and Ankylosing Spondylitis

The usual dose is two 375- or 500-milligram tablets taken once a day. Your doctor will adjust your dose. You should not take more than three 500-milligram tablets daily.

Pain, Menstrual Cramps, Acute Tendinitis and Bursitis

The starting dose is two 500-milligram tablets taken once a day. For a short time, the doctor may increase the dose to three 500-milligram tablets daily.

Acute Gout

The usual dose is two to three 500-milligram tablets taken together on the first day, then two 500-milligram tablets once daily until the attack subsides.

It is not known whether Naprelan is safe for children.

ALEVE

1 tablet or caplet every 8 to 12 hours, to a maximum of 3 per day. For those over age 65, no more than 1 tablet or caplet every 12 hours. Not recommended for children under 12.

Overdosage

Any medication taken in excess can cause symptoms of overdose. If you suspect an overdose of Anaprox, seek medical attention immediately.

■ *The symptoms of Anaprox overdose may include:*
Drowsiness, heartburn, indigestion, nausea, vomiting

Brand name:

ANASPAZ

See Levsin, page 683.

Generic name:

ANASTROZOLE

See Arimidex, page 86.

Brand name:

ANEXSIA

See Vicodin, page 1403.

Brand name:

ANOLOR 300

See Fioricet, page 518.

Brand name:

ANSAID

Pronounced: AN-sed
Generic name: Flurbiprofen

Why is this drug prescribed?
Ansaid, a nonsteroidal anti-inflammatory drug, is used to relieve the inflammation, swelling, stiffness, and joint pain associated with rheumatoid arthritis and osteoarthritis (the most common form of arthritis).

Most important fact about this drug
You should have frequent checkups with your doctor if you take Ansaid regularly. Ulcers or internal bleeding can occur without warning.

How should you take this medication?
Your doctor may ask you to take Ansaid with food or an antacid.

Take this medication exactly as prescribed by your doctor.

If you are using Ansaid for arthritis, it should be taken regularly.

■ *If you miss a dose...*
   Take the forgotten dose as soon as you remember. If it is almost time for your next dose, skip the one you missed and go back to your regular schedule. Never take 2 doses at the same time.

■ *Storage instructions...*
Store at room temperature.

What side effects may occur?
Side effects cannot be anticipated. If any develop or change in intensity, inform your doctor as soon as possible. Only your doctor can determine if it is safe for you to continue taking Ansaid.

■ *More common side effects may include:*
Abdominal pain, diarrhea, general feeling of illness, headache, indigestion, nausea, swelling due to fluid retention, urinary tract infection

■ *Less common or rare side effects may include:*
Altered sense of smell, anemia, anxiety, asthma, blood in the urine, bloody diarrhea, bruising, chills and fever, confusion, conjunctivitis (pinkeye), constipation, depression, dizziness, feeling of illness, gas, heart failure, hepatitis, high blood pressure, hives, inflammation of the nose or mouth, inflammation of the stomach, insomnia, itching, kidney failure, lack of coordination, memory loss, nervousness, nosebleed, peptic ulcer, pins and needles, rash, ringing in the ears, sensitivity of skin to light, severe allergic reaction, skin inflammation with or without sores and crusting, sleepiness, stomach and intestinal bleeding, swelling of throat, tremor, twitching, vision changes, vomiting, vomiting blood, weakness, weight changes, welts, yellow eyes and skin

Why should this drug not be prescribed?
If you are sensitive to or have ever had an allergic reaction to Ansaid, aspirin, or similar drugs such as Motrin, or if you have had asthma attacks caused by aspirin or other drugs of this type, you should not take this medication. Fatal attacks have occurred in people allergic to this drug. Make sure your doctor is aware of any drug reactions you have experienced.

Special warnings about this medication
This drug should be used with caution if you have kidney or liver disease. Kidney problems are most likely to develop in such people, as well as in those with heart failure, those taking water pills, and older adults.

If you have asthma, take Ansaid with extra caution. Do not take aspirin or similar drugs while taking Ansaid, unless your doctor tells you to do so.

Ansaid can cause vision problems. If you experience a change in your vision, inform your doctor. Blurred and/or decreased vision has occurred while taking this medication.

Ansaid slows the clotting process. If you are taking blood-thinning medication, this drug should be taken with caution.

This drug can increase water retention. If you have heart disease or high blood pressure, use with caution.

If you want to take Ansaid for pain less serious than that of arthritis, be sure to discuss the risks of using this drug with your doctor.

Possible food and drug interactions
when taking this medication

If Ansaid is taken with certain other drugs, the effects of either could be increased, decreased, or altered. It is especially important to check with your doctor before combining Ansaid with the following:

Antacids
Aspirin
Beta blockers such as the blood pressure medications Inderal and Tenormin
Blood thinners such as Coumadin
Cimetidine (Tagamet)
Methotrexate (Rheumatrex)
Oral diabetes drugs such as Micronase
Ranitidine (Zantac)
Water pills such as Lasix and Bumex

Special information
if you are pregnant or breastfeeding

The effects of Ansaid during pregnancy have not been adequately studied. If you are pregnant or plan to become pregnant, inform your doctor immediately. In particular, you should not use Ansaid in late pregnancy, as it can affect the developing baby's circulatory system. Ansaid appears in breast milk and could affect a nursing infant. If this medication is essential to your health, your doctor may advise you to discontinue breastfeeding until your treatment is finished.

Recommended dosage

ADULTS

Rheumatoid Arthritis or Osteoarthritis:

The usual starting dosage is a total of 200 to 300 milligrams a day, divided into 2, 3, or 4 smaller doses (usually 3 or 4 for rheumatoid arthritis). Your doctor will tailor the dose to suit your needs, but you should not take more than 100 milligrams at any one time or more than 300 milligrams in a day.

CHILDREN

The safety and effectiveness of Ansaid have not been established in children.

OLDER ADULTS

Older people are among those most apt to develop kidney problems while taking this drug.

Your doctor will determine the dosage according to your needs.

Overdosage

Any medication taken in excess can cause symptoms of overdose. If you suspect an overdose of Ansaid, seek medical attention immediately.

- *The symptoms of Ansaid overdose may include:*
  Agitation, change in pupil size, coma, disorientation, dizziness, double vision, drowsiness, headache, nausea, semiconsciousness, shallow breathing, stomach pain

Category:

ANTACIDS

Brand names: Gaviscon, Maalox, Mylanta, Rolaids, Tums

Why is this drug prescribed?

Available under a number of brand names, antacids are used to relieve the uncomfortable symptoms of acid indigestion, heartburn, gas, and sour stomach.

Most important fact about this drug

Do not take antacids for longer than 2 weeks or in larger than recommended doses unless directed by your doctor. If your symptoms persist, contact your doctor. Antacids should be used only for occasional relief of stomach upset.

How should you take this medication?

If you take a chewable antacid tablet, chew thoroughly before swallowing so that the medicine can work faster and be more effective. Allow Mylanta Soothing Lozenges to completely dissolve in your mouth. Shake liquids well before using.

■ *If you miss a dose...*
Take this medication only as needed or as instructed by your doctor.

■ *Storage instructions...*
Store at room temperature. Keep liquids tightly closed and protect from freezing.

What side effects may occur?
When taken as recommended, antacids are relatively free of side effects. Occasionally, one of the following symptoms may develop.

■ *Side effects may include:*
Chalky taste, constipation, diarrhea, increased thirst, stomach cramps

Why should this drug not be prescribed?
Do not take antacids if you have signs of appendicitis or an inflamed bowel; symptoms include stomach or lower abdominal pain, cramping, bloating, soreness, nausea, or vomiting.

If you are sensitive to or have ever had an allergic reaction to aluminum, calcium, magnesium, or simethicone, do not take an antacid containing these ingredients. If you are elderly and have bone problems or if you are taking care of an elderly person with Alzheimer's disease, do not use an antacid containing aluminum.

Special warnings about this medication
If you are taking any prescription drug, check with your doctor before you take an antacid. Also, tell your doctor or pharmacist about any drug allergies or medical conditions you have.

If you have kidney disease, do not take an antacid containing aluminum or magnesium. If you are on a sodium-restricted diet, do not take Gaviscon without checking first with your doctor or pharmacist.

Possible food and drug interactions
when taking this medication
If antacids are taken with certain other medications, the effects of either could be increased, decreased, or altered. It is especially important to check with your doctor before combining antacids with the following:

Cellulose sodium phosphate (Calcibind)
Isoniazid (Rifamate)
Ketoconazole (Nizoral)
Mecamylamine (Inversine)

Methenamine (Mandelamine)
Sodium polystyrene sulfonate resin (Kayexalate)
Tetracycline antibiotics (Achromycin, Minocin)

Special information
if you are pregnant or breastfeeding

As with all medications, ask your doctor or health care professional whether it is safe for you to use antacids while you are pregnant or breastfeeding.

Recommended dosage

ADULTS

Take antacids according to the following schedules, or as directed by your doctor.

Gaviscon and Gaviscon Extra Strength Relief Formula Chewable Tablets

Chew 2 to 4 tablets 4 times a day after meals and at bedtime or as needed. Follow with half a glass of water or other liquid. Do not swallow the tablets whole.

Gaviscon Extra Strength Relief Formula Liquid

Take 2 to 4 teaspoonfuls 4 times a day after meals and at bedtime. Follow with half a glass of water or other liquid.

Gaviscon Liquid

Take 1 or 2 tablespoonfuls 4 times a day after meals and at bedtime. Follow with half a glass of water.

Maalox Antacid Caplets

Take 1 caplet as needed. Swallow the tablets whole; do not chew them.

Maalox Heartburn Relief Chewable Tablets

Chew 2 to 4 tablets after meals and at bedtime. Follow with half a glass of water or other liquid.

Maalox Heartburn Relief Suspension, Maalox Magnesia and Alumina Oral Suspension, and Extra Strength Maalox Antacid Plus Anti-Gas Suspension

Take 2 to 4 teaspoonfuls 4 times a day, 20 minutes to 1 hour after meals and at bedtime.

Maalox Plus Chewable Tablets
Chew 1 to 4 tablets 4 times a day, 20 minutes to 1 hour after meals and at bedtime.

Extra Strength Maalox Antacid Plus Anti-Gas Chewable Tablets
Chew 1 to 3 tablets 20 minutes to 1 hour after meals and at bedtime.

Mylanta and Mylanta Double Strength Liquid and Chewable Tablets Antacid/Anti-Gas
Take 2 to 4 teaspoonfuls of liquid or chew 2 to 4 tablets between meals and at bedtime.

Mylanta Gelcaps
Take 2 to 4 gelcaps as needed.

Mylanta Soothing Lozenges
Dissolve 1 lozenge in your mouth. If needed, follow with a second. Repeat as needed.

Rolaids, Calcium-Rich/Sodium Free Rolaids, and Extra Strength Rolaids
Chew 1 or 2 tablets as symptoms occur. Repeat hourly if symptoms return.

Tums, Tums E-X, and Tums Anti-Gas Formula
Chew 1 or 2 tablets as symptoms occur. Repeat hourly if symptoms return. You may also hold the tablet between your gum and cheek and let it dissolve gradually.

CHILDREN

Do not give to children under 6 years of age, unless directed by your doctor.

Overdosage
Any medication taken in excess can have serious consequences. If you suspect an overdose, seek medical attention immediately.

■ *Symptoms of antacid overdose may include:*

For aluminum-containing antacids (Gaviscon, Maalox, Mylanta)
Bone pain, constipation (severe and continuing), feeling of discomfort

(continuing), loss of appetite (continuing), mood or mental changes, muscle weakness, swelling of wrists or ankles, weight loss (unusual)

For calcium-containing antacids (Mylanta, Rolaids, Tums)

Constipation (severe and continuing), difficult or painful urination, frequent urge to urinate, headache (continuing), loss of appetite (continuing), mood or mental changes, muscle pain or twitching, nausea or vomiting, nervousness or restlessness, slow breathing, unpleasant taste, unusual tiredness or weakness

For magnesium-containing antacids (Gaviscon, Maalox, Mylanta)

Difficult or painful urination, dizziness or light-headedness, irregular heartbeat, mood or mental changes, unusual tiredness or weakness

Generic name:

ANTIPYRINE, BENZOCAINE, AND GLYCERIN

See Auralgan, page 116.

Brand name:

ANTIVERT

Pronounced: AN-tee-vert
Generic name: Meclizine hydrochloride
Other brand name: Bonine

Why is this drug prescribed?
Antivert, an antihistamine, is prescribed for the management of nausea, vomiting, and dizziness associated with motion sickness.

Antivert may also be prescribed for the management of vertigo (a spinning sensation or a feeling that the ground is tilted) due to diseases affecting the vestibular system (the bony labyrinth of the ear, which contains the sensors that control your balance).

Most important fact about this drug
Antivert may cause you to become drowsy or less alert; therefore, driving a car or operating dangerous machinery is not recommended.

How should you take this medication?
Take this medication exactly as prescribed by your doctor.

■ *If you miss a dose...*
Take it as soon as you remember. If it is almost time for your next dose, skip the one you missed and go back to your regular schedule. Do not take 2 doses at the same time.

■ *Storage instructions...*
Store away from heat, light, and moisture.

What side effects may occur?
Side effects cannot be anticipated. If any develop or change in intensity, inform your doctor as soon as possible. Only your doctor can determine if it is safe for you to continue taking Antivert.

■ *More common side effects may include:*
Drowsiness, dry mouth

■ *Rare side effects may include:*
Blurred vision

Why should this drug not be prescribed?
If you are sensitive to or have ever had an allergic reaction to Antivert or similar drugs, do not take this drug. Make sure that your doctor is aware of any drug reactions you have experienced.

Special warnings about this medication
If you have asthma, glaucoma, or an enlarged prostate gland, check with your doctor before using Antivert.

**Possible food and drug interactions
when taking this medication**
Antivert may intensify the effects of alcohol. Do not drink alcohol while taking this medication.

**Special information
if you are pregnant or breastfeeding**
Studies regarding the use of Antivert in pregnant women do not indicate that this drug increases the risk of abnormalities. However, if you are pregnant or plan to become pregnant, inform your doctor before using Antivert. Check with him, too, if you are breastfeeding your baby.

Recommended dosage

ADULTS AND CHILDREN 12 AND OVER

Motion Sickness:
For protection against motion sickness, take 25 to 50 milligrams 1 hour before traveling. You may repeat the dose every 24 hours for the duration of the journey.

Vertigo:
The recommended dosage is 25 to 100 milligrams per day, divided into equal, smaller doses as determined by your doctor.

CHILDREN

The safety and effectiveness of Antivert have not been established in children under 12 years of age.

Overdosage

Any medication taken in excess can have serious consequences. If you suspect an overdose of Antivert, seek emergency medical treatment immediately.

Brand name:

ARAVA

Pronounced: ah-RAV-ah
Generic name: Leflunomide

Why is this drug prescribed?
Arava is used in the treatment of rheumatoid arthritis. It reduces the pain, stiffness, inflammation, and swelling associated with this disease, and staves off the joint damage that ultimately results.

Most important fact about this drug
You MUST NOT take Arava if you are pregnant; it can harm the developing baby. If you are still in your childbearing years, your doctor will want to see negative results from a pregnancy test before starting you on Arava. You'll also need to use reliable contraceptive measures as long as you take the drug.

If you become pregnant while taking Arava, your doctor will stop the drug immediately and prescribe a regimen of cholestyramine (Questran) in 8-gram doses 3 times a day for 11 days. Questran helps to clear Arava from the bloodstream, possibly preventing harm to the unborn child.

How should you take this medication?
Your dosage of Arava will be decreased after the first 3 days. Never take more than your doctor prescribes.

■ *If you miss a dose...*
Take it as soon as you remember. If it is almost time for your next dose, skip the one you missed and go back to your regular schedule. Do not take 2 doses at the same time.

■ *Storage instructions...*
Store at room temperature away from light.

What side effects may occur?
Side effects cannot be anticipated. If any develop or change in intensity, inform your doctor as soon as possible. Only your doctor can determine if it is safe for you to continue taking Arava.

■ *More common side effects may include:*
Abdominal pain, back pain, bronchitis, cough, diarrhea, dizziness, hair loss, headache, high blood pressure, indigestion, itching, joint disorders, loss of appetite, mouth ulcers, nausea, rash, respiratory infection, sore throat, stomach inflammation, tendon inflammation, urinary tract infection, vomiting, weakness, weight loss

■ *Less common side effects may include:*
Abscess, acne, allergic reaction, anemia, angina, anxiety, asthma, blood in the urine, blurred vision, bone pain, bruising, bursitis, cataracts, chest pain, colitis, conjunctivitis (pinkeye), constipation, cysts, depression, dermatitis, diabetes, difficulty breathing, dry mouth, dry skin, eczema, eye problems, fever, flu-like symptoms, frequent urination, fungal infection of the mouth, fungal infection of the skin, gallstones, gas, general feeling of illness, gingivitis, hair discoloration, hernia, herpes infection, hyperthyroidism, insomnia, joint pain, leg cramps, lung problems, menstrual disorders, migraine, mouth and throat inflammation, muscle aches, muscle cramps, nail disorders, nasal inflammation, nosebleeds, prostate disorder, rapid heartbeat, sinus inflammation, skin bumps, pain, painful urination, palpitations, pelvic pain, pneumonia, purple spots on skin, skin discoloration, skin tingling, skin ulcers, sleep disorders, sweating, swelling, tarry stools, taste problems, tooth problems, vaginal fungal infection, varicose veins

Why should this drug not be prescribed?
Remember that you must not take Arava if you are pregnant or plan to become pregnant. You'll also need to avoid this drug if it gives you an allergic reaction.

Special warnings about this medication
Arava is potentially damaging to the liver. Your doctor will test your liver function before starting Arava therapy, and will conduct monthly blood tests thereafter. If you have significant liver disease, including hepatitis, you'll be unable to take Arava. If you develop liver problems while taking the drug, your dose will have to be reduced or eliminated.

Theoretically, Arava may interfere with the body's ability to fight off infection. The drug is therefore not recommended for people with cancer, bone marrow problems, severe infections, AIDS, or any other immune system problems. You should also avoid immunization with live vaccines while taking Arava.

Poor kidney function can increase the amount of Arava in your system. Your doctor will prescribe the drug cautiously if you're subject to kidney problems.

Arava does not appear to cause fetal harm when taken by the father prior to conception. Nevertheless, if you plan to father a child, your doctor will instruct you to stop taking Arava and will prescribe a regimen of cholestyramine to clear Arava from your system.

**Possible food and drug interactions
when taking this medication**
If Arava is taken with certain other drugs, the effects of either could be increased, decreased, or altered. It is especially important to check with your doctor before combining Arava with the following:

Cholestyramine (Prevalite, Questran)
Methotrexate (Rheumatrex)
Nonsteroidal anti-inflammatory drugs such as Advil, Aleve, Motrin, and Naprosyn
Rifampin (Rifadin, Rifamate, Rimactane)
Tolbutamide (Orinase)

**Special information
if you are pregnant or breastfeeding**
Do not take Arava while pregnant or breastfeeding. Taken during pregnancy, the drug can cause birth defects. And although it is not known whether Arava appears in breast milk, there is good reason to suspect that it will cause serious side effects in nursing infants.

Recommended dosage

ADULTS

The recommended starting dose is one 100-milligram tablet daily for the first 3 days. The doctor will then reduce the dose to 20 milligrams a day. If side effects appear, the dose may be further decreased to 10 milligrams a day.

CHILDREN

Arava is not recommended for children less than 18 years old.

Overdosage

Little is known about the effects of an overdose. However, any medication taken in excess can have dangerous consequences. If you suspect an overdose of Arava, seek emergency medical treatment immediately.

Brand name:

ARICEPT

Pronounced: AIR-ih-sept
Generic name: Donepezil hydrochloride

Why is this drug prescribed?

Aricept is one of only two drugs that can provide some relief from the symptoms of early Alzheimer's disease. (Cognex is the other.) Alzheimer's disease causes physical changes in the brain that disrupt the flow of information and interfere with memory, thinking, and behavior. Aricept can temporarily improve brain function in some Alzheimer's sufferers, although it does not halt the progress of the underlying disease.

Most important fact about this drug

To maintain any improvement, Aricept must be taken regularly. If the drug is stopped, its benefits will soon be lost. Patience is in order when starting the drug. It can take up to 3 weeks for any positive effects to appear.

How should you take this medication?

Aricept should be taken once a day just before bedtime. Be sure it's taken every day. If Aricept is not taken regularly, it won't work. It can be taken with or without food.

■ *If you miss a dose...*
  Make it up as soon as you remember. If it is almost time for the next dose, skip the one that was missed and go back to the regular schedule. Never double the dose.

■ *Storage instructions...*
Store at room temperature.

What side effects may occur?
Side effects cannot be anticipated. If any develop or change in intensity, tell the doctor as soon as possible. Only the doctor can determine if it is safe to continue Aricept.

Side effects are more likely with higher doses. The most common are diarrhea, fatigue, insomnia, loss of appetite, muscle cramps, nausea, and vomiting. When one of these effects occurs, it is usually mild and gets better as treatment continues.

■ *Other side effects may include:*
Abnormal dreams, arthritis, bruising, depression, dizziness, fainting, frequent urination, headache, pain, sleepiness, weight loss

Why should this drug not be prescribed?
There are three reasons to avoid Aricept: an allergic reaction to the drug itself, an allergy to the group of antihistamines that includes Periactin, Optimine, and Nolahist, and an allergy to certain major tranquilizers such as Mellaril.

Special warnings about this medication
Aricept can aggravate asthma and other breathing problems, and can increase the risk of seizures. It can also slow the heartbeat and possibly cause fainting in people who have a heart condition. Contact your doctor if any of these problems occur.

In patients who have had stomach ulcers, and those who take a nonsteroidal anti-inflammatory drug such as Advil, Nuprin, or Aleve, Aricept can make stomach side effects worse. Be cautious when using Aricept and report all side effects to your doctor.

Possible food and drug interactions
when taking this medication
Aricept will increase the effects of certain anesthetics. Make sure the doctor is aware of Aricept therapy prior to any surgery.

If Aricept is taken with certain other drugs, the effects of either could be increased, decreased, or altered. It is especially important to check with your doctor before combining Aricept with the following:

Antispasmodic drugs such as Bentyl, Cogentin, and Pro-Banthine
Bethanechol chloride (Urecholine)

Carbamazepine (Tegretol)
Dexamethasone (Decadron)
Ketoconazole (Nizoral)
Phenobarbital
Phenytoin (Dilantin)
Quinidine (Quinidex)
Rifampin (Rifadin, Rifamate)

Special information
if you are pregnant or breastfeeding

Since it is not intended for women of child-bearing age, Aricept's effects during pregnancy have not been studied, and it is not known whether it appears in breast milk.

Recommended dosage

ADULTS

The usual starting dose is 5 milligrams once a day at bedtime for at least 4 to 6 weeks. Do not increase the dose during this period unless directed. The doctor may then change the dosage to 10 milligrams once a day if response to the drug warrants it.

CHILDREN

The safety and effectiveness of Aricept have not been established in children.

Overdosage

Any medication taken in excess can have serious consequences. If you suspect an overdose, seek medical attention immediately.

■ *Symptoms of Aricept overdose include:*
Collapse, convulsions, extreme muscle weakness (possibly ending in death if breathing muscles are affected), low blood pressure, nausea, salivation, slowed heart rate, sweating, vomiting

Brand name:

ARIMIDEX

Pronounced: AR-i-mi-deks
Generic name: Anastrozole

Why is this drug prescribed?

Arimidex is used to treat advanced breast cancer in postmenopausal women whose disease has spread to other parts of the body following treatment with tamoxifen (Nolvadex), another anticancer drug.

The growth of many breast cancer tumors is thought to be stimulated by estrogen. One of the hormones produced by the adrenal gland is converted to a form of estrogen by an enzyme called aromatase. Arimidex suppresses this enzyme and thereby reduces the level of estrogen circulating in the body.

Most important fact about this drug
Arimidex, like many other anticancer medications, may prolong survival and improve quality of life. To keep this medication working properly, it's important to continue taking it even when you don't feel well. If you develop bothersome side effects, call your doctor. He or she can recommend ways to reduce your discomfort.

How should you take this medication?
Take Arimidex exactly as directed.

■ *If you miss a dose...*
Take the forgotten dose if you remember within 12 hours. If it is almost time for your next dose, skip the one you missed and go back to your regular schedule. Never take 2 doses at once.

■ *Storage instructions...*
Store at room temperature.

What side effects may occur?
Side effects cannot be anticipated. If any develop or change in intensity, tell your doctor as soon as possible. Only your doctor can determine if it is safe for you to continue taking Arimidex.

■ *More common side effects may include:*
Abdominal pain, back pain, bone pain, chest pain, constipation, cough, depression, diarrhea, dizziness, dry mouth, headache, hot flashes, loss of appetite, nausea, pain, pelvic pain, "pins and needles," rash, shortness of breath, sore throat, swelling of arms and legs, vomiting, weakness, weight gain

■ *Less common or rare side effects may include:*
Accidental injury, anxiety, blood clots, breast pain, bronchitis, confusion, drowsiness, feeling of illness, fever, flu-like symptoms, fractures, hair

thinning, high blood pressure, increased appetite, infection, insomnia, itching, joint pain, muscle pain, nasal or sinus inflammation, neck pain, nervousness, sweating, urinary tract infection, vaginal bleeding, weight loss

Why should this drug not be prescribed?

Do not take Arimidex if you are pregnant.

Special warnings about this medication

Because Arimidex may raise the level of cholesterol in your blood, your doctor may periodically do blood tests to check.

Possible food and drug interactions when taking this medication

At present, no drug interactions are known.

Special information if you are pregnant or breastfeeding

If you are pregnant or plan to become pregnant, do not take Arimidex. In animal studies, this medication has caused severe birth defects, including incomplete bone formation and low birth weight; it could be poisonous to your unborn child. Arimidex also increases your chances of having a miscarriage or a stillborn baby. If you should accidentally become pregnant, tell your doctor immediately.

Because of the possibility of Arimidex passing through your breast milk to your baby, you should probably avoid breastfeeding.

Recommended dosage

ADULTS

The usual dose is a 1-milligram tablet taken once a day.

Overdosage

Although there have been no reports of Arimidex overdose, any medication taken in excess can have serious consequences. If you suspect an overdose, seek medical attention immediately.

Brand name:

ARMOUR THYROID

Pronounced: ARE-more THIGH-roid
Generic name: Natural thyroid hormones TC and TD

Why is this drug prescribed?
Armour Thyroid is prescribed when your thyroid gland is unable to produce enough hormone. It is also used to treat or prevent goiter (enlargement of the thyroid gland), and is given in a "suppression test" to diagnose an overactive thyroid.

Most important fact about this drug
Although Armour Thyroid will speed up your metabolism, it is not effective as a weight-loss drug and should not be used for that purpose. Too much Armour Thyroid may cause severe side effects, especially if you are also taking appetite suppressants.

How should you take this medication?
Take Armour Thyroid exactly as prescribed by your doctor. There is no "typical" dosage; the amount you need to take will depend on how much thyroid hormone your body is able to produce. Take no more or less than the amount your doctor prescribes. Take your dose at the same time every day for consistent effect.

Do not change brands of medication without consulting your doctor.

If you are taking Armour Thyroid to compensate for an underactive thyroid gland, you will probably need to take the medication indefinitely.

▪ *If you miss a dose...*
Take it as soon as you remember. If it is almost time for your next dose, skip the one you missed and go back to your regular schedule. Do not take 2 doses at the same time. If you miss 2 or more doses in a row, consult your doctor.

▪ *Storage instructions...*
Store at room temperature in a tightly closed container.

What side effects may occur?
Side effects are rare when Armour Thyroid is taken at the correct dosage. However, taking too much medication or increasing the dosage too quickly may lead to overstimulation of the thyroid gland.

▪ *Symptoms of overstimulation may include:*
Changes in appetite, diarrhea, fever, headache, increased heart rate, irritability, nausea, nervousness, sleeplessness, sweating, weight loss

Although children treated with Armour Thyroid may initially lose some hair, the hair loss is temporary.

Why should this drug not be prescribed?
You should not take Armour Thyroid if you have ever had an allergic reaction
to this drug, your thyroid gland is overactive, or your adrenal glands are not
making enough corticosteroid hormone.

Special warnings about this medication
If you are elderly, particularly if you suffer from angina (chest pain due to a
heart condition), you should take Armour Thyroid at a lower dosage, and
your doctor should schedule frequent checkups.

Armour Thyroid tends to aggravate symptoms of diabetes and underactive
adrenal glands. If you take medication to treat one of these disorders, your
dosage of that medication will probably need to be adjusted once you start
taking Armour Thyroid.

**Possible food and drug interactions
when taking this medication**
If you take Armour Thyroid with certain other drugs, the effect of either drug
could be increased, decreased, or altered. It is especially important to check
with your doctor before combining Armour Thyroid with the following:

Asthma medications such as Theo-Dur
Blood thinners such as Coumadin
Cholestyramine (Questran)
Colestipol (Colestid)
Estrogen preparations (including some birth control pills such as Ortho-
    Novum and Premarin)
Insulin
Oral diabetes drugs (such as Diabinese and Glucotrol)

**Special information
if you are pregnant or breastfeeding**
If you need to take Armour Thyroid because of a thyroid hormone deficiency,
you may continue using the medication during pregnancy, but your doctor
will test you regularly and may change your dosage. Once your baby is born,
you may breast-feed while continuing treatment with Armour Thyroid.

Recommended dosage

ADULTS

Your doctor will tailor the dosage of Armour Thyroid to meet your individual
requirements, taking into consideration the status of your thyroid gland and
any other medical conditions you may have.

Overdosage

An overdose of Armour Thyroid will speed up all of the body's vital processes, causing physical and mental hyperactivity, increased appetite, excessive sweating, chest pain, increased pulse rate, palpitations, nervousness, intolerance to heat, and possibly tremors or a rapid heartbeat.

Brand name:

ARTANE

Pronounced: AR-tane
Generic name: Trihexyphenidyl hydrochloride

Why is this drug prescribed?

Artane is used, in conjunction with other drugs, for the relief of certain symptoms of Parkinson's disease, a brain disorder that causes muscle tremor, stiffness, and weakness. It is also used to control certain side effects induced by antipsychotic drugs such as Thorazine and Haldol. Artane works by correcting the chemical imbalance that causes Parkinson's disease.

Most important fact about this drug

Artane is not a cure for Parkinson's disease; it merely minimizes and reduces the frequency of symptoms such as tremors.

How should you take this medication?

You may take Artane either before meals or after meals, whichever you find more convenient. Your doctor will probably start you on a small amount and increase the dosage gradually. Take Artane exactly as prescribed.

If the medication makes your mouth feel dry, try chewing gum, sucking mints, or simply sipping water.

Artane comes in tablet and liquid form. With either, you will probably need to take 3 or 4 doses a day.

Once you have reached the dosage that is best for you, your doctor may switch you to sustained-release capsules ("Sequels") which are to be taken only once or twice a day. Do not open or crush the sequels. Always swallow them whole.

- *If you miss a dose...*
  Take it as soon as you remember. If it is within 2 hours of your next dose, skip the one you missed and go back to your regular schedule. Do not take 2 doses at the same time.

■ *Storage instructions...*
Store at room temperature. Do not allow the liquid to freeze.

What side effects may occur?
Side effects cannot be anticipated. If any develop or change in intensity, inform your doctor as soon as possible. Only your doctor can determine if it is safe for you to continue taking Artane.

■ *Common side effects may include:*
Blurred vision, dry mouth, nausea, nervousness

These side effects, which appear in 30% to 50% of all people who take Artane, tend to be mild. They may disappear as your body gets used to the drug; if they persist, your doctor may want to lower your dosage slightly.

■ *Other potential side effects include:*
Agitation, bowel obstruction, confusion, constipation, delusions, difficulty urinating, dilated pupils, disturbed behavior, drowsiness, hallucinations, headache, pressure in the eye, rapid heartbeat, rash, vomiting, weakness

Why should this drug not be prescribed?
Do not take Artane if you are known to be sensitive to it or if you have ever had an allergic reaction to it or to other antiparkinson medications of this type.

Special warnings about this medication
The elderly are highly sensitive to drugs such as Artane and should use it with caution.

Artane can reduce the body's ability to perspire, one of the key ways your body prevents overheating. Avoid excess sun or exercise that also cause you to become overheated.

If you have any of the following conditions, make sure your doctor knows about them, since Artane could make them worse:

Enlarged prostate
Glaucoma
Stomach/intestinal obstructive disease
Urinary tract obstructive disease

It is important to stick to the prescribed dosage; taking larger amounts "for kicks" could lead to an overdose.

Your doctor should watch you carefully if you have heart, liver, or kidney disease or high blood pressure, and should check your eyes frequently. You should also be watched for the development of any allergic reactions.

Possible food and drug interactions
when taking this medication

If you take Artane along with any of the drugs listed below, your doctor may need to adjust the dosage of Artane, the other medication, or possibly both.

  Amantadine (Symmetrel)
  Amitriptyline (Elavil)
  Chlorpromazine (Thorazine)
  Doxepin (Sinequan)
  Haloperidol (Haldol)

Special information
if you are pregnant or breastfeeding

No specific information is available concerning the use of Artane during pregnancy or breastfeeding. If you are pregnant or plan to become pregnant while taking Artane, inform your doctor immediately.

Recommended dosage

Your doctor will individualize the dose to your needs, starting with a low dose and then increasing it gradually, especially if you are over 60 years of age.

ADULTS

Parkinson's Disease:

The usual starting dose, in tablet or liquid form, is 1 milligram on the first day.

After the first day, your doctor may increase the dose by 2 milligrams at intervals of 3 to 5 days, until you are taking a total of 6 to 10 milligrams a day.

Your total daily dose will depend upon what is found to be the most effective level. For many people, 6 to 10 milligrams is most effective. Some, however, may require a total daily dose of 12 to 15 milligrams.

Drug-Induced Parkinsonism:

Your doctor will have to determine by trial and error the size and frequency of the dose of Artane needed to control the tremors and muscle rigidity that sometimes result from commonly used tranquilizers.

The total daily dosage usually ranges between 5 and 15 milligrams, although, in some cases, symptoms have been satisfactorily controlled on as little as 1 milligram daily.

Your doctor may start you on 1 milligram of Artane a day. If your symptoms are not controlled in a few hours, he or she may slowly increase the dose until satisfactory control is achieved.

Use of Artane with Levodopa:
When Artane is used at the same time as levodopa, the usual dose of each may need to be reduced. Your doctor will adjust the dosages carefully, depending on the side effects and the degree of symptom control. Artane dosage of 3 to 6 milligrams daily, divided into equal doses, is usually adequate.

Artane Tablets and Liquid:
You will be able to handle the total daily intake of Artane tablets or liquid best if the medication is divided into 3 doses and taken at mealtimes. If you are taking high doses (more than 10 milligrams daily), your doctor may divide them into 4 parts, so that you take 3 doses at mealtimes and the fourth at bedtime.

Overdosage
Overdosage with Artane may cause agitation, delirium, disorientation, hallucinations, or psychotic episodes.

- **Other symptoms may include:**
  Clumsiness or unsteadiness, fast heartbeat, flushing of skin, seizures, severe drowsiness, shortness of breath or troubled breathing, trouble sleeping, unusual warmth

If you suspect an overdose of Artane, seek medical attention immediately.

Brand name:

ARTHROTEC

Pronounced: ARE-throw-teck
Generic ingredients: Diclofenac sodium, Misoprostol

Why is this drug prescribed?
Arthrotec is designed to relieve the symptoms of arthritis in people who are also prone to ulcers. It contains diclofenac, a nonsteroidal anti-inflammatory drug (NSAID) for control of the inflammation, swelling, stiffness, and joint

pain associated with rheumatoid arthritis and osteoarthritis. However, since NSAIDs can cause stomach ulcers in susceptible people, Arthrotec also contains misoprostol, a synthetic prostaglandin that serves to reduce the production of stomach acid, protect the stomach lining, and thus prevent ulcers.

Most important fact about this drug

Be certain to avoid taking Arthrotec during pregnancy. It can cause a miscarriage with potentially dangerous bleeding, sometimes leading to hospitalization, surgery, infertility, and even death. Arthrotec can also deform or kill the developing baby. If you haven't passed menopause, your doctor should do a pregnancy test less than 2 weeks before your therapy begins. Once you've started taking the drug, it is vitally important that you also use reliable contraceptive measures. If you do become pregnant, stop taking Arthrotec and contact your doctor immediately.

How should you take this medication?

To minimize diarrhea and related side effects, take Arthrotec with meals, exactly as prescribed. Antacids containing magnesium can make Arthrotec-induced diarrhea worse. If you need an antacid, use one containing aluminum or calcium instead. Arthrotec tablets should be swallowed whole and not chewed, crushed, or dissolved.

- *If you miss a dose...*
  If you are following a regular schedule, take the dose as soon as you remember. If it is almost time for the next one, skip the dose you missed and go back to your regular schedule. Do not take 2 doses at once.

- *Storage instructions...*
  Store at room temperature in a dry place.

What side effects may occur?

Side effects cannot be anticipated. If any develop or change in intensity, inform your doctor as soon as possible. Only your doctor can determine if it is safe for you to continue taking Arthrotec.

- *More common side effects may include:*
  Abdominal pain, acid indigestion, diarrhea, gas, nausea

- *Less common or rare side effects may include:*
  Abnormal vision or tearing, acne, anxiety, asthma, blood in the urine, breast pain, bruising, change in taste, concentration difficulties, confusion,

coughing, dark tarry stools, decreased breathing, decreased or increased urination, dehydration, depression, difficulty breathing, difficulty swallowing, difficulty urinating, disorientation, dream abnormalities, drowsiness, dry mouth, eczema, excessive or postmenopausal vaginal bleeding, eye infection, fainting, fatigue, fever, frequent urination, gout, hallucinations, hair loss, hearing impairment, hemorrhoids, high blood pressure, high blood sugar, hives, impotence, increased heart rate, increased muscle tone, increased nighttime urination, increased sweating, infection, irregular or increased menstrual bleeding, irritability, irregular heartbeat, jaundice (yellowing of the skin and eyes), joint pain, loss of appetite, low blood pressure, low blood sugar, migraine, mouth sores, muscle pain, nervousness, night blindness, nosebleed, painful menstruation, paranoia, pelvic pain, pinkeye, rapid breathing, rectal bleeding, rectal itching, seizures, sensitivity to light, skin sores, skin rash, skin swelling, stomach or intestinal bleeding, stomach ulcers, taste loss, throat swelling, throbbing heartbeat, tremor, tingling/numbness, urinary tract infection, vertigo, weakness, weight changes

Why should this drug not be prescribed?

Remember that it is essential to avoid Arthrotec during pregnancy. You should also avoid this medication if you've ever had an allergic reaction to either of its components (diclofenac and misoprostol). Avoid it, too, if you've had a reaction to any other prostaglandin medication, or to any NSAID, including aspirin. Make sure the doctor is aware of any drug reactions you've experienced.

Special warnings about this medication

Although Arthrotec is designed to protect against stomach ulcers and bleeding, they remain a possibility. Contact your doctor immediately if you notice signs of bleeding such as black tarry stools. Also call the doctor if you develop severe diarrhea, cramping, or nausea, or if milder symptoms persist for more than 7 days.

This drug should be used with caution if you have kidney problems or liver disease. Your doctor will do a blood test to monitor your liver within 4 to 8 weeks after starting Arthrotec therapy and periodically thereafter. If you develop signs of a liver problem, such as nausea, fatigue, tiredness, itching, yellowed eyes and skin, tenderness in the upper right area of your stomach, or flu-like symptoms, stop taking Arthrotec and notify your doctor at once.

Use Arthrotec cautiously if you have systemic lupus or a similar connective tissue disease. Certain rare side effects are more likely to occur. Be cautious, too, if you have heart disease or high blood pressure. Arthrotec can increase water retention. Also exercise caution if you have asthma. In some people, Arthrotec could trigger an attack.

Do not take Arthrotec if you're dehydrated (a possibility after severe vomiting or diarrhea). You should also avoid Arthrotec if you have a condition known as porphyria.

Arthrotec is not an ordinary pain reliever. It is a potent medication, and poses extreme danger during pregnancy. Never share it with anyone else.

Possible food and drug interactions
when taking this medication
If Arthrotec is taken with certain other drugs, the effects of either could be increased, decreased, or altered. It is especially important to check with your doctor before combining Arthrotec with the following:

Aspirin
Blood pressure medications such as Cardizem, Inderal, Procardia, and
 Vasotec
Cyclosporine (Neoral, Sandimmune)
Digoxin (Lanoxin)
Diuretics (Lasix, HydroDIURIL)
Glipizide (Glucotrol, Glucotrol XL)
Glyburide (Diabeta, Micronase)
Insulin
Lithium (Lithobid, Lithonate)
Magnesium-containing antacids such as Maalox and Mylanta
Methotrexate (Rheumatrex)
Phenobarbital
Prednisolone (Delta-Cortef, Pediapred, Prelone)
Warfarin (Coumadin)

Special information
if you are pregnant or breastfeeding
Arthrotec must be strictly avoided during pregnancy. If you are in your child-bearing years, your doctor will have you take your first dose on the second or third day of your menstrual period to be sure you're not pregnant. Use reliable contraception for the duration of your treatment.

Because Arthrotec appears in breast milk, your doctor may have you stop breastfeeding until your treatment is finished.

Recommended dosage

ADULTS

Osteoarthritis
The recommended dose is 50 milligrams 3 times daily.

Rheumatoid Arthritis
The recommended dose is 50 milligrams 3 or 4 times daily.

If you cannot tolerate the recommended dosage, your doctor can prescribe a dose of 50 or 75 milligrams twice daily. However, such lower dosages are less effective at preventing ulcers.

Your doctor may prescribe misoprostol (Cytotec) in addition to Arthrotec for better ulcer protection.

CHILDREN

The safety and effectiveness of Arthrotec have not been established in children below the age of 18.

Overdosage

If you suspect an overdose of Arthrotec, seek medical attention immediately.

■ *Symptoms of Arthrotec overdose may include:*
Abdominal pain, confusion, diarrhea, difficulty breathing, digestive discomfort, drowsiness, fever, lack of muscle tone, low blood pressure, tremors, seizures, slow heartbeat, throbbing heartbeat, vomiting

Brand name:

ASACOL

See Rowasa, page 1152.

Generic name:

ASPIRIN

Pronounced: ASS-per-in
Brand names: Empirin, Ecotrin, Genuine Bayer, Halfprin

Why is this drug prescribed?

Aspirin is an anti-inflammatory pain medication (analgesic) that is used to relieve headaches, toothaches, and minor aches and pains, and to reduce fever. It also temporarily relieves the minor aches and pains of arthritis, muscle aches, colds, flu, and menstrual discomfort. In some patients, a small daily dose of aspirin may be used to ensure sufficient blood flow to the brain and prevent stroke. Aspirin may also be taken to decrease recurrence of a heart attack or other heart problems.

Most important fact about this drug

Aspirin should not be used during the last 3 months of pregnancy unless specifically prescribed by a doctor. It may cause problems in the unborn child or complications during delivery.

How should you take this medication?

Do not take more than the recommended dose.

Do not use aspirin if it has a strong, vinegar-like odor.

If aspirin upsets your stomach, use of a coated or buffered brand may reduce the problem.

Do not chew or crush sustained-release brands, such as Bayer time-release aspirin, or pills coated to delay breakdown of the drug, such as Ecotrin. To make them easier to swallow, take them with a full glass of water.

■ *If you miss a dose...*
   Take it as soon as you remember. If it is almost time for your next dose, skip the one you missed and go back to your regular schedule. Never take 2 doses at the same time.

■ *Storage instructions...*
   Store at room temperature.

What side effects may occur?

Side effects cannot be anticipated. If any develop or change in intensity, inform your doctor as soon as possible. Only your doctor can determine if it is safe for you to continue using aspirin.

■ *Side effects may include:*
   Heartburn, nausea and/or vomiting, possible involvement in formation of stomach ulcers and bleeding, small amounts of blood in stool, stomach pain, stomach upset

Why should this drug not be prescribed?

Do not take aspirin if you are allergic to it, if you have asthma, ulcers or ulcer symptoms, or if you are taking a medication that affects the clotting of your blood, unless specifically told to do so by your doctor.

Special warnings about this medication

Aspirin should not be given to children or teenagers for flu symptoms or chickenpox. Aspirin has been associated with the development of Reye's syndrome, a dangerous disorder characterized by disorientation, and lethargy leading to coma.

If you have a continuous or high fever, or a severe or persistent sore throat, especially with a high fever, vomiting and nausea, consult your doctor. It could indicate a more serious illness.

If pain persists for more than 10 days or if redness or swelling appears at the site of inflammation, consult your doctor immediately.

If you experience ringing in the ears, hearing loss, upset stomach, or dizziness, consult your doctor before taking more aspirin.

Check with your doctor before giving aspirin for arthritis or rheumatism to a child under 12.

Possible food and drug interactions
when taking this medication

If aspirin is taken with certain other drugs, the effects of either could be increased, decreased, or altered. It is especially important to check with your doctor before combining aspirin with the following:

Acetazolamide (Diamox)
ACE-inhibitor-type blood pressure medications such as Capoten
Anti-gout medications such as Zyloprim
Arthritis medications such as Motrin and Indocin
Blood thinners such as Coumadin
Certain diuretics such as Lasix
Diabetes medications such as DiaBeta and Micronase
Diltiazem (Cardizem)
Dipyridamole (Persantine)
Insulin
Seizure medications such as Depakene
Steroids such as prednisone

Special information
if you are pregnant or breastfeeding

The use of aspirin during pregnancy should be discussed with your doctor. Aspirin should not be used during the last 3 months of pregnancy unless specifically indicated by your doctor. It may cause problems in the fetus and complications during delivery. Aspirin may appear in breast milk and could affect a nursing infant. Ask your doctor whether it is safe to take aspirin while you are breastfeeding.

Recommended dosage

ADULTS

Treatment of Minor Pain and Fever
The usual dose is 1 or 2 tablets every 3 to 4 hours up to 6 times a day.

Prevention of Stroke
The usual dose is 1 tablet 4 times daily or 2 tablets 2 times a day.

Prevention of Heart Attack
The usual dose is 1 tablet daily. Your physician may suggest that you take a larger dose, however. If you use Halfprin low-strength tablets (162 milligrams), adjust dosage accordingly.

CHILDREN

Consult your doctor.

Overdosage
Any medication used in excess can have serious consequences. If you suspect symptoms of an aspirin overdose, seek medical treatment immediately.

Brand name:

ASPIRIN FREE ANACIN

See Tylenol, page 1362.

Generic name:

ASPIRIN WITH CODEINE

See Empirin with Codeine, page 470.

Brand name:

ASTELIN

Pronounced: AST-eh-linn
Generic name: Azelastine hydrochloride

Why is this drug prescribed?
Astelin is an antihistamine nasal spray. It is prescribed for the relief of hay fever symptoms such as itchy, runny nose and sneezing.

Most important fact about this drug
Astelin can cause drowsiness. Do not drive a car, operate machinery, or undertake any other activity that requires mental alertness until you know how the drug affects you. Avoid combining Astelin with alcohol, antihistamines, and other drugs that slow the central nervous system; worse drowsiness could result.

How should you take this medication?
Use Astelin nasal spray only as prescribed. Avoid spraying in the eyes.

Before initial use, prime the pump by depressing it 4 times, or until a fine mist appears. When 3 or more days have elapsed since the last use, you should reprime the pump with 2 strokes, or until a fine mist appears.

Relief of symptoms usually occurs within 3 hours and lasts up to 12 hours.

■ *If you miss a dose...*
Take the forgotten dose as soon as you remember. If it is almost time for your next dose, skip the one you missed and go back to your regular schedule. Never double your dose.

■ *Storage instructions...*
Store the bottle in an upright position at room temperature with the nasal pump tightly closed. Do not freeze.

What side effects may occur?
Side effects cannot be anticipated. If any develop or change in intensity, inform your doctor as soon as possible. Only your doctor can determine if it is safe for you to continue taking Astelin.

■ *Common side effects may include:*
Bitter taste, drowsiness, headache, nasal burning, sneezing, sore throat

■ *Less common side effects may include:*
Abdominal pain, abnormal thinking, allergic reaction, anxiety, back pain, blood in the urine, breast pain, constipation, coughing, depression, dizziness, dry mouth, eye problems, fatigue, frequent urination, flu-like symptoms, flushing, herpes simplex infection, high blood pressure, increased appetite, laryngitis, loss of menstruation, loss of the sense of personal identity, loss of sensitivity to touch, mouth and tongue sores, muscle pain, nasal inflammation, nausea, nervousness, nosebleed, overactivity, pain in arms and legs, pinkeye, rapid heartbeat, skin problems, sleep disturbances, stomach and intestinal inflammation, taste loss, throat burning, vertigo, viral infection, vomiting, watery eyes, weight gain, wheezing

Why should this drug not be prescribed?
If you are sensitive to or have ever had an allergic reaction to Astelin or any of its ingredients, you should not take this medication.

Special warnings about this medication
Remember that Astelin makes some people drowsy. See "Most important fact about this drug" for precautions to take.

If you have a kidney condition, make sure the doctor is aware of it. Your dosage of Astelin may have to be reduced.

Possible food and drug interactions
If Astelin is taken with certain other drugs, the effects of either could be increased, decreased, or altered. It is especially important to check with your doctor before combining Astelin with the following:

Alcohol
Drugs that slow the nervous system, including codeine, phenobarbital, and Restoril
Cimetidine (Tagamet)
Ketoconazole (Nizoral)

Special information
if you are pregnant or breastfeeding
The effects of Astelin during pregnancy have not been adequately studied. If you are pregnant or plan to become pregnant, inform your doctor immediately. Because of the possibility of harming the developing baby, you may need to give up the medication. It is not known if Astelin appears in breast milk. Your doctor may want you to stop breastfeeding while using this drug.

Recommended dosage

ADULTS

The usual dose for adults and children 12 years of age and older is 2 sprays into each nostril twice a day.

CHILDREN

The safety and effectiveness of Astelin have not been established in children under 12 years of age.

Overdosage
A severe overdose is unlikely, and would probably cause no other symptoms than extreme drowsiness. However, if you suspect an overdose, it's still wise to seek medical attention immediately.

Generic name:

ASTEMIZOLE

See Hismanal, page 590.

Brand name:

ATARAX

Pronounced: AT-a-raks
Generic name: Hydroxyzine hydrochloride
Other brand name: Vistaril

Why is this drug prescribed?

Atarax is an antihistamine used to relieve the symptoms of common anxiety
and tension and, in combination with other medications, to treat anxiety that
results from physical illness. It also relieves itching from allergic reactions
and can be used as a sedative before and after general anesthesia.
Antihistamines work by decreasing the effects of histamine, a chemical the
body releases that narrows air passages in the lungs and contributes to
inflammation. Antihistamines reduce itching and swelling and dry up
secretions from the nose, eyes, and throat.

Most important fact about this drug

Atarax is not intended for long-term use (more than 4 months). Your doctor
should re-evaluate the prescription periodically.

How should you take this medication?

Take this medication exactly as prescribed by your doctor.

- *If you miss a dose...*
  Take it as soon as you remember. If it is almost time for your next dose,
  skip the one you missed and go back to your regular schedule. Do not take
  2 doses at once.

- *Storage instructions...*
  Store tablets and syrup away from heat, light, and moisture. Keep the
  syrup from freezing.

What side effects may occur?

Side effects cannot be anticipated. If any develop or change in intensity,
inform your doctor as soon as possible. Only your doctor can determine if it
is safe for you to continue taking Atarax.

Drowsiness, the most common side effect of Atarax, is usually temporary and may disappear in a few days or when dosage is reduced. Other side effects include dry mouth, twitches, tremors, and convulsions. The last two usually occur with higher than recommended doses of Atarax.

Why should this drug not be prescribed?

Atarax should not be taken in early pregnancy or if you are sensitive to or have ever had an allergic reaction to it. Make sure your doctor is aware of any drug reactions you have experienced.

Special warnings about this medication

Atarax increases the effects of drugs that depress the activity of the central nervous system. If you are taking narcotics, non-narcotic analgesics, or barbiturates in combination with Atarax, their dosage should be reduced.

This medication can cause drowsiness. Driving or operating dangerous machinery or participating in any hazardous activity that requires full mental alertness is not recommended until you know how you react to Atarax.

Possible food and drug interactions
when taking this medication

Atarax may increase the effects of alcohol. Avoid alcohol while taking this medication.

If Atarax is taken with certain other drugs, the effects of either could be increased, decreased, or altered. It is especially important to check with your doctor before combining Atarax with the following:

  Barbiturates such as Seconal and Phenobarbital
  Narcotics such as Demerol and Percocet
  Non-narcotic analgesics such as Motrin and Tylenol

Special information
if you are pregnant or breastfeeding

Although the effects of Atarax during pregnancy have not been adequately studied in humans, birth defects have appeared in animal studies with this medication. You should not take Atarax in early pregnancy. If you are pregnant or plan to become pregnant, inform your doctor immediately. Atarax may appear in breast milk and could affect a nursing infant. If this medication is essential to your health, your doctor may advise you to discontinue breastfeeding until your treatment is finished.

Recommended dosage

When treatment begins with injections, it can be continued in tablet form. Your doctor will adjust your dosage based on your response to the drug.

FOR ANXIETY AND TENSION

Adults

The usual dose is 50 to 100 milligrams 4 times per day.

Children under Age 6

The total dose is 50 milligrams daily, divided into several smaller doses.

Children over Age 6

The total dose is 50 to 100 milligrams daily, divided into several smaller doses.

FOR ITCHING DUE TO ALLERGIC CONDITIONS

Adults

The usual dose is 25 milligrams 3 or 4 times a day.

Children under Age 6

The total dose is 50 milligrams daily, divided into several smaller doses.

Children over Age 6

The total dose is 50 to 100 milligrams daily, divided into several smaller doses.

BEFORE AND AFTER GENERAL ANESTHESIA

Adults

The usual dose is 50 to 100 milligrams.

Children

The usual dose is 0.6 milligram per 2.2 pounds of body weight.

Overdosage

Any medication taken in excess can have serious consequences. If you suspect an overdose of Atarax, seek medical attention immediately.

The most common symptom of Atarax overdose is excessive calm; your blood pressure may drop, although it is not likely.

Generic name:

ATENOLOL

See Tenormin, page 1278.

Generic name:

ATENOLOL WITH CHLORTHALIDONE

See Tenoretic, page 1275.

Brand name:

ATIVAN

Pronounced: AT-i-van
Generic name: Lorazepam

Why is this drug prescribed?

Ativan is used in the treatment of anxiety disorders and for short-term (up to 4 months) relief of the symptoms of anxiety. It belongs to a class of drugs known as benzodiazepines.

Most important fact about this drug

Tolerance and dependence can develop with the use of Ativan. You may experience withdrawal symptoms if you stop using it abruptly. Only your doctor should advise you to discontinue or change your dose.

How should you take this drug?

Take this medication exactly as prescribed by your doctor.

■ *If you miss a dose...*
If it is within an hour or so of the scheduled time, take the forgotten dose as soon as you remember. Otherwise, skip the dose and go back to your regular schedule. Do not take 2 doses at once.

■ *Storage instructions...*
Store at room temperature in a tightly closed container, away from light.

What side effects may occur?
Side effects cannot be anticipated. If any develop or change in intensity, inform your doctor as soon as possible. Only your doctor can determine if it is safe for you to continue taking Ativan.

If you experience any side effects, it will usually be at the beginning of your treatment; they will probably disappear as you continue to take the drug, or if your dosage is reduced.

■ *More common side effects may include:*
   Dizziness, sedation (excessive calm), unsteadiness, weakness

■ *Less common or rare side effects may include:*
   Agitation, change in appetite, depression, eye function disorders, head-ache, memory impairment, mental disorientation, nausea, skin problems, sleep disturbance, stomach and intestinal disorders

■ *Side effects due to rapid decrease or abrupt withdrawal of Ativan:*
   Abdominal and muscle cramps, convulsions, depressed mood, inability to fall or stay asleep, sweating, tremors, vomiting

Why should this drug not be prescribed?
If you are sensitive to or have ever had an allergic reaction to Ativan or similar drugs such as Valium, you should not take this medication.

Also avoid Ativan if you have the eye disease acute narrow-angle glaucoma.

Anxiety or tension related to everyday stress usually does not require treatment with Ativan. Discuss your symptoms thoroughly with your doctor.

Special warnings about this medication
Ativan may cause you to become drowsy or less alert; therefore, driving or operating dangerous machinery or participating in any hazardous activity that requires full mental alertness is not recommended.

If you are severely depressed or have suffered from severe depression, consult with your doctor before taking this medication.

If you have decreased kidney or liver function, use of this drug should be discussed with your doctor.

If you are an older person or if you have been using Ativan for a prolonged period of time, your doctor will watch you closely for stomach and upper intestinal problems.

Possible food and drug interactions
when taking this medication
Ativan may intensify the effects of alcohol. Avoid alcohol while taking this medication.

If Ativan is taken with certain other drugs, the effects of either could be increased, decreased, or altered. It is especially important to check with your doctor before combining Ativan with barbiturates (phenobarbital, Seconal, Amytal) or sedative-type medications such as Valium and Halcion.

Special information
if you are pregnant or breastfeeding
Do not take Ativan if you are pregnant or planning to become pregnant. There is an increased risk of birth defects. It is not known whether Ativan appears in breast milk. If this medication is essential to your health, your doctor may advise you to discontinue breastfeeding until your treatment is finished.

Recommended dosage
ADULTS

The usual recommended dosage is a total of 2 to 6 milligrams per day divided into smaller doses. The largest dose should be taken at bedtime. The daily dose may vary from 1 to 10 milligrams.

Anxiety
The usual starting dose is a total of 2 to 3 milligrams per day taken in 2 or 3 smaller doses.

Insomnia Due to Anxiety
A single daily dose of 2 to 4 milligrams may be taken, usually at bedtime.

CHILDREN

The safety and effectiveness of Ativan have not been established in children under 12 years of age.

OLDER ADULTS

The usual starting dosage for older adults and those in a weakened condition should not exceed a total of 1 to 2 milligrams per day, divided into smaller doses, to avoid oversedation. This dose can be adjusted by your doctor as needed.

Overdosage
Any medication taken in excess can have serious consequences. An overdose of Ativan can be fatal, though this is rare. If you suspect an overdose, seek medical attention immediately.

- *The symptoms of Ativan overdose may include:*
  Coma, confusion, drowsiness, hypnotic state, lack of coordination, low blood pressure, sluggishness

Generic name:

ATORVASTATIN

See Lipitor, page 700.

Brand name:

ATRETOL

See Tegretol, page 1264.

Brand name:

ATROVENT

Pronounced: AT-row-vent
Generic name: Ipratropium bromide

Why is this drug prescribed?
Atrovent inhalation aerosol and solution are prescribed for long-term treatment of bronchial spasms (wheezing) associated with chronic obstructive pulmonary disease, including chronic bronchitis and emphysema. When inhaled, Atrovent opens the air passages, allowing more oxygen to reach the lungs.

Atrovent nasal spray relieves runny nose. The 0.03% spray is used for year-round runny nose due to allergies and other causes. The 0.06% spray is prescribed for runny nose due to colds. The spray does not relieve nasal congestion or sneezing.

Most important fact about this drug
Atrovent inhalation aerosol and solution are not for initial use in acute attacks of bronchial spasm when fast action is needed.

How should you take this medication?
Atrovent inhalation aerosol and solution are not intended for occasional use.

To get the most benefit from this drug, you must use it consistently throughout your course of treatment, as prescribed by your doctor.

The nasal spray pump must be primed; your doctor will show you how.

■ *If you miss a dose...*
Take it as soon as you remember. If it is almost time for your next dose, skip the one you missed and go back to your regular schedule. Do not take 2 doses at once.

■ *Storage instructions...*
All forms of Atrovent may be stored at room temperature. Do not freeze.

Keep the nasal spray tightly closed.

What side effects may occur?
Side effects cannot be anticipated. If any develop or change in intensity, inform your doctor as soon as possible. Only your doctor can determine if it is safe for you to continue taking Atrovent.

INHALATION AEROSOL AND SOLUTION

■ *More common side effects may include:*
Blurred vision, cough, dizziness, dry mouth, fluttering heartbeat, headache, irritation from aerosol, nausea, nervousness, rash, stomach and intestinal upset, worsening of symptoms

■ *Less common or rare side effects may include:*
Allergic reactions, constipation, coordination difficulty, difficulty in urinating, drowsiness, fatigue, flushing, hives, hoarseness, inability to fall or stay asleep, increased heart rate, itching, low blood pressure, loss of hair, mouth sores, sharp eye pain, swelling of the tongue, lips, and face, tightening of the throat, tingling sensation, tremors

NASAL SPRAY

■ *Side effects may include:*
Blurred vision, change in taste, conjunctivitis ("pinkeye"), cough, dizziness, dry mouth/ throat, eye irritation, headache, hoarseness, increased runny nose or nasal inflammation, inflamed nasal ulcers, nasal congestion, nasal dryness, nasal irritation/itching/burning, nasal tumors, nausea, nosebleed, posterior nasal drip, pounding heartbeat, ringing in the ears, skin rash, sneezing, sore throat, swollen nose, thirst, upper respiratory infection

Why should this drug not be prescribed?

If you are sensitive to or have ever had an allergic reaction to Atrovent or any of its ingredients, or to soybeans, soy lecithin, or peanuts, you should not take this medication.

You should also avoid Atrovent if you are allergic to drugs based on atropine. Make sure your doctor is aware of any drug reactions you have experienced.

Special warnings about this medication

An immediate allergic reaction (hives, swelling, rash, wheezing) is possible when you first use this drug.

Unless you are directed to do so by your doctor, do not take this medication if you have the eye condition called narrow-angle glaucoma (high pressure inside the eye), an enlarged prostate, or obstruction in the neck of the bladder.

Keep Atrovent away from your eyes. It can cause blurred vision, pain, or even narrow-angle glaucoma.

If you develop eye pain, blurred vision, very dry nose, or nosebleeds after using the nasal spray, call your doctor.

Possible food and drug interactions
when taking this medication

No interactions have been reported.

Special information
if you are pregnant or breastfeeding

The effects of Atrovent during pregnancy have not been adequately studied. If you are pregnant or plan to become pregnant, inform your doctor immediately. It is not known whether Atrovent appears in breast milk. If this drug is essential to your health, your doctor may advise you to stop nursing your baby until your treatment is finished.

Recommended dosage

AEROSOL OR SOLUTION

The usual starting dose is 2 inhalations, 4 times per day. Additional inhalations may be taken, but the total should not exceed 12 in 24 hours. Not for use in children under 12.

NASAL SPRAY 0.03%

The usual dose is 2 sprays in each nostril 2 or 3 times a day. Not for use in children under 6.

NASAL SPRAY 0.06%

The usual adult dose is 2 sprays in each nostril 3 or 4 times a day. The recommended dose for children age 5 to 11 is 2 sprays in each nostril 3 times a day. Do not use this strength for more than 4 days and do not give it to children under 5.

Overdosage

There is no information on specific symptoms of Atrovent overdose. However, any drug taken in excess can have serious consequences. If you suspect an overdose of Atrovent, seek medical attention immediately.

Brand name:

A/T/S

See Erythromycin, Topical, page 487.

Brand name:

AUGMENTIN

Pronounced: awg-MENT-in
Generic ingredients: Amoxicillin, Clavulanate potassium

Why is this drug prescribed?

Augmentin is used in the treatment of lower respiratory, middle ear, sinus, skin, and urinary tract infections that are caused by certain specific bacteria. These bacteria produce a chemical enzyme called beta lactamase that makes some infections particularly difficult to treat.

Most important fact about this drug

If you are allergic to either penicillin or cephalosporin antibiotics in any form, consult your doctor *before taking Augmentin*. You may be allergic to it, and if a reaction occurs, it could be extremely severe. If you take the drug and feel signs of a reaction, seek medical attention immediately.

How should you take this medication?

Augmentin should be taken every 8 or 12 hours, depending on the dosage strength. It may be taken with or without food, but taking it with meals or snacks will help prevent stomach upset. Be sure to take all the medicine your doctor has prescribed, even if you begin to feel better.

Shake the suspension well. Use a dosing spoon or medicine dropper to give a child the medication; rinse the spoon or dropper after each use.

■ *If you miss a dose...*
Take it as soon as you remember. If it is almost time for the next dose, and you take 2 doses a day, take the one you missed and the next dose 5 to 6 hours later. If you take 3 doses a day, take the one you missed and the next dose 2 to 4 hours later. Then go back to your regular schedule.

■ *Storage instructions...*
Store the suspension under refrigeration and discard after 10 days. Store tablets away from heat, light, and moisture.

What side effects may occur?
Side effects cannot be anticipated. If any develop or change in intensity, inform your doctor as soon as possible. Only your doctor can determine if it is safe for you to continue taking Augmentin.

■ *More common side effects may include:*
Diarrhea/loose stools, nausea, skin rashes and hives

■ *Less common side effects may include:*
Abdominal discomfort, anemia, arthritis, black "hairy" tongue, blood disorders, fever, gas, headache, indigestion, intestinal inflammation, itching, itching or burning of the vagina, joint pain, muscle pain, skin inflammation, skin peeling, sores and inflammation in the mouth and on the tongue and gums, stomach inflammation, vomiting, yeast infection

■ *Rare side effects may include:*
Agitation, anxiety, behavioral changes, blood in the urine, change in liver function, confusion, convulsions, dizziness, hyperactivity, insomnia, kidney problems

Why should this drug not be prescribed?
If you are sensitive to or have ever had an allergic reaction to any penicillin medication, do not take this drug.

Also avoid taking Augmentin if it has ever given you liver problems or yellowing of the skin and eyes.

Special warnings about this medication

Augmentin and other penicillin-like medicines are generally safe; however, anyone with liver, kidney, or blood disorders is at increased risk when using this drug. Alternative choices may be available to your doctor.

If you have diabetes and test your urine for the presence of sugar, you should ask your doctor or pharmacist if this medication will interfere with the type of test you use.

Allergic reactions to this medication can be serious and possibly fatal. Let your doctor know about previous allergic reactions to medicines, food, or other substances before using Augmentin. If you experience a reaction, report it to your doctor immediately and seek medical treatment.

If you develop diarrhea while taking Augmentin, inform your doctor. It could be a sign of a potentially dangerous form of bowel inflammation.

Some formulations of Augmentin contain phenylalanine. If you have the hereditary disease phenylketonuria, check with your doctor or pharmacist before taking this drug.

Possible food and drug interactions
when taking this medication

Augmentin may react with the antigout medication Benemid, resulting in changes in blood levels. A reaction with another antigout drug, Zyloprim, may cause a rash. Notify your doctor if you are taking either of these drugs.

Special information
if you are pregnant or breastfeeding

The effects of Augmentin during pregnancy have not been adequately studied. Because there may be risk to the developing baby, doctors usually recommend Augmentin to pregnant women only when the benefits of therapy outweigh any potential danger. Augmentin appears in breast milk and could affect a nursing infant. If Augmentin is essential to your health, your doctor may advise you to stop nursing your baby until your treatment with this drug is finished.

Recommended dosage

ADULTS

The usual adult dose is one 500-milligram tablet every 12 hours or one 250-milligram tablet every 8 hours. For more severe infections and infections of the respiratory tract, the dose should be one 875-milligram tablet every 12 hours or one 500-milligram tablet every 8 hours. It is essential that you take this medicine according to your doctor's directions.

CHILDREN LESS THAN 3 MONTHS OLD

Children in this age group take 30 milligrams per 2.2 pounds of body weight per day, divided into 2 doses and taken every 12 hours.

CHILDREN OLDER THAN 3 MONTHS

For middle ear infections, sinus inflammation, lower respiratory tract infections, and more severe infections, the usual dose of the 200- or 400-milligram suspension is 45 milligrams per 2.2 pounds per day, in 2 doses, every 12 hours, and of the 125- or 250-milligram suspension, 40 milligrams per 2.2 pounds per day, in 3 doses, every 8 hours.

For less severe infections, the usual dose is 25 milligrams of the 200- or 400-milligram suspension for each 2.2 pounds of weight per day, divided into 2 doses, every 12 hours, or 20 milligrams of the 125- or 250-milligram suspension per 2.2 pounds per day, divided into 3 doses, every 8 hours.

Children weighing 88 pounds or more will take the adult dosage.

Overdosage
Augmentin is generally safe; however, large amounts may cause overdose symptoms. Suspected overdoses of Augmentin must be treated immediately; contact your physician or an emergency room.

Symptoms of Augmentin overdose may include:
Diarrhea, drowsiness, kidney problems, overactivity, rash, stomach and abdominal pain, vomiting.

Brand name:

AURALGAN

Pronounced: Aw-RAL-gan
Generic ingredients: Antipyrine, Benzocaine, Glycerin
Other brand name: Auroto Otic

Why is this drug prescribed?
Auralgan is prescribed to reduce the inflammation and congestion and relieve the pain and discomfort of severe middle ear infections. This drug may be used in combination with an antibiotic for curing the infection.

Auralgan is also used to remove excessive or impacted earwax.

Most important fact about this drug
Discard this product 6 months after the dropper is first placed in the drug solution.

How should you use this medication?
Use this medication exactly as prescribed. Administer as follows:

1. Warm the drops to body temperature by holding the bottle in your hand for a few minutes.
2. Shake the bottle.
3. Lie on your side or tilt the affected ear up.
4. Gently pull the earlobe up.
5. Administer the prescribed number of drops.
6. Avoid touching the dropper to the ear.
7. Keep the ear tilted up for about 5 to 7 minutes.

Do not rinse the dropper; replace it in the bottle after each use. Hold the dropper assembly by the screw cap and, without squeezing the rubber bulb, insert the dropper into the bottle and screw down tightly.

■ *If you miss a dose...*
   Use it as soon as you remember. If it is almost time for your next dose, skip the one you missed and go back to your regular schedule.

■ *Storage instructions...*
   Store at room temperature.

What side effects may occur?
Side effects cannot be anticipated. If any develop or change in intensity, inform your doctor as soon as possible. For Auralgan, no specific side effects have been reported.

Why should this drug not be prescribed?
If you are sensitive to or allergic to any of the ingredients contained in Auralgan or similar drugs, you should not take this medication. Make sure your doctor is aware of any drug reactions you have experienced.

Unless directed to do so by your doctor, do not use this medication if you have a punctured eardrum.

Special warnings about this medication
Notify your doctor if irritation occurs or if you develop an allergic reaction to this medication.

Possible food and drug interactions
when taking this medication

No food or drug interactions have been reported.

Special information
if you are pregnant or breastfeeding

The effects of Auralgan during pregnancy have not been adequately studied. If you are pregnant or plan to become pregnant, notify your doctor immediately. It is not known whether Auralgan appears in breast milk. If this medication is essential to your health, your doctor may advise you to discontinue breastfeeding until your treatment is finished.

Recommended dosage

ADULTS AND CHILDREN

Acute Otitis Media (Severe Middle Ear Infection):

Apply the medication drop by drop into the ear, permitting the solution to run along the wall of the ear canal until it is filled. Avoid touching the ear with the dropper. Then moisten a piece of cotton dressing material, such as gauze, with Auralgan and insert it into the opening of the ear. Repeat every 1 to 2 hours until pain and congestion are relieved.

Removal of Earwax:

Apply Auralgan drop by drop into the ear 3 times daily for 2 or 3 days to help detach and remove earwax from the wall of the ear canal.

After the wax has been removed, Auralgan is useful for drying out the canal or relieving discomfort.

Before and after the removal of earwax, cotton dressing material such as gauze should be moistened with Auralgan and inserted into the opening of the ear following use of the medication.

Overdosage

No information on overdosage with Auralgan is available.

Generic name:

AURANOFIN

See Ridaura, page 1132.

Brand name:

AUROTO OTIC

See Auralgan, page 116.

Brand name:

AVAPRO

Pronounced: AVE-ah-pro
Generic name: Irbesartan

Why is this drug prescribed?

Avapro is used to treat high blood pressure. A member of the new family of drugs called angiotensin II receptor antagonists, it works by preventing the hormone angiotensin II from narrowing the blood vessels, an action that tends to raise blood pressure. Avapro may be prescribed alone or with other blood pressure medications.

Most important fact about this drug

You must take Avapro regularly for it to be effective. Since blood pressure declines gradually, it may be a couple of weeks before you get the full benefit of Avapro, and you must continue taking it even if you are feeling well. Avapro does not cure high blood pressure, it merely keeps it under control.

How should you take this medication?

Take your dose of Avapro around the same time every day, with or without food.

■ If you miss a dose...
  Take it as soon as you remember. If it is almost time for your next dose, skip the one you missed and go back to your regular schedule. Do not take 2 doses at the same time.

■ Storage instructions...
  Store at room temperature.

What side effects may occur?

Side effects cannot be anticipated. If any develop or change in intensity, tell your doctor as soon as possible. Only your doctor can determine if it is safe for you to continue taking Avapro.

- *More common side effects may include:*
  Diarrhea, fatigue, respiratory tract infection

- *Less common side effects may include:*
  Heartburn, indigestion

- *Rare side effects may include:*
  Abdominal bloating, arthritis, bronchitis, bruising, bursitis, chest pain, chills, congestion, constipation, depression, difficulty breathing, drowsiness, ear infection, ear pain, emotional disturbances, eye infection, eye problems, face swelling, face reddening, fainting, fever, flushing, gas, gout, hearing problems, heart attack, heart failure, heart murmur, hives, irregular heartbeat, itching, joint stiffness, muscle aches, muscle cramps, muscle weakness, nose bleeds, numbness, oral sores, prostate problems, sex drive changes, sexual dysfunction, skin inflammation, skin tingling, sleep problems, stomach and intestinal inflammation, stroke, swelling, tremor, urination problems, vision problems, wheezing

Why should this drug not be prescribed?
If Avapro gives you an allergic reaction, you will not be able to use this drug.

Special warnings about this medication
In rare cases, Avapro can cause a severe drop in blood pressure. The problem is more likely if your body's supply of water has been depleted by dialysis treatments or high doses of diuretics. Symptoms include light-headedness, dizziness, and faintness, and are more likely when you first start taking the drug. Call your doctor if they occur. You may need to have your dose adjusted.

If you have kidney disease, Avapro must be used with caution.

Possible food and drug interactions
when taking this medication
The chances of an interaction with Avapro are low. Check with your doctor, however, before combining it with tolbutamide (Orinase).

Special information if you are pregnant or breastfeeding
Avapro can cause injury or even death to the unborn child when used during the last 6 months of pregnancy. As soon as you learn you're pregnant, stop taking Avapro and call your doctor.

It is not known whether Avapro appears in breast milk, but because of potential risks to the newborn, it's considered best to avoid using the drug while breastfeeding. You and your doctor should decide whether to give up nursing or discontinue Avapro.

Recommended dosage

ADULTS

The recommended starting dose of Avapro is 150 milligrams once a day. If your blood pressure remains elevated, your dose will be gradually increased to 300 milligrams once a day.

If you are being treated with hemodialysis or high doses of diuretics, you'll be started at a lower dose of 75 milligrams once a day.

Overdosage

There has been little experience with overdosage of drugs such as Avapro. However, the most likely results would be low blood pressure and an abnormally slow or rapid heartbeat. If you suspect an overdose, seek medical attention immediately.

Brand name:

AVENTYL

See Pamelor, page 943.

Brand name:

AVITA

See Retin-A and Renova, page 1114.

Brand name:

AXID

Pronounced: AK-sid
Generic name: Nizatidine

Why is this drug prescribed?

Axid is prescribed for the treatment of duodenal ulcers and noncancerous stomach ulcers. Full-dose therapy for these problems lasts no longer than 8 weeks. However, your doctor may prescribe Axid at a reduced dosage after a duodenal ulcer has healed. The drug is also prescribed for the heartburn and the inflammation that result when acid stomach contents flow backward into the esophagus. Axid belongs to a class of drugs known as histamine H_2 blockers.

Most important fact about this drug
Although Axid can be used for up to 8-12 weeks, most ulcers are healed within 4 weeks of therapy.

How should you take this medication?
Take this medication exactly as prescribed by your doctor.

▪ *If you miss a dose...*
Take it as soon as you remember. If it is almost time for your next dose, skip the one you missed and go back to your regular schedule. Do not take 2 doses at once.

▪ *Storage instructions...*
Store at room temperature.

What side effects may occur?
Side effects cannot be anticipated. If any develop or change in intensity, inform your doctor as soon as possible. Only your doctor can determine if it is safe for you to continue taking Axid.

▪ *More common side effects may include:*
Abdominal pain, diarrhea, dizziness, gas, headache, indigestion, inflammation of the nose, nausea, pain, sore throat, vomiting, weakness

▪ *Less common or rare side effects may include:*
Abnormal dreams, anxiety, back pain, chest pain, constipation, dimmed vision, dry mouth, fever, inability to sleep, increased cough, infection, itching, loss of appetite, muscle pain, nervousness, rash, sleepiness, stomach/intestinal problems, tooth problems

Why should this drug not be prescribed?
If you are sensitive to or have ever had an allergic reaction to Axid or similar drugs such as Zantac, you should not take this medication. Make sure your doctor is aware of any drug reactions you have experienced.

Special warnings about this medication
Axid could mask a stomach malignancy. If you continue to have any problems, notify your doctor.

If you have moderate to severe kidney disease, your doctor will reduce your dosage.

**Possible food and drug interactions
when taking this medication**
If Axid is taken with certain other drugs, the effects of either could be increased, decreased, or altered. It is especially important to check with your doctor before combining Axid with aspirin, especially in high doses.

**Special information
if you are pregnant or breastfeeding**
The effects of Axid during pregnancy have not been adequately studied. If you are pregnant or plan to become pregnant, inform your doctor immediately. Axid appears in breast milk and could affect a nursing infant. If this medication is essential to your health, your doctor may advise you to discontinue breastfeeding until your treatment with this medication is finished.

Recommended dosage

ADULTS

Active Duodenal Ulcer:
The usual dose is 300 milligrams once a day at bedtime, but your doctor may have you take 150 milligrams twice a day.

Active Noncancerous Stomach Ulcer:
The usual dose is 150 milligrams twice a day or 300 milligrams once a day at bedtime.

Maintenance of a Healed Duodenal Ulcer:
The usual dose is 150 milligrams once a day at bedtime.

If you have moderate to severe kidney disease, your doctor will prescribe a lower dose.

CHILDREN

The safety and effectiveness of Axid have not been established in children.

Overdosage
No specific information on Axid overdose is available. However, any medication taken in excess can have serious consequences. If you suspect an overdose of Axid, seek medical attention immediately.

Generic name:

AZATADINE WITH PSEUDOEPHEDRINE

See Trinalin Repetabs, page 1350.

Generic name:

AZELAIC ACID

See Azelex, page 124.

Generic name:

AZELASTINE

See Astelin, page 101.

Brand name:

AZELEX

Pronounced: AY-zuh-lecks
Generic name: Azelaic acid

Why is this drug prescribed?
Azelex helps clear up mild to moderate acne. The skin eruptions and inflammation of acne typically begin during puberty, when oily secretions undergo an increase.

Most important fact about this drug
You should keep using Azelex regularly, even if you see no immediate improvement. It takes up to 4 weeks for Azelex to show results.

How should you use this medication?
Use Azelex once in the morning and again in the evening. Wash the areas to be treated and pat dry. Apply a thin film of Azelex and gently but thoroughly massage it into the skin. Wash your hands afterwards.

Do not put bandages or dressings over the treated areas. Avoid getting Azelex in the eyes, mouth, or nose. If any of the cream does get into your eyes, wash it out with large amounts of water. Call your doctor if your eyes remain irritated.

■ *If you miss a dose...*
  Apply it as soon as you remember. If it is almost time for the next dose, skip the one you missed and go back to your regular schedule.

■ *Storage instructions...*
  Store at room temperature. Protect from freezing.

What side effects may occur?
Side effects cannot be anticipated. If any develop or change in intensity, inform your doctor as soon as possible. Only your doctor can determine if it is safe for you to continue using Azelex.

■ *More common side effects may include:*
  Burning, itching, stinging, tingling

■ *Rare side effects may include:*
  Dryness, inflammation, irritation, peeling, rash, redness

Why should this drug not be prescribed?
Do not use Azelex if it causes an allergic reaction.

Special warnings about this medication
Azelex may cause some itching, burning, or stinging when you first begin treatment. You can expect this to stop as treatment continues. If it doesn't, you should check with your doctor. You may have to cut back to a single application daily, or even temporarily stop using this medication.

Azelex has been known to occasionally have a bleaching effect on the skin. Report any abnormal changes in skin color to your doctor.

**Possible food and drug interactions
when using this medication**
No interactions have been reported.

**Special information
if you are pregnant or breastfeeding**
The effects of Azelex during pregnancy and breastfeeding have not been adequately studied. If you are pregnant or plan to become pregnant, notify your doctor immediately. Small amounts of Azelex could appear in breast milk. If you are nursing, use this medication with caution.

Recommended dosage
The usual dose is a thin film of Azelex applied twice a day.

Overdosage
An overdose is unlikely. However, if your skin becomes severely irritated, you should stop applying the medication and call your doctor.

Generic name:

AZITHROMYCIN

See Zithromax, page 1461.

Brand name:

AZMACORT

Pronounced: AZ-ma-court
Generic name: Triamcinolone acetonide
Other brand names: Nasacort, Nasacort AQ

Why is this drug prescribed?
Azmacort and Nasacort are metered-dose inhalers containing the anti-inflammatory steroid medication, triamcinolone acetonide; Nasacort AQ is a metered-dose pump spray. Azmacort is used as long-term therapy to control bronchial asthma attacks. Nasacort and Nasacort AQ are prescribed to relieve the symptoms of hay fever and other nasal allergies. Nasacort is also used in the treatment of nasal polyps (projecting masses of tissue in the nose).

Most important fact about this drug
Azmacort does not provide rapid relief in an asthma attack. Instead, it reduces the frequency and severity of attacks when taken on a regular basis. For quick relief, you must still use airway-opening medications.

How should you take this medication?
Take these drugs on a regular daily basis, exactly as prescribed. With Azmacort and Nasacort, you should begin to see improvement after a week, although it may take 2 weeks or more to achieve the greatest benefit. Nasacort AQ should begin to produce results on the first day, but will take a week to yield maximum benefit.

Shake the canister or bottle before each use. Do not use an Azmacort inhaler more than 240 times. Discard the Nasacort canister after 100 inhalations and the Nasacort AQ bottle after 120 actuations.

If the drug irritates your throat, gargling and rinsing your mouth with water after each dose can help to relieve the problem.

If you are using a bronchodilator inhalant, it should be used before the Azmacort inhalant to derive the best effects from this drug. Use of the two inhalers should be separated by several minutes.

Do not spray Nasacort directly onto the bone that separates the nostrils. Avoid spraying either medication in your eyes.

Illustrated instructions for use are available with the product.

■ *If you miss a dose...*
Use it as soon as you remember. If it is almost time for your next dose, skip the one you missed and go back to your regular schedule. Do not take 2 doses at once.

■ *Storage instructions...*
Store at room temperature. Since the contents of the aerosol inhalant are under pressure, do not puncture the container and do not use or store the medication near heat or open flame. Exposure to temperatures above 120 degrees F. may cause the container to explode.

What side effects may occur?
Side effects cannot be anticipated. If any develop or change in intensity, inform your doctor as soon as possible. Only your doctor can determine if it is safe for you to continue taking these medications.

AZMACORT

■ *More common side effects may include:*
Back pain, flu symptoms, headache, sinus inflammation, sore throat

■ *Less common side effects may include:*
Abdominal pain, bladder inflammation, bursitis, chest congestion, cough, diarrhea, dry mouth, facial swelling, hives, hoarseness, increased wheezing, irritated throat, mouth infection, muscle pain, pain, rash, sensitivity to light, severe allergic reaction, toothache, urinary tract infection, vaginal infection, voice changes, vomiting, weight gain

NASACORT

■ *More common side effects may include:*
Headache

- *Less common side effects may include:*
Dryness of the membranes lining the nose, mouth, and throat, nasal irritation, nasal and sinus congestion, nosebleeds, sneezing, throat discomfort

- *Side effects of Nasacort in children aged 6 to 11 may include:*
Cough, ear inflammation, fever, indigestion, nausea, nosebleed, throat discomfort

NASACORT AQ

- *Side effects of Nasacort AQ may include:*
Headache, nosebleed, stuffy nose

- *Side effects of Nasacort AQ in children aged 6 to 11 may include:*
Asthma, headache, infection, earache, sinus problems, vomiting

Why should this drug not be prescribed?
Do not use any of these medications if you are allergic to or sensitive to any of the ingredients. Do not use Azmacort if:

- Your asthma can be controlled with airway openers and other non-steroid medications.
- You require only occasional steroid treatment for asthma. (Azmacort is not for treatment of prolonged, severe asthma attacks where fast-acting measures are required.)
- You have bronchitis not associated with asthma.

Special warnings about this medication
Your doctor will see that your asthma is reasonably under control before starting you on Azmacort. For about a week, he or she will have you take Azmacort along with your usual dose of oral steroid. After that, you will gradually take less and less of the oral drug. If you develop joint or muscular pain, weariness, and depression, contact your doctor immediately. If you feel light-headed or find that you are losing weight, also tell your doctor.

If you are using Azmacort and your airway-opening medication is not effective during an asthma attack, contact your doctor immediately. Also get medical help immediately if your wheezing gets worse after a dose of Azmacort.

The use of triamcinolone acetonide may cause a yeast-like fungal infection in the mouth and throat (Azmacort) or nose and throat (Nasacort and Nasacort AQ). If you suspect a fungal infection, notify your doctor. Treatment with antifungal medication may be necessary.

People using steroid medications such as these are more susceptible to infection. Chickenpox and measles, for example, can be far more serious for children and for adults who have not had them. Try to avoid exposure, but if you are exposed, inform your doctor. Medication may be needed.

Switching from steroid tablet therapy to Azmacort Inhaler may allow allergic conditions to surface that were previously controlled by the tablets. These include rhinitis (inflammation of the inside of the nose), conjunctivitis (pinkeye), and eczema.

If your child is using any of these medications, your doctor will watch to be sure he or she is growing properly. If you have just had an operation, or if you are experiencing extreme stress, your doctor will watch you closely.

Use these medications with extreme caution if you have tuberculosis, an untreated infection, or a herpes infection of the eye.

If your symptoms do not improve after 3 weeks, or if they get worse, contact your doctor. If you are using Nasacort or Nasacort AQ, also notify your doctor if you develop nosebleeds or notice nasal irritation, burning, or stinging after using the medication.

Use Nasacort or Nasacort AQ with caution if you have not fully healed from nasal ulcers, or an injury to your nose. Steroids can slow wound healing, and there have been rare cases of perforation inside the nose caused by inhaled steroids.

Possible food and drug interactions when taking this medication
Inhaled steroids such as Azmacort, Nasacort, and Nasacort AQ are not recommended for long-term use while you are taking prednisone (Deltasone).

Special information if you are pregnant or breastfeeding
The effects of triamcinolone acetonide during pregnancy have not been adequately studied. If you are pregnant or plan to become pregnant, inform your doctor immediately. It is not known whether triamcinolone acetonide appears in breast milk. If this medication is essential to your health, your doctor may advise you to discontinue breastfeeding until your treatment with this medication is finished.

Recommended dosage

AZMACORT

The Azmacort Inhaler unit is for oral inhalation only.

Adults

The usual dose is 2 inhalations (about 200 micrograms), taken 3 or 4 times a day or 4 inhalations taken twice a day. The daily dose should not exceed 16 inhalations.

Children 6 to 12 Years of Age

The usual dose is 1 or 2 inhalations (100 to 200 micrograms), taken 3 or 4 times a day or 2 to 4 inhalations taken twice a day. The daily dose should not exceed 12 inhalations.

Children Under 6 Years of Age

The safety and effectiveness of this drug have not been established in children under 6 years of age.

NASACORT

Adults and Children Aged 12 and Older

The usual starting dose is 220 micrograms a day, taken as 2 sprays in each nostril once a day. (One spray is 55 micrograms.) If necessary, your doctor may increase the dose up to 440 micrograms a day, taken all at once, twice a day, or 4 times a day. Once Nasacort has started to work, your doctor may decrease the dose to 110 micrograms a day.

Children 6 Through 11 Years of Age

The usual starting dose is 2 sprays in each nostril once a day, for a total of 220 micrograms a day. Your doctor will adjust the dose to best suit the child.

Children Under 6 Years of Age

The safety and effectiveness of Nasacort in children under 6 years of age have not been established.

NASACORT AQ

Adults and Children Aged 12 and Older

The usual starting dose is 220 micrograms taken as 2 sprays in each nostril once a day. Once your symptoms are under control, your doctor may reduce the dose to 110 micrograms a day.

Children Aged 6 to 12

The recommended starting dose is 110 micrograms per day taken as 1 spray in each nostril once a day. The maximum dose is 220 micrograms per day taken as 2 sprays in each nostril once a day.

Children Under 6 Years of Age

Safety and effectiveness have not been established for children under 6.

Overdosage

Any medication taken in excess can have serious consequences. If you suspect an overdose, seek emergency medical treatment immediately.

An overdose is likely to be signaled by an increase in side effects. Accidental contact with the contents of the canister would most likely irritate your nose and give you a headache.

Overuse of Nasacort AQ may upset your stomach and intestines.

Continual overuse of Azmacort inhalation aerosol could lower your resistance; cause weakness; wasting, or swelling; and interfere with healing.

Brand name:

AZULFIDINE

Pronounced: A-ZUL-fi-deen
Generic name: Sulfasalazine

Why is this drug prescribed?

Azulfidine, an anti-inflammatory medicine, is prescribed for the treatment of mild to moderate ulcerative colitis (a long-term, progressive bowel disease) and as an added treatment in severe ulcerative colitis (chronic inflammation and ulceration of the lining of large bowel and rectum, the main symptom of which is bloody diarrhea). This medication is also prescribed to decrease severe attacks of ulcerative colitis.

Azulfidine EN-tabs are prescribed for people with ulcerative colitis who cannot take the regular Azulfidine tablet because of symptoms of stomach and intestinal irritation such as nausea and vomiting when taking the first few doses of the drug, or for those in whom a reduction in dosage does not lessen the stomach or intestinal side effects. The EN-tabs are also prescribed for people with rheumatoid arthritis who fail to get relief from salicylates (such as aspirin) or other nonsteroidal anti-inflammatory drugs (such as ibuprofen).

Most important fact about this drug
Although ulcerative colitis rarely disappears completely, the risk of recurrence can be substantially reduced by the continued use of this drug.

How should you take this medication?
Take this medication in evenly spaced, equal doses, as determined by your doctor, preferably after meals or with food to avoid stomach upset. Swallow Azulfidine EN-tabs whole.

It is important that you drink plenty of fluids while taking this medication to avoid kidney stones.

If you are taking Azulfidine EN-tabs for rheumatoid arthritis, it may take up to 12 weeks for relief to occur.

- *If you miss a dose...*
  Take it as soon as you remember. If it is almost time for your next dose, skip the one you missed and go back to your regular schedule. Do not take 2 doses at once.

- *Storage instructions...*
  Store at room temperature.

What side effects may occur?
Side effects cannot be anticipated. If any develop or change in intensity, inform your doctor as soon as possible. Only your doctor can determine if it is safe for you to continue taking Azulfidine.

- *More common side effects may include:*
  Headache, lack or loss of appetite, nausea, stomach distress, vomiting

- *Less common side effects may include:*
  Anemia, bluish discoloration of the skin, fever, hives, itching, skin rash

- *Rare side effects may include:*
  Abdominal pain, blood disorders, blood in the urine, bloody diarrhea, convulsions, diarrhea, drowsiness, hallucinations, hearing loss, hepatitis, inability to fall or stay asleep, inflammation of the mouth, intestinal inflammation, itchy skin eruptions, joint pain, kidney disorders, lack of muscle coordination, loss of hair, mental depression, red, raised rash, ringing in the ears, sensitivity to light, severe allergic reaction, skin discoloration, skin disorders, spinal cord defects, swelling around the eye, urine discoloration, vertigo

Why should this drug not be prescribed?

If you are sensitive to or have ever had an allergic reaction to Azulfidine, salicylates (aspirin), or other sulfa drugs, you should not take this medication. Make sure your doctor is aware of any drug reactions you have experienced.

Unless you are directed to do so by your doctor, do not take Azulfidine if you have an intestinal or urinary obstruction or if you have porphyria (an inherited disorder involving the substance that gives color to the skin and iris of the eyes).

Special warnings about this medication

If you have kidney or liver damage or any blood disease, your doctor will check you very carefully before prescribing Azulfidine. Deaths have been reported from allergic reactions, blood diseases, kidney or liver damage, changes in nerve and muscle impulses, and fibrosing alveolitis (inflammation of the lungs due to a thickening or scarring of tissue). Signs such as sore throat, fever, abnormal paleness of the skin, purple or red spots on the skin, or jaundice (yellowing of the skin) may be an indication of a serious blood disorder. Your doctor will do frequent blood counts and urine tests. Use caution taking Azulfidine if you have a severe allergy or bronchial asthma.

If you develop loss of appetite, nausea, or vomiting, report it immediately. The doctor may need to adjust your dosage or change the prescription.

If Azulfidine EN-tabs are eliminated undisintegrated, stop taking the drug and notify your doctor immediately. (You may lack the intestinal enzymes necessary to dissolve this medication.)

Men taking Azulfidine may experience temporary infertility and a low sperm count.

Skin and urine may become yellow-orange in color while taking Azulfidine.

In addition, prolonged exposure to the sun should be avoided.

Possible food and drug interactions
when taking this medication

If Azulfidine is taken with certain other drugs, the effects of either could be increased, decreased, or altered. It is especially important to check with your doctor before combining Azulfidine with the following:

Digoxin (Lanoxin)
Folic acid (a B-complex vitamin)

**Special information
if you are pregnant or breastfeeding**
The effects of Azulfidine during pregnancy have not been adequately studied. If you are pregnant or plan to become pregnant, inform your doctor immediately. Azulfidine is secreted in breast milk and could affect a nursing infant. If this medication is essential to your health, your doctor may advise you to discontinue breastfeeding until your treatment is finished.

Recommended dosage
Your doctor will carefully individualize your dosage and monitor your response periodically.

ULCERATIVE COLITIS

Adults
The usual recommended initial dose of Azulfidine and Azulfidine EN-tabs is 3 to 4 grams daily divided into smaller doses (intervals between nighttime doses should not exceed 8 hours). In some cases the initial dosage is set at 1 to 2 grams daily to lessen side effects. As therapy continues, the dose is usually reduced to 2 grams daily.

Children Aged 2 and Older
The usual recommended initial dose is 40 to 60 milligrams per 2.2 pounds of body weight in each 24-hour period, divided into 3 to 6 doses. For the longer term, the dose is usually reduced to 30 milligrams per 2.2 pounds of body weight in each 24-hour period, divided into 4 doses.

RHEUMATOID ARTHRITIS

Adults
The usual dose of Azulfidine EN-tabs is 2 grams a day, divided into smaller doses. Your doctor may have you start with a lower dose, then raise the dosage to 3 grams after 12 weeks.

Children
Safety and effectiveness of Azulfidine EN-tabs in juvenile rheumatoid arthritis have not been established.

Overdosage
Any medication taken in excess can have serious consequences. If you suspect an Azulfidine overdose, seek emergency medical attention immediately.

- *Symptoms of Azulfidine overdose may include:*
  Abdominal pain, convulsions, drowsiness, nausea, stomach upset, vomiting

Brand name:

BACTRIM

Pronounced: BAC-trim
Generic ingredients: Trimethoprim, Sulfamethoxazole
Other brand names: Cotrim, Septra

Why is this drug prescribed?

Bactrim, an antibacterial combination drug, is prescribed for the treatment of certain urinary tract infections, severe middle ear infections in children, long-lasting or frequently recurring bronchitis in adults that has increased in seriousness, inflammation of the intestine due to a severe bacterial infection, pneumonia in patients who have a suppressed immune system (*Pneumocystis carinii* pneumonia), and travelers' diarrhea in adults.

Most important fact about this drug

Sulfamethoxazole, an ingredient in Bactrim, is one of a group of drugs called sulfonamides, which prevent the growth of bacteria in the body. Rare but sometimes fatal reactions have occurred with use of sulfonamides. These reactions include Stevens-Johnson syndrome (severe eruptions around the mouth, anus, or eyes), progressive disintegration of the outer layer of the skin, sudden and severe liver damage, a severe blood disorder (agranulocytosis), and a lack of red and white blood cells because of a bone marrow disorder.

Notify your doctor at the first sign of an adverse reaction such as skin rash, sore throat, fever, joint pain, cough, shortness of breath, abnormal skin paleness, reddish or purplish skin spots, or yellowing of the skin or whites of the eyes.

Frequent blood counts by a doctor are recommended for patients taking sulfonamide drugs.

How should you take this medication?

It is important that you drink plenty of fluids while taking this medication in order to prevent sediment in the urine and the formation of stones.

Bactrim works best when there is a constant amount in the blood. Take Bactrim exactly as prescribed; try not to miss any doses. It is best to take doses at evenly spaced times day and night.

If you are taking Bactrim suspension, ask your pharmacist for a specially marked measuring spoon that delivers accurate doses.

■ *If you miss a dose...*
Take the forgotten dose as soon as you remember. If it is almost time for your next dose, skip the one you missed and go back to your regular schedule. Do not take 2 doses at once.

■ *Storage instructions...*
Store tablets and suspension at room temperature and protect from light. Keep tablets in a dry place. Protect the suspension from freezing.

What side effects may occur?
Side effects cannot be anticipated. If any develop or change in intensity, inform your doctor as soon as possible. Only your doctor can determine if it is safe for you to continue taking Bactrim.

■ *More common side effects may include:*
Hives, lack or loss of appetite, nausea, skin rash, vomiting

■ *Less common or rare side effects may include:*
Abdominal pain, allergic reactions, anemia, chills, convulsions, depression, diarrhea, eye irritation, fatigue, fever, hallucinations, headache, hepatitis, inability to fall or stay asleep, inability to urinate, increased urination, inflammation of heart muscle, inflammation of the mouth and/or tongue, itching, joint pain, kidney failure, lack of feeling or concern, lack of muscle coordination, loss of appetite, low blood sugar, meningitis (inflammation of the brain or spinal cord), muscle pain, nausea, nervousness, red, raised rash, redness and swelling of the tongue, ringing in the ears, scaling of dead skin due to inflammation, sensitivity to light, severe skin welts or swelling, skin eruptions, skin peeling, vertigo, weakness, yellowing of eyes and skin

Why should this drug not be prescribed?
If you are sensitive to or have ever had an allergic reaction to trimethoprim, sulfamethoxazole, or other sulfa drugs, you should not take this medication. Make sure that your doctor is aware of any drug reactions that you have experienced.

Unless you are directed to do so by your doctor, do not take this medication if you have been diagnosed as having megaloblastic anemia, which is a blood disorder due to a deficiency of folic acid.

This drug should not be given to infants less than 2 months of age.

Bactrim is not recommended for preventative or prolonged use in middle ear infections and should not be used in the treatment of streptococcal pharyngitis (strep throat) or certain other strep infections.

You should not take Bactrim if you are pregnant or nursing a baby.

Special warnings about this medication

Make sure your doctor knows if you have impaired kidney or liver function, have a folic acid deficiency, are a chronic alcoholic, are taking anticonvulsants, have been diagnosed as having malabsorption syndrome (abnormal intestinal absorption), are in a state of poor nutrition, or have severe allergies or bronchial asthma. Bactrim should be used cautiously under these conditions.

If you develop severe diarrhea, call your doctor. This drug can cause a serious intestinal inflammation.

If you have AIDS (acquired immunodeficiency syndrome) and are being treated for *Pneumocystis carinii* pneumonia, you will experience more side effects than will someone without AIDS.

Possible food and drug interactions
when taking this medication

If Bactrim is taken with certain other drugs, the effects of either could be increased, decreased, or altered. It is especially important to check with your doctor before combining Bactrim with the following:

Amantadine (Symmetrel)
Blood thinners such as Coumadin
Methotrexate (Rheumatrex)
Oral diabetes medications such as Micronase
Seizure medications such as Dilantin
Water pills (diuretics) such as HydroDIURIL

Special information
if you are pregnant or breastfeeding

Bactrim should not be taken during pregnancy. If you are pregnant or plan to become pregnant, notify your doctor immediately. Bactrim does appear in breast milk and could affect a nursing infant. It should not be taken while breastfeeding.

Recommended dosage

ADULTS

Urinary Tract Infections and Intestinal Inflammation

The usual adult dosage in the treatment of urinary tract infection is 1 Bactrim DS (double strength tablet) or 2 Bactrim tablets, or 4 teaspoonfuls (20 milliliters) of Bactrim Pediatric Suspension every 12 hours for 10 to 14 days. The dosage for inflammation of the intestine is the same but is taken for 5 days.

Worsening of Chronic Bronchitis

The usual recommended dosage is 1 Bactrim DS (double strength tablet), 2 Bactrim tablets, or 4 teaspoonfuls (20 milliliters) of Bactrim Pediatric Suspension every 12 hours for 14 days.

Pneumocystis Carinii Pneumonia

The recommended dosage is 20 milligrams of trimethoprim and 100 milligrams of sulfamethoxazole per 2.2 pounds of body weight per 24 hours divided into equal doses every 6 hours for 14 days.

Travelers' Diarrhea

The usual recommended dosage is 1 Bactrim DS (double strength tablet), 2 Bactrim tablets, or 4 teaspoonfuls (20 milliliters) of Bactrim Pediatric Suspension every 12 hours for 5 days.

CHILDREN

Urinary Tract Infections or Middle Ear Infections

The recommended dose for children 2 months of age or older, given every 12 hours for 10 days, is determined by weight. The following table is a guideline for this dosage:

22 pounds, 1 teaspoonful (5 milliliters)

44 pounds, 2 teaspoonfuls (10 milliliters) or 1 tablet

66 pounds, 3 teaspoonfuls (15 milliliters) or one-and-a-half tablets

88 pounds, 4 teaspoonfuls (20 milliliters) or 2 tablets or 1 DS tablet

Intestinal Inflammation

The recommended dose is identical to the dosage recommended for urinary tract and middle ear infections; however, it should be taken for 5 days.

Pneumocystis Carinii Pneumonia

The recommended dose, taken every 6 hours for 14 days, is determined by weight. The following table is a guideline for this dosage:

18 pounds, 1 teaspoonful (5 milliliters)

35 pounds, 2 teaspoonfuls (10 milliliters) or 1 tablet

53 pounds, 3 teaspoonfuls (15 milliliters) or one-and-a-half tablets

70 pounds, 4 teaspoonfuls (20 milliliters) or 2 tablets or 1 DS tablet

The safety of repeated use of Bactrim in children under 2 years of age has not been established.

OLDER ADULTS

There may be an increased risk of severe side effects when Bactrim is taken by older people, especially in those who have impaired kidney and/or liver function or who are taking other medication. Consult with your doctor before taking Bactrim.

Overdosage

If you suspect an overdose of Bactrim, seek emergency medical attention immediately.

■ *Symptoms of an overdose of Bactrim include:*
Blood or sediment in the urine, colic, confusion, dizziness, drowsiness, fever, headache, lack or loss of appetite, mental depression, nausea, unconsciousness, vomiting, yellowed eyes and skin

Brand name:

BACTROBAN

Pronounced: BAC-tro-ban
Generic name: Mupirocin

Why is this drug prescribed?

Bactroban is prescribed for the treatment of impetigo, a bacterial infection of the skin.

Most important fact about this drug

If the use of Bactroban does not clear your skin infection within 3 to 5 days, or if the infection becomes worse, notify your doctor.

How should you use this medication?
This drug is for external use only.

■ *If you miss a dose...*
Apply it as soon as you remember. If it is almost time for the next dose, skip the one you missed and go back to your regular schedule.

■ *Storage instructions...*
Store at room temperature.

What side effects may occur?
Side effects cannot be anticipated. If any develop or change in intensity, inform your doctor as soon as possible. Only your doctor can determine if it is safe for you to continue using Bactroban.

■ *More common side effects may include:*
Burning, pain, stinging

■ *Less common side effects may include:*
Itching

■ *Rare side effects may include:*
Abnormal redness, dry skin, inflammation of the skin, nausea, oozing, skin rash, swelling, tenderness

Why should this drug not be prescribed?
If you are sensitive to or have ever had an allergic reaction to Bactroban or similar drugs, you should not use this medication. Make sure your doctor is aware of any drug reactions you have experienced.

Special warnings about this medication
Continued or prolonged use of Bactroban may result in the growth of bacteria that do not respond to this medication and can cause a secondary infection.

This drug is not intended for use in the eyes.

If your skin shows signs of an allergic reaction or irritation, stop using Bactroban and consult your doctor.

Possible food and drug interactions
when taking this medication
There are no known interactions.

**Special information
if you are pregnant or breastfeeding**
The effects of Bactroban during pregnancy have not been adequately studied.
If you are pregnant or plan to become pregnant, inform your doctor
immediately. Bactroban may appear in breast milk and could affect a nursing
infant. Your doctor may advise you to discontinue breastfeeding until your
treatment with this medication is finished.

Recommended dosage
Apply a small amount of this medication to the affected area 3 times a day.
Cover the treated area with gauze if you want.

Overdosage
There is no information available on overdosage.

Brand name:

BAYCOL

Pronounced: BAY-call
Generic name: Cerivastatin sodium

Why is this drug prescribed?
Baycol is used, along with a diet, to bring down dangerously high cholesterol
levels when other measures have failed. Excess cholesterol in the bloodstream can lead to hardening of the arteries and heart disease. Baycol lowers
both total cholesterol and LDL ("bad") cholesterol, while raising the HDL
("good") cholesterol that tends to clear the arteries.

Most important fact about this drug
Although you can't feel any symptoms of high cholesterol, it is important to
take Baycol every day. The drug will be more effective if it is used along with
a low-fat diet and plenty of exercise.

How should you take this medication?
Take Baycol once a day, in the evening, with or without food. Your
cholesterol levels should begin to show improvement within 4 weeks.

■ *If you miss a dose...*
   Take it as soon as you remember. If it is almost time for your next dose,
   skip the one you missed and go back to your regular schedule. Do not take
   2 doses at once.

■ *Storage instructions...*
Baycol tablets should be stored at room temperature, away from moisture.

What side effects may occur?
Side effects cannot be anticipated. If any develop or change in intensity, inform your doctor as soon as possible. Only your doctor can determine if it is safe for you to continue taking Baycol.

■ *More common side effects may include:*
Diarrhea, indigestion, joint pain, runny nose, sinus problems, weakness

■ *Less common side effects may include:*
Chest pain, increased cough, insomnia, leg pain, muscle pain, swelling

Why should this drug not be prescribed?
Do not take Baycol if you are pregnant or breastfeeding; it could harm the developing baby. Also avoid Baycol if you have a liver condition or the drug gives you an allergic reaction.

Special warnings about this medication
Contact your physician immediately if you experience any unexplained muscle pain, tenderness, or weakness. Baycol has been known to trigger a muscle-wasting condition that can also affect the kidneys. The drug should be temporarily discontinued if you develop any condition that might predispose you to kidney problems, including a blood infection, low blood pressure, major surgery, injury, a severe fluid disorder, or uncontrolled seizures.

Baycol occasionally causes liver problems as well. If you've had a liver disease in the past, or you regularly drink alcoholic beverages, make sure the doctor is aware of it. Because of Baycol's potential effect on the liver, the doctor will probably test your liver function regularly.

Possible food and drug interactions
when taking this medication
If Baycol is taken with certain other drugs, the effects of either could be increased, decreased, or altered. It is especially important to check with your doctor before combining Baycol with any of the following:

Antifungal drugs such as Diflucan and Nizoral
Drugs that suppress the immune system, such as Sandimmune and
    Neoral
Erythromycin (E.E.S., E-Mycin, PCE, others)
Fibric acid derivatives such as Atromid-S
Nicotinic acid (Niacin)

Special information
if you are pregnant or breastfeeding

If you are pregnant or plan to become pregnant, stop taking Baycol immediately and inform your doctor. Baycol should not be used during pregnancy or while nursing.

Recommended dosage

ADULTS

The usual starting dose of Baycol is 300 mcg (micrograms) once a day in the evening. If you have kidney disease, the starting dose is 200 mcg.

If your doctor prescribes both Baycol and cholestyramine (Questran), take the Questran first, followed by Baycol at least 2 hours later.

CHILDREN

The safety and effectiveness of Baycol have not been established in children.

Overdosage

Little is known about Baycol overdose. However, any medication taken in excess can have serious consequences. If you suspect an overdose, seek medical treatment immediately.

Generic name:

BECLOMETHASONE

Pronounced: BECK-low-METH-ah-sone
Brand names: Beclovent Inhalation Aerosol, Beconase AQ
Nasal Spray, Beconase Inhalation Aerosol, Vancenase
AQ Nasal Spray and Double Strength Nasal Spray,
Vancenase Nasal Inhaler and PocketHaler Nasal Inhaler,
Vanceril Inhalation Aerosol and Double Strength
Inhalation Aerosol, Vanceril Inhaler

Why is this drug prescribed?

Beclomethasone is a type of steroid used for respiratory problems. Beclovent and Vanceril are prescribed for the treatment of recurring symptoms of bronchial asthma.

Beconase and Vancenase are used to relieve the symptoms of hay fever and to prevent regrowth of nasal polyps following surgical removal.

Most important fact about this drug
Beclomethasone is not a bronchodilator medication (it does not quickly open the airways); and it should not be used for relief of asthma when bronchodilators and other nonsteroid drugs prove effective. Do not expect immediate relief from beclomethasone, and do not take higher doses in an attempt to make it work. It is not intended for rapid relief, but it will help control symptoms when taken routinely.

How should you take this medication?
Beclomethasone is prescribed in an oral inhalant or a nasal spray form. Use this medication only as preventive therapy, and take only the dose prescribed.

Although some people begin to notice improvement within a day or two, it may take 1 or 2 weeks for the full benefits to appear. If there's no improvement after 3 weeks, let your doctor know.

If you are already taking a steroid in tablet form for asthma, you'll need to make a gradual transition to the oral inhalant. During the first week, you'll probably take the usual number of tablets. After that, you'll be instructed to slowly reduce the number of tablets, replacing them with the inhalant.

Be sure to take the drug regularly, even if you have no symptoms. Many people will require additional drugs to control asthma symptoms fully, but this drug may allow other drugs to be used in smaller doses.

If you are also using a bronchodilator inhalant, take it before inhaling beclomethasone. This will improve the effect of the second drug. Take the two inhalations several minutes apart.

Spray the inhalation aerosol into the air twice before you use it for the first time and when you have not used it for more than 7 days. Use it within 6 months.

Before you use Vancenase AQ 84 microgram nasal spray, press the pump 6 times or until you see a fine spray. If you don't use it for more than 4 days, reprime the pump by spraying once or until a fine spray appears.

To use the inhaler:
1. Remove the cap and hold inhaler upright.
2. Shake the inhaler thoroughly.
3. Take a drink of water to moisten the throat.
4. Breathe out as fully as you comfortably can. Hold the inhaler upright and close your lips around the mouthpiece, keeping your tongue below it.

5. While pressing down on the can, inhale deeply. Hold your breath as long as you can.
6. Take your finger off the can, remove the inhaler, and breathe out gently.
7. Allow at least 1 minute between inhalations.

Gargling and rinsing your mouth with water after each dose may help prevent hoarseness and throat irritation. Do not swallow the water after you rinse.

Clean your inhaler at least once a day by removing and rinsing the plastic case and cap in warm, running water.

Be careful to avoid spraying the medication into your eyes. This medication comes with directions. Read them carefully before using it.

■ *If you miss a dose...*
Take it as soon as you remember and take the remaining doses for that day at evenly spaced intervals. If it is time for your next dose, skip the one you missed. Never take 2 doses at the same time.

■ *Storage instructions...*
Store at room temperature in a dry place, away from heat and cold. Do not puncture the container, store it near open flame, or dispose of it in a fire or incinerator.

What side effects may occur?
Side effects cannot be anticipated. If any develop or change in intensity, inform your doctor as soon as possible. Only your doctor can determine if it is safe for you to continue taking this medication.

■ *Side effects may include:*
Cataracts, dry mouth, fluid retention, hives, hoarseness, increased pressure within the eye (glaucoma), skin rash, wheezing

■ *When using a nasal spray, other possible side effects are:*
Cough, headache, light-headedness, nasal burning, nasal and throat dryness and irritation, nausea, nose and throat infections, nosebleed, pain, pinkeye, ringing in the ears, runny nose, sneezing, sore throat, stuffy nose, tearing eyes, unpleasant—or loss of—taste and smell

Why should this drug not be prescribed?
Your doctor will prescribe beclomethasone only if your asthma cannot be controlled with bronchodilators and other nonsteroid medications.

Beclomethasone is not used for the treatment of non-asthmatic bronchitis, or for intermittent asthma therapy.

Do not use beclomethasone nasal products if you've recently had nasal ulcers, nose surgery, or an injury to the nose. It could interfere with the healing process.

If you are sensitive to or have ever had an allergic reaction to beclomethasone or other steroid drugs, you should not take this medication. Make sure that your doctor is aware of any drug reactions that you have experienced.

Although unlikely, immediate allergic reactions to beclomethasone have been known to occur.

Special warnings about this medication
When steroid drugs are taken by mouth they substitute for and decrease the body's normal ability to make its own steroids as well as its ability to respond to stress.

There is a risk of causing a serious condition called "adrenal insufficiency" when people change from steroid tablets taken by mouth to aerosol beclomethasone. Although the aerosol may provide adequate control of asthma during the changeover period, it does not provide the normal amount of steroid the body needs during acute stress situations, such as injury, surgery, and infection—particularly stomach flu. If you are being transferred from steroid tablets to beclomethasone and you experience a period of stress or a severe asthma attack, contact your doctor immediately. He may prescribe additional treatment with steroid tablets. You should also carry a warning card indicating that you may need steroid tablets during such incidents. As you continue taking beclomethasone, your doctor may conduct periodic tests to measure your adrenal function.

Transfer from steroid tablet therapy to beclomethasone aerosol may reactivate allergic conditions that were previously suppressed by the steroid tablet therapy, such as runny nose, inflamed eyelids, and eczema. Some people also experience withdrawal side effects when they switch from tablets to aerosol. Potential symptoms include joint or muscle pain, weakness, and depression. Inform your doctor if you experience any of these symptoms.

High doses of steroids can suppress your immune system. Take extra care to avoid exposure to measles or chickenpox if you have never had them or never had shots. These infections can be serious or even fatal if your immune system is below par. If you are exposed, seek medical advice immediately.

Symptoms such as mental disturbances, increased bruising, weight gain, facial swelling (moon-face), acne, menstrual irregularities, and cataracts may occur with orally inhaled steroids such as Beclovent. If you experience any of these symptoms, notify your doctor immediately.

Long-term use of steroids can slow down growth in children. If your child seems to be growing more slowly than normal, call your doctor.

If bronchodilator medications seem less effective after you start taking beclomethasone, be sure to tell your doctor. Do not abruptly stop using beclomethasone on your own.

If you have tuberculosis, a herpes infection of the eye, or any untreated infection, your doctor may not want you to use an inhaled steroid.

Special information
if you are pregnant or breastfeeding
The effects of beclomethasone in pregnancy have not been adequately studied. If you are pregnant or are planning a pregnancy, let your doctor know. Steroids do appear in breast milk and could harm your baby. Your doctor may want you to avoid breastfeeding while you are using beclomethasone.

Recommended dosage

ADULTS

Beclomethasone Oral Inhalant
The usual recommended dose for adults and children 12 years of age and over is 2 inhalations taken 3 to 4 times a day. Four inhalations taken twice daily have been shown to be effective in some people. If you have severe asthma, your doctor may advise you to start with 12 to 16 inhalations a day. Daily intake should not exceed 20 inhalations.

For the double-strength inhalation aerosol, the usual dose is 2 inhalations twice a day. If your asthma is severe, your doctor may have you start with 6 to 8 inhalations a day. The maximum daily dosage is 10 inhalations.

Beclomethasone Nasal Inhalation
For adults and children 12 years of age and over, the usual dose of Vancenase PocketHaler is 1 inhalation 2 to 4 times a day.

Beclomethasone Nasal Spray
For adults and children 12 years of age and older, the usual dosage is 1 or 2 inhalations in each nostril 2 to 4 times a day, depending on the brand. For

the double strength nasal spray, the dosage is 1 or 2 inhalations in each nostril once a day.

The usual dosage of Vancenase AQ 84 micrograms for adults and children 6 years and over is 1 or 2 inhalations in each nostril once a day.

CHILDREN

Beclomethasone Oral Inhalant

Children 6 to 12 years of age: The usual recommended dose is 1 or 2 inhalations 3 or 4 times a day. Four inhalations twice daily have been effective for some children. Daily intake should not exceed 10 inhalations.

For the double-strength inhalation aerosol, the usual dose is 2 inhalations twice daily, with a maximum of 5 inhalations a day.

Beclomethasone Nasal Inhalation

Children 6 to 12 years of age: The usual dose of Vancenase PocketHaler is 1 inhalation 3 times a day.

Beclomethasone Nasal Spray

Children 6 to 12 years of age: The usual dosage is 1 inhalation in each nostril 2 or 3 times daily. Some children may need 2 inhalations. The dosage for the double strength nasal spray is 1 or 2 inhalations in each nostril once a day.

Beclomethasone should not be given to children under the age of 6 unless advised by your doctor.

Overdosage

Any medication taken in excess can have serious consequences. The main risk in an overdose of beclomethasone is adrenal insufficiency. If you suspect an overdose, seek medical attention immediately.

Brand name:

BECLOVENT

See Beclomethasone, page 143.

Brand name:

BECONASE

See Beclomethasone, page 143.

Brand name:

BEEPEN-VK

See Penicillin V Potassium, page 971.

Brand name:

BELLATAL

See Donnatal, page 431.

Brand name:

BENADRYL

Pronounced: BEN-ah-dril
Generic name: Diphenhydramine hydrochloride

Why is this drug prescribed?

Benadryl is an antihistamine with drying and sedative effects. It relieves red, inflamed eyes caused by food allergies and the itching, swelling, and redness from hives and other rashes that are caused by mild allergic reactions. It also relieves the sneezing, coughing, runny or stuffy nose, and red, teary, itching eyes caused by seasonal allergies (hay fever) and the common cold. Antihistamines work by decreasing the effects of histamine, a chemical released in the body that narrows air passages in the lungs and contributes to inflammation. Antihistamines reduce itching and swelling and dry up secretions from the nose, eyes, and throat.

Benadryl is also used to treat allergic reactions to blood transfusions, to prevent and treat motion sickness, and, with other drugs, to treat anaphylactic shock (severe allergic reaction) and Parkinson's disease, a nerve disorder characterized by tremors, stooped posture, shuffling walk, muscle weakness, drooling, and emotional instability.

Most important fact about this drug

Antihistamines may produce excitability in children. In the elderly they may cause dizziness, excessive calm, or low blood pressure.

How should you take this medication?

Benadryl should be taken exactly as prescribed, or follow instructions on the label.

■ *If you miss a dose...*
Take it as soon as you remember. If it is almost time for your next dose, skip the one you missed and go back to your regular schedule. Do not take 2 doses at once.

■ *Storage instructions...*
Store at room temperature. Protect from moisture.

What side effects may occur?
Side effects cannot be anticipated. If any develop or change in intensity, inform your doctor as soon as possible. Only your doctor can determine if it is safe for you to continue taking Benadryl.

■ *More common side effects may include:*
Disturbed coordination, dizziness, excessive calm, increased chest congestion, sleepiness, stomach upset

■ *Less common or rare side effects may include:*
Anaphylactic shock (extreme allergic reaction), anemia, blurred vision, chills, confusion, constipation, convulsions, diarrhea, difficulty sleeping, double vision, dry mouth, nose, throat, early menstruation, excessive perspiration, excitation, fast, fluttery heartbeat, fatigue, frequent or difficult urination, headache, hives, inability to urinate, increased sensitivity to light, irregular heartbeat, irritability, loss of appetite, low blood pressure, nausea, nervousness, rapid heartbeat, rash, restlessness, ringing in the ears, stuffy nose, tightness of chest and wheezing, tingling or pins and needles, tremor, unreal or exaggerated sense of well-being, vertigo, vomiting

Why should this drug not be prescribed?
Benadryl should not be used in newborn or premature infants, or if you are breastfeeding your infant.

Do not take this medication if you are sensitive to or have ever had an allergic reaction to diphenhydramine hydrochloride or other antihistamines.

Special warnings about this medication
In general, you should use antihistamines very cautiously if you have the eye condition called narrow-angle glaucoma, narrowing of the stomach or intestine because of peptic ulcer or other stomach problems, intestinal blockage, symptoms of an enlarged prostate, or difficulty urinating due to obstruction in the bladder.

Antihistamines can make adults and children less alert and, in young children, may cause excitability.

Elderly people (60 years or older) are more likely to experience dizziness, extreme calm, and low blood pressure.

Use Benadryl cautiously if you have a history of asthma or other chronic lung disease, an over-active thyroid, high blood pressure, or heart disease.

This medication can cause drowsiness. Driving or operating dangerous machinery or participating in any hazardous activity that requires full mental alertness is not recommended until you know how you react to Benadryl.

Possible food and drug interactions
when taking this medication
Benadryl may increase the effects of alcohol, and alcohol may increase the sedative effects of Benadryl. Do not drink alcohol while taking this medication.

If Benadryl is taken with certain other drugs, the effects of either could be increased, decreased, or altered. It is especially important to check with your doctor before combining Benadryl with the following:

Antidepressant drugs known as MAO inhibitors, such as Parnate and Nardil
Sedative/hypnotics such as Halcion, Nembutal, and Seconal
Tranquilizers such as Xanax and Valium

Special information
if you are pregnant or breastfeeding
The effects of Benadryl during pregnancy have not been adequately studied. If you are pregnant or plan to become pregnant, inform your doctor immediately. Benadryl should be used during pregnancy only if clearly needed. Antihistamine therapy is not advised for nursing mothers. If this medication is essential to your health, your doctor may advise you to discontinue breastfeeding until your treatment with Benadryl is finished.

Recommended dosage
Your doctor will tailor the dosage to suit your needs. Benadryl reaches its peak effect in 1 hour, and 1 dose will continue to work for 4 to 6 hours.

ADULTS
The usual recommended dose is 25 to 50 milligrams 3 or 4 times daily. The sleep-aid dosage is 50 milligrams at bedtime.

Motion Sickness
For prevention of motion sickness, take the first dose 30 minutes before exposure to motion; take the other doses before meals and at bedtime for as long as the motion continues.

CHILDREN (OVER 20 POUNDS)

The usual dose is 12.5 to 25 milligrams, 3 to 4 times daily. A child should not take more than 300 milligrams a day.

This medication should not be used as a sleep aid for children under age 12.

Your physician will determine the best use of the drug in response to its effects on the child.

Overdosage
Any medication taken in excess can have serious consequences. If you suspect an overdose, seek medical attention immediately. Antihistamine overdose has caused hallucinations, convulsions, and death in children.

■ *Symptoms of Benadryl overdose may include:*
Central nervous system depression or stimulation, especially in children, dry mouth, fixed, dilated pupils, flushing, stomach and intestinal symptoms

Generic name:

BENAZEPRIL

See Lotensin, page 729.

Brand name:

BENTYL

Pronounced: BEN-til
Generic name: Dicyclomine hydrochloride

Why is this drug prescribed?
Bentyl is prescribed for the treatment of functional bowel/irritable bowel syndrome (abdominal pain, accompanied by diarrhea and constipation associated with stress).

Most important fact about this drug
Heat prostration (fever and heat stroke due to decreased sweating) can occur with use of this drug in hot weather. If symptoms occur, stop taking the drug and notify your doctor immediately.

How should you take this medication?

Take this medication exactly as prescribed.

■ *If you miss a dose...*

Take it as soon as you remember. If it is almost time for your next dose, skip the one you missed and go back to your regular schedule. Do not take 2 doses at once.

■ *Storage instructions...*

Store at room temperature. Keep tablets out of direct sunlight. Keep syrup away from excessive heat.

What side effects may occur?

Side effects cannot be anticipated. If any develop or change in intensity, inform your doctor as soon as possible. Only your doctor can determine if it is safe for you to continue taking Bentyl.

■ *Side effects may include:*

Blurred vision, dizziness, drowsiness, dry mouth, light-headedness, nausea, nervousness, weakness

Not all of the following side effects have been reported with dicyclomine hydrochloride, but they have been reported for similar drugs with antispasmodic action; contact your doctor if they occur.

Abdominal pain, bloated feeling, constipation, decreased sweating, difficulty in urinating, double vision, enlargement of the pupil of the eye, eye paralysis, fainting, headache, hives, impotence, inability to urinate, increased pressure in the eyes, itching, labored, difficult breathing, lack of coordination, lack or loss of appetite, nasal stuffiness or congestion, numbness, rapid heartbeat, rash, severe allergic reaction, sluggishness, sneezing, suffocation, suppression of breast milk, taste loss, temporary cessation of breathing, throat congestion, tingling, vomiting

Why should this drug not be prescribed?

If you are sensitive to or have ever had an allergic reaction to Bentyl, you should not take this medication. Make sure your doctor is aware of any drug reactions you have experienced.

Unless you are directed to do so by your doctor, do not take this drug if you have a blockage of the urinary tract, stomach, or intestines; severe ulcerative colitis (inflammatory disease of the large intestine); reflux esophagitis (inflammation of the esophagus usually caused by the backflow of acid stomach contents); glaucoma; or myasthenia gravis (a disease characterized by long-lasting fatigue and muscle weakness).

This drug should not be given to infants less than 6 months of age or used by women who are nursing an infant.

Special warnings about this medication

Bentyl may produce drowsiness or blurred vision. Therefore, driving a car, operating machinery, or participating in any activity that requires full mental alertness is not recommended.

Diarrhea may be an early symptom of a partial intestinal blockage, especially in people who have had bowel removals and an ileostomy or colostomy. If this occurs, notify your doctor immediately.

You should use this medication with caution if you have autonomic neuropathy (a nerve disorder); liver or kidney disease; hyperthyroidism; high blood pressure; coronary heart disease; congestive heart failure; rapid, irregular heartbeat; hiatal hernia (protrusion of part of the stomach through the diaphragm); or enlargement of the prostate gland.

Possible food and drug interactions
when taking this medication

If Bentyl is taken with certain other drugs, the effects of either could be increased, decreased, or altered. It is especially important to check with your doctor before combining Bentyl with the following:

Airway-opening drugs such as Proventil and Ventolin
Amantadine (Symmetrel)
Antacids such as Maalox
Antiarrhythmics such as quinidine (Quinidex)
Antiglaucoma drugs such as Pilopine
Antihistamines such as Tavist
Benzodiazepines (tranquilizers) such as Valium and Xanax
Corticosteroids such as prednisone (Deltasone)
Digoxin (the heart failure medication Lanoxin)
Major tranquilizers such as Mellaril and Thorazine
MAO inhibitors (antidepressants such as Nardil and Parnate)
Metoclopramide (the gastrointestinal stimulant Reglan)
Narcotic analgesics (pain relievers such as Demerol)
Nitrates and nitrites (heart medications such as nitroglycerin)
Tricyclic antidepressant drugs such as Elavil and Tofranil

Special information
if you are pregnant or breastfeeding

The effects of Bentyl during pregnancy have not been adequately studied. If you are pregnant or plan to become pregnant, notify your doctor. Bentyl does appear in breast milk and could affect a nursing infant. Do not use it when breastfeeding.

Recommended dosage

ADULTS

The usual dosage is 160 milligrams per day divided into 4 equal doses. Since this dose is associated with a significant incidence of side effects, your doctor may recommend a starting dose of 80 milligrams per day divided into 4 equal doses. If no side effects appear, the doctor will then increase the dose.

If this drug is not effective within 2 weeks or side effects require doses below 80 milligrams per day, your doctor may discontinue it.

Overdosage

Any medication taken in excess can have serious consequences. If you suspect an overdose, seek medical attention immediately.

- *Symptoms of a Bentyl overdose include:*
  Blurred vision, difficulty in swallowing, dilated pupils, dizziness, dryness of the mouth, headache, hot, dry skin, nausea, nerve blockage causing weakness and possible paralysis, vomiting

Brand name:

BENZAC W

See Desquam-E, page 375.

Brand name:

BENZAGEL

See Desquam-E, page 375.

Brand name:

BENZAMYCIN

Pronounced: BEN-za-MI-sin
Generic ingredients: Erythromycin, Benzoyl peroxide

Why is this drug prescribed?

A combination of the antibiotic erythromycin and the antibacterial agent benzoyl peroxide, Benzamycin is effective in stopping the bacteria that cause acne and in reducing acne infection.

Most important fact about this drug
If you experience excessive irritation, stop using Benzamycin and notify your doctor.

How should you use this medication?
Use Benzamycin 2 times per day, once in the morning and once in the evening, or as directed by your doctor.

Before applying Benzamycin, thoroughly wash the affected area with soap and warm water, rinse well, and gently pat dry. Apply Benzamycin to the entire area, not just the pimples.

■ *If you miss a dose...*
   Apply it as soon as you remember. If it is almost time for your next dose, skip the one you missed and go back to your regular schedule.

■ *Storage instructions...*
   This medication should be stored in your refrigerator in a tightly closed container and discarded after 3 months. Do not freeze.

What side effects may occur?
Very few side effects have been reported with the use of Benzamycin. However, those reported include dryness and swelling.

Occasionally, use of this medication has caused a burning sensation; eye irritation; inflammation of the face, eyes, and nose; itching; oiliness; reddened skin; skin discoloration; skin irritation and peeling; and skin tenderness.

If any side effects develop or change in intensity, inform your doctor as soon as possible. Only your doctor can determine if it is safe for you to continue using Benzamycin.

Why should this drug not be prescribed?
If you are sensitive to or have ever had an allergic reaction to erythromycin or benzoyl peroxide, or any other ingredients in Benzamycin, you should not use this medication. Make sure your doctor is aware of any drug reactions you have experienced.

Special warnings about this medication
Benzamycin Topical Gel is for external use only. Avoid contact with your eyes, nose, mouth, and all mucous membranes.

Benzamycin may bleach hair or colored fabric. Avoid contact with scalp and clothes.

As you use this antibiotic, organisms that are resistant to it may start to grow. Your doctor will have you stop using Benzamycin and will give you a medication to fight the new bacteria.

If you develop diarrhea after you start using Benzamycin, call your doctor. You may have an intestinal inflammation that could be serious.

**Possible food and drug interactions
when using this medication**
If Benzamycin is used with other acne medications, the effects of either could be increased, decreased, or altered. Always check with your doctor before combining any other prescription or over-the-counter acne remedy with Benzamycin.

**Special information
if you are pregnant or breastfeeding**
The effects of Benzamycin during pregnancy have not been adequately studied. If you are pregnant or plan to become pregnant, inform your doctor immediately. It is not known whether Benzamycin appears in breast milk, but erythromycin does if it is swallowed or injected. If this medication is essential to your health, your doctor may advise you to discontinue breastfeeding your baby until your treatment with this medication is finished.

Recommended dosage

ADULTS

Apply to affected areas twice daily, once in the morning and once in the evening.

CHILDREN

The safety and effectiveness of Benzamycin have not been established in children under 12 years of age.

Overdosage
There is no information available on overdosage.

Brand name:

BENZASHAVE

See Desquam-E, page 375.

Generic name:

BENZONATATE

See Tessalon, page 1287.

Generic name:

BENZOYL PEROXIDE

See Desquam-E, page 375.

Generic name:

BENZTROPINE

See Cogentin, page 271.

Brand name:

BETAGAN

Pronounced: BAIT-ah-gan
Generic name: Levobunolol hydrochloride

Why is this drug prescribed?
Betagan eyedrops are given to treat chronic open-angle glaucoma (increased pressure inside the eye). This medication is in a class called beta blockers. It works by lowering pressure within the eyeball.

Most important fact about this drug
Although Betagan eyedrops are applied to the eye, the medication is absorbed and may have effects in other parts of the body. If you have diabetes, asthma or other respiratory diseases, or decreased heart function, make sure your doctor is aware of the problem.

How should you use this medication?
Use Betagan eyedrops exactly as prescribed. Some people also need to use eyedrops that constrict their pupils.

Administer Betagan eyedrops as follows:
1. Wash your hands thoroughly.
2. Gently pull your lower eyelid down to form a pocket between your eye and eyelid.
3. Hold the bottle on the bridge of your nose or on your forehead.
4. Do not touch the applicator tip to any surface, including your eye.
5. Tilt your head back and squeeze the medication into your eye.
6. Close your eyes gently.
7. Keep your eyes closed for 1 to 2 minutes.
8. Wait 5 to 10 minutes before using any other eyedrops.
9. Do not rinse the dropper.

■ *If you miss a dose...*
If you take Betagan once a day, use it as soon as you remember. If you do not remember until the next day, skip the dose you missed and go back to your regular schedule. Do not take 2 doses at once. If you take Betagan 2 or more times a day, use it as soon as you remember. If it is almost time for your next dose, skip the one you missed and go back to your regular schedule. Do not take 2 doses at once.

■ *Storage instructions...*
Store at room temperature, away from light.

What side effects may occur?
Side effects from Betagan cannot be anticipated. If any develop or change in intensity, inform your doctor. Only your doctor can determine whether it is safe for you to continue using this medication. You may feel a momentary burning and stinging when you place the drops in your eyes. More rarely, you may develop an eye inflammation.

Beta blockers may cause muscle weakness; weakened muscles around the eyes may cause double vision or drooping eyelids.

■ *Other potential side effects include:*
Burning and tingling (pins and needles), chest pain, confusion, congestive heart failure, depression, diarrhea, difficult or labored breathing, dizziness, fainting, hair loss, headache, heart palpitations, hives, impotence, low blood pressure, nasal congestion, nausea, rash, skin peeling, slow or irregular heartbeat, stroke, temporary heart stoppage, vision problems, weakness, wheezing

Why should this drug not be prescribed?
Do not use Betagan if you have ever had an allergic reaction to it or are sensitive to it.

You should not use Betagan if you have any of the following conditions:

Asthma
Cardiogenic shock (shock due to insufficient heart action)
Certain heart irregularities
Heart failure
Severe chronic obstructive lung disease
Slow heartbeat (sinus bradycardia)

Special warnings about this medication

Betagan contains a sulfite preservative. In a few people, sulfites can cause an allergic reaction, which may be life-threatening. If you suffer from asthma, you are at increased risk for sulfite allergy.

Betagan may be absorbed into your bloodstream. If too much of the drug is absorbed, this may worsen asthma or other lung diseases or lead to heart failure, which sometimes happens with oral beta-blocker medications.

Beta blockers may increase the risks of anesthesia. If you are facing elective surgery, your doctor may want you to taper off Betagan prior to your operation.

Use Betagan cautiously if you have diminished lung function.

Since beta blockers may mask some signs and symptoms of low blood sugar (hypoglycemia), you should use Betagan very carefully if you have low blood sugar, or if you have diabetes and are taking insulin or an oral antidiabetic medication.

If your body tends to produce too much thyroid hormone, you should taper off Betagan very gradually rather than stopping the drug all at once. Abrupt withdrawal of any beta blocker may provoke a rush of thyroid hormone ("thyroid storm").

Do not use 2 or more beta-blocker eye medications at the same time.

Possible food and drug interactions
when taking this medication

If Betagan is used with certain other drugs, the effects of either could be increased, decreased, or altered. It is especially important to check with your doctor before combining Betagan with the following:

Calcium-blocking blood pressure medications such as Calan and
  Cardizem
Digitalis (the heart medication Lanoxin)
Epinephrine (Epifrin)

Oral beta blockers such as the blood pressure medications Inderal and
  Tenormin
Reserpine (Serpasil)

Special information
if you are pregnant or breastfeeding

The use of Betagan in pregnancy has not been adequately studied. If you are
pregnant or plan to become pregnant, notify your doctor immediately.
Betagan eyedrops should be used during pregnancy only if the benefit
justifies the potential risk to the unborn child. Since other beta-blocker
medications are known to appear in breast milk, use Betagan eyedrops with
caution if you are breastfeeding.

Recommended dosage

ADULTS

The recommended starting dose is 1 or 2 drops of Betagan 0.5% in the
affected eye(s) once a day.

The typical dose of Betagan 0.25% is 1 or 2 drops twice daily.

For more severe glaucoma, your doctor may have you use Betagan 0.5%
twice a day.

Overdosage

Overuse of Betagan eyedrops may produce symptoms of beta-blocker
overdosage—slowed heartbeat, low blood pressure, breathing difficulty,
and/or heart failure. Any medication taken in excess can have serious
consequences. If you suspect an overdose of Betagan, seek medical attention
immediately.

Generic name:

BETAINE ANHYDROUS

See Cystadane, page 322.

Generic name:

BETAMETHASONE

See Diprolene, page 416.

Generic name:

BETAXOLOL

See Betoptic, page 162.

Brand name:

BETIMOL

See Timoptic, page 1308.

Brand name:

BETOPTIC

Pronounced: bet-OP-tick
Generic name: Betaxolol hydrochloride

Why is this drug prescribed?
Betoptic Ophthalmic Solution and Betoptic S Ophthalmic Suspension contain a medication that lowers internal eye pressure and is used to treat open-angle glaucoma (high pressure of the fluid in the eye).

Most important fact about this drug
Although Betoptic, a type of drug called a beta blocker, is applied directly to the eye, it may be absorbed into the bloodstream. Because it may have effects in other parts of the body, you should use Betoptic cautiously if you have diabetes, asthma or other respiratory diseases, or decreased heart function.

How should you use this medication?
Use this medication exactly as prescribed. You may need to use other medications at the same time.

Betoptic S Suspension should be shaken well before each dose.

Administer Betoptic as follows:
1. Wash your hands thoroughly.
2. Gently pull your lower eyelid down to form a pocket between your eye and eyelid.
3. Hold the bottle on the bridge of your nose or on your forehead.

4. Do not touch the applicator tip to any surface, including your eye.
5. Tilt your head back and squeeze the medication into your eye.
6. Close your eyes gently.
7. Keep your eyes closed for 1 to 2 minutes.
8. Wait for 5 to 10 minutes before using any other eyedrops.
9. Do not rinse the dropper.

■ *If you miss a dose...*
Use it as soon as you remember. If it is almost time for your next dose, skip the one you missed and go back to your regular schedule. Do not use 2 doses at once.

■ *Storage instructions...*
Store at room temperature.

What side effects may occur?
Side effects cannot be anticipated. If any develop or change in intensity, inform your doctor as soon as possible. Only your doctor can determine if it is safe for you to continue using Betoptic.

■ *More common side effects may include:*
Temporary eye discomfort

■ *Less common or rare side effects may include:*
Allergic reactions, asthma, changes in taste or smell, congestive heart failure, decreased corneal sensitivity, dead skin, depression, difficulty breathing, difficulty sleeping or drowsiness, dizziness, hair loss, headache, hives, inflammation of the cornea, inflammation of the tongue, intolerance to light, itching, peeling skin, pupils of different sizes, red eyes and skin, slow heartbeat, sluggishness, tearing, thickening chest secretions, vertigo, wheezing

Why should this drug not be prescribed?
Do not use Betoptic if you are sensitive to or have ever had an allergic reaction to it.

People with certain heart conditions should not use Betoptic.

Special warnings about this medication

Before you use Betoptic, tell your doctor if you have any of the following:

Asthma
Diabetes
Heart disease
Thyroid disease

If you are having surgery, your doctor may advise you to gradually stop using Betoptic before you undergo general anesthesia.

This drug may lose some of its effectiveness for glaucoma after you have been taking it a long time.

Possible food and drug interactions
when using this medication

If Betoptic is used with certain other drugs, the effects of either could be increased, decreased, or altered. It is especially important to check with your doctor before combining Betoptic with the following:

Drugs that alter mood, such as Nardil and Elavil
Oral beta blockers such as Inderal and Tenormin
Reserpine (Serpasil)

Special information
if you are pregnant or breastfeeding

The effects of Betoptic during pregnancy have not been adequately studied. If you are pregnant or plan to become pregnant, inform your doctor immediately. Betoptic may appear in breast milk and could affect a nursing infant. If this medication is essential to your health, your doctor may advise you to stop breastfeeding until your treatment with Betoptic is finished.

Recommended dosage

Your doctor may have you take another medication with Betoptic or Betoptic S.

ADULTS

Betoptic
The usual recommended dose is 1 to 2 drops of Betoptic in the affected eye(s) twice daily.

Betoptic S
The usual recommended dose is 1 to 2 drops of Betoptic S in the affected eye(s) twice daily.

Overdosage
Any medication used in excess can have serious consequences. If you
suspect an overdose of Betoptic, seek medical attention immediately.

*With an oral beta blocker, symptoms of overdose might
include:*
Heart failure, low blood pressure, slow heartbeat

Brand name:

BIAXIN

Pronounced: buy-AX-in
Generic name: Clarithromycin

Why is this drug prescribed?
Biaxin, an antibiotic chemically related to erythromycin, is used to treat
certain bacterial infections of the respiratory tract, including:

Strep throat
Pneumonia
Sinusitis (inflamed sinuses)
Tonsillitis (inflamed tonsils)
Acute middle ear infections
Acute flare-ups of chronic bronchitis (inflamed airways)

Biaxin is also prescribed to treat infections of the skin. Combined with
Prilosec or Tritec (or Prevacid and amoxicillin), it is used to cure ulcers near
the exit from the stomach (duodenal ulcers) caused by *H. pylori* bacteria. It
can also be prescribed to combat *Mycobacterium avium* infections in people
with AIDS.

Biaxin is available as a tablet and as a suspension.

Most important fact about this drug
Biaxin, like any other antibiotic, works best when there is a constant amount
of drug in the blood. To keep the amount constant, try not to miss any doses.

How should you take this medication?
You may take Biaxin with or without food. Take it exactly as prescribed;
continue taking it for the full course of treatment.

Shake the suspension before each dose and use it within 14 days.

■ *If you miss a dose...*
Take it as soon as you remember. If it is almost time for your next dose, take the one you missed and take the next one 5 to 6 hours later. Then go back to your regular schedule.

■ *Storage instructions...*
Store at room temperature in a tightly closed container, away from light. Do not refrigerate the suspension.

What side effects may occur?
Side effects cannot be anticipated. If any side effects develop or change in intensity, tell your doctor immediately. Only your doctor can determine whether it is safe for you to continue taking Biaxin.

■ *Side effects may include:*
Abdominal pain/discomfort, altered sense of taste, diarrhea, headache, indigestion, nausea

Why should this drug not be prescribed?
Do not take Biaxin if you have ever had an allergic reaction to it, or if you are sensitive to it or erythromycin, or similar antibiotics such as Tao and Zithromax. Also avoid Biaxin if you have a heart condition or an imbalance in the body's water and minerals; and do not take the drug while taking Orap, Propulsid, or Seldane.

Special warnings about this medication
If you have severe kidney disease, the doctor may need to prescribe a smaller dose of Biaxin. Make sure the doctor is aware of any kidney problems you may have.

Like other antibiotics, Biaxin may cause a potentially life-threatening form of diarrhea that signals a condition called pseudomembranous colitis (inflammation of the large intestine). Mild diarrhea, a fairly common Biaxin side effect, may disappear as your body gets used to the drug. However, if Biaxin gives you prolonged or severe diarrhea, stop taking the drug and call your doctor immediately.

Possible food and drug interactions
when taking this medication
If Biaxin is taken with certain other drugs, the effects of either can be increased, decreased, or altered. It is especially important to check with your doctor before combining Biaxin with the following:

Astemizole (Hismanal)
Bromocriptine (Parlodel)
Carbamazepine (Tegretol)
Cisapride (Propulsid)
Cyclosporine (Sandimmune, Neoral)
Disopyramide (Norpace)
Fluconazole (Diflucan)
Hexobarbital
Lovastatin (Mevacor)
Phenytoin (Dilantin)
Pimozide (Orap)
Tacrolimus (Prograf)
Terfenadine (Seldane)
Theophylline (Slo-Phyllin, Theo-Dur, others)
Valproate (Depakene, Depakote)
Zidovudine (Retrovir)

Biaxin is chemically related to erythromycin. It is possible that other drugs reported to interact with erythromycin could also interact with Biaxin. They include:

Blood thinners such as Coumadin
Digoxin (Lanoxin)
Ergotamine (Cafergot)
Triazolam (Halcion)

Special information
if you are pregnant or breastfeeding

If you are pregnant or plan to become pregnant, notify your doctor immediately. Since Biaxin may have the potential to produce birth defects, it is prescribed during pregnancy only when there is no alternative. Caution is advised when using Biaxin while breastfeeding. Biaxin may appear in breast milk, as does its chemical cousin, erythromycin.

Recommended dosage

ADULTS

Ear, Nose, and Throat Infections
Your doctor will carefully tailor your individual dosage of Biaxin depending upon the type of infection and organism causing it.

The usual dose varies from 250 to 500 milligrams every 12 hours for 7 to 14 days.

Duodenal Ulcers
You can expect one of three treatment regimens:

500 milligrams of Biaxin 3 times a day for 14 days combined with 40 milligrams of Prilosec taken each morning for the first 14 days, and followed by 20 milligrams of Prilosec each morning for an additional 14 days.

500 milligrams of Biaxin 3 times a day for 14 days combined with 400 milligrams of Tritec taken twice daily for 28 days.

500 milligrams of Biaxin, 30 milligrams of Prevacid, and 1 gram of amoxicillin all taken every 12 hours for 14 days.

Mycobacterium Avium Infections
For prevention or treatment, the recommended dose is 500 milligrams twice a day.

CHILDREN

Biaxin is not recommended for children under 6 months of age.

The dose for children older than 6 months depends on how much the child weighs. Biaxin is usually given twice a day for 10 days.

Overdosage
Although no specific information is available, any medication taken in excess can have serious consequences. If you suspect an overdose of Biaxin, seek medical attention immediately.

Generic name:

BISMUTH SUBSALICYLATE, METRONIDAZOLE, AND TETRACYCLINE

See Helidac Therapy, page 587.

Brand name:

BLEPH-10

See Sodium Sulamyd, page 1206.

Brand name:

BONINE

See Antivert, page 79.

Brand name:

BRETHAIRE

See Brethine, page 169.

Brand name:

BRETHINE

Pronounced: Breath-EEN
Generic name: Terbutaline sulfate
Other brand names: Bricanyl, Brethaire

Why is this drug prescribed?
Brethine is a bronchodilator (a medication that opens the bronchial tubes), prescribed for the prevention and relief of bronchial spasms in asthma. This medication is also used for the relief of bronchial spasm associated with bronchitis and emphysema.

Most important fact about this drug
If you experience an immediate allergic reaction and a worsening of a bronchial spasm, notify your doctor immediately.

How should you take this medication?
Take this drug exactly as prescribed by your doctor.

The action of Brethine may last up to 8 hours. Do not use it more frequently than recommended.

- *If you miss a dose...*
  Take it as soon as you remember. Then take the rest of your medication for that day in evenly spaced doses. Do not take 2 doses at once.

- *Storage instructions...*
  Store at room temperature in a tightly closed container, away from light.

What side effects may occur?
Side effects cannot be anticipated. If any develop or change in intensity, inform your doctor as soon as possible. Only your doctor can determine if it is safe for you to continue taking Brethine.

- *More common side effects may include:*
  Chest discomfort, difficulty in breathing, dizziness, drowsiness, fast, fluttery heartbeat, flushed feeling, headache, increased heart rate, nausea,

nervousness, pain at injection site, rapid heartbeat, sweating, tremors, vomiting, weakness

■ *Less common side effects may include:*
Anxiety, dry mouth, muscle cramps

■ *Rare side effects may include:*
Inflamed blood vessels

Why should this drug not be prescribed?
If you are sensitive to or have ever had an allergic reaction to Brethine or similar drugs such as Ventolin, you should not take this medication. Make sure your doctor is aware of any drug reactions you have experienced.

Special warnings about this medication
When taking Brethine, you should not use other asthma medications before checking with your doctor. Only your doctor can determine what is a sufficient amount of time between doses.

Consult with your doctor before using this medication if you have diabetes, high blood pressure, or an overactive thyroid gland, or if you have had seizures at any time.

Unless you are directed to do so by your doctor, do not take this medication if you have heart disease, especially if you also have an irregular heart rate.

Possible food and drug interactions
when taking this medication
If Brethine is taken with certain other drugs, the effects of either could be increased, decreased, or altered. It is especially important to check with your doctor before combining Brethine with the following:

Antidepressant drugs known as MAO inhibitors (Nardil, Parnate, others)
Beta blockers (blood pressure medications such as Inderal and
Tenormin)
Other bronchodilators such as Proventil and Ventolin
Tricyclic antidepressant drugs such as Elavil and Tofranil

Special information
if you are pregnant or breastfeeding
The effects of Brethine during pregnancy have not been adequately studied. If you are pregnant or plan to become pregnant, inform your doctor immediately. It is not known whether Brethine appears in breast milk. If this drug is essential to your health, your doctor may advise you to stop nursing your baby until your treatment is finished.

Recommended dosage

FOR BRETHINE

Adults

The usual tablet dose is 5 milligrams taken at approximately 6-hour intervals, 3 times per day during waking hours. If side effects are excessive, your doctor may reduce your dose to 2.5 milligrams, 3 times per day.

Do not take more than 15 milligrams in a 24-hour period.

Children

This medication is not recommended for use in children below 12 years of age.

For children 12 to 15 years of age, the usual dose is 2.5 milligrams, 3 times per day, not to exceed a total of 7.5 milligrams in a 24-hour period.

FOR BRETHAIRE

The usual dosage for adults and children 12 years and older is 2 inhalations separated by a 60-second interval, repeated every 4 to 6 hours.

Overdosage

Any drug taken or used in excess can have serious consequences. Signs of a Brethine overdose are the same as the side effects. If you suspect an overdose, seek medical attention immediately.

Brand name:

BREVICON

See Oral Contraceptives, page 926.

Brand name:

BRICANYL

See Brethine, page 169.

Generic name:

BROMOCRIPTINE

See Parlodel, page 952.

Generic name:

BROMPHENIRAMINE, PHENYLPROPANOLAMINE, AND CODEINE

See Dimetane-DC, page 408.

Brand name:

BRONTEX

See Tussi-Organidin NR, page 1359.

Generic name:

BUDESONIDE

See Rhinocort, page 1129.

Generic name:

BUMETANIDE

See Bumex, page 172.

Brand name:

BUMEX

Pronounced: BYOO-meks
Generic name: Bumetanide

Why is this drug prescribed?
Bumex is used to lower the amount of excess salt and water in your body by increasing the output of urine. It is prescribed in the treatment of edema, or fluid retention, associated with congestive heart failure and liver or kidney disease. It is also occasionally prescribed, along with other drugs, to treat high blood pressure.

Most important fact about this drug
Bumex is a powerful drug. If taken in excessive amounts, it can severely decrease the levels of water and minerals, especially potassium, your body needs to function. Therefore, your doctor should monitor your dose carefully.

How should you take this medication?
Bumex can increase the frequency of urination and may cause loss of sleep if taken at night. Therefore, if you are taking a single dose of Bumex daily, it should be taken in the morning after breakfast. If you take more than one dose a day, take the last dose no later than 6:00 P.M.

■ *If you miss a dose...*
Take the forgotten dose as soon as you remember. If it is almost time for your next dose, skip the one you missed and go back to your regular schedule. Never take 2 doses at the same time.

■ *Storage instructions...*
Store at room temperature.

What side effects may occur?
Side effects cannot be anticipated. If any develop or change in intensity, inform your doctor as soon as possible. Only your doctor can determine if it is safe for you to continue taking Bumex.

■ *More common side effects may include:*
Dizziness, headache, low blood pressure, muscle cramps, nausea

■ *Signs of too much potassium loss are:*
Dry mouth, irregular heartbeat, muscle cramps or pains, unusual tiredness or weakness

■ *Less common or rare side effects may include:*
Abdominal pain, black stools, chest pain, dehydration, diarrhea, dry mouth, ear discomfort, fatigue, hearing loss, itching, joint pain, kidney failure, muscle and bone pain, nipple tenderness, premature ejaculation and difficulty maintaining erection, rapid breathing, skin rash or hives, sweating, upset stomach, vertigo, vomiting, weakness

Why should this drug not be prescribed?
Bumex should not be used if you are unable to urinate or if you are dehydrated.

If you are sensitive to or have ever had an allergic reaction to Bumex or similar drugs such as Lasix, you should not take this medication. Make sure your doctor is aware of any drug reactions you have experienced.

Special warnings about this medication
If you are allergic to sulfur-containing drugs such as sulfonamides (antibacterial drugs), check with your doctor before taking Bumex.

Bumex can decrease the number of platelets in your blood. Your doctor should monitor your blood status regularly.

Bumex can cause a loss of potassium from the body. Your doctor may recommend foods or fluids high in potassium or may want you to take a potassium supplement to help prevent this. Follow your doctor's recommendation carefully.

While taking this medication you may feel dizzy or light-headed or actually faint when getting up from a lying or sitting position. If getting up slowly does not help or if this problem continues, notify your doctor.

Possible food and drug interactions
when taking this medication

If Bumex is taken with certain other drugs, the effects of either could be increased, decreased, or altered. It is especially important to check with your doctor before combining Bumex with the following:

Blood pressure medications such as Vasotec and Tenormin
Indomethacin (Indocin) and other nonsteroidal anti-inflammatory drugs
Probenecid (Benemid)

The combination of Bumex and certain antibiotics or cisplatin (Platinol) may increase the risk of hearing loss.

Because Bumex can lower potassium levels, the combination of Bumex and digitalis or digoxin (Lanoxin) may increase the risk of changes in heartbeat.

The combination of Bumex and lithium (Lithonate) may increase the levels of lithium in the body, causing it to become poisonous.

Special information
if you are pregnant or breastfeeding

The effects of Bumex during pregnancy have not been adequately studied. If you are pregnant or plan to become pregnant, inform your doctor immediately. It is not known if this medication appears in breast milk. Your doctor may advise you to discontinue breastfeeding your baby until your treatment with Bumex is finished.

Recommended dosage

ADULTS

The usual total daily dose is 0.5 to 2.0 milligrams a day. For most people, this is taken as a single dose. However, if the initial dose is not adequate, your doctor may have you take a second and, possibly, a third dose at 4- to 5-hour intervals, up to a maximum daily dose of 10 milligrams.

For the continuing control of edema, your doctor may tell you to take Bumex on alternate days or for 3 to 4 days at a time with rest periods of 1 to 2 days in between.

If you have liver failure, your dose will be kept to a minimum and increased very carefully.

CHILDREN

The safety and effectiveness of Bumex have not been established in children below the age of 18.

Overdosage

An overdose of Bumex can lead to severe dehydration, reduction of blood volume, and severe problems with the circulatory system.

■ The signs of an overdose include:
Cramps, dizziness, lethargy (sluggishness), loss or lack of appetite, mental confusion, vomiting, weakness

If you suspect an overdose, get medical attention immediately.

Generic name:

BUPROPION FOR DEPRESSION

See Wellbutrin, page 1427.

Generic name:

BUPROPION FOR SMOKING

See Zyban, page 1481.

Brand name:

BUSPAR

Pronounced: BYOO-spar
Generic name: Buspirone hydrochloride

Why is this drug prescribed?

BuSpar is used in the treatment of anxiety disorders and for short-term relief of the symptoms of anxiety.

Most important fact about this drug
BuSpar should not be used with antidepressant drugs known as monoamine oxidase (MAO) inhibitors. Brands include Nardil and Parnate.

How should you take this medication?
Take BuSpar exactly as prescribed. Do not be discouraged if you feel no immediate effect. The full benefit of this drug may not be seen for 1 to 2 weeks after you start to take it.

■ *If you miss a dose...*
Take the forgotten dose as soon as you remember. If it is almost time for your next dose, skip the one you missed and go back to your regular schedule. Never take 2 doses at the same time.

■ *Storage instructions...*
Store at room temperature in a tightly closed container, away from light.

What side effects may occur?
Side effects cannot be anticipated. If any develop or change in intensity, inform your doctor as soon as possible. Only your doctor can determine if it is safe for you to continue taking BuSpar.

■ *More common side effects may include:*
Dizziness, dry mouth, fatigue, headache, light-headedness, nausea, nervousness, unusual excitement

■ *Less common or rare side effects may include:*
Anger/hostility, blurred vision, bone aches/pain, confusion, constipation, decreased concentration, depression, diarrhea, fast, fluttery heartbeat, incoordination, muscle pain/aches, numbness, pain or weakness in hands or feet, rapid heartbeat, rash, restlessness, stomach and abdominal upset, sweating/clamminess, tingling or pins and needles, tremor, urinary incontinence, vomiting, weakness

Why should this drug not be prescribed?
If you are sensitive to or have ever had an allergic reaction to BuSpar or similar mood-altering drugs, you should not take this medication. Make sure your doctor is aware of any drug reactions you have experienced.

Anxiety or tension related to everyday stress usually does not require treatment with BuSpar. Discuss your symptoms thoroughly with your doctor.

The use of BuSpar is not recommended if you have severe kidney or liver damage.

Special warnings about this medication

The effects of BuSpar on the central nervous system (brain and spinal cord) are unpredictable. Therefore, you should not drive or operate dangerous machinery or participate in any hazardous activity that requires full mental alertness while you are taking BuSpar.

Possible food and drug interactions
when taking this medication

Although BuSpar does not intensify the effects of alcohol, it is best to avoid alcohol while taking this medication.

If BuSpar is taken with certain other drugs, the effects of either can be increased, decreased, or altered. It is especially important to check with your doctor before combining BuSpar with the following:

The blood-thinning drug Coumadin
Haloperidol (Haldol)
MAO inhibitors (antidepressant drugs such as Nardil and Parnate)
Trazodone (Desyrel)

Special information
if you are pregnant or breastfeeding

The effects of BuSpar during pregnancy have not been adequately studied. If you are pregnant or plan to become pregnant, inform your doctor immediately. It is not known whether BuSpar appears in breast milk. If this medication is essential to your health, your doctor may advise you to discontinue breastfeeding until your treatment is finished.

Recommended dosage

ADULTS

The recommended starting dose is a total of 15 milligrams per day divided into smaller doses, usually 5 milligrams 3 times a day. Every 2 to 3 days, your doctor may increase the dosage 5 milligrams per day as needed. The daily dose should not exceed 60 milligrams.

CHILDREN

The safety and effectiveness of BuSpar have not been established in children under 18 years of age.

Overdosage

Any medication taken in excess can have serious consequences. If you suspect an overdose of BuSpar, seek medical attention immediately.

■ *The symptoms of BuSpar overdose may include:*
Dizziness, drowsiness, nausea or vomiting, severe stomach upset, unusually small pupils

Generic name:

BUSPIRONE

See BuSpar, page 175.

Generic name:

BUTALBITAL, ACETAMINOPHEN, AND CAFFEINE

See Fioricet, page 518.

Generic name:

BUTALBITAL, ASPIRIN, AND CAFFEINE

See Fiorinal, page 521.

Generic name:

BUTALBITAL, CODEINE, ASPIRIN, AND CAFFEINE

See Fiorinal with Codeine, page 524.

Generic name:

BUTOCONAZOLE

See Femstat, page 515.

Brand name:

CAFERGOT

Pronounced: KAF-er-got
Generic ingredients: Ergotamine tartrate, Caffeine

Why is this drug prescribed?
Cafergot is prescribed for the relief or prevention of vascular headaches—for example, migraine, migraine variants, or cluster headaches.

Most important fact about this drug
The excessive use of Cafergot can lead to ergot poisoning resulting in symptoms such as headache, pain in the legs when walking, muscle pain, numbness, coldness, and abnormal paleness of the fingers and toes. If this condition is not treated, it can lead to gangrene (tissue death due to decreased blood supply).

How should you take this medication?
Cafergot is available in both tablet and suppository form. Be sure to take it exactly as prescribed, remaining within the limits of your recommended dosage.

Cafergot works best if you use it at the first sign of a migraine attack. If you get warning signals of a coming migraine, take the drug before the headache actually starts.

Lie down and relax in a quiet, dark room for at least a couple of hours or until you feel better.

Avoid exposure to cold.

To use the suppositories, follow these steps:
1. If the suppository feels too soft, leave it in the refrigerator for about 30 minutes or put it, still wrapped, in ice water until it hardens.
2. Remove the foil wrapper and dip the tip of the suppository in water.
3. Lie down on your side and with a finger insert the suppository into the rectum. Hold it in place for a few moments.

■ *If you miss a dose...*
   Take this medication only when threatened with an attack.

■ *Storage instructions...*
   Store at room temperature in a tightly closed container away from light. Keep suppositories away from heat.

What side effects may occur?
Side effects cannot be anticipated. If any develop or change in intensity, inform your doctor as soon as possible. Only your doctor can determine if it is safe for you to continue taking Cafergot.

■ *Side effects may include:*
   Fluid retention, high blood pressure, itching, nausea, numbness, rapid heart rate, slow heartbeat, tingling or pins and needles, vertigo, vomiting, weakness

- *Complications caused by constriction of the blood vessels can be serious. They include:*
  Bluish tinge to the skin, chest pain, cold arms and legs, gangrene, muscle pains

Although these symptoms occur most commonly with long-term therapy at relatively high doses, they have been reported with short-term or normal doses. A few people on long-term therapy have developed heart valve problems.

Why should this drug not be prescribed?

If you are sensitive to or have ever had an allergic reaction to ergotamine tartrate, caffeine, or similar drugs, you should not take this medication. Make sure your doctor is aware of any drug reactions you have experienced.

Unless directed to do so by your doctor, do not take this medication if you have coronary heart disease, circulatory problems, high blood pressure, impaired liver or kidney function, or an infection, or if you are pregnant.

Special warnings about this medication

It is extremely important that you do not exceed your recommended dosage, especially when Cafergot is used over long periods. There have been reports of psychological dependence in people who have abused this drug over long periods of time. Discontinuance of the drug may produce withdrawal symptoms such as sudden, severe headaches.

If you experience excessive nausea and vomiting during attacks, making it impossible for you to retain oral medication, your doctor will probably tell you to use rectal suppositories.

This drug is effective only for migraine and migraine-type headaches. Do not use it for any other kind of headache.

Possible food and drug interactions
when taking this medication

If Cafergot is taken with certain other drugs, the effects of either could be increased, decreased, or altered. It is especially important to check with your doctor before combining Cafergot with the following:

Beta-blocker drugs (blood pressure medications such as Inderal and Tenormin)
Drugs that constrict the blood vessels, such as EpiPen and the oral decongestant Sudafed
Macrolide antibiotics such as PCE, E.E.S., and Biaxin
Nicotine (Nicoderm, Habitrol, others)

**Special information
if you are pregnant or breastfeeding**
Do not take Cafergot if you are pregnant. Cafergot appears in breast milk and may have serious effects in your baby. If this medication is essential for your health, your doctor may advise you to discontinue breastfeeding.

Recommended dosage
Dosage should start at the first sign of an attack.

ADULTS

Orally
The total dose for any single attack should not exceed 6 tablets.

Rectally
The maximum dose for an individual attack is 2 suppositories.

The total weekly dosage should not exceed 10 tablets or 5 suppositories.

A preventive, short-term dose may be given at bedtime to certain people, but only as prescribed by a doctor.

Overdosage
If you suspect an overdose of Cafergot, seek emergency medical treatment immediately.

■ *Symptoms of Cafergot overdose include:*
   Coma, convulsions, diminished or absent pulses, drowsiness, high or low blood pressure, numbness, shock, stupor, tingling, pain and bluish discoloration of the limbs, unresponsiveness, vomiting

Brand name:

CALAN

Pronounced: CAL-an
Generic name: Verapamil hydrochloride
*Other brand names: Calan SR, Covera-HS, Isoptin, Isoptin
   SR, Verelan*

Why is this drug prescribed?
Verapamil, the active ingredient in Calan, Covera-HS, Isoptin, and Verelan, is prescribed for the treatment of various types of angina (chest pain, caused

by clogged arteries that reduce the heart muscle's oxygen supply). It is also used for irregular heartbeat and for high blood pressure.

The sustained release formulas (SR and Verelan) are used only for the treatment of high blood pressure; the extended-release tablets (Covera-HS) are used for high blood pressure and angina and are designed to release the drug 4 to 5 hours after they are taken.

Verapamil is a type of medication called a calcium channel blocker. It eases the heart's workload by slowing down the passage of nerve impulses through it, and hence the contractions of the heart muscle. This improves blood flow through the heart and throughout the body, reduces blood pressure, corrects irregular heartbeat, and helps prevent angina pain.

Some doctors also prescribe verapamil to prevent migraine headache and asthma and to treat manic depression and panic attacks.

Most important fact about this drug
If you have high blood pressure, you must take verapamil regularly for it to be effective. Since blood pressure declines gradually, it may be several weeks before you get the full benefit of verapamil; and you must continue taking it even if you are feeling well. Verapamil does not cure high blood pressure; it merely keeps it under control.

How should you take this medication?
Calan, Isoptin, and Verelan can be taken with or without food. Calan SR and Isoptin SR should be taken with food.

Covera-HS, Calan SR, Isoptin SR, and Verelan must be swallowed whole and should not be crushed, broken, or chewed.

You may open Verelan capsules and sprinkle the pellets on a spoonful of cool applesauce. Swallow all of the mixture immediately, and then drink a glass of cool water.

Take this medication exactly as prescribed, even if you are feeling well. Try not to miss any doses. If the drug is not taken regularly, your condition can get worse.

Check with your doctor before you stop taking this drug; a slow reduction in the dose may be required.

■ *If you miss a dose...*
  Take it as soon as you remember. If it is almost time for your next dose, skip the one you missed and go back to your regular schedule. Never take 2 doses at the same time.

■ *Storage instructions...*
Store at room temperature away from heat, light, and moisture.

What side effects may occur?
Side effects cannot be anticipated. If any develop or change in intensity, inform your doctor as soon as possible. Only your doctor can determine if it is safe for you to continue taking verapamil.

■ *More common side effects may include:*
Congestive heart failure, constipation, dizziness, fatigue, fluid retention, headache, low blood pressure, nausea, rash, shortness of breath, slow heartbeat, upper respiratory infection

■ *Less common or rare side effects may include:*
Angina, blurred vision, breast development in males, bruising, chest pain, confusion, diarrhea, difficulty sleeping, drowsiness, dry mouth, excessive milk secretion, fainting, fatigue, fever and rash, flushing, hair loss, heart attack, hives, impotence, increased urination, indigestion, intestinal blockage, joint pain, lightheadedness upon standing up, limping, loss of balance, muscle cramps, pounding heartbeat, rash, ringing in the ears, shakiness, skin peeling, sleepiness, spotty menstruation, sweating, tingling or pins and needles, upset stomach

Why should this drug not be prescribed?
If you have low blood pressure or certain types of heart disease or heartbeat irregularities, you should not take verapamil. Make sure the doctor is aware of any cardiac problems you may have.

If you are sensitive to or have ever had an allergic reaction to Calan or any other brands of verapamil, or other calcium channel blockers, do not take this medication.

Special warnings about this medication
Verapamil can reduce or eliminate angina pain caused by exertion or exercise. Be sure to discuss with your doctor how much exertion is safe for you.

Verapamil may cause your blood pressure to become too low. If you experience dizziness or light-headedness, notify your doctor.

Congestive heart failure and fluid in the lungs have occurred in people taking verapamil together with other heart drugs known as beta blockers. Make sure your doctor is aware of all medications you are taking.

If you have a heart condition, liver disease, kidney disease, or Duchenne's dystrophy (the most common type of muscular dystrophy), make certain your doctor knows about it. Verapamil should be used with caution.

If you are taking Covera-HS and you have a narrowing in your stomach or intestines, be sure your doctor was aware of it when the drug was prescribed.

The outer shell of Covera-HS does not dissolve; do not worry if you see it in your stool.

Possible food and drug interactions when taking this medication

If verapamil is taken with certain other drugs, the effects of either could be increased, decreased, or altered. It is especially important to check with your doctor before combining verapamil with the following:

ACE inhibitor-type blood pressure drugs such as Capoten and Vasotec
Beta-blocker-type blood pressure drugs such as Lopressor, Tenormin, and Inderal
Vasodilator-type blood pressure drugs such as Loniten
Other high blood pressure drugs such as Minipress
Alcohol
Amiodarone (Cordarone)
Carbamazepine (Tegretol)
Chloroquine (Aralen)
Cimetidine (Tagamet)
Cyclosporine (Sandimmune, Neoral)
Dantrolene (Dantrium)
Digitalis (Lanoxin)
Disopyramide (Norpace)
Diuretics such as Lasix and HydroDIURIL
Flecainide (Tambocor)
Glipizide (Glucotrol)
Imipramine (Tofranil)
Lithium (Lithonate)
Nitrates such as Transderm Nitro and Isordil
Phenobarbital
Phenytoin (Dilantin)
Quinidine (Quinidex)
Rifampin (Rifadin)
Theophylline (Theo-Dur)

Special information
if you are pregnant or breastfeeding

The effects of verapamil during pregnancy have not been adequately studied. If you are pregnant or plan to become pregnant, inform your doctor immediately. The drug appears in breast milk and could affect a nursing infant. If this medication is essential to your health, your doctor may advise you to discontinue breastfeeding until your treatment is finished.

Recommended dosage

FOR CALAN AND ISOPTIN

Dosages of this medication must be adjusted to meet individual needs. In general, dosages of this medication should not exceed 480 milligrams per day. Your doctor will closely monitor your response to this drug, usually within 8 hours of the first dose.

Safety and effectiveness of this drug in children have not been established.

Angina

The usual initial dose is 80 to 120 milligrams, 3 times a day. Lower doses of 40 milligrams 3 times a day may be used by people who have a stronger response to this medication, such as the elderly or those with decreased liver function. The dosage may be increased by your doctor either daily or weekly until the desired response is seen.

Irregular Heartbeat

The usual dose in people who are also on digitalis ranges from 240 to 320 milligrams per day divided into 3 or 4 doses.

In those not on digitalis, doses range from a total of 240 to 480 milligrams per day divided into 3 or 4 doses.

Maximum effects of this drug should be seen in the first 48 hours of use.

High Blood Pressure

Effects of this drug on blood pressure should be seen within the first week of use. Any adjustment of this medication to a higher dose will be based on its effectiveness as determined by your doctor.

The usual dose of this drug, when used alone for high blood pressure, is 80 milligrams, 3 times per day. Total daily doses of 360 milligrams and 480 milligrams may be used. Smaller doses of 40 milligrams 3 times per day may be taken by smaller individuals and the elderly.

FOR CALAN SR, ISOPTIN SR, AND VERELAN

Dosages for high blood pressure should be adjusted to meet each individual's needs.

Adults

The usual starting dose of Calan SR and Isoptin SR is 180 milligrams taken in the morning. For Verelan, it is 240 milligrams. A lower starting dose of 120 milligrams may be taken if the person is smaller. Your doctor will monitor your response to this drug and may adjust it each week. In addition, your doctor may increase the dose and add evening doses to the morning dose, based on the effectiveness of the drug.

You should see results from the drug within a week.

Children

The safety and effectiveness of this drug in children under age 18 have not been established.

Older Adults

Your doctor may start you at a lower dose of 120 milligrams and then adjust it according to your response.

FOR COVERA-HS

Adults

The usual starting dose is 180 milligrams, taken at bedtime, for both angina and high blood pressure. Your doctor may raise the dose gradually if you need more.

Children

Safety and effectiveness in children under age 18 have not been established.

Older Adults

If you have poor kidneys, the dosage may need to be lowered.

Overdosage

Any medication taken in excess can have serious consequences. If you suspect an overdose, seek medical attention immediately.

An overdose of Calan can cause dangerously low blood pressure and life-threatening heart problems. After treatment for an overdose, you should remain under observation in the hospital for at least 48 hours, especially if you have taken the sustained-release form of the drug.

Brand name:

CALCIMAR

See Miacalcin, page 788.

Generic name:

CALCITONIN-SALMON

See Miacalcin, page 788.

Generic name:

CALCITRIOL

See Rocaltrol, page 1148.

Brand name:

CAPOTEN

Pronounced: KAP-o-ten
Generic name: Captopril

Why is this drug prescribed?

Capoten is used in the treatment of high blood pressure and congestive heart failure. When prescribed for high blood pressure, it is effective used alone or combined with diuretics. If it is prescribed for congestive heart failure, it is used in combination with digitalis and diuretics. Capoten is in a family of drugs known as "ACE (angiotensin converting enzyme) inhibitors." It works by preventing a chemical in your blood called angiotensin I from converting into a more potent form that increases salt and water retention in your body. Capoten also enhances blood flow throughout your blood vessels.

In addition, Capoten is used to improve survival in certain people who have suffered heart attacks and to treat kidney disease in diabetics.

Some doctors also prescribe Capoten for angina pectoris (crushing chest pain), Raynaud's phenomenon (a disorder of the blood vessels that causes the fingers to turn white when exposed to cold), and rheumatoid arthritis.

Most important fact about this drug

If you have high blood pressure, you must take Capoten regularly for it to be effective. Since blood pressure declines gradually, it may be several weeks before you get the full benefit of Capoten; you must continue taking it even if you are feeling well. Capoten does not cure high blood pressure; it merely keeps it under control.

How should you take this medication?
Capoten should be taken 1 hour before meals. If you are taking an antacid such as Mylanta, take it 2 hours prior to Capoten.

Take this medication exactly as prescribed. Stopping Capoten suddenly could cause your blood pressure to increase.

■ *If you miss a dose...*
Take it as soon as you remember. If it is almost time for your next dose, skip the one you missed and go back to your regular schedule. Never take 2 doses at the same time.

■ *Storage instructions...*
Store Capoten at room temperature, away from moisture, in a tightly closed container.

What side effects may occur?
Side effects cannot be anticipated. If any develop or change in intensity, inform your doctor as soon as possible. Only your doctor can determine if it is safe for you to continue taking Capoten.

■ *More common side effects may include:*
Itching, loss of taste, low blood pressure, rash

■ *Less common or rare side effects may include:*
Abdominal pain, anemia, angina pectoris (severe chest pain), blisters, blurred vision, breast development in males, cardiac arrest, changes in heart rhythm, chest pain, confusion, constipation, cough, depression, diarrhea, difficulty swallowing, dizziness, dry mouth, fatigue, fever and chills, flushing, general feeling of ill health, hair loss, headache, heart attack, heart failure, impotence, inability to sleep, indigestion, inflammation of the nose, inflammation of the tongue, labored breathing, lack of coordination, loss of appetite, lung inflammation, muscle pain and/or weakness, nausea, nervousness, pallor, palpitations, peptic ulcer, rapid heartbeat, sensitivity to light, skin inflammation, skin peeling, sleepiness, sore throat, stomach irritation, stroke, sudden fainting or loss of strength, swelling of face, lips, tongue, throat, or arms and legs, tingling or pins and needles, vomiting, weakness, wheezing, yellow eyes and skin

Why should this drug not be prescribed?

If you are sensitive to or have ever had an allergic reaction to Capoten or similar drugs such as Vasotec, you should not take this medication. Make sure that your doctor is aware of any drug reactions that you have experienced.

Special warnings about this medication

If you develop swelling of the face around your lips, tongue or throat (or of your arms and legs) or have difficulty swallowing, you should stop taking Capoten and contact your doctor immediately. You may need emergency treatment.

If you are receiving bee or wasp venom to prevent an allergic reaction to stings, use of Capoten at the same time may cause a severe allergic reaction.

If you are taking Capoten, a complete assessment of your kidney function should be done; and your kidney function should continue to be monitored. If you have kidney disease, Capoten should be used only if you have taken other blood pressure medications and your doctor has determined that the results were unsatisfactory.

Some people taking Capoten have had a severe allergic reaction during kidney dialysis.

If you are taking Capoten for your heart, be careful not to increase physical activity too quickly. Check with your doctor as to how much exercise is safe for you.

If you are taking Capoten for congestive heart failure, your blood pressure may drop temporarily after the first few doses and you may feel light-headed for a time. Your doctor should monitor you closely when you start taking the medication or when your dosage is increased.

If you are taking high doses of diuretics and Capoten, you may develop excessively low blood pressure. Your doctor may reduce your diuretic dose so that your blood pressure doesn't drop too far.

If you notice a yellow coloring to your skin or the whites of your eyes, stop taking the drug and notify your doctor immediately. You could be developing a liver problem.

Capoten may cause you to become drowsy or less alert, especially if you are also taking a diuretic at the same time. If it has this effect on you, driving or participating in any potentially hazardous activity is not recommended.

Dehydration may cause a drop in blood pressure. If you experience symptoms such as excessive perspiration, vomiting, and/or diarrhea, notify your doctor immediately.

If you develop a sore throat or fever you should contact your doctor immediately. It could indicate a more serious illness.

If you develop a persistent, dry cough, tell your doctor. It may be due to the medication and, if so, will disappear if you stop taking Capoten.

Possible food and drug interactions
when taking this medication

If Capoten is taken with certain other drugs, the effects of either could be increased, decreased, or altered. It is especially important to check with your doctor before combining Capoten with the following:

Allopurinol (Zyloprim)
Aspirin
Blood pressure drugs known as beta blockers, such as Inderal and Tenormin
Cyclosporine (Sandimmune)
Digoxin (Lanoxin)
Diuretics such as HydroDIURIL
Lithium (Lithonate)
Nitroglycerin and similar heart medicines (Nitro-Dur, Transderm-Nitro, others)
Nonsteroidal anti-inflammatory drugs such as Indocin and Feldene
Potassium preparations such as Micro-K and Slow-K
Potassium-sparing diuretics such as Aldactone and Midamor

Do not use potassium-containing salt substitutes while taking Capoten.

Special information
if you are pregnant or breastfeeding

ACE inhibitors such as Capoten have been shown to cause injury and even death to the developing baby when used in pregnancy during the second and third trimesters. If you are pregnant or plan to become pregnant, contact your doctor immediately. Capoten appears in breast milk and could affect a nursing infant. If this medication is essential to your health, your doctor may advise you to discontinue breastfeeding until your treatment is finished.

Recommended dosage

ADULTS

High Blood Pressure

The usual starting dose is 25 milligrams taken 2 or 3 times a day. If you have any problems with your kidneys or suffer from other major health problems, your starting dose may be lower. Depending on how your blood pressure responds, your doctor may increase your dose later, up to a total of 150 milligrams 2 or 3 times a day. The maximum recommended daily dose is 450 milligrams.

Heart Failure

For most people, the usual dose is 25 milligrams taken 3 times a day. A daily dosage of 450 milligrams should not be exceeded.

After a Heart Attack

The usual starting dose is 6.25 milligrams, taken once, followed by 12.5 milligrams 3 times a day. Your doctor will increase the dose over the next several days to 25 milligrams taken 3 times a day and then, over the next several weeks, to 50 milligrams 3 times a day.

Kidney Disease in Diabetes

The usual dose is 25 milligrams taken 3 times a day.

CHILDREN

The safety and effectiveness of Capoten in children have not been established.

Overdosage

Any medication taken in excess can cause symptoms of overdose. If you suspect an overdose of Capoten, seek medical attention immediately.

Light-headedness or dizziness due to a sudden drop in blood pressure is the primary effect of a Capoten overdose.

Brand name:

CAPOZIDE

Pronounced: KAP-oh-zide
Generic ingredients: Captopril, Hydrochlorothiazide

Why is this drug prescribed?

Capozide is used in the treatment of high blood pressure. It combines an ACE inhibitor with a thiazide diuretic. Captopril, the ACE inhibitor, works by preventing a chemical in your blood called angiotensin I from converting into a more potent form that increases salt and water retention in your body. Captopril also enhances blood flow throughout your blood vessels. Hydrochlorothiazide, the diuretic, helps your body produce and eliminate more urine, which helps in lowering blood pressure.

Most important fact about this drug
You must take Capozide regularly for it to be effective. Since blood pressure declines gradually, it may be several weeks before you get the full benefit of Capozide; and you must continue taking it even if you are feeling well. Capozide does not cure high blood pressure; it merely keeps it under control.

How should you take this medication?
Capozide should be taken 1 hour before meals. Take it exactly as prescribed. Stopping Capozide suddenly could cause your blood pressure to increase.

■ *If you miss a dose...*
Take it as soon as you remember. If it is almost time for your next dose, skip the one you missed and go back to your regular schedule. Never take 2 doses at the same time.

■ *Storage instructions...*
Capozide should be stored at room temperature in a tightly closed container away from moisture.

What side effects may occur?
Side effects cannot be anticipated. If any develop or change in intensity, inform your doctor as soon as possible. Only your doctor can determine if it is safe for you to continue taking Capozide.

■ *More common side effects may include:*
Itching, loss of taste, low blood pressure, rash

■ *Less common or rare side effects may include:*
Abdominal pain, anemia, angina pectoris (severe chest pain), angioedema (swelling of the arms and legs, face, lips, tongue, or throat), blurred vision, breast development in males, bronchitis, bronchospasm, changes in heart rhythm, chest pain, confusion, constipation, cough, cramping, depression, diarrhea, dizziness, dizziness upon standing up, dry mouth, fainting, fatigue, fever, flushing, general feeling of ill health, hair loss, headache, heart attack, heart failure, hepatitis, hives, inability to sleep, indigestion, impotence, inflammation of nose, inflammation of tongue, labored breathing, lack of coordination, loss of appetite, low potassium levels leading to symptoms such as dry mouth, excessive thirst, weak or irregular heartbeat, muscle pain or cramps, muscle weakness, muscle spasm, nausea, nervousness, pallor, peptic ulcer, rapid heartbeat, Raynaud's Syndrome (circulatory disorder), restlessness, sensitivity to light, severe allergic reactions, skin inflammation and/or peeling, sleepiness,

stomach irritation, stroke, tingling or pins and needles, vomiting, vertigo, weakness, wheezing, yellow eyes and skin

Why should this drug not be prescribed?

If you are sensitive to or have ever had an allergic reaction to captopril, hydrochlorothiazide, other ACE inhibitors such as Vasotec, or other thiazide diuretics such as Diuril, or if you are sensitive to other sulfonamide-derived drugs, you should not take this medication. If you have a history of angioedema (swelling of face, extremities, and throat) or inability to urinate, you should not take this medication.

Special warnings about this medication

If you develop swelling of your face around your lips, tongue, or throat, or in your arms and legs, or if you begin to have difficulty swallowing, you should contact your doctor immediately. You may need emergency treatment.

If you develop a sore throat or fever you should contact your doctor immediately. It could indicate a more serious illness.

If you are taking Capozide, your doctor will make a complete assessment of your kidney function and will continue to monitor it.

If you have impaired kidney function, Capozide should be used only if you have taken other blood pressure medications and your doctor has determined that the results were unsatisfactory.

If you have liver disease or a disease of the connective tissue called lupus erythematosus, Capozide should be used with caution. Tell your doctor immediately if you notice a yellowish color in your skin or the whites of your eyes.

If you have congestive heart failure, you should be carefully watched for low blood pressure. You should not increase your physical activity too quickly.

Excessive sweating, dehydration, severe diarrhea, or vomiting could deplete your fluids and cause your blood pressure to become too low. Be careful when exercising and in hot weather.

This drug should be used with caution if you are on dialysis. There have been reports of extreme allergic reactions during dialysis in people taking ACE-inhibitor medications such as Capozide. Your odds of an allergic reaction also increase if you are being desensitized with bee venom while you are taking Capozide.

While taking Capozide, do not use potassium-sparing diuretics (such as Moduretic), potassium supplements, or salt substitutes containing potassium without talking to your doctor first.

**Possible food and drug interactions
when taking this medication**

Capozide may intensify the effects of alcohol. Do not drink alcohol while
taking this medication.

If Capozide is taken with certain other drugs, the effects of either could be
increased, decreased, or altered. It is especially important to check with your
doctor before combining Capozide with the following:

Antigout drugs such as Zyloprim
Barbiturates such as phenobarbital or Seconal
Calcium
Cardiac glycosides such as Lanoxin
Cholestyramine (Questran)
Colestipol (Colestid)
Corticosteroids such as prednisone (Deltasone)
Diabetes medications such as Micronase and Insulin
Diazoxide (Proglycem)
Heart medications such as Lanoxin
Lithium (Lithonate)
MAO inhibitors (antidepressants such as Nardil)
Methenamine (Mandelamine)
Narcotics such as Percocet
Nitroglycerin or other nitrates such as Transderm-Nitro
Nonsteroidal anti-inflammatory drugs such as Naprosyn
Norepinephrine (Levophed)
Oral blood thinners such as Coumadin
Other blood pressure drugs such as Hytrin and Minipress
Potassium-sparing diuretics such as Moduretic
Potassium supplements such as Slow K
Probenecid (Benemid)
Salt substitutes containing potassium
Sulfinpyrazone (Anturane)

**Special information
if you are pregnant or breastfeeding**

ACE inhibitors such as Capozide have been shown to cause injury and even
death to the developing baby when used in pregnancy during the second or
third trimesters. If you are pregnant your doctor should discontinue your use
of this medication as soon as possible. If you plan to become pregnant and
are taking Capozide, contact your doctor immediately to discuss the potential
hazard to your unborn child. Capozide appears in breast milk and could affect

a nursing infant. If this medication is essential to your health, your doctor may advise you to discontinue breastfeeding until your treatment is finished.

Recommended dosage

ADULTS

Dosages of this drug are always individualized, and your doctor will determine what combination works best for you. This medication can be used in conjunction with other blood pressure medications such as beta blockers. Dosages are also adjusted for people with decreased kidney function.

The initial dose is one 25 milligram/15 milligram tablet, once a day. If this is not effective, your doctor may adjust the dosage upward every 6 weeks. In general, the daily dose of captopril should not exceed 150 milligrams. The maximum recommended daily dose of hydrochlorothiazide is 50 milligrams.

CHILDREN

The safety and effectiveness of Capozide in children have not been established. Capozide should be used in children only if other measures for controlling blood pressure have not been effective.

OLDER ADULTS

Your doctor will determine the dosage according to your particular needs.

Overdosage

Any medication taken in excess can have serious consequences. If you suspect an overdose, seek medical attention immediately.

■ *The symptoms of Capozide overdose may include:*
Coma, lethargy, low blood pressure, sluggishness, stomach and intestinal irritation and hyperactivity

Generic name:

CAPTOPRIL

See Capoten, page 187.

Generic name:

CAPTOPRIL WITH HYDROCHLOROTHIAZIDE

See Capozide, page 191.

Brand name:

CARAFATE

Pronounced: CARE-uh-fate
Generic name: Sucralfate

Why is this drug prescribed?

Carafate Tablets and Suspension are used for the short-term treatment (up to 8 weeks) of an active duodenal ulcer; Carafate Tablets are also used for longer-term therapy at a reduced dosage after a duodenal ulcer has healed.

Carafate helps ulcers heal by forming a protective coating over them.

Some doctors also prescribe Carafate for ulcers in the mouth and esophagus that develop during cancer therapy, for digestive tract irritation caused by drugs, for long-term treatment of stomach ulcers, and to relieve pain following tonsil removal.

Most important fact about this drug

A duodenal ulcer is a recurring illness. While Carafate can cure an acute ulcer, it cannot prevent other ulcers from developing or lessen their severity.

How should you take this medication?

Carafate works best when taken on an empty stomach. If you take an antacid to relieve pain, avoid doing it within one-half hour before or after you take Carafate. Always take Carafate exactly as prescribed.

- *If you miss a dose...*
  Take it as soon as you remember. If it is almost time for your next dose, skip the one you missed and go back to your regular schedule. Never take 2 doses at the same time.

- *Storage instructions...*
  Store at room temperature. Protect the suspension from freezing.

What side effects may occur?

Side effects cannot be anticipated. If any develop or change in intensity, inform your doctor as soon as possible. Only your doctor can determine if it is safe for you to continue taking Carafate.

- *More common side effects may include:*
  Constipation

■ *Less common or rare side effects may include:*
Back pain, diarrhea, dizziness, dry mouth, gas, headache, indigestion, insomnia, itching, nausea, possible allergic reactions, including hives and breathing difficulty, rash, sleepiness, stomach upset, vertigo, vomiting

Why should this drug not be prescribed?
There are no restrictions on the use of this drug.

Special warnings about this medication
If you have kidney failure or are on dialysis, the doctor will be cautious about prescribing this drug. Use of Carafate while taking aluminum-containing antacids may increase the possibility of aluminum poisoning in those with kidney failure.

Possible food and drug interactions
when taking this medication
If Carafate is taken with certain other drugs, the effects of either could be increased, decreased, or altered. It is especially important to check with your doctor before combining Carafate with the following:

Antacids such as Mylanta and Maalox
Blood-thinning drugs such as Coumadin
Cimetidine (Tagamet)
Digoxin (Lanoxin)
Drugs for controlling spasms, such as Bentyl
Ketoconazole (Nizoral)
Levothyroxine (Synthroid)
Phenytoin (Dilantin)
Quinidine (Quinidex)
Quinolone antibiotics such as Cipro and Floxin
Ranitidine (Zantac)
Tetracycline (Sumycin)
Theophylline (Theo-Dur)

Special information
if you are pregnant or breastfeeding
The effects of Carafate during pregnancy have not been adequately studied. If you are pregnant or plan to become pregnant, inform your doctor immediately. Carafate may appear in breast milk and could affect a nursing infant. If this medication is essential to your health, your doctor may advise you to discontinue breastfeeding until your treatment with this medication is finished.

Recommended dosage

ADULTS

Active Duodenal Ulcer:
The usual dose is 1 gram (1 tablet or 2 teaspoonfuls of suspension) 4 times a day on an empty stomach. Although your ulcer may heal during the first 2 weeks of therapy, Carafate should be continued for 4 to 8 weeks.

Maintenance Therapy:
The usual dose is 1 gram (1 tablet) 2 times a day.

CHILDREN

The safety and effectiveness of Carafate in children have not been established.

Overdosage

Although the risk of overdose with Carafate is low, any medication taken in excess can have serious consequences. If you suspect an overdose, seek medical attention immediately.

■ *Symptoms of overdose may include:*
Abdominal pain, indigestion, nausea, vomiting

Generic name:

CARBAMAZEPINE

See Tegretol, page 1264.

Generic name:

CARBIDOPA WITH LEVODOPA

See Sinemet CR, page 1196.

Brand name:

CARDENE

Pronounced: CAR-deen
Generic name: Nicardipine hydrochloride

Why is this drug prescribed?

Cardene, a type of medication called a calcium channel blocker, is prescribed for the treatment of chronic stable angina (chest pain usually caused by lack of oxygen to the heart resulting from clogged arteries, brought on by exertion) and for high blood pressure. When used to treat angina, Cardene is effective alone or in combination with beta-blocking medications such as Tenormin or Inderal. If it is used to treat high blood pressure, Cardene is effective alone or in combination with other high blood pressure medications. Calcium channel blockers ease the workload of the heart by slowing down its muscle contractions and the passage of nerve impulses through it. This improves blood flow through the heart and throughout the body, reducing blood pressure.

Cardene SR, a long-acting form of the drug, is prescribed only for high blood pressure.

Some doctors also prescribe Cardene to prevent migraine headache and to treat congestive heart failure. In combination with other drugs, such as Amicar, Cardene is also prescribed to manage neurological problems following certain kinds of stroke.

Most important fact about this drug

If you have high blood pressure, you must take Cardene regularly for it to be effective. Since blood pressure declines gradually, it may be several weeks before you get the full benefit of Cardene and you must continue taking it even if you are feeling well. Cardene does not cure high blood pressure; it merely keeps it under control.

How should you take this medication?

Take this medication exactly as prescribed, even if your symptoms have disappeared.

If you are taking Cardene SR, swallow the capsule whole; do not chew, crush, or divide it.

Try not to miss any doses. If Cardene is not taken regularly, your condition may worsen.

- *If you miss a dose...*
  Take it as soon as you remember. If it is almost time for the next dose, skip the one you missed and go back to your regular schedule. Do not take 2 doses at the same time.

- *Storage instructions...*
  Store at room temperature, away from light and moisture.

What side effects may occur?

Side effects cannot be anticipated. If any develop or change in intensity, inform your doctor as soon as possible. Only your doctor can determine if it is safe for you to continue taking Cardene.

■ *More common side effects may include:*
Dizziness, flushing, headache, increased chest pain (angina), indigestion, nausea, pounding or rapid heartbeat, sleepiness, swelling of feet, weakness

■ *Less common side effects may include:*
Abnormal dreaming, constipation, difficulty sleeping, drowsiness, dry mouth, excessive nighttime urination, fainting, fluid retention, muscle pain, nervousness, rash, shortness of breath, tingling or pins and needles, tremors, vomiting, vague feeling of bodily discomfort

■ *Rare side effects may include:*
Allergic reactions, anxiety, blurred vision, confusion, dizziness when standing, depression, hot flashes, increased movements, infection, inflammation of the nose, inflammation of the sinuses, impotence, joint pain, low blood pressure, more frequent urination, ringing in ears, sore throat, unusual chest pain, vertigo, vision changes

Why should this drug not be prescribed?

If you have advanced aortic stenosis (a narrowing of the aorta that causes obstruction of blood flow from the heart to the body), you should not take this medication.

If you are sensitive to or have ever had an allergic reaction to Cardene, you should not take this medication. Make sure your doctor is aware of any drug reactions you may have experienced.

Special warnings about this medication

Cardene can reduce or eliminate chest (angina) pain caused by exertion or exercise. Be sure to discuss with your doctor how much exercise or exertion is safe for you.

If you experience increased chest pain when you start taking Cardene or when your dosage is increased, contact your doctor immediately.

Your doctor will monitor your progress especially carefully if you have congestive heart failure, particularly if you are also taking a beta-blocking medication such as Tenormin or Inderal.

Cardene can cause your blood pressure to become too low, making you feel light-headed or faint. Your doctor should check your blood pressure when you start taking Cardene and continue to monitor it while your dosage is being adjusted.

If you have liver disease or decreased liver function, use this drug with caution.

Possible food and drug interactions
when taking this medication

If Cardene is taken with certain other drugs, the effects of either could be increased, decreased, or altered. It is especially important to check with your doctor before combining Cardene with the following:

Amiodarone (Cordarone)
Cimetidine (Tagamet)
Cyclosporine (Sandimmune)
Digoxin (Lanoxin)
Phenytoin (Dilantin)
Propranolol (Inderal)

Special information
if you are pregnant or breastfeeding

The effects of Cardene during pregnancy have not been adequately studied. If you are pregnant or plan to become pregnant, inform your doctor immediately. Cardene may appear in breast milk and could affect a nursing infant. If this medication is essential to your health, your doctor may advise you to discontinue breastfeeding until your treatment with Cardene is finished.

Recommended dosage

ADULTS

Angina

Your doctor will adjust the dosage according to your needs, usually beginning with 20 milligrams, 3 times a day. The usual regular dose is 20 to 40 milligrams, 3 times a day. Your physician may monitor your condition for at least 3 days before adjusting your dose.

High Blood Pressure

Your doctor will adjust the dosage to suit your needs. The starting dose of Cardene is usually 20 milligrams 3 times a day. The regular dose ranges from 20 to 40 milligrams 3 times a day.

The starting dose of Cardene SR is usually 30 milligrams 2 times a day. The regular dose ranges from 30 to 60 milligrams 2 times a day.

Your doctor may monitor your response to this medication for a few hours after the first dose, and will check your condition for at least 3 days before adjusting your dose.

CHILDREN

The safety and effectiveness of this drug in children under age 18 have not been established.

Overdosage

■ *Symptoms of Cardene overdose may include:*
Confusion, drowsiness, severe low blood pressure, slow heartbeat, slurred speech

If you suspect an overdose, seek medical attention immediately.

Brand name:

CARDIOQUIN

Pronounced: CAR-dee-o-kwin
Generic name: Quinidine polygalacturonate

Why is this drug prescribed?

Cardioquin corrects certain abnormal heart rhythms, including atrial fibrillation or flutter and life-threatening ventricular arrhythmias. It is usually prescribed only after other treatments have failed. If your condition does not improve after a reasonable period of time, your doctor may discontinue this medication and try other ways of restoring normal rhythm.

Most important fact about this drug

Before starting treatment with Cardioquin, your doctor will discuss with you the serious risks involved and weigh them against the good the drug may do. You should be closely monitored while on this medication.

How should you take this medication?

If you have certain types of high-risk heart problems, your doctor will start therapy with Cardioquin in a hospital setting where your response to the drug can be carefully monitored for the first 2 or 3 days.

Be careful to take Cardioquin exactly as directed. Never take more or less than prescribed, and try to remember every dose.

■ *If you miss a dose...*
If you remember it within 2 hours, take the missed dose immediately. If

you do not remember until later, skip the dose and go back to your regular schedule. Never take a double dose.

■ *Storage instructions...*
Store at room temperature.

What side effects may occur?
Cardioquin can cause a variety of problems, including an increase in abnormal heart rhythms that could lead to death. Be certain to report any unusual symptoms to your doctor immediately. Only your doctor can determine whether it is safe for you to continue taking Cardioquin.

■ *The most common side effects include...*
Angina-like pain (chest pain), change in sleep habits, diarrhea, fatigue, headache, light-headedness, palpitations, rash, stomach and intestinal problems, vision problems, weakness

■ *Other side effects may include:*
Anemia, anxiety, depression, eye inflammation, fainting, fever, flushing, hives, inflammation of the connective tissue, itching, joint pain, lack of coordination, liver problems, lung inflammation and other conditions, muscle pain, nervousness, psychotic reaction, reddish or purplish spots below the skin, sensitivity to light, skin inflammation and peeling, swelling of the lips and tongue or throat, tremor, vomiting, wheezing

Another possible side effect is a sensitivity reaction called cinchonism. Symptoms include confusion, delirium, diarrhea, headache, hearing loss, intolerance to light, ringing in the ears, vertigo, vision disturbances, and vomiting.

Why should this drug not be prescribed?
Cardioquin should not be prescribed for the rhythm disturbance known as heart block, and you should not take this medication if your condition warrants a pacemaker. Cardioquin should be avoided if, like people with myasthenia gravis (abnormal muscle weakness), you might be affected by drugs that control muscle spasms, such as Anaspaz and Bentyl. You should also avoid Cardioquin if you have ever had an allergic reaction to quinidine or have ever developed reddish or purplish spots below the skin while taking quinidine or quinine.

Special warnings about this medication
Cardioquin has been known to cause life-threatening abnormal heart rhythms. If you have a history of congestive heart failure or any other heart

problems, this medication should be used with caution, as it can cause low blood pressure, slowed heartbeat, or heart block.

If you have kidney or liver problems, your doctor may need to reduce your dosage. Be sure to tell your doctor about any medical conditions you have.

Possible food and drug interactions when taking this medication

Concentrations of digoxin (Lanoxin) in your blood may increase or even double when this drug is taken with Cardioquin. Your doctor may need to reduce the amount of digoxin you take.

If Cardioquin is taken with certain other drugs, the effects of either could be increased, decreased, or altered. It is especially important to check with your doctor before combining Cardioquin with the following:

Amiodarone (Cordarone)
Antidepressants in the "polycyclic" category, including Desyrel, Elavil, Ludiomil, and Tofranil
Certain medications that make your urine less acid, such as Diamox, Diuril, Dyazide, Esidrix, Maxzide, Neptazane, and sodium bicarbonate
Cimetidine (Tagamet)
Felodipine (Plendil)
Haloperidol (Haldol)
Ketoconazole (Nizoral)
Major tranquilizers such as Mellaril and Thorazine
Mexiletine (Mexitil)
Nicardipine (Cardene)
Nifedipine (Procardia)
Nimodipine (Nimotop)
Phenobarbital
Phenytoin (Dilantin)
Procainamide (Procan SR)
Propranolol (Inderal)
Rifampin (Rifadin)
Verapamil (Calan)
Warfarin (Coumadin)

Special information if you are pregnant or breastfeeding

The effects of Cardioquin during pregnancy have not been adequately studied. If you are pregnant or plan to become pregnant, tell your doctor immediately. Cardioquin does appear in breast milk and can affect a nursing infant. If this medication is essential to your health, your doctor may advise you to discontinue breastfeeding until your treatment is finished.

Recommended dosage

ADULTS

Your dose will be decided by your doctor, based on your particular heart problem and your general health. If you have a serious heart condition, your doctor will start therapy in the hospital, where you can be closely monitored. The usual starting dose is two 275-milligram tablets every 6 hours or one 275-milligram tablet every 6 to 8 hours, depending on the condition being treated. If you are able to tolerate this dosage and your condition warrants it, your doctor may increase the medication. After 2 or 3 days of close monitoring, you will be discharged and may be maintained on this dosage.

Your doctor may suggest using a Holter monitor (a device that records your heart rate 24 hours a day) to check your reaction to the drug.

CHILDREN

Quinidine has been used to treat malaria in children. However, the safety and effectiveness of this medication in children with abnormal heart rhythms has not been studied.

Overdosage

Any medication taken in excess can have serious consequences; and an overdose of Cardioquin can be fatal. If you suspect an overdose, seek medical treatment immediately.

- **Symptoms of Cardioquin overdose may include:**
  Abnormal heart rhythms, blurred and double vision, confusion, delirium, diarrhea, headache, hearing loss, intolerance to light, low blood pressure, ringing in ears, vertigo, vomiting

Brand name:

CARDIZEM

Pronounced: CAR-di-zem
Generic name: Diltiazem hydrochloride
Other brand names: Cardizem CD, Cardizem SR, Dilacor XR, Tiazac

Why is this drug prescribed?

Cardizem and Cardizem CD (a controlled release form of diltiazem) are used in the treatment of angina pectoris (chest pain usually caused by lack of oxygen to the heart due to clogged arteries) and chronic stable angina (caused by exertion). Cardizem CD is also used to treat high blood pressure. Another controlled release form, Cardizem SR, is used only in the treatment of high blood pressure. Cardizem, a calcium channel blocker, dilates blood vessels and slows the heart to reduce blood pressure and the pain of angina.

Doctors sometimes prescribe Cardizem for loss of circulation in the fingers and toes (Raynaud's Syndrome), for involuntary movements (tardive dyskinesia), and to prevent heart attack.

Tiazac and Dilacor XR are used in the treatment of high blood pressure and chronic stable angina. They may be taken alone or combined with other blood pressure medications.

Most important fact about this drug
If you are taking Cardizem for high blood pressure, remember that it does not cure the problem; it merely controls it. You may need to take a blood pressure medication for the rest of your life.

If you are taking Cardizem for angina, do not stop suddenly. This can lead to an increase in your attacks.

How should you take this medication?
Cardizem should be taken before meals and at bedtime. Cardizem CD, Cardizem SR, and Dilacor XR should be swallowed whole; do not chew, crush, or divide.

Take this medication exactly as prescribed by your doctor, even if your symptoms have disappeared.

■ *If you miss a dose...*
   If you forget to take a dose, take it as soon as you remember. If it's almost time for your next dose, skip the missed dose and go back to your regular schedule. Never take 2 doses at the same time.

■ *Storage instructions...*
   Cardizem should be stored at room temperature; protect from moisture.

What side effects may occur?
Side effects cannot be anticipated. If any develop or change in intensity, inform your doctor as soon as possible. Only your doctor can determine if it is safe for you to continue taking Cardizem.

■ *More common side effects may include:*
Abnormally slow heartbeat (more common with Cardizem SR and Cardizem CD), dizziness, fluid retention, flushing (more common with Cardizem SR and Cardizem CD), headache, nausea, rash, weakness

■ *Less common or rare side effects may include:*
Abnormal dreams, allergic reaction, altered way of walking, amnesia, anemia, angina (severe chest pain), blood disorders, congestive heart failure, constipation, cough, depression, diarrhea, difficulty sleeping, drowsiness, dry mouth, excessive urination at night, eye irritation, fainting, flu symptoms, hair loss, hallucinations, heart attack, high blood sugar, hives, impotence, increased output of pale urine, indigestion, infection, irregular heartbeat, itching, joint pain, labored breathing, loss of appetite, low blood pressure, low blood sugar, muscle cramps, nasal congestion or inflammation, nervousness, nosebleed, pain, personality change, pounding heartbeat, rapid heartbeat, reddish or purplish spots on skin, ringing in ears, sexual difficulties, skin inflammation/flaking or peeling, sensitivity to light, sleepiness, sore throat, taste alteration, thirst, tingling or pins and needles, tremor, vision changes, vomiting, welts, weight increase

Why should this drug not be prescribed?
If you suffer from "sick sinus" syndrome or second- or third-degree heart block (various types of irregular heartbeat), you should not take diltiazem unless you have a ventricular pacemaker. Also avoid diltiazem if you've just suffered a heart attack or have lung congestion.

Do not take diltiazem if you have low blood pressure or an allergy to the drug.

Special warnings about this medication
If you have congestive heart failure or suffer from kidney or liver disease, use Cardizem with caution.
This medication may cause your heart rate to become too slow. You should check your pulse regularly.

Possible food and drug interactions
when taking this medication
If Cardizem is taken with certain other drugs, the effects of either could be increased, decreased, or altered. It is especially important to check with your doctor before combining Cardizem with the following:

Beta-blockers (heart and blood pressure drugs such as Tenormin and Inderal)

Carbamazepine (Tegretol)
Cimetidine (Tagamet)
Cyclosporine (Sandimmune, Neoral)
Digoxin (Lanoxin)

Special information
if you are pregnant or breastfeeding

The effects of Cardizem during pregnancy have not been adequately studied. If you are pregnant or plan to become pregnant, inform your doctor immediately. Cardizem appears in breast milk and could affect a nursing infant. If this medication is essential to your health, your doctor may advise you to discontinue breastfeeding until your treatment with this medication is finished.

Recommended dosage

ADULTS

Dosage levels are determined by each individual's needs.

Cardizem

The average daily dosage is between 180 milligrams and 360 milligrams, divided into 3 or 4 smaller doses.

Cardizem SR

The recommended starting dosage is 60 to 120 milligrams 2 times a day, to be increased to 240 to 360 milligrams a day.

Cardizem CD

This is a once-a-day form of this drug. For high blood pressure, starting doses range from 180 to 240 milligrams; for angina, 120 to 180 milligrams.

Dilacor XR

This is another once-a-day drug. For high blood pressure, doses start at 180 to 240 milligrams and may be increased to as much as 540 milligrams. For angina, doses start at 120 milligrams and may be increased to 480 milligrams.

Tiazac

The usual starting dose for high blood pressure is 120 to 240 milligrams once a day. After the drug has taken effect—in about 2 weeks—the dose can range from 120 to 540 milligrams. For angina, once-daily doses start at 120 to 180 milligrams and may be increased to 540 milligrams if necessary.

CHILDREN
Safety and effectiveness in children have not been established.

Overdosage
Any medication taken in excess can have serious consequences. If you suspect an overdose of Cardizem, seek medical attention immediately.

- *The symptoms of Cardizem overdose may include:*
  Fainting, dizziness, and irregular pulse, heart failure, low blood pressure, very slow heartbeat

Brand name:

CARDURA

Pronounced: car-DUHR-uh
Generic name: Doxazosin mesylate

Why is this drug prescribed?
Cardura is used in the treatment of benign prostatic hyperplasia, a condition in which the prostate gland grows larger, pressing on the urethra and threatening to block the flow of urine from the bladder. The drug relieves symptoms such as a weak stream, dribbling, incomplete emptying of the bladder, frequent urination, and burning during urination.

Cardura is also used in the treatment of high blood pressure. It is effective when used alone or in combination with other blood pressure medications, such as diuretics, beta-blocking medications, calcium channel blockers or ACE inhibitors.

Doctors also prescribe Cardura, along with other drugs such as digitalis and diuretics, for treatment of congestive heart failure.

Most important fact about this drug
If you have high blood pressure, you must take Cardura regularly for it to be effective. Since blood pressure declines gradually, it may be several weeks before you get the full benefit of Cardura; and you must continue taking it even if you are feeling well. Cardura does not cure high blood pressure; it merely keeps it under control.

How should you take this medication?
This medication can be taken with or without food.

Cardura should be taken exactly as prescribed, even if your symptoms have disappeared. Try not to miss any doses. If this medication is not taken regularly, your condition may worsen.

If you have benign prostatic hyperplasia, you should see improvement in a week. Blood pressure will fall in 2 to 6 hours.

■ *If you miss a dose...*
Take it as soon as you remember. If it is almost time for your next dose, skip the one you missed and go back to your regular schedule. Never take 2 doses at the same time.

■ *Storage instructions...*
Store at room temperature.

What side effects may occur?
Side effects cannot be anticipated. If any develop or change in intensity, inform your doctor as soon as possible. Only your doctor can determine if it is safe for you to continue taking Cardura.

■ *More common side effects may include:*
Dizziness, drowsiness, fatigue, headache

■ *Less common side effects may include:*
Abdominal pain, abnormal vision, arthritis, constipation, depression, diarrhea, difficulty sleeping, dry mouth, eye pain, fluid retention, flu-like symptoms, flushing, gas, increased sweating, inability to hold urine or other urination problems, indigestion, inflammation of conjunctiva (pink-eye), itching, flushes, joint pain, lack of muscle coordination, low blood pressure, motion disorders, muscle cramps, muscle pain, muscle weakness, nasal stuffiness, nausea, nervousness, nosebleeds, pain, rash, ringing in ears, shortness of breath, thirst, tingling or pins and needles, weakness

■ *Rare side effects may include:*
Abnormal thinking, agitation, altered sense of smell, amnesia, breast pain, changeable emotions, changes in taste, chest pain, confusion, coughing, decreased sense of touch, dizziness when standing up, dry skin, earache, fainting, fecal incontinence, fever, gout, hair loss, heart attack, inability to concentrate, inability to tolerate light, increased appetite, increased thirst, infection, loss of appetite, loss of sense of personal identity, migraine headache, morbid dreams, pallor, rapid pounding heartbeat, sexual problems, sinus inflammation, slight or partial paralysis, sore throat, stroke, tremors, twitching, weight gain, weight loss, wheezing

Why should this drug not be prescribed?

Cardura should not be taken if you are sensitive to or have ever had an allergic reaction to Cardura or such drugs as Minipress or Hytrin. Make sure your doctor is aware of any drug reactions you may have experienced.

Special warnings about this medication

Cardura can cause low blood pressure, especially when you first start taking the medication and when dosage is increased. This can cause you to become faint, dizzy, or light-headed, particularly when first standing up. You should avoid driving or any hazardous tasks where injury could occur for 24 hours after taking the first dose, after your dose has been increased, or if Cardura has been stopped and then restarted.

In rare cases, men taking drugs such as Cardura have developed priapism, a painful, long-lasting erection that persists for hours. This condition can lead to impotence, so if it occurs contact your doctor right away.

If you have liver disease or are taking other medications that alter liver function, your doctor will monitor you closely when you take Cardura.

Cardura may lower blood counts. Your doctor will most likely monitor your blood counts while you are taking this medication.

This medication may cause you to become drowsy or sleepy. For this reason, too, driving or operating dangerous machinery or participating in any hazardous activity that requires full mental alertness is not recommended.

Prostate cancer has some of the same symptoms as benign prostatic hyperplasia; your doctor will want to make sure you do not have cancer before starting you on Cardura.

Possible food and drug interactions
when taking this medication

No significant interactions have been reported.

Special information
if you are pregnant or breastfeeding

The effects of Cardura during pregnancy have not been adequately studied. If you are pregnant or plan to become pregnant, inform your doctor immediately. Cardura may appear in breast milk and could affect a nursing infant. If this medication is essential to your health, your doctor may advise you to discontinue breastfeeding until your treatment with this medication is finished.

Recommended dosage

ADULTS

Your doctor will adjust the dosage to fit your needs.

The usual starting dose is 1 milligram taken once a day. To minimize the potential for dizziness or fainting associated with Cardura, which may occur between 2 and 6 hours after a dose, your doctor will monitor your blood pressure during this period and afterwards.

After the effects of the starting dose are measured, your doctor may increase the daily dose to 2 milligrams and then, if necessary, to 4 milligrams, 8 milligrams, or, in people with high blood pressure only, up to 16 milligrams. As the dose increases, the potential for side effects such as dizziness, vertigo, light-headedness, and fainting also increases.

CHILDREN

The safety and effectiveness of this drug in children have not been established.

Overdosage

Any medication taken in excess can have serious consequences. Although no specific information is available, low blood pressure is the most likely symptom of an overdose of Cardura.

If you suspect an overdose, seek medical attention immediately.

Generic name:

CARISOPRODOL

See Soma, page 1209.

Generic name:

CARVEDILOL

See Coreg, page 291.

Brand name:

CATAFLAM

See Voltaren, page 1423.

Brand name:

CATAPRES

Pronounced: KAT-uh-press
Generic name: Clonidine hydrochloride

Why is this drug prescribed?
Catapres is prescribed for high blood pressure. It is effective when used alone or with other high blood pressure medications.

Doctors also prescribe Catapres for alcohol, nicotine, or benzodiazepine (tranquilizer) withdrawal; migraine headaches; smoking cessation programs; Tourette's syndrome (tics and uncontrollable utterances); narcotic/methadone detoxification; premenstrual tension; and diabetic diarrhea.

Most important fact about this drug
If you have high blood pressure, you must take Catapres regularly for it to be effective. Since blood pressure declines gradually, it may be several weeks before you get the full benefit of Catapres; and you must continue taking it even if you are feeling well. Catapres does not cure high blood pressure; it merely keeps it under control.

How should you take this medication?
Take this medication exactly as prescribed, even if you are feeling well. Try not to miss any doses. If Catapres is not taken regularly, your condition may get worse.

The Catapres-TTS patch should be put on a hairless, clean area of the upper outer arm or chest. Normally, a new one is applied every 7 days to a new area of the skin. If the patch becomes loose, use some adhesive tape or an adhesive bandage to keep it in place.

- *If you miss a dose...*
  Take it as soon as you remember, then go back to your regular schedule. If you forget to take the medication 2 or more times in a row, or if you forget to change the transdermal patch for 3 or more days, contact your doctor.

- *Storage instructions...*
  Store at room temperature in a tightly closed container away from light.

What side effects may occur?
Side effects cannot be anticipated. If any develop or change in intensity, inform your doctor as soon as possible. Only your doctor can determine if it is safe for you to continue taking Catapres.

■ *More common side effects may include:*
Agitation, constipation, dizziness, drowsiness, dry mouth, fatigue, impotence, loss of sex drive, nausea, nervousness, sedation (calm), vomiting, weakness

■ *Less common side effects may include:*
Changes in heartbeat, excessive nighttime urination, headache, loss of appetite, mental depression, pounding heartbeat, vague bodily discomfort, weight gain

■ *Rare side effects may include:*
Abdominal pain, anxiety, behavior changes, blurred vision, breast development in males, burning eyes, congestive heart failure, constipation, delirium, dry eyes, dry nasal passages, fainting, fever, greater sensitivity to alcohol, hallucinations, heart irregularities, hepatitis, hair loss, hives, insomnia, itching, joint pain, leg cramps, little or no urination, muscle pain, pallor, restlessness, vivid dreams or nightmares

■ *Additional side effects of Catapres-TTS may include:*
Abrasions, blisters, burning or reddened skin, discolored or whitened skin, pimples, throbbing skin

Why should this drug not be prescribed?
Do not take this medication if you have ever had an allergic reaction to Catapres or to any of the components of the transdermal patch.

Special warnings about this medication
Catapres should not be stopped suddenly. Headache, nervousness, agitation, tremor, confusion, and rapid rise in blood pressure can occur. Severe reactions such as disruption of brain functions, stroke, fluid in the lungs, and death have also been reported. Your doctor should gradually reduce your dosage over several days to avoid withdrawal symptoms.

If you see redness, blistering, or a rash near the transdermal patch, call your doctor. You may need to remove the patch. If you are troubled by mild irritation before completing 7 days of use, you may remove the patch and apply a new one at a different site.

If your doctor has switched you to oral Catapres (tablet) because you had an allergic reaction, such as a rash or hives, to the transdermal skin patch, be aware that you may have a similar reaction to the Catapres tablet.

If you have severe heart or kidney disease, are recovering from a heart attack, or have a disease of the blood vessels of the brain, your doctor will prescribe Catapres with caution.

If you are taking Catapres and a beta blocker such as Inderal or Tenormin, and your doctor wants to stop your medication, the beta blocker should be stopped several days before the gradual withdrawal of Catapres.

Catapres may cause drowsiness. If it has this effect on you, avoid driving, operating dangerous machinery, or participating in any hazardous activity that requires full mental alertness.

The used Catapres-TTS patch still contains enough drug to be harmful to children and pets. Fold the patch in half with the adhesive sides together and dispose of it out of the reach of children.

Possible food and drug interactions
when taking this medication

Catapres may increase the effects of alcohol. Do not drink alcohol while taking this medication.

If Catapres is taken with certain other drugs, the effects of either could be increased, decreased, or altered. It is especially important to check with your doctor before combining Catapres with the following:

Barbiturates such as Nembutal and Seconal
Beta-blocker drugs such as the blood pressure medications Inderal and Lopressor
Calcium blockers such as the heart medications Calan and Cardizem
Digitalis
Sedatives such as Valium, Xanax, and Halcion
Tricyclic antidepressants such as Elavil and Tofranil

Special information
if you are pregnant or breastfeeding

The effects of Catapres during pregnancy have not been adequately studied. If you are pregnant or plan to become pregnant, inform your doctor immediately. Catapres appears in breast milk and could affect a nursing infant. If this medication is essential to your health, your doctor may advise you to discontinue breastfeeding until your treatment with this medication is finished.

Recommended dosage

ADULTS

The dosage will be adjusted to your individual needs.

The usual starting dose is 0.1 milligram, twice a day (usually in the morning and at bedtime).

The regular dose of Catapres is determined by increasing the daily dose by 0.1 milligram at weekly intervals until the desired response is achieved. A larger portion of the increased dose can be taken at bedtime to reduce potential side effects of drowsiness and dry mouth that may appear when you begin taking this drug.

The most common effective dosages range from 0.2 milligram to 0.6 milligram per day divided into smaller doses. The maximum effective dose is 2.4 milligrams per day; however, this dose is not usually prescribed.

Transdermal Patch

The patch comes in different strengths, and your doctor will determine which is best for you based on your blood pressure response.

People who are using another high blood pressure medication should not stop taking it abruptly when they begin using the patch, because the medication in the patch may take a few days to begin working. The other medication should be discontinued slowly as the patch begins to take effect.

CHILDREN

Safety and effectiveness of the Catapres tablets and patch in children below the age of 12 have not been established.

OLDER ADULTS

Dosages are generally as above; however, the initial dosage for an older person may be lower than the regular starting dose.

Overdosage

■ *Symptoms of Catapres overdose may include:*
Constriction of pupils of the eye, drowsiness, high blood pressure followed by a drop in pressure, irritability, low body temperature, slowed breathing, slowed heartbeat, slowed reflexes, weakness

Large overdoses can cause changes in heart function or rhythm, coma, seizures, and temporary interruptions in breathing.

Getting a patch in the mouth or swallowing one can cause an overdose.

If you suspect symptoms of a Catapres overdose, seek medical attention immediately.

Brand name:

CAVERJECT

Pronounced: CA-vur-jekt
Generic name: Alprostadil
Other brand names: Edex, Muse

Why is this drug prescribed?
Caverject is used to treat male impotence. Your doctor also may use Caverject to help diagnose the exact nature of your impotence.

Caverject and the similar brand Edex are both taken by injection. A third brand, Muse, is taken as a small suppository inserted in the penis.

Most important fact about this drug
Caverject is known to have caused extremely long-lasting erections. Serious harm can occur from such a prolonged erection, so call your doctor or seek other professional help if an erection lasts more than 4 to 6 hours. Usually the erection should last about 1 hour.

How should you use this medication?
Caverject is injected into a specific area of the penis and produces an erection within 5 to 20 minutes. Do not use Caverject more than 3 times a week. Wait at least 24 hours between use.

The first injections are performed by your doctor in the doctor's office in order to determine the proper dosage. Afterwards, you can inject Caverject yourself as needed. Your doctor will train you in the proper technique for injecting Caverject and you'll be given complete printed instructions. Follow these directions exactly and do not change the dose your doctor has determined.

Do not use a Caverject solution that appears cloudy or colored or that contains particles. Do not shake the vial.

Wash your hands thoroughly and do not touch the needle. Carefully choose the injection site as instructed by your doctor, always avoiding visible veins. Cleanse the site with an alcohol swab. With each use, alternate the side of the penis and the site of the injection.

Use the needle/syringe and vial only once, then discard them properly. Do not share needles or allow anyone else to use your medication.

Caverject comes in both 10 microgram and 20 microgram strengths. Make sure you are using a vial with the correct strength.

After injecting Edex, put pressure on the injection site for 5 minutes, or until the bleeding stops.

If you have been prescribed Muse, your doctor will instruct you in the correct way to insert the suppository. An erection should occur within 5 to 10 minutes of insertion. Do not use more than 2 suppositories in 24 hours. Discard each applicator after a single use.

■ *Storage instructions...*
Store unused packs of Caverject at room temperature for up to 3 months. Protect from freezing or from overheating.

Once the Caverject solution is mixed, you must use it immediately or discard it.

When traveling, take care to prevent exposing Caverject to freezing or excessive heat. Do not store Caverject in checked luggage or leave it in a closed car.

Muse suppositories should be stored in the refrigerator, but may be left at room temperature for up to 14 days before use. Protect the suppositories from high temperatures and direct sunlight. Carry them in a portable cooler when traveling.

What side effects may occur?
Side effects cannot be anticipated. If any develop or change in intensity, inform your doctor as soon as possible. Only your doctor can determine if it is safe for you to continue using this drug.

CAVERJECT AND EDEX

The most common side effect is mild to moderate pain in the penis during and/or after injection, reported by about one-third of users. A small amount of bleeding may occur at the injection site. Notify your doctor if you have a condition or are taking a medication that interferes with blood clotting. As with any injection, the site can become infected. Call your doctor if you notice any redness, lumps, swelling, tenderness, or curving of the erect penis.

Your doctor should examine your penis regularly if you use Caverject. Use of Caverject may result in formation of fibrous (hardened) tissue in the penis or erections at an unusual angle. If those side effects occur, inform your doctor and stop using Caverject.

■ *More common side effects may include:*
Blood-filled swelling at the site of injection, disorder of the penis (such as discoloration of the head, strange feeling, tearing of the skin), hardened tissue in the penis, pain in the penis, prolonged erection, upper respiratory infection

■ *Less common side effects may include:*
Abnormal vision, back pain, bruising at the injection site, cough, dizziness, flu symptoms, headache, heart attack, high blood pressure, infection, inflamed or enlarged prostate, injuries/fractures/abrasions/lacerations/dislocations, leg pain, nasal congestion, pain, redness, sinus inflammation, skin disorders

■ *Rare side effects may include:*
Abnormal ejaculation, bleeding at the urethra, blood in the urine, dizziness, dry mouth, extreme dilation of the pupils, fainting, fluid retention at the injection site, frequent or urgent urination, hemorrhage at the injection site, impaired urination, inflammation, irritation, itching, lack of sensation, leg cramps, low blood pressure, nausea, numbness, painful erection, pelvic pain, profuse sweating, rash on the penis, redness, sensitivity, swelling at the injection site, swelling of the head of the penis, swelling of the scrotum, testicular pain, tightness of the foreskin, warmth, weakness, yeast infection

MUSE

■ *More common side effects may include:*
Extremely low blood pressure, flu symptoms, headache, infection, pain, penis bleeding, penis burning or pain, testicular pain

■ *Less common side effects may include:*
Back pain, dizziness, leg pain, pain in the area behind the testicles, pelvic pain, rapid pulse, runny nose, swelling of leg veins

Muse may cause vaginal burning and itching in your partner.

Why should this drug not be prescribed?
Do not use Caverject if you have a condition that might result in long-lasting erections, such as sickle cell anemia, increased levels of red cells and platelets in your blood, and tumor of the bone marrow.

Men with penile implants or an unusually formed penis should not use Caverject. The drug is not for use in women, children, or men whose doctors have advised them not to have sex.

Do not use Caverject, Edex, or Muse if it causes an allergic reaction or if you have ever had a reaction to any prostaglandin drugs.

Do not use Muse for sexual intercourse with a pregnant woman unless you use a condom.

Special warnings about this medication
These drugs offer no protection from the transmission of sexually transmitted diseases, such as HIV, the virus that causes AIDS. Small amounts of bleeding at the injection or suppository site can increase the risk of transmission of blood-borne diseases such as HIV.

Because Muse has been known to cause low blood pressure and fainting, you should avoid driving and other hazardous activities after using it. When using Muse with a partner in her child-bearing years, contraception is recommended.

Possible food and drug interactions when using this medication
No interactions have been reported, but these products should not be used with other drugs that act on blood vessels, such as blood pressure medications.

You may have some bleeding at the site of injection or insertion. If you are taking anticoagulants such as heparin or Coumadin you may bleed more. Make sure that any doctor who prescribes an anticoagulant is aware that you are using one of these medications.

Recommended dosage

CAVERJECT AND EDEX

The correct dose of Caverject must be carefully determined by your doctor. Each man will need a different dose of Caverject, but the usual starting dosage is 1.25 or 2.5 micrograms, which is then increased gradually. Your doctor will adjust the dosage, particularly if it produces erections lasting longer than 1 hour.

The dosage range for Edex is 1 to 40 micrograms, given over 5 to 10 seconds.

Do not change your dosage without your doctor's approval. See your doctor every 3 months for a checkup.

MUSE

The suppositories come in four strengths, ranging from 125 to 1,000 micrograms. The 125- or 250-microgram strength is recommended at the start. Your doctor will prescribe a higher strength if necessary. Remember that you must not use more than 2 suppositories in each 24 hours.

Overdosage

No overdose of Caverject has been reported. However, any medication taken in excess can have serious consequences. The chief symptom of an overdose of this drug would be a prolonged erection. If you suspect an overdose, seek medical attention immediately.

Brand name:

CECLOR

Pronounced: SEE-klor
Generic name: Cefaclor

Why is this drug prescribed?

Ceclor, a cephalosporin antibiotic, is used in the treatment of ear, nose, throat, respiratory tract, urinary tract, and skin infections caused by specific bacteria, including staph, strep, and *E. coli*. Uses include treatment of sore or strep throat, pneumonia, and tonsillitis. Ceclor CD, an extended release form of the drug, is also used for flare-ups of chronic bronchitis.

Most important fact about this drug

If you are allergic to either penicillin or cephalosporin antibiotics in any form, consult your doctor *before taking* Ceclor. There is a possibility that you are allergic to both types of medication; and if a reaction occurs, it could be extremely severe. If you take the drug and feel signs of a reaction, seek medical attention immediately.

How should you take this medication?

Take this medication exactly as prescribed. It is important that you finish taking all of this medication to obtain the maximum benefit.

Ceclor works fastest when taken on an empty stomach. However, your doctor may ask you to take this drug with food to avoid stomach upset.

Ceclor CD should be taken with meals or at least within 1 hour of eating because it's better absorbed with food. Do not cut, crush, or chew the tablets.

Ceclor suspension should be shaken well before using.

■ *If you miss a dose...*
Take it as soon as you remember. If it is almost time for your next dose, skip the one you missed and go back to your regular schedule. Never take 2 doses at the same time.

■ *Storage instructions...*
Keep Ceclor capsules in the container they came in, tightly closed. Store at room temperature.

Refrigerate Ceclor suspension. Discard any unused portion after 14 days.

What side effects may occur?
Side effects cannot be anticipated. If any develop or change in intensity, inform your doctor as soon as possible. Only your doctor can determine if it is safe for you to continue taking Ceclor.

■ *More common side effects of Ceclor may include:*
Diarrhea, hives, itching

■ *Less common or rare side effects of Ceclor may include:*
Blood disorders (an increase in certain types of white blood cells), liver disorders, nausea, severe allergic reactions (including swelling, weakness, breathing difficulty, or fainting), skin rashes accompanied by joint pain, vaginal inflammation, vomiting

■ *More common side effects of Ceclor CD may include:*
Diarrhea, headache, nasal inflammation, nausea

■ *Less common or rare side effects of Ceclor CD may include:*
Abdominal pain, accidental injury, anxiety, asthma, back pain, bronchitis, chest pain, chills, congestive heart failure, conjunctivitis (pinkeye), constipation, dizziness, ear pain or infection, fever, fluid retention with swelling, flu symptoms, gas, hives, increased cough, indigestion, infection, inflamed sinuses, insomnia, itching, joint pain, loss of appetite, lung problems, menstrual problems, muscle pain, nausea, neck pain, nervousness, rash, sleepiness, sore throat, sweating, throbbing heartbeat, tremor,

urinary problems, vaginal inflammation or infection, vague feeling of illness, vomiting

Other problems have been reported in patients taking Ceclor, although it is not known whether the drug was the cause. Check with your doctor if you suspect a side effect.

Why should this drug not be prescribed?
If you are sensitive to or have ever had an allergic reaction to Ceclor or any other cephalosporin antibiotic, you should not take this medication. Make sure your doctor is aware of any drug reactions you have experienced.

Unless you are directed to do so by your doctor, do not take this medication if you have a history of gastrointestinal problems, particularly bowel inflammation (colitis). You may be at increased risk for side effects.

Special warnings about this medication
Ceclor may cause a false positive result with some urine sugar tests for diabetics. Your doctor can advise you of any adjustments you may need to make in your medication or diet.

Ceclor occasionally causes diarrhea. Some diarrhea medications can make this diarrhea worse. Check with your doctor before taking any diarrhea remedy.

Oral contraceptives may not work properly while you are taking Ceclor. For greater certainty, use other measures while taking Ceclor.

Possible food and drug interactions
when taking this medication
If Ceclor is taken with certain other drugs, the effects of either could be increased, decreased, or altered. It is especially important to check with your doctor before combining Ceclor with the following:

    Antacids containing magnesium or aluminum, including Gelusil, Maalox, and Mylanta (interact with Ceclor CD only)
    Certain antibiotics such as Amikin
    Certain potent diuretics such as Edecrin and Lasix
    Probenecid (Benemid)
    Warfarin (Coumadin)

Special information
if you are pregnant or breastfeeding
The effects of Ceclor during pregnancy have not been adequately studied. If you are pregnant or plan to become pregnant, this drug should be used only

when prescribed by your doctor. Ceclor appears in breast milk and could affect a nursing infant. If this medication is essential to your health, your doctor may advise you to stop nursing your baby until your treatment with Ceclor is finished.

Recommended dosage

CECLOR

Adults

The usual adult dose is 250 milligrams every 8 hours. For more severe infections (such as pneumonia), your doctor may increase the dosage.

Children

The usual daily dosage is 20 milligrams per 2.2 pounds of body weight per day divided into smaller doses and taken every 8 hours. In more serious infections, such as middle ear infection, the usual dose is 40 milligrams per 2.2 pounds of body weight per day divided into smaller doses. The total daily dose should not exceed 1 gram.

CECLOR CD

Adults: Bronchitis

The usual dose is 500 milligrams every 12 hours for 7 days.

Adults: Sore throat, Tonsillitis, and Skin Infections

The usual dose is 375 milligrams every 12 hours for 10 days (sore throat and tonsillitis) or 7 to 10 days (skin infections).

Children

Safety and effectiveness of Ceclor CD in children under age 16 have not been established.

Overdosage

■ *Symptoms of Ceclor overdose may include:*
Diarrhea, nausea, stomach upset, vomiting

If other symptoms are present, they may be related to an allergic reaction or other underlying disease. In any case, you should contact your doctor or an emergency room immediately.

Brand name:

CEDAX

Pronounced: SEE-daks
Generic name: Ceftibuten

Why is this drug prescribed?

Cedax cures mild-to-moderate bacterial infections of the throat, ear, and respiratory tract. Among these infections are strep throat, tonsillitis, and acute otitis media (middle ear infection) in children and adults. Cedax is also prescribed for acute flare-ups of chronic bronchitis in adults. Cedax is a cephalosporin antibiotic.

Most important fact about this drug

If you are allergic to either penicillin or cephalosporin antibiotics in any form, double-check with your doctor *before taking* Cedax. There is a possibility that you are allergic to both types of medication and if a reaction occurs, it could be extremely severe. (Symptoms include swelling of the face, lips, tongue, and throat, making it difficult to breathe.) If you take the drug and feel any signs of this reaction, seek medical attention immediately.

How should you take this medication?

To make certain your infection is fully cleared up, take all the Cedax your doctor prescribes, even if you begin to feel better after the first few days.

If you are using the oral suspension, it must be taken at least 2 hours before a meal or 1 hour after. Shake well before using.

■ *If you miss a dose...*
Take it as soon as you remember. If it is almost time for your next dose, skip the one you missed and go back to your regular schedule. Never take 2 doses at the same time.

■ *Storage instructions...*
Keep the oral suspension in the refrigerator, and discard any unused portion after 14 days. Capsules may be stored at room temperature.

What side effects may occur?

Side effects cannot be anticipated. If any develop or change in intensity, notify your doctor as soon as possible. Only your doctor can determine whether it is safe for you to continue taking Cedax.

ADULTS

- *More common side effects may include:*
  Diarrhea, headache, nausea

- *Less common or rare side effects in adults may include:*
  Abdominal pain, belching, breathing problems, constipation, dizziness, drowsiness, dry mouth, fatigue, fever, gas, hives, inability to speak, indigestion, itching, joint pain, loose stools, loss of appetite, painful urination, rash, stuffy nose, swollen glands, tarry stools, taste alteration, tingling, vaginal inflammation, vomiting, yeast infection, yellowish skin

CHILDREN

- *The most common side effect is:*
  Diarrhea (especially in children age 2 and under)

- *Less common or rare side effects may include:*
  Abdominal pain, agitation, blood in urine, chills and fever, dehydration, diaper rash, dizziness, fever, gas, headache, hives, increased activity, insomnia, irritability, itching, loose stools, loss of appetite, nausea, rash, vomiting

Why should this drug not be prescribed?
If you are sensitive to or have ever had an allergic reaction to Cedax, other cephalosporins, such as Keflex, or any form of penicillin, do not take this medication. Make sure your doctor is aware of any drug reactions you have experienced.

Special warnings about this medication
If you have a history of gastrointestinal disease, particularly colitis, take Cedax with caution. If you develop diarrhea while taking Cedax, check with your doctor. The problem could be a sign of a serious condition.

Tell your doctor if you have kidney problems. Your dosage may have to be lowered. If you are diabetic, be sure to tell your doctor before starting therapy with Cedax; the oral suspension contains sugar.

If new infections (called superinfections) occur, talk to your doctor. You may need to be treated with a different antibiotic.

Do not give this medication to other people or use it for other infections before checking with your doctor. The drug is not effective against every type of germ.

Possible food and drug interactions
when taking this medication

Zantac may boost the level of Cedax in your system. Check with your doctor before combining these drugs.

Special information
if you are pregnant or breastfeeding

The effects of Cedax during pregnancy have not been adequately studied. If you are pregnant or plan to become pregnant, tell your doctor immediately. Cedax may appear in breast milk and could affect a nursing infant. If this medication is essential to your health, your doctor may advise you to stop breastfeeding until your treatment is finished.

Recommended dosage

ADULTS

The usual dose is a single 400-milligram capsule once a day. People with serious kidney problems are prescribed a smaller dose.

CHILDREN

Cedax oral suspension comes in two strengths: 90 milligrams and 180 milligrams. The usual dose is 9 milligrams for each 2.2 pounds of body weight, once a day. Your doctor will specify the number of teaspoonfuls required according to the following guidelines:

Children weighing 22 pounds: one 90-milligram teaspoonful or half a 180-milligram teaspoonful.

Children weighing 44 pounds: two 90-milligram teaspoonfuls or one 180-milligram teaspoonful.

Children weighing 88 pounds: four 90-milligram teaspoonfuls or two 180-milligram teaspoonfuls.

Children weighing more than 90 pounds: 400 milligrams once a day.

Cedax has not been tested for treatment of infants less than 6 months old.

Overdosage

Although no specific information is available, an overdose of cephalosporins has been known to cause convulsions. Any medication taken in excess can have serious consequences. If you suspect an overdose of Cedax, seek medical attention immediately.

Generic name:

CEFACLOR

See Ceclor, page 221.

Generic name:

CEFADROXIL

See Duricef, page 441.

Generic name:

CEFIXIME

See Suprax, page 1228.

Generic name:

CEFPROZIL

See Cefzil, page 231.

Generic name:

CEFTIBUTEN

See Cedax, page 225.

Brand name:

CEFTIN

Pronounced: SEF-tin
Generic name: Cefuroxime axetil

Why is this drug prescribed?
Ceftin, a cephalosporin antibiotic, is prescribed for mild to moderately severe bacterial infections of the throat, lungs, ears, skin, sinuses, and urinary tract, and for gonorrhea. Ceftin tablets are also prescribed in the early stages of Lyme disease.

Most important fact about this drug
If you are allergic to either penicillin or cephalosporin antibiotics such as Ceclor, Cefzil, or Keflex, consult your doctor *before taking* Ceftin. There is a possibility that you are allergic to both types of medication; if a reaction

occurs, it could be extremely severe. If you take the drug and develop shortness of breath, a pounding heartbeat, a skin rash, or hives, seek medical attention immediately.

How should you take this medication?
Ceftin tablets can be taken on a full or empty stomach. However, it enters the bloodstream and works faster when taken after meals. Ceftin oral suspension must be taken with food. Shake the suspension well before each use.

Take this medication exactly as prescribed: It is important that you finish taking all of this medication to obtain the maximum benefit.

The crushed tablet has a strong, persistent, bitter taste. Children who cannot swallow the tablet whole should take the oral suspension. Shake the oral suspension well before each use.

■ *If you miss a dose...*
   Take it as soon as you remember. If it is almost time for your next dose skip the one you missed and go back to the regular schedule. Do not take 2 doses at once.

■ *Storage instructions...*
   Store tablets at room temperature in a tightly closed container. Protect from moisture. The oral suspension may be stored either in the refrigerator or at room temperature. Replace the cap securely after each use. Discard any unused suspension after 10 days.

What side effects may occur?
Side effects cannot be anticipated. If any develop or change in intensity, inform your doctor as soon as possible. Only your doctor can determine if it is safe for you to continue taking Ceftin.

■ *More common side effects may include:*
   Diaper rash in infants, diarrhea, nausea, vomiting

■ *Rare side effects of the tablets include:*
   Abdominal pain or cramps, chest pain, chills, gas, headache, hives, indigestion, itch, loss of appetite, mouth ulcers, rash, shortness of breath, sleepiness, swollen tongue, thirst, urinary problems, vaginitis

■ *Rare side effects of the oral suspension include:*
   Abdominal pain, cough, drooling, fever, gas, gastrointestinal infection, hyperactivity, inflamed sinuses, irritability, joint pain and swelling, rash, upper respiratory infection, urinary infection, vaginal irritation, virus infection, yeast infection

Why should this drug not be prescribed?

Ceftin should not be prescribed if you have a known allergy to cephalosporin antibiotics.

Special warnings about this medication

Inflammation of the bowel (colitis) has been reported with the use of Ceftin; therefore, if you develop diarrhea while taking this medication, notify your doctor.

Continued or prolonged use of Ceftin may result in an overgrowth of bacteria that do not respond to this medication and can cause a second infection. You should take this drug only when it is prescribed by your doctor, even if you have symptoms like those of a previous infection. Tell your doctor if you have any kidney problems. Your dosage may need to be lowered.

If you are allergic to penicillin you may also be allergic to Ceftin. Make sure your doctor is aware of any allergies you have.

Possible food and drug interactions
when taking this medication

It is important to consult your doctor before taking this drug with probenecid (Benemid), a gout medication.

If diarrhea occurs while taking Ceftin, consult your doctor before taking an antidiarrhea medication. Certain drugs, such as Lomotil, may cause your diarrhea to become worse.

Be cautious if you are taking potent water pills (diuretics) such as Lasix while on Ceftin. The combination could affect your kidneys.

Special information
if you are pregnant or breastfeeding

The effects of Ceftin during pregnancy have not been adequately studied. If you are pregnant or plan to become pregnant, inform your doctor immediately. Ceftin appears in breast milk and could affect a nursing infant. If this medication is essential to your health, your doctor may advise you to discontinue breastfeeding until your treatment with this medication is finished.

Recommended dosage

ADULTS

The usual dose for adults and children 13 years and older is 250 milligrams, 2 times a day for up to 10 days. For more severe infections the dose may be increased to 500 milligrams, 2 times a day.

Throat and Tonsil Infections
The usual dose is 125 milligrams 2 times a day for 10 days.

Urinary Tract Infection
The usual dose is 125 milligrams, 2 times a day for 7 to 10 days. This dose may be increased to 250 milligrams 2 times a day for severe infection.

Gonorrhea
The usual treatment is a single dose of 1 gram.

Early Lyme Disease
The usual dosage is 500 milligrams taken twice a day for 20 days.

CHILDREN

Ceftin oral suspension may be given to children ranging in age from 3 months to 12 years.

Your doctor will determine the dosage based on your child's weight and the type of infection being treated. Ceftin oral suspension is given twice a day for 10 days. The maximum daily dose ranges from 500 to 1000 milligrams.

Overdosage
Any medication taken in excess can have serious consequences. Overdosage with cephalosporin antibiotics can cause brain irritation leading to convulsions. If you suspect an overdose, seek medical attention immediately.

Generic name:

CEFUROXIME

See Ceftin, page 228.

Brand name:

CEFZIL

Pronounced: SEFF-zil
Generic name: Cefprozil

Why is this drug prescribed?
Cefzil, a cephalosporin antibiotic, is prescribed for mild to moderately severe bacterial infections of the throat, ear, sinuses, respiratory tract, and skin. Among these infections are strep throat, tonsillitis, bronchitis, and pneumonia.

Most important fact about this drug
If you are allergic to penicillin or cephalosporin antibiotics in any form, consult your doctor *before taking* Cefzil. An allergy to either type of medication may signal an allergy to Cefzil; and if a reaction occurs, it could be extremely severe. If you take the drug and feel signs of a reaction, seek medical attention immediately.

How should you use this medication?
Take this medication exactly as prescribed. It is important that you finish all of the medication to obtain the maximum benefit.

Cefzil works fastest when taken on an empty stomach, but can be taken with food to avoid stomach upset.

Cefzil oral suspension should be shaken well before using.

▪ *If you miss a dose...*
Take it as soon as you remember. If it is almost time for your next dose, skip the one you missed and go back to your regular schedule. Never take 2 doses at the same time.

▪ *Storage instructions...*
Store Cefzil tablets at room temperature. Keep the oral suspension in the refrigerator; discard any unused portion after 14 days.

What side effects may occur?
Side effects cannot be anticipated. If any develop or change in intensity, notify your doctor as soon as possible. Only your doctor can determine whether it is safe for you to continue taking Cefzil.

The most common side effect is nausea.

▪ *Less common or rare side effects may include:*
Abdominal pain, confusion, diaper rash, diarrhea, difficulty sleeping, dizziness, genital itching, headache, hives, hyperactivity, nervousness, rash, sleepiness, superinfection (additional infection), vaginal inflammation, vomiting, yellow eyes and skin

Although not reported for Cefzil, similar antibiotics have been known occasionally to have severe side effects such as anaphylaxis (a severe allergic reaction), skin rash with blisters, Stevens-Johnson syndrome (a rare skin condition characterized by severe blisters and bleeding in the lips, eyes, mouth, nose, and genitals), and "serum-sickness" (itchy rash, fever, and pain in the joints).

Why should this drug not be prescribed?

If you are sensitive to or have ever had an allergic reaction to Cefzil or other cephalosporin antibiotics, do not take this medication. Make sure your doctor is aware of any drug reactions you have experienced.

Special warnings about this medication

Cefzil occasionally causes colitis (inflammation of the bowel) leading to diarrhea. Some diarrhea medications can make this diarrhea worse. Check with your doctor before taking any diarrhea remedy.

Oral contraceptives may not work properly while you are taking Cefzil. For greater certainty, use other measures while taking Cefzil.

Your doctor will check your kidney function before and during your treatment with this medication.

Use Cefzil with caution if you are taking a strong diuretic, or if you have ever had stomach and intestinal disease, particularly colitis.

If new infections (called superinfections) occur, talk to your doctor. You may need to be treated with a different antibiotic.

Cefzil may alter the results of some urine sugar tests for diabetics. Your doctor can advise you of any adjustments you may need to make in your medication or diet.

Possible food and drug interactions
when taking this medication

When Cefzil is taken with certain other drugs, the effects of either could be increased, decreased, or altered. It is especially important to check with your doctor before combining Cefzil with the following:

   Certain other antibiotics such as Amikin
   Certain potent diuretics such as Edecrin and Lasix
   Oral contraceptives
   Probenecid (Benemid)
   Propantheline (Pro-Banthine)

Special information
if you are pregnant or breastfeeding

The effects of Cefzil during pregnancy have not been adequately studied. If you are pregnant or plan to become pregnant, inform your doctor immediately. Cefzil does appear in breast milk and could affect a nursing infant. If this medication is essential to your health, your doctor may advise you to stop breastfeeding until your treatment with this medication is finished.

Recommended dosage

ADULTS

Throat and Respiratory Tract Infections
The usual dose is 500 milligrams, taken once or twice a day for 10 days.

Sinus Infection
The usual dose is 250 milligrams every 12 hours for 10 days; for severe infections the dose is 500 milligrams.

Skin Infections
The dosage is usually either 250 milligrams taken 2 times a day, or 500 milligrams taken once or twice a day for 10 days.

CHILDREN 2 TO 12 YEARS OF AGE

Throat Infections and Tonsillitis
The usual dose is 7.5 milligrams for each 2.2 pounds of body weight, taken 2 times a day for 10 days.

Skin Infections
The usual dose is 20 milligrams for each 2.2 pounds of body weight, taken once a day for 10 days.

INFANTS AND CHILDREN 6 MONTHS TO 12 YEARS OF AGE

Ear Infections
The usual dose is 15 milligrams for each 2.2 pounds of body weight, taken 2 times a day for 10 days.

Sinus Infection
The usual dose is 7.5 milligrams for each 2.2 pounds of body weight every 12 hours for 10 days. For severe infections, the amount may be doubled.

Overdosage
Although no specific information is available, any medication taken in excess can have serious consequences. If you suspect an overdose of Cefzil, seek medical attention immediately.

Brand name:

CELEBREX

Pronounced: SELL-eh-breks
Generic name: Celecoxib

Why is this drug prescribed?
Celebrex relieves the pain and inflammation of osteoarthritis and rheumatoid arthritis. It is the first of a new class of nonsteroidal anti-inflammatory drugs (NSAIDs) called "COX-2 inhibitors." Like older NSAIDs such as Motrin and Naprosyn, Celebrex is believed to fight pain and inflammation by inhibiting the effect of a natural enzyme called COX-2. Unlike the older medications, however, it does not interfere with a similar substance, called COX-1, which exerts a protective effect on the lining of the stomach. Celebrex is therefore less likely to cause the bleeding and ulcers that sometimes accompany sustained use of the older NSAIDs.

Most important fact about this drug
Although Celebrex is easy on the stomach, it still poses some degree of risk—especially if you've had a stomach ulcer or gastrointestinal bleeding in the past. If you've ever had such problems, make sure the doctor is aware of it. And be sure to alert the doctor if you develop any digestive problems or black tarry stools.

How should you take this medication?
For best results, take Celebrex regularly, exactly as prescribed. You can take it with or without food.

▪ *If you miss a dose...*
  Take it as soon as you remember. If it is almost time for your next dose, skip the one you missed and go back to your regular schedule. Do not take 2 doses at the same time.

▪ *Storage instructions...*
  Store at room temperature.

What side effects may occur?
Side effects cannot be anticipated. If any develop or change in intensity, inform your doctor as soon as possible. Only your doctor can determine if it is safe for you to continue taking Celebrex.

■ *More common side effects may include:*
Abdominal pain, diarrhea, headache, indigestion, nausea, respiratory infection, sinus inflammation

■ *Less common side effects may include:*
Back pain, dizziness, gas, insomnia, rash, runny nose, sore throat, swelling

■ *Rare side effects may include:*
Allergic reactions, anxiety, belching, blurred vision, bone disorders, breast pain, breast problems, bronchitis, cataracts, chest pain, conjunctivitis (pinkeye), constipation, coughing, cysts, dark-tarry stools, deafness, depression, dermatitis, diabetes, difficult urination, difficulty breathing, difficulty swallowing, drowsiness, dry mouth, dry skin, earache, ear infection, ear ringing, eye infection, eye pain, fatigue, fever, flu symptoms, fungal infection, glaucoma (pressure in the eye), hair loss, hemorrhoids, hernia of the stomach, herpes infection, hives, hot flashes, increased appetite, increased blood pressure, increased heart rate, increased muscle tone, increased urination, infection, inflammation of the digestive tract, inflammation of the bladder, itching, joint pain or inflammation, kidney stones, laryngitis, leg cramps, liver problems, loss of appetite, loss of balance, menstrual disorders, migraine headache, mouth ulcers, muscle ache, nail disorders, neck stiffness, nerve pain, nervousness, nosebleeds, pain, painful urination, pneumonia, prostate problems, severe diarrhea, skin reaction due to sun light, skin sensitivity, skin tingling, sweating, swelling, taste disturbances, tendonitis, tiredness, tooth disorders, urinary incontinence, urinary tract infections, vaginal problems, vomiting, weakness, weight gain

Why should this drug not be prescribed?
Do not take Celebrex if you are allergic to sulfonamide drugs such as sulfadiazine, sulfisoxazole, Gantanol, and Thiosulfil. Also avoid Celebrex if you've ever suffered an asthma attack, face and throat swelling, or skin eruptions after taking aspirin or other NSAIDs. If you find that you are allergic to Celebrex, you will not be able to use it.

Special warnings about this medication
Remember to tell your doctor about any stomach ulcers or bleeding you've had in the past. Also alert your doctor if you develop any digestive problems, swelling, or rash.

If you have asthma, use Celebrex with caution. It could trigger an attack, especially if you are also sensitive to aspirin.

If you are taking a steroid medication for your arthritis, do not discontinue it abruptly when you begin therapy with Celebrex. Celebrex is not a substitute for such drugs.

Celebrex has been known to cause kidney or liver problems, particularly in people with an existing condition. If you have such a disorder, take Celebrex with caution. If you develop symptoms of liver poisoning, stop taking the drug and see your doctor immediately. Warning signs include nausea, fatigue, itching, yellowish skin, pain in the right side of the stomach, and flu-like symptoms.

If you are prone to anemia (loss of red blood cells), make sure the doctor knows about it. Celebrex occasionally fosters this problem.

Celebrex sometimes causes water retention, which can aggravate swelling, high blood pressure, and heart failure. Use this drug with caution if you have any of these conditions.

The safety and effectiveness of Celebrex have not been tested in children under 18.

Possible food and drug interactions
when taking this medication

If Celebrex is taken with certain other drugs, the effects of either could be increased, decreased, or altered. It is especially important to check with your doctor before combining Celebrex with the following:

ACE-inhibitors (a type of blood pressure and heart medication, including
    such drugs as Capoten, Vasotec, and Prinivil)
Aspirin
Blood thinning agents such as Coumadin
Fluconazole (Diflucan)
Furosemide (Lasix)
Lithium (Lithobid, Lithonate)
Thiazide diuretics (water pills) such as hydrochlorothiazide and Dyazide

Special information
if you are pregnant or breastfeeding

Celebrex can harm a developing baby if taken during the third trimester, and its safety earlier in pregnancy has not been confirmed. Take it during pregnancy only if you feel the risk is justified.

It's possible that Celebrex makes its way into breast milk (scientists aren't sure), and it could cause serious reactions in a nursing infant. If this drug is essential to your health, your doctor may advise you to discontinue breastfeeding.

Recommended dosage

ADULTS

Osteoarthritis
The recommended daily dose is 200 milligrams, taken as a single dose or in 100-milligram doses twice a day.

Rheumatoid Arthritis
The recommended dose is 100 to 200 milligrams twice a day.

Overdosage
Any medication taken in excess can have serious consequences. If you suspect an overdose, seek medical attention immediately.

■ *Symptoms of Celebrex overdose may include:*
 Breathing difficulties, coma, drowsiness, fainting, gastrointestinal bleeding, hives, itching, nausea, sluggishness, stomach pain, vomiting

Generic name:

CELECOXIB

See Celebrex, page 235.

Brand name:

CELEXA

Pronounced: sell-EX-ah
Generic name: Citalopram hydrobromide

Why is this drug prescribed?
Celexa is used to treat major depression—a stubbornly low mood that persists nearly every day for at least 2 weeks and interferes with everyday living. Symptoms may include loss of interest in your usual activities, insomnia or excessive sleeping, a change in weight or appetite, constant fidgeting or a slowdown in movement, fatigue, feelings of worthlessness or guilt, difficulty thinking or concentrating, and repeated thoughts of suicide.

Like the antidepressant medications Paxil, Prozac, and Zoloft, Celexa is thought to work by boosting serotonin levels in the brain. Serotonin, one of the nervous system's primary chemical messengers, is known to elevate mood.

Most important fact about this drug

Be careful to avoid taking Celexa for 2 weeks before or after using an antidepressant known as an MAO inhibitor. Drugs in this category include Marplan, Nardil, and Parnate. Combining Celexa with one of these medications could lead to a serious—even fatal—reaction.

How should you take this medication?

Take Celexa once a day, in the morning or evening, with or without food. Although your depression will begin to lift in 1 to 4 weeks, you should continue taking Celexa regularly. It takes several months for the medication to yield its full benefits.

■ *If you miss a dose...*
Take it as soon as you remember. If it is almost time for your next dose, skip the one you missed and go back to your regular schedule. Do not take 2 doses at the same time.

■ *Storage instructions...*
Store at room temperature.

What side effects may occur?

Side effects cannot be anticipated. If any develop or change in intensity, inform your doctor as soon as possible. Only your doctor can determine if it is safe for you to continue taking Celexa.

■ *More common side effects may include:*
Abdominal pain, agitation, anxiety, diarrhea, drowsiness, dry mouth, ejaculation disorders, fatigue, impotence, indigestion, insomnia, loss of appetite, nausea, painful menstruation, respiratory tract infection, sinus or nasal inflammation, sweating, tremor, vomiting

■ *Less common side effects may include:*
Amnesia, attempted suicide, confusion, coughing, decreased sexual drive, depression, excessive urination, fever, gas, impaired concentration, increased appetite, increased salivation, itching, joint pain, lack of emotion, loss of menstruation, low blood pressure, migraine, muscle pain, rapid heartbeat, rash, skin tingling, taste disturbances, visual disturbances, weight gain, weight loss, yawning

■ *Rare side effects may include:*
Abnormal dreams, acne, aggressive behavior, alcohol intolerance, angina (chest pain), arthritis, belching, bone pain, breast enlargement, breast pain, bronchitis, bruising, chills, conjunctivitis (pinkeye), decreased muscle

movements, delusions, dermatitis, difficulty breathing, difficulty swallowing, dizziness, drug dependence, dry eyes, dry skin, eczema, emotional instability, excessive milk flow, excessive muscle tone, eye pain, fainting, feeling of well-being, flu-like symptoms, flushing, frequent urination, gum inflammation, hair loss, hallucinations, heart attack, heart failure, hemorrhoids, high blood pressure, hives, hot flashes, inability to hold urine, inability to urinate completely, increased sex drive, increased urination, involuntary muscle movements, leg cramps, mouth sores, muscle weakness, nosebleeds, numbness, painful urination, panic, paranoia, pneumonia, psoriasis, psychosis, ringing in the ears, sensitivity to light, skin discoloration, slow heartbeat, stomach and intestinal inflammation, stroke, swelling, teeth grinding, thirst, uncontrollable muscle movements, unsteady or abnormal walk, vaginal bleeding

Why should this drug not be prescribed?

If Celexa gives you an allergic reaction, you cannot continue using it. Also remember that Celexa must never be combined with an MAO inhibitor (see Most important fact about this drug, above).

Special warnings about this medication

In recommended doses, Celexa does not seem to impair judgment or motor skills. However, a theoretical possibility of such problems remains, so you should use caution when driving or operating dangerous equipment until you are certain of Celexa's effect.

There is a slight chance that Celexa will trigger a manic episode. Use Celexa with caution if you suffer from manic-depression (bipolar disorder). Use caution, too, if you are over 60 years old, have liver or kidney problems, suffer from heart disease or high blood pressure, or have ever had seizures.

Possible food and drug interactions
when taking this medication

Celexa does not increase the effects of alcohol. Nevertheless, it's considered unwise to combine Celexa with alcohol or any other drug that affects the brain. (Be particularly careful to avoid MAO inhibitors.)

If Celexa is taken with certain other drugs, the effects of either could be increased, decreased, or altered. Tell your doctor about any prescription or over-the-counter drugs you are planning to take, and be especially certain to check with him before combining Celexa with the following:

Carbamazepine (Tegretol)
Cimetidine (Tagamet)
Erythromycin (Eryc, Ery-Tab)
Fluconazole (Diflucan)

Itraconazole (Sporanox)
Ketoconazole (Nizoral)
Lithium (Lithobid, Lithonate)
Omeprazole (Prilosec)
Other antidepressants such as Elavil, Norpramin, Pamelor, and Tofranil
Metoprolol (Lopressor)
Warfarin (Coumadin)

Special information
if you are pregnant or breastfeeding

The effects of Celexa during pregnancy have not been adequately studied, and the potential for harm has not been ruled out. If you are pregnant or plan to become pregnant while on Celexa therapy, tell your doctor immediately.

Celexa appears in breast milk and will affect the nursing infant. You should consider discontinuing either breastfeeding or Celexa. Talk with your doctor about the pros and cons of each option.

Recommended dosage

ADULTS

The recommended starting dose is 20 milligrams once a day. Dosage is usually increased to 40 milligrams once daily after at least a week has passed. Do not exceed 40 milligrams a day.

For older adults and those who have liver problems, the recommended dose is 20 milligrams once a day.

Overdosage

Any medication taken in excess can have serious consequences. If you suspect an overdose, seek medical attention immediately.

■ *Symptoms of Celexa overdose may include:*
Amnesia, bluish or purplish discoloration of the skin, coma, confusion, convulsions, dizziness, drowsiness, hyperventilation, nausea, rapid heartbeat, sweating, tremor, vomiting

Brand name:

CENTRUM

See Multivitamins, page 838.

Generic name:

CEPHALEXIN

See Keflex, page 653.

Generic name:

CERIVASTATIN

See Baycol, page 141.

Brand name:

CETECORT

See Hydrocortisone Skin Preparations, page 599.

Generic name:

CETIRIZINE

See Zyrtec, page 1494.

Generic name:

CHLORDIAZEPOXIDE

See Librium, page 694.

Generic name:

CHLORDIAZEPOXIDE WITH CLIDINIUM

See Librax, page 692.

Generic name:

CHLORHEXIDINE

See Peridex, page 985.

Generic name:

CHLOROTHIAZIDE

See Diuril, page 424.

Generic name:

CHLORPHENIRAMINE WITH PSEUDOEPHEDRINE

See Deconamine, page 353.

Generic name:

CHLORPROMAZINE

See Thorazine, page 1297.

Generic name:

CHLORPROPAMIDE

See Diabinese, page 385.

Generic name:

CHLORTHALIDONE

See Hygroton, page 605.

Generic name:

CHLORZOXAZONE

See Parafon Forte DSC, page 950.

Generic name:

CHOLESTYRAMINE

See Questran, page 1090.

Generic name:

CHOLINE MAGNESIUM TRISALICYLATE

See Trilisate, page 1346.

Brand name:

CHRONULAC SYRUP

Pronounced: KRON-yoo-lak
Generic name: Lactulose
Other brand name: Duphalac

Why is this drug prescribed?
Chronulac treats constipation. In people who are chronically constipated, Chronulac increases the number and frequency of bowel movements.

Most important fact about this drug
It may take 24 to 48 hours to produce a normal bowel movement.

How should you take this medication?
Take this medication exactly as prescribed. If you find the taste of Chronulac unpleasant, it can be mixed with water, fruit juice, or milk.

- *If you miss a dose...*
  Take the forgotten dose as soon as you remember; but do not try to "catch up" by taking a double dose.

- *Storage instructions...*
  Store at room temperature. Avoid excessive heat or direct light. The liquid may darken in color, which is normal. Do not freeze.

What side effects may occur?
Side effects cannot be anticipated. If any develop or change in intensity, inform your doctor as soon as possible. Only your doctor can determine if it is safe for you to continue taking Chronulac.

- *Side effects may include:*
  Diarrhea, gas (temporary, at the beginning of use), intestinal cramps (temporary, at the beginning of use), nausea, potassium and fluid loss, vomiting

Why should this drug not be prescribed?
Chronulac contains galactose, a simple sugar. If you are on a low-galactose diet, do not take this medication.

Special warnings about this medication
Because of its sugar content, this medication should be used with caution if you have diabetes.

If unusual diarrhea occurs, contact your doctor.

Possible food and drug interactions when taking this medication

If Chronulac is taken with certain other drugs, the effects of either could be increased, decreased, or altered. It is especially important to check with your doctor before combining Chronulac with nonabsorbable antacids such as Maalox and Mylanta.

Special information if you are pregnant or breastfeeding

The effects of Chronulac during pregnancy have not been adequately studied. If you are pregnant or plan to become pregnant, inform your doctor immediately. Chronulac may appear in breast milk and could affect a nursing infant. If this medication is essential to your health, your doctor may advise you to stop breastfeeding until your treatment is finished.

Recommended dosage

The usual dose is 1 to 2 tablespoonfuls (15 to 30 milliliters) daily. Your doctor may increase the dose to 60 milliliters a day, if necessary.

Safety and effectiveness for children have not been established.

Overdosage

Any medication taken in excess can have serious consequences. If you suspect an overdose, seek medical treatment immediately.

- *Symptoms of Chronulac overdose may include:*
  Abdominal cramps, diarrhea

Generic name:

CICLOPIROX

See Loprox, page 722.

Generic name:

CIMETIDINE

See Tagamet, page 1240.

Brand name:

CIPRO

Pronounced: SIP-roh
Generic name: Ciprofloxacin hydrochloride

Why is this drug prescribed?

Cipro is used to treat infections of the lower respiratory tract, the abdomen, the skin, the bones and joints, and the urinary tract, including cystitis (bladder inflammation) in women. It is also prescribed for severe sinus or bronchial infections, infectious diarrhea, typhoid fever, infections of the prostate gland, and some sexually transmitted diseases. Additionally, some doctors prescribe Cipro for certain serious ear infections, tuberculosis, and some of the infections common in people with AIDS.

Because Cipro is effective only for certain types of bacterial infections, before beginning treatment your doctor may perform tests to identify the specific organisms causing your infection.

Cipro is available as a tablet and an oral suspension and as a suspension to be used externally in the ear.

Most important fact about this drug

Cipro kills a variety of bacteria, and is frequently used to treat infections in many parts of the body. However, be sure to notify your doctor immediately at the first sign of a skin rash or any other allergic reaction. Although quite rare, serious and occasionally fatal allergic reactions—some following the first dose—have been reported in people receiving this type of antibacterial drug. Some reactions have been accompanied by collapse of the circulatory system, loss of consciousness, swelling of the face and throat, shortness of breath, tingling, itching, and hives.

How should you take this medication?

Cipro may be taken with or without meals but is best tolerated when taken 2 hours after a meal.

Drink plenty of fluids while taking this medication.

Cipro, like other antibiotics, works best when there is a constant amount in the blood and urine. To help keep the level constant, try not to miss any doses, and take them at evenly spaced intervals around the clock.

If you are taking the suspension, be sure to shake the bottle vigorously for 15 seconds before each dose. Swallow without chewing the microcapsules in the suspension. Do not use Cipro HC Otic suspension in your eyes, and avoid contaminating the dropper by letting it touch your ears, fingers, or other surfaces.

Warm the suspension by holding the bottle in your hand for a minute or two; putting a cold suspension into the ear can make you dizzy.

Lie down with the affected ear up, and do not get up for 30 to 60 seconds after the drops are instilled.

Throw away any suspension that remains after treatment is finished.

■ *If you miss a dose...*
Take it as soon as you remember. If it is almost time for your next dose, skip the one you missed and go back to your regular schedule. Never take 2 doses at the same time.

■ *Storage instructions...*
Cipro tablets should be stored at room temperature. Cipro suspension may be stored at room temperature or in the refrigerator. The suspension is good for 14 days. Protect Cipro HC Otic suspension from light and avoid freezing.

What side effects may occur?
Side effects cannot be anticipated. If any develop or change in intensity, inform your doctor as soon as possible. Only your doctor can determine if it is safe for you to continue taking Cipro.

■ *Most common side effect:*
Nausea

■ *Less common side effects may include:*
Abdominal pain/discomfort, diarrhea, headache, rash, restlessness, vomiting

■ *Rare side effects may include:*
Abnormal dread or fear, achiness, bleeding in the stomach and/or intestines, blood clots in the lungs, blurred vision, change in color perception, chills, confusion, constipation, convulsions, coughing up blood, decreased vision, depression, difficulty in swallowing, dizziness, double vision, drowsiness, eye pain, fainting, fever, flushing, gas, gout flare up, hallucinations, hearing loss, heart attack, hiccups, high blood pressure, hives, inability to fall or stay asleep, inability to urinate,

indigestion, intestinal inflammation, involuntary eye movement, irregular heartbeat, irritability, itching, joint or back pain, joint stiffness, kidney failure, labored breathing, lack of muscle coordination, lack or loss of appetite, large volumes of urine, light-headedness, loss of sense of identity, loss of sense of smell, mouth sores, neck pain, nightmares, nosebleed, pounding heartbeat, ringing in the ears, seizures, sensitivity to light, severe allergic reaction, skin peeling, redness, sluggishness, speech difficulties, swelling of the face, neck, lips, eyes, or hands, swelling of the throat, tender, red bumps on skin, tingling sensation, tremors, unpleasant taste, unusual darkening of the skin, vaginal inflammation, vague feeling of illness, weakness, yellowed eyes and skin

Why should this drug not be prescribed?
If you are sensitive to or have ever had an allergic reaction to Cipro or certain other antibiotics of this type, you should not take this medication. Make sure that your doctor is aware of any drug reactions that you have experienced.

Cipro HC Otic suspension should not be used on anyone whose ear drum is perforated or who has a viral infection of the ear.

Special warnings about this medication
Cipro may cause you to become dizzy or light-headed; therefore, you should not drive a car, operate dangerous machinery, or participate in any hazardous activity that requires full mental alertness until you know how the drug affects you.

Continued or prolonged use of this drug may result in a growth of bacteria that do not respond to this medication and can cause a secondary infection. Therefore, it is important that your doctor monitor your condition on a regular basis.

Cipro can cause increased pressure within the brain. Convulsions have been reported in people receiving the drug. If you experience a seizure or convulsion, notify your doctor immediately.

This medication may stimulate the central nervous system, which may lead to tremors, restlessness, light-headedness, confusion, depression, and hallucinations. If these reactions occur, consult your doctor at once. Other central nervous system reactions include nervousness, agitation, insomnia, anxiety, nightmares, and paranoia.

If you have a known or suspected central nervous system disorder such as epilepsy or hardening of the arteries in the brain, make sure your doctor knows about it when prescribing Cipro.

You may become more sensitive to light while taking this drug. Try to stay out of the sun as much as possible.

People taking Cipro have been known to suffer torn tendons. If you feel any pain or inflammation in a tendon area, stop taking the drug and call your doctor; you should rest and avoid exercise. You may need surgery to repair the tendon.

If you must take Cipro for an extended period of time, your doctor will probably order blood tests and tests for urine, kidney, and liver function.

Possible food and drug interactions
when taking this medication
Serious and fatal reactions have occurred when Cipro was taken in combination with theophylline (Theo-Dur). These reactions have included cardiac arrest, seizures, status epilepticus (continuous attacks of epilepsy with no periods of consciousness), and respiratory failure.

Products containing iron, multivitamins containing zinc, or antacids containing magnesium, aluminum, or calcium, when taken in combination with Cipro, may interfere with absorption of this medication.

Cipro may increase the effects of caffeine.

If Cipro is taken with certain other drugs, the effects of either could be increased, decreased, or altered. These drugs include:

Cyclophosphamide (Cytoxan)
Cyclosporine (Sandimmune, Neoral)
Glyburide (DiaBeta, Glynase, Micronase)
Metoprolol (Lopressor)
Phenytoin (Dilantin)
Probenecid (Benemid)
Sucralfate (Carafate)
Theophylline (Theo-Dur)
Warfarin (Coumadin)

Special information
if you are pregnant or breastfeeding
The effects of Cipro during pregnancy have not been adequately studied. If you are pregnant or plan to become pregnant, notify your doctor immediately. Cipro does appear in breast milk when it's taken internally, and could affect a nursing infant. If this medication is essential to your health, your doctor may advise you to discontinue breastfeeding your baby until your treatment is finished.

Recommended dosage

ADULTS

The length of treatment with Cipro depends upon the severity of infection. Generally, Cipro should be continued for at least 2 days after the signs and symptoms of infection have disappeared. The usual length of time is 7 to 14 days; however, for severe and complicated infections, treatment may be prolonged.

Cystitis in women is treated for 3 days.

Bone and joint infections may require treatment for 4 to 6 weeks or longer.

Infectious diarrhea may be treated for 5 to 7 days.

Typhoid fever should be treated for 10 days.

Chronic prostate inflammation should be treated for 28 days.

If you are using the oral suspension, 1 teaspoonful of 5% suspension equals 250 milligrams and 1 teaspoonful of 10% suspension equals 500 milligrams.

Urinary Tract Infections
The usual adult dosage is 250 milligrams taken every 12 hours. Complicated infections, as determined by your doctor, may require 500 milligrams taken every 12 hours.

For cystitis in women, the usual dosage is 100 milligrams every 12 hours.

Lower Respiratory Tract, Skin, Bone, and Joint Infections
The usual recommended dosage is 500 milligrams taken every 12 hours. Complicated infections, as determined by your doctor, may require a dosage of 750 milligrams taken every 12 hours.

Infectious Diarrhea; Typhoid Fever; Sinus, Prostate, and Abdominal Infections
The recommended dosage is 500 milligrams taken every 12 hours.

Gonorrhea in the Urethra or Cervix
For these sexually transmitted diseases, a single 250-milligram dose is the usual treatment.

Ear Infection
Instill 3 drops of suspension into the ear twice a day for 7 days.

CHILDREN

Safety and effectiveness of Cipro oral tablets and suspension have not been established in children and adolescents under 18 years of age.

The dosage of Cipro HC Otic suspension for children aged 1 and up is the same as for adults.

Overdosage

Any medication taken in excess can have serious consequences. If you suspect an overdose, seek medical attention immediately.

Generic name:

CIPROFLOXACIN

See Cipro, page 246.

Generic name:

CISAPRIDE

See Propulsid, page 1064.

Generic name:

CITALOPRAM

See Celexa, page 238.

Generic name:

CLARITHROMYCIN

See Biaxin, page 165.

Brand name:

CLARITIN

Pronounced: CLAR-i-tin
Generic name: Loratadine

Why is this drug prescribed?

Claritin is an antihistamine that relieves the sneezing, runny nose, stuffiness, itching, and tearing eyes caused by hay fever. It is also prescribed for relief of the swollen, red, itchy patches of skin labeled chronic hives.

Most important fact about this drug
If you have liver or kidney disease, your doctor should prescribe a lower starting dose of Claritin.

How should you take this medication?
Claritin is available in syrup, regular tablets, and rapidly dissolving tablets called Reditabs. The Reditabs should be placed on the tongue rather than swallowed. They disintegrate rapidly and can be taken with or without water.

- *If you miss a dose...*
  Take the forgotten dose as soon as you remember. If it is almost time for your next dose, skip the one you missed. Never take two doses at the same time.

- *Storage instructions...*
  Claritin can be stored at room temperature. The Reditabs should be kept in a dry place. Use them within 6 months after opening the foil pouch in which they are packed. Take each tablet immediately after removing it from its individual blister.

What side effects may occur?
Side effects cannot be anticipated. If any develop or change in intensity, inform your doctor as soon as possible. Only your doctor can determine if it is safe for you to continue taking Claritin.

- *More common side effects may include:*
  Dry mouth, fatigue, headache, sleepiness

- *Less common or rare side effects may include:*
  Abdominal discomfort or pain, abnormal dreams, agitation, anxiety, back pain, blurred vision, breast enlargement, breast pain, bronchitis, change in salivation, change in taste, chest pain, chills and fever, confusion, conjunctivitis (pinkeye), constipation, coughing, coughing up blood, decreased sensitivity to touch, decreased sex drive, depression, diarrhea, difficult or labored breathing, difficulty concentrating, difficulty speaking, discoloration of urine, dizziness, dry hair, dry skin, earache, eye pain, fainting, fever, flushing, gas, general feeling of illness, hair loss, hepatitis, high blood pressure, hives, hyperactivity, impotence, increased appetite, increased or decreased eye tearing, increased sweating, indigestion, inflammation of the mouth, insomnia, itching, joint pain, laryngitis, leg cramps, loss of appetite, low blood pressure, memory loss, menstrual changes, migraine, muscle pain, nasal congestion or dryness, nausea,

nervousness, nosebleeds, palpitations, rapid heartbeat, rash, ringing in ears, seizures, sensitivity to light, sinus inflammation, skin inflammation, sneezing, sore throat, stomach inflammation, swelling, thirst, tingling, toothache, tremor, twitching of the eye, upper respiratory infection, urinary changes, vaginal inflammation, vertigo, vomiting, weakness, weight gain, wheezing, yellow eyes and skin

Why should this drug not be prescribed?

Do not take Claritin if you are sensitive to or have ever had an allergic reaction to it. Make sure your doctor is aware of any drug reactions that you have experienced.

Special warnings about this medication

This medication may cause excessive sleepiness in people with liver or kidney disease, or older adults, and should be used with caution.

Possible food and drug interactions
when taking this medication

Although no harmful interactions with Claritin have been reported, there is a theoretical possibility of an interaction with the following drugs:

Antibiotics such as erythromycin and Biaxin
Cimetidine (Tagamet)
Ketoconazole (Nizoral)
Ranitidine (Zantac)
Theophylline (Theo-Dur)

Special information
if you are pregnant or breastfeeding

The effects of Claritin during pregnancy have not been adequately studied. If you are pregnant or plan to become pregnant, inform your doctor immediately. Claritin appears in breast milk and could affect a nursing infant. If this medication is essential to your health, your doctor may advise you to discontinue breastfeeding until your treatment with Claritin is finished.

Recommended dosage

ADULTS AND CHILDREN 6 YEARS OF AGE AND OVER

The usual dose is 10 milligrams once a day, taken as 1 tablet or 2 teaspoonfuls of syrup. In people with liver or kidney disease, the usual dose is 10 milligrams every other day.

Overdosage
Any medication taken in excess can have serious consequences. If you suspect an overdose, seek medical attention immediately.

■ *Symptoms of Claritin overdose may include:*
   Headache, rapid heartbeat, sleepiness

Brand name:

CLARITIN-D

Pronounced: CLAR-i-tin dee
Generic ingredients: Loratadine, Pseudoephedrine sulfate

Why is this drug prescribed?
Claritin-D is an antihistamine and decongestant that relieves the sneezing, runny nose, stuffiness, and itchy, tearing eyes caused by hay fever. Two versions are available: Claritin-D 12 Hour for twice-daily dosing and Claritin-D 24 Hour for once-a-day use.

Most important fact about this drug
If you have liver disease, make sure the doctor is aware of it. Claritin-D is not recommended in this situation.

How should you take this medication?
Take Claritin-D exactly as prescribed by your doctor. Do not break or chew the tablet. Take the 24-hour variety with a glass of water.

■ *If you miss a dose...*
   Take it as soon as you remember. If it is almost time for your next dose, skip the one you missed. Never take 2 doses at the same time.

■ *Storage instructions...*
   Store at room temperature.

What side effects may occur?
Side effects cannot be anticipated. If any develop or change in intensity, inform your doctor as soon as possible. Only your doctor can determine if it is safe for you to continue taking Claritin-D.

■ *More common side effects may include:*
   Coughing, dizziness, dry mouth, fatigue, insomnia, nausea, nervousness, sleepiness, sore throat

■ *Less common or rare side effects may include:*
Abnormal heart beat, abnormal skin sensations, acne, altered taste sensation, altered tear production, back pain, breathing difficulties, chest pain, conjunctivitis (pinkeye), constipation, convulsions, depression, diarrhea, difficulty speaking, distended abdomen, earache, eye pain, facial swelling, fatigue, flu-like symptoms, flushing, frequent urination, gas, high blood pressure, inability to urinate, increased sputum production, increased sweating, indigestion, itching, leg cramps, migraine headache, mood disorders, movement abnormalities, muscle pain, muscle stiffness, nasal congestion, nervousness, nosebleed, painful menstrual periods, pneumonia, ringing in ears, sinus problems, swollen mouth, thirst, toothache, tremor, upset stomach, urinary tract infection, vaginal swelling, viral infections, vision problems, vomiting, weakness, weight loss, wheezing

Why should this drug not be prescribed?
Do not take Claritin-D if you have ever had an allergic reaction to any of its ingredients.

Avoid Claritin-D if you have the eye condition called narrow-angle glaucoma, very high blood pressure, or coronary artery disease; and do not take the drug if you have difficulty urinating. Also avoid taking Claritin-D within 14 days of taking any drug classified as an MAO inhibitor, including the antidepressants Nardil and Parnate.

Do not use Claritin-D 24 Hour if you have trouble swallowing or have been diagnosed with a narrowing of the food canal (esophagus) leading to your stomach.

Special warnings about this medication
If you are taking Claritin-D and experience insomnia, dizziness, weakness, tremor, or unusual heartbeats, tell your doctor; you may be having an allergic reaction.

You must be careful using Claritin-D if you have diabetes, heart disease, an overactive thyroid gland, kidney or liver problems, or an enlarged prostate gland.

Do not use Claritin-D with over-the-counter antihistamines and decongestants.

Possible food and drug interactions
when taking this medication
Check with your doctor before combining Claritin-D with any of the following:

Blood pressure medications classified as beta blockers, such as Inderal
and Tenormin

Digoxin (Lanoxin)

MAO inhibitors, such as the antidepressants Nardil and Parnate

Mecamylamine (Inversine)

Methyldopa (Aldomet)

Reserpine

Special information
if you are pregnant or breastfeeding

The effects of Claritin-D during pregnancy have not been adequately studied.
If you are pregnant or plan to become pregnant, inform your doctor
immediately. Claritin-D may appear in breast milk. If this medication is
essential to your health, your doctor may advise you not to breastfeed until
your treatment is finished.

Recommended dosage

ADULTS AND CHILDREN 12 YEARS OF AGE AND OVER

The usual dose is 1 tablet every 12 hours for Claritin-D 12 Hour, 1 tablet a
day for Claritin-D 24 Hour. If you have kidney trouble, your doctor will start
you on 1 tablet a day (1 tablet every other day for Claritin-D 24 Hour).

Overdosage

Any medication taken in excess can have serious consequences. If you
suspect an overdose, seek medical attention immediately.

■ *Symptoms of Claritin-D overdose may include:*
Anxiety, breathing difficulty, chest pain, coma, convulsions, delusions,
difficulty urinating, fast, fluttery heartbeat, giddiness, hallucinations,
headache, insomnia, irregular heartbeat, nausea, rapid heartbeat, restlessness, sleepiness, sweating, tension, thirst, vomiting, weakness

Generic name:

CLEMASTINE

See Tavist, page 1259.

Brand name:

CLEOCIN T

Pronounced: KLEE-oh-sin tee
Generic name: Clindamycin phosphate

Why is this drug prescribed?
Cleocin T is an antibiotic used to treat acne.

Most important fact about this drug
Although applied only to the skin, some of this medication could be absorbed into the bloodstream; and it has been known to cause severe—sometimes even fatal—colitis (an inflammation of the lower bowel) when taken internally. Symptoms, which can occur a few days, weeks, or months after beginning treatment with this drug, include severe diarrhea, severe abdominal cramps, and the possibility of the passage of blood.

How should you take this medication?
Use this medication exactly as prescribed. Excessive use of Cleocin T can cause your skin to become too dry or irritated.

- *If you miss a dose...*
  Apply it as soon as you remember. If it is almost time for your next dose, skip the one you missed and go back to your regular schedule.

- *Storage instructions...*
  Store at room temperature. Keep from freezing. Store liquids in tightly closed containers.

What side effects may occur?
Side effects cannot be anticipated. If any develop or change in intensity, inform your doctor as soon as possible. Only your doctor can determine if it is safe for you to continue taking Cleocin T.

- *More common side effects may include:*
  Burning, itching, peeling skin, reddened skin, skin dryness

- *Less common or rare side effects may include:*
  Abdominal pain, bloody diarrhea, colitis, diarrhea, oily skin, skin inflammation and irritation, stomach and intestinal disturbances

Why should this drug not be prescribed?
If you are sensitive to or have ever had an allergic reaction to Cleocin T or

similar drugs, such as Lincocin, you should not use this medication. Make sure your doctor is aware of any drug reactions you have experienced.

Unless you are directed to do so by your doctor, do not take this medication if you have ever had an intestinal inflammation, ulcerative colitis, or antibiotic-associated colitis.

Special warnings about this medication

Cleocin T contains an alcohol base, which can cause burning and irritation of the eyes. It also has an unpleasant taste. Use caution when applying this medication so as not to get it in the eyes, nose, mouth, or skin abrasions. In the event of accidental contact, rinse the affected area with cool water.

Use with caution if you have hay fever, asthma, or eczema.

Possible food and drug interactions
when taking this medication

If you have diarrhea while taking Cleocin T, check with your doctor before taking an antidiarrhea medication, as certain drugs may cause your diarrhea to become worse.

The diarrhea should not be treated with the commonly used drugs that slow movement through the intestinal tract, such as Lomotil or products containing paregoric.

Special information
if you are pregnant or breastfeeding

The effects of Cleocin T during pregnancy have not been adequately studied. If you are pregnant or plan to become pregnant, inform your doctor immediately. Cleocin T may appear in breast milk and could affect a nursing infant. If this medication is essential to your health, your doctor may advise you to discontinue breastfeeding your baby until your treatment with this medication is finished.

Recommended dosage

ADULTS

Apply a thin film of gel, solution, or lotion to the affected area 2 times a day, or use a solution pledget (application pad). Discard a pledget after you have used it once; you may use more than 1 pledget for a treatment. Do not remove the pledget from its foil container until you are ready to use it.

If you are using the lotion, shake it well immediately before using.

CHILDREN

The safety and effectiveness of Cleocin T have not been established in children under 12 years of age.

Overdosage

Cleocin T can be absorbed through the skin and produce side effects in the body. If you suspect an overdose, seek medical attention immediately.

Brand name:

CLIMARA

See Estraderm, page 490.

Generic name:

CLINDAMYCIN

See Cleocin T, page 256.

Brand name:

CLINORIL

Pronounced: CLIN-or-il
Generic name: Sulindac

Why is this drug prescribed?

Clinoril, a nonsteroidal anti-inflammatory drug, is used to relieve the inflammation, swelling, stiffness, and joint pain associated with rheumatoid arthritis, osteoarthritis (the most common form of arthritis), and ankylosing spondylitis (stiffness and progressive arthritis of the spine). It is also used to treat bursitis, tendinitis, acute gouty arthritis, and other types of pain.

The safety and effectiveness of this medication in the treatment of people with severe, incapacitating rheumatoid arthritis have not been established.

Most important fact about this drug

You should have frequent checkups with your doctor if you take Clinoril regularly. Ulcers or internal bleeding can occur without warning.

How should you take this medication?

Take this medication exactly as prescribed by your doctor.

If you are using Clinoril for arthritis, it should be taken regularly.

■ *If you miss a dose...*
Take it as soon as you remember. If it is almost time for your next dose, skip the one you missed and go back to your regular schedule. Never take 2 doses at the same time.

■ *Storage instructions...*
Do not store in damp places like the bathroom.

What side effects may occur?
Side effects cannot be anticipated. If any develop or change in intensity, inform your doctor as soon as possible. Only your doctor can determine if it is safe for you to continue taking Clinoril.

■ *More common side effects may include:*
Abdominal pain, constipation, diarrhea, dizziness, gas, headache, indigestion, itching, loss of appetite, nausea, nervousness, rash, ringing in ears, stomach cramps, swelling due to fluid retention, vomiting

■ *Less common or rare side effects may include:*
Abdominal bleeding, abdominal inflammation, anemia, appetite change, bloody diarrhea, blurred vision, change in color of urine, chest pain, colitis, congestive heart failure, depression, fever, hair loss, hearing loss, hepatitis, high blood pressure, inability to sleep, inflammation of lips and tongue, kidney failure, liver failure, loss of sense of taste, low blood pressure, muscle and joint pain, nosebleed, painful urination, pancreatitis, peptic ulcer, sensitivity to light, shortness of breath, skin eruptions, sleepiness, Stevens-Johnson syndrome (blisters in the mouth and eyes), vaginal bleeding, weakness, yellow eyes and skin

Why should this drug not be prescribed?
If you are sensitive to or have ever had an allergic reaction to Clinoril, aspirin, or similar drugs, or if you have had asthma attacks caused by aspirin or other drugs of this type, you should not take this medication. Make sure that your doctor is aware of any drug reactions that you have experienced.

Special warnings about this medication
Peptic ulcers and bleeding can occur without warning.

This drug should be used with caution if you have kidney or liver disease; it can cause liver inflammation in some people.

Do not take aspirin or any other anti-inflammatory medications while taking Clinoril, unless your doctor tells you to do so.

Nonsteroidal anti-inflammatory drugs such as Clinoril can hide the signs and symptoms of an infection. Be sure your doctor knows about any infection you may have.

Clinoril can cause vision problems. If you experience a change in your vision, inform your doctor.

If you have heart disease or high blood pressure, this drug can increase water retention. Use with caution.

If you develop pancreatitis (inflammation of the pancreas), Clinoril should be stopped immediately and not restarted.

Clinoril may cause you to become drowsy or less alert. If this happens, driving or operating dangerous machinery or participating in any hazardous activity that requires full mental alertness is not recommended.

Possible food and drug interactions
when taking this medication

If Clinoril is taken with certain other drugs, the effects of either could be increased, decreased, or altered. It is especially important to check with your doctor before combining Clinoril with the following:

Aspirin
Blood thinners such as Coumadin
Cyclosporine (Sandimmune)
Diflunisal (Dolobid)
Dimethyl sulfoxide (DMSO)
Lithium
Loop diuretics such as Lasix
Methotrexate
Oral diabetes medications
Other nonsteroidal anti-inflammatory drugs (Aleve, Motrin, others)
The antigout medication Benemid

Special information
if you are pregnant or breastfeeding

The effects of Clinoril during pregnancy have not been adequately studied; drugs of this class are known to cause birth defects. If you are pregnant or plan to become pregnant, inform your doctor immediately. Clinoril may appear in breast milk and could affect a nursing infant. If this medication is essential to your health, your doctor may advise you to discontinue breastfeeding until your treatment with Clinoril is finished.

Recommended dosage

ADULTS

Osteoarthritis, Rheumatoid Arthritis, Ankylosing Spondylitis

Starting dosage is 150 milligrams 2 times a day. Take with food. Doses should not exceed 400 milligrams per day.

Acute Gouty Arthritis or Arthritic Shoulder and Joint Condition

400 milligrams daily taken in doses of 200 milligrams 2 times a day.

For acute painful shoulder, therapy lasting 7 to 14 days is usually adequate.

For acute gouty arthritis, therapy lasting 7 days is usually adequate.

The lowest dose that proves beneficial should be used.

CHILDREN

The safety and effectiveness of Clinoril have not been established in children.

Overdosage

Any medication taken in excess can cause symptoms of overdose. If you suspect an overdose, seek medical attention immediately.

■ *Symptoms of Clinoril overdose may include:*
 Coma, low blood pressure, reduced output of urine, stupor

Generic name:

CLOBETASOL

See Temovate, page 1269.

Brand name:

CLOMID

See Clomiphene Citrate, page 262.

Generic name:

CLOMIPHENE CITRATE

Pronounced: KLAHM-if-een SIT-rate
Brand names: Clomid, Serophene

Why is this drug prescribed?
Clomiphene is prescribed for the treatment of ovulatory failure in women who wish to become pregnant and whose husbands are fertile and potent.

Most important fact about this drug
Properly timed sexual intercourse is very important to increase the chances of conception. The likelihood of conception diminishes with each succeeding course of treatment. Your doctor will determine the need for continuing therapy after the first course. If you do not ovulate after 3 courses or do not become pregnant after 3 ovulations, your doctor will stop the therapy.

How should you take this medication?
Take this medication exactly as prescribed by your doctor.

■ *If you miss a dose...*
Take it as soon as you remember. If it is time for your next dose, take the 2 doses together and go back to your regular schedule. If you miss more than 1 dose, contact your doctor.

■ *Storage instructions...*
Store at room temperature in a tightly closed container, away from light, moisture, and excessive heat.

What side effects may occur?
Side effects occur infrequently and generally do not interfere with treatment at the recommended dosage of clomiphene. They tend to occur more frequently at higher doses and during long-term treatment.

■ *More common side effects include:*
Abdominal discomfort, enlargement of the ovaries, hot flushes

■ *Less common side effects include:*
Abnormal uterine bleeding, breast tenderness, depression, dizziness, fatigue, hair loss, headache, hives, inability to fall or stay asleep, increased urination, inflammation of the skin, light-headedness, nausea, nervousness, ovarian cysts, visual disturbances, vomiting, weight gain

Why should this drug not be prescribed?
If you are pregnant or think you may be, do not take this drug.

Unless directed to do so by your doctor, do not use this medication if you have an uncontrolled thyroid or adrenal gland disorder, an abnormality of the brain such as a pituitary gland tumor, a liver disease or a history of liver problems, abnormal uterine bleeding of undetermined origin, ovarian cysts, or enlargement of the ovaries not caused by polycystic ovarian syndrome (a hormonal disorder causing lack of ovulation).

Special warnings about this medication

Your doctor will evaluate you for normal liver function and normal estrogen levels before considering you for treatment with clomiphene.

Your doctor will also examine you for pregnancy, ovarian enlargement, or cyst formation prior to treatment with this drug and between each treatment cycle. He or she will do a complete pelvic examination before each course of this medication.

Clomiphene treatment increases the possibility of multiple births; also, birth defects have been reported following treatment to induce ovulation with clomiphene, although no direct effects of the drug on the unborn child have been established.

Because blurring and other visual symptoms may occur occasionally with clomiphene treatment, you should be cautious about driving a car or operating dangerous machinery, especially under conditions of variable lighting.

If you experience visual disturbances, notify your doctor immediately. Symptoms of visual disturbance may include blurring, spots or flashes, double vision, intolerance to light, decreased visual sharpness, loss of peripheral vision, and distortion of space. Your doctor may recommend a complete evaluation by an eye specialist.

Ovarian hyperstimulation syndrome (or OHSS, enlargement of the ovary) has occurred in women receiving treatment with clomiphene. OHSS may progress rapidly and become serious. The early warning signs are severe pelvic pain, nausea, vomiting, and weight gain. Symptoms include abdominal pain, abdominal enlargement, nausea, vomiting, diarrhea, weight gain, difficult or labored breathing, and less urine production. If you experience any of these warning signs or symptoms, notify your doctor immediately.

To lessen the risks associated with abnormal ovarian enlargement during treatment with clomiphene, the lowest effective dose should be prescribed. Women with the hormonal disorder, polycystic ovarian syndrome, may be unusually sensitive to certain hormones and may respond abnormally to usual doses of this drug. If you experience pelvic pain, notify your doctor. He may discontinue your use of clomiphene until the ovaries return to pretreatment size.

Because the safety of long-term treatment with clomiphene has not been established, your doctor will not prescribe more than about 6 courses of therapy. Prolonged use may increase the risk of a tumor in the ovaries.

Possible food and drug interactions
when taking this medication
No food or drug interactions have been reported.

Special information
if you are pregnant or breastfeeding
If you become pregnant, notify your doctor immediately. You should not be taking this drug while you are pregnant.

Recommended dosage
The recommended dosage for the first course of treatment is 50 milligrams (1 tablet) daily for 5 days. If ovulation does not appear to have occurred, your doctor may try up to 2 more times.

Overdosage
Taking any medication in excess can have serious consequences. If you suspect an overdose of clomiphene, contact your doctor immediately.

Generic name:

CLOMIPRAMINE

See Anafranil, page 62.

Generic name:

CLONAZEPAM

See Klonopin, page 657.

Generic name:

CLONIDINE

See Catapres, page 213.

Generic name:

CLOPIDOGREL

See Plavix, page 1011.

Generic name:

CLORAZEPATE

See Tranxene, page 1332.

Generic name:

CLOTRIMAZOLE

See Gyne-Lotrimin, page 576.

Generic name:

CLOTRIMAZOLE WITH BETAMETHASONE

See Lotrisone, page 735.

Generic name:

CLOZAPINE

See Clozaril, page 266.

Brand name:

CLOZARIL

Pronounced: KLOH-zah-ril
Generic name: Clozapine

Why is this drug prescribed?
Clozaril is given to help people with severe schizophrenia who have failed to respond to standard treatments. Clozaril is not a cure, but it can help some people return to more normal lives.

Most important fact about this drug
Even though it does not produce some of the disturbing side effects of other antipsychotic medications, Clozaril may cause agranulocytosis, a potentially lethal disorder of the white blood cells. Because of the risk of agranulocytosis, anyone who takes Clozaril is required to have a blood test once a week for the first 6 months. The drug is carefully controlled so that those taking it must get their weekly blood test before receiving the following week's supply of medication. If your blood counts have been acceptable for the 6-month period, you will need to have your blood tested only every other week thereafter. Anyone whose blood test results are abnormal will be taken off

CLOZARIL / 267

Clozaril either temporarily or permanently, depending on the results of an additional 4 weeks of testing.

How should you take this medication?

Take Clozaril exactly as directed by your doctor. Because of the significant risk of serious side effects associated with this drug, your doctor will periodically reassess the need for continued Clozaril therapy. Clozaril is distributed *only* through the Clozaril Patient Management System, which ensures regular white blood cell testing, monitoring, and pharmacy services prior to delivery of your next supply.

Clozaril may be taken with or without food.

■ *If you miss a dose...*
Take it as soon as you remember. If it is almost time for your next dose, skip the one you missed and go back to your regular schedule. Do not take 2 doses at once.

If you stop taking Clozaril for more than 2 days, do not start taking it again without consulting your physician.

■ *Storage instructions...*
Store at room temperature.

What side effects may occur?

Side effects cannot be anticipated. If any develop or change in intensity, inform your doctor as soon as possible. Only your doctor can determine if it is safe for you to continue taking Clozaril.

The most feared side effect is agranulocytosis, a dangerous drop in the number of a certain kind of white blood cell. Symptoms include fever, lethargy, sore throat, and weakness. If not caught in time, agranulocytosis can be fatal. That is why all people who take Clozaril must have a blood test every week. About 1 percent develop agranulocytosis and must stop taking the drug.

Seizures are another potential side effect, occurring in some 5 percent of people who take Clozaril. The higher the dosage, the greater the risk of seizures.

■ *More common side effects may include:*
Abdominal discomfort, agitation, confusion, constipation, disturbed sleep, dizziness, drowsiness, dry mouth, fainting, fever, headache, heartburn, high blood pressure, inability to sit down, loss or slowness of muscle movement, low blood pressure, nausea, nightmares, rapid heartbeat and other heart conditions, restlessness, rigidity, salivation, sedation, sweating, tremors, vertigo, vision problems, vomiting, weight gain

■ *Less common side effects may include:*
Anemia, angina (severe, crushing chest pain), anxiety, appetite increase, blocked intestine, blood clots, bloodshot eyes, bluish tinge in the skin, breast pain or discomfort, bronchitis, bruising, chest pain, chills or chills and fever, constant involuntary eye movement, coughing, delusions, depression, diarrhea, difficult or labored breathing, difficulty swallowing, dilated pupils, disorientation, dry throat, ear disorders, ejaculation problems, excessive movement, eyelid disorder, fast, fluttery heartbeat, fatigue, fluid retention, frequent urination, hallucinations, heart problems, hives, hot flashes, impacted stool, impotence, inability to fall asleep or stay asleep, inability to hold urine, inability to urinate, increase or decrease in sex drive, involuntary movement, irritability, itching, jerky movements, joint pain, lack of coordination, laryngitis, lethargy, light-headedness (especially when rising quickly from a seated or lying position), loss of appetite, loss of speech, low body temperature, memory loss, muscle pain or ache, muscle spasm, muscle weakness, nosebleed, numbness, pain in back, neck, or legs, painful menstruation, pallor, paranoia, pneumonia or pneumonia-like symptoms, poor coordination, rapid breathing, rash, runny nose, shakiness, shortness of breath, skin inflammation, redness, scaling, slow heartbeat, slurred speech, sneezing, sore or numb tongue, speech difficulty, stomach pain, stuffy nose, stupor, stuttering, swollen salivary glands, thirst, throat discomfort, tics, twitching, urination problems, vaginal infection, vaginal itch, a vague feeling of being sick, weakness, wheezing, yellow skin and eyes

Why should this drug not be prescribed?
Clozaril is considered a somewhat risky medication because of its potential to cause agranulocytosis and seizures. It should be taken only by people whose condition is serious, and who have not been helped by more traditional antipsychotic medications such as Haldol or Mellaril.

You should not take Clozaril if:

■ You have a bone marrow disease or disorder;
■ You have epilepsy that is not controlled;
■ You ever developed an abnormal white blood cell count while taking Clozaril;
■ You are currently taking some other drug, such as Tegretol, that could cause a decrease in white blood cell count or a drug that could affect the bone marrow;
■ You have ever had an allergic reaction to any of its ingredients.

Special warnings about this medication
Clozaril can cause drowsiness, especially at the start of treatment. For this

reason, and also because of the potential for seizures, you should not drive, swim, climb, or operate dangerous machinery while you are taking this medication, at least in the early stages of treatment.

Even though you will have blood tests weekly for the first 6 months of treatment and every other week after that, you should stay alert for early symptoms of agranulocytosis: weakness, lethargy, fever, sore throat, a general feeling of illness, a flu-like feeling, or ulcers of the lips, mouth, or other mucous membranes. If any such symptoms develop, tell your doctor immediately.

Especially during the first 3 weeks of treatment, you may develop a fever. If you do, notify your doctor.

While taking Clozaril, do not drink alcohol or use drugs of any kind, including over-the-counter medicines, without first checking with your doctor.

If you take Clozaril, you must be monitored especially closely if you have either the eye condition called narrow-angle glaucoma or an enlarged prostate; Clozaril could make these conditions worse.

On rare occasions, Clozaril can cause intestinal problems—constipation, impaction, or blockage—that can, in extreme cases, be fatal.

Especially when you begin taking Clozaril, you may feel light-headed upon standing up, to the point where you pass out.

If you have kidney, liver, lung, or heart disease, or a history of seizures or prostate problems, you should discuss these with your doctor before taking Clozaril. Nausea, vomiting, loss of appetite, and a yellow tinge to your skin and eyes are signs of liver trouble; call your doctor immediately if you develop these symptoms.

Drugs such as Clozaril can sometimes cause a set of symptoms called Neuroleptic Malignant Syndrome. Symptoms include high fever, muscle rigidity, irregular pulse or blood pressure, rapid heartbeat, excessive perspiration, and changes in heart rhythm. Your doctor will have you stop taking Clozaril while this condition is being treated.

There is also a risk of developing tardive dyskinesia, a condition of involuntary, slow, rhythmical movements. It happens more often in older adults, especially older women.

Clozaril has been known to occasionally raise blood sugar levels, causing unusual hunger, thirst, and weakness, along with excessive urination. If you develop these symptoms, alert your doctor. You may have to switch to a different medication.

In very rare instances, Clozaril may also cause a blood clot in the lungs. If you develop severe breathing problems or chest pain, call your doctor immediately.

Possible food and drug interactions
when taking this medication

If Clozaril is taken with certain other drugs, the effects of either could be increased, decreased, or altered. It is especially important to check with your doctor before combining Clozaril with the following:

Alcohol
Antidepressants such as Prozac and Zoloft
Antipsychotic drugs such as Thorazine and Mellaril
Blood pressure medications such as Aldomet and Hytrin
Cimetidine (Tagamet)
Digitoxin (Crystodigin)
Digoxin (Lanoxin)
Drugs that depress the central nervous system such as phenobarbital and Seconal
Drugs that contain atropine such as Donnatal and Levsin
Epilepsy drugs such as Tegretol and Dilantin
Epinephrine (EpiPen)
Erythromycin (E-Mycin, Eryc, others)
Fluvoxamine (Luvox)
Heart rhythm stabilizers such as Quinidex and Tambocor
Tranquilizers such as Valium and Xanax
Warfarin (Coumadin and Panwarfin)

Special information
if you are pregnant or breastfeeding

The effects of Clozaril during pregnancy have not been adequately studied. If you are pregnant or plan to become pregnant, inform your doctor immediately. Clozaril treatment should be continued during pregnancy only if absolutely necessary. You should not breastfeed if you are taking Clozaril, since the drug may appear in breast milk.

Recommended dosage

ADULTS

Your doctor will carefully individualize your dosage and monitor your response regularly.

The usual recommended initial dose is half of a 25-milligram tablet (12.5 milligrams) 1 or 2 times daily. Your doctor may increase the dosage in increments of 25 to 50 milligrams a day to achieve a daily dose of 300 to 450 milligrams by the end of 2 weeks. Dosage increases after that will be only once or twice a week and will be no more than 100 milligrams each time. The most you can take is 900 milligrams a day divided into 2 or 3 doses.

Your doctor will determine long-term dosage depending upon your response and results of the regular blood tests.

CHILDREN

Safety and efficacy have not been established for children up to 16 years of age.

Overdosage
Any medication taken in excess can have serious consequences. If you suspect an overdose, seek emergency medical attention immediately.

■ *Symptoms of overdose with Clozaril may include:*
Coma, delirium, drowsiness, excess salivation, low blood pressure, faintness, pneumonia, rapid heartbeat, seizures, shallow breathing or absence of breathing

Brand name:

COGENTIN

Pronounced: co-JEN-tin
Generic name: Benztropine mesylate

Why is this drug prescribed?
Cogentin is given to help relieve the symptoms of "parkinsonism": the muscle rigidity, tremors, and difficulties with posture and balance that occur in Parkinson's disease and that sometimes develop as unwanted side effects of antipsychotic drugs such as Haldol and Thorazine.

Cogentin is an "anticholinergic" medication, a drug that controls spasms. It reduces the symptoms of parkinsonism, but it is not a cure.

Most important fact about this drug
When starting Cogentin, you may not feel its effect for 2 or 3 days. Symptoms caused by drugs such as Haldol and Thorazine are often temporary, so if drug-induced parkinsonism is your problem, you may need to take Cogentin for only a couple of weeks.

How should you take this medication?
Take Cogentin exactly as prescribed. Unlike some of the other antiparkinson-

ian medications, Cogentin acts over a long period of time. It is thus particularly suitable as a bedtime medication because it lasts through the night. Taken at bedtime, it may help a person regain enough muscle control to move and roll over during sleep and to arise unaided in the morning.

Cogentin causes dry mouth. Sucking on sugarless hard candy or sipping water can relieve this problem.

Cogentin can reduce the ability to sweat, one of the key ways your body prevents overheating. Avoid excess sun or exercise that may cause overheating.

■ *If you miss a dose...*
Take it as soon as you remember. If it is within 2 hours of your next dose, skip the one you missed and go back to your regular schedule. Do not take 2 doses at once.

■ *Storage instructions...*
Store away from heat, light, and moisture.

What side effects may occur?
Side effects cannot be anticipated. If any develop or change in intensity, inform your doctor as soon as possible. Only your doctor can determine if it is safe for you to continue taking Cogentin.

■ *Side effects may include:*
Blurred vision, bowel blockage, confusion, constipation, depression, dilated pupils, disorientation, dry mouth, fever, hallucinations, heat stroke, impaired memory, inability to urinate, listlessness, nausea, nervousness, numbness in fingers, painful urination, rapid heartbeat, rash, vomiting

Why should this drug not be prescribed?
Do not take Cogentin if you are sensitive to it or if you have ever had an allergic reaction to it or to any similar antispasmodic medication.

Do not take Cogentin if you have an eye condition called angle-closure glaucoma.

Some people who take certain antipsychotic medications develop tardive dyskinesia, a syndrome of involuntary movements of the mouth, jaw, arms, and legs. Cogentin should not be given to treat tardive dyskinesia; it will not help, and it may make the condition worse.

Cogentin should not be given to children under the age of 3; it should be used with caution in older children.

Special warnings about this medication

Do not drive or operate dangerous machinery while taking Cogentin, since the drug may impair your mental or physical abilities.

Be sure to tell your doctor if you have ever had tachycardia (excessively rapid heartbeats) or if you have an enlarged prostate; you will require especially close monitoring while taking Cogentin in these cases.

Tell your doctor if Cogentin produces weakness in particular muscle groups. For example, if you have been suffering from neck rigidity and Cogentin suddenly causes your neck to relax so much that it feels weak, you may be taking more Cogentin than you need.

If you have been taking another antiparkinsonism drug, do not stop taking it abruptly when you start taking Cogentin. If you are to stop taking the other drug, your doctor will have you taper off gradually.

Cogentin has a drying effect on the mouth and other moist tissues. If you take it along with another drug that also has a drying effect, you are at risk for anhidrosis (inability to sweat), heat stroke, and even death from hyperthermia (high fever). Chronic illness, alcoholism, central nervous system (brain and spinal cord) disease, or heavy manual labor in a hot environment can increase this risk. In hot weather, your doctor may lower your dosage of Cogentin.

Possible food and drug interactions
when taking this medication

When taken simultaneously with an antipsychotic medication (Thorazine, Stelazine, Haldol, others) or a tricyclic antidepressant medication (Elavil, Norpramin, Tofranil, others), Cogentin has occasionally caused bowel blockage or heat stroke that proved dangerous or even fatal. If you are taking Cogentin along with an antipsychotic or with a tricyclic antidepressant, tell your doctor immediately if you begin to have any stomach or bowel complaint, fever, or heat intolerance.

Antacids, such as Tums, Maalox, and Mylanta, may decrease the effects of Cogentin. Do not take them within 1 hour of taking Cogentin.

Certain other drugs may also interact with Cogentin. Consult your doctor before combining Cogentin with any of the following:

Amantadine (Symmetrel)
Doxepin (Sinequan)
Antihistamines such as Benadryl and Tavist
Other anticholinergic agents such as Bentyl

Special information
if you are pregnant or breastfeeding

If you are pregnant or plan to become pregnant, inform your doctor immediately. No information is available about the safety of taking Cogentin during pregnancy or while you are breastfeeding.

Recommended dosage

Your doctor will individualize the dose of Cogentin, taking into consideration your age and weight, the condition being treated, the presence of other diseases, and any physical disorder.

In general, the usual oral dose is 1 to 2 milligrams a day, but it can range from 0.5 to 6 milligrams a day.

Overdosage

Any medication taken in excess can have serious consequences. If you suspect symptoms of an overdose of Cogentin, seek medical attention immediately. Symptoms of overdose may include any of those listed in the "side effects section" (see page 250) or any of the following:

Blurred vision, confusion, coma, constipation, convulsions, delirium, difficulty swallowing or breathing, dilated pupils, dizziness, dry mouth, flushed, dry skin, glaucoma, hallucinations, headache, high blood pressure, high body temperature, inability to sweat, listlessness, muscle weakness, nausea, nervousness, numb fingers, painful urination, palpitations, rapid heartbeat, rash, shock, uncoordinated movements, vomiting

Brand name:

CO-GESIC

See Vicodin, page 1403.

Brand name:

COGNEX

Pronounced: COG-necks
Generic name: Tacrine hydrochloride

Why is this drug prescribed?

Cognex is used for the treatment of mild to moderate Alzheimer's disease. This progressive, degenerative disorder causes physical changes in the brain that disrupt the flow of information and affect memory, thinking, and behavior. As someone caring for a person with Alzheimer's, you should be aware that Cognex is not a cure, but has helped some people.

Most important fact about this drug
Do not abruptly stop Cognex treatment, or reduce the dosage, without consulting the doctor. A sudden reduction can cause the person you are caring for to become more disturbed and forgetful. Taking more Cognex than the doctor advises can also cause serious problems. Do not change the dosage of Cognex unless instructed by the doctor.

How should you take this medication?
This medication will work better if taken at regular intervals, usually 4 times a day. Cognex is best taken between meals; however, if it is irritating to the stomach, the doctor may advise taking it with meals. If Cognex is not taken regularly, as the doctor directs, the condition may get worse.

■ *If you miss a dose...*
Give the forgotten dose as soon as possible. If it is within 2 hours of the next dose, skip the missed dose and go back to the regular schedule. Do not double the doses.

■ *Storage instructions...*
Store at room temperature away from moisture.

What side effects may occur?
Side effects cannot be anticipated. If any develop or change in intensity, tell the doctor as soon as possible. Only the doctor can determine if it is safe to continue giving Cognex.

■ *More common side effects may include:*
Abdominal pain, abnormal thinking, agitation, anxiety, chest pain, clumsiness or unsteadiness, confusion, constipation, coughing, depression, diarrhea, dizziness, fatigue, flushing, frequent urination, gas, headache, inflamed nasal passages, insomnia, indigestion, liver function disorders, loss of appetite, muscle pain, nausea, rash, sleepiness, upper respiratory infection, urinary tract infection, vomiting, weight loss

■ *Less common side effects may include:*
Back pain, hallucinations, hostile attitude, purple or red spots on the skin, skin discoloration, tremor, weakness

Be sure to report any symptoms that develop while on Cognex therapy. You should alert the doctor if the person you are caring for develops nausea, vomiting, loose stools, or diarrhea at the start of therapy or when the dosage is increased. Later in therapy, be on the lookout for rash or fever, yellowing of the eyes and skin, or changes in the color of the stool.

Why should this drug not be prescribed?

People who are sensitive to or have ever had an allergic reaction to Cognex (including symptoms such as rash or fever) should not take this medication. Before starting treatment with Cognex, it is important to discuss any medical problems with the doctor. If during previous Cognex therapy the person you are caring for developed jaundice (yellow skin and eyes), which signals that something is wrong with the liver, Cognex should not be used again.

Special warnings about this medication

Use Cognex with caution if the person you are caring for has a history of liver disease, certain heart disorders, stomach ulcers, or asthma.

Because of the risk of liver problems when taking Cognex, the doctor will schedule blood tests every other week to monitor liver function from at least the fourth week to the sixteenth week of treatment. After 16 weeks, blood tests will be given monthly for 2 months and every 3 months after that. If the person you are caring for develops any liver problems, the doctor may temporarily discontinue Cognex treatment until further testing shows that the liver has returned to normal. If the doctor resumes Cognex treatment, regular blood tests will be conducted again. Blood tests should be performed every other week for at least the first 16 weeks at the beginning of Cognex treatment in order to monitor liver function. If no significant changes in liver function have been observed, monitoring may be decreased to monthly for 2 months and every 3 months thereafter.

Before having any surgery, including dental surgery, tell the doctor that the person is being treated with Cognex.

Cognex can cause seizures, and may cause difficulty urinating.

Possible food and drug interactions
when taking this medication

If Cognex is taken with certain other drugs, the effects of either could be increased, decreased, or altered. It is especially important that you check with your doctor before combining Cognex with the following:

Antispasmodic drugs such as Bentyl and Levsin
Bethanechol chloride (Urecholine)
Cimetidine (Tagamet)
Fluvoxamine (Luvox)
Muscle stimulants such as Mestinon, Mytelase, and Prostigmin
Nonsteroidal anti-inflammatory drugs such as Aleve, Motrin, and
    Naprosyn
The Parkinson's medications Artane and Cogentin
Theophylline (Theo-Dur)

Special information
if you are pregnant or breastfeeding
The effects of Cognex during pregnancy have not been studied; and it is not known whether Cognex appears in breast milk.

Recommended dosage

ADULTS

The usual starting dose is 10 milligrams 4 times a day, for at least 4 weeks. Do not increase the dose during this 4-week period unless directed by your doctor.

Depending on your tolerance of the drug, dosage may then be increased at 4-week intervals, first to 20 milligrams, then to 30, and finally to 40, always taken 4 times a day.

CHILDREN

The safety and effectiveness of Cognex have not been established in children.

Overdosage

Any medication taken in excess can have serious consequences. If you suspect an overdose, seek medical attention immediately.

- *Symptoms of Cognex overdose include:*
  Collapse, convulsions, extreme muscle weakness, possibly ending in death (if breathing muscles are affected), low blood pressure, nausea, salivation, slowed heart rate, sweating, vomiting.

Brand name:

COLACE

Pronounced: KOH-lace
Generic name: Docusate sodium
Other brand name: Sof-Lax

Why is this drug prescribed?
Colace, a stool softener, promotes easy bowel movements without straining. It softens the stool by mixing in fat and water.

Colace is helpful for people who have had recent rectal surgery, people with heart problems, high blood pressure, hemorrhoids, or hernias, and women who have just had babies.

Colace Microenema is used to relieve occasional constipation.

Most important fact about this drug

Colace is for short-term relief only, unless your doctor directs otherwise. It usually takes a day or two for the drug to achieve its laxative effect; some people may need to wait 4 or 5 days. Sof-Lax Overnight works in 6 to 12 hours. Colace Microenema works in 2 to 15 minutes.

How should you take this medication?

To conceal the drug's bitter taste, take Colace liquid in half a glass of milk or fruit juice; it can be given in infant formula. The proper dosage of this medication may also be added to a retention or flushing enema.

For Colace Microenema:

1. Lubricate the tip by pushing out a drop of the medication.
2. Slowly insert the full length of the nozzle into the rectum. (Stop halfway for children aged 3 to 12 years of age.)
3. Squeeze out the contents of the tube.
4. Remove the nozzle before you release your grip on the tube.

■ *If you miss a dose...*
Take this medication only as needed.

■ *Storage instructions...*
Store at room temperature. Keep from freezing.

What side effects may occur?

Side effects are unlikely. The main ones reported are bitter taste, throat irritation, and nausea (mainly associated with use of the syrup and liquid). Rash has occurred.

Why should this drug not be prescribed?

There are no known reasons this drug should not be prescribed.

Special warnings about this medication

Do not use this product if you have any abdominal pain, nausea, or vomiting, unless your doctor advises it. Do not take this product if you are taking mineral oil. If you have noticed a change in your bowel habits that has lasted for 2 weeks, ask your doctor before you use this product. If you bleed from the rectum or you do not have a bowel movement after using this product, stop using it and call your doctor; you may have a more serious condition. Do not use any laxative for more than a week without your doctor's approval.

Possible food and drug interactions when taking this medication

No interactions have been reported with Colace.

Special information
if you are pregnant or breastfeeding
If you are pregnant, plan to become pregnant, or are breastfeeding your baby, notify your doctor before using this medication.

Recommended dosage
Your doctor will adjust the dosage according to your needs.

You will be using higher doses at the start of treatment with Colace. You should see an effect on stools 1 to 3 days after the first dose.

Colace Microenema should produce a bowel movement in 2 to 15 minutes.

ADULTS AND CHILDREN 12 AND OLDER

The suggested daily dosage of Colace is 50 to 200 milligrams.

In enemas, add 50 to 100 milligrams of Colace or 5 to 10 milliliters of Colace liquid to a retention or flushing enema, as prescribed by your doctor.

For Colace Microenema, use the entire contents of the tube.

CHILDREN UNDER 12

The suggested daily dosage of Colace for children 6 to 12 years of age is 40 to 120 milligrams; for children 3 to 6, it is 20 to 60 milligrams; for children under 3, it is 10 to 40 milligrams.

Colace Microenema should not be given to children under 3.

Overdosage
Overdose is unlikely with normal use of Colace. If you or your child should accidentally take too much, call your doctor or a Poison Control Center.

Brand name:

COLESTID

Pronounced: Koh-LESS-tid
Generic name: Colestipol hydrochloride

Why is this drug prescribed?
Colestid, in conjunction with diet, is used to help lower high levels of cholesterol in the blood. It is available in plain and orange-flavored granules and in tablet form.

Most important fact about this drug
Accidentally inhaling Colestid granules may cause serious effects. To avoid this, NEVER take them in their dry form. Colestid granules should always be mixed with water or other liquids BEFORE you take them.

How should you take this medication?
Colestid granules should be mixed with liquids such as:
  Carbonated beverages (may cause stomach or intestinal discomfort)
  Flavored drinks
  Milk
  Orange juice
  Pineapple juice
  Tomato juice
  Water

Colestid may also be mixed with:
  Milk used on breakfast cereals
  Pulpy fruit (such as crushed peaches, pears, or pineapple) or fruit
    cocktail
  Soups with a high liquid content (such as chicken noodle or tomato)

To take Colestid granules with beverages:
1. Measure at least 3 ounces of liquid into a glass.
2. Add the prescribed dose of Colestid to the liquid.
3. Stir until Colestid is completely mixed (it will not dissolve) and then drink the mixture.
4. Pour a small amount of the beverage into the glass, swish it around, and drink it. This will help make sure you have taken all the medication.

Swallow Colestid tablets whole, one at a time. Do not cut, chew, or crush them. Take the tablets with plenty of water or other liquid.

■ *If you miss a dose...*
   Take the forgotten dose as soon as you remember. If it is almost time for the next dose, skip the one you missed and go back to your regular schedule. Never try to "catch up" by doubling the dose.

■ *Storage instructions...*
   Store Colestid granules and tablets at room temperature.

What side effects may occur?
Side effects cannot be anticipated. If any develop or change in intensity, inform your doctor as soon as possible. Only your doctor can determine if it is safe for you to continue taking Colestid.

- *Most common side effects:*
Constipation, worsening of hemorrhoids

- *Less common or rare side effects may include:*
Abdominal bloating or distention/cramping/pain, arthritis, diarrhea, dizziness, fatigue, gas, headache, hives, joint pain, loss of appetite, muscle pain, nausea, shortness of breath, skin inflammation, vomiting, weakness

- *Additional side effects from regular Colestid granules may include:*
Anxiety, belching, drowsiness, vertigo

- *Additional side effects from Flavored Colestid granules or Colestid tablets may include:*
Aches and pains in arms and legs, angina (crushing chest pain), backache, bleeding hemorrhoids, blood in the stool, bone pain, chest pain, heartburn, indigestion, insomnia, light-headedness, loose stools, migraine, rapid heartbeat, rash, sinus headache, swelling of hands or feet

Why should this drug not be prescribed?
You should not be using Colestid if you are allergic to it or any of its components.

Special warnings about this medication
Before starting treatment with Colestid, you should:

- Be tested (and treated) for diseases that may contribute to increased blood cholesterol, such as an underactive thyroid gland, diabetes, nephrotic syndrome (a kidney disease), dysproteinemia (a blood disease), obstructive liver disease, and alcoholism.
- Be on a diet plan (approved by your doctor) that stresses low-cholesterol foods and weight loss (if necessary).

Because certain medications may increase cholesterol, you should tell your doctor all of the medications you use.

Colestid may prevent the absorption of vitamins such as A, D, and K. Long-term use of Colestid may be connected to increased bleeding from a lack of vitamin K. Taking vitamin K_1 will help relieve this condition and prevent it in the future.

Your cholesterol and triglyceride levels should be checked regularly while you are taking Colestid.

Colestid may cause or worsen constipation. Dosages should be adjusted by your doctor. You may need to increase your intake of fiber and fluid. A stool softener also may be needed occasionally. People with coronary artery disease should be especially careful to avoid constipation. Hemorrhoids may be worsened by constipation related to Colestid.

If you have phenylketonuria (a hereditary disease caused by your body's inability to handle the amino acid phenylalanine), be aware that Flavored Colestid granules contain phenylalanine.

Possible food and drug interactions when taking this medication

Colestid may delay or reduce the absorption of other drugs. Allow as much time as possible between taking Colestid and taking other medications. Other drugs should be taken at least 1 hour before or 4 hours after taking Colestid.

If Colestid is taken with certain other drugs, the effects of either could be increased, decreased, or altered. It is especially important to check with your doctor before combining Colestid with the following:

Chlorothiazide (Diuril)
Digitalis (Lanoxin)
Folic acid and vitamins such as A, D, and K
Furosemide (Lasix)
Gemfibrozil (Lopid)
Hydrochlorothiazide (HydroDIURIL)
Hydrocortisone (Anusol-HC, Cortisporin, others)
Penicillin G, including brands such as Pentids
Phosphate supplements
Propranolol (Inderal)
Tetracycline drugs such as Sumycin

Special information if you are pregnant or breastfeeding

The effects of Colestid during pregnancy have not been adequately studied. If you are pregnant or planning to become pregnant, or plan to breastfeed, check with your doctor. Since Colestid interferes with the absorption of fat soluble vitamins A, D, and K it may affect both the mother and the nursing infant.

Recommended dosage

ADULTS

One packet or 1 level scoopful of Flavored Colestid granules contains 5 grams of Colestipol.

The usual starting dose is 1 packet or 1 level scoopful once or twice a day. Your doctor may increase this by 1 dose a day every month or every other month, up to 6 packets or 6 level scoopfuls taken once a day or divided into smaller doses.

If you are taking Colestid tablets, the usual starting dose is 2 grams (2 tablets) once or twice a day. Your doctor may increase the dose every month or every other month, to a maximum of 16 grams a day, taken once a day or divided into smaller doses.

CHILDREN

The safety and effectiveness of Colestid have not been established for children.

Overdosage

Overdoses of Colestid have not been reported. If an overdose occurred, the most likely harmful effect would be obstruction of the stomach and/or intestines. If you suspect an overdose, seek medical help immediately.

Generic name:

COLESTIPOL

See Colestid, page 279.

Generic name:

COLISTIN, NEOMYCIN, HYDROCORTISONE, AND THONZONIUM

See Coly-Mycin S Otic, page 284.

Brand name:

COLY-MYCIN S OTIC

Pronounced: KOH-lee-MY-sin ESS OH-tic
Generic ingredients: Colistin sulfate, Neomycin sulfate,
  Hydrocortisone acetate, Thonzonium bromide

Why is this drug prescribed?
Coly-Mycin S Otic is a liquid suspension used to treat ear infections. Colistin sulfate and neomycin sulfate are antibiotics used to treat the bacterial infection itself, while hydrocortisone acetate is a steroid that helps reduce the inflammation, swelling, itching, and other skin reactions associated with an ear infection; thonzonium bromide facilitates the drug's effects.

Most important fact about this drug
As with other antibiotics, long-term treatment may encourage other infections. Therefore, if your ear infection does not improve within a week, your physician may want to change your medication.

How should you use this medication?
Use Coly-Mycin S Otic for the full course of treatment (but no more than 10 days) even if you start to feel better in a few days.

Shake well before using.

The external ear canal should be thoroughly cleaned and dried with a sterile cotton swab (applicator). The person should lie with the infected ear facing up. Pull the earlobe down and back (for children) or up and back (for adults) to straighten the ear canal. Drop the suspension into the ear. The person should lie in this position for 5 minutes to help the drops penetrate into the ear. If necessary, this procedure should be repeated for the other ear. To keep the medicine from leaking out, you can gently insert a sterile cotton plug.

If you prefer, a sterile cotton wick or plug may be inserted into the ear canal and then soaked with the Coly-Mycin S Otic suspension. This cotton wick should be moistened every 4 hours with more suspension and replaced at least once every 24 hours.

Avoid touching the dropper to the ear or other surfaces.

■ *If you miss a dose...*
  Apply it as soon as you remember. If it is almost time for your next dose, skip the one you missed and go back to your regular schedule.

■ *Storage instructions...*
Store at room temperature; avoid prolonged exposure to high temperatures.

What side effects may occur?
No specific side effects have been reported; however, neomycin (an ingredient in Coly-Mycin S Otic) may be associated with an increased risk of allergic skin reaction.

Why should this drug not be prescribed?
You should not take this drug if you have had an allergic reaction to any of the ingredients, or if you suffer from herpes simplex, vaccinia (cowpox), or varicella (chickenpox).

Special warnings about this medication
Treatment should not continue for more than 10 days.

If you warm Coly-Mycin S Otic before applying, do not heat the suspension to above body temperature, since this will lessen its potency. Warm the drops by holding the bottle in your hand for a few minutes.

If an allergic reaction occurs, you should stop using Coly-Mycin S Otic immediately. Your doctor may also recommend that future treatment with kanamycin, paromomycin, streptomycin, and possibly gentamicin be avoided, since you may also be allergic to these medications.

Use Coly-Mycin S Otic with care if you have a perforated eardrum or chronic otitis media (inflammation of the middle ear).

**Possible food and drug interactions
when using this medication**
No interactions have been reported.

**Special information
if you are pregnant or breastfeeding**
The effects of Coly-Mycin S Otic during pregnancy have not been adequately studied. If you are pregnant or plan to become pregnant, inform your doctor immediately. Coly-Mycin S Otic may appear in breast milk and could affect a nursing infant. If this medication is essential to your health, your doctor may advise you to stop breastfeeding until your treatment is finished.

Recommended dosage

ADULTS

The usual dose is 5 drops (when using the supplied measured dropper) or 4 drops (when using the dropper-bottle container) in the affected ear, 3 or 4 times daily.

INFANTS AND CHILDREN

The usual dose is 4 drops (when using the supplied measured dropper) or 3 drops (when using the dropper-bottle container) in the affected ear 3 or 4 times daily.

Please see the "How should you use this medication?" section on page 262 for more information on applying Coly-Mycin S Otic.

Overdosage

Although no specific information is available, any medication taken in excess can have serious consequences. If you suspect an overdose of Coly-Mycin S Otic, seek medical treatment immediately.

Brand name:

COMPAZINE

Pronounced: KOMP-ah-zeen
Generic name: Prochlorperazine

Why is this drug prescribed?

Compazine is used to control severe nausea and vomiting. It is also used to treat symptoms of mental disorders such as schizophrenia, and is occasionally prescribed for anxiety.

Most important fact about this drug

Compazine may cause tardive dyskinesia—involuntary muscle spasms and twitches in the face and body. This condition may be permanent. It appears to be most common among the elderly, especially women. Ask your doctor for information about this possible risk.

How should you take this medication?

Never take more Compazine than prescribed. It can increase the risk of serious side effects.

If you are using the suppository form of Compazine and find it is too soft to insert, you can chill it in the refrigerator for about 30 minutes or run cold water over it before removing the wrapper.

To insert a suppository, first remove the wrapper and moisten the suppository with cold water. Then lie down on your side and use a finger to push the suppository well up into the rectum.

■ *If you miss a dose...*
Take the forgotten dose as soon as you remember. If it is almost time for the next dose, skip the one you missed and go back to your regular schedule. Never try to "catch up" by doubling the dose.

■ *Storage instructions...*
Store at room temperature. Protect from heat and light.

What side effects may occur?
Side effects cannot be anticipated. If any develop or change in intensity, inform your doctor as soon as possible. Only your doctor can determine if it is safe for you to continue taking Compazine.

■ *Side effects may include:*
Abnormal muscle rigidity, abnormal secretion of milk, abnormal sugar in urine, abnormalities of posture and movement, agitation, anemia, appetite changes, asthma, blurred vision, breast development in males, chewing movements, constipation, convulsions, difficulty swallowing, discolored skin tone, dizziness, drooling, drowsiness, dry mouth, ejaculation problems, exaggerated reflexes, fever, fluid retention, head arched backward, headache, heart attack, heels bent back on legs, high or low blood sugar, hives, impotence, inability to urinate, increased psychotic symptoms, increased weight, infection, insomnia, intestinal obstruction, involuntary movements of arms, hands, legs, and feet, involuntary movements of face, tongue, and jaw, irregular movements, jerky movements, jitteriness, light sensitivity, low blood pressure, mask-like face, menstrual irregularities, narrowed or dilated pupils, nasal congestion, nausea, pain in the shoulder and neck area, painful muscle spasm, parkinsonism-like symptoms, persistent, painful erections, pill-rolling motion, protruding tongue, puckering of the mouth, puffing of the cheeks, rigid arms, feet, head, and muscles, rotation of eyeballs or state of fixed gaze, shock, shuffling gait, skin peeling, rash and inflammation, sore throat, mouth, and gums, spasms in back, feet and ankles, jaw, and neck, swelling and itching skin, swelling in throat, tremors, yellowed eyes and skin

Why should this drug not be prescribed?
Do not take Compazine if you are sensitive to or have ever had an allergic reaction to prochlorperazine or other phenothiazine drugs such as Thorazine, Prolixin, Triavil, Mellaril, or Stelazine.

Special warnings about this medication

Never take large amounts of alcohol, barbiturates, or narcotics when taking Compazine. Serious problems can result.

If you suddenly stop taking Compazine, you may experience a change in appetite, dizziness, nausea, vomiting, and tremors. Follow your doctor's instructions closely when discontinuing this drug.

Make sure the doctor knows if you are being treated for a brain tumor, intestinal blockage, heart disease, glaucoma, or an abnormal blood condition such as leukemia, or if you are exposed to extreme heat or pesticides.

This drug may impair your ability to drive a car or operate potentially dangerous machinery. Do not participate in any activities that require full alertness if you are unsure about your ability.

While taking Compazine, try to stay out of the sun. Use sun block and wear protective clothing. Your eyes may become more sensitive to sunlight, too, so keep sunglasses handy.

Compazine interferes with your ability to shed extra heat. Be cautious in hot weather.

Compazine may cause false-positive pregnancy tests.

Possible food and drug interactions
when taking this medication

If Compazine is taken with certain other drugs, the effects of either could be increased, decreased, or altered. It is especially important to check with your doctor before combining Compazine with the following:

Antiseizure drugs such as Dilantin and Tegretol
Anticoagulants such as Coumadin
Guanethidine (Ismelin)
Lithium (Lithobid, Eskalith)
Narcotic painkillers such as Demerol and Tylenol with Codeine
Other central nervous system depressants such as Xanax, Valium,
    Seconal, Halcion
Propranolol (Inderal)
Thiazide diuretics such as Dyazide

Special information
if you are pregnant or breastfeeding

Compazine is not usually recommended for pregnant women. However, your doctor may prescribe it for severe nausea and vomiting if the potential benefits of the drug outweigh the potential risks. Compazine appears in breast milk and may affect a nursing infant. If this drug is essential to your health, your doctor may recommend that you stop breastfeeding until your treatment is finished.

Recommended dosage

ADULTS

To Control Severe Nausea and Vomiting

Tablets: The usual dosage is one 5-milligram or 10-milligram tablet 3 or 4 times a day.

"Spansule" Capsules: The usual starting dose is one 15-milligram capsule on getting out of bed or one 10-milligram capsule every 12 hours.

The usual rectal dosage (suppository) is 25 milligrams, taken 2 times a day.

For Non-Psychotic Anxiety

Tablets: The usual dose is 5 milligrams, taken 3 or 4 times a day.

"Spansule" capsule: The usual starting dose is one 15-milligram capsule on getting up or one 10-milligram capsule every 12 hours.

Treatment should not continue for longer than 12 weeks, and daily doses should not exceed 20 milligrams.

Relatively Mild Psychotic Disorders

The usual dose is 5 or 10 milligrams, taken 3 or 4 times daily.

Moderate to Severe Psychotic Disorders

Dosages usually start at 10 milligrams, taken 3 or 4 times a day. If needed, dosage may be gradually increased; 50 to 75 milligrams daily has been helpful for some people.

More Severe Psychotic Disorders

Dosages may range from 100 to 150 milligrams per day.

CHILDREN

Children under 2 years of age or weighing less than 20 pounds should not be given Compazine. If a child becomes restless or excited after taking Compazine, do not give the child another dose.

For Severe Nausea and Vomiting

An oral or rectal dose of Compazine is usually not needed for more than 1 day.

Children 20 to 29 Pounds
The usual dose is 2½ milligrams 1 or 2 times daily. Total daily amount should not exceed 7.5 milligrams.

Children 30 to 39 Pounds
The usual dose is 2½ milligrams 2 or 3 times daily. Total daily amount should not exceed 10 milligrams.

Children 40 to 85 Pounds
The usual dose is 2½ milligrams 3 times daily, or 5 milligrams 2 times daily.

Total daily amount should not exceed 15 milligrams.

For Psychotic Disorders

Children 2 to 5 Years Old
The starting oral or rectal dose is 2½ milligrams 2 or 3 times daily. Do not exceed 10 milligrams the first day and 20 milligrams thereafter.

Children 6 to 12 Years Old
The starting oral or rectal dose is 2½ milligrams 2 or 3 times daily. Do not exceed 10 milligrams the first day and 25 milligrams thereafter.

OLDER ADULTS

In general, older people take lower dosages of Compazine. Because they may develop low blood pressure while taking the drug, the doctor should monitor them closely. Older people (especially women) may be more susceptible to tardive dyskinesia—a possibly permanent condition. Tardive dyskinesia causes involuntary muscle spasms and twitches in the face and body. Consult your doctor for more information about these potential risks.

Overdosage
An overdose of Compazine can be fatal. If you suspect an overdose, seek medical help immediately.

■ *Symptoms of Compazine overdose may include:*
Agitation, coma, convulsions, dry mouth, extreme sleepiness, fever, intestinal blockage, irregular heart rate, restlessness

Generic name:

CONJUGATED ESTROGENS

See Premarin, page 1036.

Brand name:

COREG

Pronounced: KOE-regg
Generic name: Carvedilol

Why is this drug prescribed?
Coreg lowers blood pressure and increases the output of the heart. It is prescribed for both congestive heart failure and high blood pressure. It is often used with other drugs.

Most important fact about this drug
In some people, Coreg causes a drop in blood pressure when they first stand up, resulting in dizziness or even fainting. If this happens, sit or lie down and notify your doctor. Taking the drug with food reduces the chance of this problem. Even so, during the first month of therapy, or after a change in your dose, be careful about driving and operation of dangerous machinery.

How should you take this medication?
Take Coreg twice a day with food. If you are taking the drug for high blood pressure, there should be improvement within 7 to 14 days.

■ *If you miss a dose...*
Take it as soon as you remember. If it is almost time for your next dose, skip the one you missed and go back to your regular schedule. Do not take 2 doses at once.

■ *Storage instructions...*
Coreg should be stored at room temperature, away from light and moisture. Keep the container tightly closed.

What side effects may occur?
Side effects cannot be anticipated. If any develop or change in intensity, inform your doctor as soon as possible. Only your doctor can determine if it is safe for you to continue taking Coreg.

■ *More common side effects may include:*
Abdominal pain, back pain, bronchitis, chest pain, diarrhea, dizziness, fainting, fatigue, fever, gout, headache, increased blood sugar levels, joint pain, low blood pressure, muscle aches, nausea, pain, respiratory infection, sinus problems, slow heartbeat, sore throat, swelling, urinary infection, vision changes, vomiting, weight gain

■ *Less common side effects may include:*
Allergy, blood in urine, dark stools, dehydration, feeling of illness, gum disease, high blood pressure, impotence, increased sweating, infection, lack of sensitivity to touch, reddish or purplish spots, runny nose, shortness of breath, sleepiness, tingling or numbness, trouble sleeping, vertigo

■ *Rare side effects may include:*
Abnormal thinking, anemia, asthma, changeable emotions, convulsions, decreased sex drive in males, diabetes, digestive bleeding, dry mouth, hair loss, hearing problems, heart problems, impaired concentration, increased urination, itching, memory loss, migraine, nervousness, paralysis, rapid heartbeat, rash, ringing in ears, sensitivity to light, skin flaking, slow movement, wheezing, worsening of depression

Why should this drug not be prescribed?
Avoid Coreg if you have asthma, certain serious heart conditions, or liver disease. Do not take the drug if it causes an allergic reaction.

Special warnings about this medication
Coreg sometimes aggravates chronic bronchitis and emphysema. If you have either condition, make sure the doctor is aware of it. You'll need to use the drug cautiously. Report any weight gain or shortness of breath to your doctor immediately.

Liver damage is a rare side effect of the drug. Notify your doctor immediately if you develop these signs of liver disorder: appetite loss, dark urine, flu-like symptoms, itching, pain in your side, or yellowing of the skin. You will need to be switched from Coreg.

Make sure your doctor knows if you have diabetes or low blood sugar. Coreg can interfere with the effectiveness of diabetes drugs and can cover up the symptoms of low blood sugar. Monitor your blood sugar regularly, and report any changes to your doctor.

When Coreg is taken for heart failure, there is a slight chance that it will interfere with the kidneys. If this reaction seems likely, the doctor will monitor your kidney function and, if necessary, change your dosage—or take you off the drug.

Under no circumstances should you abruptly stop taking this drug on your own. Your symptoms could return with a vengeance; and if you have an overactive thyroid, those symptoms could be aggravated as well. The doctor will taper you off the drug gradually, if need be. Notify the doctor if you miss even a few doses of Coreg.

If you wear contact lenses, you should know that Coreg can dry your eyes.

Possible food and drug interactions when taking this medication

If Coreg is taken with certain other drugs, the effects of either could be increased, decreased, or altered. It is especially important to check with your doctor before combining Coreg with any of the following:

Calcium channel blockers (blood pressure and heart medications such as Calan, Cardizem, Isoptin, and Verelan)
Cimetidine (Tagamet)
Clonidine (Catapres)
Diabetes pills such as Diabinese, Glucophage, and Rezulin
Drugs classified as MAO inhibitors, including the antidepressants Nardil and Parnate
Digoxin (Lanoxin)
Fluoxetine (Prozac)
Insulin
Paroxetine (Paxil)
Propafenone (Rythmol)
Quinidine (Quinaglute)
Reserpine (Ser-Ap-Es)
Rifampin (Rifadin)

Special information
if you are pregnant or breastfeeding

Coreg has not been adequately studied in pregnant women; and it is not known whether the drug appears in breast milk. If you are pregnant or plan to become pregnant, check with your doctor immediately.

Recommended dosage

ADULTS

Hypertension

The starting dose is 6.25 milligrams twice a day with food. Your doctor may raise the dosage every 1 or 2 weeks to a maximum of 50 milligrams a day.

Congestive heart failure

The starting dose is 3.125 milligrams twice a day with food. Your doctor may increase the dosage every 2 weeks. The maximum dosage for people weighing under 187 pounds is 50 milligrams a day; for those over 187 pounds, the maximum is 100 milligrams a day.

CHILDREN

The safety and effectiveness of Coreg have not been studied in children under 18.

Overdosage

Any medication taken in excess can have serious consequences. If you suspect an overdose, seek medical treatment immediately.

■ *Symptoms of Coreg overdose may include:*
Breathing difficulties, loss of consciousness, seizures, heart problems, slow heartbeat, very low blood pressure, vomiting

Brand name:

CORGARD

Pronounced: CORE-guard
Generic name: Nadolol

Why is this drug prescribed?

Corgard is used in the treatment of angina pectoris (chest pain, usually caused by lack of oxygen to the heart due to clogged arteries) and to reduce high blood pressure.

When prescribed for high blood pressure, it is effective when used alone or in combination with other high blood pressure medications. Corgard is a type of drug known as a beta blocker. It decreases the force and rate of heart contractions, reducing the heart's demand for oxygen and lowering blood pressure.

Most important fact about this drug

If you have high blood pressure, you must take Corgard regularly for it to be effective. Since blood pressure declines gradually, it may be several weeks before you get the full benefit of Corgard; and you must continue taking it even if you are feeling well. Corgard does not cure high blood pressure; it merely keeps it under control.

How should you take this medication?

Corgard can be taken with or without food. Take it exactly as prescribed even if your symptoms have disappeared.

Try not to miss any doses. Corgard is taken once a day. If it is not taken regularly, your condition may worsen.

■ *If you miss a dose...*
Take it as soon as you remember. If it is within 8 hours of your next scheduled dose, skip the one you missed and go back to your regular schedule. Never take 2 doses at the same time.

■ *Storage instructions...*
Store at room temperature, away from light and heat, in a tightly closed container.

What side effects may occur?
Side effects cannot be anticipated. If any develop or change in intensity, inform your doctor as soon as possible. Only your doctor can determine if it is safe for you to continue taking Corgard.

■ *More common side effects may include:*
Change in behavior, changes in heartbeat, dizziness or light-headedness, mild drowsiness, slow heartbeat, weakness or tiredness

■ *Less common or rare side effects may include:*
Abdominal discomfort, asthma-like symptoms, bloating, confusion, constipation, cough, decreased sex drive, diarrhea, dry eyes, dry mouth, dry skin, facial swelling, gas, headache, heart failure, impotence, indigestion, itching, loss of appetite, low blood pressure, nasal stuffiness, nausea, rash, ringing in ears, slurred speech, vision changes, vomiting, weight gain

Why should this drug not be prescribed?
If you have a slow heartbeat, bronchial asthma, certain types of heartbeat irregularity, cardiogenic shock (shock due to inadequate blood supply from the heart), or active heart failure, you should not take this medication.

Special warnings about this medication
If you have a history of congestive heart failure, your doctor will prescribe Corgard with caution.

Corgard should not be stopped suddenly. This can cause increased chest pain and even a heart attack. Dosage should be gradually reduced.

If you suffer from asthma, chronic bronchitis, emphysema, seasonal allergies or other bronchial conditions, or kidney or liver disease, this medication should be used with caution.

Ask your doctor if you should check your pulse while taking Corgard. It can cause your heartbeat to become too slow.

This medication may mask the symptoms of low blood sugar or alter blood sugar levels. If you are diabetic, discuss this with your doctor.

This medication may cause you to become drowsy or less alert; therefore, driving or operating dangerous machinery or participating in any hazardous activity that requires full mental alertness is not recommended until you know how you respond to this medication.

Notify your doctor or dentist that you are taking Corgard if you have a medical emergency or before you have surgery or dental treatment.

Possible food and drug interactions when taking this medication

If Corgard is taken with certain other drugs, the effects of either could be increased, decreased, or altered. It is especially important to check with your doctor before combining Corgard with the following:

Antidiabetic drugs, including insulin and oral drugs such as Micronase
Certain blood pressure drugs such as Diupres and Ser-Ap-Es
Epinephrine (EpiPen)

Special information if you are pregnant or breastfeeding

The effects of Corgard during pregnancy have not been adequately studied. If you are pregnant or plan to become pregnant, inform your doctor immediately. Corgard appears in breast milk and could affect a nursing infant. If this medication is essential to your health, your doctor may advise you to discontinue breastfeeding until your treatment with this medication is finished.

Recommended dosage

ADULTS

Dosage is tailored to each individual's needs.

Angina Pectoris

The usual starting dose is 40 milligrams once daily. The usual long-term dose is 40 or 80 milligrams, once a day. Doses up to 160 or 240 milligrams, once a day, may be needed.

High Blood Pressure
The usual starting dose is 40 milligrams once daily.

The usual long-term dose is 40 or 80 milligrams, once a day. Doses up to 240 or 320 milligrams, once a day, may be needed.

CHILDREN

The safety and effectiveness of Corgard have not been established in children.

Overdosage
Any medication taken in excess can have serious consequences. If you suspect an overdose, seek medical attention immediately.

■ *The symptoms of Corgard overdose may include:*
Difficulty in breathing, heart failure, low blood pressure, slow heartbeat

Brand name:

CORMAX

See Temovate, page 1269.

Brand name:

CORTISPORIN OPHTHALMIC SUSPENSION

Pronounced: KORE-ti-SPORE-in
Generic ingredients: Polymyxin B sulfate, Neomycin
*   sulfate, Hydrocortisone*

Why is this drug prescribed?
Cortisporin Ophthalmic Suspension is a combination of the steroid drug, hydrocortisone, and two antibiotics. It is prescribed to relieve inflammatory conditions such as irritation, swelling, redness, and general eye discomfort, and to treat superficial bacterial infections of the eye.

Most important fact about this drug
Prolonged use of this medication may increase pressure within the eye, leading to potential damage to the optic nerve and visual problems. Prolonged use also may suppress your immune response and thus increase the hazard of secondary eye infections. Your doctor should measure your eye pressure periodically if you are using this product for 10 days or longer.

How should you use this medication?

To help clear up your infection completely, use this medication exactly as prescribed for the full time of treatment, even if your symptoms have disappeared.

Administer the eyedrops as follows:

1. Shake the dropper bottle well.
2. Wash your hands thoroughly.
3. Gently pull your lower eyelid down to form a pocket between your eye and eyelid.
4. Hold the bottle on the bridge of your nose or on your forehead.
5. Tilt your head back and squeeze the medication into your eye.
6. Do not touch the applicator tip to any surface, including your eye.
7. Close your eyes gently, and keep them closed for 1 to 2 minutes.
8. Do not rinse the dropper.
9. Wait 5 to 10 minutes before using any other eyedrops.

If you do not improve after 2 days, your doctor should re-evaluate your case.

Do not share this medication with anyone else; you may spread the infection.

■ *If you miss a dose...*
Apply it as soon as you remember. If it is almost time for your next dose, skip the one you missed and go back to your regular schedule.

■ *Storage instructions...*
Store at room temperature. Keep tightly closed and protect from freezing.

What side effects may occur?

Side effects cannot be anticipated. If any develop or change in intensity, inform your doctor as soon as possible. Only your doctor can determine if it is safe for you to continue using Cortisporin.

■ *Side effects may include:*
Cataract formation (results in blurred vision), delayed wound healing, increased eye pressure (with possible development of glaucoma and, infrequently, optic nerve damage), irritation when drops are instilled, local allergic reactions (itching, swelling, redness), other infections (particularly fungal infections of the cornea and bacterial eye infections), severe allergic reactions

Why should this drug not be prescribed?

Cortisporin should not be used if you have certain viral or fungal diseases of the eye, including inflammation of the cornea caused by herpes simplex, chickenpox, or cowpox, or if you are sensitive to or have ever had an allergic reaction to any of its ingredients.

Special warnings about this medication

Remember that steroids such as hydrocortisone may hide the existence of an infection or worsen an existing one.

If you are using this medication for more than 10 days, your doctor should routinely check your eye pressure. If you already have high pressure within the eye (glaucoma), use this medication cautiously.

Neomycin, one of the ingredients in Cortisporin, may cause an allergic reaction—usually itching, redness, and swelling—or failure to heal. If you develop any of these signs, stop using Cortisporin; the symptoms should quickly subside. If the condition persists or gets worse, or if a rash or allergic reaction develops, call your doctor immediately. You are more likely to be sensitive to neomycin if you are sensitive to the following antibiotics: kanamycin, paromomycin, streptomycin, and possibly gentamicin.

The use of steroids in the eye can prolong and worsen many viral infections of the eye, including herpes simplex. Use this medication with extreme caution if you have this infection.

If you develop a sensitivity to Cortisporin, avoid other topical medications that contain neomycin.

Eye products that are not handled properly can become contaminated with bacteria that cause eye infections. If you use a contaminated product, you can seriously damage your eyes, even to the point of blindness.

Possible food and drug interactions
when taking this medication

No interactions have been reported.

Special information
if you are pregnant or breastfeeding

Although the effects of Cortisporin during pregnancy have not been adequately studied, steroids should be used during pregnancy only if the benefits outweigh the dangers to the fetus. If you are pregnant or plan to become pregnant, inform your doctor immediately. Hydrocortisone, when taken orally, appears in breast milk. Since medication may be absorbed into the bloodstream when it is applied to the eye, your doctor may advise you to stop breastfeeding until your treatment with Cortisporin is finished.

Recommended dosage

ADULTS

The usual recommended dose is 1 or 2 drops in the affected eye every 3 or 4 hours, depending on the severity of the condition. Cortisporin may be used more often if necessary.

Overdosage

Any medication used in excess can have serious consequences. If you suspect an overdose of Cortisporin Ophthalmic Suspension, seek medical treatment immediately.

Brand name:

CORZIDE

Pronounced: CORE-zide
Generic ingredients: Nadolol, Bendroflumethiazide

Why is this drug prescribed?

Corzide is a combination drug used in the treatment of high blood pressure. It combines a beta blocker and a thiazide diuretic. Nadolol, the beta blocker, decreases the force and rate of heart contractions thereby reducing blood pressure. Bendroflumethiazide, the diuretic, helps your body produce and eliminate more urine, which also helps in lowering blood pressure.

Most important fact about this drug

You must take Corzide regularly for it to be effective. Since blood pressure declines gradually, it may be several weeks before you get the full benefit of Corzide; and you must continue taking it even if you are feeling well. Corzide does not cure high blood pressure; it merely keeps it under control.

How should you take this medication?

Corzide may be taken with or without food. Take it exactly as prescribed, even if your symptoms have disappeared.

Try not to miss any doses. Corzide is taken once a day. If this medication is not taken regularly, your condition may worsen.

■ *If you miss a dose...*
Take it as soon as you remember. If it's within 8 hours of your next scheduled dose, skip the one you missed and go back to your regular schedule. Never take 2 doses at the same time.

■ *Storage instructions...*
   Store at room temperature, away from heat, in a tightly closed container.

What side effects may occur?
Side effects cannot be anticipated. If any develop or change in intensity, inform your doctor as soon as possible. Only your doctor can determine if it is safe for you to continue taking Corzide.

■ *More common side effects may include:*
   Asthma-like symptoms, changes in heart rhythm, cold hands and feet, dizziness, fatigue, low blood pressure, low potassium levels (symptoms include dry mouth, excessive thirst, weak or irregular heartbeat, muscle pain or cramps), slow heartbeat

■ *Less common or rare side effects may include:*
   Abdominal discomfort, anemia, bloating, blurred vision, certain types of irregular heartbeat, change in behavior, constipation, cough, diarrhea, dry mouth, eyes, or skin, facial swelling, gas, headache, heart failure, hepatitis, impotence, indigestion, inflammation of the pancreas, itching, loss of appetite, lowered sex drive, muscle spasm, nasal stuffiness, nausea, rash, ringing in ears, sedation, sensitivity to light, slurred speech, sweating, tingling or pins and needles, vertigo, vomiting, weakness, weight gain, wheezing, yellowed eyes and skin

Why should this drug not be prescribed?
If you have bronchial asthma, slow heartbeat, certain heartbeat irregularities (heart block), inadequate blood supply to the circulatory system (cardiogenic shock), active congestive heart failure, inability to urinate, or if you are sensitive to or have ever had an allergic reaction to Corzide, its ingredients, or similar drugs, you should not take this medication.

Special warnings about this medication
If you have a history of congestive heart failure, your doctor will prescribe Corzide with caution.

Corzide should not be stopped suddenly. This can cause increased chest pain and even a heart attack. Dosage should be gradually reduced.

If you suffer from asthma, seasonal allergies, emphysema or other bronchial conditions, or kidney or liver disease, this medication should be used with caution.

Ask your doctor if you should check your pulse while taking Corzide. It can cause your heartbeat to become too slow.

Corzide may mask the symptoms of low blood sugar or alter blood sugar levels. If you are diabetic, discuss this with your doctor.

This medication can cause you to become drowsy or less alert; therefore, activity that requires full mental alertness is not recommended until you know how you respond to this medication.

Notify your doctor or dentist that you are taking Corzide if you have a medical emergency, or before you have surgery or dental treatment.

Possible food and drug interactions when taking this medication

Corzide may intensify the effects of alcohol. Do not drink alcohol while taking this medication.

If Corzide is taken with any other drug, the effects of either could be increased, decreased, or altered. It is especially important to check with your doctor before combining Corzide with the following:

Amphotericin B
Antidepressant drugs known as MAO inhibitors, such as Nardil and Parnate
Antidiabetic drugs, including insulin and oral drugs such as Micronase
Antigout drugs such as Benemid
Barbiturates such as phenobarbital
Blood thinners such as Coumadin
Calcium salt
Certain blood pressure drugs such as Diupres and Ser-Ap-Es
Cholestyramine (Questran)
Colestipol (Colestid)
Diazoxide (Proglycem)
Digitalis medications such as Lanoxin
Lithium (Lithonate)
Methenamine (Mandelamine)
Narcotics such as Percocet
Nonsteroidal anti-inflammatory drugs, such as Motrin, Naprosyn, and Nuprin
Other antihypertensives such as Vasotec
Steroid medications such as prednisone
Sulfinpyrazone (Anturane)

Special information if you are pregnant or breastfeeding

The effects of Corzide during pregnancy have not been adequately studied. If you are pregnant or plan to become pregnant, inform your doctor immediately. Corzide appears in breast milk and could affect a nursing infant. If this medication is essential to your health, your doctor may advise you to discontinue breastfeeding until your treatment with Corzide is finished.

Recommended dosage

ADULTS

Dosages of this drug are always tailored to the individual's needs.

The usual dose is 1 Corzide 40/5 milligram tablet per day or, if necessary, 1 Corzide 80/5 milligram tablet per day. Your doctor may gradually add another high blood pressure medication to this drug.

CHILDREN

The safety and effectiveness of Corzide have not been established in children.

Overdosage

Any medication taken in excess can have serious consequences. If you suspect an overdose, seek medical attention immediately.

■ *The symptoms of Corzide overdose may include:*
Abdominal irritation, central nervous system depression, coma, extremely slow heartbeat, heart failure, lethargy, low blood pressure, wheezing

Brand name:

COTRIM

See Bactrim, page 135.

Brand name:

COUMADIN

Pronounced: COO-muh-din
Generic name: Warfarin sodium

Why is this drug prescribed?

Coumadin is an anticoagulant (blood thinner). It is prescribed to:

Prevent and/or treat a blood clot that has formed within a blood vessel or in the lungs.

Prevent and/or treat blood clots associated with certain heart conditions or replacement of a heart valve.

Aid in the prevention of blood clots that may form in blood vessels anywhere in the body after a heart attack.

Reduce the risk of death, another heart attack, or stroke after a heart attack.

Most important fact about this drug

The most serious risks associated with Coumadin treatment are hemorrhage (severe bleeding resulting in the loss of a large amount of blood) in any tissue or organ and, less frequently, the destruction of skin tissue cells (necrosis) or gangrene. The risk of hemorrhage usually depends on the dosage and length of treatment with this drug.

Hemorrhage and necrosis have been reported to result in death or permanent disability. Severe necrosis can lead to the removal of damaged tissue or amputation of a limb. Necrosis appears to be associated with blood clots located in the area of tissue damage and usually occurs within a few days of starting Coumadin treatment.

How should you take this medication?

The objective of treatment with a blood-thinner is to control the blood-clotting process without causing severe bleeding, so that a clot does not form and cut off the blood supply necessary for normal body function. Therefore, it is very important that you take this medication exactly as prescribed by your doctor and that your doctor monitor your condition on a regular basis. Be especially careful to stick to the exact dosage schedule your doctor prescribes.

Effective treatment with minimal complications depends on your cooperation and communication with the doctor.

Do not take or discontinue any other medication unless directed to do so by your doctor. Avoid alcohol, salicylates such as aspirin, larger than usual amounts of foods rich in vitamin K (including liver, vegetable oil, egg yolks, and green leafy vegetables), which can counteract the effect of Coumadin, or any other drastic change in diet.

Note that Coumadin often turns urine reddish-orange.

You should carry an identification card that indicates you are taking Coumadin.

- *If you miss a dose...*
  Take the forgotten dose as soon as you remember, then go back to your regular schedule. If you do not remember until the next day, skip the dose. Never try to "catch up" by doubling the dose. Keep a record for your doctor of any doses you miss.

- *Storage instructions...*
Coumadin can be stored at room temperature. Close the container tightly and protect from light.

What side effects may occur?
Side effects cannot be anticipated. If any develop or change in intensity, inform your doctor as soon as possible. Only your doctor can determine if it is safe for you to continue taking Coumadin.

- *More common side effects may include:*
Hemorrhage: Signs of severe bleeding resulting in the loss of large amounts of blood depend upon the location and extent of bleeding. Symptoms include: chest, abdomen, joint, muscle, or other pain; difficult breathing or swallowing; dizziness; headache; low blood pressure; numbness and tingling; paralysis; shortness of breath; unexplained shock; unexplained swelling; weakness

- *Less common side effects may include:*
Abdominal pain and cramping, allergic reactions, diarrhea, fatigue, feeling cold and chills, feeling of illness, fever, fluid retention and swelling, gas and bloating, hepatitis, hives, intolerance to cold, itching, lethargy, liver damage, loss of hair, nausea, necrosis (gangrene), pain, purple toes, rash, severe or long-lasting inflammation of the skin, taste changes, vomiting, yellowed skin and eyes

Why should this drug not be prescribed?
This drug should not be used for any condition where the danger of hemorrhage may be greater than the potential benefits of treatment. Unless directed to do so by your doctor, do not take this medication if one of the following conditions or situations applies to you:

A tendency to hemorrhage
Alcoholism
An abnormal blood condition
Aneurysm (balloon-like swelling of a blood vessel) in the brain or heart
Bleeding tendencies associated with: ulceration or bleeding of the stomach, intestines, respiratory tract, or the genital or urinary system
Eclampsia (a rare and serious pregnancy disorder producing life-threatening convulsions), or preeclampsia (a toxic condition— including headache, high blood pressure, and swelling of the legs and feet—that can lead to eclampsia)
Excessive bleeding of brain blood vessels
Inflammation, due to bacterial infection, of the membrane that lines the inside of the heart

Inflammation of the sac that surrounds the heart or an escape of fluid from the heart sac

Malignant hypertension (extremely elevated blood pressure that damages the inner linings of blood vessels, the heart, spleen, kidneys, and brain)

Pregnancy

Recent or contemplated surgery of the central nervous system (brain and spinal cord) or eye

Spinal puncture or any procedure that can cause uncontrollable bleeding

Threatened miscarriage

Allergy to any of the drug's ingredients

Special warnings about this medication

Treatment with blood thinners may increase the risk that fatty plaque will break away from the wall of an artery and lodge at another point, causing the blockage of a blood vessel. If you notice any of the following symptoms, contact your doctor immediately:

Abdominal pain; abrupt and intense pain in the leg, foot, or toes; blood in the urine; bluish mottling of the skin of the legs and hands; foot ulcers; gangrene; high blood pressure; muscle pain; "purple toes syndrome" (see below); rash; or thigh or back pain.

If you have any of the following conditions, tell your doctor. He or she will have to consider the risks against the benefits before giving you Coumadin.

An infectious disease or intestinal disorder

A history of recurrent blood clot disorders in you or your family

An implanted catheter

Dental procedures

Inflammation of a blood vessel

Moderate to severe high blood pressure

Moderate to severe kidney or liver dysfunction

Polycythemia vera (blood disorder)

Severe diabetes

Surgery or injury that leaves large raw surfaces

Trauma or injury that may result in internal bleeding

Purple toes syndrome can occur when taking Coumadin, usually 3 to 10 weeks after the start of anticoagulation therapy. Symptoms include dark purplish or mottled color of the toes that turns white when pressure is applied and fades when you elevate your legs, pain and tenderness of the toes, and change in intensity of the color over a period of time. If any of these symptoms develop, notify your doctor immediately.

If you are taking Coumadin, your doctor should periodically check the time it takes for your blood to start the clotting process (prothrombin time). Numerous factors such as travel and changes in diet, environment, physical state, and medication may alter your response to treatment with an anticoagulant. Clotting time should also be monitored after your release from the hospital and whenever other medications are started, discontinued, or taken sporadically.

While taking Coumadin, avoid activities and sports that could cause an injury. Remain cautious after you stop taking Coumadin. It will continue to work for 2 to 5 days.

If you have congestive heart failure, you may become more sensitive to Coumadin and may need to have your dosage reduced. Your doctor will have you tested regularly.

Notify your doctor if any illness, such as diarrhea, infection, or fever develops; if any unusual symptoms, such as pain, swelling, or discomfort, appear; or if you see prolonged bleeding from cuts, increased menstrual flow, vaginal bleeding, nosebleeds, bleeding of gums from brushing, unusual bleeding or bruising, red or dark brown urine, red or tarry black stool, headache, dizziness, or weakness.

Possible food and drug interactions when taking this medication

Coumadin can interact with a very wide variety of drugs, both prescription and over-the-counter. Check with your doctor before taking ANY other medication or vitamin product.

Special information if you are pregnant or breastfeeding

Coumadin should not be taken by women who are or may become pregnant since the drug may cause fatal hemorrhage in the developing baby. There have also been reports of birth malformations, low birth weight, and retarded growth in children born to mothers treated with Coumadin during pregnancy. Spontaneous abortions and stillbirths are also known to occur. If you become pregnant while taking this drug, inform your doctor immediately. Coumadin may appear in breast milk and could affect a nursing infant. If this medication is essential to your health, your doctor may advise you to stop nursing your baby until your treatment with this drug is finished.

Recommended dosage

ADULTS

The administration and dosage of Coumadin must be individualized by your doctor according to your sensitivity to the drug.

A common starting dosage of Coumadin tablets for adults is 2 to 5 milligrams per day. Individualized daily dosage adjustments are based on the results of tests that determine the amount of time it takes for the blood clotting process to begin.

A maintenance dose of 2 to 10 milligrams per day is satisfactory for most people. The duration of treatment will be determined by your physician.

CHILDREN

Although Coumadin has been widely used in children below the age of 18, its safety and effectiveness for this purpose have not been formally established.

Overdosage
Signs and symptoms of Coumadin overdose reflect abnormal bleeding.

■ *Symptoms of abnormal bleeding include:*
Blood in stools or urine, excessive menstrual bleeding, black stools, reddish or purplish spots on skin, excessive bruising, persistent bleeding from superficial injuries

If you suspect an overdose, seek emergency medical treatment immediately.

Brand name:

COVERA-HS

See Calan, page 181.

Brand name:

COZAAR

Pronounced: CO-zahr
Generic name: Losartan potassium

Why is this drug prescribed?
Cozaar is used in the treatment of high blood pressure. It is effective when used alone or with other high blood pressure medications, such as diuretics that help the body get rid of water.

Cozaar is the first of a new class of blood pressure medications called angiotensin II receptor antagonists. Cozaar works, in part, by preventing the hormone angiotensin II from constricting the blood vessels, which tends to raise blood pressure.

Most important fact about this drug

You must take Cozaar regularly for it to be effective. Since blood pressure declines gradually, it may be several weeks before you get the full benefit of Cozaar, and you must continue taking it even if you are feeling well. Cozaar does not cure high blood pressure; it merely keeps it under control.

How should you take this medication?

Cozaar can be taken with or without food.

Take it at the same time each day. For example, if you take the medication every morning before or after breakfast, you will establish a regular routine and be less likely to forget your dose.

■ *If you miss a dose...*
Take it as soon as possible. If it is almost time for your next dose, skip the missed dose and go back to your regular schedule.

■ *Storage instructions...*
Store at room temperature. Keep in a tightly closed container, away from light.

What side effects may occur?

Side effects cannot be anticipated. If any develop or change in intensity, tell your doctor as soon as possible. Only your doctor can determine if it is safe for you to continue taking Cozaar.

■ *More common side effects may include:*
Cough, dizziness, upper respiratory infection

■ *Less common and rare side effects may include:*
Back and leg pain, diarrhea, indigestion, insomnia, muscle cramps or pain, nasal congestion, sinus problems, swelling of face, lips, throat, and tongue

Why should this drug not be prescribed?

Do not take Cozaar when you are pregnant. Avoid it if you have ever had an allergic reaction to it.

Special warnings about this medication

Cozaar can cause low blood pressure, especially if you are also taking a diuretic. You may feel light-headed or faint, especially during the first few days of therapy. If these symptoms occur, contact your doctor. Your dosage may need to be adjusted or discontinued. Be sure you know how you react to Cozaar before you drive or operate machinery.

Excessive sweating, dehydration, severe diarrhea, or vomiting could make you lose too much water, causing a severe drop in blood pressure. Call your doctor if you experience any of these symptoms. Be sure to tell your doctor about any medical conditions you have, especially liver or kidney disease.

Possible food and drug interactions when taking this medication

If Cozaar is taken with certain other drugs, the effects of either could be increased, decreased, or altered. It is especially important to check with your doctor before taking Cozaar with the following:

Ketoconazole (Nizoral)
Troleandomycin (Tao)

Special information if you are pregnant or breastfeeding

Drugs such as Cozaar can cause injury or even death to the unborn child when used in the second or third trimester of pregnancy. Stop taking Cozaar as soon as you know you are pregnant. If you are pregnant or plan to become pregnant, tell your doctor before taking Cozaar. Cozaar may appear in breast milk and could affect the nursing infant. If this medication is essential to your health, your doctor may advise you to stop breastfeeding while you are taking Cozaar.

Recommended dosage

ADULTS

The usual starting dose is 50 milligrams once daily. However, Cozaar can also be taken twice daily, with total daily doses ranging from 25 milligrams to 100 milligrams. If your blood pressure does not respond, your doctor may increase your dose or add a low-dose diuretic to your regimen.

People taking diuretics and people with liver problems
The usual starting dose is 25 milligrams daily. Your doctor may adjust your dosage according to your response.

CHILDREN

The safety and effectiveness of Cozaar in children have not been studied.

Overdosage

Any medication taken in excess can have serious consequences. If you suspect an overdose, seek medical attention immediately. Information concerning Cozaar overdosage is limited. However, hypotension (low blood pressure) and abnormally rapid or slow heartbeat may be signs of an overdose.

Brand name:

CREON

See Pancrease, page 947.

Brand name:

CRIXIVAN

Pronounced: CRIX-i-van
Generic name: Indinavir sulfate

Why is this drug prescribed?
Crixivan is used in the treatment of human immunodeficiency virus (HIV) infection. HIV causes the immune system to break down so that it can no longer fight off other infections. This leads to the fatal disease known as acquired immune deficiency syndrome (AIDS).

HIV thrives by taking over the immune system's vital CD4 cells (white blood cells) and using their inner workings to make additional copies of itself. Crixivan belongs to a class of HIV drugs called protease inhibitors, which work by interfering with an important step in the virus's reproductive cycle. Although Crixivan cannot eliminate HIV already present in the body, it can reduce the amount of virus available to infect other cells.

Crixivan can be taken alone or in combination with other HIV drugs such as Retrovir. Because Crixivan and Retrovir attack the virus in different ways, the combination is likely to be more effective than either drug alone.

Most important fact about this drug
It is important that you drink at least 48 ounces (4 soda-can sized glasses) of liquid daily while taking Crixivan. If you do not get enough liquid, you may develop kidney stones and have to temporarily stop taking Crixivan or even discontinue it altogether.

How should you take this medication?
Take this medication exactly as prescribed by your doctor. Do not share this medication with anyone and do not take more than your recommended dosage.

To ensure maximum absorption, do not take Crixivan with food. Instead, take it with water 1 hour before or 2 hours after a meal. (Crixivan may also be taken with liquids such as skim milk, juice, coffee, or tea, or even with a light meal such as dry toast with jelly, juice, and coffee with skim milk and sugar, or corn flakes with skim milk and sugar.)

■ *If you miss a dose...*
Skip it and take the next dose at the regularly scheduled time. Do not double the dose.

■ *Storage instructions...*
Crixivan capsules are sensitive to moisture. Store Crixivan at room temperature in the original container and leave the drying agent in the bottle to keep the medication dry. Keep the container tightly closed.

What side effects may occur?
Side effects cannot be anticipated. If any develop or change in intensity, inform your doctor as soon as possible. Only your doctor can determine if it is safe for you to continue taking Crixivan.

■ *Possible side effects may include:*
Abdominal pain, anemia, back pain, blood in the urine, changes in taste, diarrhea, discolored skin, dizziness, drowsiness, dry skin and mouth, fatigue, general feeling of illness, headache, indigestion, insomnia, kidney stones, liver problems, loss of appetite, nausea, pain in the side, rash, vomiting, weakness, yellow skin or eyes

Why should this drug not be prescribed?
If you suffer a severe allergic reaction to Crixivan or any of its ingredients, you should not take this medication.

Special warnings about this medication
Although Crixivan reduces the amount of HIV in the blood and increases the white blood cell count, its long-term effect on survival is still unknown. The virus remains in the body, and you will continue to face the possibility of complications, including opportunistic infections (rare infections that develop when the immune system falters) such as certain types of pneumonia, tuberculosis, and fungal infection. Therefore, it is important that you remain under the care of a doctor and keep all your follow-up appointments.

Crixivan is not a cure for HIV infection, and it does not reduce the risk of transmission of HIV to others through sexual contact or blood contamination. Therefore, you should continue to avoid practices that could spread HIV.

Check with your doctor if you have liver disease, particularly cirrhosis of the liver, before using Crixivan. Because there is little information concerning the use of this drug in people with kidney disease or severe liver disease, be sure to tell your doctor if you have either condition.

Protease inhibitors such as Crixivan have been known to trigger diabetes (high blood sugar levels) or worsen existing diabetes. If you have diabetes, the dosages of your diabetes medications may have to be adjusted.

Cases of liver failure and death have occurred in patients treated with Crixivan and other medications. If you have a liver problem, particularly cirrhosis of the liver, make sure the doctor is aware of it. Kidney problems are also a possibility, so alert the doctor if you have any type of kidney disease.

Some patients have developed severe anemia (loss of red blood cells) while taking Crixivan. If this problem surfaces, you will have to stop taking the drug.

If you have hemophilia, you should also be aware that spontaneous bleeding has occurred in hemophilia victims taking protease inhibitors such as Crixivan.

Possible food and drug interactions
when taking this medication

Do not take Crixivan with rifampin (Rifadin); it reduces Crixivan's effectiveness. Also avoid the following medications while taking Crixivan. The combination may cause serious or life-threatening effects.

Astemizole (Hismanal)
Cisapride (Propulsid)
Ergot-based drugs such as Cafergot
Midazolam (Versed)
Terfenadine (Seldane)
Triazolam (Halcion)

Crixivan may also interact with certain other drugs, and the effects of either could be increased, decreased, or altered. It is especially important to check with your doctor before combining Crixivan with the following:

Carbamazepine (Tegretol)
Clarithromycin (Biaxin)
Dexamethasone (Decadron)
Didanosine (Videx)
Fluconazole (Diflucan)

Isoniazid (Nydrazid)
Ketoconazole (Nizoral)
Ortho-Novum
Phenobarbital
Phenytoin (Dilantin)
Quinidine (Quinidex)
Rifabutin (Mycobutin)
Trimethoprim (Bactrim, Trimpex, Septra)

Avoid drinking grapefruit juice while taking Crixivan. This kind of juice can reduce the drug's effectiveness.

Be sure to tell your doctor and pharmacist about all medications you are taking, both prescription and over-the-counter. Alert them, too, when you *stop* taking a medication.

Special information
if you are pregnant or breastfeeding
The effects of Crixivan during pregnancy have not been adequately studied. If you are pregnant or plan to become pregnant, tell your doctor immediately. Do not breastfeed your baby. HIV appears in breast milk and can infect a nursing infant.

Recommended dosage

ADULTS

The recommended dose of Crixivan is 800 milligrams (two 400-milligram capsules) every 8 hours. Your doctor may lower the dose to 600 milligrams every 8 hours if you have mild-to-moderate liver problems due to cirrhosis or if you are also taking ketoconazole. If you have been prescribed another HIV drug along with Crixivan, take it as directed.

CHILDREN

The safety and effectiveness of Crixivan for use in children have not been established.

Overdosage
There is no information presently available on Crixivan overdose. However, any medication taken in excess can have serious consequences. If you suspect an overdose, seek emergency medical treatment immediately.

Brand name:

CROLOM

Pronounced: CROW-lum
Generic name: Cromolyn sodium

Why is this drug prescribed?

Crolom is an eyedrop that relieves the itching, tearing, discharge, and redness caused by seasonal and chronic allergies. The drug works by preventing certain cells in the body from releasing histamine and other substances that can cause an allergic reaction.

Most important fact about this drug

In order for Crolom to work properly, you must continue to use it every day at regular intervals even if your symptoms have disappeared. It can take up to 6 weeks for your condition to clear up.

How should you use this medication?

Use Crolom exactly as directed by your doctor. Do not use more or less than required and apply it only when scheduled.

To administer Crolom, follow these steps:

1. Wash your hands thoroughly.
2. Gently pull your lower eyelid down to form a pocket between your eye and the lid.
3. Drop the medicine into this pocket. Let go of the eyelid and gently close the eye. Do not blink. Keep your eyes closed for a minute or two.
4. Do not touch the applicator tip to your eye or any other surface. This could lead to infection.
5. Do not rinse the dropper.

■ *If you miss a dose...*
Use it as soon as possible. Then go back to your regular schedule.

■ *Storage instructions...*
Keep the container tightly closed and away from light. Store at room temperature.

What side effects may occur?

You may experience temporary burning or stinging in the eye after you apply Crolom.

- *Rare side effects may include:*
  Dryness around the eye, eye irritation, inflammation of the eyelids, itchy eyes, puffy eyes, styes, watery eyes

Why should this drug not be prescribed?
If you have ever had an allergic reaction to cromolyn sodium, avoid this medication.

Special warnings about this medication
Do not wear soft contact lenses while you are using Crolom.

If your symptoms do not begin to improve, alert your doctor.

Possible food and drug interactions with the medication
No interactions have been reported.

Special information if you are pregnant or breastfeeding
There are no studies on use of Crolom with pregnant women. If you are pregnant or plan to become pregnant, tell your doctor. Crolom should be used during pregnancy only if clearly needed. It is not known whether Crolom appears in human breast milk. If you are nursing and need to use Crolom, use it with caution.

Recommended dosage

ADULTS AND CHILDREN

Put 1 or 2 drops into each eye 4 to 6 times a day at evenly spaced intervals.

It is not known whether Crolom is safe and effective for children under 4 years.

Overdosage
Although there is no information on Crolom overdose, any medication taken in excess can have serious consequences. If you suspect an overdose, seek medical attention immediately.

Generic name:

CROMOLYN, INHALED

See Intal, page 645.

Generic name:

CROMOLYN, OCULAR

See Crolom, page 315.

Generic name:

CYCLOBENZAPRINE

See Flexeril, page 532.

Brand name:

CYCLOCORT

Pronounced: SIKE-low-court
Generic name: Amcinonide

Why is this drug prescribed?
Cyclocort is prescribed for the relief of the inflammatory and itchy symptoms of skin disorders that are responsive to corticosteroid treatment.

Most important fact about this drug
When you use Cyclocort, you inevitably absorb some of the medication through your skin and into the bloodstream. Too much absorption can lead to unwanted side effects elsewhere in the body. To keep this problem to a minimum, avoid using large amounts of Cyclocort over large areas, and do not cover it with airtight dressings such as plastic wrap or adhesive bandages unless specifically told to by your doctor.

How should you use this medication?
Use this medication exactly as prescribed by your doctor. It is for use only on the skin. Be careful to keep it out of your eyes.

Apply Cyclocort sparingly. Rub it in gently.

■ *If you miss a dose...*
Apply the forgotten dose as soon as you remember. Use the remaining doses for that day at evenly spaced intervals. Never try to "catch up" by doubling the amount applied.

■ *Storage instructions...*
Cyclocort can be stored at room temperature. Protect from freezing.

What side effects may occur?

Side effects cannot be anticipated. If any develop or change in intensity, inform your doctor as soon as possible. Only your doctor can determine if it is safe for you to continue taking Cyclocort.

■ *More common side effects may include:*
Burning, itching, soreness, stinging

■ *Less common or rare side effects may include:*
Dryness, excessive growth of hair, infection, inflammation of hair follicles, inflammation of the skin around the mouth, irritation, prickly heat, skin eruptions resembling acne, softening of the skin, stretch marks

Why should this drug not be prescribed?

If you are sensitive to or have ever had an allergic reaction to amcinonide or other steroid medications, you should not use Cyclocort. Make sure your doctor is aware of any drug reactions you have experienced.

Special warnings about this medication

Do not use this drug for any disorder other than the one for which it was prescribed.

The use of tight-fitting diapers or plastic pants is not recommended for a child being treated in the diaper area. These garments may act as airtight dressings or bandages.

The treated skin area should not be bandaged, covered, or wrapped unless you have been directed to do so by your doctor.

If an irritation or allergic reaction develops while you are using Cyclocort, notify your doctor.

Possible food and drug interactions
when taking this medication

No interactions with food or other drugs have been reported.

Special information
if you are pregnant or breastfeeding

The effects of Cyclocort during pregnancy have not been adequately studied. If you are pregnant or plan to become pregnant, inform your doctor immediately. It is not known whether this medication appears in breast milk. If this drug is essential to your health, your doctor may advise you to discontinue breastfeeding until your treatment is finished.

Recommended dosage

ADULTS

Apply a thin film of Cyclocort to the affected area 2 or 3 times a day, depending on the severity of the condition.

Cyclocort lotion may be applied to the affected areas, particularly hairy areas, 2 times per day. The lotion should be rubbed in completely, and the area should not be washed and should be protected from clothing until the lotion has dried.

Your doctor may recommend airtight bandages or dressings if you are being treated for psoriasis (a skin disorder characterized by patches of red, dry, scale-covered skin) or other stubborn skin conditions. If an infection develops, stop bandaging the area.

CHILDREN

Topical use of Cyclocort on children should be limited to the smallest amount that is effective. Long-term treatment may interfere with children's growth and development.

Overdosage

A severe overdosage is unlikely with the use of Cyclocort; however, long-term or prolonged use can produce side effects throughout the body (see "Most important fact about this drug" on page 295).

Generic name:

CYCLOPHOSPHAMIDE

See Cytoxan, page 328.

Generic name:

CYCLOSPORINE

See Sandimmune, page 1164.

Brand name:

CYCRIN

See Provera, page 1078.

Brand name:

CYLERT

Pronounced: SIGH-lert
Generic name: Pemoline

Why is this drug prescribed?

Cylert is used to help treat children who have attention deficit disorder with hyperactivity. However, this condition does not always require drug treatment. Drugs such as Cylert should be taken as part of a comprehensive treatment plan offering psychological and educational support to help the child become more stable.

Children who have attention deficit disorder with hyperactivity may show signs of:

Emotional mood swings
Hyperactivity
Impulsive actions
Moderate to severe distractibility
Short attention span

Most important fact about this drug

Because long-term use of drugs such as Cylert may affect a child's growth, your doctor will monitor your child carefully if he or she is taking this drug for an extended period.

How should you take this medication?

Cylert should be taken once a day, in the morning.

■ *If you miss a dose...*
Have your child take it as soon as you remember, then go back to the regular schedule. If you do not remember it until the next day, skip the missed dose and go back to the regular schedule. Do not give 2 doses at once.

■ *Storage instructions...*
Store at room temperature.

What side effects may occur?

Side effects cannot be anticipated. If any develop or change in intensity, inform your doctor as soon as possible. Only your doctor can determine if it is safe for your child to continue taking Cylert.

- *More common side effects may include:*
  Insomnia

- *Less common side effects may include:*
  Dizziness, drowsiness, hallucinations, headache, hepatitis and other liver problems, increased irritability, involuntary, fragmented movements of the face, eyes, lips, tongue, arms, and legs, loss of appetite, mild depression, nausea, seizures, skin rash, stomachache, suppressed growth, uncontrolled vocal outbursts (such as grunts, shouts, and obscene language), weight loss, yellowing of skin or eyes

- *Rare side effects may include:*
  A rare form of anemia with symptoms such as bleeding gums, bruising, chest pain, fatigue, headache, nosebleeds, and abnormal paleness

Why should this drug not be prescribed?
Your child should not be using Cylert if he or she is allergic to it or if he or she has liver problems.

Special warnings about this medication
Cylert may cause dizziness. Warn your child to be careful climbing stairs or participating in activities that require mental alertness.

Although there have been no reports that Cylert is physically addictive, it is chemically similar to a class of drugs that are potentially addictive. Make sure your child takes no more than the prescribed dosage.

Remember that children who take this drug on a long-term basis should be carefully monitored for signs of stunted growth.

Use Cylert cautiously if your child has kidney problems.

Psychotic children who take Cylert may experience increasingly disordered thoughts and behavioral disturbances.

Possible food and drug interactions
when taking this medication
If Cylert is taken with certain other drugs, the effects of either could be increased, decreased, or altered. It is especially important to check with your doctor before combining Cylert with the following:

Seizure medications such as Tegretol
Other drugs that affect the central nervous system (brain and spinal cord) such as Ritalin

Special information
if you are pregnant or breastfeeding

This drug is for use only in children, and its effects in pregnancy have not been adequately studied. Cylert should be used during pregnancy only if it is clearly necessary. The drug may appear in breast milk and affect the baby.

Recommended dosage

The recommended beginning dose is 37.5 milligrams daily. Dosages may be gradually increased if needed. Most children take doses ranging from 56.25 to 75 milligrams a day. The maximum recommended daily dose of Cylert is 112.5 milligrams. Significant improvement is gradual and may not be apparent until the third or fourth week of treatment with Cylert.

Your doctor may occasionally stop treatment with Cylert to see whether behavioral problems return and whether further treatment with Cylert is necessary.

Overdosage

Any medication taken in excess can have serious consequences. If you suspect an overdose, seek medical help immediately.

■ *Symptoms of Cylert overdose may include:*
Agitation, coma, confusion, convulsions, delirium, dilated pupils, exaggerated feeling of well-being, extremely high temperature, flushing, hallucinations, headache, high blood pressure, increased heart rate, increased reflex reactions, muscle twitches, sweating, tremors, vomiting

Generic name:

CYPROHEPTADINE

See Periactin, page 982.

Brand name:

CYSTADANE

Pronounced: SIST-uh-dane
Generic name: Betaine anhydrous

Why is this drug prescribed?

Cystadane is prescribed to reduce dangerously high blood levels of the naturally occurring amino acid homocysteine. Excessive levels of homocysteine can lead to formation of clots within your blood vessels, brittle bones (osteoporosis), other bone abnormalities, and dislocation of the lens of the eye. Homocysteine is also linked with an increased risk of heart disease and heart attack.

When homocysteine levels are so high that the substance appears in the urine, the condition is called homocystinuria. The problem is usually the result of an inherited lack of the enzymes needed to process homocysteine and generally shows up within the first months or years of life. Early signs of homocystinuria include delays in development, failure to thrive, seizures, and sluggishness.

Most important fact about this drug
The active ingredient in Cystadane (betaine) is found in our bodies and in foods such as beets, cereals, seafood, and spinach. Your doctor may prescribe Cystadane along with vitamin B_6 (pyridoxine), vitamin B_{12} (cobalamin), and folate. All of these dietary substances aid in the proper processing of homocysteine.

How should you take this medication?
Take Cystadane exactly as directed. To avoid forgetting a dose, try to get in the habit of taking it at the same time each day.

Cystadane will start to work within a week, and should have your condition completely under control within a month. You can continue therapy indefinitely; people have taken betaine for years without a problem.

■ *If you miss a dose...*
Take the forgotten dose as soon as you remember. If it is almost time for your next dose, skip the one you missed and go back to your regular schedule.

■ *Storage instructions...*
Store Cystadane at room temperature and protect from moisture. Keep the bottle tightly closed.

What side effects may occur?
Side effects of Cystadane are minimal. If any develop or change in intensity, inform your doctor as soon as possible. Only your doctor can determine whether it is safe for you to continue taking Cystadane.

■ *Side effects may include:*
Diarrhea, nausea, odor, stomach and intestinal problems, possible mental changes

Why should this drug not be prescribed?
There are no known reasons for avoiding Cystadane.

Special warnings about this medication
Do not use the powder if it does not completely dissolve in water, or if it makes a colored solution.

Possible food and drug interactions
when taking this medication
No interactions have been reported.

Special information
if you are pregnant or breastfeeding
The effects of Cystadane during pregnancy have not been studied. If you are pregnant or plan to become pregnant, check with your doctor immediately. It is not known whether Cystadane appears in breast milk. If this medication is essential to your health, your doctor may advise you to avoid breastfeeding.

Recommended dosage
Shake the bottle of Cystadane before removing the cap. Measure the number of scoops your doctor has prescribed by using the scoop provided.

ADULTS

The usual dosage is 3 scoops (3 grams) mixed with 4 to 6 ounces of water twice a day (6 grams daily). Make sure the powder is completely dissolved before drinking. Drink immediately after mixing.

The doctor will gradually increase your dosage until your homocysteine levels are under control. Dosages of up to 20 grams daily are sometimes necessary.

CHILDREN

In children less than 3 years old, the usual starting dose is 100 milligrams per 2.2 pounds of body weight per day. Each week, the doctor will increase the daily dose by 100 milligrams per 2.2 pounds until homocysteine levels are normal.

Overdosage
There have been no reported cases of overdose with Cystadane. However, a massive overdose could be dangerous. If you suspect an overdose, seek medical attention immediately.

Brand name:

CYTOTEC

Pronounced: SITE-oh-tek
Generic name: Misoprostol

Why is this drug prescribed?

Cytotec, a synthetic prostaglandin (hormone-like substance), reduces the production of stomach acid and protects the stomach lining. People who take nonsteroidal anti-inflammatory drugs (NSAIDs) may be given Cytotec tablets to help prevent stomach ulcers.

Aspirin and other NSAIDs such as Motrin, Naprosyn, Feldene, and others, which are widely used to control the pain and inflammation of arthritis, are generally hard on the stomach. If you must take an NSAID for a prolonged period of time, and if you are elderly or have ever had a stomach ulcer, your doctor may want you to take Cytotec for as long as you take the NSAID.

Most important fact about this drug

You must not become pregnant while using Cytotec. This drug causes uterine contractions that could lead to a miscarriage. If you do have a miscarriage, there is a risk that it might be incomplete. This could lead to bleeding, hospitalization, surgery, infertility, or even death. It is vitally important to use reliable contraception while taking Cytotec.

How should you take this medication?

Take Cytotec with meals, exactly as prescribed.

Take Cytotec for the full course of NSAID treatment, even if you notice no stomach problems.

Take the final dosage at bedtime.

■ *If you miss a dose...*
Take it as soon as you remember. If it is almost time for your next dose, skip the one you missed and go back to your regular schedule. Do not take 2 doses at once.

■ *Storage instructions...*
Store at room temperature in a dry place.

What side effects may occur?

Cytotec may cause abdominal cramps, diarrhea, and/or nausea, especially during the first few weeks of treatment. These symptoms may disappear as your body gets used to the drug. Taking Cytotec with food can help minimize diarrhea. If you have prolonged difficulty (more than 8 days), or if you have severe diarrhea, cramping, or nausea, call your doctor.

■ *Other side effects may include:*
Constipation, gas, indigestion, headache, heavy menstrual bleeding, menstrual disorder, menstrual pain or cramps, paleness, spotting (light bleeding between menstrual periods), stomach or intestinal bleeding, vomiting

Cytotec may cause uterine bleeding even if you have gone through menopause. However, postmenopausal bleeding could be a sign of some other gynecological problem. If you experience any such bleeding while taking Cytotec, notify your doctor at once.

Why should this drug not be prescribed?
Do not take Cytotec if you are sensitive to or have ever had an allergic reaction to it or to another prostaglandin medication.

Do not take Cytotec if you are pregnant or might become pregnant while taking it.

Special warnings about this medication
Since Cytotec may cause diarrhea, you should use this drug very cautiously if you have inflammatory bowel disease or any other condition in which the loss of fluid caused by diarrhea would be particularly dangerous.

To reduce the risk of diarrhea, take Cytotec with food and avoid taking it with a magnesium-containing antacid, such as Di-Gel, Gelusil, Maalox, Mylanta, and others. Have frequent medical checkups.

Never give Cytotec to anyone else; the dosage might be wrong, and if the other person is pregnant, the drug might harm the unborn baby or cause a miscarriage.

Possible food and drug interactions
when taking this medication
Cytotec does not interfere with arthritis medications such as aspirin and ibuprofen.

Special information
if you are pregnant or breastfeeding
If you are pregnant or plan to become pregnant, inform your doctor immediately. Because Cytotec can cause miscarriage, it should not be taken

during pregnancy. If you are a woman of childbearing age, you should not take Cytotec unless you have thoroughly discussed the risks with your doctor and believe you are able to take effective contraceptive measures.

You will need to take a pregnancy test about 2 weeks before starting to take Cytotec. To be sure you are not pregnant at the start of Cytotec treatment, your doctor will have you take your first dose on the second or third day of your menstrual period.

Even the most scrupulous contraceptive measures sometimes fail. If you believe you may have become pregnant while taking Cytotec, stop taking the drug and contact your doctor immediately.

It is not known if Cytotec appears in breast milk. Because of the potential for severe diarrhea in a nursing infant, your doctor may have you stop breastfeeding until your treatment is finished.

Recommended dosage

ADULTS

The recommended oral dose of Cytotec for the prevention of NSAID-induced stomach ulcers is 200 micrograms 4 times daily with food. Take the last dose of the day at bedtime.

If you cannot tolerate this dosage, your doctor can prescribe a dose of 100 micrograms.

Your should take Cytotec for the duration of NSAID therapy, as prescribed by your doctor.

For People with Kidney Impairment

You will not normally need an adjustment in the dosing schedule, but your doctor can reduce the dosage if you have trouble handling the usual dose.

Overdosage

Any medication taken in excess can have serious consequences. If you suspect symptoms of an overdose of Cytotec, seek medical attention immediately.

- *Symptoms of Cytotec overdose may include:*
  Abdominal pain, breathing difficulty, convulsions, diarrhea, fever, heart palpitations, low blood pressure, sedation (extreme drowsiness), slowed heartbeat, stomach or intestinal discomfort, tremors

Brand name:

CYTOXAN

Pronounced: sigh-TOKS-an
Generic name: Cyclophosphamide

Why is this drug prescribed?

Cytoxan, an anticancer drug, works by interfering with the growth of malignant cells. It may be used alone but is often given with other anticancer medications.

Cytoxan is used in the treatment of the following types of cancer:

Breast cancer
Leukemias (cancers affecting the white blood cells)
Malignant lymphomas (Hodgkin's disease or cancer of the lymph
    nodes)
Multiple myeloma (a malignant condition or cancer of the plasma cells)
Advanced mycosis fungoides (cancer of the skin and lymph nodes)
Neuroblastoma (a malignant tumor of the adrenal gland or sympathetic
    nervous system)
Ovarian cancer (adenocarcinoma)
Retinoblastoma (a malignant tumor of the retina)

In addition, Cytoxan may sometimes be given to children who have "minimal change" nephrotic syndrome (kidney damage resulting in loss of protein in the urine) and who have not responded well to treatment with steroid medications.

Most important fact about this drug

Cytoxan may cause bladder damage, probably from toxic byproducts of the drug that are excreted in the urine. Potential problems include bladder infection with bleeding and fibrosis of the bladder.

While you are being treated with Cytoxan, drink 3 or 4 liters of fluid a day to help prevent bladder problems. The extra fluid will dilute your urine and make you urinate frequently, thus minimizing the Cytoxan byproducts' contact with your bladder.

How should you take this medication?

Take Cytoxan exactly as prescribed. You will undergo frequent blood tests, and the doctor will adjust your dosage depending on the evolution of your white blood cell count; a dosage reduction is necessary if the count drops below a certain level. You will also have frequent urine tests to check for blood in the urine, a sign of bladder damage.

Take Cytoxan on an empty stomach. If you have severe stomach upset, then you may take it with food.

If you are unable to swallow the tablet form, you may be given an oral solution made from the injectable form of Cytoxan and Aromatic Elixir. This solution should be used within 14 days.

■ *If you miss a dose...*
Do not take the dose you missed. Go back to your regular schedule and contact your doctor. Do not take 2 doses at once.

■ *Storage instructions...*
Store tablets at room temperature. Store the oral solution in the refrigerator.

What side effects may occur?
Side effects cannot be anticipated. If any develop or change in intensity, inform your doctor immediately. Only your doctor can determine if it is safe for you to continue using Cytoxan.

One possible Cytoxan side effect is the development of a secondary cancer, typically of the bladder, lymph nodes, or bone marrow. A secondary cancer may occur up to several years after the drug is given.

Cytoxan can lower the activity of your immune system, making you more vulnerable to infection.

Noncancerous bladder problems may occur during Cytoxan therapy (see "Most important fact about this drug" section, page 306).

■ *More common side effects may include:*
Loss of appetite, nausea and vomiting, temporary hair loss

■ *Less common or rare side effects may include:*
Abdominal pain, anemia, bleeding, inflamed colon, darkening of skin and changes in fingernails, decreased sperm count, diarrhea, fever, impaired wound healing, mouth sores, new tumor growth, prolonged impairment of fertility or temporary sterility in men, rash, severe allergic reaction, temporary failure to menstruate, yellowing of eyes and skin

Why should this drug not be prescribed?
Do not take this medication if you have ever had an allergic reaction to it.

Also, tell your doctor if you have ever had an allergic reaction to another alkylating anticancer drug such as Alkeran, CeeNU, Emcyt, Leukeran, Myleran, or Zanosar.

In adults, Cytoxan should not be given for "minimal change" nephrotic syndrome or any other kidney disease.

Also, Cytoxan should not be given to anyone who is unable to produce normal blood cells because the bone marrow—where blood cells are made—is not functioning well.

Special warnings about this medication
You are at increased risk for toxic side effects from Cytoxan if you have any of the following conditions:

Blood disorder (low white blood cell or platelet count)
Bone marrow tumors
Kidney disorder
Liver disorder
Past anticancer therapy
Past X-ray therapy

Possible food and drug interactions
when taking this medication
If Cytoxan is taken with certain other drugs, the effects of either could be increased, decreased, or altered. It is especially important to check with your doctor before combining Cytoxan with the following:

Anticancer drugs such as Adriamycin
Allopurinol (the gout medicine Zyloprim)
Phenobarbital

If you take adrenal steroid hormones because you have had your adrenal glands removed, you are at increased risk for toxic effects from Cytoxan; your dosage of both steroids and Cytoxan may need to be modified.

Special information
if you are pregnant or breastfeeding
If you are pregnant or plan to become pregnant, inform your doctor immediately. When taken during pregnancy, Cytoxan can cause defects in the unborn baby. Women taking Cytoxan should use effective contraception. Cytoxan does appear in breast milk. A new mother will need to choose between taking this drug and nursing her baby.

Recommended dosage

ADULTS AND CHILDREN

Malignant Diseases
Your doctor will tailor your dosage according to your condition and other drugs taken with Cytoxan.

The recommended oral dosage range is 1 to 5 milligrams per 2.2 pounds of body weight per day.

CHILDREN

"Minimal Change" Nephrotic Syndrome
The recommended oral dosage is 2.5 to 3 milligrams per 2.2 pounds of body weight per day for a period of 60 to 90 days.

Overdosage
Although there is no specific information on Cytoxan overdose, any medication taken in excess can have serious consequences. If you suspect an overdose of Cytoxan, seek medical attention immediately.

Brand name:

DALMANE

Pronounced: DAL-main
Generic name: Flurazepam hydrochloride

Why is this drug prescribed?
Dalmane is used for the relief of insomnia, defined as difficulty falling asleep, waking up frequently at night, or waking up early in the morning. It can be used by people whose insomnia keeps coming back and in those who have poor sleeping habits. It belongs to a class of drugs known as benzodiazepines.

Most important fact about this drug
Tolerance and dependence can occur with the use of Dalmane. You may experience withdrawal symptoms if you stop using this drug abruptly. Discontinue or change your dose only in consultation with your doctor.

How should you take this medication?
Take this medication exactly as prescribed.

■ *If you miss a dose...*
Take the dose you missed as soon as you remember, if it is within an hour or so of the scheduled time. If you do not remember it until later, skip the dose you missed and go back to your regular schedule. Do not take 2 doses at once.

■ *Storage instructions...*
Store away from heat, light, and moisture.

What side effects may occur?
Side effects cannot be anticipated. If any develop or change in intensity, inform your doctor as soon as possible. Only your doctor can determine if it is safe for you to continue taking Dalmane.

■ *More common side effects may include:*
Dizziness, drowsiness, falling, lack of muscular coordination, light-headedness, staggering

■ *Less common or rare side effects may include:*
Apprehension, bitter taste, blurred vision, body and joint pain, burning eyes, chest pains, confusion, constipation, depression, diarrhea, difficulty in focusing, dry mouth, exaggerated feeling of well-being, excessive salivation, excitement, faintness, flushes, genital and urinary tract disorders, hallucinations, headache, heartburn, hyperactivity, irritability, itching, loss of appetite, low blood pressure, nausea, nervousness, rapid, fluttery heartbeat, restlessness, shortness of breath, skin rash, slurred speech, stimulation, stomach and intestinal pain, stomach upset, sweating, talkativeness, vomiting, weakness

■ *Side effects due to rapid decrease or abrupt withdrawal from Dalmane:*
Abdominal and muscle cramps, convulsions, depressed mood, inability to fall asleep or stay asleep, sweating, tremors, vomiting

Why should this drug not be prescribed?
If you are sensitive to or have had an allergic reaction to Dalmane or similar drugs such as Valium, you should not take this medication. Make sure your doctor is aware of any drug reactions you have experienced.

Special warnings about this medication

Dalmane will cause you to become drowsy or less alert; therefore, you should not drive or operate dangerous machinery or participate in any hazardous activity that requires full mental alertness after taking Dalmane.

If you are severely depressed or have suffered from severe depression, consult with your doctor before taking this medication.

If you have decreased kidney or liver function or chronic respiratory or lung disease, discuss use of this drug with your doctor.

**Possible food and drug interactions
when taking this medication**

Alcohol intensifies the effects of Dalmane. Do not drink alcohol while taking this medication.

If Dalmane is taken with certain other drugs, the effects of either could be increased, decreased, or altered. It is especially important to check with your doctor before combining Dalmane with the following:

Antidepressants such as Elavil and Tofranil
Antihistamines such as Benadryl and Tavist
Barbiturates such as Seconal and phenobarbital
Major tranquilizers such as Mellaril and Thorazine
Narcotic painkillers such as Demerol and Tylenol with Codeine
Sedatives such as Xanax and Halcion
Tranquilizers such as Librium and Valium

**Special information
if you are pregnant or breastfeeding**

Do not take Dalmane if you are pregnant or planning to become pregnant. There is an increased risk of birth defects. This drug may appear in breast milk and could affect a nursing infant. If this medication is essential to your health, your doctor may advise you to discontinue breastfeeding until your treatment with Dalmane is finished.

Recommended dosage

ADULTS

The usual recommended dose is 30 milligrams at bedtime; however, 15 milligrams may be all that is necessary. Your doctor will adjust the dose to your needs.

CHILDREN

Safety and effectiveness of Dalmane have not been established in children under 15 years of age.

OLDER ADULTS

Your doctor will limit the dosage to the smallest effective amount to avoid oversedation, dizziness, confusion, or lack of muscle coordination. The usual starting dose is 15 milligrams.

Overdosage

Any medication taken in excess can cause symptoms of overdose. If you suspect an overdose of Dalmane, seek medical attention immediately.

■ *The symptoms of Dalmane overdose may include:*
Coma, confusion, low blood pressure, sleepiness

Brand name:

DARVOCET-N

Pronounced: DAR-voe-set en
Generic ingredients: Propoxyphene napsylate,
  Acetáminophen
Other brand names: Darvon-N (propoxyphene napsylate),
  Darvon (propoxyphene hydrochloride), Darvon
  Compound-65 (propoxyphene hydrochloride, aspirin, and
  caffeine)

Why is this drug prescribed?

Darvocet-N and Darvon Compound-65 are mild narcotic analgesics prescribed for the relief of mild to moderate pain, with or without fever.

Darvon-N and Darvon are prescribed for the relief of mild to moderate pain.

Most important fact about this drug

You can build up tolerance to, and become dependent on, these drugs if you take them in higher than recommended doses over long periods of time.

How should you take this medication?

Take these drugs exactly as prescribed. Do not increase the amount you take without your doctor's approval. Do not take them for any reason other than those for which they are prescribed. Do not give them to others who may have similar symptoms.

■ *If you miss a dose...*
Take it as soon as you remember. If it is almost time for your next dose, skip the one you missed and go back to your regular schedule. Do not take 2 doses at once.

■ *Storage instructions...*
Store at room temperature.

What side effects may occur?
Side effects cannot be anticipated. If any develop or change in intensity, inform your doctor as soon as possible. Only your doctor can determine if it is safe for you to continue taking one of these medications.

■ *More common side effects may include:*
Drowsiness, dizziness, nausea, sedation, vomiting

If these side effects occur, it may help if you lie down after taking the medication.

■ *Less common side effects may include:*
Abdominal pain, constipation, feelings of elation or depression, hallucinations, headache, kidney problems, light-headedness, liver problems, minor visual disturbances, skin rashes, weakness, yellowed eyes and skin

Why should this drug not be prescribed?
If you are sensitive to or have ever had an allergic reaction to propoxyphene, any of the other ingredients in these drugs, or other pain relievers of this type, you should not take this medication. Make sure your doctor is aware of any drug reactions you have experienced.

Special warnings about this medication
These medicines may cause you to become drowsy or less alert; therefore, you should not drive or operate dangerous machinery or participate in any hazardous activity that requires full mental alertness until you know how the drug affects you.

If you have a kidney or liver disorder, consult your doctor before taking Darvocet-N.

Darvon Compound-65 contains aspirin and caffeine. If you have an ulcer or a blood clotting problem, consult your doctor before taking this medication. Aspirin may irritate the stomach lining and could cause bleeding.

Because there is a possible association between aspirin and the severe neurological disorder known as Reye's syndrome, children and teenagers with chickenpox or flu should not take Darvon Compound-65 unless prescribed by a doctor.

Aspirin may cause asthma attacks. If you have had an asthma attack while taking aspirin, consult your doctor before you take Darvon Compound-65.

Possible food and drug interactions
when taking this medication

The propoxyphene in these drugs slows down the central nervous system and intensifies the effects of alcohol. Heavy use of alcohol with this drug may cause overdose symptoms. Therefore, limit or avoid use of alcohol while you are taking this medication.

If these medications are taken with certain other drugs, the effects of either could be increased, decreased, or altered. It is especially important to check with your doctor before combining them with the following:

Antiseizure medications such as Tegretol
Antidepressant drugs such as Elavil
Antihistamines such as Benadryl
Muscle relaxants such as Flexeril
Narcotic pain relievers such as Demerol
Sleep aids such as Halcion
Tranquilizers such as Xanax and Valium
Warfarin-like drugs such as Coumadin

The use of these drugs with propoxyphene can lead to potentially fatal overdose symptoms.

Severe neurologic disorders, including coma, have occurred with the use of propoxyphene in combination with Tegretol.

The use of anticoagulants (blood thinners such as Coumadin) in combination with Darvon Compound-65 may cause bleeding. If you are taking an anticoagulant, consult your doctor before taking this drug.

The use of aspirin with drugs for gout may alter the effects of the antigout medication. Consult your doctor before taking Darvon Compound-65.

Special information
if you are pregnant or breastfeeding

Do not take these medications if you are pregnant or planning to become pregnant unless you are directed to do so by your doctor. Temporary drug dependence may occur in newborns when the mother has taken this drug consistently in the weeks before delivery. The use of Darvon Compound-65 (which contains aspirin) during pregnancy may cause problems in the developing baby or complications during delivery. Do not take it during the last 3 months of pregnancy. Darvocet-N does appear in breast milk. However, no adverse effects have been found in nursing infants.

Recommended dosage

ADULTS

These medicines may be taken every 4 hours as needed for pain. The usual doses are:

Darvocet-N 50: 2 tablets

Darvocet-N 100: 1 tablet

Darvon: 1 capsule

Darvon Compound-65: 1 capsule

Your doctor may lower the total daily dosage if you have kidney or liver problems.

The most you should take of Darvon or Darvon Compound-65 is 6 capsules a day.

CHILDREN

The safety and effectiveness of Darvocet-N have not been established in children.

OLDER ADULTS

Your doctor may lengthen the time between doses.

Overdosage

Any medication taken in excess can have serious consequences. If you suspect an overdose, seek medical attention immediately.

- *Symptoms of a propoxyphene overdose may include:*
  Bluish tinge to the skin, coma, convulsions, decreased or difficult breathing to the point of temporary stoppage, decreased heart function, extreme sleepiness, irregular heartbeat, low blood pressure, pinpoint pupils becoming dilated later, stupor

- *Additional symptoms of overdose with Darvocet-N:*
  Abdominal pain, excessive sweating, general feeling of illness, kidney failure, liver problems, loss of appetite, nausea, vomiting

■ *Additional symptoms of overdose with Darvon Compound-65:*
Confusion, deafness, excessive perspiration, headache, mental dullness, nausea, rapid breathing, rapid pulse, ringing in the ears, vertigo, vomiting

Extreme overdosage may lead to unconsciousness and death.

Brand name:

DARVON

See Darvocet-N, page 334.

Brand name:

DARVON COMPOUND-65

See Darvocet-N, page 334.

Brand name:

DARVON-N

See Darvocet-N, page 334.

Brand name:

DAYPRO

Pronounced: DAY-pro
Generic name: Oxaprozin

Why is this drug prescribed?
Daypro is a nonsteroidal anti-inflammatory drug used to relieve the inflammation, swelling, stiffness, and joint pain associated with rheumatoid arthritis and osteoarthritis (the most common kind of arthritis).

Most important fact about this drug
You should have frequent check-ups with your doctor if you take Daypro regularly. Ulcers and internal bleeding can occur without warning.

How should you take this medication?
Take Daypro with a full glass of water. If the drug upsets your stomach, your doctor may recommend taking Daypro with food, milk, or an antacid, even though food may delay onset of relief.

It will also help to prevent irritation in your upper digestive tract if you avoid lying down for about 20 minutes after taking Daypro.

Take this medication exactly as prescribed.

■ *If you miss a dose...*
Try to take Daypro at the same time each day—for example, after breakfast. If you forget to take a dose and remember later in the day, you can still take it. If you completely forget to take your medication, do *not* double the dose the next day to make up for the missed dose. You should get back on your normal schedule as soon as possible.

■ *Storage instructions...*
Store at room temperature in a tightly closed container, away from light.

What side effects may occur?
Side effects cannot be anticipated. If any develop or change in intensity, tell your doctor as soon as possible. Only your doctor can decide if it is safe for you to continue taking Daypro.

■ *More common side effects may include:*
Constipation, diarrhea, indigestion, nausea, rash

■ *Less common side effects may include:*
Abdominal pain, confusion, depression, frequent or painful urination, gas, loss of appetite, ringing in the ears, sleep disturbances, sleepiness, vomiting

■ *Rare side effects may include:*
Anaphylaxis (a severe allergic reaction), anemia, blood in the urine, blood pressure changes, blurred vision, bruising, changes in kidney and liver function, decreased menstrual flow, fluid retention, general feeling of illness, hemorrhoidal or rectal bleeding, hepatitis, hives, inflammation of the mouth, inflammation of the pancreas, irritated eyes, itching, peptic ulcerations, respiratory infection, sensitivity to light, stomach and intestinal bleeding, weight gain or loss, weakness

Why should this drug not be prescribed?
If you are sensitive to or have ever had an allergic reaction to Daypro, or if you have ever developed asthma, nasal tumors, or other allergic reactions due to aspirin or other nonsteroidal anti-inflammatory drugs, you should not take this medication. Make sure your doctor is aware of any drug reactions you have experienced.

Special warnings about this medication

Use Daypro with caution if you have kidney or liver disease.

Do not take aspirin or any other anti-inflammatory medications while taking Daypro, unless your doctor tells you to do so.

Daypro can increase water retention. Use with caution if you have heart disease or high blood pressure.

If you are taking Daypro for an extended period, your doctor should check your blood for anemia.

Daypro can prolong bleeding time. If you are taking a blood-thinning medication, use Daypro with caution.

Daypro may cause sensitivity to sunlight. Avoid prolonged exposure to the sun. Use sunscreens and wear protective clothing.

Do not use Daypro if you are planning to have surgery in the immediate future.

Possible food and drug interactions
when taking this medication

If you take Daypro with certain other drugs, the effects of either medication could be increased, decreased, or altered. It is especially important to check with your doctor before combining Daypro with the following medications:

Aspirin
Beta-blocking blood pressure medications such as Inderal and Tenormin
Blood thinners such as Coumadin
Digitalis and digoxin (Lanoxin)
Diuretics such as Lasix and Midamor
Lithium (Lithonate)
Ulcer drugs such as Tagamet and Zantac

Avoid alcoholic beverages while taking Daypro.

Special information
if you are pregnant or breastfeeding

The effects of Daypro during pregnancy have not been adequately studied. If you are pregnant or plan to become pregnant, tell your doctor immediately. Since the effects of Daypro on nursing infants are not known, tell your doctor if you are nursing or plan to nurse. If Daypro treatment is necessary for your health, your doctor may tell you to discontinue nursing until your treatment is finished.

Recommended dosage

ADULTS

Your doctor will adjust the dose based on your needs.

Rheumatoid Arthritis

The usual daily dose is 1200 milligrams (two 600-milligram caplets) once a day.

Osteoarthritis

The usual starting dose for moderate to severe osteoarthritis is 1200 milligrams (two 600-milligram caplets) once a day.

The most you should take in a day is 1800 milligrams divided into smaller doses, or 26 milligrams per 2.2 pounds of body weight, whichever is lower.

CHILDREN

The safety and efficacy of Daypro in children have not been determined.

Overdosage

If you take too much of any medication, it can have serious consequences. If you suspect an overdose, seek medical attention immediately.

■ *Symptoms of Daypro overdose may include:*
Coma, drowsiness, fatigue, nausea, pain in the stomach, stomach and intestinal bleeding, vomiting

Acute kidney failure, high blood pressure, and a slowdown in breathing have occurred rarely.

Brand name:

DDAVP

Pronounced: dee-dee-ai-vee-pee
Generic name: Desmopressin acetate
Other brand name: Stimate

Why is this drug prescribed?

DDAVP nasal spray, nose drops, and tablets are given to prevent or control the frequent urination and loss of water associated with diabetes insipidus (a rare condition characterized by very large quantities of diluted urine and excessive thirst). They are also used to treat frequent passage of urine and increased thirst in people with certain brain injuries, and those who have undergone surgery in the pituitary region of the brain. DDAVP nasal spray and nose drops are also prescribed to help stop some types of bed-wetting.

Stimate nasal spray is used to stop bleeding in certain types of hemophilia (failure of the blood to clot).

Most important fact about this drug
When taking DDAVP, elderly and young people in particular should limit their fluid intake to no more than what satisfies thirst. Although extremely rare, there is a possibility of water intoxication, in which reduced sodium levels in the blood can lead to seizures.

How should you use this medication?
Use DDAVP exactly as prescribed. The spray and drops are for nasal use only; never swallow the medication or allow the liquid to run into your mouth.

Your doctor may increase or decrease your dosage, depending on how you respond to DDAVP. Your response will be judged by how long you are able to sleep without having to get up to urinate and how much urine your kidneys produce.

The DDAVP nasal spray pump bottle accurately delivers 50 doses of the medication. After the 50th dose, the amount of medication that comes out with each spray will no longer be a full dose. When this happens, throw the bottle away even if it is not completely empty.

Stimate nasal spray delivers 25 doses; the same instructions apply. The Stimate nasal spray pump must be primed before you use it for the first time: Press down 4 times.

Since the DDAVP spray bottle delivers only a standard-sized dose, those who need more or less medication should use the nose drops instead of the spray.

If nasal congestion, scars, or swelling inside the nose make it difficult to absorb DDAVP, your doctor may temporarily stop the drug or give you tablets or an injectable form. If you are switched to tablets, you should start taking them 12 hours after you last used the nasal spray or nose drops.

■ *If you miss a dose...*
   Take the forgotten dose as soon as you remember. If you take 1 dose a day and don't remember until the next day, skip the dose. If you take DDAVP more than once a day and it is almost time for the next dose, skip the one

you missed and go back to your regular schedule. Never try to "catch up" by doubling the dose.

- *Storage instructions...*
  The drops should be stored in the refrigerator. If you are traveling, they will stay fresh at room temperature for up to 3 weeks.

The tablets and nasal spray can be kept at room temperature. Protect the tablets from heat and light.

What side effects may occur?
Too high a dosage of DDAVP nasal spray or drops may produce headache, nausea, mild abdominal cramps, stuffy nose, irritation of the nose, or flushing. These symptoms will probably disappear when the dosage is reduced. Some people have complained of nosebleed, sore throat, cough, or a cold or other upper respiratory infections after taking DDAVP nasal spray or drops.

- *Other potential side effects include:*
  Abdominal pain, chills, conjunctivitis (pinkeye), depression, dizziness, inability to produce tears, leg rash, nostril pain, rash, stomach or intestinal upset, swelling around the eyes, weakness

- *Side effects of Stimate nasal spray may include:*
  Agitation, chest pain, chills, dizziness, fluid retention and swelling, indigestion, inflammation of the penis, insomnia, itchy or light-sensitive eyes, pain, pounding heartbeat, rapid heartbeat, sleepiness, vomiting, warm feeling

Why should this drug not be prescribed?
Do not use DDAVP if you are sensitive to or have ever had an allergic reaction to any of its ingredients.

Special warnings about this medication
If you have cystic fibrosis or any other condition in which there is fluid and electrolyte imbalance, you should use DDAVP with extreme caution.

Because DDAVP may cause a rise in blood pressure, use this medication cautiously if you have high blood pressure and/or coronary artery disease. Your blood pressure could also fall temporarily. If you continue to experience bleeding after using Stimate nasal spray, contact your doctor.

**Possible food and drug interactions
when taking this medication**

If DDAVP is taken with certain other drugs, the effects of either could be increased, decreased, or altered. It is especially important to check with your doctor before combining DDAVP with the following:

Any drug used to increase blood pressure
Clofibrate (Atromid-S)
Glyburide (Micronase)
Epinephrine (EpiPen)

**Special information
if you are pregnant or breastfeeding**

If you are pregnant or plan to become pregnant, inform your doctor immediately. Although DDAVP is not known to cause birth defects, it should be used with caution. DDAVP should be taken during pregnancy only if clearly needed. DDAVP is not believed to appear in breast milk. However, check with your doctor before using the drug while breastfeeding.

Recommended dosage

Your doctor will carefully tailor your dosage to meet your individual needs.

CENTRAL CRANIAL DIABETES INSIPIDUS

DDAVP Nasal Spray and Nose Drops

Adults: The usual recommended dosage range is 0.1 to 0.4 milliliter daily, either as a single dose or divided into 2 or 3 doses. Most adults require 0.2 milliliter per day divided into 2 doses.

Children: The usual dosage range for children aged 3 months to 12 years is 0.05 to 0.3 milliliter daily, either as a single dose or divided into 2 doses.

DDAVP Tablets

Adults and Children Aged 4 and Over: The usual starting dose is half of a 0.1-milligram tablet twice a day. Your doctor will adjust the dose to suit you. You will eventually take 0.1 to 1.2 milligrams a day, divided into smaller doses.

PRIMARY NOCTURNAL ENURESIS (BEDWETTING)

DDAVP Nasal Spray/Nose Drops

Children 6 Years of Age and Older: The usual recommended dose is 20 micrograms or 0.2 milliliter at bedtime. Dosage requirements range from 10 to 40 micrograms. One-half the dose should be taken in each nostril.

HEMOPHILIA

Stimate Nasal Spray

To stop bleeding, the usual dose is one 150-microgram spray in each nostril. If you use the spray more frequently than every 48 hours, you may find you are not responding as well as you should to the drug.

Overdosage

An overdose of DDAVP may cause abdominal cramps, flushing, headache, or nausea. If you suspect an overdose of DDAVP, seek medical attention immediately.

Brand name:

DECADRON TABLETS

Pronounced: DECK-uh-drohn
Generic name: Dexamethasone

Why is this drug prescribed?

Decadron, a corticosteroid drug, is used to reduce inflammation and relieve symptoms in a variety of disorders, including rheumatoid arthritis and severe cases of asthma. It may be given to people to treat primary or secondary adrenal cortex insufficiency (lack of sufficient adrenal hormone). It is also given to help treat the following disorders:

Severe allergic conditions such as drug-induced allergies
Blood disorders such as various anemias
Certain cancers (along with other drugs)
Skin diseases such as severe psoriasis
Collagen (connective tissue) diseases such as systemic lupus
    erythematosus
Digestive tract disease such as ulcerative colitis
High serum levels of calcium associated with cancer
Fluid retention due to nephrotic syndrome (a condition in which damage
    to the kidneys causes the body to lose protein in the urine)
Eye diseases such as allergic conjunctivitis
Lung diseases such as tuberculosis (along with other drugs)

Most important fact about this drug

Decadron lowers your resistance to infections and can make them harder to treat. Decadron may also mask some of the signs of an infection, making it difficult for your doctor to diagnose the actual problem.

How should you take this medication?
Decadron should be taken exactly as prescribed by your doctor.

If you are taking large doses, your doctor may advise you to take Decadron with meals and to take antacids between meals, to prevent a peptic ulcer from developing.

Check with your doctor before stopping Decadron abruptly. If you have been taking the drug for a long time, you may need to reduce your dose gradually over a period of days or weeks.

The lowest possible dose should always be used, and as symptoms subside, dosage should be reduced gradually.

- *If you miss a dose...*
  Take the forgotten dose as soon as you remember. If it is almost time for the next dose, skip the one you missed and go back to your regular schedule. Never try to "catch up" by doubling the dose.

- *Storage instructions...*
  There are no special storage requirements.

What side effects may occur?
Side effects cannot be anticipated. If any develop or change in intensity, inform your doctor as soon as possible. Only your doctor can determine if it is safe for you to continue taking Decadron.

- *Side effects may include:*
  Abdominal distention, allergic reactions, blood clots, bone fractures and degeneration, bruises, cataracts, congestive heart failure, convulsions, "cushingoid" symptoms (moon face, weight gain, high blood pressure, emotional disturbances, growth of facial hair in women), excessive hairiness, fluid and salt retention, general feeling of illness, glaucoma, headache, hiccups, high blood pressure, hives, increased appetite, increased eye pressure, increased pressure in head, increased sweating, increases in amounts of insulin or hypoglycemic medications needed in diabetes, inflammation of the esophagus, inflammation of the pancreas, irregular menstruation, loss of muscle mass, low potassium levels in blood (leading to symptoms such as dry mouth, excessive thirst, weak or irregular heartbeat, and muscle pain or cramps), muscle weakness, nausea, osteoporosis, peptic ulcer, perforated small and large bowel, poor healing of wounds, protruding eyeballs, suppression of growth in children, thin skin, tiny red or purplish spots on the skin, torn tendons, vertigo, weight gain

Why should this drug not be prescribed?
Decadron should not be used if you have a fungal infection, or if you are sensitive or allergic to any of its ingredients.

Special warnings about this medication
Decadron can alter the way your body responds to unusual stress. If you are injured, need surgery, or develop an acute illness, inform your doctor. Your dosage may need to be increased.

Corticosteroids such as Decadron can lower your resistance to infection. Diseases such as measles and chickenpox can be serious and even fatal in adults. Likewise, a simple case of threadworm can run rampant, producing life-threatening complications. If you are taking Decadron and are exposed to chickenpox or measles—or suspect a case of threadworm—notify your doctor immediately. Symptoms of threadworm include stomach pain, vomiting, and diarrhea.

Do not get a smallpox vaccination or any other immunizations while taking Decadron, especially in high doses. The vaccination might not take, and could do harm to the nervous system.

Decadron may reactivate a dormant case of tuberculosis. If you have inactive tuberculosis and must take Decadron for an extended period, your doctor will prescribe anti-TB medication as well.

When you stop taking Decadron after long-term therapy, you may develop withdrawal symptoms such as fever, muscle or joint pain, and a feeling of illness.

Long-term use of Decadron may cause cataracts, glaucoma, and eye infections.

If you have any of the following conditions, make sure your doctor knows about it:

Allergy to any cortisone-like drug
Cirrhosis
Diabetes
Diverticulitis
Eye infection (herpes simplex)
Glaucoma
High blood pressure
Impaired thyroid function
Kidney disease
Myasthenia gravis (a muscle disorder)

Osteoporosis (brittle bones)
Peptic ulcer
Recent heart attack
Tuberculosis
Ulcerative colitis

Steroids may alter male fertility.

This medication can aggravate existing emotional problems or cause emotional disturbances. Symptoms range from an exaggerated sense of well-being and difficulty sleeping to mood swings and psychotic episodes. If you experience any changes in mood, contact your doctor.

If you have recently been to the tropics or are suffering from diarrhea with no apparent cause, inform your doctor before taking Decadron.

Possible food and drug interactions
when taking this medication

If Decadron is taken with certain other drugs, the effects of either could be increased, decreased, or altered. It is especially important to check with your doctor before combining Decadron with the following:

Aspirin
Blood-thinning medications such as Coumadin
Ephedrine (a decongestant in drugs such as Marax and Rynatuss)
Indomethacin (Indocin)
Phenobarbital
Phenytoin (Dilantin)
Rifampin (Rifadin, Rimactane)
Water pills that pull potassium out of the system, such as HydroDIURIL

Special information
if you are pregnant or breastfeeding

The effects of Decadron during pregnancy have not been adequately studied. If you are pregnant or plan to become pregnant, inform your doctor immediately. Infants born to mothers who have taken substantial doses of corticosteroids during pregnancy should be carefully watched for adrenal problems. Corticosteroids appear in breast milk and can suppress growth in infants. If Decadron is essential to your health, your doctor may advise you to stop breastfeeding until your treatment with Decadron is finished.

Recommended dosage

ADULTS

Your doctor will tailor your individual dose to the condition being treated. Initial doses range from 0.75 milligram to 9 milligrams a day.

After the drug produces a satisfactory response, your doctor will gradually lower the dose to the minimum effective level.

Overdosage

Reports of overdose with this medication are rare. However, if you suspect an overdose, seek medical treatment immediately.

Brand name:

DECADRON TURBINAIRE AND RESPIHALER

Pronounced: DECK-ah-drahn tur-bin-AIR and RESS-pi-hail-er
Generic name: Dexamethasone sodium phosphate
Other brand name: Dexacort

Why is this drug prescribed?

Decadron is a synthetic adrenocortical steroid (a hormone created in the laboratory). Decadron Turbinaire is used to treat hay fever and other nasal allergies, and to assist in the treatment of nasal polyps. Decadron Respihaler is prescribed for bronchial asthma in people who need sustained treatment.

Most important fact about this drug

Decadron lowers your resistance to infections and can make them harder to treat. Decadron may also mask some of the signs of an infection, making it difficult for your doctor to diagnose the actual problem.

How should you take this medication?

These medications come with directions. Read them carefully before using the medicine. To work, the medications must be used exactly as directed.

If you are using the Decadron Respihaler, gargling and rinsing your mouth with water after each dose may help prevent hoarseness and throat irritation. Do not swallow the water after you rinse.

■ *If you miss a dose...*
Take the forgotten dose as soon as possible and take the remaining doses for that day at evenly spaced intervals. If it is time for your next dose, skip the one you missed. Never take a double dose.

■ *Storage instructions...*
Store Decadron at room temperature. Since the contents are under pressure, keep the container away from fire or extreme heat.

What side effects may occur?
Side effects cannot be anticipated. If any develop or change in intensity, inform your doctor as soon as possible. Only your doctor can determine whether it is safe to continue using Decadron.

■ *More common side effects of Decadron Turbinaire may include:*
Nasal dryness and irritation

■ *Less common side effects of Decadron Turbinaire may include:*
Bronchial asthma, headache, hives, light-headedness, loss of smell, nausea, nosebleeds, perforated nasal septum (dividing wall of the nose), rebound nasal congestion

■ *Side effects of Decadron Respihaler may include:*
Coughing, fungal infections in the throat, hoarseness, throat irritation

■ *Side effects that may occur when Decadron is absorbed into the bloodstream:*
Abdominal distention, abnormal skin redness, allergic reactions, blood clots, bruising, cataracts, congestive heart failure, convulsions, development of Cushing's syndrome (moon face, emotional disturbances, high blood pressure, weight gain, and growth of facial and body hair in women), diabetes, emotional disturbances, excessive hairiness, fractures of the long bones, fractures of the vertebrae, fragile skin, glaucoma, headache, hiccups, high blood pressure, hives, increased appetite, increased eye pressure, increased pressure in head), increased sweating, loss of muscle mass, menstrual irregularities, muscle weakness, nausea, osteoporosis, perforated small or large bowel, poor wound healing, potassium loss, protruding eyeballs, reddish or purplish spots on the skin, ruptured tendons, salt and fluid retention, stomach ulcer, ulcer of the esophagus, vague feeling of weakness, vertigo, weight gain

Why should this drug not be prescribed?

Do not use Decadron if you have a fungal infection or if you have ever had an allergic reaction or are sensitive to any cortisone-like medication such as Beclovent. Decadron Turbinaire should not be used if you have tuberculosis or a nasal condition caused by a virus or a fungus, or if you have herpes simplex infection of the eye. Decadron Respihaler should not be used if tests show that you have a yeast infection (*Candida albicans*).

Special warnings about this medication

Decadron does not expand the bronchial passages, and should be used for asthma only if bronchodilators and other asthma medications are not effective. Decadron does not provide rapid relief of symptoms, but does help to control asthma when taken routinely.

Decadron can alter the way your body responds to unusual stress. If you are injured, need surgery, or develop an acute illness, tell your doctor. Your dosage may need to be increased.

If you develop an infection of the throat or voice box while using the Decadron Respihaler, stop using the Respihaler and notify your doctor. You will need medication.

Corticosteroids such as Decadron may mask the symptoms of infection and make you more susceptible to infections. Diseases such as chickenpox and measles can be serious and even fatal in adults who have never had these illnesses. If you are using Decadron Turbinaire or Respihaler and are exposed to chickenpox or measles, notify your doctor immediately. Do not get a smallpox vaccination or any other immunizations while taking Decadron, especially in high doses. The vaccination might not take, and could do harm to the nervous system.

Using Decadron for a long time may cause cataracts, glaucoma, and eye infections.

Large doses of Decadron may raise blood pressure and increase salt and water retention. If this happens, your doctor may tell you to restrict salt in your diet.

Decadron should be used with extreme caution if you have dormant tuberculosis or test positive for tuberculosis. Decadron may reactivate the disease.

When you stop taking Decadron after long-term therapy, you may develop withdrawal symptoms such as fever, muscle or joint pain, and weakness.

Decadron should be used with care if you have an underactive thyroid or cirrhosis.

Your doctor will prescribe the lowest possible dose to control your condition, and reduce your dosage of Decadron gradually. Do not suddenly stop taking it.

Decadron may aggravate existing emotional problems or cause emotional disturbances. Symptoms range from euphoria (an exaggerated sense of well-being) and difficulty sleeping to mood swings, personality changes, severe depression, and psychotic episodes. If you experience any changes in mood, call your doctor.

Decadron should be used with care if you have ulcerative colitis, diverticulitis (an inflammation of the digestive tract), peptic ulcer, kidney disease, high blood pressure, osteoporosis, or myasthenia gravis (muscle weakness, especially in the face and neck), or if you have recently had a heart attack.

Long-term therapy with Decadron may affect the growth and development of children and should be carefully checked by your doctor. Decadron Turbinaire is not recommended for children under 6 years of age.

If you have recently been to the tropics or are suffering from diarrhea with no apparent cause, inform your doctor before using Decadron.

Possible food and drug interactions
when taking this medication
If Decadron is taken with certain other drugs, the effects of either could be increased, decreased, or altered. It is especially important to check with your doctor before combining Decadron with the following:

Aspirin
Blood thinners such as Coumadin
Ephedrine
Phenytoin (Dilantin)
Phenobarbital (Bellergal-S, Donnatal, others)
Potassium-depleting diuretics such as Dyazide and Esidrix
Rifampin (Rifadin, Rimactane)

Special information
if you are pregnant or breastfeeding
The effects of Decadron during pregnancy have not been adequately studied. If you are pregnant or plan to become pregnant, inform your doctor immediately. Infants born to mothers who have taken substantial doses of steroids during pregnancy may have problems with their adrenal glands. Corticosteroids appear in breast milk and could affect infant growth or cause other damaging effects. Decadron is not recommended for nursing mothers. If Decadron is essential to your health, your doctor may advise you to stop breastfeeding until your treatment with Decadron is finished.

Recommended dosage
TURBINAIRE

Adults
The usual initial dosage is 2 sprays in each nostril, 2 or 3 times a day.

Children (6 to 12 Years of Age)
The usual initial dosage is 1 or 2 sprays in each nostril 2 times a day, depending on age.

Dosage should be gradually reduced when improvement occurs. The maximum daily dosage for adults is 12 sprays and for children, 8 sprays. Therapy should be stopped as soon as possible. If symptoms return, your doctor may start the medication again.

RESPIHALER

Adults
The recommended initial dose is 3 inhalations, 3 or 4 times a day.

Children
The recommended initial dose is 2 inhalations, 3 or 4 times a day.

Dosage should be gradually reduced when improvement occurs. The maximum daily dosage for adults is 3 inhalations per dose, 12 inhalations per day; and for children, 2 inhalations per dose, 8 inhalations per day.

Overdosage
There have been rare reports of toxicity (poisoning) and death following steroid overdose. If you suspect Decadron overdose, seek medical treatment immediately.

Brand name:

DECONAMINE

Pronounced: dee-CON-uh-meen
Generic ingredients: Chlorpheniramine maleate,
*   d-Pseudoephedrine hydrochloride*

Why is this drug prescribed?
Deconamine is an antihistamine and decongestant used for the temporary relief of persistent runny nose, sneezing, and nasal congestion caused by upper respiratory infections (the common cold), sinus inflammation, or hay

fever. It is also used to help clear nasal passages and shrink swollen membranes and to drain the sinuses and relieve sinus pressure.

Most important fact about this drug
Deconamine may cause you to become drowsy or less alert. You should not drive or operate machinery or participate in any activity that requires full mental alertness until you know how you react to Deconamine.

How should you take this medication?
If Deconamine makes you nervous or restless, or you have trouble sleeping, take the last dose of the day a few hours before you go to bed. Take Deconamine exactly as prescribed.

Antihistamines can make your mouth and throat dry. It may help to suck on hard candy, chew gum, or melt bits of ice in your mouth.

- *If you miss a dose...*
  Take it as soon as you remember. If it is almost time for your next dose, skip the one you missed and go back to your regular schedule. Never take 2 doses at once.

- *Storage instructions...*
  Store at room temperature.

What side effects may occur?
Side effects cannot be anticipated. If any develop or change in intensity, inform your doctor as soon as possible. Only your doctor can determine if it is safe for you to continue taking Deconamine.

The most common side effect is mild to moderate drowsiness.

- *Less common or rare side effects may include:*
  Anaphylactic shock (extreme allergic reaction), anemia, anxiety, blurred vision, breathing difficulty, chills, confusion, constipation, convulsion, diarrhea, difficulty sleeping, difficulty in carrying out movements, disturbed coordination, dizziness, double vision, dry mouth, nose, and throat, early menstruation, exaggerated sense of well being, excessive perspiration, excitation, fatigue, extreme calm (sedation), fear, frequent or difficult urination, hallucinations, headache, hives, hysteria, increased chest congestion, irregular heartbeat, irritability, light-headedness, loss of appetite, low blood pressure, nausea, nervousness, painful urination, pallor, pounding heartbeat, rapid heartbeat, restlessness, ringing in ears, sensitivity to light, skin rash, stomach upset or pain, stuffy nose,

tenseness, tightness of chest, tingling or numbness, tremor, unusual bleeding or bruising, vertigo, vomiting, weakness, wheezing

Why should this drug not be prescribed?

Do not use Deconamine if you have severe high blood pressure or severe heart disease, are taking an antidepressant drug known as an MAO inhibitor (Nardil, Parnate, others), or are sensitive to or have ever had an allergic reaction to antihistamines or decongestants.

Special warnings about this medication

Use Deconamine with extreme caution if you have the eye condition called glaucoma, peptic ulcer or stomach obstructions, an enlarged prostate, or difficulty urinating.

Also use caution if you have bronchial asthma, emphysema, chronic lung disease, high blood pressure, heart disease, diabetes, or an overactive thyroid.

Deconamine may cause excitability, especially in children.

Possible food and drug interactions
when taking this medication

Alcohol increases the sedative effect of Deconamine. Avoid it while taking this medication.

If Deconamine is taken with certain other drugs, the effects of either may be increased, decreased, or altered. It is especially important to check with your doctor before combining Deconamine with the following:

Antidepressant drugs such as the MAO inhibitors Nardil and Parnate
Asthma medications such as Ventolin and Proventil
Bromocriptine (Parlodel)
Mecamylamine (Inversine)
Methyldopa (Aldomet)
Narcotic pain killers such as Demerol and Percocet
Phenytoin (Dilantin)
Reserpine (Ser-Ap-Es, others)
Sleep aids such as Halcion and Seconal
Tranquilizers such as Valium and Xanax

Special information
if you are pregnant or breastfeeding

The effects of Deconamine during pregnancy have not been adequately studied. If you are pregnant or plan to become pregnant, notify your doctor immediately. Deconamine appears in breast milk and could affect a nursing infant. If this medication is essential to your health, your doctor may advise you to discontinue breastfeeding until your treatment with Deconamine is finished.

Recommended dosage

DECONAMINE TABLETS

Adults and Children over 12 Years
The usual dosage is 1 tablet 3 or 4 times daily.

Children under 12 Years
Use Deconamine Syrup or Chewable Tablets instead of the tablets.

DECONAMINE SYRUP

Adults and Children over 12 Years
The usual dose is 1 to 2 teaspoonfuls (5 to 10 milliliters) 3 or 4 times daily.

Children 6 to 12 Years
The usual dose is ½ to 1 teaspoonful (2.5 to 5 milliliters) 3 or 4 times daily, not to exceed 4 teaspoonfuls in 24 hours.

Children 2 to 6 Years
The usual dose is ½ teaspoonful (2.5 milliliters) 3 or 4 times daily, not to exceed 2 teaspoonfuls in 24 hours.

Children under 2 Years
Use as directed by your doctor.

DECONAMINE SR CAPSULES

Adults and Children over 12 Years
The usual dose is 1 capsule every 12 hours.

Children under 12 Years
Use Deconamine Syrup or Chewable Tablets instead of the capsules.

DECONAMINE CHEWABLE TABLETS

Adults
The usual dose is 2 tablets 3 or 4 times a day.

Children 6 to 12 Years
The usual dose is 1 tablet 3 or 4 times a day.

Children 2 to 6 Years
The usual dose is ½ tablet 3 or 4 times a day.

Overdosage
Any medication taken in excess can have serious consequences. If you suspect an overdose, seek medical attention immediately.

■ *Symptoms of Deconamine overdose include:*
Convulsions, diminished alertness, hallucinations, severe drowsiness, severe dryness of mouth, nose, and throat, shortness of breath/difficulty breathing, sleep problems, slow or rapid heartbeat, tremors

Brand name:

DELTASONE

Pronounced: DELL-tuh-zone
Generic name: Prednisone
Other brand name: Orasone

Why is this drug prescribed?
Deltasone, a steroid drug, is used to reduce inflammation and alleviate symptoms in a variety of disorders, including rheumatoid arthritis and severe cases of asthma. It may be given to treat primary or secondary adrenal cortex insufficiency (lack of sufficient adrenal hormone in the body). It is used in treating all of the following:

Abnormal adrenal gland development
Allergic conditions (severe)
Blood disorders
Certain cancers (along with other drugs)
Diseases of the connective tissue including systemic lupus
    erythematosus
Eye diseases of various kinds
Flare-ups of multiple sclerosis
Fluid retention due to "nephrotic syndrome" (a condition in which
    damage to the kidneys causes protein to be lost in the urine)
Lung diseases, including tuberculosis
Meningitis (inflamed membranes around the brain)

Prevention of organ rejection
Rheumatoid arthritis and related disorders
Severe flare-ups of ulcerative colitis or enteritis (inflammation of the
    intestines)
Skin diseases
Thyroid gland inflammation
Trichinosis (with complications)

Most important fact about this drug
Deltasone lowers your resistance to infections and can make them harder to
treat. Deltasone may also mask some of the signs of an infection, making it
difficult for your doctor to diagnose the actual problem.

How should you take this medication?
Take Deltasone exactly as prescribed. Dosages are kept to an absolute
minimum.

If you need long-term Deltasone treatment, your doctor may prescribe
alternate-day therapy, in which you take the medication only every other
morning. The "resting day" gives your adrenal glands a chance to produce
some hormone naturally so they will not lose the ability.

If you have been taking Deltasone for a period of time, you will probably need
an increased dosage of the medication before, during, and after any stressful
situation. Always consult your doctor if you are anticipating stress and think
you may need a temporary dosage increase.

When stopping Deltasone treatment, tapering off is better than quitting
abruptly. Your doctor will probably have you decrease the dosage very
gradually over a period of days or weeks.

You should take Deltasone with food to avoid stomach upset.

If you are on alternate-day therapy or have been prescribed a single daily
dose, take Deltasone in the morning with breakfast (about 8 AM). If you have
been prescribed several doses per day, take them at evenly spaced intervals
around the clock.

Patients on long-term Deltasone therapy should wear or carry identification.

▪ *If you miss a dose...*
    If you take your dose once a day, take it as soon as you remember. If you
    don't remember until the next day, skip the one you missed.

If you take several doses a day, take the forgotten dose as soon as you remember and then go back to your regular schedule. If you don't remember until your next dose, double the dose you take.

If you take your dose every other day, and you remember it the same morning, take it as soon as you remember, then go back to your regular schedule. If you don't remember until the afternoon, do not take a dose until the following morning, then skip a day.

■ *Storage instructions...*
Store at room temperature.

What side effects may occur?
Side effects cannot be anticipated. If any develop or change in intensity, inform your doctor as soon as possible. Only your doctor can determine if it is safe for you to continue taking Deltasone.

Deltasone may cause euphoria, insomnia, mood changes, personality changes, psychotic behavior, or severe depression. It may worsen any existing emotional instability.

At a high dosage, Deltasone may cause fluid retention and high blood pressure. If this happens, you may need a low-salt diet and a potassium supplement.

With prolonged Deltasone treatment, eye problems may develop (e.g., a viral or fungal eye infection, cataracts, or glaucoma).

If you take Deltasone over the long term, the buildup of adrenal hormones in your body may cause a condition called Cushing's syndrome, marked by weight gain, a "moon-faced" appearance, thin, fragile skin, muscle weakness, brittle bones, and purplish stripe marks on the skin. Women are more vulnerable to this problem than men. Alternate-day therapy may help prevent its development.

■ *Other potential side effects from Deltasone include:*
Bone fractures, bruising, bulging eyes, congestive heart failure, convulsions, distended abdomen, face redness, glaucoma, headache, hives and other allergic-type reactions, increased pressure inside eyes or skull, inflamed esophagus or pancreas, irregular menstrual periods, muscle weakness or disease, osteoporosis, peptic ulcer, poor healing of wounds, stunted growth (in children), sweating, thin, fragile skin, vertigo

Why should this drug not be prescribed?
Do not take Deltasone if you have ever had an allergic reaction to it.

You should not be treated with Deltasone if you have a body-wide fungus infection, such as candidiasis or cryptococcosis.

Special warnings about this medication
Do not get a smallpox vaccination or any other immunization while you are taking Deltasone. The vaccination might not "take," and could do harm to the nervous system.

Deltasone may reactivate a dormant case of tuberculosis. If you have inactive TB and must take Deltasone for an extended time, you should be given anti-TB medication as well.

If you have an underactive thyroid gland or cirrhosis of the liver, your doctor will probably need to prescribe Deltasone for you at a lower-than-average dosage.

If you have an eye infection caused by the herpes simplex virus, Deltasone should be used with great caution; there is a potential danger that the cornea will become perforated.

A few people taking Deltasone develop Kaposi's sarcoma, a form of cancer; it may disappear when the drug is stopped.

Deltasone should also be taken with caution if you have any of the following conditions:

Diverticulitis or other disorder of the intestine
High blood pressure
Kidney disorder
Myasthenia gravis (a muscle-weakness disorder)
Osteoporosis (brittle bones)
Peptic ulcer
Ulcerative colitis (inflammation of the bowel)

Long-term treatment with Deltasone may stunt growth. If this medication is given to a child, the youngster's growth should be monitored carefully.

Diseases such as chickenpox or measles can be very serious or even fatal in both children and adults who are taking this drug. Try to avoid exposure to these diseases.

Possible food and drug interactions
when taking this medication
Deltasone may decrease your carbohydrate tolerance or activate a latent case of diabetes. If you are already taking insulin or oral medication for diabetes,

make sure your doctor knows this; you may need an increased dosage while you are being treated with Deltasone.

If you have a blood-clotting disorder caused by a vitamin K deficiency and are taking Deltasone, check with your doctor before you use aspirin.

You may be at risk of convulsions if you take the immunosuppressant drug cyclosporine (Sandimmune) while being treated with Deltasone.

If Deltasone is taken with certain other drugs, the effects of either could be increased, decreased, or altered. Check with your doctor before combining Deltasone with any of the following:

Amphotericin B (Fungizone)
Blood thinners such as Coumadin
Carbamazepine (Tegretol)
Estrogen drugs such as Premarin
Ketoconazole (Nizoral)
Oral contraceptives
Phenobarbital (Donnatal, others)
Phenytoin (Dilantin)
Potent diuretics such as Lasix
Rifampin (Rifadin)
Troleandomycin (Tao)

Special information
if you are pregnant or breastfeeding
If you are pregnant or plan to become pregnant, inform your doctor immediately. Deltasone should be taken during pregnancy or while breast-feeding only if clearly needed and only if the benefit outweighs the potential risks to the child.

Recommended dosage
Dosage is determined by the condition being treated and your response to the drug. Typical starting doses can range from 5 milligrams to 60 milligrams a day. Once you respond to the drug, your doctor will lower the dose gradually to the minimum effective amount. For treatment of acute attacks of multiple sclerosis, doses of as much as 200 milligrams per day may be given for a week, followed by 80 mg every other day for a month.

Overdosage
Long-term high doses of Deltasone may produce Cushing's syndrome (see "side effects" section). Although no specific information is available

regarding short-term overdosage, any medication taken in excess can have serious consequences. If you suspect an overdose of Deltasone, seek medical attention immediately.

Brand name:

DEMEROL

Pronounced: DEM-er-awl
Generic name: Meperidine hydrochloride

Why is this drug prescribed?
Demerol, a narcotic analgesic, is prescribed for the relief of moderate to severe pain.

Most important fact about this drug
Do not take Demerol if you are currently taking drugs known as MAO inhibitors or have used them in the previous 2 weeks. Drugs in this category include the antidepressants Nardil and Parnate. When taken with Demerol, they can cause unpredictable, severe, and occasionally fatal reactions.

How should you take this medication?
Take Demerol exactly as prescribed. Do not increase the amount or length of time you take this drug without your doctor's approval.

If you are using Demerol in syrup form, take each dose in a half glass of water.

■ *If you miss a dose...*
Take it as soon as you remember. If it is almost time for your next dose, skip the one you missed and go back to your regular schedule. Never take 2 doses at once.

■ *Storage instructions...*
Store at room temperature. Protect from heat.

What side effects may occur?
Side effects cannot be anticipated. If any develop or change in intensity, inform your doctor as soon as possible. Only your doctor can determine if it is safe for you to continue taking Demerol.

DRUG IDENTIFICATION GUIDE

ACCOLATE

ZAFIRLUKAST
ZENECA

20 MG

ACCUPRIL

QUINAPRIL HCL
PARKE-DAVIS

5 MG

10 MG

20 MG

40 MG

ACCUTANE

ISOTRETINOIN
ROCHE

10 MG

20 MG

40 MG

ACHROMYCIN V

TETRACYCLINE HCL
LEDERLE

250 MG

500 MG

ACTIGALL

URSODIOL
NOVARTIS

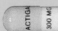

300 MG

ADALAT CC

NIFEDIPINE
BAYER

30 MG   60 MG

90 MG

ADDERALL

AMPHETAMINE
SHIRE RICHWOOD

10 MG

20 MG

ADIPEX-P

PHENTERMINE HCL
GATE

37.5 MG

ALDACTAZIDE

**SPIRONOLACTONE/
HYDROCHLOROTHIAZIDE**
G. D. SEARLE

25 MG / 25 MG

50 MG / 50 MG

ALDACTONE

SPIRONOLACTONE
G. D. SEARLE

25 MG

50 MG

100 MG

ALDOMET

METHYLDOPA
MERCK

125 MG

250 MG

500 MG

ALLEGRA

FEXOFENADINE
HOECHST MARION ROUSSEL

60 MG

ALTACE

RAMIPRIL
HOECHST MARION ROUSSEL

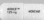

1.25 MG

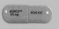

2.5 MG

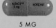

5 MG

10 MG

ALUPENT

METAPROTERENOL SULFATE
BOEHRINGER INGELHEIM

10 MG

AMARYL

GLIMEPIRIDE
HOECHST MARION ROUSSEL

1 MG

2 MG

4 MG

AMBIEN

ZOLPIDEM TARTRATE
G. D. SEARLE

5 MG   10 MG

AMERGE

NARATRIPTAN HCL
GLAXO WELLCOME

1 MG

2.5 MG

AMOXIL

AMOXICILLIN
SMITHKLINE BEECHAM

250 MG

500 MG

125 MG
CHEWABLE

250 MG
CHEWABLE

500 MG

875 MG

ANAFRANIL

CLOMIPRAMINE HCL
NOVARTIS

25 MG

50 MG

75 MG

ANAPROX

NAPROXEN SODIUM
ROCHE

275 MG

ANEXSIA

HYDROCODONE BITARTRATE/ ACETAMINOPHEN
MALLINCKRODT

5 MG / 500 MG

7.5 MG / 650 MG

ANSAID

FLURBIPROFEN
PHARMACIA & UPJOHN

50 MG

100 MG

ANTIVERT

MECLIZINE HCL
ROERIG

12.5 MG

25 MG

50 MG

ARAVA

LEFLUNOMIDE
HOECHST MARION ROUSSEL

10 MG

20 MG

100 MG

ARICEPT

DONEPEZIL HCL
PFIZER

5 MG   10 MG

ARIMIDEX

ANASTROZOLE
ZENECA

1 MG

ARMOUR THYROID

THYROID
FOREST

30 MG

60 MG

ARTANE

TRIHEXYPHENIDYL HCL
LEDERLE

2 MG

5 MG

ARTHROTEC	AUGMENTIN	AVAPRO
DICLOFENAC/MISOPROTOL G.D. SEARLE	**AMOXICILLIN/** **CLAVULANATE POTASSIUM** SMITHKLINE BEECHAM	**IRBESARTAN** BRISTOL-MYERS SQUIBB

50 MG / 200 MCG

75 MG / 200 MCG

ASACOL

MESALAMINE
PROCTER & GAMBLE

400 MG
DELAYED-RELEASE TABLETS

ATARAX

HYDROXYZINE HCL
ROERIG

10 MG   25 MG

50 MG   100 MG

ATIVAN

LORAZEPAM
WYETH-AYERST

0.5 MG   1 MG   2 MG

250 MG / 125 MG

500 MG / 125 MG

875 MG/125 MG

125 MG/31.25 MG
CHEWABLE

200 MG/28.5 MG
CHEWABLE

250 MG/62.5 MG
CHEWABLE

400 MG/57 MG
CHEWABLE

75 MG

150 MG

300 MG

AXID

NIZATIDINE
ELI LILLY

150 MG

300 MG

AZULFIDINE EN-TABS

SULFASALAZINE
PHARMACIA & UPJOHN

500 MG

BACTRIM

SULFAMETHOXAZOLE/
TRIMETHOPRIM
ROCHE

400 MG / 80 MG

BAYCOL

CERIVASTATIN SODIUM
BAYER

0.2 MG   0.3 MG

BENTYL

DICYCLOMINE HCL
HOECHST MARION ROUSSEL

10 MG

20 MG

BIAXIN

CLARITHROMYCIN
ABBOTT

250 MG

500 MG

BRETHINE

TERBUTALINE SULFATE
NOVARTIS

2.5 MG   5 MG

BRICANYL

TERBUTALINE SULFATE
HOECHST MARION ROUSSEL

2.5 MG

5 MG

BRONTEX

**CODEINE PHOSPHATE /
GUAIFENESIN**
KENWOOD

10 MG / 300 MG

BUMEX

BUMETANIDE
ROCHE

0.5 MG

1 MG

2 MG

BUSPAR

BUSPIRONE HCL
BRISTOL-MYERS SQUIBB

5 MG

10 MG

15 MG

CALAN

VERAPAMIL HCL
G. D. SEARLE

40 MG

80 MG

120 MG

CAPOTEN

CAPTOPRIL
BRISTOL-MYERS SQUIBB

12.5 MG   25 MG

50 MG

100 MG

CAPOZIDE

**CAPTOPRIL/
HYDROCHLOROTHIAZIDE**
BRISTOL-MYERS SQUIBB

25 MG/15 MG

25 MG/25 MG

50 MG/15 MG

50 MG/25 MG

CARAFATE

SUCRALFATE
HOECHST MARION ROUSSEL

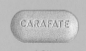

1 GM

CARDENE

NICARDIPINE HCL
ROCHE

20 MG

30 MG

CARDIZEM

DILTIAZEM HCL
HOECHST MARION ROUSSEL

30 MG

60 MG

90 MG

120 MG

CARDURA

DOXAZOSIN MESYLATE
ROERIG

1 MG

2 MG

4 MG

CARDURA

8 MG

CATAFLAM

DICLOFENAC POTASSIUM
NOVARTIS

50 MG

CATAPRES

CLONIDINE HCL
BOEHRINGER INGELHEIM

0.1 MG   0.2 MG

0.3 MG

CECLOR

CEFACLOR
ELI LILLY

250 MG

500 MG

CEDAX

CEFTIBUTEN
SCHERING

400 MG

CEFTIN

CEFUROXIME AXETIL
GLAXO WELLCOME

125 MG

250 MG

500 MG

CEFZIL

CEFPROZIL
BRISTOL-MYERS SQUIBB

250 MG

500 MG

CELEXA

CITALOPRAM HYDROBROMIDE
FOREST

20 MG

40 MG

CELEBREX

CELECOXIB
PFIZER

100 MG

200 MG

CIPRO

CIPROFLOXACIN HCL
BAYER

250 MG

500 MG

750 MG

CLARITIN

LORATADINE
SCHERING

10 MG

CLARITIN D

**LORATADINE/
PSEUDOEPHEDRINE SULFATE**
SCHERING

5 MG/120 MG

CLINORIL

SULINDAC
MERCK

150 MG

200 MG

CLOMID

CLOMIPHENE CITRATE
HOECHST MARION ROUSSEL

50 MG

CLOZARIL

CLOZAPINE
NOVARTIS

25 MG   100 MG

COGENTIN

BENZTROPINE MESYLATE
MERCK

0.5 MG

1 MG

2 MG

COGNEX

TACRINE HCL
PARKE-DAVIS

10 MG

20 MG

30 MG

40 MG

COLACE

DOCUSATE SODIUM
ROBERTS

50 MG

100 MG

COLESTID

COLESTIPOL HCL
PHARMACIA & UPJOHN

1 GM

COMPAZINE

PROCHLORPERAZINE
SMITHKLINE BEECHAM

5 MG

10 MG

10 MG
SUSTAINED RELEASE

15 MG
SUSTAINED RELEASE

COREG

CARVEDILOL
SMITHKLINE BEECHAM

3.125 MG

6.25 MG

12.5 MG

25 MG

CORGARD

NADOLOL
BRISTOL-MYERS SQUIBB

20 MG   40 MG

80 MG

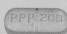

120 MG

160 MG

COUMADIN

WARFARIN SODIUM
DUPONT PHARMA

1 MG   2 MG

2.5 MG   3 MG

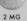

4 MG   5 MG

6 MG   7.5 MG

10 MG

COZAAR

LOSARTAN POTASSIUM
MERCK

25 MG

50 MG

CRIXIVAN

INDINAVIR SULFATE
MERCK

200 MG

400 MG

CYCRIN

MEDROXYPROGESTERONE ACETATE
ESI LEDERLE

2.5 MG   5 MG

10 MG

CYLERT

PEMOLINE
ABBOTT

18.75 MG   37.5 MG

75 MG   37.5 MG
            CHEWABLE

CYTOTEC

MISOPROSTOL
G. D. SEARLE

100 MCG   200 MCG

CYTOXAN

CYCLOPHOSPHAMIDE
BRISTOL MYERS
SQUIBB ONCOLOGY

25 MG   50 MG

DALMANE

FLURAZEPAM HCL
ROCHE

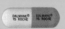

15 MG

30 MG

DARVOCET-N 100

**ACETAMINOPHEN/
PROPOXYPHENE NAPSYLATE**
ELI LILLY

650 MG/100 MG

DARVON

PROPOXYPHENE HCL
ELI LILLY

65 MG

DARVON COMPOUND-65

**PROPOXYPHENE HCL/
ASPIRIN/CAFFEINE**
ELI LILLY

65 MG/389 MG/32.4 MG

DAYPRO

OXAPROZIN
G. D. SEARLE

600 MG

DECADRON

DEXAMETHASONE
MERCK

0.5 MG 0.75 MG 4 MG

DELTASONE

PREDNISONE
PHARMACIA & UPJOHN

5 MG   10 MG

20 MG

DEMEROL

MEPERIDINE HCL
SANOFI

50 MG   100 MG

DEPAKENE

VALPROIC ACID
ABBOTT

250 MG

DEPAKOTE

DIVALPROEX SODIUM
ABBOTT

125 MG

125 MG

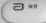

250 MG

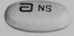

500 MG

DESOGEN

DESOGESTREL / ETHINYL ESTRADIOL
ORGANON

0.15 MG/0.03 MG

DESYREL

TRAZODONE HCL
APOTHECON

50 MG   100 MG

150 MG
DIVIDOSE

300 MG
DIVIDOSE

DEXEDRINE

DEXTROAMPHETAMINE SULFATE
SMITHKLINE BEECHAM

5 MG

15 MG
EXTENDED RELEASE

DIABETA

GLYBURIDE
HOECHST MARION ROUSSEL

1.25 MG

2.5 MG

5 MG

DIABINESE

CHLORPROPAMIDE
PFIZER

100 MG   250 MG

DIAMOX

ACETAZOLAMIDE
LEDERLE

125 MG   250 MG

500 MG

DIDRONEL

ETIDRONATE DISODIUM
PROCTER & GAMBLE

200 MG

400 MG

DIFLUCAN

FLUCONAZOLE
ROERIG

50 MG   100 MG

150 MG   200 MG

DILANTIN

PHENYTOIN
PARKE-DAVIS

30 MG

100 MG

50 MG
CHEWABLE

DILAUDID

HYDROMORPHONE HCL
KNOLL

2 MG   4 MG

8 MG

DIOVAN

VALSARTAN
NOVARTIS

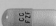

80 MG

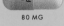

160 MG

DIPENTUM

OLSALAZINE SODIUM
PHARMACIA & UPJOHN

250 MG

DISALCID

SALSALATE
3M

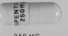

500 MG

500 MG

750 MG

DITROPAN

OXYBUTYNIN CHLORIDE
HOECHST MARION ROUSSEL

5 MG

DIURIL

CHLOROTHIAZIDE
MERCK

250 MG

500 MG

DOLOBID

DIFLUNISAL
MERCK

250 MG

500 MG

DONNATAL

**BELLADONNA ALKALOIDS/
PHENOBARBITAL**
A. H. ROBINS

EXTENDED RELEASE

DORAL

QUAZEPAM
WALLACE

7.5 MG   15 MG

DORYX

DOXYCYCLINE HYCLATE
PARKE-DAVIS

100 MG

DURICEF

**CEFADROXIL
MONOHYDRATE**
BRISTOL-MYERS SQUIBB

500 MG

1 WGM

DYAZIDE

**HYDROCHLOROTHIAZIDE /
TRIAMTERENE**
SMITHKLINE BEECHAM

25 MG / 37.5 MG

DYCILL

DICLOXACILLIN SODIUM
SMITHKLINE BEECHAM

250 MG

500 MG

DYNABAC

DIRITHROMYCIN
SANOFI

250 MG

DYNACIRC

ISRADIPINE
NOVARTIS

2.5 MG

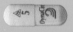

5 MG

E.E.S. 400 FILMTAB

**ERYTHROMYCIN
ETHYLSUCCINATE**
ABBOTT

400 MG

E-MYCIN

ERYTHROMYCIN
KNOLL

250 MG

333 MG

EFFEXOR

VENLAFAXINE HCL
WYETH-AYERST

25 MG

37.5 MG

50 MG

75 MG

100 MG

ELAVIL

AMITRIPTYLINE HCL
ZENECA

10 MG   25 MG

50 MG   75 MG

100 MG

150 MG

ELDEPRYL

SELEGILINE HCL
SOMERSET

5 MG

ENTEX LA

**PHENYLPROPANOLAMINE
HCL/GUAIFENESIN**
DURA

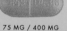

75 MG / 400 MG

EPITOL

CARBAMAZEPINE
TEVA

200 MG

EPIVIR

LAMIVUDINE
GLAXO WELLCOME

150 MG

EQUANIL

MEPROBAMATE
WYETH-AYERST

200 MG

400 MG

ERYPED CHEWABLE

ERYTHROMYCIN ETHYLSUCCINATE
ABBOTT

200 MG

ERY-TAB

ERYTHROMYCIN
ABBOTT

250 MG

333 MG

500 MG

ERYC

ERYTHROMYCIN
PARKE-DAVIS

250 MG
DELAYED-RELEASE

ERYTHROMYCIN FILMTAB

ERYTHROMYCIN
ABBOTT

250 MG

500 MG

ESGIC

BUTALBITAL / ACETAMINOPHEN / CAFFEINE
FOREST

50 MG /325 MG /40 MG

ESGIC PLUS

BUTALBITAL / ACETAMINOPHEN/ CAFFEINE
FOREST

50 MG /500 MG /40 MG

ESIDRIX

HYDROCHLOROTHIAZIDE
NOVARTIS

25 MG

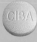

50 MG

ESKALITH

LITHIUM CARBONATE
SMITHKLINE BEECHAM

300 MG

ESTRACE

ESTRADIOL
BRISTOL-MYERS SQUIBB

0.5 MG

1 MG

2 MG

EULEXIN

FLUTAMIDE
SCHERING

125 MG

FAMVIR

FAMCICLOVIR
SMITHKLINE BEECHAM

500 MG

FASTIN

PHENTERMINE HCL
SMITHKLINE BEECHAM

30 MG

FELBATOL

FELBAMATE
WALLACE

04 | 30

400 MG

04 | 31

600 MG

FELDENE

PIROXICAM
PRATT

FELDENE | PFIZER 322

10 MG

FELDENE | PFIZER 323

20 MG

FIORICET

**ACETAMINOPHEN/
BUTALBITAL/CAFFEINE**
NOVARTIS

325 MG / 50 MG/ 40 MG

FIORICET W/CODEINE

**ACETAMINOPHEN/
BUTALBITAL/CAFFEINE/
CODEINE**
NOVARTIS

325 MG / 50 MG /
40 MG / 30 MG

FIORINAL

**BUTALBITAL/ASPIRIN/
CAFFEINE**
NOVARTIS

FIORINAL

50 MG / 325 MG / 40 MG

FIORINAL | FIORINAL
78-139 | 78-163

50 MG / 325 MG / 40 MG

FIORINAL W/CODEINE

**BUTALBITAL/ASPIRIN/
CAFFEINE/CODEINE**
NOVARTIS

S·F·C | SANDOZ 78-107

50 MG / 325 MG/
40 MG / 30 MG

FLAGYL

METRONIDAZOLE
G.D. SEARLE

SEARLE 1831

250 MG

FLAG | 375 m

375 MG

FLAGYL

500 MG

FLEXERIL

CYCLOBENZAPRINE HCL
MERCK

MSD 931

10 MG

FLOMAX

TAMSULOSIN HCL
BOEHRINGER INGELHEIM

Flomax 0.4 mg | BI 58

0.4 MG

FLOXIN

OFLOXACIN
ORTHO-MCNEIL

FLOXIN 200

200 MG

FLOXIN 300

300 MG

FLOXIN 400

400 MG

FORTOVASE

SAQUINAVIR
ROCHE

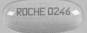
ROCHE 0246

200 MG

FOSAMAX

ALENDRONATE SODIUM
MERCK

10 MG   40 MG

FULVICIN-P/G

GRISEOFULVIN
SCHERING

250 MG

330 MG

GLUCOPHAGE

METFORMIN HCL
BRISTOL-MYERS SQUIBB
COMPANY

500 MG

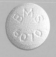

850 MG

GLUCOTROL

GLIPIZIDE
PRATT

5 MG   10 MG

GLYNASE PRESTAB

GLYBURIDE , MICRONIZED
PHARMACIA & UPJOHN

1.5 MG

3 MG

6 MG

GRISACTIN

GRISEOFULVIN
WYETH-AYERST

250 MG

500 MG

GRISACTIN ULTRA

GRISEOFULVIN
WYETH-AYERST

250 MG

330 MG

HALCION

TRIAZOLAM
PHARMACIA & UPJOHN

0.125 MG   0.25 MG

HALDOL

HALOPERIDOL
ORTHO-MCNEIL

0.5 MG   1 MG

2 MG   5 MG

10 MG   20 MG

HISMANAL

ASTEMIZOLE
JANSSEN

10 MG

HIVID

ZALCITABINE
ROCHE

0.375 MG

0.750 MG

HYDERGINE

ERGOLOID MESYLATES
NOVARTIS

1 MG

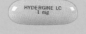

1 MG

HYDRODIURIL

HYDROCHLOROTHIAZIDE
MERCK

25 MG

50 MG

100 MG

HYGROTON

CHLORTHALIDONE
RHONE-POULENC RORER

25 MG   50 MG

HYZAAR

LOSARTAN POTASSIUM /
HYDROCHLOROTHIAZIDE
MERCK

50 MG / 12.5 MG

HYTRIN

TERAZOSIN HCL
ABBOTT

1 MG   2 MG

5 MG   10 MG

ILOSONE

ERYTHROMYCIN ESTOLATE
DISTA

250 MG

IMDUR

ISOSORBIDE MONONITRATE
KEY

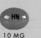

60 MG

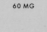

120 MG

IMITREX

SUMATRIPTAN SUCCINATE
GLAXO WELLCOME

25 MG   50 MG

IMODIUM

LOPERAMIDE HCL
JANSSEN

2 MG

INDERAL

PROPRANOLOL HCL
WYETH-AYERST

10 MG   20 MG

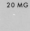

40 MG   60 MG

80 MG

INDERIDE

PROPRANOLOL HCL/
HYDROCHLOROTHIAZIDE
WYETH-AYERST

40 MG / 25 MG

80 MG / 25 MG

INDOCIN

INDOMETHACIN
MERCK

25 MG

50 MG

75 MG

IONAMIN

PHENTERMINE RESIN
MEDEVA

15 MG

30 MG

ISMO

ISOSORBIDE MONONITRATE
WYETH-AYERST

20 MG

ISOPTIN

VERAPAMIL HCL
KNOLL

40 MG   80 MG

120 MG

ISORDIL

ISOSORBIDE DINITRATE
WYETH-AYERST

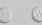

2.5 MG   5 MG   10 MG
SUBLINGUAL

5 MG   10 MG

20 MG

30 MG

40 MG

40 MG
EXTENDED RELEASE

K-DUR

POTASSIUM CHLORIDE
KEY

10 MEQ

20 MEQ

KAON-CL 10

POTASSIUM CHLORIDE
SAVAGE

10 MEQ

KEFLEX

CEPHALEXIN
DISTA

250 MG

500 MG

KEFTAB

CEPHALEXIN HCL
EL LILLY

500 MG

KLONOPIN

CLONAZEPAM
ROCHE

0.5 MG

1 MG

2 MG

KLOR-CON

POTASSIUM CHLORIDE
UPSHER-SMITH

8 MEQ

10 MEQ

LAMICTAL

LAMOTRIGINE
GLAXO WELLCOME

25 MG

100 MG

150 MG

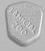

200 MG

LANOXIN

DIGOXIN
GLAXO WELLCOME

0.125 MG   0.25 MG

LASIX

FUROSEMIDE
HOECHST MARION ROUSSEL

20 MG

40 MG

80 MG

LEDERCILLIN VK

PENICILLIN V POTASSIUM
LEDERLE

250 MG

500 MG

LESCOL

FLUVASTATIN SODIUM
NOVARTIS

20 MG

40 MG

LEVOTHROID

LEVOTHYROXINE SODIUM
FOREST

50 MCG   100 MCG

150 MCG

LEVLEN

**LEVONORGESTREL/
ETHINYL ESTRADIOL**
BERLEX

0.15 MG/0.03 MG

LEVOXYL

LEVOTHYROXINE SODIUM
JONES MEDICAL

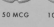

50 MCG   100 MCG

150 MCG

LEVAQUIN

LEVOFLOXACIN
ORTHO-MCNEIL

250 MG

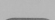

500 MG

LEVSIN

HYOSCYAMINE SULFATE
SCHWARZ

0.125 MG

LEVSIN / SL

HYOSCYAMINE SULFATE
SCHWARZ

0.125 MG

LEVSINEX

HYOSCYAMINE SULFATE
SCHWARZ

0.375 MG

LEXXEL

**ENALAPRIL MALEATE /
FELODIPINE**
ASTRA

5 MG / 5 MG

LIBRAX

**CHLORDIAZEPOXIDE HCL/
CLIDINIUM BROMIDE**
ICN

5 MG/2.5 MG

LIBRIUM

CHLORDIAZEPOXIDE HCL
ICN

5 MG

10 MG

25 MG

LIPITOR

ATORVASTATIN CALCIUM
PARKE DAVIS

10 MG

20 MG

40 MG

LITHONATE

LITHIUM CARBONATE
SOLVAY

SOLVAY   7512

300 MG

LITHOTABS

LITHIUM CARBONATE
SOLVAY

300 MG

LODINE

ETODOLAC
WYETH-AYERST

200 MG

300 MG

400 MG

LOMOTIL

**DIPHENOXYLATE HCL
ATROPINE SULFATE**
G. D. SEARLE

2.5 MG / 0.025 MG

LOPID

GEMFIBROZIL
PARKE-DAVIS

600 MG

LOPRESSOR

METOPROLOL TARTRATE
NOVARTIS

50 MG

100 MG

LORABID

LORACARBEF
ELI LILLY

200 MG

400 MG

LORCET PLUS

**HYDROCODONE
BITARTRATE/
ACETAMINOPHEN**
FOREST

7.5 MG / 650 MG

LORTAB

**HYDROCODONE BITARTRATE /
ACETAMINOPHEN**
UCB

2.5 MG / 500 MG

5 MG / 500 MG

7.5 MG / 500 MG

LOTENSIN

BENAZEPRIL HCL
NOVARTIS

5 MG   10 MG

20 MG   40 MG

LOTENSIN HCT

**BENAZEPRIL HCL/
HYDROCHLOROTHIAZIDE USP**
NOVARTIS

5 MG/6.25 MG

10 MG/12.5 MG

20 MG/12.5 MG

20 MG/25 MG

LOTREL

**AMLODIPINE /
BENAZEPRIL HCL**
NOVARTIS

2.5 MG / 10 MG

5 MG / 10 MG

5 MG / 20 MG

LOZOL

INDAPAMIDE
RHONE-POULENC RORER

1.25 MG   2.5 MG

LURIDE SF LOZI-TABS

SODIUM FLUORIDE
COLGATE ORAL

1 MG

LUVOX

FLUVOXAMINE MALEATE
SOLVAY

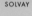

50 MG

100 MG

MACRODANTIN

NITROFURANTOIN
PROCTER & GAMBLE

25 MG

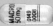

50 MG

100 MG

MACROBID

NITROFURANTOIN MONOHYDRATE / MACROCRYSTALS
PROCTER & GAMBLE

75 MG / 25 MG

MATERNA

VITAMINS & MINERALS
LEDERLE

MAVIK

TRANDOLAPRIL
KNOLL

1 MG   2 MG

4 MG

MAXALT

RIZATRIPTAN BENZOATE
MERCK

5 MG   10 MG

MAXAQUIN

LOMEFLOXACIN HCL
UNIMED

400 MG

MAXZIDE

TRIAMTERENE / HYDROCHLOROTHIAZIDE
BERTEK

37.5 MG / 25 MG

75 MG / 50 MG

MEDROL

METHYLPREDNISOLONE
PHARMACIA & UPJOHN

2 MG   4 MG

8 MG   16 MG

MELLARIL

THIORIDAZINE HCL
NOVARTIS

25 MG   50 MG

100 MG   150 MG

200 MG

MERIDIA

SIBUTRAMINE
KNOLL

5 MG

10 MG

15 MG

METHERGINE

METHYLERGONOVINE MALEATE
NOVARTIS

0.2 MG

METHOTREXATE SODIUM

METHOTREXATE SODIUM
LEDERLE

2.5 MG

MEVACOR

LOVASTATIN
MERCK

10 MG

20 MG

40 MG

MEXITIL

MEXILETINE HCL
BOEHRINGER INGELHEIM

150 MG

200 MG

250 MG

MICRO-K EXTENCAPS

POTASSIUM CHLORIDE
A. H. ROBINS

8 MEQ

10 MEQ

MICRONASE

GLYBURIDE
PHARMACIA & UPJOHN

1.25 MG

2.5 MG

5 MG

MIDRIN

**ISOMETHEPTENE MUCATE/
DICHLORALPHENAZONE/
ACETAMINOPHEN**
CARRICK

65 MG / 100 MG / 325 MG

MILTOWN

MEPROBAMATE
WALLACE

200 MG

400 MG

MINIPRESS

PRAZOSIN HCL
PFIZER

1 MG

2 MG

5 MG

MINOCIN

MINOCYCLINE HCL
LEDERLE

50 MG

100 MG

MIRAPEX

**PRAMIPEXOLE
DIHYDROCHLORIDE**
PHARMACIA & UPJOHN

0.125 MG   0.25 MG

0.5 MG

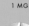

1 MG

1.5 MG

MODURETIC

**AMILORIDE HCL/
HYDROCHLOROTHIAZIDE**
MERCK

5 MG / 50 MG

MONOKET

ISOSORBIDE MONONITRATE
SCHWARZ

10 MG

20 MG

MONOPRIL

FOSINOPRIL SODIUM
BRISTOL-MYERS SQUIBB

10 MG

20 MG

MOTRIN

IBUPROFEN
PHARMACIA & UPJOHN

400 MG

600 MG

800 MG

MS CONTIN

MORPHINE SULFATE
PURDUE FREDERICK

15 MG   30 MG

60 MG   100 MG

200 MG

MYSOLINE

PRIMIDONE
WYETH-AYERST

50 MG

250 MG

NAPROSYN

NAPROXEN
ROCHE

250 MG

375 MG

500 MG

NARDIL

PHENELZINE SULFATE
PARKE-DAVIS

15 MG

NAVANE

THIOTHIXENE
ROERIG

5 MG

10 MG

NEORAL

CYCLOSPORINE
NOVARTIS

25 MG

100 MG

NEPTAZANE

METHAZOLAMIDE
STORZ / LEDERLE

25 MG   50 MG

NEURONTIN

GABAPENTIN
PARKE-DAVIS

100 MG

300 MG

400 MG

NILANDRON

NILUTAMIDE
HOECHST MARION ROUSSEL

50 MG

NIZORAL

KETOCONAZOLE
JANSSEN

200 MG

NOLVADEX

TAMOXIFEN CITRATE
ZENECA

10 MG   20 MG

NORGESIC

ORPHENADRINE CITRATE/ ASPIRIN/CAFFEINE
3M

25 MG / 385 MG / 30 MG

NORGESIC FORTE

ORPHENADRINE CITRATE/ ASPIRIN/ CAFFEINE
3M

50 MG / 770 MG / 60 MG

NOROXIN

NORFLOXACIN
MERCK

400 MG

NORMODYNE

LABETALOL HCL
SCHERING

100 MG

200 MG

300 MG

NORPACE

DISOPYRAMIDE PHOSPHATE
G. D. SEARLE

100 MG

150 MG

NORPRAMIN

DESIPRAMINE HCL
HOECHST MARION ROUSSEL

10 MG   25 MG

50 MG   75 MG

100 MG   150 MG

NORVASC

AMLODIPINE BESYLATE
PFIZER

2.5 MG   5 MG

10 MG

■ *More common side effects may include:*
Dizziness, light-headedness, nausea, sedation, sweating, vomiting

If any of these side effects occur, it may help if you lie down after taking the medication.

■ *Less common or rare side effects may include:*
Agitation, constipation, difficulty urinating, disorientation, dry mouth, fainting, fast heartbeat, feeling of elation or depression, flushing of the face, hallucinations, headache, hives, impairment of physical performance, itching, low blood pressure, mental sluggishness or clouding, palpitations, rashes, restlessness, severe convulsions, slow heartbeat, tremors, troubled and slowed breathing, uncoordinated muscle movements, visual disturbances, weakness

Why should this drug not be prescribed?
If you are sensitive to or have ever had an allergic reaction to Demerol or other narcotic painkillers, you should not use this medication. Make sure your doctor is aware of any drug reactions you have experienced.

Do not take Demerol with MAO inhibitors such as Nardil and Parnate.

Special warnings about this medication
Demerol may affect you both mentally and physically. You should not drive a car, operate machinery, or perform any other potentially hazardous activities until you know how the drug affects you.

You can build up tolerance to, and both mental and physical dependence on, Demerol if you take it repeatedly. If you have ever had a problem with drug abuse, consult with your doctor before taking this drug.

Use Demerol with caution if you have a severe liver or kidney disorder, hypothyroidism (underactive thyroid gland), Addison's disease (adrenal gland failure), an enlarged prostate, a urethral stricture (narrowing of the tube leading from the bladder), a head injury, a severe abdominal condition, or an irregular heartbeat, or if you have ever had convulsions.

Be very careful taking this drug if you are having a severe asthma attack, if you have frequently recurring lung disease, if you are unable to inhale or exhale extra air when needed, or if you have any pre-existing breathing difficulties.

Because Demerol may cause unusually slow or troubled breathing and may increase the pressure from fluid surrounding the brain and spinal cord, this drug should be used by people with head injury only if the doctor considers it absolutely necessary.

Demerol may make you feel light-headed or dizzy when you get up from lying down.

Before having surgery, make sure the doctor knows you are taking Demerol.

Possible food and drug interactions
when taking this medication

Demerol slows brain activity and intensifies the effects of alcohol. Do not drink alcohol while taking this medication.

If Demerol is taken with certain other drugs, the effects of either could be increased, decreased, or altered. It is especially important to check with your doctor before combining Demerol with the following:

Antidepressant drugs such as Elavil, Tofranil
Antihistamines such as Benadryl
Cimetidine (Tagamet)
Major tranquilizers such as Mellaril and Thorazine
MAO inhibitors such as the antidepressant drugs Nardil and Parnate
Other narcotic painkillers such as Percocet and Tylenol with Codeine
Phenytoin (Dilantin)
Sedatives such as Halcion and Restoril
Tranquilizers such as Xanax and Valium

Special information
if you are pregnant or breastfeeding

Do not take Demerol if you are pregnant or planning to become pregnant unless you are directed to do so by your doctor. Demerol appears in breast milk and could affect a nursing infant. If this medication is essential to your health, your doctor may advise you to discontinue breastfeeding your baby until your treatment is finished.

Recommended dosage

ADULTS

The usual dosage of Demerol is 50 milligrams to 150 milligrams every 3 or 4 hours, determined according to your response and the severity of the pain.

CHILDREN

The usual dosage is 0.5 milligram to 0.8 milligram per pound of body weight, taken every 3 or 4 hours, as determined by your doctor.

OLDER ADULTS
Your doctor may reduce the dosage.

Overdosage
- **Symptoms of Demerol overdose include:**
  Bluish discoloration of the skin, cold and clammy skin, coma or extreme sleepiness, limp, weak muscles, low blood pressure, slow heartbeat, troubled or slowed breathing

  With severe overdose, a person may stop breathing, have a heart attack, and even die.

If you suspect an overdose, seek emergency medical treatment immediately.

Brand name:

DEMULEN

See Oral Contraceptives, page 926.

Brand name:

DENAVIR

Pronounced: DEN-a-veer
Generic name: Penciclovir

Why is this drug prescribed?
Denavir cream is used to treat recurrent cold sores on the lips and face. It works by interfering with the growth of the herpes virus responsible for the sores.

Most important fact about this drug
You should begin applying Denavir at the first hint of a developing cold sore. The drug will not cure herpes, but it will reduce pain and may speed healing.

How should you use this medication?
Avoid using Denavir cream in or near the eyes; it can irritate them. Apply it only to sores on the lips and face.

- **If you miss a dose...**
  Apply it as soon as you remember. If it is almost time for your next dose, skip the one you missed and go back to your regular schedule.

■ *Storage instructions...*
Store at room temperature; avoid freezing.

What side effects may occur?
Reactions to Denavir are quite rare. If any develop or change in intensity, inform your doctor as soon as possible. Only your doctor can determine if it is safe for you to continue using this medication.

■ *Side effects may include:*
Headache, numbing of the skin, rash, skin reaction where the cream was applied, taste alteration

Why should this drug not be prescribed?
If you have ever had an allergic reaction to any of the ingredients in Denavir, you should not use this medication.

Special warnings about this medication
It is not known whether Denavir is effective for people with weak immune systems.

Possible food and drug interactions when using this medication
No interactions with Denavir cream have been reported.

Special information if you are pregnant or breastfeeding
The effects of Denavir during pregnancy have not been adequately studied. If you are pregnant or plan to become pregnant, inform your doctor immediately. Researchers do not know whether this drug will appear in breast milk after external application. For safety's sake, your doctor may advise you to discontinue breastfeeding your baby until your treatment with Denavir is finished.

Recommended dosage

ADULTS

Apply cream every 2 hours, while awake, for 4 days.

CHILDREN

The safety and effectiveness of this drug in children have not been established.

Overdosage
There have been no reported overdoses of this medication. Even if the cream is accidentally swallowed, it is unlikely to cause a harmful reaction.

Brand name:

DEPAKENE

Pronounced: DEP-uh-keen
Generic name: Valproic acid

Why is this drug prescribed?
Depakene, an epilepsy medicine, is used to treat certain types of seizures and convulsions. It may be prescribed alone or with other anticonvulsant medications.

Most important fact about this drug
Depakene can cause serious liver damage, especially during the first 6 months of treatment. Children under 2 years of age are the most vulnerable, especially if they are also taking other anticonvulsant medicines and have certain other disorders such as mental retardation. The risk of liver damage decreases with age; but you should always be alert for the following symptoms: loss of seizure control, weakness, dizziness, drowsiness, a general feeling of ill health, facial swelling, loss of appetite, vomiting, and yellowing of the skin and eyes. If you suspect a liver problem, call your doctor immediately.

How should you take this medication?
If Depakene irritates your digestive system, take it with food. To avoid irritating your mouth and throat, swallow Depakene capsules whole; do not chew them.

- *If you miss a dose...*
  If you take 1 dose a day, take the dose you missed as soon as you remember. If you do not remember until the next day, skip the dose you missed and go back to your regular schedule.

  If you take more than 1 dose a day and you remember the missed dose within 6 hours of the scheduled time, take it immediately. Take the rest of the doses for that day at equally spaced intervals. Never take 2 doses at once.

■ *Storage instructions...*
Store at room temperature.

What side effects may occur?
Side effects cannot be anticipated. If any develop or change in intensity, inform your doctor as soon as possible. Only your doctor can determine if it is safe for you to continue taking Depakene.

■ *More common side effects may include:*
Indigestion, nausea, vomiting

■ *Less common or rare side effects may include:*
Abdominal cramps, aggression, anemia, bleeding, blood disorders, breast enlargement, breast milk not associated with pregnancy or nursing, bruising, changes in behavior, coma, constipation, depression, diarrhea, difficulty in speaking, dizziness, double vision, drowsiness, emotional upset, excessive urination (mainly children), fever, growth failure in children, hair loss (temporary), hallucinations, headache, involuntary eye movements, involuntary jerking or tremors, irregular menstrual periods, itching, lack of coordination, liver disease, loss of bladder control, loss of or increased appetite, overactivity, rash, rickets (mainly children), sedation, sensitivity to light, skin eruptions or peeling, spots before the eyes, swelling of the arms and legs due to fluid retention, swollen glands, weakness, weight loss or gain

Why should this drug not be prescribed?
You should not take this drug if you have liver disease or your liver is not functioning properly, or if you have had an allergic reaction to it.

Special warnings about this medication
Remember that liver failure is possible when taking Depakene (see "Most important fact about this drug"). Your doctor should test your liver function at regular intervals.

Because of the potential for side effects involving blood disorders, your doctor will probably test your blood before prescribing Depakene and at regular intervals while you are taking it. Bruising, hemorrhaging, or clotting disorders usually mean the dosage should be reduced or the drug should be stopped altogether.

Since Depakene may cause drowsiness, you should not drive a car, operate heavy machinery, or engage in hazardous activity until you know how you react to the drug.

Do not abruptly stop taking this medicine without first consulting your doctor. A gradual reduction in dosage is usually required.

This drug can also increase the effect of painkillers and anesthetics. Before any surgery or dental procedure, make sure the doctor knows you are taking Depakene.

Possible food and drug interactions
when taking this medication

If Depakene is taken with certain other drugs, the effects of either could be increased, decreased, or altered. It is especially important to check with your doctor before combining Depakene with the following:

Aspirin
Barbiturates such as phenobarbital and Seconal
Blood-thinning drugs such as Coumadin and Dicumarol
Carbamazepine (Tegretol)
Clonazepam (Klonopin)
Felbamate (Felbatol)
Oral contraceptives
Phenytoin (Dilantin)
Primidone (Mysoline)

Extreme drowsiness and other serious effects may occur if Depakene is taken with alcohol or other central nervous system depressants such as Halcion, Restoril, or Xanax.

Special information
if you are pregnant or breastfeeding

If taken during pregnancy, Depakene may harm the baby. The drug is not recommended for pregnant women unless the benefits of therapy clearly outweigh the risks. In fact, women in their childbearing years should take Depakene only if it has been shown to be essential in the control of seizures. Since Depakene appears in breast milk, nursing mothers should use it only with caution.

Recommended dosage

The usual starting dose is 15 milligrams per 2.2 pounds of body weight per day. Your doctor may increase the dose at weekly intervals by 5 to 10 milligrams per 2.2 pounds per day until seizures are controlled or side effects become too severe. The daily dose should not exceed 60 milligrams per 2.2 pounds per day.

Overdosage
Any medication taken in excess can have serious consequences. An overdose of Depakene can be fatal. If you suspect an overdose, seek medical help immediately.

■ *Symptoms of Depakene overdose may include:*
Coma, extreme drowsiness, heart problems

Brand name:

DEPAKOTE

Pronounced: DEP-uh-coat
Generic name: Divalproex sodium (Valproic acid)

Why is this drug prescribed?
Depakote, in both tablet and capsule form, is used to treat certain types of seizures and convulsions. It may be prescribed alone or with other epilepsy medications.

The tablets are also used to control the manic episodes—periods of abnormally high spirits and energy—that occur in bipolar disorder (manic depression).

The tablet form is also prescribed to prevent migraine headaches.

Most important fact about this drug
Depakote can cause serious liver damage, especially during the first 6 months of treatment. Children under 2 years of age are the most vulnerable, especially if they are also taking other anticonvulsant medicines and have certain other disorders such as mental retardation. The risk of liver damage decreases with age; but you should always be alert for the following symptoms: loss of seizure control, weakness, dizziness, drowsiness, a general feeling of ill health, facial swelling, loss of appetite, vomiting, and yellowing of the skin and eyes. If you suspect a liver problem, call your doctor immediately.

How should you take this medication?
Take the tablet with water and swallow it whole (don't chew it or crush it). It has a special coating to avoid upsetting your stomach.

If you are taking the sprinkle capsule, you can swallow it whole or open it and sprinkle the contents on a teaspoon of soft food such as applesauce or pudding. Swallow it immediately, without chewing. The sprinkle capsules are large enough to be opened easily.

Depakote can be taken with meals or snacks to avoid stomach upset. Take it exactly as prescribed.

■ *If you miss a dose...*
If you take Depakote once a day, take your dose as soon as you remember. If you don't remember until the next day, skip the missed dose and return to your regular schedule. Never take 2 doses at the same time.

If you take more than one dose a day, take your dose right away if it's within 6 hours of the scheduled time, and take the rest of the day's doses at equal intervals during the day. Never take 2 doses at the same time.

■ *Storage instructions...*
Store at room temperature.

What side effects may occur?
Side effects cannot be anticipated. If any develop or change in intensity, inform your doctor as soon as possible. Because Depakote is often used with other antiseizure drugs, it may not be possible to determine whether a side effect is due to Depakote alone. Only your doctor can determine if it is safe for you to continue taking Depakote.

■ *More common side effects may include:*
Abdominal pain, abnormal thinking, breathing difficulty, bronchitis, bruising, constipation, depression, diarrhea, dizziness, emotional changeability, fever, flu symptoms, hair loss, headache, incoordination, indigestion, infection, insomnia, loss of appetite, memory loss, nasal inflammation, nausea, nervousness, ringing in the ears, sleepiness, sore throat, tremor, vision problems, vomiting, weakness, weight loss or gain

■ *Less common or rare side effects may include:*
Abnormal dreams, abnormal milk secretion, abnormal walk, aggression, anemia, anxiety, back pain, behavior problems, belching, bleeding, blood disorders, bone pain, breast enlargement, chest pain, chills, coma, confusion, coughing up blood, dental abscess, drowsiness, dry skin, ear or hearing problems, excessive urination (mainly children) or other urination problems, eye problems, feeling of illness, gas, growth failure in children, hallucinations, heart palpitations, high blood pressure, hostility, increased appetite, increased cough, involuntary rapid movement of eyeball, irregular or painful menstruation, itching, jerky movements, lack of muscular coordination, leg cramps, liver problems, loss of bladder or bowel control, muscle or joint pain, muscle weakness, neck pain, nosebleed, overactivity, pneumonia, rickets (mainly children), sedation, seeing "spots before your

eyes," sensitivity to light, sinus inflammation, skin eruptions or peeling, skin rash, speech difficulties, stomach and intestinal disorders, swelling of arms and legs due to fluid retention, swollen glands, taste changes, tingling or pins and needles, twitching, urinary problems, vertigo

Why should this drug not be prescribed?
You should not take this medication if you have liver disease or your liver is not functioning well.

If you are sensitive to or have ever had an allergic reaction to Depakote, you should not take this medication.

Special warnings about this medication
This medication can severely damage the liver (see "Most important fact about this drug").

Depakote causes some people to become drowsy or less alert. You should not drive or operate dangerous machinery or participate in any hazardous activity that requires full mental alertness until you are certain the drug does not have this effect on you.

Do not abruptly stop taking this medicine without first consulting your doctor. A gradual reduction in dosage is usually required.

Depakote prolongs the time it takes blood to clot, which increases your chances of serious bleeding.

This drug can also increase the effect of painkillers and anesthetics. Before any surgery or dental procedure, make sure the doctor knows you are taking Depakote.

If you are taking Depakote to prevent migraine, remember that it will not cure a headache once it has started.

Some coated particles from the capsules may appear in your stool. This is to be expected, and need not worry you.

Possible food and drug interactions
when taking this medication
Depakote depresses activity of the central nervous system, and may increase the effects of alcohol. Do not drink alcohol while taking this medication.

If Depakote is taken with certain other drugs, the effects of either could be increased, decreased, or altered. It is especially important to check with your doctor before combining Depakote with the following:

Aspirin
Barbiturates such as phenobarbital and Seconal

Blood thinners such as Coumadin
Cyclosporine (Sandimmune, Neoral)
Oral contraceptives
Other seizure medications, including carbamazepine (Tegretol),
    clonazepam (Klonopin), ethosuximide (Zarontin), felbamate (Felbatol),
    phenytoin (Dilantin), and Primidone (Mysoline)
Sleep aids such as Halcion
Tranquilizers such as Valium and Xanax

Special information
if you are pregnant or breastfeeding

Depakote may produce birth defects if it is taken during pregnancy. If you are pregnant or plan to become pregnant, inform your doctor immediately. Depakote appears in breast milk and could affect a nursing infant. If Depakote is essential to your health, your doctor may advise you to discontinue breastfeeding until your treatment with this medication is finished.

Recommended dosage

EPILEPSY

Dosage for adults and children is determined by body weight. The usual recommended starting dose is 10 to 15 milligrams per 2.2 pounds per day, depending on the type of seizure. Your doctor may increase the dose at 1-week intervals by 5 to 10 milligrams per 2.2 pounds per day until your seizures are controlled or the side effects become too severe. The most you should take is 60 milligrams per 2.2 pounds per day. If your total dosage is more than 250 milligrams a day, your doctor will divide it into smaller individual doses.

MANIC EPISODES

The usual starting dose for those aged 18 and over is 750 milligrams a day, divided into smaller doses. Your doctor will adjust the dose for best results.

MIGRAINE PREVENTION

The usual starting dose for those aged 16 and over is 250 milligrams twice a day. Your doctor will adjust the dose, up to a maximum of 1,000 milligrams a day. The drug has not been tested for migraine in adults over age 65.

Overdosage

Any medication taken in excess can have serious consequences. An overdose of Depakote can be fatal. If you suspect an overdose, seek medical attention immediately.

■ *Symptoms of Depakote overdose may include:*
Coma, extreme sleepiness, heart problems

Brand name:

DERMACORT

See Hydrocortisone Skin Preparations, page 599.

Generic name:

DESIPRAMINE

See Norpramin, page 906.

Generic name:

DESMOPRESSIN

See DDAVP, page 341.

Brand name:

DESOGEN

See Oral Contraceptives, page 926.

Generic name:

DESONIDE

See Tridesilon, page 1343.

Brand name:

DESOWEN

See Tridesilon, page 1343.

Generic name:

DESOXIMETASONE

See Topicort, page 1326.

Brand name:

DESQUAM-E

Pronounced: DES-kwam ee
Generic name: Benzoyl peroxide
Other brand names: Benzac W, Benzagel, BenzaShave,
   Triaz

Why is this drug prescribed?
Desquam-E gel is used to treat various types of acne. It can be used alone or with other treatments, including antibiotics and products that contain retinoic acid, sulfur, or salicylic acid.

Most important fact about this drug
Significant clearing of the skin should occur after 2 to 3 weeks of treatment with Desquam-E.

How should you use this medication?
Cleanse the affected area thoroughly before applying the medication. Desquam-E should then be gently rubbed in.

- *If you miss a dose...*
   Apply it as soon as you remember. Then go back to your regular schedule.

- *Storage instructions...*
   Store at room temperature.

What side effects may occur?
Side effects cannot be anticipated. If any develop or change in intensity, notify your doctor as soon as possible. Only your doctor can determine whether it is safe for you to continue using Desquam-E.

- *Side effects may include:*
   Allergic reaction (itching, rash in area where the medication was applied), excessive drying (red and peeling skin and possible swelling)

Why should this drug not be prescribed?
Do not use Desquam-E if you are sensitive to or allergic to benzoyl peroxide or any other components of the drug.

Special warnings about this medication
Desquam-E is for external use only. Avoid contact with your eyes, nose, lips, or throat. If the drug does touch these areas accidentally, rinse with water.

If you are sensitive to medications derived from benzoic acid (including certain topical anesthetics) or to cinnamon, you may also be sensitive to Desquam-E.

If your skin becomes severely irritated, stop using the drug and call your doctor.

Desquam-E can bleach or discolor hair or colored fabric.

Stay out of the sun as much as possible, and use a sunscreen.

Possible food and drug interactions when using this medication
When used with sunscreens containing PABA (para-aminobenzoic acid), Desquam-E may cause temporary skin discoloration.

Special information if you are pregnant or breastfeeding
The effects of Desquam-E during pregnancy have not been adequately studied. It should be used only if clearly needed. If you are pregnant or plan to become pregnant, inform your doctor immediately. This medication may appear in breast milk and could affect a nursing infant. If this medication is essential to your health, your doctor may advise you to stop breastfeeding until your treatment with Desquam-E is finished.

Recommended dosage

ADULTS AND CHILDREN 12 YEARS AND OVER

Gently rub Desquam-E gel into all affected areas once or twice a day. If you are fair-skinned or live in an excessively dry climate, you should probably start with one application a day. You can continue to use Desquam-E for as long as your doctor thinks it is necessary.

Overdosage
Overdosage of Desquam-E can result in excessive scaling of the skin, reddening skin, or swelling due to fluid retention. Any medication taken in excess can have serious consequences. If you suspect an overdose, seek medical attention.

Brand name:

DESYREL

Pronounced: DES-ee-rel
Generic name: Trazodone hydrochloride

Why is this drug prescribed?
Desyrel is prescribed for the treatment of depression.

Most important fact about this drug
Desyrel does not provide immediate relief. It may take up to 4 weeks before you begin to feel better, although most patients notice improvement within 2 weeks.

How should you take this medication?
Take Desyrel shortly after a meal or light snack. You may be more apt to feel dizzy or light-headed if you take the drug before you have eaten.

Desyrel may cause dry mouth. Sucking on a hard candy, chewing gum, or melting bits of ice in your mouth can relieve the problem.

- *If you miss a dose...*
  Take it as soon as you remember. If it is within 4 hours of your next dose, skip the one you missed and go back to your regular schedule. Never take 2 doses at once.

- *Storage instructions...*
  Store at room temperature in a tightly closed container away from light and excessive heat.

What side effects may occur?
Side effects cannot be anticipated. If any develop or change in intensity, inform your doctor as soon as possible. Only your doctor can determine if it is safe for you to continue taking Desyrel.

- *More common side effects may include:*
  Abdominal or stomach disorder, aches or pains in muscles and bones, anger or hostility, blurred vision, brief loss of consciousness, confusion, constipation, decreased appetite, diarrhea, dizziness or light-headedness, drowsiness, dry mouth, excitement, fainting, fast or fluttery heartbeat, fatigue, fluid retention and swelling, headache, inability to fall or stay asleep, low blood pressure, nasal or sinus congestion, nausea, nervousness, nightmares or vivid dreams, tremors, uncoordinated movements, vomiting, weight gain or loss

- *Less common or rare side effects may include:*
  Allergic reactions, anemia, bad taste in mouth, blood in the urine, chest pain, delayed urine flow, decreased concentration, decreased sex drive,

disorientation, ejaculation problems, excess salivation, gas, general feeling of illness, hallucinations or delusions, high blood pressure, impaired memory, impaired speech, impotence, increased appetite, increased sex drive, menstrual problems, more frequent urination, muscle twitches, numbness, prolonged erections, red, tired, itchy eyes, restlessness, ringing in the ears, shortness of breath, sweating or clammy skin, tingling or pins and needles

Why should this drug not be prescribed?

If you are sensitive to or have ever had an allergic reaction to Desyrel or similar drugs, you should not take this medication. Make sure your doctor is aware of any drug reactions you have experienced.

Special warnings about this medication

Desyrel may cause you to become drowsy or less alert and may affect your judgment. Therefore, you should not drive or operate dangerous machinery or participate in any hazardous activity that requires full mental alertness until you know how this drug affects you.

Desyrel has been associated with priapism, a persistent, painful erection of the penis. Men who experience prolonged or inappropriate erections should stop taking this drug and consult their doctor.

Notify your doctor or dentist that you are taking this drug if you have a medical emergency, and before you have surgery or dental treatment. Your doctor will ask you to stop using the drug if you are going to have elective surgery.

Be careful taking this drug if you have heart disease. Desyrel can cause irregular heartbeats.

Possible food and drug interactions when taking this medication

Desyrel may intensify the effects of alcohol. Do not drink alcohol while taking this medication.

If Desyrel is taken with certain other drugs, the effects of either could be increased, decreased, or altered. It is especially important to check with your doctor before combining Desyrel with the following:

Antidepressant drugs known as MAO inhibitors, including Nardil and Parnate
Barbiturates such as Seconal
Central nervous system depressants such as Demerol and Halcion
Chlorpromazine (Thorazine)

Digoxin (Lanoxin)
Drugs for high blood pressure such as Catapres and Wytensin
Other antidepressants such as Prozac and Norpramin
Phenytoin (Dilantin)
Warfarin (Coumadin)

Special information
if you are pregnant or breastfeeding

The effects of Desyrel during pregnancy have not been adequately studied. If you are pregnant or planning to become pregnant, inform your doctor immediately. This medication may appear in breast milk. If treatment with this drug is essential to your health, your doctor may advise you to discontinue breastfeeding your baby until your treatment is finished.

Recommended dosage

ADULTS

The usual starting dosage is a total of 150 milligrams per day, divided into 2 or more smaller doses. Your doctor may increase your dose by 50 milligrams per day every 3 or 4 days. Total dosage should not exceed 400 milligrams per day, divided into smaller doses. Once you have responded well to the drug, your doctor may gradually reduce your dose. Because this medication makes you drowsy, your doctor may tell you to take the largest dose at bedtime.

CHILDREN

The safety and effectiveness of Desyrel have not been established in children below 18 years of age.

Overdosage

Any medication taken in excess can have serious consequences. An overdose of Desyrel in combination with other drugs can be fatal.

■ *Symptoms of a Desyrel overdose may include:*
Breathing failure, drowsiness, irregular heartbeat, prolonged, painful erection, seizures, vomiting

If you suspect an overdose, seek medical attention immediately.

Brand name:

DEXACORT

See Decadron Turbinaire and Respihaler, page 349.

Generic name:

DEXAMETHASONE

See Decadron Tablets, page 345.

Generic name:

DEXAMETHASONE SODIUM PHOSPHATE

See Decadron Turbinaire and Respihaler, page 349.

Generic name:

DEXAMETHASONE WITH NEOMYCIN

See Neodecadron Ophthalmic Ointment and Solution, page 862.

Brand name:

DEXEDRINE

Pronounced: DEX-eh-dreen
Generic name: Dextroamphetamine sulfate

Why is this drug prescribed?
Dexedrine, a stimulant drug available in tablet or sustained-release capsule form, is prescribed to help treat the following conditions:

1. Narcolepsy (recurrent "sleep attacks")
2. Attention deficit disorder with hyperactivity. (The total treatment program should include social, psychological, and educational guidance along with Dexedrine.)

Most important fact about this drug
Because it is a stimulant, this drug has high abuse potential. The stimulant effect may give way to a letdown period of depression and fatigue. Although the letdown can be relieved by taking another dose, this soon becomes a vicious circle.

If you habitually take Dexedrine in doses higher than recommended, or if you take it over a long period of time, you may eventually become dependent on the drug and suffer from withdrawal symptoms when it is unavailable.

How should you take this medication?
Take Dexedrine exactly as prescribed. If it is prescribed in tablet form, you may need up to 3 doses a day. Take the first dose when you wake up; take the next 1 or 2 doses at intervals of 4 to 6 hours. You can take the sustained-release capsules only once a day.

Do not take Dexedrine late in the day, since this could cause insomnia. If you experience insomnia or loss of appetite while taking this drug, notify your doctor; you may need a lower dosage.

It is likely that your doctor will periodically take you off Dexedrine to determine whether you still need it.

Do not chew or crush the sustained-release form, Dexedrine Spansules.

Do not increase the dosage, except on your doctor's advice.

Do not use Dexedrine to improve mental alertness or stay awake. Do not share it with others.

■ *If you miss a dose...*
If you take 1 dose a day, take it as soon as you remember, but not within 6 hours of going to bed. If you do not remember until the next day, skip the dose you missed and go back to your regular schedule.

If you take 2 or 3 doses a day, take the dose you missed if it is within an hour or so of the scheduled time. Otherwise, skip the dose and go back to your regular schedule. Never take 2 doses at once.

■ *Storage instructions...*
Store at room temperature in a tightly closed container, away from light.

What side effects may occur?
Side effects cannot be anticipated. If any develop or change in intensity, inform your doctor as soon as possible. Only your doctor can determine if it is safe for you to continue taking Dexedrine.

■ *More common side effects may include:*
Excessive restlessness, overstimulation

■ *Other side effects may include:*
Changes in sex drive, constipation, diarrhea, dizziness, dry mouth, exaggerated feeling of well-being or depression, headache, heart palpitations, high blood pressure, hives, impotence, loss of appetite, rapid

heartbeat, sleeplessness, stomach and intestinal disturbances, tremors, uncontrollable twitching or jerking, unpleasant taste in the mouth, weight loss

■ *Effects of chronic heavy abuse of Dexedrine may include:* Hyperactivity, irritability, personality changes, schizophrenia-like thoughts and behavior, severe insomnia, severe skin disease

Why should this drug not be prescribed?

Do not take Dexedrine if you are sensitive to or have ever had an allergic reaction to it.

Do not take Dexedrine for at least 14 days after taking a monoamine oxidase inhibitor (MAO inhibitor) such as the antidepressants Nardil and Parnate. Dexedrine and MAO inhibitors may interact to cause a sharp, potentially life-threatening rise in blood pressure.

Your doctor will not prescribe Dexedrine for you if you suffer from any of the following conditions:

Agitation
Cardiovascular disease
Glaucoma
Hardening of the arteries
High blood pressure
Overactive thyroid gland
Substance abuse

Special warnings about this medication

Be aware that one of the inactive ingredients in Dexedrine is a yellow food coloring called tartrazine (Yellow No. 5). In a few people, particularly those who are allergic to aspirin, tartrazine can cause a severe allergic reaction.

Dexedrine may impair judgment or coordination. Do not drive or operate dangerous machinery until you know how you react to the medication.

There is some concern that Dexedrine may stunt a child's growth. For the sake of safety, any child who takes Dexedrine should have his or her growth monitored.

Possible food and drug interactions when taking this medication

If Dexedrine is taken with certain foods or drugs, the effects of either could be increased, decreased, or altered. It is especially important to check with your doctor before combining Dexedrine with the following:

- *Substances that dampen the effects of Dexedrine:*
  Ammonium chloride
  Chlorpromazine (Thorazine)
  Fruit juices
  Glutamic acid hydrochloride
  Guanethidine (Ismelin)
  Haloperidol (Haldol)
  Lithium carbonate (Lithonate)
  Methenamine (Urised)
  Reserpine (Diupres)
  Sodium acid phosphate
  Vitamin C (as ascorbic acid)

- *Substances that boost the effects of Dexedrine:*
  Acetazolamide (Diamox)
  MAO inhibitors such as Nardil and Parnate
  Propoxyphene (Darvon)
  Sodium bicarbonate (baking soda)
  Thiazide diuretics such as Diuril

- *Substances that have decreased effect when taken with Dexedrine:*
  Antihistamines such as Benadryl
  Blood pressure medications such as Catapres, Hytrin, and Minipress
  Ethosuximide (Zarontin)
  Veratrum alkaloids (found in certain blood pressure drugs)

- *Substances that have increased effect when taken with Dexedrine:*
  Antidepressants such as Norpramin and Vivactil
  Meperidine (Demerol)
  Norepinephrine (Levophed)
  Phenobarbital
  Phenytoin (Dilantin)

Special information
if you are pregnant or breastfeeding

The effects of Dexedrine during pregnancy have not been adequately studied.
If you are pregnant or plan to become pregnant, inform your doctor
immediately. Babies born to women taking Dexedrine may be premature or
have low birth weight. They may also be depressed, agitated, or apathetic
due to withdrawal symptoms. Since Dexedrine appears in breast milk, it
should not be taken by a nursing mother.

Recommended dosage

Take no more Dexedrine than your doctor prescribes. Intake should be kept to the lowest level that proves effective.

NARCOLEPSY

Adults

The usual dose is 5 to 60 milligrams per day, divided into smaller, equal doses.

Children

Narcolepsy seldom occurs in children under 12 years of age; however, when it does, Dexedrine may be used.

The suggested initial dose for children between 6 and 12 years of age is 5 milligrams per day. Your doctor may increase the daily dose in increments of 5 milligrams at weekly intervals until it becomes effective.

Children 12 years of age and older will be started with 10 milligrams daily. The daily dosage may be raised in increments of 10 milligrams at weekly intervals until effective. If side effects such as insomnia or loss of appetite appear, the dosage will probably be reduced.

ATTENTION DEFICIT DISORDER WITH HYPERACTIVITY

This drug is not recommended for children under 3 years of age.

Children from 3 to 5 Years of Age

The usual starting dose is 2.5 milligrams daily, in tablet form. Your doctor may raise the daily dosage by 2.5 milligrams at weekly intervals until the drug becomes effective.

Children 6 Years of Age and Older

The usual starting dose is 5 milligrams once or twice a day. Your doctor may raise the dose by 5 milligrams at weekly intervals until he or she is satisfied with the response. Only in rare cases will the child take more than 40 milligrams per day.

The doctor may prescribe "Spansule" capsules for your child. They are taken once a day.

Your child should take the first dose when he or she wakes up; the remaining 1 or 2 doses are taken at intervals of 4 to 6 hours. Your doctor may interrupt the schedule occasionally to see if behavioral symptoms come back enough to require continued therapy.

Overdosage

An overdose of Dexedrine can be fatal. If you suspect an overdose, seek medical attention immediately.

- ■ *Symptoms of an acute Dexedrine overdose may include:*
  Abdominal cramps, assaultiveness, coma, confusion, convulsions, depression, diarrhea, fatigue, hallucinations, high fever, heightened reflexes, high or low blood pressure, irregular heartbeat, nausea, panic, rapid breathing, restlessness, tremor, vomiting

Generic name:

DEXTROAMPHETAMINE

See Dexedrine, page 380.

Brand name:

DIABETA

See Micronase, page 794.

Brand name:

DIABINESE

Pronounced: dye-AB-in-eez
Generic name: Chlorpropamide

Why is this drug prescribed?

Diabinese is an oral antidiabetic medication used to treat Type II (non-insulin-dependent) diabetes. Diabetes occurs when the body fails to produce enough insulin or is unable to use it properly. Insulin is believed to work by helping sugar penetrate the cell wall so it can be used by the cell.

There are two forms of diabetes: Type I insulin-dependent and Type II non-insulin-dependent. Type I usually requires insulin injection for life, while Type II diabetes can usually be treated by dietary changes and oral antidiabetic medications such as Diabinese. Apparently, Diabinese controls diabetes by stimulating the pancreas to secrete more insulin. Occasionally, Type II diabetics must take insulin injections on a temporary basis, especially during stressful periods or times of illness.

Most important fact about this drug
Always remember that Diabinese is an aid to, not a substitute for, good diet and exercise. Failure to follow a sound diet and exercise plan can lead to serious complications, such as dangerously high or low blood sugar levels. Remember, too, that Diabinese is *not* an oral form of insulin, and cannot be used in place of insulin.

How should you take this medication?
Ordinarily, your doctor will ask you to take a single daily dose of Diabinese each morning with breakfast. However, if this upsets your stomach, he or she may ask you to take Diabinese in smaller doses throughout the day.

To prevent low blood sugar levels (hypoglycemia):

- You should understand the symptoms of hypoglycemia
- Know how exercise affects your blood sugar levels
- Maintain an adequate diet
- Keep a source of quick-acting sugar with you all the time

- *If you miss a dose...*
  Take it as soon as you remember. If it is almost time for the next dose, skip the one you missed and go back to your regular schedule. Do not take 2 doses at the same time.

- *Storage instructions...*
  Store at room temperature.

What side effects may occur?
Side effects cannot be anticipated. If any develop or change in intensity, inform your doctor as soon as possible. Only your doctor can determine if it is safe for you to continue taking Diabinese.

Side effects from Diabinese are rare and seldom require discontinuation of the medication.

- *More common side effects include:*
  Diarrhea, hunger, itching, loss of appetite, nausea, stomach upset, vomiting

- *Less common or rare side effects may include:*
  Anemia and other blood disorders, hives, inflammation of the rectum and colon, sensitivity to light, yellowing of the skin and eyes

Diabinese, like all oral antidiabetics, can cause hypoglycemia (low blood sugar). The risk of hypoglycemia is increased by missed meals, alcohol, other medications, and excessive exercise. To avoid hypoglycemia, closely follow the dietary and exercise regimen suggested by your physician.

■ *Symptoms of mild hypoglycemia may include:*
Cold sweat, drowsiness, fast heartbeat, headache, nausea, nervousness

■ *Symptoms of more severe hypoglycemia may include:*
Coma, pale skin, seizures, shallow breathing

Contact your doctor immediately if these symptoms of severe low blood sugar occur.

Why should this drug not be prescribed?
You should not take Diabinese if you have ever had an allergic reaction to it.

Do not take Diabinese if you are suffering from diabetic ketoacidosis (a life-threatening medical emergency caused by insufficient insulin and marked by excessive thirst, nausea, fatigue, pain below the breastbone, and a fruity breath).

Special warnings about this medication
It's possible that drugs such as Diabinese may lead to more heart problems than diet treatment alone, or diet plus insulin. If you have a heart condition, you may want to discuss this with your doctor.

If you are taking Diabinese, you should check your blood and urine periodically for the presence of abnormal sugar levels.

Remember that it is important that you closely follow the diet and exercise regimen established by your doctor.

Even people with well-controlled diabetes may find that stress, illness, surgery, or fever results in a loss of control. If this happens, your doctor may recommend that Diabinese be discontinued temporarily and insulin used instead.

In addition, the effectiveness of any oral antidiabetic, including Diabinese, may decrease with time. This may occur because of either a diminished responsiveness to the medication or a worsening of the diabetes.

Possible food and drug interactions
when taking this medication
When you take Diabinese with certain other drugs, the effects of either could be increased, decreased, or altered. It is important that you consult with your doctor before taking Diabinese with the following:

Anabolic steroids
Aspirin in large doses
Barbiturates such as Seconal
Beta-blocking blood pressure medications such as Inderal and Tenormin
Calcium-blocking blood pressure medications such as Cardizem and
    Procardia
Chloramphenicol (Chloromycetin)
Coumarin (Coumadin)
Diuretics such as Diuril and HydroDIURIL
Epinephrine (EpiPen)
Estrogen medications such as Premarin
Isoniazid (Nydrazid)
Major tranquilizers such as Mellaril and Thorazine
MAO inhibitor-type antidepressants such as Nardil and Parnate
Nicotinic acid (Nicobid, Nicolar)
Nonsteroidal anti-inflammatory agents such as Advil, Motrin, Naprosyn,
    and Nuprin
Oral contraceptives
Phenothiazines
Phenylbutazone
Phenytoin (Dilantin)
Probenecid (Benemid, ColBENEMID)
Steroids such as prednisone
Sulfa drugs such as Bactrim and Septra
Thyroid medications such as Synthroid

Avoid alcohol since excessive alcohol consumption can cause low blood
sugar, breathlessness, and facial flushing.

Special information
if you are pregnant or breastfeeding
The effects of Diabinese during pregnancy have not been adequately
established. If you are pregnant or plan to become pregnant you should
inform your doctor immediately. Since studies suggest the importance of
maintaining normal blood sugar (glucose) levels during pregnancy, your
physician may prescribe injected insulin.

To minimize the risk of low blood sugar (hypoglycemia) in newborn babies,
Diabinese, if prescribed during pregnancy, should be discontinued at least 1
month before the expected delivery date.

Since Diabinese appears in breast milk, it is not recommended for nursing
mothers. If diet alone does not control glucose levels, then insulin should be
considered.

Recommended dosage
Dosage levels are determined by each individual's needs.

ADULTS

Usually, an initial daily dose of 250 milligrams is recommended for stable, middle-aged, non-insulin-dependent diabetics. After 5 to 7 days, your doctor may adjust this dosage in increments of 50 to 125 milligrams every 3 to 5 days to achieve the best benefit. People with mild diabetes may respond well to daily doses of 100 milligrams or less of Diabinese, while those with severe diabetes may require 500 milligrams daily. Maintenance doses above 750 milligrams are not recommended.

OLDER ADULTS

People who are old, malnourished, or debilitated and those with impaired kidney and liver function usually take an initial dose of 100 to 125 milligrams.

CHILDREN

Safety and effectiveness have not been established.

Overdosage

An overdose of Diabinese can cause low blood sugar (see "What side effects may occur?" for symptoms).

Eating sugar or a sugar-based product will often correct the condition. If you suspect an overdose, seek medical attention immediately.

Brand name:

DIAMOX

Pronounced: DYE-uh-mocks
Generic name: Acetazolamide

Why is this drug prescribed?
Diamox controls fluid secretion. It is used in the treatment of glaucoma (excessive pressure in the eyes), epilepsy (for both brief and unlocalized seizures), and fluid retention due to congestive heart failure or drugs. It is also used to prevent or relieve the symptoms of acute mountain sickness in climbers attempting a rapid climb and those who feel sick even though they are making a gradual climb.

Most important fact about this drug
This drug is considered to be a sulfa drug because of its chemical properties. Although rare, severe reactions have been reported with sulfa drugs. If you develop a rash, bruises, sore throat, or fever contact your doctor immediately.

How should you take this medication?
Take this medication exactly as prescribed by your doctor.

■ *If you miss a dose...*
Take it as soon as you remember. If it is almost time for your next dose, skip the one you missed and go back to your regular schedule. Never take 2 doses at the same time.

■ *Storage instructions...*
Store at room temperature.

What side effects may occur?
Side effects cannot be anticipated. If any develop or change in intensity, inform your doctor as soon as possible. Only your doctor can determine if it is safe for you to continue taking Diamox.

■ *More common side effects may include:*
Change in taste, diarrhea, increase in amount or frequency of urination, loss of appetite, nausea, ringing in the ears, tingling or pins and needles in hands or feet, vomiting

■ *Less common or rare side effects may include:*
Anemia, black or bloody stools, blood in urine, confusion, convulsions, drowsiness, fever, hives, liver dysfunction, nearsightedness, paralysis, rash, sensitivity to light, severe allergic reaction, skin peeling

Why should this drug not be prescribed?
Your doctor will not prescribe this medication for you if your sodium or potassium levels are low, or if you have kidney or liver disease, including cirrhosis.

Diamox should not be used as a long-term treatment for the type of glaucoma called chronic noncongestive angle-closure glaucoma.

Special warnings about this medication
Be very careful about taking high doses of aspirin if you are also taking Diamox. Effects of this combination can range from loss of appetite, sluggishness, and rapid breathing to unresponsiveness; the combination can be fatal.

If you have emphysema or other breathing disorders, use this drug with caution.

If you are taking Diamox to help in rapid ascent of a mountain, you must still come down promptly if you show signs of severe mountain sickness.

Possible food and drug interactions
when taking this medication

If Diamox is taken with certain other drugs, the effects of either could be increased, decreased, or altered. It is especially important to check with your doctor before combining Diamox with the following:

Amitriptyline (Elavil)
Amphetamines such as Dexedrine
Aspirin
Cyclosporine (Sandimmune)
Lithium (Lithonate)
Methenamine (Urex)
Oral diabetes drugs such as Micronase
Quinidine (Quinidex)

Special information
if you are pregnant or breastfeeding

The effects of Diamox during pregnancy have not been adequately studied. If you are pregnant or plan to become pregnant, inform your doctor immediately. Diamox may appear in breast milk and could affect a nursing infant. If this medication is essential to your health, your doctor may advise you to discontinue breastfeeding until your treatment with Diamox is finished.

Recommended dosage

ADULTS

This medication is available in both oral and injectable form. Dosages are for the oral form only.

Glaucoma

This medication is used as an addition to regular glaucoma treatment. Dosages for open-angle glaucoma range from 250 milligrams to 1 gram per 24 hours in 2 or more smaller doses. Your doctor will supervise your dosage and watch the effect of this medication carefully if you are using it for glaucoma. In secondary glaucoma and before surgery in acute congestive (closed-angle) glaucoma, the usual dosage is 250 milligrams every 4 hours or, in some cases, 250 milligrams twice a day. Some people may take 500 milligrams to start, and then 125 or 250 milligrams every 4 hours. The injectable form of this drug is occasionally used in acute cases.

The usual dosage of Diamox Sequels (sustained-release capsules) is 1 capsule (500 milligrams) twice a day, usually in the morning and evening.

Your doctor may adjust the dosage, as needed.

Epilepsy

The daily dosage is 8 to 30 milligrams per 2.2 pounds of body weight in 2 or more doses. Typical dosage may range from 375 to 1,000 milligrams per day. Your doctor will adjust the dosage to suit your needs; Diamox can be used with other anticonvulsant medication.

Congestive Heart Failure

The usual starting dosage to reduce fluid retention in people with congestive heart failure is 250 milligrams to 375 milligrams per day or 5 milligrams per 2.2 pounds of body weight, taken in the morning. Diamox works best when it is taken every other day—or 2 days on, 1 day off—for this condition.

Edema Due to Medication

The usual dose is 250 milligrams to 375 milligrams daily for 1 or 2 days, alternating with a day of rest.

Acute Mountain Sickness

The usual dose is 500 milligrams to 1,000 milligrams a day in 2 or more doses, using either tablets or sustained-release capsules. Doses of this medication are often begun 1 or 2 days before attempting to reach high altitudes.

CHILDREN

The safety and effectiveness of Diamox in children have not been established. However, doses of 8 milligrams to 30 milligrams per 2.2 pounds of body weight have been used in children with various forms of epilepsy.

Overdosage

There is no specific information available on Diamox overdose, but any medication taken in excess can have serious consequences. If you suspect an overdose, seek medical attention immediately.

Generic name:

DIAZEPAM

See Valium, page 1385.

Generic name:

DICLOFENAC

See Voltaren, page 1423.

Generic name:

DICLOFENAC WITH MISOPROSTOL

See Arthrotec, page 94.

Generic name:

DICYCLOMINE

See Bentyl, page 152.

Generic name:

DIDANOSINE

See Videx, page 1409.

Generic name:

DIETHYLPROPION

See Tenuate, page 1282.

Brand name:

DIFFERIN

Pronounced: DIFF-er-in
Generic name: Adapalene

Why is this drug prescribed?
Differin is prescribed for the treatment of acne.

Most important fact about this drug
Differin makes your skin more sensitive to sunlight. While using this product, keep your exposure to the sun at a minimum, and protect yourself with sunscreen and clothing. Never apply Differin to sunburned skin.

How should you use this medication?
Differin should be applied once a day at bedtime. Wash the affected areas, then apply a thin layer of the gel. Avoid eyes, lips, and nostrils.

Use Differin exactly as prescribed. Applying excessive amounts or using the gel more than once a day will not produce better results and may cause severe redness, peeling, and discomfort.

■ *If you miss a dose...*
Don't try to make it up. Simply return to your regular schedule on the following day.

■ *Storage instructions...*
Store at room temperature.

What side effects may occur?
Side effects cannot be anticipated. If any develop or change in intensity, inform your doctor as soon as possible. Only your doctor can determine if it is safe for you to continue using Differin.

Side effects are most likely to occur during the first 2 to 4 weeks and usually diminish with continued treatment. If side effects are severe, your doctor may advise you to reduce the frequency of use or discontinue the drug entirely. Side effects disappear when the drug is stopped.

■ *Side effects may include...*
Acne flare-ups, burning, dryness, irritation, itching, redness, scaling, stinging, sunburn

Why should this drug not be prescribed?
Do not use Differin if you are sensitive to adapalene or any other components of the gel.

Special warnings about this medication
If you have an allergic reaction or severe irritation, stop using the medication and call your doctor.

Remember that Differin increases sensitivity to sunlight. Take measures to protect yourself from overexposure. Wind and cold weather may also be irritating.

Do not apply Differin to cuts, abrasions, eczema, or sunburned skin.

In the first few weeks of treatment, your acne may actually seem to get worse. This just means the medication is working on hidden acne sores. Continue using the product. It can take as much as 8 to 12 weeks before you start to see improvement in your condition.

Differin has not been tested for children under 12 years old.

Possible food and drug interactions
when using this medication

Avoid using Differin with any other product that can irritate the skin, such as medicated soaps and cleansers, soaps and cosmetics that have a strong drying effect, and products with high concentrations of alcohol, astringents, spices, and lime.

Special caution is necessary if you have used, or are currently using, any skin product containing sulfur, resorcinol, or salicylic acid. Do not use such a product with Differin. If you have used one of these products recently, do not begin Differin treatment until the effects of the other product have subsided.

Special information
if you are pregnant or breastfeeding

The effects of Differin during pregnancy and breastfeeding have not been adequately studied. If you are pregnant or plan to become pregnant, notify your doctor immediately. It is not known whether Differin appears in breast milk. If you are nursing and need to use Differin, your doctor may advise you to discontinue breastfeeding while using the medication.

Recommended dosage

The usual dose is a thin film applied over the acne-affected area just before bedtime.

Overdosage

Any medication taken in excess can have serious consequences. Overuse of Differin can cause redness, peeling, and discomfort. If you suspect an overdose, check with your doctor immediately.

Generic name:

DIFLORASONE

See Psorcon, page 1086.

Brand name:

DIFLUCAN

Pronounced: Dye-FLEW-can
Generic name: Fluconazole

Why is this drug prescribed?

Diflucan is used to treat fungal infections called candidiasis (also known as thrush or yeast infections). These include vaginal infections, throat infections, and fungal infections elsewhere in the body, such as infections of the urinary tract, peritonitis (inflammation of the lining of the abdomen), and pneumonia. Diflucan is also prescribed to guard against candidiasis in some people receiving bone marrow transplants, and is used to treat meningitis (brain or spinal cord inflammation) caused by another type of fungus.

In addition, Diflucan is now being prescribed for fungal infections in kidney and liver transplant patients, and fungal infections in patients with AIDS.

Most important fact about this drug
Strong allergic reactions to Diflucan, although rare, have been reported. Symptoms may include hives, itching, swelling, sudden drop in blood pressure, difficulty breathing or swallowing, diarrhea, or abdominal pain. If you experience any of these symptoms, notify your doctor immediately.

How should you take this medication?
You can take Diflucan with or without meals.

Take this medication exactly as prescribed, and continue taking it for as long as your doctor instructs. You may begin to feel better after the first few days; but it takes weeks or even months of treatment to completely cure certain fungal infections.

- *If you miss a dose...*
  Take the forgotten dose as soon as you remember. However, if it is almost time for your next dose, skip the one you missed and return to your regular schedule. Do not take double doses.

- *Storage instructions...*
  Diflucan tablets should be stored at normal room temperature. Avoid exposing them to temperatures above 86°F.

What side effects may occur?
Side effects cannot be anticipated. If any develop or change in intensity, inform your doctor as soon as possible. Only your doctor can determine if it is safe for you to continue taking Diflucan.

The most common side effect for people taking more than one dose is nausea.

For women taking a single dose to treat vaginal infection, the most common side effects are abdominal pain, diarrhea, headache, and nausea; changes in taste, dizziness, and indigestion may occur less often.

- *Less common side effects may include:*
  Abdominal pain, diarrhea, headache, skin rash, vomiting

Why should this drug not be prescribed?

Do not take Diflucan if you are sensitive to any of its ingredients or have ever had an allergic reaction to similar drugs, such as Nizoral. Make sure your doctor is aware of any drug reactions you have experienced.

Special warnings about this medication

Your doctor will watch your liver function carefully while you are taking Diflucan.

If your immunity is low and you develop a rash, your doctor should monitor your condition closely. You may have to stop taking Diflucan if the rash gets worse.

Possible food and drug interactions
when taking this medication

If Diflucan is taken with certain other drugs, the effects of either could be increased, decreased, or altered. It is especially important to check with your doctor before combining Diflucan with the following:

   Blood-thinning drugs such as Coumadin
   Antidiabetic drugs such as Orinase, DiaBeta, and Glucotrol
   Astemizole (Hismanal)
   Cisapride (Propulsid)
   Cyclosporine (Sandimmune, Neoral)
   Hydrochlorothiazide (HydroDIURIL)
   Phenytoin (Dilantin)
   Rifampin (Rifadin)
   Terfenadine (Seldane)
   Ulcer medications such as Tagamet

Special information
if you are pregnant or breastfeeding

The effects of Diflucan during pregnancy have not been adequately studied. If you are pregnant or plan to become pregnant, inform your doctor immediately. Diflucan appears in breast milk and could affect a nursing infant. If this medication is essential to your health, your doctor may advise you to stop breastfeeding until your treatment with Diflucan is finished.

Recommended dosage

ADULTS

For vaginal infections
The usual treatment is a single 150-milligram dose.

For throat infections

The usual dose for candidiasis of the mouth and throat is 200 milligrams on the first day, followed by 100 milligrams once a day. You should see results in a few days, but treatment should continue for at least 2 weeks to avoid a relapse. For candidiasis of the esophagus (gullet) the usual dose is 200 milligrams on the first day, followed by 100 milligrams once a day. Treatment should continue for a minimum of 3 weeks and for at least 2 weeks after symptoms have stopped.

For systemic (bodywide) infections

Doses of up to 400 milligrams per day are sometimes prescribed.

For cryptococcal meningitis

The usual dose is 400 milligrams on the first day, followed by 200 milligrams once a day. Treatment should continue for 10 to 12 weeks once tests of spinal fluid come back negative. For AIDS patients, a 200-milligram dose taken once a day is recommended to prevent relapse.

Prevention of candidiasis during bone marrow transplantation

The usual dose is 400 milligrams once a day.

If you have kidney disease, your doctor may have to reduce your dosage.

CHILDREN

For throat infections

The usual dose for candidiasis of the mouth and throat is 6 milligrams for each 2.2 pounds of the child's weight on the first day, and 3 milligrams per 2.2 pounds once a day after that.

The duration of treatment is the same as that for adults.

For systemic (bodywide) infections

The drug has been given at 6 to 12 milligrams per 2.2 pounds of weight per day.

For cryptococcal meningitis

The usual dose is 12 milligrams per 2.2 pounds of body weight per day on the first day, and 6 milligrams per 2.2 pounds per day after that. Treatment will last 10 to 12 weeks after the fungus disappears.

Overdosage

Any medication taken in excess can have serious consequences. If you suspect an overdose, seek medical treatment immediately.

■ *Symptoms of Diflucan overdose may include:*
Hallucinations, paranoia

Generic name:

DIFLUNISAL

See Dolobid, page 427.

Generic name:

DIGOXIN

See Lanoxin, page 669.

Generic name:

DIHYDROCODEINE, ASPIRIN, AND CAFFEINE

See Synalgos-DC, page 1234.

Generic name:

DIHYDROERGOTAMINE

See Migranal, page 800.

Brand name:

DILACOR XR

See Cardizem, page 205.

Brand name:

DILANTIN

Pronounced: dye-LAN-tin
Generic name: Phenytoin sodium

Why is this drug prescribed?

Dilantin is an antiepileptic drug, prescribed to control grand mal seizures (a type of seizure in which the individual experiences a sudden loss of consciousness immediately followed by generalized convulsions) and temporal lobe seizures (a type of seizure caused by disease in the cortex of the temporal [side] lobe of the brain affecting smell, taste, sight, hearing, memory, and movement).

Dilantin may also be used to prevent and treat seizures occurring during and after neurosurgery (surgery of the brain and spinal cord).

Most important fact about this drug
If you have been taking Dilantin regularly, do not stop abruptly. This may precipitate prolonged or repeated epileptic seizures without any recovery of consciousness between attacks—a condition called status epilepticus that can be fatal if not treated promptly.

How should you take this medication?
It is important that you strictly follow the prescribed dosage regimen and tell your doctor about any condition that makes it impossible for you to take Dilantin as prescribed.

If you are given Dilantin Oral Suspension, shake it well before using. Use the specially marked measuring spoon, a plastic syringe, or a small measuring cup to measure each dose accurately.

Swallow Dilantin Kapseals whole. Dilantin Infatabs can be either chewed thoroughly and then swallowed, or swallowed whole. The Infatabs are not to be used for once-a-day dosing.

Do not change from one form of Dilantin to another without consulting your doctor. Different products may not work the same way.

Depending on the type of seizure disorder, your doctor may give you another drug with Dilantin.

■ *If you miss a dose...*
If you take one dose a day, take the dose you missed as soon as you remember. If you do not remember until the next day, skip the missed dose and go back to your regular schedule. Do not take 2 doses at once.

If you take more than 1 dose a day, take the missed dose as soon as possible. If it is within 4 hours of your next dose, skip the one you missed and go back to your regular schedule. Do not take 2 doses at once.

If you forget to take your medication 2 or more days in a row, check with your doctor.

■ *Storage instructions...*
Store at room temperature away from light and moisture.

What side effects may occur?
Side effects cannot be anticipated. If any develop or change in intensity, inform your doctor as soon as possible. Only your doctor can determine whether it is safe for you to continue taking Dilantin.

■ *More common side effects may include:*
Decreased coordination, involuntary eye movement, mental confusion, slurred speech

■ *Other side effects may include:*
Abnormal hair growth, abnormal muscle tone, blood disorders, coarsening of facial features, constipation, dizziness, enlargement of lips, fever, headache, inability to fall asleep or stay asleep, joint pain, nausea, nervousness, overgrowth of gum tissue, Peyronie's disease (a disorder of the penis that causes the penis to bend on an angle during erection, often making intercourse painful or difficult), rapid and spastic involuntary movement, skin peeling or scaling, skin rash, tremors, twitching, vomiting, yellowing of skin and eyes

Why should this drug not be prescribed?
If you have ever had an allergic reaction to or are sensitive to phenytoin or similar epilepsy medications such as Peganone or Mesantoin, do not take Dilantin. Make sure your doctor is aware of any drug reactions you have experienced.

Special warnings about this medication
Tell your doctor if you develop a skin rash. If the rash is scale-like, characterized by reddish or purplish spots, or consists of (fluid-filled) blisters, your doctor may stop Dilantin and prescribe an alternative treatment. If the rash is more like measles, your doctor may have you stop taking Dilantin until the rash is completely gone.

Because Dilantin is processed by the liver, people with impaired liver function, older adults, and those who are seriously ill may show early signs of drug poisoning.

Practicing good dental hygiene minimizes the development of gingival hyperplasia (excessive formation of the gums over the teeth) and its complications.

Avoid drinking alcoholic beverages while taking Dilantin.

Possible food and drug interactions when taking this medication

If Dilantin is taken with certain other drugs, the effects of either could be increased, decreased, or altered. It is especially important to check with your doctor before combining Dilantin with the following:

Alcohol
Amiodarone (Cordarone)
Antacids containing calcium
Blood-thinning drugs such as Coumadin
Chloramphenicol (Chloromycetin)
Chlordiazepoxide (Librium)
Diazepam (Valium)
Dicumarol
Digitoxin (Crystodigin)
Disulfiram (Antabuse)
Doxycycline (Vibramycin)
Estrogens such as Premarin
Felbamate (Felbatol)
Fluoxetine (Prozac)
Furosemide (Lasix)
Isoniazid (Nydrazid)
Major tranquilizers such as Mellaril and Thorazine
Methylphenidate (Ritalin)
Molindone hydrochloride (Moban)
Oral contraceptives
Phenobarbital
Quinidine (Quinidex)
Reserpine (Diupres)
Rifampin (Rifadin)
Salicylates such as aspirin
Seizure medications such as Depakene, Depakote, Tegretol, and Zarontin
Steroid drugs such as prednisone (Deltasone)
Sucralfate (Carafate)
Sulfa drugs such as Gantrisin
Theophylline (Theo-Dur, others)
Tolbutamide (Orinase)
Trazodone (Desyrel)
Ulcer medications such as Tagamet and Zantac

Tricyclic antidepressants (such as Elavil, Norpramin, and others) may cause seizures in susceptible people, making a dosage adjustment of Dilantin necessary.

Hyperglycemia (high blood sugar) may occur in people taking Dilantin, which blocks the release of insulin. People with diabetes may experience increased blood sugar levels due to Dilantin.

Abnormal softening of the bones may occur in people taking Dilantin because of Dilantin's interference with vitamin D metabolism.

Special information
if you are pregnant or breastfeeding
If you are pregnant or plan to become pregnant, inform your doctor immediately. Because of the possibility of birth defects with antiepileptic drugs such as Dilantin, you may need to discontinue the drug. Do not, however, stop taking it without first consulting your doctor. Dilantin appears in breast milk; breastfeeding is not recommended during treatment with this drug.

Recommended dosage
Dosage is tailored to each individual's needs. Your doctor will monitor blood levels of the drug closely, particularly when switching you from one drug to another.

ADULTS

Standard Daily Dosage
If you have not had any previous treatment, your doctor will have you take one 100-milligram Dilantin capsule 3 times daily to start.

On a continuing basis, most adults need 1 capsule 3 to 4 times a day. Your doctor may increase that dosage to 2 capsules 3 times a day, if necessary.

Once-A-Day Dosage
If your seizures are controlled on 100-milligram Dilantin capsules 3 times daily, your doctor may allow you to take the entire 300 milligrams as a single dose once daily.

CHILDREN

The starting dose is 5 milligrams per 2.2 pounds of body weight per day, divided into 2 or 3 equal doses; the most a child should take is 300 milligrams a day. The regular daily dosage is usually 4 to 8 milligrams per 2.2 pounds. Children over 6 years of age and adolescents may need the minimum adult dose (300 milligrams per day).

Overdosage

An overdose of Dilantin can be fatal. If you suspect an overdose, seek medical attention immediately.

■ *Symptoms of Dilantin overdose may include:*
Coma, difficulty in pronouncing words correctly, involuntary eye movement, lack of muscle coordination, low blood pressure, nausea, sluggishness, slurred speech, tremors, vomiting

Brand name:

DILAUDID

Pronounced: Dye-LAW-did
Generic name: Hydromorphone hydrochloride

Why is this drug prescribed?

Dilaudid, a narcotic analgesic, is prescribed for the relief of moderate to severe pain such as that due to:

Biliary colic (pain caused by an obstruction in the gallbladder or bile duct)
Burns
Cancer
Heart attack
Injury (soft tissue and bone)
Renal colic (sharp lower back and groin pain usually caused by the passage of a stone through the ureter)
Surgery

Most important fact about this drug

High dose tolerance leading to mental and physical dependence can occur with the use of Dilaudid when it is taken repeatedly. Physical dependence (need for continual doses to prevent withdrawal symptoms) can occur after only a few days of narcotic use, although it usually takes several weeks.

How should you take this medication?

Take Dilaudid exactly as prescribed by your doctor. Never increase the amount you take without your doctor's approval.

■ *If you miss a dose...*
Take the forgotten dose as soon as you remember. If it is almost time for the next dose, skip the one you missed and go back to your regular schedule. Never try to "catch up" by doubling the dose.

■ *Storage instructions...*
Tablets and liquid should be stored at room temperature. Protect from light and extreme cold or heat. Suppositories should be stored in the refrigerator.

What side effects may occur?
Side effects cannot be anticipated. If any develop or change in intensity, inform your doctor as soon as possible. Only your doctor can determine if it is safe for you to continue taking Dilaudid.

■ *More common side effects may include:*
Anxiety, constipation, dizziness, drowsiness, fear, impairment of mental and physical performance, inability to urinate, mental clouding, mood changes, nausea, restlessness, sedation, sluggishness, troubled and slowed breathing, vomiting

■ *Less common side effects may include:*
Agitation, blurred vision, chills, cramps, diarrhea, difficulty urinating, disorientation, double vision, dry mouth, exaggerated feelings of depression or well-being, failure of breathing or heartbeat, faintness/fainting, flushing, hallucinations, headache, increased pressure in the head, insomnia, involuntary eye movements, itching, light-headedness, loss of appetite, low or high blood pressure, muscle rigidity or tremor, muscle spasms of the throat or air passages, palpitations, rashes, shock, slow or rapid heartbeat, small pupils, sudden dizziness on standing, sweating, taste changes, tingling and/or numbness, tremor, uncoordinated muscle movements, visual disturbances, weakness

Why should this drug not be prescribed?
If you are sensitive to or have ever had an allergic reaction to Dilaudid or narcotic pain killers you should not take this medication. Make sure that your doctor is aware of any drug reactions that you have experienced.

Special warnings about this medication
Dilaudid may impair the mental and/or physical abilities required for the performance of potentially hazardous tasks such as driving a car or operating machinery.

Dilaudid should be used with caution if you are in a weakened condition or if you have a severe liver or kidney disorder, hypothyroidism (underactive thyroid gland), Addison's disease (adrenal gland failure), an enlarged prostate, a urethral stricture (narrowing of the urethra), low blood pressure or a head injury.

Dilaudid suppresses the cough reflex; therefore, the doctor will be cautious about prescribing Dilaudid after an operation or for patients with a lung disease.

High doses of Dilaudid may produce labored or slowed breathing. This drug also affects centers that control breathing rhythm and may produce irregular breathing. People who already have breathing difficulties should be very careful about taking Dilaudid.

Narcotics such as Dilaudid may mask or hide the symptoms of sudden or severe abdominal conditions, making diagnosis and treatment difficult.

If you are prone to convulsions, your doctor may not prescribe Dilaudid. It can make seizures worse.

Possible food and drug interactions
when taking this medication

Dilaudid is a central nervous system depressant and intensifies the effects of alcohol. Do not drink alcohol while taking this medication.

If Dilaudid is taken with certain other drugs, the effects of either could be increased, decreased, or altered. It is especially important to check with your doctor before combining Dilaudid with the following:

Antiemetics (drugs that prevent or lessen nausea and vomiting such as
    Compazine and Phenergan)
Antihistamines such as Benadryl
General anesthetics
Other central nervous system depressants such as Nembutal, Restoril
Other narcotic analgesics such as Demerol and Percocet
Phenothiazines such as Thorazine
Sedative/hypnotics such as Valium, Halcion
Tranquilizers such as Xanax
Tricyclic antidepressants such as Elavil and Tofranil

Special information
if you are pregnant or breastfeeding

Do not take Dilaudid if you are pregnant or plan to become pregnant unless you are directed to do so by your doctor. Drug dependence occurs in newborns when the mother has taken narcotic drugs regularly during pregnancy. Withdrawal signs include irritability and excessive crying, tremors, overactive reflexes, increased breathing rate, increased stools, sneezing, yawning, vomiting, and fever. Dilaudid may appear in breast milk and could affect a nursing infant. If this medication is essential to your health, your doctor may advise you to discontinue breastfeeding your baby until your treatment is finished.

Recommended dosage

ADULTS

Tablets
The usual starting dose of Dilaudid tablets is 2 to 4 milligrams every 4 to 6 hours as determined by your doctor. Severity of pain, your individual response, and your size are used to determine your exact dosage.

Liquid
The usual dose of Dilaudid liquid is ½ to 2 teaspoonfuls every 3 to 6 hours. In some cases, the dosage may be higher.

Suppositories
Dilaudid suppositories (3 milligrams) may provide relief for a longer period of time. The usual adult dose is 1 suppository inserted rectally every 6 to 8 hours or as directed by your doctor.

CHILDREN

The safety and effectiveness of Dilaudid have not been established in children.

OLDER ADULTS

Be very careful when using Dilaudid. Your doctor will prescribe a dose individualized to suit your needs.

Overdosage

■ *Symptoms of Dilaudid overdose include:*
Bluish tinge to skin, cold and clammy skin, constricted pupils, coma, extreme sleepiness progressing to a state of unresponsiveness, labored or slowed breathing, limp, weak muscles, low blood pressure, slow heart rate

In severe overdosage, the patient may stop breathing. Shock, heart attack, and death can occur.

If you suspect an overdose, seek emergency medical treatment immediately.

Generic name:

DILTIAZEM

See Cardizem, page 205.

Brand name:

DIMETANE-DC

Pronounced: DYE-meh-tayne DEE SEE
Generic ingredients: Brompheniramine maleate,
    Phenylpropanolamine hydrochloride, Codeine phosphate

Why is this drug prescribed?

Dimetane-DC cough syrup is an antihistamine/decongestant/cough suppressant combination that relieves coughs and nasal congestion caused by allergies and the common cold. Brompheniramine, the antihistamine, reduces itching and dries up secretions from the nose, eyes, and throat. Phenylpropanolamine, the decongestant, clears nasal stuffiness and makes breathing easier. Codeine calms a cough.

Most important fact about this drug

Dimetane-DC may cause you to become drowsy or less alert. You should not drive or operate dangerous machinery or participate in any hazardous activity that requires full mental alertness until you know how you react to Dimetane-DC.

How should you take this medication?

Take this medication exactly as prescribed.

Do not exceed the directed dosage.

- *If you miss a dose...*
  Take it as soon as you remember. If it is almost time for your next dose, skip the one you missed and go back to your regular schedule. Do not take 2 doses at once.

- *Storage instructions...*
  Store at room temperature in a tightly closed container, away from light.

What side effects may occur?

Side effects cannot be anticipated. If any side effects develop or change in intensity, tell your doctor as soon as possible. Only your doctor can determine whether it is safe for you to continue taking Dimetane-DC.

- *More common side effects may include:*
  Dizziness/light-headedness, drowsiness, dry mouth, nose, and throat, sedation, thickening of phlegm

■ *Less common or rare side effects may include:*
Anemia, constipation, convulsions, diarrhea, difficulty sleeping, difficulty urinating, disturbed coordination, exaggerated sense of well-being or depression, frequent urination, headache, high blood pressure, hives, increased sensitivity to light, irregular heartbeat, irritability, itching, loss of appetite, low blood pressure, nausea, nervousness, rash, shortness of breath, stomach upset, tightness in chest, tremor, vision changes, vomiting, weakness, wheezing

Why should this drug not be prescribed?
This medication should not be given to children under 2 years of age or used by nursing mothers.

Do not take Dimetane-DC if you have severe high blood pressure or heart disease, or if you are taking antidepressant drugs known as MAO inhibitors (Nardil, Parnate). Dimetane-DC is not for treatment of asthma or other breathing disorders. Avoid Dimetane-DC if you have ever had an allergic reaction to it or are sensitive to any of its ingredients.

Special warnings about this medication
Use Dimetane-DC cautiously if you have, or have ever had, bronchial asthma, the eye condition called narrow-angle glaucoma, stomach, intestinal, or bladder obstruction, diabetes, high blood pressure, heart disease, or thyroid disease.

Codeine can cause drug dependence and tolerance with continued use; your doctor will monitor your use of this drug carefully.

Antihistamines can make young children excited.

Possible food and drug interactions
when taking this medication
Dimetane-DC may increase the effects of alcohol. Do not drink alcohol while taking this medication.

If Dimetane-DC is taken with certain other drugs, the effects of either drug could be increased, decreased, or altered. It is especially important to check with your doctor before combining Dimetane-DC with the following:

MAO inhibitor-type antidepressant drugs such as Nardil and Parnate
Medications for high blood pressure such as Aldomet
Sedatives/hypnotics such as phenobarbital, Halcion, and Seconal
Tranquilizers such as Xanax, BuSpar, Librium, and Valium

Special information
if you are pregnant or breastfeeding

No information is available about the safety of Dimetane-DC during pregnancy. If you are pregnant or plan to become pregnant, inform your doctor immediately.

Dimetane-DC should not be taken if you are breastfeeding. If Dimetane-DC is essential to your health, your doctor may advise you to stop breastfeeding until your treatment is finished.

Recommended dosage

Do not take more than 6 doses in 24 hours.

ADULTS AND CHILDREN 12 YEARS OLD AND OVER

The recommended dosage is 2 teaspoonfuls every 4 hours.

CHILDREN 6 TO UNDER 12 YEARS OLD

The usual dosage is 1 teaspoonful every 4 hours.

CHILDREN 2 TO UNDER 6 YEARS OLD

The dosage is one-half teaspoonful every 4 hours.

Overdosage

An overdose of antihistamines may cause hallucinations, convulsions, and death, especially in infants and small children. If you suspect an overdose, seek medical treatment immediately.

- *Symptoms of Dimetane-DC overdose may include:*
  Anxiety, breathing difficulty, convulsions, delirium, depression, dilated pupils, excessive excitement or stimulation, extreme sleepiness leading to loss of consciousness, hallucinations, heart attack, high blood pressure, irregular heartbeat, rapid heartbeat, restlessness, tremors

Brand name:

DIOVAN

Pronounced: DYE-oh-van
Generic name: Valsartan
Other brand name: Diovan HCT

Why is this drug prescribed?
Diovan is one of a new class of blood pressure medications called angiotensin II receptor antagonists. Diovan works by preventing the hormone angiotensin II from narrowing the blood vessels, which tends to raise blood pressure. Diovan may be prescribed alone or with other blood pressure medications, such as diuretics that help the body get rid of excess water. Diovan HCT provides just such a combination. It contains Diovan plus the common diuretic hydrochlorothiazide.

Most important fact about this drug
You must take Diovan regularly for it to be effective. Since blood pressure declines gradually, it may be several weeks before you get the full benefit of Diovan, and you must continue taking it even if you are feeling well. Diovan does not cure high blood pressure; it merely keeps it under control.

How should you take this medication?
Diovan and Diovan HCT can be taken with or without food. Try to get in the habit of taking the medicine at the same time each day—for example, before or after breakfast. You'll be less likely to forget your dose.

■ *If you miss a dose...*
Take it as soon as possible. If it is almost time for your next dose, skip the one you missed and go back to your regular schedule. Never take 2 doses at the same time.

■ *Storage instructions...*
Store at room temperature. Keep in a tightly closed container, away from moisture.

What side effects may occur?
Side effects cannot be anticipated. If any develop or change in intensity, tell your doctor as soon as possible. Only your doctor can determine if it is safe for you to continue taking Diovan or Diovan HCT.

■ *More common side effects may include:*
Cold or flu, cough, diarrhea, dizziness, fatigue, headache, sore throat

■ *Less common side effects may include:*
Abdominal pain, back pain, chest pain, headache, respiratory tract infection, sinus inflammation

Why should this drug not be prescribed?

Do not take Diovan or Diovan HCT while pregnant. Avoid both drugs if they cause an allergic reaction, and do not take Diovan HCT if you have ever had an allergic reaction to a Sulfa drug such as Bactrim or Septra. Also avoid Diovan HCT if you have trouble urinating.

Special warnings about this medication

In rare cases, Diovan and Diovan HCT can cause a severe drop in blood pressure. The problem is more likely if your body's supply of water has been depleted by high doses of diuretics. Symptoms include light-headedness or faintness, and are more likely when you first start taking the drug. Diovan HCT can also cause dry mouth, weakness, drowsiness, muscle cramps, nausea, and vomiting. Call your doctor if any of these symptoms occur. You may need to have your dosage adjusted.

Use Diovan HCT with caution if you have a history of allergy or bronchial asthma, or suffer from the condition called lupus erythematosus. Report a rapid or irregular pulse to your doctor.

If you have liver or kidney disease, Diovan and Diovan HCT must be used with caution. Be sure the doctor is aware of either problem. Also let the doctor know if you suffer from gout or diabetes.

The safety and effectiveness of Diovan and Diovan HCT have not been studied in children.

Possible food and drug interactions
when taking this medication

There have been no reports of significant interactions with Diovan. However, the hydrochlorothiazide in Diovan HCT may interact with a variety of drugs. Be sure to check with your doctor before combining Diovan HCT with the following:

Alcohol
Cholestyramine (Questran)
Colestipol (Colestid)
Corticosteroids such as hydrocortisone and prednisone
Glipizide (Glucotrol)
Glyburide (Diabeta, Micronase)
Insulin
Lithium (Lithobid, Lithonate)
Non-steroidal anti-inflammatory drugs such as Advil, Aleve, Motin, and
    Naprosyn
Other blood pressure medications such as Cardizem, Lopressor, and
    Procardia

Phenobarbital
Narcotic drugs such as morphine or codeine products

Special information
if you are pregnant or breastfeeding

Drugs such as Diovan and Diovan HCT can cause injury or even death to the unborn child when used during the last 6 months of pregnancy. As soon as you find out that you're pregnant, stop taking the drug and call your doctor. Both of these drugs may also appear in breast milk and could affect the nursing infant. If the medication is essential to your health, your doctor may advise you to avoid breastfeeding while you are taking Diovan or Diovan HCT.

Recommended dosage

DIOVAN

The usual starting dose is 80 milligrams once a day. If your blood pressure does not go down, your doctor may increase the dose or add a diuretic to your regimen. The maximum recommended dose is 320 milligrams a day.

DIOVAN HCT

The usual starting dose when switching from Diovan to Diovan HCT is one 80 milligram/12.5 milligram tablet daily. Daily dosage may be increased to a maximum of 160 milligrams of valsartan and 25 milligrams of hydrochlorothiazide.

Overdosage

There has been little experience with overdosage. However, the most likely results would be extremely low blood pressure and an abnormally slow or rapid heartbeat. If you suspect an overdose, seek medical attention immediately.

Brand name:

DIPENTUM

Pronounced: dye-PENT-um
Generic name: Olsalazine sodium

Why is this drug prescribed?

Dipentum is an anti-inflammatory drug used to maintain long-term freedom from symptoms of ulcerative colitis (chronic inflammation and ulceration of the large intestine and rectum). It is prescribed for people who cannot take sulfasalazine (Azulfidine).

Most important fact about this drug

If you have kidney disease, Dipentum could cause further damage. You'll need regular checks on your kidney function, so be sure to keep all regular appointments with your doctor.

How should you take this medication?

Take Dipentum for as long as your doctor has directed, even if you feel better.

Take Dipentum with food.

- ■ *If you miss a dose...*
  Take it as soon as you remember. If it is almost time for your next dose, skip the one you missed and go back to your regular schedule. Do not take 2 doses at once.

- ■ *Storage instructions...*
  Store at room temperature.

What side effects may occur?

Side effects cannot be anticipated. If any develop or change in intensity, inform your doctor as soon as possible. Only your doctor can determine if it is safe for you to continue taking Dipentum.

Diarrhea or loose stools are the most common side effects.

- ■ *Other side effects may include:*
  Abdominal pain/cramping, bloating, depression, dizziness, drowsiness, headache, heartburn, indigestion, inflammation of the mouth, insomnia, joint pain, light-headedness, loss of appetite, nausea, rectal bleeding, skin itching, skin rash, sluggishness, upper respiratory infection, vertigo, vomiting

Rare cases of hepatitis have been reported in people taking Dipentum. Symptoms may include aching muscles, chills, fever, headache, joint pain, loss of appetite, vomiting, and yellowish skin.

Why should this drug not be prescribed?

You should not be using Dipentum if you are allergic to salicylates such as aspirin.

Special warnings about this medication

If diarrhea occurs, contact your doctor.

Possible food and drug interactions
when taking this medication
If Dipentum is taken with certain other drugs, the effects of either could be increased, decreased, or altered. It is especially important to check with your doctor before combining Dipentum with warfarin (Coumadin).

Special information
if you are pregnant or breastfeeding
The effects of Dipentum in pregnancy have not been adequately studied. Pregnant women should use Dipentum only if the possible gains warrant the possible risks to the unborn child. Women who breastfeed an infant should use Dipentum cautiously, because it is not known whether this drug appears in breast milk and what effect it might have on a nursing infant.

Recommended dosage

ADULTS

The usual dose is a total of 1 gram per day, divided into 2 equal doses.

CHILDREN

Safety and effectiveness have not been established in children.

Overdosage
There have been no reports of Dipentum overdose. However, should you suspect one, seek medical help immediately.

Generic name:

DIPHENHYDRAMINE

See Benadryl, page 149.

Generic name:

DIPHENOXYLATE WITH ATROPINE

See Lomotil, page 711.

Generic name:

DIPIVEFRIN

See Propine, page 1062.

Brand name:

DIPROLENE

Pronounced: dye-PROH-leen
Generic name: Betamethasone dipropionate

Why is this drug prescribed?
Diprolene, a synthetic cortisone-like steroid available in cream, gel, lotion, or ointment form, is used to treat certain itchy rashes and other inflammatory skin conditions.

Most important fact about this drug
When you use Diprolene, you inevitably absorb some of the medication through your skin and into the bloodstream. Too much absorption can lead to unwanted side effects elsewhere in the body. To keep this problem to a minimum, avoid using large amounts of Diprolene over large areas, and do not cover it with airtight dressings such as plastic wrap or adhesive bandages.

How should you use this medication?
Apply Diprolene in a thin film, exactly as prescribed by your doctor. A typical regimen is 1 or 2 applications per day. Do not use the medication for longer than prescribed.

Diprolene is for use only on the skin. Be careful to keep it out of your eyes.

Once you have applied Diprolene, never cover the skin with an airtight bandage or other tight dressing.

For a fungal or bacterial skin infection, you will need antifungal or antibacterial medication in addition to Diprolene. If improvement is not prompt, you should stop using Diprolene until the infection is visibly clearing.

- *If you miss a dose...*
  Apply it as soon as you remember. If it is almost time for the next dose, skip the one you missed and go back to your regular schedule.

- *Storage instructions...*
  Store at room temperature.

What side effects may occur?
Side effects cannot be anticipated. A possible side effect of Diprolene is stinging or burning of the skin where the medication is applied.

■ *Other side effects on the skin may include:*
Acne-like eruptions, atrophy, "broken" capillaries (fine reddish lines), cracking or tightening, dryness, infected hair follicles, irritation, itching, prickly heat, rash, redness, sensitivity

Diprolene can be absorbed and produce side effects elsewhere in the body; see the "Overdosage" section on page 396.

Why should this drug not be prescribed?
Do not use Diprolene if you are sensitive to it or have ever had an allergic reaction to it.

Special warnings about this medication
Do not use Diprolene to treat any condition other than the one for which it was prescribed.

Possible food and drug interactions when using this medication
No interactions have been reported.

Special information if you are pregnant or breastfeeding
It is not known whether Diprolene, when applied to skin, causes any problem during pregnancy or while breastfeeding. Nevertheless, let your doctor know if you are pregnant or are planning to become pregnant.

Recommended dosage

ADULTS

Diprolene products are not to be used with airtight dressings.

Cream or ointment
Apply a thin film to the affected skin areas once or twice daily. Treatment should be limited to 45 grams per week.

Lotion
Apply a few drops of Diprolene Lotion to the affected area once or twice daily and massage lightly until the lotion disappears.

Treatment must be limited to 14 days; do not use any more than 50 milliliters per week.

Gel
Apply a thin layer of Diprolene Gel to the affected area once or twice daily and rub in gently and completely.

Treatment must be limited to 14 days; do not use any more than 50 grams per week.

CHILDREN

Use of Diprolene Gel, Lotion, Ointment, and AF Cream is not recommended for children under 12 years of age. For those 12 and over, use no more than necessary to obtain results.

Overdosage

With copious or prolonged use of Diprolene, hormone absorbed into the bloodstream may cause high blood sugar, sugar in the urine, and a group of symptoms called Cushing's syndrome.

■ *Symptoms of Cushing's syndrome may include:*
Acne, depression, high blood pressure, humped upper back, insomnia, moon-faced appearance, muscle weakness, obese trunk, paranoia, stretch marks, susceptibility to bruising, fractures, infections, retardation of growth, delayed weight gain, wasted limbs

Cushing's syndrome may also trigger the development of diabetes mellitus. Left uncorrected, the syndrome may become serious. If you suspect your use of Diprolene has led to this problem, seek medical attention immediately.

Generic name:

DIPYRIDAMOLE

See Persantine, page 987.

Generic name:

DIRITHROMYCIN

See Dynabac, page 446.

Brand name:

DISALCID

Pronounced: dye-SAL-sid
Generic name: Salsalate

Why is this drug prescribed?

Disalcid, a nonsteroidal anti-inflammatory drug, is used to relieve the symptoms of rheumatoid arthritis, osteoarthritis (the most common form of arthritis), and other rheumatic disorders (conditions that involve pain and inflammation in joints and the tissues around them).

Most important fact about this drug
Disalcid contains salicylate, an ingredient that may be associated with the development of Reye's syndrome (a disorder that causes abnormal brain and liver function). It occurs mostly in children who have taken aspirin or other medications containing salicylate to relieve symptoms of the flu or chickenpox. Do not take Disalcid if you have flu symptoms or chickenpox.

How should you take this medication?
Take Disalcid exactly as prescribed. Food may slow its absorption. However, your doctor may ask you to take Disalcid with food in order to avoid stomach upset.

■ *If you miss a dose...*
Take it as soon as you remember. If it is almost time for your next dose, skip the one you missed and go back to your regular schedule. Never take 2 doses at once.

■ *Storage instructions...*
Store at room temperature. Keep out of the reach of children.

What side effects may occur?
Side effects cannot be anticipated. If any develop or change in intensity, inform your doctor as soon as possible. Only your doctor can determine if it is safe for you to continue taking Disalcid.

■ *Side effects may include:*
Hearing impairment, nausea, rash, ringing in the ears, vertigo

Why should this drug not be prescribed?
Disalcid should not be taken if you are sensitive to or have ever had an allergic reaction to salsalate.

Special warnings about this medication
Use Disalcid with extreme caution if you have chronic kidney disease or a peptic ulcer.

Salicylates occasionally cause asthma in people who are sensitive to aspirin. Although Disalcid contains a salicylate, it is less likely than aspirin to cause this reaction.

Possible food and drug interactions
when taking this medication

If Disalcid is taken with certain other drugs, the effects of either could be increased, decreased, or altered. It is especially important to check with your doctor before combining Disalcid with the following:

ACE inhibitor-type blood pressure drugs such as Capoten and Vasotec

Acetazolamide (Diamox)

Aspirin and other drugs containing salicylates such as Bufferin and Empirin

Blood-thinning medications such as Coumadin

Medications for gout such as Zyloprim and Benemid

Methotrexate (Rheumatrex)

Naproxen (Anaprox, Naprosyn)

Oral diabetes drugs such as Glucotrol and Tolinase

Penicillin (Pen-Vee K)

Phenytoin (Dilantin)

Steroids such as Deltasone and Decadron

Sulfinpyrazone (Anturane)

Thyroid medications such as Synthroid

Special information
if you are pregnant or breastfeeding

The effects of Disalcid during pregnancy have not been adequately studied. If you are pregnant or plan to become pregnant, inform your doctor immediately. Disalcid may appear in breast milk and could affect a nursing infant. If this medication is essential to your health, your doctor may advise you to stop breastfeeding until your treatment with Disalcid is finished.

Recommended dosage

You may not feel the full benefit of this medication for 3 to 4 days.

ADULTS

The usual dosage is 3,000 milligrams daily, divided into smaller doses as follows:

(1) 2 doses of two 750-milligram tablets

(2) 2 doses of three 500-milligram tablets or capsules

(3) 3 doses of two 500-milligram tablets or capsules

CHILDREN

Safety and effectiveness of Disalcid use in children have not been established.

OLDER ADULTS

A lower dosage may be sufficient to achieve desired blood levels without the more common side effects.

Overdosage

Any medication taken in excess can have serious consequences. Deaths have occurred from salicylate overdose. If you suspect an overdose, seek medical treatment immediately.

■ *Symptoms of Disalcid overdose may include:*
Confusion, dehydration, diarrhea, drowsiness, headache, high body temperature, hyperventilation, ringing in the ears, sweating, vertigo, vomiting

Generic name:

DISOPYRAMIDE

See Norpace, page 903.

Brand name:

DITROPAN

Pronounced: DYE-tro-pan
Generic name: Oxybutynin chloride

Why is this drug prescribed?

Ditropan relaxes the bladder muscle and reduces spasms. It is used to treat the urgency, frequency, leakage, incontinence, and painful or difficult urination caused by a neurogenic bladder (altered bladder function due to a nervous system abnormality).

Most important fact about this drug

Ditropan can cause heat prostration (fever and heat stroke due to decreased sweating) in high temperatures. If you live in a hot climate or will be exposed to high temperatures, take appropriate precautions.

How should you take this medication?

Take this medication exactly as prescribed.

Ditropan can make your mouth dry. Sucking hard candies or melting bits of ice in your mouth can remedy the problem.

■ *If you miss a dose...*
Take the forgotten dose as soon as you remember. If it is almost time for your next dose, skip the one you missed and go back to your regular schedule. Never take 2 doses at once.

■ *Storage instructions...*
Keep this medication in a tightly closed container and store it at room temperature. Protect the syrup from direct light.

What side effects may occur?
Side effects cannot be anticipated. If any develop or change in intensity, inform your doctor as soon as possible. Only your doctor can determine if it is safe for you to continue taking Ditropan.

■ *Side effects may include:*
Constipation, decreased production of tears, decreased sweating, difficulty falling or staying asleep, dilation of the pupil of the eye, dim vision, dizziness, drowsiness, dry mouth, eye paralysis, hallucinations, impotence, inability to urinate, nausea, palpitations, rapid heartbeat, rash, restlessness, suppression of milk production, weakness

Why should this drug not be prescribed?
You should not take Ditropan if you have certain types of untreated glaucoma (excessive pressure in the eye), partial or complete blockage of the gastrointestinal tract, or paralytic ileus (obstructed bowel). Ditropan should also be avoided if you have severe colitis (inflamed colon), myasthenia gravis (abnormal muscle weakness), or urinary tract obstruction. This drug is usually not prescribed for the elderly or debilitated.

Do not take this medication if you are sensitive or have ever had an allergic reaction to it. Make sure your doctor is aware of any allergic reactions you have experienced.

Special warnings about this medication
If you have an ileostomy or colostomy (an artificial opening to the bowel) and develop diarrhea while taking Ditropan, inform your doctor immediately.

Ditropan may cause drowsiness or blurred vision. Driving or operating dangerous machinery or participating in any hazardous activity that requires full mental alertness is not recommended until you know how this medication affects you.

Your doctor will prescribe Ditropan with caution if you have liver disease, kidney disease, or a nervous system disorder.

Ditropan may aggravate the symptoms of overactive thyroid, heart disease or congestive heart failure, irregular or rapid heartbeat, high blood pressure, or enlarged prostate.

Possible food and drug interactions when taking this medication

If Ditropan is taken with certain other drugs, the effects of either may be increased, decreased or altered. It is especially important to check with your doctor before combining Ditropan with alcohol or sedatives such as Halcion or Restoril because increased drowsiness may occur.

Special information if you are pregnant or breastfeeding

The effects of Ditropan during pregnancy have not been adequately studied. If you are pregnant or plan to become pregnant, inform your doctor immediately. Ditropan may appear in breast milk and could affect a nursing infant. If this medication is essential to your health, your doctor may advise you to stop breastfeeding until your treatment is finished.

Recommended dosage

ADULTS

Tablets
The usual dose is one 5 milligram tablet taken 2 to 3 times a day. You should not take more than 4 tablets a day.

Syrup
The usual dose is one teaspoonful 2 to 3 times a day, but not more than 4 times a day.

CHILDREN OVER 5 YEARS OF AGE

Tablets
The usual dose is one 5 milligram tablet taken twice a day. The most a child should take is 3 tablets a day.

Syrup
The usual dose is one teaspoonful 2 times a day, but not more than 3 times a day.

Ditropan is not recommended for children under 5 years of age.

Overdosage

Any medication taken in excess can have serious consequences. If you suspect an overdose, seek medical attention immediately.

■ *Symptoms of Ditropan overdose may include:*
Coma, convulsions, delirium, difficulty breathing, fever, flushing, hallucinations, irritability, low or high blood pressure, nausea, paralysis, rapid heartbeat, restlessness, tremor, vomiting

Brand name:

DIURIL

Pronounced: DYE-your-il
Generic name: Chlorothiazide

Why is this drug prescribed?

Diuril is used in the treatment of high blood pressure and other conditions that require the elimination of excess fluid (water) from the body. These conditions include congestive heart failure, cirrhosis of the liver, corticosteroid and estrogen therapy, and kidney disease. When used for high blood pressure, Diuril can be used alone or with other high blood pressure medications. Diuril contains a form of thiazide, a diuretic that prompts your body to eliminate more fluid, which helps lower blood pressure.

Most important fact about this drug

If you have high blood pressure, you must take Diuril regularly for it to be effective. Since blood pressure declines gradually, it may be several weeks before you get the full benefit of Diuril; and you must continue taking it even if you are feeling well. Diuril does not cure high blood pressure; it merely keeps it under control.

How should you take this medication?

Take Diuril exactly as prescribed. Stopping Diuril suddenly could cause your condition to worsen.

■ *If you miss a dose...*
Take it as soon as you remember. If it is almost time for your next dose, skip the one you missed and go back to your regular schedule. Never take 2 doses at the same time.

■ *Storage instructions...*
Store at room temperature in a tightly closed container. Protect from moisture and freezing.

What side effects may occur?
Side effects cannot be anticipated. If any develop or change in intensity, inform your doctor as soon as possible. Only your doctor can determine if it is safe for you to continue taking Diuril.

■ *Side effects may include:*
Abdominal cramps, anemia, changes in blood sugar, constipation, diarrhea, difficulty breathing, dizziness, dizziness on standing up, fever, fluid in lungs, hair loss, headache, high levels of sugar in urine, hives, hypersensitivity reactions, impotence, inflammation of the pancreas, inflammation of the salivary glands, light-headedness, loss of appetite, low blood pressure, low potassium (leading to symptoms such as dry mouth, excessive thirst, weak or irregular heartbeat, muscle pain or cramps), lung inflammation, muscle spasms, nausea, rash, reddish or purplish spots on skin, restlessness, sensitivity to light, Stevens-Johnson syndrome, stomach irritation, stomach upset, tingling or pins and needles, vertigo, vision changes, vomiting, weakness, yellow eyes and skin

Why should this drug not be prescribed?
If you are unable to urinate, you should not take this medication. If you are sensitive to or have ever had an allergic reaction to Diuril or other thiazide-type diuretics, or if you are sensitive to sulfa drugs, you should not take this medication.

Special warnings about this medication
Diuretics can cause your body to lose too much potassium. Signs of an excessively low potassium level include muscle weakness and rapid or irregular heartbeat. To boost your potassium level, your doctor may recommend eating potassium-rich foods or taking a potassium supplement.

If you are taking Diuril, your doctor will do a complete assessment of your kidney function and continue to monitor it. Use with caution if you have severe kidney disease.

If you have liver disease, diabetes, gout, or the connective tissue disease lupus erythematosus, your doctor will prescribe Diuril cautiously.

If you have bronchial asthma or a history of allergies you may be at greater risk for an allergic reaction to this medication.

Dehydration, excessive sweating, severe diarrhea, or vomiting could deplete your body's fluids and lower your blood pressure too much. Be careful when exercising and in hot weather.

Notify your doctor or dentist that you are taking Diuril if you have a medical emergency, and before you have surgery or dental treatment.

Possible food and drug interactions
when taking this medication

Diuril may increase the effects of alcohol. Do not drink alcohol while taking it.

If Diuril is taken with certain other drugs, the effects of either may be increased, decreased, or altered. It is especially important to check with your doctor before combining Diuril with the following:

Barbiturates such as phenobarbital and Seconal
Cholesterol-lowering drugs such as Questran and Colestid
Drugs to treat diabetes such as insulin and Micronase
Lithium (Lithonate)
Narcotic painkillers such as Percocet
Nonsteroidal anti-inflammatory drugs such as Naprosyn and Motrin
Norepinephrine (Levophed)
Other drugs for high blood pressure such as Capoten and Procardia XL
Steroids such as prednisone

Special information
if you are pregnant or breastfeeding

The effects of Diuril during pregnancy have not been adequately studied. If you are pregnant or plan to become pregnant, inform your doctor immediately. Diuril appears in breast milk and could affect a nursing infant. If this medication is essential to your health, your doctor may advise you to discontinue breastfeeding until your treatment is finished.

Recommended dosage

ADULTS

Diuril comes in tablets, an oral suspension, and an intravenous preparation, reserved for emergencies. Dosages below are for the oral preparations.

Swelling due to excess water

The usual dose is 0.5 to 1 gram 1 or 2 times per day. Your doctor may have you take this medication on alternate days or on some other on-off schedule.

High Blood Pressure

The starting dose is 0.5 gram to 1 gram per day, taken as one dose or two or more smaller doses. Your doctor will adjust the dosage to suit your needs.

CHILDREN

Dosages for children are adjusted according to weight, generally 10 milligrams per pound of body weight daily in 2 doses.

Under 6 months
Dosage may be up to 15 milligrams per pound of body weight per day in 2 doses.

Under 2 years
The usual dosage is 125 milligrams to 375 milligrams per day in 2 doses. The liquid form of this drug may be used in children under 2 years of age at ½ to 1½ teaspoons (2.5 to 7.5 milliliters) per day.

2 to 12 years
The usual dosage is 375 milligrams to 1 gram daily in 2 doses. The liquid form of this medication may be used in children 2 to 12 years at 1½ to 4 teaspoons (7.5 milliliters to 20 milliliters) per day.

Overdosage
Any medication taken in excess can have serious consequences. If you suspect an overdose, seek medical attention immediately.

■ *Signs of Diuril overdose may include:*
  Dehydration and symptoms of low potassium (dry mouth, excessive thirst, weak or irregular heartbeat, muscle pain or cramps)

Generic name:

DIVALPROEX SODIUM

See Depakote, page 370.

Generic name:

DOCUSATE

See Colace, page 277.

Brand name:

DOLOBID

Pronounced: DOLL-oh-bid
Generic name: Diflunisal

Why is this drug prescribed?
Dolobid, a nonsteroidal anti-inflammatory drug, is used to treat mild to moderate pain and relieve the inflammation, swelling, stiffness, and joint

pain associated with rheumatoid arthritis and osteoarthritis (the most common form of arthritis).

Most important fact about this drug

You should have frequent checkups with your doctor if you take Dolobid regularly. Ulcers or internal bleeding can occur without warning.

How should you take this medication?

Dolobid should be taken with food or food together with an antacid, and with a full glass of water or milk. Never take it on an empty stomach.

Tablets should be swallowed whole, not chewed or crushed.

Take this medication exactly as prescribed by your doctor. If you are using Dolobid for arthritis, it should be taken regularly.

- *If you miss a dose...*
  Take it as soon as you remember. If it is almost time for your next dose, skip the one you missed and go back to your regular schedule. Never take 2 doses at the same time.

- *Storage instructions...*
  Do not store in damp places like the bathroom.

What side effects may occur?

Side effects cannot be anticipated. If any develop or change in intensity, inform your doctor as soon as possible. Only your doctor can determine if it is safe for you to continue taking Dolobid.

- *More common side effects may include:*
  Abdominal pain, constipation, diarrhea, dizziness, fatigue, gas, headache, inability to sleep, indigestion, nausea, rash, ringing in ears, sleepiness, vomiting

- *Less common or rare side effects may include:*
  Abdominal bleeding, anemia, blurred vision, confusion, depression, disorientation, dry mouth and nose, fluid retention, flushing, hepatitis, hives, inflammation of lips and tongue, itching, kidney failure, light-headedness, loss of appetite, nervousness, painful urination, peptic ulcer, pins and needles, protein or blood in urine, rash, sensitivity to light, skin eruptions, Stevens-Johnson syndrome, vertigo, weakness, yellow eyes and skin

Why should this drug not be prescribed?
If you are sensitive to or have had an allergic reaction to Dolobid, aspirin, or similar drugs, or if you have had asthma attacks caused by aspirin or other drugs of this type, you should not take this medication. Make sure that your doctor is aware of any drug reactions that you have experienced.

Special warnings about this medication
Peptic ulcers and bleeding can occur without warning.

This drug should be used with caution if you have kidney or liver disease; and it can cause liver inflammation in some people.

Do not take aspirin or any other anti-inflammatory medications while taking Dolobid, unless your doctor tells you to do so.

Nonsteroidal anti-inflammatory drugs such as Dolobid can hide the signs and symptoms of infection. Be sure your doctor knows about any infection you may have.

Dolobid can cause vision problems. If you experience any changes in your vision, inform your doctor.

Dolobid may prolong bleeding time. If you are taking blood-thinning medication, take Dolobid with caution.

If you have heart disease or high blood pressure, use Dolobid with caution. It can increase water retention.

Dolobid may cause you to become drowsy or less alert; therefore, driving or operating dangerous machinery or participating in any hazardous activity that requires full mental alertness is not recommended.

Possible food and drug interactions
when taking this medication
If Dolobid is taken with certain other drugs, the effects of either could be increased, decreased, or altered. It is especially important to check with your doctor before combining Dolobid with the following:

Acetaminophen (Tylenol)
Antacids taken regularly
Aspirin
Cyclosporine (Sandimmune)
Methotrexate (Rheumatrex)
Oral anticoagulants (blood thinners)
Other nonsteroidal anti-inflammatory drugs (Advil, Motrin, Naprosyn, others)

The arthritis medication sulindac (Clinoril)
The diuretic hydrochlorothiazide

Special information
if you are pregnant or breastfeeding

The effects of Dolobid during pregnancy have not been adequately studied. If you are pregnant or plan to become pregnant, inform your doctor immediately. Dolobid appears in breast milk and could affect a nursing infant. If this medication is essential to your health, your doctor may advise you to discontinue breastfeeding until your treatment with Dolobid is finished.

Recommended dosage

ADULTS

Mild to Moderate Pain

Starting dose is 1,000 milligrams, followed by 500 milligrams every 8 to 12 hours, depending on the individual. Your physician may adjust your dosage according to your age and weight, and the severity of your symptoms.

Osteoarthritis and Rheumatoid Arthritis

The usual dose is 500 to 1,000 milligrams per day in 2 doses of 250 milligrams or 500 milligrams. Use no more than necessary to relieve the pain.

The maximum recommended dosage is 1,500 milligrams per day.

CHILDREN

Safety and effectiveness of Dolobid have not been established in children under 12 years of age. The drug is not recommended for this age group.

Overdosage

Any medication taken in excess can cause symptoms of overdose. If you suspect an overdose, seek medical attention immediately.

■ *Symptoms of Dolobid overdose may include:*
Abnormally rapid heartbeat, coma, diarrhea, disorientation, drowsiness, hyperventilation, nausea, ringing in the ears, stupor, sweating, vomiting

Generic name:

DONEPEZIL

See Aricept, page 84.

Brand name:

DONNATAL

Pronounced: DON-nuh-tal
Generic ingredients: Phenobarbital, Hyoscyamine sulfate,
Atropine sulfate, Scopolamine hydrobromide
Other brand name: Bellatal

Why is this drug prescribed?

Donnatal is a mild antispasmodic medication; it has been used with other drugs for relief of cramps and pain associated with various stomach, intestinal, and bowel disorders, including irritable bowel syndrome, acute colitis, and duodenal ulcer.

One of its ingredients, phenobarbital, is a mild sedative.

Most important fact about this drug

Phenobarbital, one of the ingredients of Donnatal, can be habit-forming. If you have ever been dependent on drugs, do not take Donnatal.

How should you take this medication?

Take Donnatal one-half hour to 1 hour before meals. Use it exactly as prescribed.

- *If you miss a dose...*
  Take it as soon as you remember. If it is almost time for your next dose, skip the one you missed and go back to your regular schedule. Never take 2 doses at the same time.

- *Storage instructions...*
  Store at room temperature in a tightly closed container. Protect from light.

What side effects may occur?

Side effects cannot be anticipated. If any develop or change in intensity, inform your doctor as soon as possible. Only your doctor can determine if it is safe for you to continue taking Donnatal.

- *Side effects may include:*
  Agitation, allergic reaction, bloated feeling, blurred vision, constipation, decreased sweating, difficulty sleeping, difficulty urinating, dilation of the pupil of the eye, dizziness, drowsiness, dry mouth, excitement, fast or

fluttery heartbeat, headache, hives, impotence, muscular and bone pain, nausea, nervousness, rash, reduced sense of taste, suppression of lactation, vomiting, weakness

Why should this drug not be prescribed?
Do not take Donnatal if you suffer from the eye condition called glaucoma, diseases that block the urinary or gastrointestinal tracts, or myasthenia gravis, a condition in which the muscles become progressively paralyzed. Also, you should not use Donnatal if you have intestinal atony (loss of strength in the intestinal muscles), unstable cardiovascular status, severe ulcerative colitis (chronic inflammation and ulceration of the bowel), or hiatal hernia (a rupture in the diaphragm above the stomach). You should also avoid Donnatal if you have acute intermittent porphyria—a disorder of the metabolism in which there is severe abdominal pain and sensitivity to light.

If you are sensitive to or have ever had an allergic reaction to Donnatal, its ingredients, or similar drugs, you should not take this medication. Also avoid Donnatal if phenobarbital makes you excited or restless, instead of calming you down. Make sure your doctor is aware of any drug reactions you have experienced.

Special warnings about this medication
Be cautious in using Donnatal if you suffer from high blood pressure, overactive thyroid (hyperthyroidism), irregular or rapid heartbeat, or heart, kidney, or liver disease.

Donnatal can decrease sweating. If you are exercising or are subjected to high temperatures, be alert for heat prostration.

If you develop diarrhea, especially if you have an ileostomy or colostomy (artificial openings to the bowel), check with your doctor.

If you have a gastric ulcer, use this medication with caution.

Donnatal may cause you to become drowsy or less alert. You should not drive or operate dangerous machinery or participate in any hazardous activity that requires full mental alertness until you know how this drug affects you.

Possible food and drug interactions
when taking this medication
Donnatal may intensify the effects of alcohol. Check with your doctor before using alcohol with this medication.

Avoid taking antacids within 1 hour of a dose of Donnatal; they may reduce its effectiveness.

If Donnatal is taken with certain other drugs, the effects of either could be increased, decreased, or altered. It is especially important to check with your doctor before combining Donnatal with the following:

Antidepressants such as Elavil and Tofranil
Antidepressants known as MAO inhibitors, including Nardil and Parnate
Antihistamines such as Benadryl
Antispasmodic drugs such as Bentyl and Cogentin
Barbiturates such as Seconal
Blood-thinning drugs such as Coumadin
Diarrhea medications containing Kaolin or attapulgite
Digitalis (Lanoxin)
Narcotics such as Percocet
Potassium (Slow-K, K-Dur, others)
Steroids such as Medrol and Deltasone
Tranquilizers such as Valium

Special information
if you are pregnant or breastfeeding

The effects of Donnatal during pregnancy have not been adequately studied. If you are pregnant or plan to become pregnant, this drug should be used only when prescribed by your doctor. It is not known whether Donnatal appears in breast milk. If this medication is essential to your health, your doctor may advise you to discontinue breastfeeding until your treatment is finished.

Recommended dosage

ADULTS

Your doctor will adjust the dosage to your needs.

Tablets or Capsules
The usual dosage is 1 or 2 tablets or capsules, 3 or 4 times a day.

Liquid
The usual dosage is 1 or 2 teaspoonfuls, 3 or 4 times a day.

Donnatal Extentabs
The usual dosage is 1 tablet every 12 hours. Your doctor may tell you to take 1 tablet every 8 hours, if necessary.

CHILDREN

Dosage of the elixir is determined by body weight; it can be given every 4 to 6 hours. Follow your doctor's instructions carefully when giving this medication to a child.

Overdosage

Any medication taken in excess can cause symptoms of overdose. If you suspect an overdose, seek medical attention immediately.

■ *The symptoms of Donnatal overdose may include:*
Blurred vision, central nervous system stimulation, difficulty swallowing, dilated pupils, dizziness, dry mouth, headache, hot and dry skin, nausea, vomiting

Brand name:

DORAL

Pronounced: DOHR-al
Generic name: Quazepam

Why is this drug prescribed?

Doral, a sleeping medication available in tablet form, is taken as short-term treatment for insomnia. Symptoms of insomnia may include difficulty falling asleep, frequent awakenings throughout the night, or very early morning awakening.

Most important fact about this drug

Doral is a chemical cousin of Valium and is potentially addictive. Over time, your body will get used to the prescribed dosage of Doral, and you will no longer derive any benefit from it. If you were to increase the dosage against medical advice, the drug would again work as a sleeping pill—but only until your body adjusted to the higher dosage. This is a vicious circle that can lead to addiction. To avoid this danger, use Doral only as prescribed.

How should you take this medication?

Take Doral exactly as prescribed by your doctor—one dose per day, at bedtime. Keep in touch with your doctor; if you respond very well, it may be possible to cut your dosage in half after the first few nights. The older or more run-down you are, the more desirable it is to try for this early dosage reduction.

If you have been taking Doral regularly for 6 weeks or so, you may experience withdrawal symptoms if you stop suddenly, or even if you reduce the dosage without specific instructions on how to do it. Always follow your doctor's advice for tapering off gradually from Doral.

■ *If you miss a dose...*
Take this medication only if needed.

■ *Storage instructions...*
Store at room temperature, away from moisture.

What side effects may occur?
Side effects cannot be anticipated. If any develop or change in intensity, inform your doctor as soon as possible. Only your doctor can determine if it is safe for you to continue taking Doral.

■ *More common side effects may include:*
Drowsiness during the day, headache

■ *Less common side effects may include:*
Changes in sex drive, dizziness, dry mouth, fatigue, inability to urinate, incontinence, indigestion, irregular menstrual periods, irritability, muscle spasms, slurred or otherwise abnormal speech, yellowed eyes and skin

In rare instances, Doral produces agitation, sleep disturbances, hallucinations, or stimulation—exactly the opposite of the desired effect. If this should happen to you, tell your doctor; he or she will take you off the medication.

Why should this drug not be prescribed?
Do not take Doral if you are sensitive to it, or if you have ever had an allergic reaction to it or to another Valium-type medication.

You should not take Doral if you know or suspect that you have sleep apnea (short periods of interrupted breathing that occur during sleep).

You should not take Doral if you are pregnant.

Special warnings about this medication
Because Doral may decrease your daytime alertness, do not drive, climb, or operate dangerous machinery until you find out how the drug affects you. In some cases, Doral's sedative effect may last for several days after the last dose.

If you are suffering from depression, Doral may make your depression worse.

If you have ever abused alcohol or drugs, you are at special risk for addiction to Doral.

Never increase the dosage of Doral on your own. Tell your doctor right away if the medication no longer seems to be working.

Possible food and drug interactions
when taking this medication

If Doral is taken with certain other drugs, the effects of either could be increased, decreased, or altered. It is especially important to check with your doctor before combining Doral with the following:

Antihistamines such as Benadryl
Antiseizure medications such as Dilantin and Tegretol
Mood-altering medications such as Thorazine and Clozaril
Other central nervous system depressants such as Xanax and Valium

Do not drink alcohol while taking Doral; it can increase the drug's effects.

Special information
if you are pregnant or breastfeeding

Because Doral may cause harm to the unborn child, it should not be taken during pregnancy. If you want to have a baby, tell your doctor, and plan to discontinue taking Doral before getting pregnant.

Babies whose mothers are taking Doral at the time of birth may experience withdrawal symptoms from the drug. Such babies may be "floppy" (flaccid) instead of having normal muscle tone.

Since Doral does appear in breast milk, you should not take this medication if you are nursing a baby.

Recommended dosage

ADULTS

The recommended initial dose is 15 milligrams daily. Your doctor may later reduce this dosage to 7.5 milligrams.

CHILDREN

Safety and efficacy of Doral in children under 18 years old have not been established.

OLDER ADULTS

You may be more sensitive to this drug, and the doctor may reduce the dosage after only 1 or 2 nights.

Overdosage

Any medication taken in excess can have serious consequences. If you suspect an overdose of Doral, seek medical attention immediately.

- *Symptoms of an overdose of Doral may include:*
  Coma, confusion, extreme sleepiness

Brand name:

DORYX

Pronounced: DORE-icks
Generic name: Doxycycline hyclate
Other brand names: Vibramycin, Vibra-Tabs

Why is this drug prescribed?

Doxycycline is a broad-spectrum tetracycline antibiotic used against a wide variety of bacterial infections, including Rocky Mountain spotted fever and other fevers caused by ticks, fleas, and lice; urinary tract infections; trachoma (chronic infections of the eye); and some gonococcal infections in adults. It is also used with other medications to treat severe acne and amoebic dysentery (diarrhea caused by severe parasitic infection of the intestines).

Doxycycline may also be taken for the prevention of malaria on foreign trips of less than 4 months' duration.

Occasionally doctors prescribe doxycycline to treat early Lyme disease and to prevent "traveler's diarrhea." These are not yet officially approved uses for this drug.

Most important fact about this drug

Children under 8 years old and women in the last half of pregnancy should not take this medication. It may cause developing teeth to become permanently discolored (yellow-gray-brown).

How should you take this medication?

Take doxycycline with a full glass of water or other liquid to avoid irritating your throat or stomach. Doxycycline can be taken with or without food. However, if the medicine does upset your stomach, you may wish to take it with a glass of milk or after you have eaten. Doxycycline tablets should be swallowed whole.

Take this medication exactly as prescribed by your doctor, even if your symptoms have disappeared.

If you are taking an oral suspension form of doxycycline, shake the bottle well before using. Do not use outdated doxycycline.

■ *If you miss a dose...*
Take the forgotten dose as soon as you remember. If it is almost time for the next dose, put it off for several hours after taking the missed dose. Specifically, if you are taking one dose a day, take the next one 10 to 12 hours after the missed dose. If you are taking two doses a day, take the next one 5 to 6 hours after the missed dose. If you are taking three doses a day, take the next one 2 to 4 hours after the missed dose. Then return to your regular schedule.

■ *Storage instructions...*
Doxycycline can be stored at room temperature. Protect from light and excessive heat.

What side effects may occur?
Side effects cannot be anticipated. If any develop or change in intensity, inform your doctor as soon as possible. Only your doctor can determine if it is safe for you to continue taking doxycycline.

■ *More common side effects may include:*
Angioedema (chest pain; swelling of face, around lips, tongue and throat, arms and legs; difficulty swallowing), bulging foreheads in infants, diarrhea, difficulty swallowing, discolored teeth in infants and children (more common during long-term use of tetracycline), inflammation of the tongue, loss of appetite, nausea, rash, rectal or genital itching, severe allergic reaction (hives, itching, and swelling), skin sensitivity to light, vomiting

■ *Less common or rare side effects may include:*
Aggravation of lupus erythematosus (disease of the connective tissue), skin inflammation and peeling, throat inflammation and ulcerations

Why should this drug not be prescribed?
If you are sensitive to or have ever had an allergic reaction to doxycycline or drugs of this type, you should not take this medication. Make sure your doctor is aware of any drug reactions that you have experienced.

Special warnings about this medication
As with other antibiotics, treatment with doxycycline may result in a growth of bacteria that do not respond to this medication and can cause a secondary infection.

Bulging foreheads in infants and headaches in adults have occurred. These symptoms disappeared when doxycycline was discontinued.

You may become more sensitive to sunlight while taking doxycycline. Be careful if you are going out in the sun or using a sunlamp. If you develop a skin rash, notify your doctor immediately.

Birth control pills that contain estrogen may not be as effective while you are taking tetracycline drugs. Ask your doctor or pharmacist if you should use another form of birth control while taking doxycycline.

Doxycycline syrup (Vibramycin) contains a sulfite that may cause allergic reactions in certain people. This reaction happens more frequently to people with asthma.

**Possible food and drug interactions
when taking this medication**
If doxycycline is taken with certain other drugs, the effects of either could be increased, decreased, or altered. It is especially important to check with your doctor before combining doxycycline with the following:

Antacids containing aluminum, calcium, or magnesium, and iron-
  containing preparations such as Maalox, Mylanta, and others
Barbiturates such as phenobarbital
Bismuth subsalicylate (Pepto-Bismol)
Blood-thinning medications such as Coumadin
Carbamazepine (Tegretol)
Oral contraceptives
Penicillin (V-Cillin K, Pen-Vee K, others)
Phenytoin (Dilantin)
Sodium bicarbonate

**Special information
if you are pregnant or breastfeeding**
Doxycycline should not be used during pregnancy. Tetracycline can damage developing teeth during the last half of pregnancy. If you are pregnant or plan to become pregnant, inform your doctor immediately. Tetracyclines such as doxycycline appear in breast milk and can affect a nursing infant. If this medication is essential to your health, your doctor may advise you to discontinue breastfeeding until your treatment is finished.

Recommended dosage

ADULTS

The usual dose of oral doxycycline is 200 milligrams on the first day of treatment (100 milligrams every 12 hours) followed by a maintenance dose of 100 milligrams per day. The maintenance dose may be taken as a single dose or as 50 milligrams every 12 hours.

Your doctor may prescribe 100 milligrams every 12 hours for severe infections such as chronic urinary tract infection.

For Uncomplicated Gonorrhea (Except Anorectal Infections in Men)
The usual dose is 100 milligrams by mouth, twice a day for 7 days. An alternate, single-day treatment is 300 milligrams, followed in 1 hour by a second 300-milligram dose.

For Primary and Secondary Syphilis
The usual dose is 200 milligrams a day, divided into smaller, equal doses for 14 days.

For Prevention of Malaria
The usual dose is 100 milligrams a day. Treatment should begin 1 to 2 days before travel to the area where malaria is found, then continue daily during travel in the area and 4 weeks after leaving.

CHILDREN

For children above 8 years of age, the recommended dosage schedule for those weighing 100 pounds or less is 2 milligrams per pound of body weight, divided into 2 doses, on the first day of treatment, followed by 1 milligram per pound of body weight given as a single daily dose or divided into 2 doses on subsequent days.

For more severe infections, up to 2 milligrams per pound of body weight may be used.

For prevention of malaria, the recommended dose is 2 milligrams per 2.2 pounds of body weight up to 100 milligrams.

For children over 100 pounds, the usual adult dose should be used.

Overdosage
Any medication taken in excess can have serious consequences. If you suspect an overdose, seek medical treatment immediately.

Generic name:

DOXAZOSIN

See Cardura, page 209.

Generic name:

DOXEPIN

See Sinequan, page 1200.

Generic name:

DOXYCYCLINE

See Doryx, page 437.

Brand name:

DUPHALAC

See Chronulac Syrup, page 244.

Brand name:

DURICEF

Pronounced: DUHR-i-sef
Generic name: Cefadroxil monohydrate

Why is this drug prescribed?
Duricef, a cephalosporin antibiotic, is used in the treatment of nose, throat, urinary tract, and skin infections that are caused by specific bacteria, including staph, strep, and *E. coli.*

Most important fact about this drug
If you are allergic to either penicillin or cephalosporin antibiotics in any form, consult your doctor *before taking* Duricef. An allergy to either type of medication may signal an allergy to Duricef; and if a reaction occurs, it could be extremely severe. If you take the drug and feel signs of a reaction, seek medical attention immediately.

How should you take this medication?
Take this medication exactly as prescribed. It is important that you finish all of it to obtain the maximum benefit.

■ *If you miss a dose...*
Take it as soon as you remember. If it is almost time for the next dose, and you take it once a day, take the one you missed and the next dose 10 to 12 hours later. If you take 2 doses a day, take the one you missed and the

next dose 5 to 6 hours later. If you take it 3 or more times a day, take the one you missed and the next dose 2 to 4 hours later. Then go back to your regular schedule.

■ *Storage information...*
Store at room temperature.

What side effects may occur?
Side effects cannot be anticipated. If any develop or change in intensity, inform your doctor as soon as possible. Only your doctor can determine if it is safe for you to continue taking Duricef.

■ *More common side effects may include:*
Diarrhea

■ *Less common or rare side effects may include:*
Inflammation of the bowel (colitis), nausea, redness and swelling of skin, skin rash and itching, vaginal inflammation, vomiting

Why should this drug not be prescribed?
If you are sensitive to or have ever had an allergic reaction to a cephalosporin antibiotic, you should not take Duricef.

Special warnings about this medication
If you have allergies, particularly to drugs, or often develop diarrhea when taking other antibiotics, you should tell your doctor before taking Duricef.

Use with caution if you have a history of gastrointestinal disease, particularly inflammation of the bowel (colitis).

Continued or prolonged use of Duricef may result in a growth of bacteria that do not respond to this medication and can cause a second infection.

Possible food and drug interactions
when taking this medication
No significant interactions have been reported.

Special information
if you are pregnant or breastfeeding
The effects of Duricef during pregnancy have not been adequately studied. If you are pregnant or plan to become pregnant, inform your doctor immediately. Duricef may appear in breast milk and could affect a nursing infant. If this medication is essential to your health, your doctor may advise you to stop nursing your baby until your treatment time with Duricef is finished.

Recommended dosage

ADULTS

Urinary Tract Infections
The usual dosage for uncomplicated infections is a total of 1 to 2 grams per day in a single dose or 2 smaller doses. For all other urinary tract infections, the usual dosage is a total of 2 grams per day taken in 2 doses.

Skin and Skin Structure Infections
The usual dose is a total of 1 gram per day in a single dose or 2 smaller doses.

Throat Infections—Strep Throat and Tonsillitis:
The usual dosage is a total of 1 gram per day in a single dose or 2 smaller doses for 10 days.

CHILDREN

For urinary tract and skin infections, the usual dose is 30 milligrams per 2.2 pounds of body weight per day, divided into 2 doses and taken every 12 hours. For throat infections, the recommended dose per day is 30 milligrams per 2.2 pounds of body weight in a single dose or 2 smaller doses. In the treatment of strep throat, the dose should be taken for at least 10 days.

OLDER ADULTS

Your dose may be reduced by your doctor.

Overdosage

Duricef is generally safe. However, large amounts may cause seizures or the side effects listed above. If you suspect an overdose of Duricef, seek medical attention immediately.

Brand name:

DYAZIDE

Pronounced: DYE-uh-zide
Generic ingredients: Hydrochlorothiazide, Triamterene
Other brand names: Maxzide, Maxzide-25 MG

Why is this drug prescribed?

Dyazide is a combination of diuretic drugs used in the treatment of high blood pressure and other conditions that require the elimination of excess fluid from the body. When used for high blood pressure, Dyazide can be taken alone or with other high blood pressure medications. Diuretics help your body produce and eliminate more urine, which helps lower blood pressure. Triamterene, one of the ingredients of Dyazide, helps to minimize the potassium loss that can be caused by the other component, hydrochlorothiazide. Maxzide and Maxzide-25 MG contain the same combination of ingredients.

Most important fact about this drug

If you have high blood pressure, you must take Dyazide regularly for it to be effective. Since blood pressure declines gradually, it may be several weeks before you get the full benefit of Dyazide; and you must continue taking it even if you are feeling well. Dyazide does not cure high blood pressure; it merely keeps it under control.

How should you take this medication?

Dyazide should be taken early in the day. To avoid stomach upset, take it with food.

- *If you miss a dose...*
  Take it as soon as you remember. If it is almost time for the next dose, skip the one you missed and go back to your regular schedule. Do not take 2 doses at the same time.

- *Storage instructions...*
  Store at room temperature, away from light.

What side effects may occur?

Side effects cannot be anticipated. If any occur or change in intensity, inform your doctor as soon as possible. Only your doctor can determine if it is safe for you to continue taking Dyazide.

- *Side effects may include:*
  Abdominal pain, anemia, breathing difficulty, change in potassium level (causing symptoms such as numbness, tingling, muscle weakness, slow heart rate, shock), constipation, diabetes, diarrhea, dizziness, dizziness when standing up, dry mouth, fatigue, headache, hives, impotence, irregular heartbeat, kidney stones, muscle cramps, nausea, rash, sensitivity to light, strong allergic reaction (localized hives, itching, and swelling or, in severe cases, shock), vomiting, weakness, yellow eyes and skin

Why should this drug not be prescribed?
If you are unable to urinate or have any serious kidney disease, if you have high potassium levels in your blood, or if you are taking other drugs that prevent loss of potassium, you should not take Dyazide.

If you are sensitive to or have ever had an allergic reaction to triamterene (Dyrenium), hydrochlorothiazide (Oretic), or sulfa drugs such as Gantrisin you should not take this medication.

Special warnings about this medication
When taking Dyazide, do not use potassium-containing salt substitutes. Take potassium supplements only if specifically directed to by your doctor. Your potassium level should be checked frequently.

If you are taking Dyazide and have kidney disease, your doctor should monitor your kidney function closely.

If you have liver disease, diabetes, cirrhosis of the liver, heart failure, or kidney stones, this medication should be used with care.

Possible food and drug interactions
when taking this medication
Dyazide should be used with caution if you are taking a type of blood pressure medication called an ACE inhibitor, such as Vasotec or Capoten.

If Dyazide is taken with certain other drugs, the effects of either could be increased, decreased, or altered. It is especially important to check with your doctor before combining Dyazide with the following:

Blood-thinning medications such as Coumadin
Corticosteroids such as Deltasone
Drugs for diabetes such as Micronase
Gout medications such as Zyloprim
Laxatives
Lithium (Lithonate)
Methenamine (Urised)
Nonsteroidal anti-inflammatory drugs such as Indocin and Dolobid
Other drugs that minimize potassium loss or contain potassium
Other high blood pressure medications such as Minipress
Salt substitutes containing potassium
Sodium polystyrene sulfonate (Kayexalate)

Special information
if you are pregnant or breastfeeding
The effects of Dyazide during pregnancy have not been adequately studied. If you are pregnant or plan to become pregnant, inform your doctor immediate-

ly. Dyazide appears in breast milk and could affect a nursing infant. If this medication is essential to your health, your doctor may advise you to discontinue breastfeeding until your treatment is finished.

Recommended dosage

ADULTS

The usual dose of Dyazide is 1 or 2 capsules once daily, with appropriate monitoring of blood potassium levels by your doctor. The usual dose of Maxizide is 1 tablet daily. The recommendation for Maxizde-25 MG is 1 or 2 tablets daily taken in a single dose.

CHILDREN

Safety and effectiveness in children have not been established.

Overdosage

Any medication taken in excess can have serious consequences. If you suspect an overdose, seek medical treatment immediately.

■ *Symptoms of Dyazide overdose may include:*
Fever, flushed face, nausea, production of large amounts of pale urine, vomiting, weakness, weariness

Brand name:

DYNABAC

Pronounced: DYE-na-bak
Generic name: Dirithromycin

Why is this drug prescribed?
Dynabac cures certain mild-to-moderate skin infections and respiratory infections such as strep throat, tonsillitis, pneumonia, and flare-ups of chronic bronchitis. Dynabac is part of the same family of drugs as the commonly prescribed antibiotic erythromycin.

Most important fact about this drug
Serious and sometimes fatal reactions have occurred in people who combined other erythromycin-type antibiotics with Seldane or Hismanal. If you are taking either of these drugs and have a heart condition, particularly irregular heart rhythms, do not take Dynabac.

How should you take this medication?

Take Dynabac with food or within 1 hour after a meal. Swallow the tablet whole; do not crush, chew, or break it.

To make sure your infection is completely cured, it's important to finish your entire prescription, even if you begin to feel better after the first few days. If you stop taking this medicine too soon, your symptoms may return.

■ *If you miss a dose...*
Take it as soon as you remember. If you don't remember until the next day, skip the forgotten dose and go back to your regular schedule. Never try to "catch up" by doubling the dose.

■ *Storage instructions...*
Store Dynabac at room temperature.

What side effects may occur?

Side effects cannot be anticipated. If any develop or change in intensity, tell your doctor as soon as possible. Only your doctor can determine if it is safe for you to continue taking Dynabac.

■ *More common side effects may include:*
Abdominal pain, diarrhea, headache, nausea, vomiting

■ *Less common side effects may include:*
Dizziness/vertigo, gas, hives, increased cough, insomnia, itching, pain, rash, shortness of breath, stomach and intestinal disturbances, weakness

■ *Rare side effects may include:*
Abnormal stools, allergic reaction, anxiety, constipation, coughing up blood, dehydration, depression, dry mouth, fainting, fever, fluid retention, flu-like symptoms, frequent urination, inflammation of the stomach and intestines, loss of appetite, mouth sores, muscle pain, neck pain, nervousness, nosebleeds, painful menstruation, "pins and needles," pounding heartbeat, rapid breathing, reduced vision or other eye problems, ringing in ears, sleepiness, sweating, swelling of hands and feet, taste alteration, thirst, tremor, vaginal fungus, vaginal inflammation

Why should this drug not be prescribed?

If you have ever had an allergic reaction to Dynabac or to similar antibiotics such as erythromycin (E.E.S., PCE, and others), do not take this medication.

Special warnings about this medication

Dynabac, like certain other antibiotics, may cause a potentially life-threatening form of diarrhea called pseudomembranous colitis. A mild case may clear up on its own when the drug is stopped. For a more severe case, your doctor may need to prescribe fluids, electrolytes, and another antibiotic.

Possible food and drug interactions
when taking this medication

If Dynabac is taken with certain other drugs, the effects of either could be increased, decreased, or altered. It is especially important to check with your doctor before combining Dynabac with the following:

Antacids (Maalox, Mylanta)
Cimetidine (Tagamet)
Ranitidine (Zantac)
Terfenadine (Seldane)
Theophylline drugs such as Bronkodyl, Slo-Phyllin, Theo-Dur, and others

The following medications can interact with the related drug erythromycin:

Astemizole (Hismanal)
Blood-thinning drugs such as Coumadin
Bromocriptine (Parlodel)
Carbamazepine (Tegretol)
Cyclosporine (Sandimmune)
Digoxin (Lanoxin)
Disopyramide (Norpace)
Ergot-containing drugs such as Cafergot and D.H.E.
Lovastatin (Mevacor)
Phenytoin (Dilantin)
Triazolam (Halcion)
Valproate (Depakene, Depakote)

Special information
if you are pregnant or breastfeeding

If you are pregnant or plan to become pregnant, tell your doctor immediately. You should take Dynabac during pregnancy only if it is clearly needed. It is not known whether Dynabac appears in breast milk. If this medication is essential to your health, your doctor may advise you to stop breastfeeding until your treatment is finished.

Recommended dosage

ADULTS AND CHILDREN 12 AND OVER

Bronchitis and Skin Infections
The usual dose is 500 milligrams (2 tablets) once a day for 7 days.

Pneumonia
The usual dose is 500 milligrams (2 tablets) once a day for 14 days.

Strep Throat and Tonsillitis
The usual dose is 500 milligrams (2 tablets) once a day for 10 days.

CHILDREN UNDER 12 YEARS OF AGE

The safety and effectiveness of Dynabac in children under the age of 12 have not been established.

Overdosage

Any medication taken in excess can have serious consequences. If you suspect an overdose, seek medical attention immediately.

- *Symptoms of Dynabac overdose may include...*
  Diarrhea, nausea, stomach problems, vomiting

Brand name:

DYNACIN

See Minocin, page 810.

Brand name:

DYNACIRC

Pronounced: DYE-na-serk
Generic name: Isradipine
Other brand name: DynaCirc CR

Why is this drug prescribed?

DynaCirc, a type of medication called a calcium channel blocker, is prescribed for the treatment of high blood pressure. It is effective when used alone or with a thiazide-type diuretic to flush excess water from the body. Calcium channel blockers ease the workload of the heart by slowing down the passage of nerve impulses through the heart muscle, thereby slowing the beat. This improves blood flow through the heart and throughout the body and reduces blood pressure. A controlled-release version of this drug (DynaCirc CR) maintains lower blood pressure for 24 hours.

Most important fact about this drug

You must take DynaCirc regularly for it to be effective. Since blood pressure declines gradually, it may be several weeks before you get the full benefit of DynaCirc; and you must continue taking it even if you are feeling well. DynaCirc does not cure high blood pressure; it merely keeps it under control.

How should you take this medication?

Take this medication exactly as prescribed, even if your symptoms have disappeared. Try not to miss any doses. If DynaCirc is not taken regularly, your condition may worsen.

Swallow the capsule or tablet whole, without crushing or chewing it.

■ *If you miss a dose...*
  Take it as soon as you remember. If it is almost time for your next dose, skip the one you missed and go back to your regular schedule. Never take 2 doses at the same time.

■ *Storage instructions...*
  Store at room temperature, away from light, in a tightly closed container.

What side effects may occur?

Side effects cannot be anticipated. If any develop or change in intensity, inform your doctor as soon as possible. Only your doctor can determine if it is safe for you to continue taking DynaCirc.

■ *More common side effects may include:*
  Dizziness, fluid retention, flushing, headache, pounding heartbeat

■ *Less common side effects may include:*
  Chest pain, diarrhea, fatigue, nausea, rapid heartbeat, rash, shortness of breath, stomach upset, unusually frequent urination, vomiting, weakness

■ *Rare side effects may include:*
  Constipation, cough, decreased sex drive, depression, difficulty sleeping, drowsiness, dry mouth, excessive sweating, fainting, changes in heartbeat, heart attack, heart failure, hives, impotence, itching, leg and foot cramps, low blood pressure, nervousness, numbness, severe dizziness, sluggishness, stroke, throat discomfort, tingling or pins and needles, vision changes

Why should this drug not be prescribed?
If you are sensitive to or have ever had an allergic reaction to DynaCirc or other calcium channel blockers such as Vascor and Procardia, you should not take this medication. Tell your doctor about any drug reactions you have experienced.

Special warnings about this medication
DynaCirc can cause your blood pressure to become too low. If you feel light-headed or faint, contact your doctor.

This medication should be carefully monitored if you have congestive heart failure, especially if you are also taking a beta-blocking medication such as Tenormin or Inderal.

Before having surgery, including dental surgery, tell the doctor that you are taking DynaCirc.

**Possible food and drug interactions
when taking this medication**
If DynaCirc is taken with certain other drugs, the effects of either could be increased, decreased, or altered. It is especially important to check with your doctor before combining DynaCirc with the following:

Beta-blocking blood pressure drugs such as Tenormin, Inderal, and
    Lopressor
Cimetidine (Tagamet)
Rifampin (Rifadin)

**Special information
if you are pregnant or breastfeeding**
The effects of DynaCirc during pregnancy have not been adequately studied. If you are pregnant or plan to become pregnant, consult your doctor immediately. DynaCirc may appear in breast milk and could affect a nursing infant. If this medication is essential to your health, your doctor may advise you to discontinue breastfeeding until your treatment with DynaCirc is finished.

Recommended dosage

DYNACIRC

Your dosage will be adjusted to meet your individual needs.

The usual starting dose is 2.5 milligrams, 2 times a day, either alone or in combination with a thiazide diuretic drug. DynaCirc may lower blood pressure 2 to 3 hours after taking the first dose, but the full effect of the drug may not take place for 2 to 4 weeks.

After a 2- to 4-week trial, your doctor may increase the dosage by 5 milligrams per day every 2 to 4 weeks until a maximum dose of 20 milligrams per day is reached. Side effects may increase or become more common after a 10-milligram dose.

If you are an older adult or have kidney or liver disease, you should still begin treatment with a 2.5-milligram dose 2 times per day; however, your doctor will monitor you closely, since your condition may alter the effects of this drug.

DYNACIRC CR

The usual starting dose is 5 milligrams once a day, either alone or in combination with a thiazide diuretic. A starting dose of 5 milligrams once a day is also recommended for older adults and those with mild liver and kidney problems.

As with regular DynaCirc, the dosage may be increased to a maximum of 20 milligrams per day.

Overdosage
Although there is little information on DynaCirc, overdose has resulted in sluggishness, low blood pressure, and rapid heartbeat. The symptoms of overdose with other calcium channel blockers include drowsiness, severe low blood pressure, and rapid heartbeat.

If you suspect a DynaCirc overdose, seek medical attention immediately.

Generic name:

ECHOTHIOPHATE

See Phospholine Iodide, page 1001.

Brand name:

EC-NAPROSYN

See Naprosyn, page 849.

Generic name:

ECONAZOLE

See Spectazole Cream, page 1212.

Brand name:

ECOTRIN

See Aspirin, page 98.

Brand name:

EDEX

See Caverject, page 217.

Brand name:

E.E.S.

See Erythromycin, Oral, page 482.

Brand name:

EFFEXOR

Pronounced: ef-ECKS-or
Generic name: Venlafaxine hydrochloride
Other brand name: Effexor XR

Why is this drug prescribed?

Effexor is prescribed for the treatment of depression—that is, a continuing depression that interferes with daily functioning. The symptoms usually include changes in appetite, sleep habits, and mind/body coordination, decreased sex drive, increased fatigue, feelings of guilt or worthlessness, difficulty concentrating, slowed thinking, and suicidal thoughts.

Effexor must be taken 2 or 3 times daily. An extended-release form, Effexor XR, permits once-a-day dosing.

Most important fact about this drug

Serious, sometimes fatal reactions have occurred when Effexor is used in combination with other drugs known as MAO inhibitors, including the antidepressants Nardil and Parnate. Never take Effexor with one of these drugs; and do not begin therapy with Effexor within 14 days of discontinuing treatment with one of them. Also, allow at least 7 days between the last dose of Effexor and the first dose of an MAO inhibitor.

How should you take this medication?

Take Effexor with food, exactly as prescribed. It may take several weeks before you begin to feel better. Your doctor should check your progress periodically.

Take Effexor XR once at the same time each day. Swallow the capsule whole with water. Do not divide, crush, or chew it.

■ *If you miss a dose...*
It is not necessary to make it up. Skip the missed dose and continue with your next scheduled dose. Do not take 2 doses at once.

■ *Storage instructions...*
Store in a tightly closed container at room temperature. Protect from excessive heat and moisture.

What side effects may occur?

Side effects cannot be anticipated. If any develop or change in intensity, tell your doctor as soon as possible. Only your doctor can determine if it is safe for you to continue taking Effexor.

■ *More common side effects may include:*
Abnormal dreams, abnormal ejaculation/orgasm, anxiety, blurred vision, chills, constipation, diarrhea, dizziness, dry mouth, extreme muscle tension, flushing, frequent urination, gas, headache, impotence, inability to sleep, indigestion, loss of appetite, nausea, nervousness, prickling or burning sensation, rash, sleepiness, sweating, tremor, vomiting, weakness, yawning

■ *Less common side effects may include:*
Abnormal thinking, abnormal vision, accidental injury, agitation, belching, blood in the urine, bronchitis, bruising, changeable emotions, chest pain, confusion, decreased sex drive, depression, difficult or painful urination, difficulty in breathing, difficulty swallowing, dilated pupils, ear pain, high or low blood pressure, inflammation of the vagina, injury, itching, lack of orgasm, light-headedness on standing up, lockjaw, loss of touch with reality, menstrual problems, migraine headache, neck pain, orgasm disturbance, rapid heartbeat, ringing in the ears, taste changes, twitching, vague feeling of illness, vertigo, weight loss or gain

■ *Rare side effects may include:*
Abnormally slow movements, abnormal movements, abnormal sensitivity to sound, abnormal speech, abortion, abuse of alcohol, acne, alcohol

intolerance, allergic reaction, anemia, angina pectoris (crushing chest pain), apathy, appendicitis, arthritis, asthma, bad breath, black stools, bleeding gums, blocked intestine, blood clots, blood clots in the lungs, blood disorders, bluish color to the skin, body odor, bone disease and/or pain (including osteoporosis), breast enlargement or swelling, breast pain, brittle nails, bulging eyes, cancerous growth, cataracts, changed sense of smell, chest congestion, cold hands and feet, colitis (inflamed bowel), confusion, conjunctivitis ("pinkeye"), coughing up blood, deafness, delusions, depression, diabetes, double vision, drug withdrawal symptoms, dry eyes, dry skin, ear infection, eczema, enlarged abdomen, enlarged thyroid gland, exaggerated feeling of well-being, excessive hair growth, excessive menstrual flow, eye disorders, eye pain, fainting, fungus infection, gallstones, glaucoma, gout, hair discoloration, hair loss, hallucinations, hangover effect, heart disorders, hemorrhoids, hepatitis, herpes infections, high cholesterol, hives, hostility, hyperventilation (fast, deep breathing), inability to communicate, increased mucus, increased physical activity, increased salivation, increased sensitivity to touch, increased sex drive, inflammation of the stomach, intestines, anus and rectum, gums, tongue, eyelid, or inner ear, intolerance to light, involuntary eye movements, irregular or slow heartbeat, kidney disorders, lack of menstruation, large amounts of urine, laryngitis, loss of consciousness, loss of muscle movement, low or high blood sugar, menstrual problems, middle ear infection, mouth fungus, mouth sores, muscle spasms, muscle weakness, nosebleeds, over- and underactive thyroid gland, overdose, paranoia, pelvic pain, pinpoint pupils, "pins and needles" around the mouth, pneumonia, prolonged erection, psoriasis, rectal hemorrhage, reduced menstrual flow, restlessness, secretion of milk, seizures, sensitivity to light, skin disorders, skin eruptions or hemorrhage, skin inflammation, sleep disturbance, soft stools, stiff neck, stomach or peptic ulcer, stroke, stupor, sugar in the urine, swelling due to fluid retention, swollen or discolored tongue, taste loss, temporary failure to breathe, thirst, twisted neck, ulcer, unconsciousness, uncoordinated movements, urgent need to urinate, urination at night, uterine and vaginal hemorrhage, varicose veins, voice changes, vomiting blood, yellowed eyes and skin

Why should this drug not be prescribed?
Never take Effexor while taking other drugs known as MAO inhibitors. (See "Most important fact about this drug.") Also avoid this drug if it has ever given you an allergic reaction.

Special warnings about this medication
Your doctor will prescribe Effexor with caution if you have high blood pressure, heart, liver, or kidney disease or a history of seizures or mania

(extreme agitation or excitability). You should discuss all of your medical problems with your doctor before taking Effexor.

Effexor may cause you to feel drowsy or less alert and may affect your judgment. Therefore, avoid driving or operating dangerous machinery or participating in any hazardous activity that requires full mental alertness until you know how this drug affects you.

If you have ever been addicted to drugs, tell your doctor before you start taking Effexor.

If you develop a skin rash or hives while taking Effexor, notify your doctor.

Do not stop taking the drug without consulting your doctor. If you stop suddenly, you may have withdrawal symptoms, even though this drug does not seem to be habit-forming. Your doctor will have you taper off gradually.

The safety and effectiveness of Effexor have not been established in children under 18 years of age.

Possible food and drug interactions
when taking this medication
Combining Effexor with MAO inhibitors could cause a fatal reaction. (See "Most important fact about this drug.")

Although Effexor does not interact with alcohol, the manufacturer recommends avoiding alcohol while taking this medication.

If you have high blood pressure or liver disease, or are elderly, check with your doctor before combining Effexor with cimetidine (Tagamet).

Effexor does not interact with Lithium or Valium. However, you should consult your doctor before combining Effexor with other drugs that affect the central nervous system, including narcotic painkillers, sleep aids, tranquilizers, antipsychotic medicines such as Haldol, and other antidepressants such as Tofranil.

Special information
if you are pregnant or breastfeeding
The effects of Effexor during pregnancy have not been adequately studied. If you are pregnant or are planning to become pregnant, tell your doctor immediately. Effexor should be used during pregnancy only if clearly needed. Effexor may appear in breast milk. If this medication is essential to your health, your doctor may tell you to discontinue breastfeeding your baby until your treatment with Effexor is finished.

Recommended dosage

EFFEXOR

The usual starting dose is 75 milligrams a day, divided into 2 or 3 smaller doses, and taken with food. If needed, your doctor may gradually increase your daily dose in steps of no more than 75 milligrams at a time up to a maximum of 375 milligrams per day.

If you have kidney or liver disease or are taking other medications, your doctor will adjust your dosage accordingly.

EFFEXOR XR

The usual starting dose is 75 milligrams once daily, although some people begin with a dose of 37.5 milligrams for the first 4 to 7 days. Your doctor may gradually increase the dose, in steps of no more than 75 milligrams, up to a maximum of 225 milligrams daily. As with regular Effexor, the doctor will make adjustments in your dosage if you have kidney or liver disease.

Overdosage

An overdose of Effexor, combined with other drugs or alcohol, can be fatal. If you suspect an overdose, seek medical attention immediately.

- *Symptoms of Effexor overdose include:*
  Convulsions, rapid heartbeat, sleepiness

Brand name:

EFUDEX

Pronounced: EFF-you-decks
Generic name: Fluorouracil

Why is this drug prescribed?

Efudex is prescribed for the treatment of actinic or solar keratoses (small red horny growths or flesh-colored wartlike growths caused by overexposure to ultraviolet radiation or the sun). Such growths may develop into skin cancer. When conventional methods are impractical—as when the affected sites are hard to get at—Efudex is useful in the treatment of superficial basal cell carcinomas, or slow-growing malignant tumors of the face usually found at the edge of the nostrils, eyelids, or lips. Efudex is available in cream and solution forms.

Most important fact about this drug

If you use an airtight dressing to cover the skin being treated, there may be inflammatory reactions in the normal skin around the treated area. If it is necessary to cover the treated area, use a porous gauze dressing to avoid skin reactions.

How should you take this medication?

Use care when applying Efudex around the eyes, nose, and mouth. Wash your hands immediately after applying this medication.

- *If you miss a dose...*

  Apply it as soon as you remember. If more than a few hours have passed, skip the dose you missed and go back to your regular schedule. If you miss more than 1 dose, contact your doctor.

- *Storage instructions...*

  Store away from heat, light, and moisture.

What side effects may occur?

Side effects cannot be anticipated. If any develop or change in intensity, inform your doctor as soon as possible. Only your doctor can determine if it is safe for you to continue using Efudex.

- *More common side effects may include:*

  Burning, discoloration of the skin, itching, pain

- *Less common side effects may include:*

  Allergic skin inflammation, pus, scaling, scarring, soreness, swelling, tenderness

Why should this drug not be prescribed?

If you are sensitive to or have ever had an allergic reaction to Efudex or similar drugs, you should not take this medication. Make sure your doctor is aware of any drug reactions you have experienced.

Special warnings about this medication

Avoid prolonged exposure to ultraviolet rays while you are under treatment with Efudex.

Skin may be unsightly during treatment with this drug and, in some cases, for several weeks after treatment has ended.

If your solar keratoses do not clear up with use of this drug, your doctor will probably order a biopsy (removal of a small amount of tissue to be examined under a microscope) to confirm the skin disease.

Your doctor will perform follow-up biopsies if you are being treated for superficial basal cell carcinoma.

Possible food and drug interactions
when taking this medication
There are no reported food or drug interactions.

Special information
if you are pregnant or breastfeeding
The effects of Efudex during pregnancy have not been adequately studied. If you are pregnant, plan to become pregnant, or are breastfeeding your baby, consult your doctor immediately.

Recommended dosage
When Efudex is applied to affected skin, the skin becomes abnormally red, blisters form, and the surface skin wears away. A lesion or sore forms at the affected site, and the diseased or cancerous skin cells die before a new layer of skin forms.

ADULTS

Actinic or Solar Keratosis
Apply cream or solution 2 times a day in an amount sufficient to cover the affected area. Continue using the medication until the inflammatory response reaches the stage where the skin wears away, a sore or lesion forms, and the skin cells die; your doctor will then have you stop using the medication. The usual length of treatment is from 2 to 4 weeks. You may not see complete healing of the affected area for 1 to 2 months after ending the treatment.

Superficial Basal Cell Carcinomas
You should use only the 5% strength of this medication. Twice a day, apply enough cream or solution to cover the affected area. Continue the treatment for at least 3 to 6 weeks; it may take 10 to 12 weeks of application before the lesions are gone.

Your doctor will want to monitor your condition to make sure it has been cured.

Overdosage
Although no specific information is available on Efudex overdosage, any medication used in excess can have serious consequences. If you suspect an overdosage, seek medical attention immediately.

Brand name:

ELAVIL

Pronounced: ELL-uh-vil
Generic name: Amitriptyline hydrochloride

Why is this drug prescribed?
Elavil is prescribed for the relief of symptoms of mental depression. It is a member of the group of drugs called tricyclic antidepressants. Some doctors also prescribe Elavil to treat bulimia (an eating disorder), to control chronic pain, to prevent migraine headaches, and to treat a pathological weeping and laughing syndrome associated with multiple sclerosis.

Most important fact about this drug
You may need to take Elavil regularly for several weeks before it becomes fully effective. Do not skip doses, even if they seem to make no difference or you feel you don't need them.

How should you take this medication?
Take Elavil exactly as prescribed. You may experience side effects, such as mild drowsiness, early in therapy. However, they usually disappear after a few days. Beneficial effects may take as long as 30 days to appear.

Elavil may cause dry mouth. Sucking a hard candy, chewing gum, or melting bits of ice in your mouth can provide relief.

■ *If you miss a dose...*
Take it as soon as you remember. If it is almost time for your next dose, skip the one you missed and go back to your regular schedule. Never take 2 doses at the same time.

If you take a single daily dose at bedtime, do not make up for it in the morning. It may cause side effects during the day.

■ *Storage instructions...*
Keep Elavil in a tightly closed container. Store at room temperature. Protect from light and excessive heat.

What side effects may occur?
Side effects cannot be anticipated. If any develop or change in intensity, inform your doctor as soon as possible. Only your doctor can determine if it is safe for you to continue taking Elavil.

■ *Side effects may include:*
Abnormal movements, anxiety, black tongue, blurred vision, breast development in males, breast enlargement, coma, confusion, constipation, delusions, diarrhea, difficult or frequent urination, difficulty in speech, dilation of pupils, disorientation, disturbed concentration, dizziness on getting up, dizziness or light-headedness, drowsiness, dry mouth, excessive or spontaneous flow of milk, excitement, fatigue, fluid retention, hair loss, hallucinations, headache, heart attack, hepatitis, high blood pressure, high fever, high or low blood sugar, hives, impotence, inability to sleep, increased or decreased sex drive, increased perspiration, increased pressure within the eye, inflammation of the mouth, intestinal obstruction, irregular heartbeat, lack or loss of coordination, loss of appetite, low blood pressure, nausea, nightmares, numbness, rapid and/or fast, fluttery heartbeat, rash, red or purple spots on skin, restlessness, ringing in the ears, seizures, sensitivity to light, stomach upset, strange taste, stroke, swelling due to fluid retention in the face and tongue, swelling of testicles, swollen glands, tingling and pins and needles in the arms and legs, tremors, vomiting, weakness, weight gain or loss, yellowed eyes and skin

■ *Side effects due to rapid decrease or abrupt withdrawal from Elavil include:*
Headache, nausea, vague feeling of bodily discomfort

■ *Side effects due to gradual dosage reduction may include:*
Dream and sleep disturbances, irritability, restlessness

These side effects do not signify an addiction to the drug.

Why should this drug not be prescribed?
If you are sensitive to or have ever had an allergic reaction to Elavil or similar drugs such as Norpramin and Tofranil, you should not take this medication. Make sure your doctor is aware of any drug reactions you have experienced.

Do not take Elavil while taking other drugs known as MAO inhibitors. Drugs in this category include the antidepressants Nardil and Parnate.

Unless you are directed to do so by your doctor, do not take this medication if you are recovering from a heart attack.

Special warnings about this medication

Do not stop taking Elavil abruptly, especially if you have been taking large doses for a long time. Your doctor probably will want to decrease your dosage gradually. This will help prevent a possible relapse and will reduce the possibility of withdrawal symptoms.

Elavil may make your skin more sensitive to sunlight. Try to stay out of the sun, wear protective clothing, and apply a sun block.

Elavil may cause you to become drowsy or less alert; therefore, you should not drive or operate dangerous machinery or participate in any hazardous activity that requires full mental alertness until you know how this drug affects you.

While taking this medication, you may feel dizzy or light-headed or actually faint when getting up from a lying or sitting position. If getting up slowly doesn't help or if this problem continues, notify your doctor.

Use Elavil with caution if you have ever had seizures, urinary retention, glaucoma or other chronic eye conditions, a heart or circulatory system disorder, or liver problems. Be cautious, too, if you are receiving thyroid medication. You should discuss all of your medical problems with your doctor before starting Elavil therapy.

Before having surgery, dental treatment, or any diagnostic procedure, tell the doctor that you are taking Elavil. Certain drugs used during surgery, such as anesthetics and muscle relaxants, and drugs used in certain diagnostic procedures may react badly with Elavil.

Possible food and drug interactions
when taking this medication

Elavil may intensify the effects of alcohol. Do not drink alcohol while taking this medication.

If Elavil is taken with certain other drugs, the effects of either could be increased, decreased, or altered. It is especially important that you consult with your doctor before taking Elavil in combination with the following:

Airway-opening drugs such as Sudafed and Proventil
Antidepressants that raise serotonin levels, such as Paxil, Prozac, and Zoloft
Other antidepressants, such as Asendin
Antihistamines such as Benadryl and Tavist
Barbiturates such as phenobarbital
Certain blood pressure medicines such as Catapres and Ismelin
Cimetidine (Tagamet)

Disulfiram (Antabuse)
Drugs that control spasms, such as Bentyl and Donnatal
Estrogen drugs such as Premarin and oral contraceptives
Ethchlorvynol (Placidyl)
Major tranquilizers such as Mellaril and Thorazine
MAO inhibitors, such as Nardil and Parnate
Medications for irregular heartbeat, such as Tambocor and Rythmol
Painkillers such as Demerol and Percocet
Parkinsonism drugs such as Cogentin and Larodopa
Quinidine (Quinidex)
Seizure medications such as Tegretol and Dilantin
Sleep medicines such as Halcion and Dalmane
Thyroid hormones (Synthroid)
Tranquilizers such as Librium and Xanax
Warfarin (Coumadin)

Special information
if you are pregnant or breastfeeding

The effects of Elavil during pregnancy have not been adequately studied. If you are pregnant or planning to become pregnant, inform your doctor immediately. This medication appears in breast milk. If Elavil is essential to your health, your doctor may advise you to discontinue breastfeeding until your treatment is finished.

Recommended dosage

ADULTS

The usual starting dosage is 75 milligrams per day divided into 2 or more smaller doses. Your doctor may gradually increase this dose to 150 milligrams per day. The total daily dose is generally never higher than 200 milligrams.

Alternatively, your doctor may want you to start with 50 milligrams to 100 milligrams at bedtime. He or she may increase this bedtime dose by 25 or 50 milligrams up to a total of 150 milligrams a day.

For long-term use, the usual dose ranges from 40 to 100 milligrams taken once daily, usually at bedtime.

CHILDREN

Use of Elavil is not recommended for children under 12 years of age.

The usual dose for adolescents 12 years of age and over is 10 milligrams, 3 times a day, with 20 milligrams taken at bedtime.

OLDER ADULTS

The usual dose is 10 milligrams taken 3 times a day, with 20 milligrams taken at bedtime.

Overdosage
An overdose of Elavil can prove fatal.

- *Symptoms of Elavil overdose may include:*
  Abnormally low blood pressure, confusion, convulsions, dilated pupils and other eye problems, disturbed concentration, drowsiness, hallucinations, impaired heart function, rapid or irregular heartbeat, reduced body temperature, stupor, unresponsiveness or coma

- *Symptoms contrary to the effect of this medication are:*
  Agitation, extremely high body temperature, overactive reflexes, rigid muscles, vomiting

If you suspect an overdose, seek medical attention immediately.

Brand name:

ELDEPRYL

Pronounced: ELL-dep-rill
Generic name: Selegiline hydrochloride

Why is this drug prescribed?
Eldepryl is prescribed along with Sinemet (levodopa/carbidopa) for people with Parkinson's disease. It is used when Sinemet no longer seems to be working well. Eldepryl has no effect when taken by itself; it works only in combination with Larodopa (levodopa) or Sinemet.

Parkinson's disease, which causes muscle rigidity and difficulty with walking and talking, involves the progressive degeneration of a particular type of nerve cell. Early on, Larodopa or Sinemet alone may alleviate the symptoms of the disease. In time, however, these medications work less well; their effectiveness seems to switch on and off at random, and the individual may begin to experience side effects such as involuntary movements and "freezing" in mid-motion.

Eldepryl may be prescribed at this stage of the disease to help restore the effectiveness of Larodopa or Sinemet. When you begin to take Eldepryl, you may need a reduced dosage of the other medication.

Most important fact about this drug
Eldepryl belongs to a class of drugs known as MAO inhibitors. These drugs can interact with certain foods—including aged cheeses and meats, pickled herring, beer, and wine—to cause a life-threatening surge in blood pressure. At the dose recommended for Eldepryl, this interaction is not a problem. But for safety's sake, you may want to watch your diet; and you should never take more Eldepryl than the doctor prescribed.

How should you take this medication?
Take Eldepryl and your other Parkinson's medication exactly as prescribed.

■ *If you miss a dose...*
Take it as soon as you remember. If you do not remember until late afternoon or evening, skip the dose you missed and go back to your regular schedule. Never take 2 doses at once.

■ *Storage instructions...*
Store at room temperature.

What side effects may occur?
Side effects cannot be anticipated. If any develop or change in intensity, inform your doctor as soon as possible. Only your doctor can determine if it is safe for you to continue taking Eldepryl.

■ *Side effects may include:*
Abdominal pain, abnormal movements, abnormally fast walking, aches, agitation, angina (crushing chest pain), anxiety, apathy, asthma, back pain, behavior or mood changes, bleeding from the rectum, blurred vision, burning lips and mouth or throat, chills, confusion, constipation, delusions, depression, diarrhea, difficulty swallowing, disorientation, dizziness, double vision, drowsiness, dry mouth, excessive urination at night, eyelid spasm, facial grimace, facial hair, fainting, falling down, freezing, frequent urination, general feeling of illness, hair loss, hallucinations, headache, heartburn, heart palpitations, heart rhythm abnormalities, "heavy leg," high blood pressure, hollow feeling, inability to carry out purposeful movements, inability to urinate, increased or excessive sweating, increased tremor, insomnia, involuntary movements, irritability, lack of appetite, leg pain, lethargy, light-headedness upon standing up, loss of balance, low blood pressure, lower back pain, migraine, muscle cramps, nausea, nervousness, numbness in toes/fingers, overstimulation, pain over the eyes, personality change, poor appetite, rapid heartbeat, rash, restlessness (desire to keep moving), ringing in the ears, sensitivity to

light, sexual problems, shortness of breath, sleep disturbance, slow heartbeat, slow urination, slowed body movements, speech problems, stiff neck, stomach and intestinal bleeding, swelling of the ankles or arms and legs, taste disturbance, tension, tiredness, twitching, urinary problems, vertigo, vivid dreams or nightmares, vomiting, weakness, weight loss

Why should this drug not be prescribed?
Do not take Eldepryl if you are sensitive to or have ever had an allergic reaction to it. Do not take narcotic painkillers such as Demerol while you are taking Eldepryl.

Special warnings about this medication
Never take Eldepryl at a higher dosage than prescribed; doing so could put you at risk for a dangerous rise in blood pressure. If you develop a severe headache or any other unusual symptoms, contact your doctor immediately.

You may suffer a severe reaction if you combine Eldepryl with tricyclic antidepressants such as Elavil and Tofranil, or with antidepressants that affect serotonin levels, such as Prozac and Paxil. Wait at least 14 days after taking Eldepryl before beginning therapy with any of these drugs. If you have been taking antidepressants such as Prozac and Paxil, you should wait at least 5 weeks before taking Eldepryl. This much time is needed to clear the antidepressant completely from your system.

Possible food and drug interactions
when taking this medication
If Eldepryl is taken with certain other drugs, the effects of either could be increased, decreased, or altered. It is especially important to check with your doctor before combining Eldepryl with the following:

Antidepressant medications that raise serotonin levels, such as Paxil, Prozac, and Zoloft
Antidepressant medications classified as tricyclics, such as Elavil and Tofranil
Narcotic painkillers such as Demerol, Percocet, and Tylenol with Codeine

Eldepryl may worsen side effects caused by your usual dosage of levodopa.

Special information
if you are pregnant or breastfeeding
The effects of Eldepryl during pregnancy have not been adequately studied. If you are pregnant or plan to become pregnant, inform your doctor immediately. Although Eldepryl is not known to cause specific birth defects, it should

not be taken during pregnancy unless it is clearly needed. It is not known whether Eldepryl appears in breast milk. As a general rule, a nursing mother should not take any drug unless it is clearly necessary.

Recommended dosage

ADULTS

The recommended dose of Eldepryl is 10 milligrams per day divided into 2 smaller doses of 5 milligrams each, taken at breakfast and lunch. There is no evidence of additional benefit from higher doses, and they increase the risk of side effects.

CHILDREN

The use of Eldepryl in children has not been evaluated.

Overdosage

Although no specific information is available about Eldepryl overdosage, it is assumed, because of chemical similarities, that the symptoms would resemble those of overdose with an MAO inhibitor antidepressant.

- *Symptoms of MAO inhibitor overdose may include:*
  Agitation, chest pain, clammy skin, coma, convulsions, dizziness, drowsiness, extremely high fever, faintness, fast and irregular pulse, hallucinations, headache (severe), high blood pressure, hyperactivity, inability to breathe, irritability, lockjaw, low blood pressure (severe), shallow breathing, spasm of the entire body, sweating

It is important to note that after a large overdose, symptoms may not appear for up to 12 hours and may not reach their full force for 24 hours or more. An overdose can be fatal. If you suspect an Eldepryl overdose, seek medical attention immediately. Hospitalization is recommended, with continuous observation and monitoring for at least 2 days.

Brand name:

ELOCON

Pronounced: ELL-oh-con
Generic name: Mometasone furoate

Why is this drug prescribed?

Elocon is a cortisone-like steroid available in cream, ointment, and lotion form. It is used to treat certain itchy rashes and other inflammatory skin conditions.

Most important fact about this drug
When you use Elocon, you inevitably absorb some of the medication through your skin and into the bloodstream. Too much absorption can lead to unwanted side effects elsewhere in the body. To keep this problem to a minimum, avoid using large amounts of Elocon over large areas, and do not cover it with airtight dressings such as plastic wrap or adhesive bandages unless specifically told to by your doctor.

How should you use this medication?
Apply a thin film of the cream or ointment or a few drops of the lotion to the affected skin once a day. Massage it in until it disappears.

Elocon is for use only on the skin. Be careful to keep it out of your eyes.

For the most effective and economical use of Elocon lotion, hold the tip of the bottle very close to (but not touching) the affected skin and squeeze the bottle gently.

Once you have applied Elocon, never cover the skin with an airtight bandage, a tight diaper, plastic pants, or any other airtight dressing. This could encourage excessive absorption of the medication into your bloodstream.

Be careful not to use Elocon for a longer time than prescribed. If you do, you may disrupt your ability to make your own natural adrenal corticoid hormones (hormones secreted by the outer layer of the adrenal gland).

■ *If you miss a dose...*
  Apply it as soon as you remember. If it is almost time for your next dose, skip the one you missed and go back to your regular schedule.

■ *Storage instructions...*
  Store at room temperature.

What side effects may occur?
Side effects cannot be anticipated. If any develop or change in intensity, notify your doctor as soon as possible. Only your doctor can determine if it is safe for you to continue using Elocon.

■ *Side effects may include:*
  Acne-like pimples, allergic skin rash, boils, burning, damaged skin, dryness, excessive hairiness, infected hair follicles, infection of the skin, irritation, itching, light colored patches on skin, prickly heat, rash around the mouth, skin atrophy and wasting, softening of the skin, stretch marks, tingling or stinging

Why should this drug not be prescribed?
Do not use Elocon if you have ever had an allergic reaction to it or any other steroid medication.

Special warnings about this medication
Remember, Elocon is for external use only. Avoid getting it into your eyes. Do not use it to treat anything other than the condition for which it was prescribed.

If your skin becomes irritated, call your doctor.

If you have any kind of skin infection, tell your doctor before you start using Elocon.

Do not use Elocon on your face, underarms, or groin area unless your doctor tells you to.

If your condition doesn't improve in 2 weeks, call your doctor.

**Possible food and drug interactions
when using this medication**
No interactions have been noted.

**Special information
if you are pregnant or breastfeeding**
If you are pregnant or plan to become pregnant, inform your doctor immediately. Elocon should not be used during pregnancy unless the benefit outweighs the potential risk to the unborn child.

You should not use Elocon while breastfeeding, since absorbed hormone could make its way into the breast milk and perhaps harm the nursing baby. If you are a new mother, you should contact your doctor, who will help you decide between breastfeeding and using Elocon.

Recommended dosage

ADULTS

Apply once daily.

CHILDREN

Use should be limited to the least amount necessary. Use of steroids over a long period of time may interfere with growth and development.

Elocon cream and ointment may be used for children aged 2 and older, but not for more than 3 weeks.

Overdosage

With extensive or long-term use of Elocon, hormone absorbed into the bloodstream may cause a group of symptoms called Cushing's syndrome.

■ *Symptoms of Cushing's syndrome may include:*
Acne, depression, excessive hair growth, high blood pressure, humped upper back, insomnia, moon-faced appearance, obese trunk, paranoia, stretch marks, wasted limbs, stunted growth (in children), susceptibility to bruising, fractures, and infections

Cushing's syndrome may also trigger diabetes mellitus.

If it is left uncorrected, Cushing's syndrome may become serious. If you suspect your long-term use of Elocon has led to this problem, seek medical attention immediately.

Brand name:

EMPIRIN

See Aspirin, page 98.

Brand name:

EMPIRIN WITH CODEINE

Pronounced: EM-pir-in with KOE-deen
Generic ingredients: Aspirin, Codeine phosphate

Why is this drug prescribed?

Empirin with Codeine is a narcotic pain reliever and anti-inflammatory medication. It is prescribed for mild, moderate, and moderate to severe pain.

Most important fact about this drug

Codeine can be habit-forming when taken over a long period of time or in high doses. Do not take more of the drug, or use it for a longer period of time than your doctor has indicated.

How should you take this medication?

Take Empirin with Codeine with food or a full glass of milk or water to reduce stomach irritation. Take it exactly as prescribed.

■ *If you miss a dose...*
Take it as soon as you remember. If it is almost time for your next dose, skip the one you missed and go back to your regular schedule. Never take 2 doses at once.

■ *Storage instructions...*
Store at room temperature in a dry place; protect from light.

What side effects may occur?
Side effects cannot be anticipated. If any develop or change in intensity, inform your doctor as soon as possible. Only your doctor can determine if it is safe for you to continue using Empirin with Codeine.

■ *More common side effects may include:*
Constipation, dizziness, drowsiness, light-headedness, nausea, shallow breathing, vomiting

■ *Less common side effects may include:*
Abdominal pain, aggravation of peptic ulcer, anaphylactic shock (severe allergic reaction), asthma, bruising or bleeding, confusion, dizziness, drowsiness, exaggerated sense of well-being or depression, excessive bleeding following injury or surgery, fatigue, headache, hearing problems, heartburn, hives, indigestion, itching, nausea, rapid heartbeat, ringing in ears, runny nose, skin rashes, sweating, thirst, vision problems, vomiting, weakness

Why should this drug not be prescribed?
Empirin with Codeine should not be used if you: are sensitive or allergic to aspirin or codeine, experience severe bleeding, have a blood clotting disorder or severe vitamin K deficiency, are taking blood-thinning medications, have a peptic ulcer or have liver damage. Children or teenagers with symptoms of chickenpox or the flu should not take Empirin with Codeine because of the danger of contracting Reye's syndrome, a condition characterized by nausea, vomiting, and lethargy and disorientation deepening to coma.

Special warnings about this medication
Aspirin can cause severe allergic reactions including anaphylactic shock (difficulty breathing, bluish skin color caused by lack of oxygen, fever, rash or hives, irregular pulse, convulsions, or collapse).

Aspirin can cause bleeding if you have a peptic ulcer, open sores in the stomach or intestines, or a bleeding disorder. It may also prolong bleeding time after an injury or surgery.

Codeine can hide symptoms of serious abdominal conditions.

Use codeine with care if you have a head or brain injury. It can slow your breathing, make you drowsy, and increase pressure in your head.

Be careful taking Empirin with Codeine if you are elderly or in a weakened condition or have severe kidney or liver disease, gallstones or gallbladder disease, a breathing disorder, an irregular heartbeat, an inflamed stomach or intestines, an underactive thyroid gland, Addison's disease (a disorder of the adrenal glands), or an enlarged prostate or narrowing of the urethra.

Use aspirin with care if you have ever had any allergies. Sensitivity reactions are relatively common in people with asthma and nasal polyps (swollen growths in the nose).

Empirin with Codeine may make you drowsy or less alert. Be careful driving, operating machinery, or using appliances that require full mental alertness until you know how you react to this medication.

Remember, this medication can be habit-forming and should be taken exactly as prescribed. Do not take more of the medication, or use it more often, than your doctor has indicated.

Possible food and drug interactions when taking this medication

The effects of alcohol may be increased if taken with Empirin with Codeine. Avoid using alcohol while taking this medication.

If Empirin with Codeine is taken with certain other drugs, the effects of either could be increased, decreased, or altered. It is especially important to check with your doctor before combining Empirin with Codeine with the following:

Blood thinners such as Coumadin
Furosemide (Lasix)
Insulin
MAO inhibitors such as the antidepressants Parnate and Nardil
Mercaptopurine
Methotrexate (Rheumatrex)
Nonsteroidal anti-inflammatory drugs such as Advil, Motrin, and Indocin
Oral diabetes medications such as Diabinese and Tolinase
Other narcotic analgesics such as Percodan and Tylox

Para-amino salicylic acid
Penicillin
Probenecid (Benemid)
Sedatives such as phenobarbital and Nembutal
Steroids such as Medrol and prednisone
Sulfa drugs such as Azo Gantrisin and Septra
Sulfinpyrazone (Anturane)
Tranquilizers such as Xanax and Valium
Vitamin C

Special information
if you are pregnant or breastfeeding

The effects of Empirin with Codeine during pregnancy have not been adequately studied. If you are pregnant or plan to become pregnant, inform your doctor immediately. Aspirin and codeine appear in small amounts in breast milk and may affect a nursing infant. If this medication is essential to your health, your doctor may advise you to stop breastfeeding until your treatment with this medication is finished.

Recommended dosage

Dosage is determined by the severity of your pain and your response to this medication. Your doctor may prescribe more than the usual recommended dose if your pain is severe or if you are no longer getting enough pain relief from the dose you have been taking.

The usual adult dose for Empirin with Codeine No. 3 is 1 or 2 tablets every 4 hours as needed. The usual adult dose for Empirin with Codeine No. 4 is 1 tablet every 4 hours as required.

Overdosage

- *In adults, symptoms of Empirin with Codeine overdose may include:*
  Bluish skin color due to lack of oxygen, circulatory collapse, clammy skin, coma, constricted pupils, delirium, delusions, difficult or labored breathing, double vision, excitability, flabby muscles, garbled speech, hallucinations, restlessness, skin eruptions, slow and shallow breathing, stupor, vertigo

- *In children, symptoms of Empirin with Codeine overdose may include:*
  Confusion, convulsions, dehydration, difficulty hearing, dim vision, dizziness, drowsiness, extremely high body temperature, headache, nausea, rapid breathing, ringing in ears, sweating, thirst, vomiting

If you suspect an overdose, seek medical treatment immediately.

Brand name:

E-MYCIN

See Erythromycin, Oral, page 482.

Generic name:

ENALAPRIL

See Vasotec, page 1395.

Generic name:

ENALAPRIL WITH FELODIPINE

See Lexxel, page 688.

Generic name:

ENALAPRIL WITH HYDROCHLOROTHIAZIDE

See Vaseretic, page 1391.

Brand name:

ENBREL

Pronounced: EN-brell
Generic name: Etanercept

Why is this drug prescribed?

Enbrel is used to treat the symptoms of moderate to severe rheumatoid arthritis when other drugs have proved inadequate. It is the first in a new class of drugs designed to block the action of tumor necrosis factor (TNF), a naturally occurring protein responsible for much of the joint inflammation that plagues the victims of rheumatoid arthritis.

In clinical trials, Enbrel provided the majority of patients with significant relief. In addition, it can be taken along with other drugs commonly used to treat rheumatoid arthritis, including methotrexate (Rheumatrex), steroids such as hydrocortisone and prednisone, nonsteroidal anti-inflammatory drugs such as Motrin and Naprosyn, aspirin, and other pain-killers.

Most important fact about this drug

TNF plays a significant role in the immune system, so blocking its action could, in theory, undermine your resistance. Enbrel does not appear to do this; people taking it have not experienced an increase in serious infections or cancer. Nevertheless, caution is advisable if you have a chronic infection or your immune system has already been weakened by HIV or drugs such as Imuran, Prograf, Cellcept, Neoral, and Sandimmune. For the same reason, children with juvenile rheumatoid arthritis should be brought up to date with all immunizations before starting Enbrel therapy.

How should you take this medication?
Enbrel is given by injection under the skin of the thigh, abdomen, or upper arm. Your doctor will instruct you in the proper injection technique and supervise your first injection in the office. You should rotate injection sites and make each new injection at least 1 inch from an older one. Never inject into areas where the skin is tender, bruised, red, or hard.

Never reuse a syringe. Throw it away in a puncture-proof container immediately after using it.

■ *If you miss a dose...*
Take it as soon as you remember. If it is almost time for your next dose, skip the one you missed and return to your regular schedule. Do not take 2 doses at once.

■ *Storage instructions...*
Store Enbrel powder in the refrigerator. Do not freeze. After mixing Enbrel powder with sterile water, you should inject it as soon as possible. If you can't inject it immediately, it can be stored in the refrigerator for up to 6 hours.

What side effects may occur?
Side effects cannot be anticipated. If any develop or change in intensity inform your doctor as soon as possible. Only your doctor can determine if it is safe for you to continue taking Enbrel.

■ *More common side effects may include:*
Abdominal pain, cough, dizziness, headache, indigestion, infection, injection site reaction, rash, respiratory problems, respiratory tract infection, sinus and nasal inflammation, sore, throat, weakness

■ *Less common side effects may include:*
Bursitis, chest pain, depression, difficulty breathing, gallbladder problems, heart attack, heart failure, high or low blood pressure, stomach and intestinal bleeding, stroke

Why should this drug not be prescribed?
If Enbrel gives you an allergic reaction, you will not be able to continue using it. Do not take it if you are suffering from a serious infection.

Special warnings about this medication
If you develop a serious infection, stop taking Enbrel and call your doctor.

Possible food and drug interactions
when taking this medication
No drug interactions have been reported. Do not get any live-type vaccinations while taking Enbrel.

Special information
if you are pregnant or breastfeeding
The effects of Enbrel during pregnancy have not been studied. If you are pregnant or plan to become pregnant, inform your doctor immediately.

It is not known whether Enbrel appears in breast milk, but because there is a possible risk to the infant, you should either give up nursing while taking Enbrel or discontinue the drug. Discuss the problem with your doctor.

Recommended dosage

ADULTS

The recommended dose is 25 milligrams injected under the skin twice a week.

CHILDREN 4 YEARS OLD AND OVER

Dosage is determined by weight. The safety of Enbrel has not been studied in children less than 4 years old.

Overdosage
High doses of Enbrel do not appear to have any toxic effects. Nevertheless, if you suspect an overdose, you should notify your doctor.

Generic name:

ENOXACIN

See Penetrex, page 968.

Brand name:

ENTEX LA

Pronounced: ENN-teks ELL AI
Generic ingredients: Guaifenesin, Phenylpropanolamine
hydrochloride
Other brand name: Exgest LA

Why is this drug prescribed?

Entex LA is used to treat bronchitis, the common cold, sinus inflammation, nasal congestion, and sore throat.

Entex LA is a combination of two medications, phenylpropanolamine (a decongestant) and guaifenesin (an expectorant), specially formulated to deliver prolonged action. Phenylpropanolamine helps reduce congestion in the nasal passages, while guaifenesin breaks up mucus in the lower respiratory tract, making it easier to clear the passages.

Most important fact about this drug

Certain medical conditions can affect your use of Entex LA. If you have heart disease, high blood pressure, or diabetes, make sure the doctor knows about it. The phenylpropanolamine in Entex LA can raise blood pressure and speed up the heart, and can put you at a greater risk of heart or blood-vessel disease if you are diabetic.

How should you take this medication?

You may break Entex LA tablets in half to make them easier to swallow, but you must not chew or crush them.

▪ *If you miss a dose...*
 Take it as soon as you remember. If it is almost time for your next dose, skip the one you missed and go back to your regular schedule. Never take 2 doses at once.

▪ *Storage instructions...*
 Store at room temperature in a tightly closed container, away from light.

What side effects may occur?

Side effects cannot be anticipated. If any develop or change in intensity, inform your doctor as soon as possible. Only your doctor can determine if it is safe for you to continue taking Entex LA.

■ *Side effects may include:*
Difficulty urinating (in men with an enlarged prostate), headache, inability to sleep or difficulty sleeping, irritated stomach, nausea, nervousness, restlessness

Why should this drug not be prescribed?
You should not use Entex LA if you have severe high blood pressure, are sensitive to other stimulating drugs such as Dristan Decongestant, or take antidepressant medications known as MAO inhibitors, including Nardil and Parnate.

Special warnings about this medication
Use Entex LA cautiously if you have any of the following conditions:

Diabetes
Glaucoma (excessive pressure in the eyes)
Heart disease
High blood pressure
Hyperthyroidism (excessive thyroid gland activity)
Prostate enlargement

Possible food and drug interactions
when taking this medication
Do not take Entex LA if you are taking a medication classified as an MAO inhibitor, including the antidepressants Nardil and Parnate. Avoid other stimulating drugs such as Proventil, Ventolin, and many decongestants. Interactions can also occur with the following:

Bromocriptine (Parlodel)
Methyldopa (Aldomet)

Special information
if you are pregnant or breastfeeding
The effects of Entex LA during pregnancy have not been adequately studied. If you are pregnant or plan to become pregnant, notify your doctor immediately. It is not known whether Entex LA appears in breast milk. If this medication is essential to your health, your doctor may advise you to discontinue breastfeeding until treatment with this drug is finished.

Recommended dosage

ADULTS AND CHILDREN 12 YEARS AND OLDER

The usual dosage is 1 tablet every 12 hours.

CHILDREN 6 TO 12 YEARS OLD

The usual dosage is one-half tablet every 12 hours.

The safety and effectiveness of Entex LA have not been established in children under the age of 6.

Overdosage

Any medication taken in excess can have serious consequences. If you suspect an overdose, seek medical help immediately.

- *Symptoms of Entex LA overdose may include:*
  Coma, convulsions, high blood pressure

Brand name:

EPITOL

See Tegretol, page 1264.

Brand name:

EPIVIR

Pronounced: EPP-ih-veer
Generic name: Lamivudine

Why is this drug prescribed?

Epivir is one of the drugs used to fight infection with the human immunodeficiency virus (HIV), the deadly cause of AIDS. Doctors turn to Epivir as the infection gets worse. The drug is taken along with Retrovir, another HIV medication.

HIV does its damage by slowly destroying the immune system, eventually leaving the body defenseless against infections. Like other drugs for HIV, Epivir interferes with the virus's ability to reproduce. This staves off the collapse of the immune system.

Most important fact about this drug

The Epivir/Retrovir combination does not completely eliminate HIV or totally restore the immune system. There is still a danger of serious infections, so you should be sure to see your doctor regularly for monitoring and tests.

How should you take this medication?

It's important to keep adequate levels of Epivir in your bloodstream at all times, so you need to keep taking this medication regularly, just as prescribed, even when you're feeling better.

■ *If you miss a dose...*
Take it as soon as you remember. If it is almost time for the next dose, skip the one you missed and go back to your regular schedule. Do not take 2 doses at once.

■ *Storage instructions...*
Store at room temperature. Keep the bottle tightly closed.

What side effects may occur?

Side effects cannot be anticipated. If any develop or change in intensity, inform your doctor as soon as possible. Only your doctor can determine if it is safe for you to continue taking Epivir.

■ *Side effects may include:*
Abdominal cramps and pains, chills, cough, depression, diarrhea, dizziness, fatigue, fever, general feeling of illness, hair loss, headache, hives, insomnia and other sleep problems, itching, joint pain, lost appetite, muscle and bone pain, nasal problems, nausea, skin rashes, stomach upset, vomiting, weakness

Why should this drug not be prescribed?

If Epivir gives you an allergic reaction, you cannot take this drug.

Special warnings about this medication

Remember that Epivir does not eliminate HIV from the body. The infection can still be passed to others through sexual contact or blood contamination.

The Epivir/Retrovir combination should be given to a child with a history of pancreatitis (inflammation of the pancreas) only when there is no alternative. If any signs of a pancreas problem develop while the child is taking this combination, treatment should be stopped immediately. The chief signs of pancreatitis are bouts of severe abdominal pain—usually lasting for days—accompanied by nausea and vomiting.

If you have the chronic liver disease hepatitis B, as well as HIV infection, the hepatitis B may come back when you stop taking Epivir.

Possible food and drug interactions
when taking this medication

Check with your doctor before combining Epivir with Bactrim or Septra.

While no other interactions with Epivir have been reported, its companion drug, Retrovir, can interact with a number of medications.

Special information
if you are pregnant or breastfeeding

The effects of Epivir during pregnancy have not been adequately studied, but there is reason to suspect some risk. If you are pregnant or plan to become pregnant, notify your doctor immediately.

Since HIV can be passed to your baby through breast milk, you should not plan on breastfeeding.

Recommended dosage

ADULTS

The usual dose (either tablets or liquid) is 150 milligrams twice daily. Your doctor may adjust the dosage if you have kidney problems or weigh less than 110 pounds.

CHILDREN UNDER 12 YEARS OF AGE

The usual dose is 4 milligrams per 2.2 pounds of body weight twice a day, up to a maximum of 150 milligrams twice daily.

Overdosage

The symptoms of Epivir overdose are unknown at this time. However, any medication taken in excess can have serious consequences. If you suspect an overdose, seek medical attention immediately.

Brand name:

EQUANIL

See Miltown, page 804.

Generic name:

ERGOLOID MESYLATES

See Hydergine, page 596.

Generic name:

ERGOTAMINE WITH CAFFEINE

See Cafergot, page 178.

Brand name:

ERYC

See Erythromycin, Oral, page 482.

Brand name:

ERYCETTE

See Erythromycin, Topical, page 487.

Brand name:

ERY-TAB

See Erythromycin, Oral, page 482.

Brand name:

ERYTHROCIN

See Erythromycin, Oral, page 482.

Generic name:

ERYTHROMYCIN, ORAL

Pronounced: er-ITH-row MY-sin
Brand names: E.E.S., E-Mycin, ERYC, Ery-Tab,
  Erythrocin, Ilosone, PCE

Why is this drug prescribed?
Erythromycin is an antibiotic used to treat many kinds of infections, including:

Acute pelvic inflammatory disease
Gonorrhea
Intestinal parasitic infections
Legionnaires' disease
Pinkeye
Skin infections
Syphilis
Upper and lower respiratory tract infections
Urinary tract infections
Whooping cough

Erythromycin is also prescribed to prevent infections of the heart (rheumatic fever and bacterial endocarditis) in people who are allergic to penicillin and who have congenital or rheumatic heart disease.

Most important fact about this drug
Erythromycin, like any other antibiotic, works best when there is a constant amount of drug in the blood. To help keep the drug amount constant, it is important not to miss any doses. Also, it is advisable to take the doses at evenly spaced times around the clock.

How should you take this medication?
Your doctor may advise you to take erythromycin at least 1 hour before or 2 hours after meals. If the drug upsets your stomach, taking it with meals may help. Ask your doctor whether this is advisable for you.

Chewable forms of erythromycin should be crushed or chewed before being swallowed.

Delayed-release brands and tablets and capsules that are coated to slow their breakdown should be swallowed whole. Do not crush or break. If you are not sure about the form of erythromycin you are taking, ask your pharmacist.

The liquid should be shaken well before each use.

■ *If you miss a dose...*
Take it as soon as you remember. If it is almost time for your next dose, and you take 2 doses a day, space the missed dose and the next dose 5 to 6 hours apart; if you take 3 or more doses a day, space the missed dose and the next one 2 to 4 hours apart. Never take 2 doses at the same time.

■ *Storage instructions...*
The liquid form of erythromycin should be kept in the refrigerator; use E.E.S. within 10 days. Do not freeze. Store tablets and capsules at room temperature.

What side effects may occur?
Side effects cannot be anticipated. If any develop or change in intensity, inform your doctor as soon as possible. Only your doctor can determine whether it is safe to continue taking this medication.

- *More common side effects may include:*
  Abdominal pain, diarrhea, loss of appetite, nausea, vomiting

- *Less common side effects may include:*
  Hives, rash, skin eruptions, yellow eyes and skin

- *Rare side effects may include:*
  Hearing loss (temporary), inflammation of the large intestine, irregular heartbeat, severe allergic reaction, skin reddening

Why should this drug not be prescribed?
You should not use erythromycin if you have ever had an allergic reaction to it or are sensitive to it. Erythromycin should not be used with Seldane, Hismanal, or Propulsid.

Special warnings about this medication
If you have ever had liver disease, consult your doctor before taking erythromycin.

If a new infection (called superinfection) develops, talk to your doctor. You may need to be treated with a different antibiotic.

This drug may cause a severe form of intestinal inflammation. If you develop diarrhea, contact your doctor immediately. If you have myasthenia gravis (muscle weakness), it can be aggravated by erythromycin.

Possible food and drug interactions
when taking this medication
If erythromycin is taken with certain other drugs, the effects of either could be increased, decreased, or altered. It is especially important to check with your doctor before combining erythromycin with the following:

Astemizole (Hismanal)
Blood-thinning drugs such as Coumadin
Bromocriptine (Parlodel)
Carbamazepine (Tegretol)
Cisapride (Propulsid)
Cyclosporine (Sandimmune, Neoral)
Digoxin (Lanoxin)

Dihydroergotamine (D.H.E. 45)
Disopyramide (Norpace)
Ergotamine (Cafergot)
Hexobarbital
Lovastatin (Mevacor)
Seizure medications such as Depakane, Depakote, and Dilantin
Tacrolimus (Prograf)
Terfenadine (Seldane)
Theophylline (Theo-Dur)
Triazolam (Halcion)

Special information
if you are pregnant or breastfeeding
If you are pregnant or plan to become pregnant, inform your doctor immediately. Erythromycin appears in breast milk and could affect a nursing infant. If this medication is essential to your health, your doctor may advise you to discontinue breastfeeding until your treatment is finished.

Recommended dosage
Dosage instructions are determined by the type (and severity) of infection being treated and may vary slightly for different brands of erythromycin. The following are recommended dosages for PCE, one of the most commonly prescribed brands.

ADULTS

Streptococcal Infections
The usual dose is 333 milligrams every 8 hours, or 500 milligrams every 12 hours. Depending on the severity of the infection, the dose may be increased to a total of 4 grams a day. However, when the daily dosage is larger than 1 gram, twice-a-day doses are not recommended, and the drug should be taken more often in smaller doses.

To treat streptococcal infections of the upper respiratory tract (tonsillitis or strep throat), erythromycin should be taken for at least 10 days.

To Prevent Bacterial Endocarditis (Inflammation and Infection of the Heart Lining and Valves) in Those Allergic to Penicillin
The oral regimen is 800 milligrams to 1 gram of erythromycin taken 1 to 2 hours before dental surgery or surgical procedures of the upper respiratory tract, followed by 400 to 500 milligrams 6 hours later.

Urinary Tract Infections Due to Chlamydia Trachomatis During Pregnancy

The usual dosage is 500 milligrams of erythromycin orally 4 times a day or 666 milligrams every 8 hours on an empty stomach for at least 7 days. For women who cannot tolerate this regimen, a decreased dose of 500 milligrams every 12 hours or 333 milligrams every 8 hours a day should be used for at least 14 days.

For Those with Uncomplicated Urinary, Reproductive Tract, or Rectal Infections Caused by Chlamydia Trachomatis When Tetracycline Cannot Be Taken

The usual oral dosage is 500 milligrams of erythromycin 4 times a day or 666 milligrams every 8 hours for at least 7 days.

For Those with Nongonococcal Urethral Infections When Tetracycline Cannot Be Taken

The usual dosage is 500 milligrams of erythromycin by mouth 4 times a day or 666 milligrams orally every 8 hours for at least 7 days.

Acute Pelvic Inflammatory Disease Caused by Neisseria Gonorrhoeae

The usual treatment is three days of intravenous erythromycin followed by 500 milligrams orally every 12 hours or 333 milligrams orally every 8 hours for 7 days.

Syphilis

The usual dosage is 30 to 40 grams divided into smaller doses over a period of 10 to 15 days.

Intestinal Infections

The usual dosage is 500 milligrams every 12 hours, or 333 milligrams every 8 hours, for 10 to 14 days.

Legionnaires' Disease

The usual dosage ranges from 1 to 4 grams daily, divided into smaller doses.

CHILDREN

Age, weight, and severity of the infection determine the correct dosage.

The usual dosage is from 30 to 50 milligrams daily for each 2.2 pounds of body weight, divided into equal doses for 10 to 14 days.

For more severe infections, this dosage may be doubled, but it should not exceed 4 grams per day.

Children weighing over 44 pounds should follow the recommended adult dose schedule.

For prevention of bacterial endocarditis, the children's dosage is 10 milligrams per 2.2 pounds of body weight 2 hours before dental work or surgery, followed by 5 milligrams per 2.2 pounds 6 hours later.

Overdosage
Any medication taken in excess can have serious consequences. If you suspect an overdose, seek medical help immediately.

- *Symptoms of erythromycin overdose may include:*
  Diarrhea, nausea, stomach cramps, vomiting

Generic name:

ERYTHROMYCIN, TOPICAL

Pronounced: err-rith-ro-MY-sin
Brand names: A/T/S, Erycette, T-Stat

Why is this drug prescribed?
Topical erythromycin (applied directly to the skin) is used for the treatment of acne.

Most important fact about this drug
For best results, you should continue the treatment for as long as prescribed, even if your acne begins to clear up. This medicine is not an instant cure.

How should you use this medication?
Use exactly as prescribed by your doctor.

Thoroughly wash the affected area with soap and water and pat dry before applying medication.

Moisten the applicator or pad with the medication and lightly spread it over the affected area. A/T/S Topical Gel should not be rubbed in.

- *If you miss a dose...*
  Apply the forgotten dose as soon as you remember. If it is almost time for the next application, skip the one you missed and go back to your regular schedule.

- *Storage instructions...*
  This medicine can be stored at room temperature.

What side effects may occur?
Side effects cannot be anticipated. If any develop or change in intensity, inform your doctor as soon as possible. Only your doctor can determine if it is safe for you to continue using topical erythromycin.

■ *Side effects may include:*
 Burning sensation, dryness, hives, irritation of the eyes, itching, oiliness, peeling, scaling, tenderness, unusual redness of the skin

Why should this drug not be prescribed?
Erythromycin should not be used if you are sensitive to or have ever had an allergic reaction to any of the ingredients.

Special warnings about this medication
This type of erythromycin is for external use only. Do not use it in the eyes, nose, or mouth.

If the acne does not improve after 6 to 8 weeks of treatment, or if it gets worse, stop using the topical erythromycin preparation and call your doctor.

The use of antibiotics can stimulate the growth of other bacteria that are resistant to the antibiotic you are taking. If new infections (called superinfections) occur, talk to your doctor. You may need to be treated with a different antibiotic drug.

If you develop diarrhea, let your doctor know right away. Drugs such as erythromycin can cause a potentially serious intestinal inflammation.

The use of other topical acne medications in combination with topical erythromycin may cause irritation, especially with the use of peeling, scaling, or abrasive medications.

The safety and effectiveness of A/T/S and Erycette have not been established in children.

**Possible food and drug interactions
when using this medication**
If topical erythromycin is used with certain other drugs, the effects of either could be increased, decreased, or altered. It is especially important to check with your doctor before combining topical erythromycin with other topical acne medications.

**Special information
if you are pregnant or breastfeeding**
The effects of topical erythromycin during pregnancy have not been adequately studied. If you are pregnant or plan to become pregnant, inform

your doctor immediately. Erythromycin may appear in breast milk and could affect a nursing infant. If this medication is essential to your health, your doctor may advise you to stop breastfeeding until your treatment with erythromycin is finished.

Recommended dosage
Apply solution to the affected area 2 times a day. Moisten the applicator or a pad, then spread over the affected area. Use additional pads as needed. Apply gel products as a thin film over the affected area once or twice a day.

Make sure the area is thoroughly washed with soap and water and patted dry before applying medication. Thoroughly wash your hands after application of the medication.

Reducing the frequency of applications may reduce peeling and drying.

Overdosage
Although overdosage is unlikely, any medication used in excess can have serious consequences. If you suspect an overdose, seek medical treatment immediately.

Generic name:

ERYTHROMYCIN WITH BENZOYL PEROXIDE

See Benzamycin, page 155.

Generic name:

ERYTHROMYCIN WITH SULFISOXAZOLE

See Pediazole, page 964.

Brand name:

ERYZOLE

See Pediazole, page 964.

Brand name:

ESGIC

See Fioricet, page 518.

Brand name:

ESIDRIX

See HydroDIURIL, page 601.

Brand name:

ESKALITH

See Lithonate, page 704.

Generic name:

ESTAZOLAM

See ProSom, page 1069.

Brand name:

ESTRACE

See Estraderm, page 490.

Brand name:

ESTRADERM

Pronounced: ESS-tra-derm
Generic name: Estradiol
Other brand names: Alora, Climara, Estrace, Vivelle

Why is this drug prescribed?

Estraderm and other estrogen patches such as Alora, Climara, and Vivelle are used to reduce symptoms of menopause, including feelings of warmth in face, neck, and chest, and the sudden intense episodes of heat and sweating known as "hot flashes." Estrace tablets are also prescribed for this purpose, and another form of estrogen—Estrace vaginal cream—is prescribed to relieve dry, itchy external genitals and vaginal irritation. And some doctors prescribe estrogen for teenagers who fail to mature at the usual rate.

Along with diet, calcium supplements, and exercise, Estraderm patches are also prescribed to prevent osteoporosis, a condition in which the bones become brittle and easily broken. Estrace tablets are also used for this purpose.

All forms of this drug are used to treat low levels of estrogen in certain people. In addition, Climara patches are used to treat abnormal bleeding from the uterus in some cases, and Estrace tablets are used to provide relief in breast or prostate cancer.

Most important fact about this drug
Because estrogens have been linked with increased risk of endometrial cancer (cancer in the lining of the uterus), it is essential to have regular checkups and to report any unusual vaginal bleeding to your doctor immediately.

How should you take this medication?

ESTRADERM, ALORA, CLIMARA, AND VIVELLE

Each patch is individually sealed in a protective pouch and is applied directly to the skin.

A stiff protective liner covers the adhesive side of the patch. Remove the liner by sliding it sideways between your thumb and index finger. Holding the patch at one edge, remove the protective liner and discard it. Try to avoid touching the adhesive. Use immediately after removing the liner. If you are using Alora or Vivelle, peel off one side of the protective liner and discard it. Use the other half of the liner as a handle until you have applied the sticky area, then fold back the remaining side of the patch, pull off the rest of the liner, and smooth the second half of the patch onto your skin.

Apply the adhesive side to a clean, dry area of your skin on the trunk of your body (including the buttocks and abdomen). Do not apply to your breasts or waist. Firmly press the patch in place with the palm of your hand for about 10 seconds, to make sure the edges are flat against your skin. When first using Alora, start on the lower abdomen. Climara is applied only to the abdomen and is pressed in place with the fingers.

Contact with water during bathing, swimming, or showering will not affect the patch.

The application site must be rotated. Allow an interval of at least 1 week between applications to a particular site.

Alora, Estraderm, and Vivelle patches should be replaced twice a week.

ESTRACE

Estrace Tablets are taken orally.

If you are using Estrace vaginal cream, follow these steps to apply:
1. Load the supplied applicator to the fill line.
2. Lie on your back with your knees drawn up.
3. Gently insert the applicator high into the vagina. Release the medicine by pushing the plunger.
4. Withdraw the applicator.
5. Wash the applicator with soap and water.

■ *If you miss a dose...*
  If you forget to apply a new patch when you are supposed to, do it as soon as you remember. If it is almost time to change patches anyway, skip the one you missed and go back to your regular schedule. Do not apply more than one patch at a time.

  If you miss a dose of the tablets, take it as soon as you remember. If it is almost time for your next dose, skip the one you missed and go back to your regular schedule. Do not take 2 doses at once.

■ *Storage instructions...*
  Store patches at room temperature, in their sealed pouches. Store Estrace at room temperature in a tightly closed container; keep away from light.

What side effects may occur?
Side effects cannot be anticipated. If any develop or change in intensity, notify your doctor as soon as possible. Only your doctor can determine if it is safe for you to continue taking Estraderm.

■ *The most common side effect is:*
  Skin redness and irritation at the site of the patch.

■ *Less common or rare side effects may include:*
  Abdominal cramps, bloating, breakthrough bleeding, breast enlargement, breast tenderness, change in cervical secretions, change in menstrual flow, change in sex drive, change in weight, darkening of skin, dizziness, fluid retention, growth of benign fibroid tumors in the uterus, headache, intolerance to contact lenses, migraine, nausea, rash, severe allergic reaction, vaginal bleeding (more common at higher doses), vomiting, yellowing of eyes and skin

■ *Other side effects reported with estradiol include:*
  Abnormal withdrawal bleeding, certain cancers, cardiovascular disease, depression, excessive growth of hair, gallbladder disease, hair loss, high blood pressure, reddened skin, twitching, vaginal yeast infection

Why should this drug not be prescribed?
Estraderm should not be used if you are sensitive to or have ever had an allergic reaction to any of its components.

Estrogens should not be used if you have ever had breast or uterine cancer or a tumor promoted by estrogen. Also avoid estrogens if you are pregnant or think you are pregnant, if you have abnormal, undiagnosed genital bleeding, or if you have blood clots or a blood clotting disorder.

Special warnings about this medication
The risk of cancer of the uterus increases when estrogen is used for a long time or taken in large doses. There also may be increased risk of breast cancer in women who take estrogen for an extended period of time or in high doses.

Women who take estrogen after menopause are more likely to develop gallbladder disease.

Tell your doctor if you have any problems with your circulation.

Estrogen also increases the risk of blood clots. These blood clots can cause stroke, heart attack, or other serious disorders.

While taking Estraderm, get in touch with your doctor right away if you notice any of the following:

Abdominal pain, tenderness, or swelling
Abnormal bleeding of the vagina
Breast lumps
Coughing up blood
Pain in your chest or calves
Severe headache, dizziness, or faintness
Skin irritation, redness, or rash
Sudden shortness of breath
Vision changes
Yellowing of the skin or eyes

A complete medical and family history should be taken by your doctor before starting any estrogen therapy.

In general, you should not take estrogen for more than 1 year without another physical examination by your doctor.

Estraderm may cause fluid retention in some people. If you have asthma, epilepsy, migraine, or heart or kidney disease, use this medication cautiously.

Estrogen therapy may cause uterine bleeding or breast pain.

Possible food and drug interactions when taking this medication

If you take certain other drugs while using Estraderm, the effects of either could be increased, decreased, or altered. It is especially important to check with your doctor before taking the following:

Barbiturates such as phenobarbital and Seconal
Blood thinners such as Coumadin
Dantrolene (Dantrium)
Epilepsy drugs such as Tegretol and Dilantin
Rifampin (Rifadin)
Steroids such as Deltasone
Tricyclic antidepressants such as Elavil and Tofranil

Special information
if you are pregnant or breastfeeding

Estrogens should not be used during pregnancy or immediately after childbirth. Use of estrogens during pregnancy has been linked to reproductive tract problems in the children. If you are pregnant or plan to become pregnant, notify your doctor immediately. Estraderm may appear in breast milk and could affect a nursing infant. Estrogens decrease the quantity and quality of breast milk. If this medication is essential to your health, your doctor may advise you to discontinue breastfeeding until your treatment is finished.

Recommended dosage

SYMPTOMS OF MENOPAUSE

After starting your therapy, the doctor will prescribe a higher dose if necessary, but should try decreasing the dose or discontinuing the medication every 3 to 6 months.

Estraderm, Alora, and Vivelle

The usual starting dose is one 0.05 milligram patch applied to the skin 2 times a week.

Estrace

The usual starting dose is 1 or 2 milligrams a day; you will take the tablets for 3 weeks and then have 1 week off for each cycle.

Climara

The usual starting dose for all uses is one 0.5 milligram patch applied to the skin once a week. You will use the patch for 3 weeks, then have 1 week off.

PREVENTION OF OSTEOPOROSIS

Estraderm
The usual starting dose is 0.05 milligram per day.

Estrace
The usual dose is 0.5 milligram taken every day for 23 days, followed by 5 days off.

LOW ESTROGEN LEVELS

Estrace
The usual starting dose is 1 or 2 milligrams a day.

Alora
The usual starting dose is one 0.05 milligram patch applied twice a week.

RELIEF IN BREAST CANCER

Estrace
The usual dose is 10 milligrams 3 times a day for at least 3 months.

RELIEF IN PROSTATE CANCER

Estrace
The usual dose is 1 to 2 milligrams 3 times a day.

VAGINAL ITCHING AND DRYNESS

Estrace Vaginal Cream
The usual dosage is 2 to 4 grams (marked on the applicator) inserted into the vagina once a day, for 1 to 2 weeks. The dosage and frequency may be reduced after your condition improves.

To prevent recurrence, a dosage of 1 gram 1 to 3 times a week is recommended.

Overdosage
Any medication taken in excess can have serious consequences. If you suspect an overdose, seek medical attention immediately.

■ *Symptoms of Estraderm overdose may include:*
Nausea, vomiting, withdrawal bleeding

Generic name:

ESTRADIOL

See Estraderm, page 490.

Generic name:

ESTRADIOL VAGINAL RING

See Estring, page 496.

Brand name:

ESTRING

Pronounced: ESST-ring
Generic name: Estradiol vaginal ring

Why is this drug prescribed?

Estring is an estrogen replacement system for relief of the vaginal problems that often occur after menopause, including vaginal dryness, burning, and itching, and difficult or painful intercourse. Estring is also prescribed for postmenopausal urinary problems such as difficulty urinating or urinary urgency.

Most important fact about this drug

Because estrogen replacement therapy is not advisable if you are in any danger of developing cancer, your doctor should take a complete medical and family history—and do a complete physical exam—before prescribing Estring. As a general rule, you should have an examination at least once a year while using Estring.

How should you use this medication?

Each Estring is left in place for 3 months. Press the Estring into an oval and insert it as deeply as possible into the upper third of the vagina. The exact position is unimportant as long as you don't feel the ring. If the ring causes discomfort, it is probably not far enough inside.

If the ring slips down into the lower part of the vagina, push it back up with your finger. If it falls out, rinse it in warm water and reinsert it. When replacing the ring, simply hook a finger through it and pull it out.

■ If you miss a dose...
   If the ring is not replaced after 90 days, the dose of estrogen will gradually decline and your symptoms will return.

■ *Storage instructions...*
   Store at room temperature.

What side effects may occur?
Side effects cannot be anticipated. If any develop or change in intensity, tell your doctor as soon as possible. Only your doctor can determine if it is safe for you to continue using Estring.

■ *More common side effects may include:*
   Abdominal pain, arthritis, back pain, flu-like symptoms, headaches, insomnia, joint pain, nausea, sinus inflammation, upper respiratory tract infections, vaginal discharge, vaginal discomfort or pain, vaginal inflammation or bleeding, yeast infection

■ *Less common side effects may include:*
   Abnormal bleeding from the uterus, allergic reaction, bone pain, breast pain, bronchitis, chest pain, diarrhea, fainting, family stress, gas, genital itching or eruptions, hemorrhoids, hot flashes, inability to hold urine, indigestion, middle ear infection, migraine, painful urination, skin inflammation, sore throat, stomach inflammation, swelling of legs, toothache, urinary tract infection

Why should this drug not be prescribed?
Do not use Estring if there is any chance that you have breast cancer or any other cancer stimulated by estrogen. Also avoid Estring if there is a possibility that you are pregnant. Do not use Estring if you have unexplained genital bleeding, and avoid it in the event of an allergic reaction.

Special warnings about this medication
Estrogen replacement therapy is associated with a slight increase in the chances of heart disease, high blood pressure, gallbladder disease, certain forms of cancer, and excessive calcium levels. Estrogen is also suspected of increasing the risk of breast cancer, although this remains controversial.

Any vaginal infection should be cleared up before you begin Estring therapy. If an infection develops after you begin, you'll need to remove the ring during treatment.

If you have a liver problem, Estring should be used with caution. Make sure your doctor is aware of the situation.

Possible food and drug interactions
when using this medication
No interactions have been reported, but Estring should be removed during treatment with other vaginally administered drugs.

Special information
if you are pregnant or breastfeeding
Estring must not be used during pregnancy and is not intended for nursing mothers.

Recommended dosage
Insert a new ring every 3 months.

Overdosage
An overdose from Estring is unlikely. An oral overdose of estrogen could be expected to cause the symptoms listed below.

■ *Symptoms of estrogen overdose may include:*
Nausea, vomiting, vaginal bleeding

Generic name:

ESTROPIPATE

See Ogen, page 917.

Generic name:

ETANERCEPT

See Enbrel, page 474.

Generic name:

ETODOLAC

See Lodine, page 708.

Brand name:

EULEXIN

Pronounced: you-LEKS-in
Generic name: Flutamide

Why is this drug prescribed?
Eulexin is used along with drugs such as Lupron to treat prostate cancer. Eulexin belongs to a class of drugs known as antiandrogens. It blocks the effect of the male hormone testosterone. Giving Eulexin with Lupron, which reduces the body's testosterone levels, is one way of treating prostate

cancer. For some forms of prostate cancer, radiation therapy is given along with the drugs.

Most important fact about this drug
Taking Eulexin and Lupron together is essential in this form of treatment. You should not interrupt their doses or stop taking either of these medications without consulting your doctor.

How should you take this medication?
Take Eulexin exactly as prescribed. Do not use more or less, and do not take it more often than instructed.

■ *If you miss a dose...*
Take it as soon as you remember. If it is almost time for your next dose, skip the one you missed and go back to your regular schedule. Never take 2 doses at once.

■ *Storage instructions...*
Store at room temperature.

What side effects may occur?
Side effects cannot be anticipated. If any develop or change in intensity, inform your doctor immediately. Since Eulexin is always given with another antiandrogen drug, when a side effect develops, it is difficult to know which drug is responsible. Only your doctor can determine if it is safe for you to continue taking Eulexin.

■ *More common side effects may include:*
Breast tissue swelling and tenderness, diarrhea, hot flashes, impotence, loss of sex drive, nausea, vomiting

■ *Less common side effects may include:*
Confusion, decreased sexual ability, jaundice and liver damage, rash, sun sensitivity (rashes, blisters upon exposure to sun), urine discoloration (amber or yellow-green)

When the drugs are used along with radiation therapy, additional side effects may include bladder inflammation, bleeding from the rectum, blood in the urine, and intestinal problems.

Why should this drug not be prescribed?
Do not take Eulexin if you have ever had an allergic reaction to it or are sensitive to it or to any of the colorings or other inactive ingredients in the capsules.

Special warnings about this medication

Eulexin may cause liver damage in some people. Your doctor will do blood tests to check your liver function before you start treatment with Eulexin, and at regular intervals thereafter. If a liver problem does develop, you may need to take less Eulexin or stop taking the drug altogether. Report any signs or symptoms that might suggest liver damage to your doctor right away. Warning signs include dark urine, itching, flu-like symptoms, jaundice (a yellowing of the skin and eyes), persistent appetite loss, and persistent tenderness on the right side of the upper abdomen.

Possible food and drug interactions
when taking this medication

If you are already taking the anticoagulant drug warfarin (Coumadin), you will need to be monitored especially closely after treatment with Eulexin begins. Your doctor may need to lower your dosage of warfarin.

Recommended dosage

The recommended adult Eulexin dosage is 2 capsules 3 times a day at 8-hour intervals for a total daily dosage of 750 milligrams.

Overdosage

You may notice breast development or tenderness with an overdose of Eulexin. Any medication taken in excess can have serious consequences. If you suspect an overdose, seek medical attention immediately.

Brand name:

EVISTA

Pronounced: Eve-IST-ah
Generic name: Raloxifene hydrochloride

Why is this drug prescribed?

Evista is prescribed to prevent osteoporosis, the brittle-bone disease that strikes some women after menopause. A variety of factors promote osteoporosis. The more factors that apply to you, the greater your chances of developing the disease. These factors include:

Caucasian or Asian descent
Slender build
Early menopause
Smoking
Drinking
A diet low in calcium

An inactive lifestyle
Osteoporosis in the family

Most important fact about this drug

Like estrogen, Evista reduces bone loss and increases bone density. However, Evista does not have estrogen-like effects on the uterus and breasts, and therefore is unlikely to increase the risk of cancer, as estrogen therapy sometimes can do.

Although Evista has been shown to increase bone density over the course of a two-year study, its longer-term ability to prevent bone fractures has not yet been proven.

How should you use this medication?

Take Evista once daily, at any time, with or without food. Take calcium and vitamin D supplements as well, if you do not get enough in your diet. Avoid alcohol and tobacco. Do weight-bearing exercises to strengthen your bones.

■ *If you miss a dose...*
Take it as soon as you remember. If it is almost time for your next dose, skip the one you missed and go back to your regular schedule. Never take a double dose.

■ *Storage instructions...*
Store at room temperature.

What side effects may occur?

Evista has one very positive side effect: It lowers total cholesterol and LDL ("bad") cholesterol. It does not affect HDL ("good") cholesterol or triglyceride levels.

The unwanted side effects of Evista cannot be predicted. If any develop or change in intensity, inform your doctor as soon as possible. Only your doctor can determine if it is safe for you to continue taking Evista.

■ *More common side effects may include:*
Abdominal pain, arthritis, breast pain, chest pain, depression, fever, flu symptoms, gas, gynecological problems, hot flashes, increased cough, indigestion, infection, inflammation of the throat and sinus passages, insomnia, joint pain, leg cramps, muscle ache, nausea, rash, stomach and intestinal problems, sweating, swelling, urinary tract infection, vomiting, weight gain

■ *Less common side effects may include:*
Laryngitis, migraine, pneumonia

Why should this drug not be prescribed?

Evista is not for use by women who are—or could become—pregnant. You should also avoid this drug if you have a history of blood clot formation, including deep vein thrombosis (blood clot in the legs), pulmonary embolism (blood clot in the lungs), and retinal vein thrombosis (blood clot in the retina of the eye), since Evista increases the risk of clots. Avoid the drug, too, if it gives you an allergic reaction.

Special warnings about this medication

Because of Evista's tendency to promote clots, you should not take it during long periods of immobilization such as recovery from surgery or prolonged bed rest, or for 72 hours beforehand. If you are scheduled for surgery, make sure the doctor is aware that you are taking Evista.

For the same reason, if you are going on a trip where your movement will be restricted, make a point of periodically getting up and walking around.

Evista is not needed prior to menopause and shouldn't be taken until menopause has passed. It has not been studied in premenopausal women and its use is not recommended.

Use Evista with caution if you have congestive heart failure, a liver condition, or cancer. Be cautious, too, if you've had breast cancer in the past; the drug's effect in this situation is unknown.

If you develop unusual uterine bleeding or breast problems while taking Evista, tell your doctor immediately.

Evista will not cure hot flashes. (In fact, it may cause them.) Nevertheless, never combine Evista with estrogen hormones.

Possible food and drug interactions
when taking this medication

If Evista is taken with certain other drugs, the effects of either could be increased, decreased, or altered. It is especially important to check with your doctor before combining Evista with the following:

Cholestyramine (Questran)
Clofibrate (Atromid-S)
Diazepam (Valium)
Diazoxide (Proglycem)
Ibuprofen (Advil, Motrin, Nuprin)
Indomethacin (Indocin)
Naproxen (Aleve, Anaprox, Naprosyn)
Warfarin (Coumadin)

**Special information
if you are pregnant or breastfeeding**
Evista can harm a developing baby. Do not use if you are or may become pregnant. Also avoid breastfeeding while taking Evista.

Recommended dosage

POSTMENOPAUSAL WOMEN

The recommended dosage is one 60-milligram tablet once a day.

Overdosage
There have not been any reports of overdose with Evista. However, any medication taken in excess can have serious consequences. If you suspect an overdose, seek medical attention immediately.

Brand name:

EXGEST LA

See Entex LA, page 477.

Generic name:

FAMCICLOVIR

See Famvir, below.

Generic name:

FAMOTIDINE

See Pepcid, page 975.

Brand name:

FAMVIR

*Pronounced: FAM-veer
Generic name: Famciclovir*

Why is this drug prescribed?
Famvir tablets are used to treat herpes zoster, commonly referred to as "shingles," in adults. Shingles is a painful rash with raised, red pimples on the trunk of the body, usually the back. Because it is caused by the same virus that causes chickenpox, only people who have had chickenpox can get

shingles. When prescribed for shingles, Famvir works best in people age 50 or over.

Famvir is also prescribed to treat attacks of genital herpes and to prevent future flare-ups. For people with HIV infections, it is used as a treatment for both genital and oral herpes.

Most important fact about this drug

Famvir is most effective if started within the first 48 hours after shingles first appears; treatment should be started at the first sign or symptom of genital herpes. Famvir treatment may not be effective if it is delayed more than 72 hours after the herpes zoster rash first appears or more than 6 hours after genital herpes becomes evident. Thus, it is important to see your doctor as soon as possible after symptoms appear.

How should you take this medication?

For maximum benefit, take Famvir for the full time of treatment, even if your symptoms begin to clear up. Do not, however, take Famvir more often or for a longer time than your doctor directs.

You may take Famvir with meals or in between.

■ *If you miss a dose...*
Take the forgotten dose as soon as you remember. If it is almost time for your next dose, skip the one you missed and go back to your regular schedule. Never take two doses at the same time.

■ *Storage instructions...*
Store at room temperature.

What side effects may occur?

Side effects cannot be anticipated. If any develop or change in intensity, inform your doctor as soon as possible. Only your doctor can determine if it is safe for you to continue taking Famvir.

■ *More common side effects may include:*
Constipation, diarrhea, dizziness, fatigue, fever, headache, nausea, vomiting

■ *Less common side effects may include:*
Abdominal pain, back pain, chills and fever, gas, indigestion, injury, insomnia, irritated sinuses, itching, joint pain, loss of appetite, pain, prickling or burning sensation of the skin, sleepiness, sore throat, upper respiratory infection

There have been infrequent cases of hallucinations, hives, and rash, and some people—especially older adults—may experience confusion, including delirium and disorientation.

Why should this drug not be prescribed?

Do not take Famvir if you are sensitive to it or have ever had an allergic reaction to it. Also avoid Famvir if you are sensitive to Denavir (penciclovir cream).

Special warnings about this medication

Famvir speeds healing of shingles and genital herpes, but it is not a cure. It may not prevent transmission of genital herpes to others, so you should avoid sexual intercourse whenever you have symptoms of the disease.

If you have any kidney problems, be sure your doctor knows about them before prescribing Famvir for you.

Possible food and drug interactions
when taking this medication

If Famvir is taken with certain other drugs, the effects of either could be increased, decreased, or altered. It is especially important to check with your doctor before combining Famvir with probenecid (Benemid), a drug used to treat gout (a type of arthritis).

Special information
if you are pregnant or breastfeeding

The effects of Famvir during pregnancy have not been adequately studied. If you are pregnant or plan to become pregnant, inform your doctor immediately. Famvir should be used during pregnancy only when the benefit to the mother clearly outweighs the potential risk to the baby. Famvir may appear in breast milk, and could affect a nursing infant. If this drug is essential to your health, your doctor may advise you to discontinue breastfeeding until your treatment with Famvir is finished.

Recommended dosage

ADULTS

Herpes Zoster
The usual adult dose is 500 milligrams every 8 hours for 7 days.

Recurrent Genital Herpes Treatment
The usual dose is 125 milligrams twice a day for 5 days.

Recurrent Genital Herpes Prevention
The usual dose is 250 milligrams twice a day for up to one year. Famvir therapy to prevent genital herpes has not been tested for periods exceeding one year.

Recurrent Oral or Genital Herpes in HIV-infected Individuals
The usual dose is 500 milligrams twice a day for 7 days. Smaller doses are prescribed for people with damaged kidneys.

CHILDREN

Safety and effectiveness in children under the age of 18 have not been established.

Overdosage
Any medication taken in excess can have serious consequences. If you suspect an overdose, seek medical attention immediately.

Brand name:

FASTIN

Pronounced: FAS-tin
Generic name: Phentermine hydrochloride
Other brand names: Adipex-P, Ionamin, Oby-Cap

Why is this drug prescribed?
Fastin, an appetite suppressant, is prescribed for short-term use (a few weeks) as part of an overall diet plan for weight reduction. Fastin should be used along with a behavior modification program.

Most important fact about this drug
Take Fastin only as directed by your doctor. Do not combine it with the weight-loss drug fenfluramine (Pondimin); this combination can cause dangerously high blood pressure in the lungs or damage to the valves in the heart. Do not take it more often or for a longer time than your doctor has ordered. Fastin can lose its effectiveness after a few weeks.

How should you take this medication?
Take Fastin about 2 hours after breakfast. Do not take it late in the evening because it may keep you from sleeping.

Take Adipex-P before breakfast or up to 2 hours after breakfast. Tablets can be broken in half, if necessary.

Take Ionamin before breakfast or 10 to 14 hours before you go to bed. Ionamin capsules should be swallowed whole.

- *If you miss a dose...*
  Skip the missed dose completely; then take the next dose at the regularly scheduled time.

- *Storage instructions...*
  Store at room temperature.

What side effects may occur?
Side effects cannot be anticipated. If any develop or change in intensity, inform your doctor as soon as possible. Only your doctor can determine if it is safe for you to continue taking this medication.

- *Side effects may include:*
  Changes in sex drive, constipation, diarrhea, dizziness, dry mouth, exaggerated feelings of depression or elation, headache, high blood pressure, hives, impotence, inability to fall or stay asleep, increased heart rate, overstimulation, restlessness, stomach or intestinal problems, throbbing heartbeat, tremors, unpleasant taste

Why should this drug not be prescribed?
If you are sensitive to or have ever had an allergic reaction to phentermine hydrochloride or other drugs that stimulate the nervous system, you should not take this medication. Make sure your doctor is aware of any drug reactions you have experienced.

Do not take this drug if you have hardening of the arteries, symptoms of heart or blood vessel disease, an overactive thyroid gland, the eye condition known as glaucoma, or moderate to severe high blood pressure. Also avoid this drug if you are agitated, have ever abused drugs, or have taken an MAO inhibitor, including antidepressant drugs such as Nardil and Parnate, within the last 14 days.

Special warnings about this medication
Fastin may affect your ability to perform potentially hazardous activities. Therefore, you should be extremely careful if you have to drive a car or operate machinery.

You can become psychologically dependent on this drug. Consult your doctor if you rely on this drug to maintain a state of well-being.

If you stop taking Fastin suddenly after you have taken high doses for a long time, you may find you are extremely fatigued or depressed, or that you have trouble sleeping.

If you continually take too much of any appetite suppressant it can cause severe skin disorders, a pronounced inability to fall or stay asleep, irritability, hyperactivity, and personality changes.

Even if your blood pressure is only mildly high, be careful taking this drug.

Possible food and drug interactions
when taking this medication

Remember that this drug should never be combined with the weight-loss drug fenfluramine (Pondimin); very dangerous side effects could result. This drug may also react badly with alcohol. Avoid alcoholic beverages while you are taking it.

If Fastin is taken with certain other drugs, the effects of either can be increased, decreased, or altered. It is especially important that you check with your doctor before combining Fastin with the following:

Drugs that boost serotonin levels, such as the antidepressants Luvox, Paxil, Prozac, and Zoloft

Drugs classified as MAO inhibitors, including the antidepressants Nardil and Parnate

Diabetes medications such as insulin and Micronase

High blood pressure medications such as guanethidine (Ismelin)

Special information
if you are pregnant or breastfeeding

The effects of Fastin during pregnancy have not been adequately studied. If you are pregnant, plan to become pregnant, or are breastfeeding, notify your doctor immediately.

Recommended dosage

ADULTS

Fastin or Oby-Cap

The usual dosage is 1 capsule approximately 2 hours after breakfast. One capsule should suppress your appetite for 12 to 14 hours.

Adipex-P
The usual dose is 1 capsule or tablet a day, taken before breakfast or up to 2 hours after breakfast. Some people need only half a tablet each day. Others may find it more effective to take half a tablet twice daily.

Ionamin
The usual dose is 1 capsule a day, taken before breakfast or 10 to 14 hours before bedtime.

CHILDREN

This drug is not recommended for use in children under 12 years of age.

Overdosage
Any medication taken in excess can have serious consequences. An overdose of Fastin can be fatal. If you suspect an overdose, seek emergency medical treatment immediately.

- *Symptoms of Fastin overdose may include:*
  Abdominal cramps, aggressiveness, confusion, diarrhea, exaggerated reflexes, hallucinations, high or low blood pressure, irregular heartbeat, nausea, panic states, rapid breathing, restlessness, tremors, vomiting

Fatigue and depression may follow the stimulant effects of Fastin.

In cases of fatal poisoning, convulsions and coma usually precede death.

Generic name:

FELBAMATE

See Felbatol, page 509.

Brand name:

FELBATOL

Pronounced: FELL-ba-tohl
Generic name: Felbamate

Why is this drug prescribed?
Felbatol, a relatively new epilepsy medication, is used alone or with other drugs to treat partial seizures with or without generalization (seizures in which consciousness may be retained or lost). It is also used with other

medications to treat seizures associated with Lennox-Gastaut syndrome (a childhood condition characterized by brief loss of awareness and muscle tone).

Felbatol is prescribed only when other medications have failed to control severe cases of epilepsy.

Most important fact about this drug
When taking Felbatol, be alert for signs of a very rare but dangerous side effect called aplastic anemia, in which the red blood cell count declines drastically. Warning signs include weakness, fatigue, and a tendency to easily bruise or bleed. Be on the watch, also, for signs of liver problems such as yellowing of the skin or eyes. There have been reports of fatal cases of liver failure among people taking Felbatol.

How should you take this medication?
Take this medication exactly as prescribed by your doctor. Felbatol should not be stopped suddenly. This could increase the frequency of your seizures.

If you are taking Felbatol liquid, shake well before using.

■ *If you miss a dose...*
Take the forgotten dose as soon as you remember. If it is almost time for your next dose, skip the one you missed and go back to your regular schedule. Never take a double dose.

■ *Storage instructions...*
Felbatol should be stored in a tightly closed container, at room temperature, away from excessive heat and moisture.

What side effects may occur?
Side effects cannot be anticipated. If any develop or change in intensity, notify your doctor as soon as possible. Only your doctor can determine if it is safe for you to continue taking Felbatol.

■ *Side effects in adults taking Felbatol alone may include:*
Acne, anxiety, constipation, diarrhea, double vision, ear infection, facial swelling, fatigue, headache, inability to fall or stay asleep, indigestion, loss of appetite, menstrual irregularities, nausea, nasal inflammation, rash, upper respiratory infection, urinary tract infection, vomiting, weight decrease

■ *Side effects in adults taking Felbatol with other medication may include:*
Abdominal pain, abnormal stride, abnormal taste, abnormal vision, anxiety, chest pain, constipation, depression, diarrhea, dizziness, double vision, dry mouth, fatigue, fever, headache, inability to fall or stay asleep, indigestion, lack of muscle coordination, loss of appetite, muscle pain, nausea, nervousness, pins and needles, rash, sinus inflammation, sleepiness, sore throat, stupor, tremor, upper respiratory infection, vomiting

■ *Side effects in children taking Felbatol with other medication may include:*
Abnormal stride, abnormal thinking, abnormally small pupils (pinpoint pupils), constipation, coughing, diarrhea, ear infection, fatigue, fever, headache, hiccups, inability to control urination, inability to fall or stay asleep, indigestion, lack of muscle coordination, loss of appetite, mood changes, nausea, nervousness, pain, rash, red or purple spots on skin, sleepiness, sore throat, taste changes, unstable emotions, upper respiratory infection, vomiting, weight decrease

Why should this drug not be prescribed?
If you are sensitive to or have ever had an allergic reaction to Felbatol or similar drugs, or if you have ever had any blood abnormalities or liver problems, do not take this medication. Make sure your doctor is aware of any drug reactions you have experienced.

Special warnings about this medication
Remember to watch for signs of aplastic anemia. (See "Most important fact about this drug.") If you have ever had liver problems, be sure to tell your doctor.

Expect your doctor to monitor your response carefully when you start taking Felbatol and to check your liver function every 1 or 2 weeks.

Possible food and drug interactions when taking this medication
If you are taking Felbatol with certain other drugs, the effects of either could be increased, decreased, or altered. It is especially important to check with your doctor before combining Felbatol with other epilepsy drugs, such as Dilantin, Depakene, Depakote, Tegretol, and phenobarbital.

Special information
if you are pregnant or breastfeeding

The effects of Felbatol during pregnancy have not been adequately studied. If you are pregnant or plan to become pregnant, inform your doctor immediately. Felbatol appears in breast milk and could affect a nursing infant. If this medication is essential to your health, your doctor may advise you to discontinue breastfeeding until your treatment is finished.

Recommended dosage

ADULTS 14 YEARS OF AGE AND OVER

Whether Felbatol is taken alone or with other antiepileptic drugs, the usual starting dose is 1,200 milligrams per day divided into smaller doses and taken 3 or 4 times daily. Your doctor may gradually increase your daily dose to as much as 3,600 milligrams.

If you are already taking a drug to control your epilepsy, your doctor will reduce its dosage when you add Felbatol.

CHILDREN WITH LENNOX-GASTAUT SYNDROME (2 TO 14 YEARS)

The usual dose is 15 milligrams per 2.2 pounds of body weight per day divided into smaller doses taken 3 or 4 times daily. Your doctor may gradually increase your child's dose to 45 milligrams per 2.2 pounds of body weight per day. The doctor will reduce the amount of any other epilepsy drug your child is taking when starting Felbatol.

Overdosage

Any medication taken in excess can have serious consequences. If you suspect an overdose, seek medical treatment immediately.

■ *Symptoms of Felbatol overdose may include:*
  Mild stomach upset, unusually fast heartbeat

Brand name:

FELDENE

Pronounced: FELL-deen
Generic name: Piroxicam

Why is this drug prescribed?

Feldene, a nonsteroidal anti-inflammatory drug, is used to relieve the inflammation, swelling, stiffness, and joint pain associated with rheumatoid arthritis and osteoarthritis (the most common form of arthritis). It is prescribed both for sudden flare-ups and for long-term treatment.

Most important fact about this drug

In a few patients on long-term therapy, Feldene can cause stomach ulcers and bleeding. Warning signs include severe abdominal or stomach cramps, pain or burning in the stomach, and black, tarry stools. Inform your doctor immediately if you develop any of these symptoms.

How should you take this medication?

To avoid digestive side effects, take Feldene with food or an antacid, and with a full glass of water. Never take it on an empty stomach.

Take this medication exactly as prescribed by your doctor. Avoid alcohol and aspirin while taking this drug.

■ *If you miss a dose...*
If you forget to take a dose, take it as soon as you remember. If it is almost time for your next dose, skip the one you missed and go back to your regular schedule Never take 2 doses at the same time.

■ *Storage instructions...*
Store at room temperature. Protect from light and heat.

What side effects may occur?

Side effects cannot be anticipated. If any develop or change in intensity, inform your doctor as soon as possible. Only your doctor can determine if it is safe for you to continue taking Feldene.

■ *More common side effects may include:*
Abdominal pain or discomfort, anemia, constipation, diarrhea, dizziness, fluid retention, gas, general feeling of ill health, headache, heartburn, indigestion, inflammation inside the mouth, itching, loss of appetite, nausea, rash, ringing in ears, sleepiness, stomach upset, vertigo

■ *Less common or rare side effects may include:*
Abdominal bleeding, severe allergic reactions, angioedema (swelling of lips, face, tongue and throat), black stools, blood in the urine, blurred vision, bruising, colicky pain, congestive heart failure (worsening of), depression, dry mouth, eye irritations, fatigue, fever, flu-like symptoms, hepatitis, high blood pressure, hives, inability to sleep, joint pain, labored breathing, low or high blood sugar, nervousness, nosebleed, serum sickness (fever, painful joints, enlarged lymph nodes, skin rash), skin

allergy to sunlight, skin eruptions, Stevens-Johnson syndrome (blisters in the mouth and eyes), sweating, swollen eyes, vomiting, vomiting blood, weight loss or gain, wheezing, worsening of angina, yellow eyes and skin

Why should this drug not be prescribed?

If you are sensitive to or have ever had an allergic reaction to Feldene, aspirin, or similar drugs, or if you have had asthma attacks caused by aspirin or other drugs of this type, you should not take this medication. Make sure that your doctor is aware of any drug reactions that you have experienced.

Special warnings about this medication

If you have heart disease, or high blood pressure, or other conditions that cause fluid retention, use this drug with caution. Feldene can increase water retention.

This drug should be used with caution if you have kidney or liver disease; it can cause liver inflammation in some people.

Drugs such as Feldene may cause eye disturbances in some people. If you develop visual problems, notify your eye doctor.

Possible food and drug interactions
when taking this medication

If Feldene is taken with certain other drugs, the effects of either could be increased, decreased, or altered. It is especially important to check with your doctor before combining Feldene with the following:

Anticoagulants (blood thinners such as Coumadin)
Aspirin
Lithium

Special information
if you are pregnant or breastfeeding

Feldene is not recommended for use in nursing mothers or pregnant women. If you are pregnant or plan to become pregnant, inform your doctor immediately.

Recommended dosage

ADULTS

Rheumatoid Arthritis and Osteoarthritis:
The usual dose is 20 milligrams a day in one dose. Your doctor may want you to divide this dose into smaller ones. You will not feel Feldene's full effects

for 7 to 12 days, although some relief of symptoms will start to occur soon after you take the medication.

CHILDREN
The safety and effectiveness of Feldene have not been established in children.

Overdosage
Although there are no specific symptoms of a Feldene overdose, any medication taken in excess can have serious consequences. If you suspect an overdose, seek medical attention immediately.

Generic name:

FELODIPINE

See Plendil, page 1014.

Brand name:

FEMSTAT

Pronounced: FEM-stat
Generic name: Butoconazole nitrate

Why is this drug prescribed?
Femstat Vaginal Cream cures yeast-like fungal infections of the vulva and vagina.

Most important fact about this drug
To obtain maximum benefit, it is important that you continue to use Femstat Vaginal Cream during menstruation and that you finish using all of the medication, even if your symptoms have disappeared.

How should you use this medication?
Use this medication exactly as prescribed. To keep it from getting on your clothing, wear a sanitary napkin. Do not use a tampon; it will absorb the drug. Do not douche unless your doctor tells you to do so.

While using Femstat, wear cotton underwear or pantyhose with a cotton crotch. Avoid synthetic fabrics such as rayon and nylon.

To apply Femstat:
1. Following the instructions, fill the applicator that comes with the vaginal

cream to the level indicated; the cream also comes in a prefilled applicator.
2. Lie on your back with your knees drawn up.
3. Gently insert the applicator high into the vagina and push the plunger.
4. Withdraw the applicator and discard it.

To avoid reinfection, refrain from intercourse during treatment or ask your partner to use a condom.

■ *If you miss a dose...*
Insert it as soon as you remember. If it is almost time for your next dose, skip the one you missed and go back to your regular schedule.

■ *Storage instructions...*
Store at room temperature, away from heat. Do not freeze.

What side effects may occur?
Side effects cannot be anticipated. If any develop or change in intensity, inform your doctor as soon as possible. Only your doctor can determine if it is safe for you to continue using Femstat.

■ *Side effects may include:*
Itching of the fingers, soreness, swelling, vaginal discharge, vulvar itching, vulvar or vaginal burning

Why should this drug not be prescribed?
If you are sensitive to or have ever had an allergic reaction to butoconazole nitrate or any other ingredients in Femstat Cream, you should not use this medication. Make sure your doctor is aware of any drug reactions you have experienced.

Special warnings about this medication
If your symptoms persist, or if you become irritated or have an allergic reaction while using this medication, notify your doctor.

If this is the first time you have had vaginal itching and discomfort, see your doctor before using Femstat to be sure it is the right medication to use.

Do not use Femstat Cream if you have abdominal pain, a fever, or a vaginal discharge with a foul odor; instead, see your doctor.

If your infection doesn't clear up in 3 days, call your doctor. The problem may not be a yeast infection.

If your symptoms come back within 2 months, call your doctor. It could be a sign of pregnancy or a condition such as AIDS or diabetes.

Do not use this product if you have diabetes, have tested positive for HIV, or have AIDS.

Femstat Cream may damage condoms and diaphragms. Employ another method of birth control while you are using this product.

This product is for vaginal use only. Avoid getting it in your eyes or mouth.

**Possible food and drug interactions
when taking this medication**
No interactions with other drugs have been reported.

**Special information
if you are pregnant or breastfeeding**
You should not use Femstat if you are pregnant or think you may be pregnant. It is not known whether this drug appears in breast milk. If Femstat is essential to your health, your doctor may advise you to discontinue breastfeeding until your treatment is finished.

Recommended dosage

ADULTS

The recommended dose is 1 applicatorful of cream inserted in the vagina at bedtime for 3 days.

CHILDREN

Femstat Cream should not be used by girls under 12 years of age.

Overdosage
No overdosage has been reported.

Generic name:

FEXOFENADINE

See Allegra, page 36.

Generic name:

FINASTERIDE FOR BALDNESS

See Propecia, page 1060.

Generic name:

FINASTERIDE FOR PROSTATE PROBLEMS

See Proscar, page 1067.

Brand name:

FIORICET

Pronounced: fee-OAR-i-set
Generic ingredients: Butalbital, Acetaminophen, Caffeine
Other brand names: Anolor 300, Esgic, Esgic-Plus

Why is this drug prescribed?

Fioricet, a strong, non-narcotic pain reliever and relaxant, is prescribed for the relief of tension headache symptoms caused by muscle contractions in the head, neck, and shoulder area. It combines a sedative barbiturate (butalbital), a non-aspirin pain reliever (acetaminophen), and caffeine.

Most important fact about this drug

Mental and physical dependence can occur with the use of barbiturates such as butalbital when these drugs are taken in higher than recommended doses over long periods of time.

How should you take this medication?

Take Fioricet exactly as prescribed. Do not increase the amount you take without your doctor's approval.

■ *If you miss a dose...*
Take it as soon as you remember. If it is almost time for your next dose, skip the one you missed and go back to your regular schedule. Never take 2 doses at the same time.

■ *Storage instructions...*
Store at room temperature in a tight, light-resistant container.

What side effects may occur?

Side effects cannot be anticipated. If any develop or change in intensity, inform your doctor as soon as possible. Only your doctor can determine if it is safe for you to continue taking Fioricet.

■ *More common side effects may include:*
Abdominal pain, dizziness, drowsiness, intoxicated feeling, light-headedness, nausea, sedation, shortness of breath, vomiting

■ *Less common or rare side effects may include:*
Agitation, allergic reactions, constipation, depression, difficulty swallowing, dry mouth, earache, exaggerated feeling of well-being, excessive sweating, excessive urination, excitement, fainting, fatigue, fever, flatulence, headache, heartburn, heavy eyelids, high energy, hot spells, itching, leg pain, mental confusion, muscle fatigue, numbness, rapid heartbeat, ringing in the ears, seizure, shaky feeling, skin redness and/or peeling, sluggishness, stuffy nose, tingling

Why should this drug not be prescribed?
If you are sensitive to or have ever had an allergic reaction to barbiturates, acetaminophen, or caffeine, you should not take this medication. Make sure that your doctor is aware of any drug reactions that you have experienced.

Unless you are directed to do so by your doctor, do not take this medication if you have porphyria (an inherited metabolic disorder affecting the liver or bone marrow).

Special warnings about this medication
Fioricet may cause you to become drowsy or less alert; therefore, driving or operating dangerous machinery or participating in any hazardous activity that requires full mental alertness is not recommended until you know your response to this drug.

If you are being treated for severe depression or have a history of severe depression or drug abuse, consult with your doctor before taking Fioricet.

Use this drug with caution if you are elderly or in a weakened condition, if you have liver or kidney problems, or if you have severe abdominal trouble.

Possible food and drug interactions
when taking this medication
Butalbital slows the central nervous system (CNS) and intensifies the effects of alcohol and other CNS depressants. Use of alcohol with this drug may also cause overdose symptoms. Avoid alcoholic beverages while taking Fioricet.

If Fioricet is taken with certain other drugs, the effects of either could be increased, decreased, or altered. It is especially important to check with your doctor before combining Fioricet with the following:

Antihistamines such as Benadryl
Drugs known as monoamine oxidase inhibitors, including the antidepressants Nardil and Parnate
Drugs to treat depression such as Elavil
Major tranquilizers such as Haldol and Thorazine

Muscle relaxants such as Flexeril
Narcotic pain relievers such as Darvon
Sleep aids such as Halcion
Tranquilizers such as Xanax and Valium

Special information
if you are pregnant or breastfeeding

If you are pregnant or plan to become pregnant, inform your doctor immediately. Fioricet can affect a developing baby. It also appears in breast milk. If this medication is essential to your health, your doctor may advise you to discontinue breastfeeding your baby until your treatment is finished.

Recommended dosage

ADULTS

The usual dose of Fioricet is 1 or 2 tablets taken every 4 hours as needed. Do not exceed a total dose of 6 tablets per day.

The usual dose of Esgic-Plus is 1 tablet every 4 hours as needed. Do not take more than 6 tablets a day.

CHILDREN

The safety and effectiveness of Fioricet have not been established in children under 12 years of age.

OLDER ADULTS

Fioricet may cause excitement, depression, and confusion in older people. Therefore, your doctor will prescribe a dose individualized to suit your needs.

Overdosage

Symptoms of Fioricet overdose can be due to its barbiturate or its acetaminophen component.

■ *Symptoms of barbiturate poisoning may include:*
Coma, confusion, drowsiness, low blood pressure, shock, slow or troubled breathing

Overdose due to the acetaminophen component of Fioricet may cause kidney and liver damage, blood disorders, or coma due to low blood sugar. Massive doses may cause liver failure.

- *Symptoms of liver damage include:*
  Excess perspiration, feeling of bodily discomfort, nausea, vomiting

If you suspect an overdose, seek emergency medical treatment immediately.

Brand name:

FIORINAL

Pronounced: fee-OR-i-nahl
Generic ingredients: Butalbital, Aspirin, Caffeine

Why is this drug prescribed?
Fiorinal, a strong, non-narcotic pain reliever and muscle relaxant, is prescribed for the relief of tension headache symptoms caused by stress or muscle contraction in the head, neck, and shoulder area. It combines a non-narcotic, sedative barbiturate (butalbital) with a pain reliever (aspirin) and a stimulant (caffeine).

Most important fact about this drug
Barbiturates such as butalbital can be habit-forming if you take them over long periods of time.

How should you take this medication?
For best relief, take Fiorinal as soon as a headache begins.

Take the medication with a full glass of water or food to reduce stomach irritation. Do not take this medication if it has a strong odor of vinegar.

Take Fiorinal exactly as prescribed. Do not increase the amount you take without your doctor's approval, or take the drug for longer than prescribed.

- *If you miss a dose...*
  If you take Fiorinal on a regular schedule, take the forgotten dose as soon as you remember. If it is almost time for your next dose, skip the one you missed and go back to your regular schedule. Do not take 2 doses at once.

- *Storage instructions...*
  Store at room temperature. Keep the container tightly closed.

What side effects may occur?
Side effects cannot be anticipated. If any develop or change in intensity, inform your doctor as soon as possible. Only your doctor can determine if it is safe for you to continue taking Fiorinal.

- *More common side effects may include:*
  Dizziness, drowsiness

- *Less common or rare side effects may include:*
  Gas, light-headedness, nausea, skin problems, vomiting

Why should this drug not be prescribed?

If you are sensitive to or have ever had an allergic reaction to barbiturates, aspirin, caffeine, or other sedatives and pain relievers, you should not take this medication. The aspirin in Fiorinal, in particular, can cause a severe reaction in someone allergic to it. Make sure your doctor is aware of any drug reactions you have experienced.

Unless you are directed to do so by your doctor, do not take this medication if you have porphyria (an inherited metabolic disorder affecting the liver or bone marrow).

Because aspirin, when given to children and teenagers suffering from flu or chickenpox, can cause a dangerous neurological disease called Reye's syndrome, do not use Fiorinal under these circumstances.

Fiorinal contains aspirin. If you have a stomach (peptic) ulcer or a disorder affecting the blood clotting process, you should not take Fiorinal. Aspirin may irritate the stomach lining and may cause bleeding.

Special warnings about this medication

Fiorinal may make you drowsy or less alert; therefore, you should not drive or operate dangerous machinery or participate in any hazardous activity that requires full mental alertness until you know your response to this drug.

Taking more of this drug than your doctor has prescribed may cause dependence and symptoms of overdose.

Be especially careful with Fiorinal if you are an older person or in a weakened condition, if you have any kidney, liver, or intestinal problems or an enlarged prostate gland, or if you have had a head injury. Also be cautious if you have a thyroid problem, blood clotting difficulties, or a urinary disorder.

Possible food and drug interactions
when taking this medication

Butalbital decreases the activity of the central nervous system and intensifies the effects of alcohol. Avoid drinking alcohol while you are taking Fiorinal.

If Fiorinal is taken with certain other drugs, the effects of either could be increased, decreased, or altered. It is especially important to check with your doctor before combining Fiorinal with the following:

Acetazolamide (Diamox)
Beta-blocking blood pressure drugs such as Inderal and Tenormin
Blood-thinning drugs such as Coumadin
Drugs known as MAO inhibitors, such as the antidepressants Nardil and Parnate
Insulin
Mercaptopurine (Purinethol)
Methotrexate (Rheumatrex)
Narcotic pain relievers such as Darvon and Percocet
Nonsteroidal anti-inflammatory drugs such as Naprosyn, Motrin
Oral contraceptives
Oral diabetes drugs such as Micronase
Probenecid (Benemid)
Sleep aids such as Halcion and Nembutal
Steroid medications such as prednisone
Sulfinpyrazone (Anturane)
Theophylline (Theo-Dur, others)
Tranquilizers such as Librium, Valium, and Xanax
Valproic acid (Depakene, Depakote)

Special information
if you are pregnant or breastfeeding

The effects of Fiorinal during pregnancy have not been adequately studied. If you are pregnant or plan to become pregnant, inform your doctor immediately. If you take aspirin late in your pregnancy it could cause bleeding in you or your baby, or could delay the baby's birth. Aspirin, butalbital, and caffeine appear in breast milk. If this medication is essential to your health, your doctor may advise you to discontinue breastfeeding until your treatment with this medication is finished.

Recommended dosage

ADULTS

The usual dose of Fiorinal is 1 or 2 tablets or capsules taken every 4 hours. You should not take more than 6 tablets or capsules in a day.

CHILDREN

The safety and effectiveness of Fiorinal have not been established in children.

Overdosage
Any medication taken in excess can have serious consequences. If you suspect an overdose, seek medical attention immediately.

■ *Symptoms of an overdose of Fiorinal are mainly attributed to its barbiturate component. These symptoms may include:*
Coma, confusion, drowsiness, low blood pressure, shock, slow or troubled breathing

■ *Symptoms attributed to the aspirin and caffeine components of Fiorinal may include:*
Abdominal pain, deep, rapid breathing, delirium, high fever, inability to fall or stay asleep, rapid or irregular heartbeat, restlessness, ringing in the ears, seizures, tremor, vomiting

Brand name:

FIORINAL WITH CODEINE

Pronounced: fee-OR-i-nahl with KO-deen
Generic ingredients: Butalbital, Codeine phosphate, Aspirin, Caffeine

Why is this drug prescribed?
Fiorinal with Codeine, a strong narcotic pain reliever and muscle relaxant, is prescribed for the relief of tension headache caused by stress and muscle contraction in the head, neck, and shoulder area. It combines a sedative-barbiturate (butalbital), a narcotic pain reliever and cough suppressant (codeine), a non-narcotic pain and fever reliever (aspirin), and a stimulant (caffeine).

Most important fact about this drug
Barbiturates such as butalbital and narcotics such as codeine can be habit-forming when taken in higher than recommended doses over long periods of time.

How should you take this medication?
Take Fiorinal with Codeine with a full glass of water or food to reduce stomach irritation. Do not take this medication if it has a strong odor of vinegar.

Take Fiorinal with Codeine exactly as prescribed. Do not increase the amount you take without your doctor's approval.

Do not take it more frequently than your doctor has prescribed.

■ *If you miss a dose...*
If you take the drug on a regular schedule, take the forgotten dose as soon as you remember. If it is almost time for your next dose, skip the one you missed and go back to your regular schedule. Do not take 2 doses at once.

■ *Storage instructions...*
Store at room temperature. Keep the container tightly closed.

What side effects may occur?
Side effects cannot be anticipated. If any develop or change in intensity, inform your doctor as soon as possible. Only your doctor can determine if it is safe for you to continue taking Fiorinal with Codeine.

■ *More common side effects may include:*
Abdominal pain, dizziness, drowsiness, nausea

■ *Additional side effects, which can be caused by this drug's components, may include:*
Anemia, blocked air passages, hepatitis, high blood sugar, internal bleeding, intoxicated feeling, irritability, kidney damage, lack of clotting, light-headedness, peptic ulcer, stomach upset, tremors

Why should this drug not be prescribed?
If you are sensitive to or have ever had an allergic reaction to butalbital, codeine, aspirin, caffeine, or other pain relievers, you should not take this medication. Make sure your doctor is aware of any drug reactions you have experienced.

Unless you are directed to do so by your doctor, do not take this medication if you have: a tendency to bleed too much, severe vitamin K deficiency, severe liver damage, nasal polyps (growths or nodules), asthma due to aspirin or other nonsteroidal anti-inflammatory drugs such as Motrin, swelling due to fluid retention, peptic ulcer, or porphyria (an inherited metabolic disorder affecting the liver and bone marrow).

Because aspirin, when given to children and teenagers with chickenpox or flu, can cause a dangerous neurological disease called Reye's syndrome, do not use Fiorinal with Codeine under these circumstances.

Special warnings about this medication

Fiorinal with Codeine may make you drowsy or less alert; therefore, you should not drive or operate dangerous machinery or participate in any hazardous activity that requires full mental alertness until you know how this drug affects you.

Codeine may cause unusually slow or troubled breathing and may increase the pressure caused by fluid surrounding the brain and spinal cord in people with head injury. Codeine also affects brain and spinal cord function and makes it hard for the doctor to see how people with head injuries are doing.

If you have chronic (long-lasting or frequently recurring) tension headaches and your prescribed dose of Fiorinal with Codeine does not relieve the pain, consult with your doctor. Taking more of this drug than your doctor has prescribed may cause dependence and symptoms of overdose.

Aspirin can cause internal bleeding in people with ulcers or bleeding disorders.

Codeine can hide signs of severe abdominal problems.

If you have ever developed dependence on a drug, consult with your doctor before taking Fiorinal with Codeine.

If you are being treated for a kidney, liver, or blood clotting disorder, consult with your doctor before taking Fiorinal with Codeine.

If you are older or in a weakened condition, be very careful taking Fiorinal with Codeine. You should also be careful if you have Addison's disease (an adrenal gland disorder), if you have difficulty urinating, if your prostate gland is enlarged, or if your thyroid gland is not working well.

Possible food and drug interactions
when taking this medication

Fiorinal with Codeine reduces the activity of the central nervous system and intensifies the effects of alcohol. Use of alcohol with this drug may also cause overdose symptoms. Therefore, use of alcohol should be avoided.

If Fiorinal with Codeine is taken with certain other drugs, the effects of either could be increased, decreased, or altered. It is especially important to check with your doctor before combining Fiorinal with Codeine with the following:

Acetazolamide (Diamox)
Antidepressant drugs such as Elavil, Nardil, and Parnate
Antigout medications such as Benemid and Anturane
Antihistamines such as Benadryl
Beta-blocking blood pressure drugs such as Inderal and Tenormin

Blood-thinning drugs such as Coumadin
Divalproex (Depakote)
Insulin
6-Mercaptopurine (Purinethol)
Methotrexate (Rheumatrex)
Narcotic pain relievers such as Darvon and Vicodin
Nonsteroidal anti-inflammatory drugs such as Motrin and Indocin
Oral contraceptives
Oral diabetes drugs such as Micronase
Sleep aids such as Nembutal and Halcion
Steroid drugs such as prednisone
Theophylline (Theo-Dur, others)
Tranquilizers such as Librium, Xanax, and Valium
Valproic acid (Depakene)

Special information
if you are pregnant or breastfeeding

The effects of Fiorinal with Codeine during pregnancy have not been adequately studied. If you are pregnant or plan to become pregnant, inform your doctor immediately. Butalbital, aspirin, caffeine, and codeine appear in breast milk. If this medication is essential to your health, your doctor may advise you to discontinue breastfeeding until your treatment with this medication is finished.

Recommended dosage

ADULTS

The usual dose of Fiorinal with Codeine is 1 or 2 capsules taken every 4 hours. Do not take more than 6 capsules per day.

CHILDREN

The safety and effectiveness of butalbital have not been established in children under 12 years of age.

Overdosage

Symptoms of an overdose of Fiorinal with Codeine are mainly attributed to its barbiturate and codeine ingredients.

■ *Symptoms attributed to the barbiturate ingredient of Fiorinal with Codeine may include:*
Coma, confusion, dizziness, drowsiness, low blood pressure, shock, slow or troubled breathing

- *Symptoms attributed to the codeine ingredient of Fiorinal with Codeine may include:*
  Convulsions, loss of consciousness, pinpoint pupils, troubled and slowed breathing

- *Symptoms attributed to the aspirin ingredient of Fiorinal with Codeine may include:*
  Abdominal pain, deep, rapid breathing, delirium, high fever, restlessness, ringing in the ears, seizures, vomiting

Though caffeine poisoning occurs only at very high doses, it can cause delirium, insomnia, irregular heartbeat, rapid heartbeat, restlessness, and tremor.

If you suspect an overdose of Fiorinal with Codeine, seek emergency medical treatment immediately.

Brand name:

FLAGYL

Pronounced: FLAJ-ill
Generic name: Metronidazole
Other brand name: Protostat

Why is this drug prescribed?
Flagyl is an antibacterial drug prescribed for certain vaginal and urinary tract infections in men and women; amebic dysentery and liver abscess; and infections of the abdomen, skin, bones and joints, brain, lungs, and heart caused by certain bacteria.

Most important fact about this drug
Do not drink alcoholic beverages while taking Flagyl. The combination can cause abdominal cramps, nausea, vomiting, headaches, and flushing. It can also change the taste of the alcoholic beverage. When you have stopped taking Flagyl, wait at least 72 hours (3 days) before consuming any alcohol. Also avoid over-the-counter medications containing alcohol, such as certain cough and cold products.

How should you take this medication?
Flagyl works best when there is a constant amount in the blood. Take your doses at evenly spaced intervals, day and night, and try to avoid missing any.

If you are being treated for the sexually transmitted genital infection called trichomoniasis, your doctor may want to treat your partner at the same time, even if there are no symptoms. Try to avoid sexual intercourse until the infection is cured. If you do have sex, use a condom.

Flagyl can be taken with or without food. It may cause dry mouth. Hard candy, chewing gum, or bits of ice can help to relieve the problem.

■ *If you miss a dose...*
Take it as soon as you remember. If it is almost time for your next dose skip the one you missed and go back to your regular schedule. Do not take 2 doses at once.

■ *Storage instructions...*
Store at room temperature. Protect from light.

What side effects may occur?
Side effects cannot be anticipated. If any develop or change in intensity, tell your doctor immediately. Only your doctor can determine whether it is safe for you to continue taking Flagyl.

Two serious side effects that have occurred with Flagyl are seizures and numbness or tingling in the arms, legs, hands, and feet. If you experience either of these symptoms, stop taking the medication and call your doctor immediately.

■ *More common side effects may include:*
Abdominal cramps, constipation, diarrhea, headache, loss of appetite, nausea, upset stomach, vomiting

■ *Less common side effects may include:*
Blood disorders, confusion, dark urine, decreased sex drive, depression, difficulty sleeping, dizziness, dry mouth (or vagina or vulva), fever, flushing, furry tongue, hives, inability to hold urine, increased production of pale urine, inflamed mouth or tongue, inflammation of the rectum, irritability, lack of muscle coordination, metallic taste, occasional joint pain, pain during sexual intercourse, painful or difficult urination, pelvic pressure, rash, stuffy nose, vertigo, weakness, yeast infection (candida) in vagina

Why should this drug not be prescribed?
Flagyl should not be used during the first 3 months of pregnancy to treat vaginal infections. Do not take Flagyl if you have ever had an allergic reaction to or are sensitive to metronidazole or similar drugs. Tell your doctor about any drug reactions you have experienced.

Special warnings about this medication

If you experience seizures or numbness or tingling in your arms, legs, hands, or feet, remember that you should stop taking Flagyl and call your doctor immediately.

If you have liver disease, make sure the doctor is aware of it. Flagyl should be used with caution.

Active or undiagnosed yeast infections may appear or worsen when you take Flagyl.

Possible food and drug interactions when taking this medication

Do not drink alcohol while taking Flagyl and for at least 72 hours after your last dose.

If Flagyl is taken with certain other drugs, the effects of either could be increased, decreased, or altered. It is especially important to check with your doctor before combining Flagyl with any of the following:

Blood thinners such as Coumadin
Cholestyramine (Questran)
Cimetidine (Tagamet)
Disulfiram (Antabuse)
Lithium (Lithonate)
Phenobarbital
Phenytoin (Dilantin)

Special information if you are pregnant or breastfeeding

The effects of Flagyl in pregnancy have not been adequately studied. If you are pregnant or plan to become pregnant, notify your doctor. This medication should be used during pregnancy only if it is clearly needed. Flagyl appears in breast milk and could affect a nursing infant. If Flagyl is essential to your health, your doctor may advise you to stop breastfeeding until your treatment is finished.

Recommended dosage

ADULT

Trichomoniasis

One-day treatment: 2 grams of Flagyl, taken as a single dose or divided into 2 doses (1 gram each) taken in the same day.

Seven-day course of treatment: 250 milligrams 3 times daily for 7 consecutive days.

Acute Intestinal Amebiasis (Acute Amebic Dysentery)
The usual dose is 750 milligrams taken by mouth 3 times daily for 5 to 10 days.

Amebic Liver Abscess
The usual dose is 500 milligrams or 750 milligrams taken by mouth 3 times daily for 5 to 10 days.

Anaerobic Bacterial Infections
The usual adult oral dosage is 7.5 milligrams per 2.2 pounds of body weight every 6 hours.

CHILDREN

Amebiasis
The usual dose is 35 to 50 milligrams for each 2.2 pounds of body weight per day, divided into 3 doses taken for 10 days.

The safety and efficacy of Flagyl for any other condition in children have not been established.

OLDER ADULTS

Your doctor will test to see how much medication is in your blood and will adjust your dosage if necessary.

Overdosage
Any medication taken in excess can have serious consequences. If you suspect an overdose, seek medical treatment immediately.

■ *Symptoms of Flagyl overdose may include:*
  Lack of muscle coordination, nausea, vomiting

Generic name:

FLAVOXATE

See Urispas, page 1383.

Generic name:

FLECAINIDE

See Tambocor, page 1248.

Brand name:

FLEXERIL

Pronounced: FLEX-eh-rill
Generic name: Cyclobenzaprine hydrochloride

Why is this drug prescribed?

Flexeril is a muscle relaxant prescribed to relieve muscle spasms resulting from injuries such as sprains, strains, or pulls. Combined with rest and physical therapy, Flexeril provides relief of muscular stiffness and pain.

Most important fact about this drug

Flexeril is not a substitute for the physical therapy, rest, or exercise that your doctor orders for proper healing. Although Flexeril relieves the pain of strains and sprains, it is not useful for other types of pain.

How should you take this medication?

Flexeril may be taken with or without food.

Flexeril should be used only for short periods (no more than 3 weeks). Since the type of injury that Flexeril treats should improve in a few weeks, there is no reason to use it for a longer period.

Flexeril may cause dry mouth. Sucking a hard candy, chewing gum, or melting ice chips in your mouth can provide temporary relief.

- *If you miss a dose...*
  Take it as soon as you remember, if it is within an hour or so of your scheduled time. If you do not remember until later, skip the missed dose and go back to your regular schedule. Do not take 2 doses at once.

- *Storage instructions...*
  Store away from heat, light, and moisture.

What side effects may occur?

Side effects cannot be anticipated. If any develop or change in intensity, inform your doctor as soon as possible. Only your doctor can determine if it is safe for you to continue taking Flexeril.

■ *More common side effects may include:*
Dizziness, drowsiness, dry mouth

■ *Less common or rare side effects may include:*
Abnormal heartbeats, abnormal sensations, abnormal thoughts or dreams, agitation, anxiety, bloated feeling, blurred vision, confusion, constipation, convulsions, decreased appetite, depressed mood, diarrhea, difficulty falling or staying asleep, difficulty speaking, disorientation, double vision, excitement, fainting, fatigue, fluid retention, gas, hallucinations, headache, heartburn, hepatitis, hives, increased heart rate, indigestion, inflammation of the stomach, itching, lack of coordination, liver diseases, loss of sense of taste, low blood pressure, muscle twitching, nausea, nervousness, palpitations, rash, ringing in the ears, severe allergic reaction, stomach and intestinal pain, sweating, swelling of the tongue or face, thirst, tingling in hands or feet, tremors, unpleasant taste in the mouth, urinating more or less than usual, vague feeling of bodily discomfort, vertigo, vomiting, weakness, yellow eyes and skin

Why should this drug not be prescribed?
You should not take this drug if you are taking an antidepressant drug known as an MAO inhibitor (such as Nardil or Parnate) or have taken an MAO inhibitor within the last 2 weeks. Also avoid Flexeril if you have ever had an allergic reaction to it, or if your thyroid gland is overactive.

In addition, you should not take Flexeril if you have recently had a heart attack or if you have congestive heart failure, or suffer from irregular heartbeat.

Special warnings about this medication
Flexeril may cause you to become drowsy or less alert; therefore, you should not drive or operate dangerous machinery or participate in any hazardous activity that requires full mental alertness until you know how this drug affects you.

You should use Flexeril with caution if you have ever been unable to urinate or if you have ever had the eye condition called glaucoma.

Possible food and drug interactions
when taking this medication
Serious, potentially fatal reactions may occur if you take Flexeril with an antidepressant drug known as an MAO inhibitor (such as Nardil or Parnate) or if it has been less than 2 weeks since you last took an MAO inhibitor. You should closely follow your doctor's advice regarding discontinuation of MAO inhibitors before taking Flexeril.

Avoid alcoholic beverages while taking Flexeril.

If Flexeril is taken with certain other drugs, the effects of either could be increased, decreased, or altered. It is especially important to check with your doctor before combining Flexeril with the following:

   Antispasmodic drugs such as Donnatal or Bentyl
   Barbiturates such as phenobarbital
   Guanethidine (Esimil, Ismelin) and other high blood pressure drugs
   Other drugs that slow the central nervous system, such as Halcion and Xanax

Special information
if you are pregnant or breastfeeding

The effects of Flexeril during pregnancy have not been adequately studied. If you are pregnant or plan to become pregnant, inform your doctor immediately. It is not known if Flexeril appears in breast milk. However, cyclobenzaprine is related to tricyclic antidepressants, and some of those drugs do appear in breast milk. If this medication is essential to your health, your doctor may advise you to discontinue breastfeeding your baby until your treatment is finished.

Recommended dosage

ADULTS

The usual dose is 10 milligrams 3 times a day. You should not take more than 60 milligrams a day.

CHILDREN

Safety and effectiveness of Flexeril have not been established for children under the age of 15.

Overdosage

Any medication taken in excess can have serious consequences. If you suspect a Flexeril overdose, seek medical attention immediately.

■ *Symptoms of Flexeril overdose may include:*
   Agitation, coma, confusion, congestive heart failure, convulsions, dilated pupils, disturbed concentration, drowsiness, hallucinations, high or low temperature, increased heartbeats, irregular heart rhythms, muscle stiffness, overactive reflexes, severe low blood pressure, stupor, vomiting

High doses also may cause any of the conditions listed in "What side effects may occur?"

Brand name:

FLOMAX

Pronounced: FLOW-maks
Generic name: Tamsulosin hydrochloride

Why is this drug prescribed?
Flomax is used to treat the symptoms of an enlarged prostate—a condition technically known as benign prostatic hyperplasia or BPH. The walnut-sized prostate gland surrounds the urethra (the duct that drains the bladder). If the gland becomes enlarged, it can squeeze the urethra, interfering with the flow of urine. This can cause difficulty in starting urination, a weak flow of urine, and the need to urinate urgently or more frequently. Flomax doesn't shrink the prostate. Instead, it relaxes the muscle around it, freeing the flow of urine and decreasing urinary symptoms.

Most important fact about this drug
Flomax can cause dizziness, especially when you first stand up. Be careful about driving, operating machinery, and performing any other hazardous task until you know how you react to the drug.

How should you take this medication?
Take Flomax once daily, half an hour after the same meal each day. Do not crush, chew, or open the capsule.

- *If you miss a dose...*
  Take it as soon as you remember. If it is almost time for your next dose, skip the one you missed and go back to your regular schedule. Do not take 2 doses at once.

If you miss several doses in a row, resume treatment with a dose of 1 capsule daily and check with your doctor on how to proceed.

- *Storage instructions...*
  Store at room temperature.

What side effects may occur?
Side effects cannot be anticipated. If any develop or change in intensity, inform your doctor as soon as possible. Only your doctor can determine if it is safe for you to continue taking Flomax.

- *More common side effects may include:*
  Abnormal ejaculation, back pain, chest pain, cough, diarrhea, dizziness, headache, infection, nausea, runny nose, sinus problems, sleepiness, sore throat, weakness

■ *Less common side effects may include:*
Decreased sex drive, dental problems, insomnia, vision problems

■ *Rare side effects may include:*
Fainting, low blood pressure upon standing, vertigo

Why should this drug not be prescribed?
If Flomax gives you an allergic reaction, you cannot take the drug.

Special warnings about this medication
Remember that, in a few men, Flomax can cause a drop in blood pressure upon first standing up, which in turn can lead to dizziness or fainting. Avoid driving and other hazardous tasks for 12 hours after your first dose or a dosage increase, and be careful to stand up slowly until you're sure the drug won't make you dizzy. If you do become dizzy, sit down until it passes.

Possible food and drug interactions
when taking this medication
If Flomax is taken with certain other drugs, the effects of either could be increased, decreased, or altered. It is especially important to check with your doctor before combining Flomax with any of the following:

Blood pressure drugs classified as alpha-blockers, such as Catapres
Cimetidine (Tagamet)
Warfarin (Coumadin)

Special information
if you are pregnant or breastfeeding
Flomax is for use only by men.

Recommended dosage

ADULT MEN

The recommended starting dose of Flomax is 1 capsule (0.4 milligram) daily, half an hour following the same meal each day. Your doctor may increase the dose to 2 capsules (0.8 milligram) once a day if needed.

Overdosage
Any medication taken in excess can have serious consequences. If you suspect an overdose, seek medical treatment immediately.

■ *Symptoms of Flomax overdose may include:*
Dizziness, fainting, headache

Brand name:

FLONASE

See Fluticasone, page 542.

Brand name:

FLOVENT

See Fluticasone, page 542.

Brand name:

FLOXIN

Pronounced: FLOCKS-in
Generic name: Ofloxacin

Why is this drug prescribed?

Floxin is an antibiotic. It has been used effectively to treat lower respiratory tract infections, including chronic bronchitis and pneumonia, sexually transmitted diseases (except syphilis), pelvic inflammatory disease, and infections of the urinary tract, prostate gland, and skin.

Most important fact about this drug

Floxin kills a variety of bacteria, and is frequently used to treat infections in many parts of the body. However, you should stop taking the drug and notify your doctor immediately at the first sign of a skin rash or any other allergic reaction. Although quite rare, serious and occasionally fatal allergic reactions have been reported, some after only one dose. Signs of an impending reaction include swelling of the face and throat, shortness of breath, difficulty swallowing, rapid heartbeat, tingling, itching, and hives.

How should you take this medication?

You may take Floxin with or without food. Be sure to drink plenty of fluids while taking this medication.

Do not take mineral supplements, vitamins with iron or minerals, or antacids containing calcium, aluminum, or magnesium within 2 hours of taking Floxin.

Take Floxin exactly as prescribed. You need to complete the full course of therapy to obtain best results and decrease the risk of a recurrence of the infection.

■ *If you miss a dose...*
Take it as soon as you remember. If it is almost time for your next dose, skip the one you missed and go back to your regular schedule. Never take 2 doses at the same time.

■ *Storage instructions...*
Store at room temperature in a tightly closed container.

What side effects may occur?
Side effects cannot be anticipated. If any develop or change in intensity, inform your doctor as soon as possible. Only your doctor can determine if it is safe for you to continue taking Floxin.

■ *More common side effects may include:*
Diarrhea, difficulty sleeping, dizziness, headache, itching of genital area in women, nausea, vaginal inflammation, vomiting

■ *Less common or rare side effects may include:*
Abdominal pain and cramps, aggressiveness or hostility, agitation, anemia, anxiety, asthma, blood in the urine, blurred vision, body pain, bruising, burning or rash of the female genitals, burning sensation in the upper chest, changeable emotions, changes in thinking and perception, chest pain, confusion, conjunctivitis (pinkeye), continual runny nose, constipation, cough, decreased appetite, depression, difficult or labored breathing, disorientation, disturbed dreams, disturbed sense of smell, double vision, dry mouth, exaggerated sense of well-being, excessive perspiration, fainting, fatigue, fear, fever, fluid retention, frequent urination, gas, hallucinations, hearing disturbance or loss, hepatitis, hiccups, high or low blood pressure, high or low blood sugar, hives, inability to urinate, increased urination, indigestion, inflammation of the colon, inflammation or rupture of tendons, intolerance to light, involuntary eye movement, itching, joint pain, kidney problems, lack of coordination, light-headedness, liver problems, menstrual changes, muscle pain, nervousness, nightmares, nosebleed, pain, pain in arms and legs, painful or difficult urination, purple or red areas/spots on the skin, rapid heartbeat, rash, reddened skin, restlessness, ringing in the ears, seizures, sensitivity to light, severe allergic reaction, skin inflammation and flaking or eruptions, sleepiness, sleep problems, sore mouth or throat, speech difficulty, Stevens-Johnson syndrome (severe skin eruptions), stomach and intestinal upset or bleeding, taste distortion, thirst, throbbing or fluttering heartbeat, tingling or pins and needles, tremor, unexplained bleeding from the uterus, vaginal discharge, vaginal yeast infection, vague feeling of illness, vertigo, visual disturbances, weakness, weight loss, yellowing of eyes and skin

Why should this drug not be prescribed?

Do not take Floxin if you are sensitive to or have ever had an allergic reaction to it or other quinolone antibiotics such as Cipro and Noroxin.

Special warnings about this medication

Floxin, used in high doses for short periods of time, may hide or delay the symptoms of syphilis, but is not effective in treating syphilis. If you are taking Floxin for gonorrhea, your doctor will test you for syphilis and then perform a follow-up test after 3 months of treatment.

Convulsions, increased pressure in the head, psychosis, tremors, restlessness, light-headedness, nervousness, confusion, depression, nightmares, insomnia, and hallucinations have occasionally been reported with this type of antibiotic. If you experience any of these symptoms, stop taking the drug and contact your doctor immediately.

Floxin can cause a rupture in the muscle tendons in your hand, shoulder, or heel. If you notice any pain and inflammation in a tendon, rest and avoid exercise until you have seen your doctor.

If you are prone to seizures due to kidney disease, a brain disorder, or epilepsy, make sure your doctor knows about it. Floxin should be used with caution under these conditions.

If you have liver or kidney disease, your doctor will watch you closely while you are taking Floxin.

Avoid being in the sun too much; you can develop sun poisoning while you are taking Floxin.

Floxin may make you feel dizzy or light-headed. Be careful driving, operating machinery, or doing any activity that requires full mental alertness until you know how you react to this medication.

Safety has not been established for children under 18 years of age.

Possible food and drug interactions
when taking this medication

If Floxin is taken with certain other drugs, the effects of either could be increased, decreased, or altered. It is especially important to check with your doctor before combining Floxin with the following:

Antacids containing calcium, magnesium, or aluminum
Blood thinners such as Coumadin
Calcium supplements such as Caltrate
Cyclosporine (Sandimmune, Neoral)
Insulin

Iron supplements such as Feosol
Multivitamins containing zinc
Nonsteroidal anti-inflammatory drugs such as Motrin and Naprosyn
Oral diabetes drugs such as Diabinese and Micronase
Sucralfate (Carafate)
Theophylline-containing drugs, such as Theo-Dur

Special information
if you are pregnant or breastfeeding

The effects of Floxin during pregnancy have not been adequately studied. If
you are pregnant or plan to become pregnant, inform your doctor immediately. This medication should not be used during pregnancy unless your doctor
has determined that the benefit to you outweighs the risk to the unborn
baby. Floxin appears in breast milk and could affect a nursing infant. If this
medication is essential to your health, your doctor may advise you to stop
breastfeeding until your treatment with Floxin is finished.

Recommended dosage

LOWER RESPIRATORY TRACT INFECTIONS

Worsening of Chronic Bronchitis
The usual dose is 400 milligrams every 12 hours for 10 days, for a total daily
dose of 800 milligrams.

Pneumonia
The usual dose is 400 milligrams every 12 hours for 10 days, for a total daily
dose of 800 milligrams.

SEXUALLY TRANSMITTED DISEASES

Gonorrhea
The usual dose is 400 milligrams taken once.

Infections of the Cervix or Urethra
The usual dose is 300 milligrams every 12 hours for 7 days, for a total daily
dose of 600 milligrams.

PELVIC INFLAMMATORY DISEASE

The usual dose is 400 milligrams every 12 hours for 10 to 14 days, for a
total daily dose of 800 milligrams.

MILD TO MODERATE SKIN INFECTIONS

The usual dose is 400 milligrams every 12 hours for 10 days, for a total daily
dose of 800 milligrams.

URINARY TRACT INFECTIONS

Bladder Infections
The usual dose is 200 milligrams every 12 hours for a total daily dose of 400 milligrams. This dose is taken for 3 days for infections due to *E. coli* or *K. pneumoniae*. For infections due to other microbes, it is taken for 7 days.

Complicated Urinary Tract Infections
The usual dose is 200 milligrams every 12 hours for 10 days, for a total daily dose of 400 milligrams.

Prostatitis
The usual dose is 300 milligrams every 12 hours for 6 weeks, for a total daily dose of 600 milligrams.

Overdosage
Although no specific information is available, any medication taken in excess can have serious consequences. If you suspect an overdose, seek medical treatment immediately.

Generic name:

FLUCONAZOLE

See Diflucan, page 395.

Generic name:

FLUNISOLIDE

See AeroBid, page 21.

Generic name:

FLUOCINONIDE

See Lidex, page 697.

Generic name:

FLUOROMETHOLONE

See FML, page 547.

Generic name:

FLUOROURACIL

See Efudex, page 457.

Generic name:

FLUOXETINE

See Prozac, page 1082.

Generic name:

FLURAZEPAM

See Dalmane, page 331.

Generic name:

FLURBIPROFEN

See Ansaid, page 72.

Generic name:

FLUTAMIDE

See Eulexin, page 498.

Generic name:

FLUTICASONE

Pronounced: flue-TICK-uh-zone
Brand names: Flonase, Flovent, Flovent Rotadisk

Why is this drug prescribed?
Flonase nasal spray is a remedy for the stuffy, runny, itchy nose that plagues many allergy-sufferers. It can be used either for seasonal attacks of hay fever or for year-round allergic conditions. Flonase is a steroid medication. It works by relieving inflammation within the nasal passages.

The Flovent and Flovent Rotadisk oral inhalers are used to prevent flare-ups of asthma. (They will not, however, relieve an acute attack.) They sometimes serve as a replacement for the steroid tablets that many people take to control asthma.

Most important fact about this drug

Fluticasone is not an instant cure. It may take a few days for the medication to start working; and you need to keep taking it regularly in order to maintain its benefits. While you are waiting for fluticasone to take effect, neither increase the dose nor stop taking the medication.

How should you take this medication?

Flonase is taken in the nostrils. First, blow your nose. Then shake the spray bottle gently, tilt your head back, press one nostril closed, and insert the tip of the bottle a short way into the other nostril. Spray once, pull the tip of the bottle away from your nose, and inhale deeply through the treated nostril. Repeat with the other nostril.

Flovent inhalation aerosol is taken orally. Shake the canister before each use. Take a deep breath and exhale. Then, as you begin to inhale, put your lips around the mouthpiece and depress the canister. Rinse your mouth with water after each use of the inhaler. Avoid spraying the contents in your eyes.

Flovent Rotadisk inhalation powder is also taken orally. Assemble the Rotadisk Diskhaler according to package instructions. To use, exhale, then place the Diskhaler mouthpiece between your teeth (without biting down) and close your lips firmly around it. (Be careful to avoid covering the small air holes on either side of the mouthpiece.) Breath in through your mouth as deeply as you can, then hold your breath while you remove the Diskhaler. Continue to hold your breath as long as you comfortably can, up to a maximum of 10 seconds.

■ *If you miss a dose...*
   Take it as soon as you remember. If it is almost time for your next dose, skip the one you missed and go back to your regular schedule. Do not take 2 doses at once.

■ *Storage instructions...*
   Flonase may be stored at room temperature or in the refrigerator.

Flovent inhalation aerosol may be stored at room temperature away from sunlight, or in the refrigerator.

Flovent Rotadisk inhalation powder should be stored at room temperature in a dry place. Use the Rotadisk blisters within 2 months after opening the foil overwrap or before the expiration date, whichever comes first. Do not puncture the blisters until you are ready to use them in the Diskhaler.

What side effects may occur?
Side effects cannot be anticipated. If any develop or change in intensity, inform your doctor as soon as possible. Only your doctor can determine if it is safe for you to continue taking fluticasone.

■ *Side effects may include:*
Back problems, bad taste in mouth, bronchitis, congestion, diarrhea, dizziness, dry mouth, dry nose, eye problems, fever, flu, headache, hives, hoarseness, indigestion, mouth infection, nasal congestion, nasal irritation or burning, nasal sores, nausea, nosebleeds, respiratory tract infection, runny nose, sinus problems, sneezing, sore throat, vomiting

Why should this drug not be prescribed?
If you have ever had an allergic reaction to Flonase or similar steroid inhalants such as Flovent, you should not take this medication.

Flovent is not to be used to treat status asthmaticus or acute asthma attacks.

Special warnings about this medication
If your symptoms do not improve after the first few days of fluticasone therapy, check with your doctor. Never take more than the recommended dose. High doses of steroid medications such as fluticasone can cause a condition known as Cushing's syndrome. Warning signs of this problem include weight gain and changes in the appearance of the face.

If you are being switched from an oral steroid tablet to fluticasone, you may experience joint pain, muscle pain, weakness, depression, or fatigue while your body adjusts to the absence of steroid tablets and increases its own production of steroids. You may also experience eye inflammation, eczema, arthritis, and nasal inflammation.

People taking steroid medications run an increased risk of infections such as chickenpox and measles. If you are exposed to someone with either of these diseases and you have neither had the infection nor been vaccinated against it, contact your physician immediately.

In rare cases, fluticasone can also cause a fungal infection in the nose and throat. And steroid treatment can also make an existing infection worse. Be sure the doctor is aware of any infections you may have, including TB and viral infections of the eye.

Steroid medications can stunt growth. If your child is on fluticasone therapy, the doctor should periodically check height and weight.

If you develop wheezing and an asthma attack after inhaling Flovent, use an emergency medicine such as an inhaled bronchodilator and call your doctor immediately. Also alert your doctor immediately if emergency medications fail to work as well once you've started Flovent therapy.

In rare cases, inhaled steroids such as Flovent have caused cataracts or increased pressure in the eye (glaucoma). Alert your doctor if you suffer from either problem.

If you have recently had a nasal injury or ulcer, or had surgery on your nose, you should wait until you are fully healed before using Flonase.

Possible food and drug interactions
when taking this medication
The risk of developing Cushing's syndrome and other side effects increases when you take other steroid medications while using fluticasone. Prednisone and dexamethasone are examples of oral steroid medications. Certain other asthma inhalers, skin creams, eye drops, and ear drops also may contain steroids.

Also be sure to check with your doctor before combining fluticasone with ketoconazole (Nizoral).

Special information
if you are pregnant or breastfeeding
The effects of this drug during pregnancy have not been adequately studied. If you are pregnant or plan to become pregnant, inform your doctor immediately. It is not known whether fluticasone appears in breast milk. If the drug is essential to your health, your doctor may advise you to stop nursing until your treatment is finished.

Recommended dosage

FLONASE

Adults
The usual starting dose is 2 sprays in each nostril once daily. (Some doctors may prescribe 1 spray in each nostril every 12 hours.) Once your symptoms are under control, your doctor may reduce the dose to 1 spray in each nostril once daily.

Children
Flonase is not recommended for children under the age of 12 unless advised by your doctor. For adolescents, the recommended starting dose is 1 spray in each nostril once a day. If symptoms do not improve in a few days, the dose can be increased to 2 sprays in each nostril once a day, then reduced again once symptoms have subsided.

FLOVENT INHALATION AEROSOL

Adults and children 12 and over
If you are currently using an inhaled bronchodilator, the recommended starting dose is 88 micrograms twice a day. The maximum dose is 440 micrograms twice a day.

If you are currently using another steroid inhaler, the starting dose ranges from 88 to 220 micrograms twice daily. The maximum dose is 440 micrograms twice a day.

If you are taking oral steroid tablets, the doctor will start you at 880 micrograms of Flovent twice a day. He will slowly decrease your dose of steroid tablets, then lower your dose of Flovent.

Children under 12
Flovent inhalation aerosol is not recommended.

FLOVENT ROTADISK INHALATION POWDER

Adults and children 12 and over
If you are currently using an inhaled bronchodilator, the recommended starting dose is 100 micrograms twice a day. The maximum dose is 500 micrograms twice a day.

If you are currently using another steroid inhaler, the starting dose ranges from 100 to 250 micrograms twice daily. The maximum dose is 500 micrograms twice a day.

If you are taking oral steroid tablets, the doctor will start you at 1000 micrograms of Flovent twice a day. He will slowly decrease your dose of steroid tablets, then lower your dose of Flovent.

Children 4 to 11 years old
For children already taking an inhaled bronchodilator or steroid, the recommended starting dose is 50 micrograms twice daily. The maximum dose is 100 micrograms twice a day.

Children under 4
Flovent Rotadisk is not recommended.

Overdosage
Any medication taken in excess can have serious consequences. If you habitually use too much fluticasone, you run the risk of developing Cushing's syndrome (see "Special warnings about this medication").

Generic name:

FLUVASTATIN

See Lescol, page 676.

Generic name:

FLUVOXAMINE

See Luvox, page 744.

Brand name:

FML

Generic name: Fluorometholone

Why is this drug prescribed?
FML is a steroid (cortisone-like) eye ointment that is used to treat inflammation of the eyelid and the eye itself.

Most important fact about this drug
Do not use FML more often or for a longer period of time than your doctor orders. Overuse can increase the risk of side effects and lead to eye damage. Also, if your eye problems return, do not use any leftover FML without first consulting your doctor.

How should you use this medication?
FML may increase the chance of infection from contact lenses. Your doctor may advise you to stop wearing your contacts while using this medication.

Use FML exactly as prescribed. Do not stop until your doctor advises you to do so. To avoid spreading infection, do not let anyone else use your prescription.

To administer FML eyedrops:
1. Wash your hands thoroughly.
2. Shake well before using.
3. Gently pull your lower eyelid down to form a pocket between your eye and eyelid.
4. Hold the eyedrop bottle on the bridge of your nose or on your forehead.
5. Do not touch the applicator tip to any surface, including your eye.
6. Tilt your head back and squeeze the medication into your eye.
7. Close your eyes gently. Keep them closed for 1 to 2 minutes.
8. Do not rinse the dropper.
9. Wait for 5 to 10 minutes before using a second eye medication.

- *If you miss a dose...*
  Apply it as soon as you remember. If it is almost time for your next dose, skip the one you missed and return to your regular schedule. Do not apply a double dose.

- *Storage instructions...*
  Store at room temperature. Protect from extreme heat.

What side effects may occur?
Side effects cannot be anticipated. If any develop or change in intensity, inform your doctor as soon as possible. Only your doctor can determine if it is safe for you to continue using FML.

- *Side effects may include:*
  Allergic reactions, blurred vision, burning/stinging, cataract formation, corneal ulcers, dilation of the pupil, drooping eyelids, eye inflammation and infection including pinkeye, eye irritation, glaucoma, increased eye pressure, slow wound healing, taste alterations

Why should this drug not be prescribed?
Do not use FML if you have ever had an allergic reaction to or are sensitive to fluorometholone or similar drugs (anti-inflammatories and steroids) such as Decadron. Tell your doctor about any drug reactions you have experienced.

FML is not prescribed for patients with certain viral, fungal, and bacterial infections of the eye.

Special warnings about this medication
Prolonged use of FML may result in glaucoma (elevated pressure in the eye causing optic nerve damage and loss of vision), cataract formation (an eye

disorder causing the lens of the eye to cloud up), or the development or worsening of eye infections.

Steroids such as FML have been known to cause punctures when used in the presence of diseases that cause thinning of the cornea or the sclera (tough, opaque covering at the back of the eyeball).

The use of a corticosteroid medication could hide the presence of a severe eye infection or cause the infection to become worse.

Internal pressure of the eye should be checked frequently by your doctor.

This medication should be used with caution after cataract surgery.

If pain or inflammation lasts longer than 48 hours, or becomes worse, discontinue use of FML and notify your doctor.

Possible food and drug interactions when taking this medication

No interactions with food or other drugs have been reported.

Special information if you are pregnant or breastfeeding

The effects of FML in pregnancy have not been adequately studied. If you are pregnant or plan to become pregnant, tell your doctor immediately. FML may appear in breast milk and could affect a nursing infant. If using FML is essential to your health, your doctor may advise you to stop breastfeeding until your treatment is finished.

Recommended dosage

ADULTS

FML Ointment

Apply a small amount of ointment (a ½-inch ribbon) between the lower eyelid and eyeball 1 to 3 times a day. During the first 24 to 48 hours, your doctor may increase the dosage to 1 application every 4 hours.

FML Liquifilm

Place 1 drop of suspension between the lower eyelid and eyeball 2 to 4 times a day. During the first 24 to 48 hours, the dosage may be increased to 1 application every 4 hours.

CHILDREN

The safety and effectiveness of FML have not been established in children under 2 years of age.

Overdosage
Overdosage with FML will not ordinarily cause severe problems. If FML is accidentally swallowed, drink fluids to dilute the medication.

Brand name:

FORTOVASE

Pronounced: FORT-o-vace
Generic name: Saquinavir

Why is this drug prescribed?
Fortovase is used in the treatment of advanced human immunodeficiency virus (HIV) infection. HIV causes the immune system to break down so that it can no longer fight off other infections. This leads to the fatal disease known as acquired immune deficiency syndrome (AIDS).

Fortovase belongs to a new class of HIV drugs called protease inhibitors, which work by interfering with an important step in the virus's reproductive cycle. Fortovase is used in combination with other HIV drugs called nucleoside analogues (Retrovir or Hivid, for example). The combination produces an increase in the immune system's vital CD4 cells (white blood cells) and reduces the amount of virus in the bloodstream.

Most important fact about this drug
Fortovase will not cure an HIV infection. You will continue to face the possibility of complications, including opportunistic infections (rare infections that develop only when the immune system falters, such as certain types of pneumonia, tuberculosis, and fungal infections). Therefore, it is important that you remain under the care of a doctor and keep all your follow-up appointments.

How should you take this medication?
Take this medication exactly as prescribed by your doctor. Do not share this medication with anyone and do not exceed your recommended dosage. Take Fortovase with a meal or within 2 hours afterwards. This allows the drug to be properly absorbed by your body. Your doctor will perform laboratory tests before you start therapy with Fortovase and at regular intervals during your therapy to see how you are reacting to the medication.

■ *If you miss a dose...*
Take it as soon as possible. If it is almost time for your next dose, skip the one you missed and go back to your regular schedule. Never take a double dose.

■ *Storage instructions...*
Store Fortovase in the refrigerator in a tightly closed bottle. The capsules should be used within 3 months if they've been allowed to reach room temperature.

What side effects may occur?
Side effects cannot be anticipated. If any develop or change in intensity, tell your doctor as soon as possible. Only your doctor can determine if it is safe for you to continue taking Fortovase.

■ *Possible side effects may include:*
Abdominal discomfort and pain, appetite disturbance, depression, diarrhea, dizziness, fatigue, gas, headache, indigestion, mouth sores, muscle and bone pain, nausea, numbness in the arms and legs, tingling or "pins and needles" sensation, vomiting, weakness

Why should this drug not be prescribed?
If you suffer an allergic reaction to Fortovase or any of its components, you will not be able to use this drug.

Special warnings about this medication
Fortovase has been studied for only a limited period of time and only in patients with advanced HIV infections. Its long-term effects are still unknown.

It is known, however, that Fortovase may increase blood sugar levels. If you have diabetes, be sure to let the doctor know. Your dosage of diabetes medication may need adjustment.

Fortovase may aggravate liver problems and should be used with caution if you have such liver disorders as hepatitis or cirrhosis. It may also cause bleeding in people with hemophilia type A or B.

This medication does not reduce the risk of transmission of HIV to others through sexual contact or blood contamination. Therefore, you should continue to avoid practices that could give HIV to others.

Possible food and drug interactions
when taking this medication
If Fortovase is taken with certain other drugs, the effects of either could be increased, decreased, or altered. It is especially important to check with your doctor before combining Fortovase with the following:

Astemizole (Hismanal)
Carbamazepine (Tegretol)

Certain migraine drugs, including D.H.E. 45 injection, Cafergot, Ergostat, and Migranal Nasal Spray
Cisapride (Propulsid)
Clarithromycin (Biaxin)
Delavirdine (Rescriptor)
Dexamethasone (Decadron)
Indinavir (Crixivan)
Ketoconazole (Nizoral)
Midazolam (Versed)
Nelfinavir (Viracept)
Nevirapine (Viramune)
Phenobarbital (Donnatal)
Phenytoin (Dilantin)
Rifabutin (Mycobutin)
Rifampin (Rifadin)
Ritonavir (Norvir)
Terfenadine (Seldane)
Triazolam (Halcion)

Be sure to tell your doctor and pharmacist about all the medications (both prescription and over-the-counter) that you are presently taking. Alert them, too, whenever you *stop* taking a medication.

Special information
if you are pregnant or breastfeeding
The effects of Fortovase during pregnancy have not been adequately studied. If you are pregnant or plan to become pregnant, tell your doctor immediately. Do not breastfeed. HIV appears in breast milk and can be passed to a nursing infant.

Recommended dosage

ADULTS

The recommended dosage is 1200 milligrams (six 200-milligram capsules), taken 3 times a day with a meal or within 2 hours afterwards. Daily doses lower than 1200 milligrams 3 times a day are not recommended, since they will not have the same antiviral activity. You should also be taking Retrovir, Hivid, or another antiviral drug as directed.

CHILDREN

The safety and effectiveness of Fortovase in children younger than 16 years of age have not been established.

Overdosage
There have been no reports of Fortovase poisoning. However, any medication taken in excess can have serious consequences. If you suspect an overdose, seek emergency medical treatment immediately.

Brand name:

FOSAMAX

Pronounced: FAH-suh-max
Generic name: Alendronate sodium

Why is this drug prescribed?
Fosamax is prescribed for the treatment of osteoporosis, the brittle-bone disease, in postmenopausal women and for Paget's disease, a painful weakening of the bones.

Most important fact about this drug
For Fosamax to be effective, you must take the tablets without food or other medications, exactly as directed.

How should you use this medication?
Fosamax is effective only when each tablet is taken with a full glass of water first thing in the morning, at least 30 minutes before the first food, beverage, or other medication. If you can wait longer before eating or drinking, the medication will be absorbed better. Do not lie down for at least 30 minutes after taking Fosamax and avoid chewing or sucking on the tablet; it can cause mouth sores.

You should take calcium and vitamin D supplements if you don't get enough in your diet. Avoid smoking and alcohol. Weight-bearing exercise can also strengthen bones.

■ *If you miss a dose...*
Take it as soon as you remember it. If it is almost time for the next dose, skip the one you missed and go back to your regular schedule.

■ *Storage instructions...*
Keep the container tightly closed and store at room temperature.

What side effects may occur?
Side effects cannot be anticipated. If any develop or change in intensity, inform your doctor as soon as possible. Only your doctor can determine if it is safe for you to continue using Fosamax.

- *More common side effects may include:*
  Abdominal pain, bone and joint pain, constipation, diarrhea, indigestion, muscle pain, nausea

- *Less common side effects may include:*
  Abdominal distention, acid backup, difficulty in swallowing, esophageal ulcers, gas, headache, vomiting

- *Rare side effects may include:*
  Changes in taste, inflammation of the stomach, rash, skin redness

Why should this drug not be prescribed?

You should not take Fosamax if the calcium level in your blood is low. Avoid Fosamax if it causes an allergic reaction.

Special warnings about this medication

Fosamax is not recommended for women on hormone replacement therapy, or for women with kidney problems.

Be sure to tell your doctor if you have trouble swallowing or have any digestive disease.

Possible food and drug interactions
when taking this medication

Combining aspirin with a Fosamax dose of more than 10 milligrams per day will increase the likelihood of stomach upset.

Calcium supplements such as Caltrate, antacids such as Riopan, and some other oral medications will interfere with the absorption of Fosamax, so wait at least 30 minutes after taking Fosamax before you take anything else.

Special information
if you are pregnant or breastfeeding

The effects of Fosamax during pregnancy and breastfeeding have not been adequately studied. If you are pregnant or plan to become pregnant, notify your doctor immediately. It is not known whether Fosamax appears in breast milk. The drug is not recommended for nursing mothers.

Recommended dosage

POSTMENOPAUSAL OSTEOPOROSIS

The usual dose is 10 milligrams once a day. Treatment continues for years.

PAGET'S DISEASE

The usual dose is 40 milligrams once a day for 6 months.

Overdosage

Any medication taken in excess can have serious consequences. If you suspect an overdose, seek medical attention immediately.

- *Symptoms of Fosamax overdose may include:*
  Heartburn, inflammation of the esophagus or stomach, ulcer, upset stomach

Generic name:

FOSFOMYCIN

See Monurol, page 828.

Generic name:

FOSINOPRIL

See Monopril, page 824.

Brand name:

FULVICIN P/G

See Gris-PEG, page 572.

Generic name:

FUROSEMIDE

See Lasix, page 673.

Generic name:

GABAPENTIN

See Neurontin, page 867.

Brand name:

GANTRISIN

Pronounced: GAN-tris-in
Generic name: Sulfisoxazole acetyl

Why is this drug prescribed?
Gantrisin is a children's medication prescribed for the treatment of severe, repeated, or long-lasting urinary tract infections. These include pyelonephritis (bacterial kidney inflammation), pyelitis (inflammation of the part of the kidney that drains urine into the ureter), and cystitis (inflammation of the bladder).

This drug is also used to treat bacterial meningitis, and is prescribed as a preventive measure for children who have been exposed to meningitis.

Some middle ear infections are treated with Gantrisin in combination with penicillin or erythromycin.

Toxoplasmosis (parasitic disease transmitted by infected cats, their feces or litter boxes, and by undercooked meat) can be treated with Gantrisin in combination with pyrimethamine (Daraprim).

Malaria that does not respond to the drug chloroquine (Aralen) can be treated with Gantrisin in combination with other drug treatment.

Gantrisin is also used in the treatment of bacterial infections such as trachoma and inclusion conjunctivitis (eye infections), nocardiosis (bacterial disease affecting the lungs, skin, and brain), and chancroid (venereal disease causing enlargement and ulceration of lymph nodes in the groin).

Most important fact about this drug
Notify your doctor at the first sign of a reaction such as skin rash, sore throat, fever, joint pain, cough, shortness of breath, or other breathing difficulties, abnormal skin paleness, reddish or purplish skin spots or yellowing of the skin or whites of the eyes.

Rare but severe reactions, sometimes fatal, have occurred with the use of sulfa drugs such as Gantrisin. These reactions include sudden and severe liver damage, agranulocytosis (a severe blood disorder), and Stevens-Johnson syndrome (severe blistering).

Children taking sulfa drugs such as Gantrisin should have frequent blood counts.

How should you take this medication?

Be sure your child takes Gantrisin exactly as prescribed. It is important that the child drink plenty of fluids while taking this medication in order to prevent crystals in the urine and the formation of stones.

Gantrisin is available as a suspension and should be shaken well before each dose. To ensure an accurate dose, ask your pharmacist for a specially marked measuring spoon.

Gantrisin, like other antibacterials, works best when there is a constant amount in the blood and urine. To help keep a constant level, try to make sure that your child does not miss any doses and takes them at evenly spaced intervals, around the clock.

- *If you miss a dose...*
  Give it as soon as you remember. If it is almost time for the next dose, skip the one you missed and go back to the regular schedule. Never take 2 doses at the same time.

- *Storage instructions...*
  Keep this medication in the container it came in, tightly closed. Store it at room temperature, away from moist places and direct light.

What side effects may occur?

Side effects cannot be anticipated. If any develop or change in intensity, inform your doctor as soon as possible. Only your doctor can determine if it is safe for your child to continue taking Gantrisin.

- *Side effects may include:*
  Abdominal bleeding, abdominal pain, allergic reactions, anemia and other blood disorders, angioedema (swelling of face, lips, tongue and throat), anxiety, bluish discoloration of the skin, chills, colitis, convulsions, cough, dark, tarry stools, depression, diarrhea, disorientation, dizziness, drowsiness, enlarged salivary glands, enlarged thyroid, exhaustion, fainting, fatigue, fever, flushing, gas, hallucinations, headache, hearing loss, hepatitis, hives, inability to fall or stay asleep, inability to urinate, increased urination, inflammation of the mouth or tongue, itching, joint pain, kidney failure, lack of feeling or concern, lack of muscle coordination, lack or loss of appetite, low blood sugar, muscle pain, nausea, palpitations, presence of blood or crystals in urine, rapid heartbeat, reddish or purplish skin spots, retention of urine, ringing in the ears, sensitivity to light, serum sickness (fever, painful joints, enlarged lymph nodes, skin

rash), severe skin welts or swelling, shortness of breath, skin eruptions, skin rash, swelling due to fluid retention, tingling or pins and needles, vertigo, vomiting, weakness, yellow eyes and skin

Why should this drug not be prescribed?

If your child is sensitive to or has ever had an allergic reaction to Gantrisin or other sulfa drugs, do not use this medication. Make sure your doctor is aware of any drug reactions the child has experienced.

Except in rare cases, doctors do not prescribe Gantrisin for infants less than 2 months of age. In addition, Gantrisin should never be taken by women at the end of pregnancy or those nursing a baby under 2 months.

Special warnings about this medication

If your child has impaired kidney or liver function, or severe allergies or bronchial asthma, make sure your doctor knows about it. Caution should be exercised when taking Gantrisin.

An analysis of urine and kidney function should be performed by your doctor during treatment with Gantrisin, especially if your child has a kidney problem.

If your child develops a skin rash, stop Gantrisin therapy and call your doctor. Also notify the doctor if your child develops diarrhea.

Possible food and drug interactions
when taking this medication

If Gantrisin is taken with certain other drugs, the effects of either could be increased, decreased, or altered. It is especially important to check with your doctor before combining this drug with the following:

Blood-thinning drugs such as Coumadin
Methotrexate, an anticancer drug
Oral diabetes drugs such as Micronase

Special information
if you are pregnant or breastfeeding

There are no adequate and well controlled studies in pregnant women. This medication should never be used during pregnancy unless the doctor has determined that the benefits outweigh the potential risks. Gantrisin appears in breast milk. If this medication is essential, the doctor may recommend against breastfeeding until treatment with this drug is finished.

Recommended dosage

CHILDREN

This medication should not be prescribed for infants under 2 months of age except in the treatment of congenital toxoplasmosis (a parasitic infection contracted by pregnant women and passed along to the fetus).

The usual dose for children 2 months of age or older is 150 milligrams per 2.2 pounds of body weight divided into 4 to 6 doses taken over 24 hours.

The usual starting dose is one-half of the regular dose, or 75 milligrams per 2.2 pounds of body weight divided into 4 to 6 doses taken over 24 hours. Doses should not exceed 6 grams over 24 hours.

Gantrisin pediatric suspension supplies a half-gram (500 milligrams) in each teaspoonful.

Overdosage

Any medication taken in excess can have serious consequences. If you suspect an overdose, seek emergency medical treatment immediately.

- *Symptoms of an overdose of Gantrisin include:*
  Blood or sediment in the urine, blue tinge to the skin, colic, dizziness, drowsiness, fever, headache, lack or loss of appetite, nausea, unconsciousness, vomiting, yellowing of skin and whites of eyes

Brand name:

GARAMYCIN OPHTHALMIC

Pronounced: gar-uh-MY-sin
Generic name: Gentamicin sulfate

Why is this drug prescribed?

Garamycin Ophthalmic, an antibiotic, is applied to the eye for treatment of infections such as conjunctivitis (pinkeye) and other eye infections.

Most important fact about this drug

To help clear up your infection completely, keep using Garamycin eyedrops or ointment for the full time of treatment, even if your symptoms have disappeared. Do not allow anyone else to use this medication, and do not save it for use on another infection.

How should you use this medication?
Use this medication exactly as prescribed. To administer Garamycin, follow these steps:

Eyedrops
1. Wash your hands thoroughly.
2. Gently pull your lower eyelid down to form a pocket between your eye and the lid.
3. Brace the eyedrop bottle on your forehead or on the bridge of your nose.
4. Do not touch the applicator tip to your eye or any other surface.
5. Close your eyes gently and keep them closed for a minute or two.
6. Do not rinse the dropper.
7. If you are using a second type of eyedrop, wait 5 to 10 minutes before applying it.

Eye Ointment
1. Wash your hands thoroughly.
2. Pull your lower eyelid down away from the eye to form a pocket.
3. Squeeze a thin strip of ointment into the pouch.
4. Avoid touching the tip of the tube to your eye or any other surface.
5. Close your eyes for a couple of minutes.
6. Wipe the tip of the tube with tissue and immediately replace the cap tightly.

Your vision may be blurred for a few minutes following application of the ointment.

- ■ *If you miss a dose...*
  Apply it as soon as you remember. If it is almost time for your next dose, skip the one you missed and go back to your regular schedule.

- ■ *Storage instructions...*
  Store away from heat and light. Do not freeze.

What side effects may occur?
Occasional eye irritation—with itching, redness and swelling—may occur with use of the eyedrops.

Occasional burning or stinging in the eye may occur with use of the ointment.

Why should this drug not be prescribed?

If you are sensitive to or have ever had an allergic reaction to Garamycin or certain other antibiotics, such as Tobrex, you should not take this medication. Make sure your doctor is aware of any drug reactions you have experienced.

Special warnings about this medication

Continued or prolonged use of this drug may result in a growth of bacteria or fungi that do not respond to this medication and can cause a second infection. Should this occur, notify your doctor.

Ophthalmic ointments may slow corneal healing.

Possible food and drug interactions
with this medication

No interactions have been reported.

Special information
if you are pregnant or breastfeeding

There are no special recommendations for this medication. If you are pregnant or plan to become pregnant, ask your doctor for the best advice in your personal situation.

Recommended dosage

ADULTS AND CHILDREN

Garamycin Ophthalmic Solution

Put 1 or 2 drops into the affected eye every 4 hours. For severe infections, your doctor may increase your dosage up to a maximum of 2 drops once every hour.

Garamycin Ophthalmic Ointment

Apply a thin strip—about one-third inch—of ointment to the affected eye 2 or 3 times a day.

Overdosage

Although there is no information on overdose with Garamycin Ophthalmic products, any medication taken in excess can have serious consequences. If you suspect an overdose, seek medical attention immediately.

Brand name:

GAVISCON

See Antacids, page 75.

Generic name:

GEMFIBROZIL

See Lopid, page 715.

Brand name:

GENORA

See Oral Contraceptives, page 926.

Generic name:

GENTAMICIN

See Garamycin Ophthalmic, page 559.

Brand name:

GENUINE BAYER

See Aspirin, page 98.

Generic name:

GLIMEPIRIDE

See Amaryl, page 47.

Generic name:

GLIPIZIDE

See Glucotrol, page 567.

Brand name:

GLUCOPHAGE

Pronounced: GLEW-co-faje
Generic name: Metformin hydrochloride

Why is this drug prescribed?
Glucophage is an oral antidiabetic medication used to treat Type II (noninsulin-dependent) diabetes. Diabetes develops when the body proves unable to burn sugar and the unused sugar builds up in the bloodstream. Glucophage lowers the amount of sugar in your blood by decreasing sugar production and absorption and helping your body respond better to its own insulin, which promotes the burning of sugar. It does not, however, increase the body's production of insulin.

Most important fact about this drug
Always remember that Glucophage is an aid to, not a substitute for, good diet and exercise. Failure to follow a sound diet and exercise plan can lead to serious complications such as dangerously high or low blood sugar levels. Remember, too, that Glucophage is not an oral form of insulin and cannot be used in place of insulin.

How should you take this medication?
Do not take more or less of this medication than directed by your doctor. Glucophage should be taken with food to reduce the possibility of nausea or diarrhea, especially during the first few weeks of therapy.

- *If you miss a dose...*
  Take it as soon as you remember. If it is almost time for your next dose, skip the one you missed and go back to your regular schedule. Never take 2 doses at the same time.

- *Storage instructions...*
  Store it at room temperature.

What side effects may occur?
Side effects cannot be anticipated. If any develop or change in intensity, tell your doctor as soon as possible. Only your doctor can determine if it is safe for you to continue taking Glucophage.

If side effects from Glucophage occur, they usually happen during the first few weeks of therapy. Most side effects are minor and will go away after you've taken Glucophage for a while.

■ *More common side effects may include:*
Abdominal bloating, diarrhea, gas, loss of appetite, metallic or unpleasant taste, nausea, vomiting

Glucophage, unlike other oral antidiabetics, does not usually cause hypoglycemia (low blood sugar). However, hypoglycemia remains a possibility, especially in older, weak, and undernourished people and those with kidney, liver, adrenal, or pituitary gland problems. The risk of hypoglycemia can be increased by missed meals, alcohol, other medications, fever, trauma, infection, surgery, or excessive exercise. To avoid hypoglycemia, you should closely follow the dietary and exercise plan suggested by your physician. If you feel hypoglycemia coming on, get some fast-acting sugar, such as a 4 to 6 ounce glass of fruit juice.

Glucophage can cause a serious side effect called lactic acidosis, a buildup of lactic acid in the blood. This problem is most likely to occur in people whose liver or kidneys are not working well. Although the condition is rare, it can be fatal. Lactic acidosis is a medical emergency that must be treated in a hospital.

■ *Symptoms of lactic acidosis may include:*
Feeling very weak, tired, or uncomfortable, feeling cold, dizzy, or lightheaded, increasing sleepiness, muscle pain, slow or irregular heartbeat, trouble breathing, unexpected or unusual stomach discomfort

If you notice these symptoms, stop taking Glucophage and call your doctor right away.

Why should this drug not be prescribed?
Avoid Glucophage if it has ever given you an allergic reaction.

If you have congestive heart failure, do not take Glucophage. This condition increases your risk of developing lactic acidosis.

Do not take Glucophage if you are suffering from acute or chronic metabolic acidosis, including diabetic ketoacidosis (a life-threatening medical emergency caused by insufficient insulin and marked by excessive thirst, nausea, fatigue, pain below the breastbone, and fruity breath).

You should not take Glucophage for 2 days before and after having an X-ray procedure with an injectable contrast agent (radioactive iodine). Also, if you are going to have surgery, except minor surgery, you should stop taking Glucophage. Once you have resumed normal food and fluid intake, your doctor will tell you when you can go back to therapy with Glucophage.

If you have kidney or liver disease or develop serious conditions such as a heart attack, severe infection, or a stroke, do not take Glucophage.

You should not take Glucophage if you are seriously dehydrated, having lost a large amount of fluid from severe vomiting, diarrhea, or high fever.

Special warnings about this medication

Before you start therapy with Glucophage, and at least once a year thereafter, your doctor will do a complete assessment of your kidney function. If you develop kidney problems while on Glucophage, your doctor will discontinue this medication. If you are an older person, you will need to have your kidney function monitored more frequently, and your doctor may want to start you at a lower dosage.

If you are taking Glucophage, you should check your blood or urine periodically for abnormal sugar (glucose) levels. Your doctor will do annual blood checks to see if Glucophage is causing a vitamin B_{12} deficiency or any other blood problem.

It's possible that drugs such as Glucophage may lead to more heart problems than diet treatment alone, or diet plus insulin. If you have a heart condition, you may want to discuss this with your doctor. The effectiveness of any oral antidiabetic, including Glucophage, may decrease with time. This may be due to either a diminished responsiveness to the medication or a worsening of the diabetes.

Possible food and drug interactions
when taking this medication

If Glucophage is taken with certain other drugs, the effects of either could be increased, decreased, or altered. It is especially important to check with your doctor before combining Glucophage with the following:

Amiloride (Moduretic)
Calcium channel blockers (heart medications) such as Calan, Isoptin, and Procardia
Cimetidine (Tagamet)
Decongestant, airway-opening drugs such as Sudafed and Ventolin
Digoxin (Lanoxin)
Estrogens such as Premarin
Furosemide (Lasix) and other diuretics
Isoniazid (Rifamate), a drug used for tuberculosis
Major tranquilizers such as Thorazine
Morphine
Niacin (Slo-Niacin, Nicobid)
Oral contraceptives
Phenytoin (Dilantin)
Procainamide (Procan SR)

Quinidine (Quinidex)
Quinine
Ranitidine (Zantac)
Steroids such as prednisone (Deltasone)
Thyroid hormones (Synthroid)
Trimethoprim (Bactrim, Trimpex)
Vancomycin (Vancocin HCl)

Do not drink too much alcohol, since excessive alcohol consumption can cause low blood sugar and alcohol enhances some effects of this drug.

Special information
if you are pregnant or breastfeeding

If you are pregnant or plan to become pregnant, tell your doctor immediately. Glucophage should not be taken during pregnancy. Since studies suggest the importance of maintaining normal blood sugar (glucose) levels during pregnancy, your doctor may prescribe insulin injections instead.

It is not known whether Glucophage appears in human breast milk. Therefore, women should discuss with their doctors whether to discontinue the medication or to stop breastfeeding. If the medication is discontinued and if diet alone does not control glucose levels, then your doctor may consider insulin injections.

Recommended dosage
Your doctor will tailor your dosage to your individual needs.

ADULTS

The usual starting dose is one 500-milligram tablet twice a day, taken with morning and evening meals. Your doctor may increase your daily dose by 500 milligrams at weekly intervals, based on your response. Daily doses of greater than 2,500 milligrams are not recommended. An alternative starting dose is one 850-milligram tablet a day, taken with the morning meal. Your doctor may increase this by 850 milligrams at 14-day intervals, to a maximum of 2,550 milligrams a day.

The usual maintenance dose ranges from 1,500 to 2,550 milligrams daily.

OLDER ADULTS

Older people and those who are malnourished or in a weakened state are generally given lower doses of Glucophage because their kidneys may be weaker, making side effects more likely.

CHILDREN

The safety and effectiveness of Glucophage have not been established in children.

Overdosage

An overdose of Glucophage can cause lactic acidosis. (See "What Side Effects May Occur?") If you suspect a Glucophage overdose, seek emergency treatment immediately.

Brand name:

GLUCOTROL

Pronounced: GLUE-kuh-troll
Generic name: Glipizide
Other brand name: Glucotrol XL

Why is this drug prescribed?

Glucotrol is an oral antidiabetic medication used to treat Type II (non-insulin-dependent) diabetes. In diabetics either the body does not make enough insulin or the insulin that is produced no longer works properly.

There are actually two forms of diabetes: Type I insulin-dependent and Type II non-insulin-dependent. Type I usually requires insulin injections for life, while Type II diabetes can usually be treated by dietary changes and/or oral antidiabetic medications such as Glucotrol. Apparently, Glucotrol controls diabetes by stimulating the pancreas to secrete more insulin. Occasionally, Type II diabetics must take insulin injections on a temporary basis, especially during stressful periods or times of illness.

Most important fact about this drug

Always remember that Glucotrol is an aid to, not a substitute for, good diet and exercise. Failure to follow a sound diet and exercise plan can lead to serious complications, such as dangerously high or low blood sugar levels. Remember, too, that Glucotrol is *not* an oral form of insulin, and cannot be used in place of insulin.

How should you take this medication?

In general, to achieve the best control over blood sugar levels, Glucotrol should be taken 30 minutes before a meal. However, the exact dosing schedule as well as the dosage amount must be determined by your physician.

Glucotrol XL should be taken with breakfast. Swallow the tablets whole; do not chew, crush, or divide them. Do not be alarmed if you notice something that looks like a tablet in your stool—it will be the empty shell that has been eliminated.

■ *If you miss a dose...*
Take it as soon as you remember. If it is almost time for your next dose, skip the one you missed and go back to your regular schedule. Never take 2 doses at the same time.

■ *Storage instructions...*
Glucotrol should be stored at room temperature and protected from moisture and humidity.

What side effects may occur?
Side effects from Glucotrol are rare and seldom require discontinuation of the medication.

■ *More common side effects may include:*
Constipation, diarrhea, dizziness, drowsiness, gas, headache, hives, itching, low blood sugar, nervousness, sensitivity to light, skin rash and eruptions, stomach pain, tremor

■ *Less common or rare side effects may include:*
Anemia and other blood disorders, yellow eyes and skin

Glucotrol and Glucotrol XL, like all oral antidiabetic drugs, can cause low blood sugar. This risk is increased by missed meals, alcohol, other medications, and/or excessive exercise. To avoid low blood sugar, you should closely follow the dietary and exercise regimen suggested by your physician.

■ *Symptoms of mild low blood sugar may include:*
Blurred vision, cold sweats, dizziness, fast heartbeat, fatigue, headache, hunger, light-headedness, nausea, nervousness

■ *Symptoms of more severe low blood sugar may include:*
Coma, disorientation, pale skin, seizures, shallow breathing

Ask your doctor what steps you should take if you experience mild hypoglycemia. If symptoms of severe low blood sugar occur, contact your doctor immediately. Severe hypoglycemia should be considered a medical emergency, and·prompt medical attention is essential.

Why should this drug not be prescribed?
You should not take Glucotrol if you have had an allergic reaction to it previously.

Glucotrol will be stopped if you are suffering from diabetic ketoacidosis (a life-threatening medical emergency caused by insufficient insulin and marked by excessive thirst, nausea, fatigue, pain below the breastbone, and a fruity breath).

Special warnings about this medication
It's possible that drugs such as Glucotrol may lead to more heart problems than diet treatment alone, or diet plus insulin. If you have a heart condition, you may want to discuss this with your doctor.

If you are taking Glucotrol, you should check your blood and urine periodically for the presence of abnormal sugar (glucose) levels.

Even people with well-controlled diabetes may find that injury, infection, surgery, or fever results in a lack of control over their diabetes. In these cases, the physician may recommend that you stop taking Glucotrol temporarily and use insulin instead.

Glucotrol may not work well in patients with poor kidney or liver function.

In addition, the effectiveness of any oral antidiabetic, including Glucotrol, may decrease with time. This may occur because of either a diminished responsiveness to the medication or a worsening of the diabetes.

Be careful taking the extended-release form of the drug, Glucotrol XL, if you have any narrowing in your stomach or intestines. Also, if you have any stomach or intestinal disease, Glucotrol XL may not work as well.

Possible food and drug interactions
when taking this medication
It is essential that you closely follow your physician's dietary guidelines and that you inform your physician of any medication, either prescription or nonprescription, that you are taking. Specific medications that affect Glucotrol include:

Airway-opening drugs such as Sudafed
Antacids such as Mylanta
Aspirin
Chloramphenicol (Chloromycetin)
Cimetidine (Tagamet)
Clofibrate (Atromid-S)

Corticosteroids such as prednisone (Deltasone)
Diuretics such as HydroDIURIL
Estrogens such as Premarin
Fluconazole (Diflucan)
Gemfibrozil (Lopid)
Heart and blood pressure medications called beta blockers such as Tenormin and Lopressor
Heart medications called calcium channel blockers such as Cardizem and Procardia XL
Isoniazid (Nydrazid)
Itraconazole (Sporanox)
MAO inhibitors (antidepressant drugs such as Nardil)
Major tranquilizers such as Thorazine and Mellaril
Miconazole (Monistat)
Nicotinic acid (Nicobid)
Nonsteroidal anti-inflammatory drugs such as Motrin
Oral contraceptives
Phenytoin (Dilantin)
Probenecid (Benemid)
Rifampin (Rifadin)
Sulfa drugs such as Bactrim
Thyroid medications such as Synthroid
Warfarin (Coumadin)

Alcohol must be used carefully, since excessive alcohol consumption can cause low blood sugar.

Special information
if you are pregnant or breastfeeding

The effects of Glucotrol during pregnancy have not been adequately studied. Therefore, if you are pregnant, or planning to become pregnant, you should take Glucotrol only on the advice of your physician. Since studies suggest the importance of maintaining normal blood sugar (glucose) levels during pregnancy, your physician may prescribe insulin during pregnancy. To minimize the risk of low blood sugar in newborn babies, Glucotrol, if taken during pregnancy, should be discontinued at least one month before the expected delivery date. Although it is not known if Glucotrol appears in breast milk, other oral antidiabetics do. Because of the potential for hypoglycemia in nursing infants, your doctor may advise you either to discontinue Glucotrol or to stop nursing. If Glucotrol is discontinued and if diet alone does not control glucose levels, your doctor may prescribe insulin.

Recommended dosage

Dosage levels must be determined by each patient's needs.

ADULTS

Glucotrol
The usual recommended starting dose is 5 milligrams taken before breakfast. Depending upon blood glucose response, your doctor may increase the initial dose in increments of 2.5 to 5 milligrams. The maximum recommended daily dose is 40 milligrams; total daily dosages above 15 milligrams are usually divided into 2 equal doses that are taken before meals.

Glucotrol XL
The usual starting dose is 5 milligrams each day at breakfast. After 3 months, your doctor may increase the dose to 10 milligrams daily. The maximum recommended daily dose is 20 milligrams.

CHILDREN

The safety and effectiveness of this drug in children have not been established.

OLDER ADULTS

Older people or those with liver disease usually start Glucotrol therapy with 2.5 milligrams. They can start Glucotrol XL treatment with 5 milligrams.

Overdosage
An overdose of Glucotrol can cause low blood sugar. (See side effects section for symptoms.) Eating sugar or a sugar-based product will often correct the condition. Otherwise, seek medical attention immediately.

Generic name:

GLYBURIDE

See Micronase, page 794.

Brand name:

GLYNASE

See Micronase, page 794.

Brand name:

GRISACTIN

See Gris-PEG, page 572.

Generic name:

GRISEOFULVIN

See Gris-PEG, page 572.

Brand name:

GRIS-PEG

Pronounced: GRISS-peg
Generic name: Griseofulvin
Other brand names: Grisactin, Fulvicin P/G

Why is this drug prescribed?
Gris-PEG is prescribed for the treatment of the following ringworm infections:

Athlete's foot
Barber's itch (inflammation of the facial hair follicles)
Ringworm of the body
Ringworm of the groin and thigh
Ringworm of the nails
Ringworm of the scalp

Because Gris-PEG is effective for only certain types of fungal infections, before treatment your doctor may perform tests to identify the source of infection.

Most important fact about this drug
To clear up your infection completely, continue taking Gris-PEG as prescribed until your doctor tells you to stop. Although some improvement may appear within a few days, you need to take Gris-PEG for an extended period.

How should you take this medication?
To minimize stomach irritation and help your body absorb the drug, take Gris-PEG at meal times or with food or whole milk. If you are on a low fat diet, check with your doctor.

Observe good hygiene during treatment to help control infection and prevent reinfection.

■ *If you miss a dose...*
Take it as soon as you remember. If it is almost time for your next dose, skip the one you missed and go back to your regular schedule. Do not take 2 doses at once.

■ *Storage instructions...*
Store at room temperature in a tightly closed container. Protect from light.
Keep the liquid from freezing.

What side effects may occur?
Side effects cannot be anticipated. If any develop or change in intensity,
inform your doctor as soon as possible. Only your doctor can determine if it
is safe for you to continue taking Gris-PEG.

■ *More common side effects may include:*
Hives, skin rashes

■ *Less common side effects may include:*
Confusion, diarrhea, dizziness, fatigue, headache, impairment of performance of routine activities, inability to fall or stay asleep, nausea, oral
thrush (mouth inflammation), upper abdominal pain, vomiting

■ *Rare side effects may include:*
Menstrual irregularities, swelling, itching, and shedding of areas of skin,
tingling sensation in hands and feet

Why should this drug not be prescribed?
If you are sensitive to or have ever had an allergic reaction to Gris-PEG or
other drugs of this type, you should not take this medication. Make sure your
doctor is aware of any drug reactions you have experienced.

Unless you are directed to do so by your doctor, do not take this medication if
you have liver damage or porphyria (an inherited disorder of the liver or bone
marrow).

Do not take Gris-PEG while pregnant.

Special warnings about this medication
Gris-PEG is similar to penicillin. Although penicillin-sensitive people have
used Gris-PEG without difficulty, notify your doctor if you are sensitive to or
allergic to penicillin.

Because Gris-PEG can make you sensitive to light, avoid exposure to intense
natural or artificial sunlight.

Notify your doctor if you develop lupus erythematosus (a form of
rheumatism) or a lupus-like condition. Signs and symptoms of lupus include
arthritis, red butterfly rash over the nose and cheeks, tiredness, weakness,
sensitivity to sunlight, and skin eruptions.

If you are being treated with Gris-PEG for an extended period of time, your doctor should perform regular tests, including periodic monitoring of kidney function, liver function, and blood cell production.

Gris-PEG has not been proved safe and effective for the prevention of fungal infections.

Gris-PEG may decrease the effectiveness of birth-control pills. Use additional protection while you are taking Gris-PEG.

Men should wait at least 6 months after finishing therapy with griseofulvin before they father a child.

Women should avoid becoming pregnant while they are taking the drug.

Possible food and drug interactions
when taking this medication
Gris-PEG may intensify the effects of alcohol. If you drink alcohol while taking this medication, your heart may start beating faster and your skin may be flushed.

If Gris-PEG is taken with certain other drugs, the effects of either could be increased, decreased, or altered. It is especially important to check with your doctor before combining Gris-PEG with the following:

Blood-thinning drugs such as Coumadin
Barbiturates such as phenobarbital
Oral contraceptives

Special information
if you are pregnant or breastfeeding
Do not take Gris-PEG if you are pregnant. If you become pregnant while taking this drug, notify your doctor immediately. There is a potential hazard to the developing baby.

If you are breastfeeding, consult with your doctor before taking Gris-PEG.

Recommended dosage
The usual treatment periods for various ringworm infections are:

Ringworm of the scalp—4 to 6 weeks
Ringworm of the body—2 to 4 weeks
Athlete's foot—4 to 8 weeks

The usual treatment period, depending on the rate of growth, for ringworm of the fingernails is at least 4 months and for ringworm of the toenails at least 6 months.

ADULTS

Ringworm of the Body, Groin and Thigh, Scalp
The usual dosage is 375 milligrams a day taken as a single dose or divided into smaller doses, as determined by your doctor.

Athlete's Foot, Ringworm of the Nails
The usual dosage is 750 milligrams a day divided into smaller doses, as determined by your doctor.

CHILDREN

A single daily dose is effective in children with ringworm of the scalp.

The usual dosage is 3.3 milligrams per pound of body weight per day. This means that children weighing 35 to 60 pounds will take 125 to 187.5 milligrams a day, and children weighing more than 60 pounds will take 187.5 to 375 milligrams a day.

No dosage has been established for children 2 years of age and under.

Overdosage
Any medication taken in excess can have dangerous consequences. If you suspect an overdose of Gris-PEG, seek emergency medical treatment immediately.

Generic name:

GUAIFENESIN WITH CODEINE

See Tussi-Organidin NR, page 1359.

Generic name:

GUAIFENESIN WITH PHENYLPROPANOLAMINE

See Entex LA, page 477.

Generic name:

GUANABENZ

See Wytensin, page 1431.

Generic name:

GUANFACINE

See Tenex, page 1272.

Brand name:

GYNE-LOTRIMIN

Pronounced: GUY-nuh-LOW-trim-in
Generic name: Clotrimazole
Other brand names: Lotrimin, Mycelex, Mycelex-7

Why is this drug prescribed?
Clotrimazole, the active ingredient in these medications, is used to treat fungal infections. In preparations for the skin, it is effective against ringworm, athlete's foot, and jock itch. In vaginal creams and tablets, it is used against vaginal yeast infections. In lozenge form, it is prescribed to treat oral yeast infections and to prevent them in people with weak immune systems.

Most important fact about this drug
Keep using this medicine for the full time of treatment, even if the infection seems to have disappeared. If you stop too soon, the infection could return. You should continue using the vaginal forms of this medicine even during your menstrual period.

How should you take this medication?
Keep all forms of this medicine away from your eyes.

Before applying the skin preparations, be sure to wash your hands. Massage the medication gently into the affected area and the surrounding skin.

If you are taking Mycelex troches, place the lozenge in your mouth and let it dissolve slowly for 15 to 30 minutes. Do not chew the lozenge or swallow it whole.

If you are using a vaginal cream or tablet, use the following administration technique:

1. Load the applicator to the fill line with cream, or unwrap a tablet, wet it with warm water, and place it in the applicator as shown in the instructions you receive with the product.
2. Lie on your back with your knees drawn up.
3. Gently insert the applicator high into the vagina and push the plunger.

4. Withdraw the applicator and discard it if disposable, or wash with soap and water.

To keep the vaginal medication from getting on your clothing, wear a sanitary napkin. Do not use a tampon because it will absorb the medicine. Wear underwear or pantyhose with a cotton crotch—avoid synthetic fabrics such as nylon or rayon. Do not douche unless your doctor tells you to do so.

■ *If you miss a dose...*
  Make up for it as soon as you remember. If it is almost time for the next dose, skip the one you missed and go back to your regular schedule.

■ *Storage instructions...*
  Store at room temperature, away from heat, light, and moisture.

What side effects may occur?
Side effects cannot be anticipated. If any develop or change in intensity, inform your doctor as soon as possible. Only your doctor can determine if it is safe for you to continue using this medication.

■ *Side effects may include:*
  Blistering, burning, hives, irritated skin, itching, peeling, reddened skin, stinging, swelling due to fluid retention

■ *Side effects of clotrimazole vaginal preparations may include:*
  Abdominal/stomach cramps/pain, burning/irritation of penis of sexual partner, headache, pain during sexual intercourse, skin rash, hives, vaginal burning, vaginal irritation, vaginal itching, vaginal soreness during sexual intercourse

An unpleasant mouth sensation has been reported by some people taking Mycelex.

Why should this drug not be prescribed?
You should not be using this medication if you have had an allergic reaction to any of its ingredients.

Special warnings about this medication
Contact your doctor if you experience increased skin irritations (such as redness, itching, burning, blistering, swelling, or oozing).

Check with your doctor before using this medication on a child.

In general, if your symptoms have not improved within 2 to 4 weeks of treatment, notify your doctor.

Clotrimazole vaginal preparations should not be used if you have abdominal pain, fever, or a foul-smelling vaginal discharge. Contact your doctor immediately.

While using the vaginal preparations, either avoid sexual intercourse or make sure your partner uses a condom. This will prevent reinfection. Oils used in some vaginal preparations can weaken latex condoms or diaphragms. To find out whether you can use your medication with latex products, check with your pharmacist.

**Possible food and drug interactions
when taking this medication**
None have been reported.

**Special information
if you are pregnant or breastfeeding**
The use of clotrimazole during the first trimester of pregnancy has not been adequately studied. It should be used during the first trimester only if clearly needed. Do not use clotrimazole at any time during pregnancy without the advice and supervision of your doctor.

It is not known whether clotrimazole appears in breast milk. Nursing mothers should use this medication cautiously and only when clearly needed.

Recommended dosage
LOTRIMIN

Adults and Children

Wash your hands before and after you use Lotrimin. Apply in the morning and evening. Use enough Lotrimin to massage into the affected area.

Symptoms usually improve during the first week of treatment with Lotrimin.

GYNE-LOTRIMIN CREAM

Adults

Fill the applicator with the cream and insert 1 applicatorful into the vagina every day, preferably at bedtime. Repeat this procedure for 7 consecutive days.

MYCELEX TROCHE

Adults

The recommended dosage is 1 troche slowly dissolved in the mouth 5 times daily for 14 consecutive days. For prevention, the recommended dose is 1 troche 3 times daily.

Overdosage

Although any medication used in excess can have serious consequences, an overdose of clotrimazole is unlikely. If you suspect an overdose, however, seek medical help immediately.

Brand name:

HABITROL

See Nicotine Patches, page 870.

Brand name:

HALCION

Pronounced: HAL-see-on
Generic name: Triazolam

Why is this drug prescribed?

Halcion is used for short-term treatment of insomnia. It is a member of the benzodiazepine class of drugs, many of which are used as tranquilizers.

Most important fact about this drug

Sleep problems are usually temporary, requiring treatment for only a short time, usually 1 or 2 days and no more than 1 to 2 weeks. Insomnia that lasts longer than this may be a sign of another medical problem. If you find you need this medicine for more than 7 to 10 days, be sure to check with your doctor.

How should you take this medication?

Take this medication exactly as directed; never take more than your doctor has prescribed.

As with all prescription medications, never share Halcion with anyone else.

To help avoid upset stomach, Halcion can be taken with food.

■ *If you miss a dose...*
Take Halcion only as needed.

■ *Storage instructions...*
Keep this medication in the container it came in, tightly closed, and out of reach of children. Store it at room temperature.

What side effects may occur?
Side effects cannot be anticipated. If any develop or change in intensity, inform your doctor as soon as possible. Only your doctor can determine if it is safe for you to continue taking Halcion.

■ *More common side effects may include:*
Coordination problems, dizziness, drowsiness, headache, light-headedness, nausea/vomiting, nervousness

■ *Less common or rare side effects may include:*
Aggressiveness, agitation, behavior problems, burning tongue, changes in sexual drive, chest pain, confusion, congestion, constipation, cramps/pain, delusions, depression, diarrhea, disorientation, dreaming abnormalities, drowsiness, dry mouth, exaggerated sense of well-being, excitement, fainting, falling, fatigue, hallucinations, impaired urination, inappropriate behavior, incontinence, inflammation of the tongue and mouth, irritability, itching, loss of appetite, loss of sense of reality, memory impairment, memory loss (e.g., traveler's amnesia), menstrual irregularities, morning "hangover" effects, muscle spasms in the shoulders or neck, nightmares, rapid heart rate, restlessness, ringing in the ears, skin inflammation, sleep disturbances including insomnia, sleepwalking, slurred or difficult speech, stiff awkward movements, taste changes, tingling or pins and needles, tiredness, visual disturbances, weakness, yellowing of the skin and whites of the eyes

Why should this drug not be prescribed?
You should not take this drug if you are pregnant or if you have had an allergic reaction to it or to other benzodiazepine drugs such as Valium.

Also avoid Halcion if you are taking the antifungal medications Nizoral or Sporanox, or the antidepressant Serzone.

Special warnings about this medication
When Halcion is used every night for more than a few weeks, it loses its effectiveness to help you sleep. This is known as tolerance. Also, it can cause dependence, especially when it is used regularly for longer than a few weeks or at high doses.

Abrupt discontinuation of Halcion should be avoided, since it has been associated with withdrawal symptoms (convulsions, cramps, tremor, vomiting, sweating, feeling ill, perceptual problems, and insomnia). A gradual dosage tapering schedule is usually recommended for patients taking more than the lowest dose of Halcion for longer than a few weeks. The usual treatment period is 7 to 10 days.

If you develop unusual and disturbing thoughts or behavior during treatment with Halcion, you should discuss them with your doctor immediately.

"Traveler's amnesia" has been reported by patients who took Halcion to induce sleep while traveling. To avoid this condition, do not take Halcion on an overnight airplane flight of less than 7 to 8 hours.

You may suffer increased anxiety during the daytime while taking Halcion.

When you first start taking Halcion, until you know whether the medication will have any "carry over" effect the next day, use extreme care while doing anything that requires complete alertness such as driving a car or operating machinery.

After discontinuing the drug, you may experience a "rebound insomnia" for the first 2 nights—that is, insomnia may be worse than before you took the sleeping pill.

You should be aware that anterograde amnesia (forgetting events after an injury) has been associated with benzodiazepine drugs such as Halcion.

You should be cautious about using this drug if you have liver or kidney problems, lung problems, or a tendency to temporarily stop breathing while you are asleep.

**Possible food and drug interactions
when taking this medication**
Avoid alcoholic beverages and grapefruit juice.

If Halcion is taken with certain other drugs, the effects of either could be increased, decreased, or altered. It is especially important to check with your doctor before combining Halcion with the following:

Amiodarone (Cordarone)
Antidepressant medications, including "tricyclic" drugs such as Elavil and such MAO inhibitors as Nardil and Parnate
Antihistamines such as Benadryl and Tavist
Barbiturates such as phenobarbital and Seconal
Cimetidine (Tagamet)
Clarithromycin (Biaxin)

Cyclosporine (Sand-immune Neoral)
Diltiazem (Cardizem)
Ergotamine (Cafergot)
Erythromycin (E.E.S., PCE, E-Mycin, others)
Fluvoxamine (Luvox)
Isoniazid (Nydrazid)
Itraconazole (Nizoral)
Ketoconazole (Sporanox)
Narcotic painkillers such as Demerol
Major tranquilizers such as Mellaril and Thorazine
Nefazodone (Serzone)
Nicardipine (Cardene)
Nifedipine (Adalat)
Other tranquilizers such as BuSpar, Valium, and Xanax
Oral contraceptives
Paroxetine (Paxil)
Ranitidine (Zantac)
Seizure medications such as Dilantin and Tegretol
Sertraline (Zoloft)
Verapamil (Calan)

Special information
if you are pregnant or breastfeeding

Since benzodiazepines have been associated with damage to the developing baby, you should not take Halcion if you are pregnant, think you may be pregnant, or are planning to become pregnant; or if you are breastfeeding.

Recommended dosage

ADULTS

The usual dose is 0.25 milligram before bedtime. The dose should never be more than 0.5 milligram.

CHILDREN

Safety and effectiveness for children under the age of 18 have not been established.

OLDER ADULTS

To decrease the possibility of oversedation, dizziness, or impaired coordination, the usual starting dose is 0.125 milligram. This may be increased to 0.25 milligram if necessary.

Overdosage

Any medication taken in excess can have serious consequences. Severe overdosage of Halcion can be fatal. If you suspect an overdose, seek medical help immediately.

■ *Symptoms of Halcion overdose may include:*
Apnea (temporary cessation of breathing), coma, confusion, excessive sleepiness, problems in coordination, seizures, shallow or difficult breathing, slurred speech

Brand name:

HALDOL

Pronounced: HAL-dawl
Generic name: Haloperidol

Why is this drug prescribed?

Haldol is used to reduce the symptoms of mental disorders such as schizophrenia. It is also prescribed to control tics (uncontrolled muscle contractions of face, arms, or shoulders) and the unintended utterances that mark Gilles de la Tourette's syndrome. In addition, it is used in short-term treatment of children with severe behavior problems, including hyperactivity and combativeness.

Some doctors also prescribe Haldol to relieve severe nausea and vomiting caused by cancer drugs, to treat drug problems such as LSD flashback and PCP intoxication, and to control symptoms of hemiballismus, a condition that causes involuntary writhing of one side of the body.

Most important fact about this drug

Haldol may cause tardive dyskinesia—a condition characterized by involuntary muscle spasms and twitches in the face and body. This condition can be permanent, and appears to be most common among the elderly, especially women. Ask your doctor for information about this possible risk.

How should you take this medication?

Haldol may be taken with food or after eating. If taking Haldol in a liquid concentrate form, you will need to dilute it with milk or water.

You should not take Haldol with coffee, tea, or other caffeinated beverages, or with alcohol.

Haldol causes dry mouth. Sucking on a hard candy or ice chips may help alleviate the problem.

- *If you miss a dose...*
  Take it as soon as you remember. Take the rest of the doses for that day at equally spaced intervals. Do not take 2 doses at once.

- *Storage instructions...*
  Store away from heat, light, and moisture in a tightly closed container. Do not freeze the liquid.

What side effects may occur?
Side effects cannot be anticipated. If any side effects develop or change in intensity, inform your doctor as soon as possible. Only your doctor can determine if it is safe for you to continue taking Haldol.

- *Side effects may include:*
  Abnormal secretion of milk, acne-like skin reactions, agitation, anemia, anxiety, blurred vision, breast pain, breast development in males, cataracts, catatonic (unresponsive) state, chewing movements, confusion, constipation, coughing, deeper breathing, dehydration, depression, diarrhea, dizziness, drowsiness, dry mouth, epileptic seizures, exaggerated feeling of well-being, exaggerated reflexes, excessive perspiration, excessive salivation, hair loss, hallucinations, headache, heat stroke, high fever, high or low blood pressure, high or low blood sugar, impotence, inability to urinate, increased sex drive, indigestion, involuntary movements, irregular menstrual periods, irregular pulse, lack of muscular coordination, liver problems, loss of appetite, muscle spasms, nausea, Parkinson-like symptoms, persistent abnormal erections, physical rigidity and stupor, protruding tongue, puckering of mouth, puffing of cheeks, rapid heartbeat, restlessness, rigid arms, feet, head, and muscles, rotation of eyeballs, sensitivity to light, skin rash, skin eruptions, sleeplessness, sluggishness, swelling of breasts, twitching in the body, neck, shoulders, and face, vertigo, visual problems, vomiting, wheezing or asthma-like symptoms, yellowing of skin and whites of eyes

Why should this drug not be prescribed?
You should not take Haldol if you have Parkinson's disease or are sensitive to or allergic to the drug.

Special warnings about this medication
You should use Haldol cautiously if you have ever had breast cancer, a severe heart or circulatory disorder, chest pain, the eye condition known as glaucoma, seizures, or any drug allergies.

Temporary muscle spasms and twitches may occur if you suddenly stop taking Haldol. Follow your doctor's instructions closely when discontinuing the drug.

This drug may impair your ability to drive a car or operate potentially dangerous machinery. Do not participate in any activities that require full alertness if you are unsure of your reaction to Haldol.

Haldol may make your skin more sensitive to sunlight. When spending time in the sun, use a sunscreen or wear protective clothing.

Avoid exposure to extreme heat or cold. Haldol interferes with the body's temperature-regulating mechanism, so you could become overheated or suffer severe chills.

Possible food and drug interactions when taking this medication
Extreme drowsiness and other potentially serious effects can result if Haldol is combined with alcohol, narcotics, painkillers, sleeping medications, or other drugs that slow down the central nervous system.

If Haldol is taken with certain other drugs, the effects of either could be increased, decreased, or altered. It is especially important to check with your doctor before combining Haldol with the following:

Antiseizure drugs such as Dilantin or Tegretol
Antispasmodic drugs such as Bentyl and Cogentin
Blood-thinning medications such as Coumadin
Certain antidepressants, including Elavil, Tofranil, and Prozac
Epinephrine (EpiPen)
Lithium (Lithonate)
Methyldopa (Aldomet)
Propranolol (Inderal)
Rifampin (Rifadin)

Special information if you are pregnant or breastfeeding
The effects of Haldol during pregnancy have not been adequately studied. Pregnant women should use Haldol only if clearly needed. If you are pregnant or plan to become pregnant, inform your doctor immediately. Haldol should not be used by women who are breastfeeding an infant.

Recommended dosage

ADULTS

Moderate Symptoms
The usual dosage is 1 to 6 milligrams daily. This amount should be divided into 2 or 3 smaller doses.

Severe Symptoms
The usual dosage is 6 to 15 milligrams daily, divided into 2 or 3 smaller doses.

CHILDREN

Children younger than 3 years old should not take Haldol.

For children between the ages of 3 and 12, weighing approximately 33 to 88 pounds, doses should start at 0.5 milligram per day. Your doctor will increase the dose if needed.

For Psychotic Disorders
The daily dose may range from 0.05 milligram to 0.15 milligram for every 2.2 pounds of body weight.

For Non-Psychotic Behavior Disorders and Tourette's Syndrome
The daily dose may range from 0.05 milligram to 0.075 milligram for every 2.2 pounds of body weight.

OLDER ADULTS

In general, older people take dosages of Haldol in the lower ranges. Older adults (especially older women) may be more susceptible to tardive dyskinesia—a possibly irreversible condition marked by involuntary muscle spasms and twitches in the face and body. Consult your doctor for information about these potential risks.

Doses may range from 1 to 6 milligrams daily.

Overdosage
Any medication taken in excess can have serious consequences. If you suspect an overdose, seek medical help immediately.

- *Symptoms of Haldol overdose may include:*
  Catatonic (unresponsive) state, coma, decreased breathing, low blood pressure, rigid muscles, sedation, tremor, weakness

Brand name:

HALFPRIN

See Aspirin, page 98.

Generic name:

HALOPERIDOL

See Haldol, page 583.

Brand name:

HELIDAC THERAPY

Pronounced: HEL-i-dak
Generic ingredients: Bismuth subsalicylate, Metronidazole,
Tetracycline hydrochloride

Why is this drug prescribed?
Helidac is a drug combination that cures the infection responsible for most stomach ulcers. Although ulcers used to be blamed on stress and spicy food, doctors now know that a germ called *Helicobacter pylori* is the actual culprit in a majority of cases.

Most important fact about this drug
You need to take all of the Helidac pills 4 times each day for 14 days. (You should also be taking an acid blocker such as Zantac, Pepcid, or Tagamet.) If you fail to stick to this regimen, the infection may not be cured.

How should you take this medication?
There are four pills in each dose of Helidac. The two pink tablets (bismuth subsalicylate) should be chewed and swallowed. The white tablet (metronidazole) and the orange and white capsule (tetracycline) should be swallowed whole. Be sure to drink plenty of fluid with each dose—and especially at bedtime—to prevent irritation.

- *If you miss a dose...*
  Take the next dose at the appointed time and continue with your regular schedule until the medication is used up. Do not try to "catch up" by doubling a dose. If you miss more than four doses, contact your physician.

■ *Storage instructions...*
Store at room temperature.

What side effects may occur?
Side effects cannot be anticipated. If any develop or change in intensity, inform your doctor as soon as possible. Only your doctor can determine if it is safe for you to continue taking Helidac.

■ *More common side effects may include:*
Abdominal pain, diarrhea, nausea

■ *Less common side effects may include:*
Appetite loss, black bowel movements, constipation, dizziness, insomnia, pain, prickly feeling, rectal discomfort, upper respiratory infection, vomiting, weakness

■ *Rare side effects may include:*
Arthritis, bleeding in the stomach or intestines, dry mouth, fainting, gas, general feeling of illness, heart attack, high blood pressure, indigestion, inflamed mouth or tongue, nervousness, rash, sensitivity to light, trouble swallowing

Why should this drug not be prescribed?
Do not take Helidac if you have ever had an allergic reaction to any of the following medications:

Aspirin
Pepto-Bismol (bismuth subsalicylate)
Flagyl (metronidazole)
Tetracycline
Vibramycin (doxycycline)

Helidac is not for use by children and pregnant or nursing women. The tetracycline part of the therapy can harm a developing baby, stunt a child's growth, and interfere with tooth development.

You should also avoid Helidac if you have kidney or liver disease.

Special warnings about this medication
Don't be alarmed if your tongue and/or bowel movements turn black while you are taking Helidac. This a harmless side effect of the bismuth subsalicylate part of the therapy.

The tetracycline part of Helidac therapy increases the risk of getting a bad sunburn. Limit your exposure to the sun. If you notice a reddening of your skin, stop taking Helidac and call your doctor.

If you develop a headache and blurred vision, numbness and tingling in the arms and legs, or seizures, stop taking Helidac and call your doctor immediately. Also report any infection that develops and be sure your doctor is aware of any infection or blood disorder you already have.

Possible food and drug interactions
when taking this medication

Combining aspirin with Helidac sometimes causes ringing in the ears. If this happens, check with your doctor. You may need to temporarily stop taking aspirin.

During Helidac therapy, alcoholic beverages can cause abdominal cramps, nausea, vomiting, headache, and flushing. Avoid alcohol until at least 1 day after finishing Helidac.

For 1 hour before and 2 hours after each dose of Helidac, avoid eating dairy products. They can interfere with the medication's absorption.

Since Helidac can interfere with oral contraceptives, you should use an additional form of birth control during Helidac therapy.

Certain other drugs may also interact. Check with your doctor before combining Helidac with any of the following:

Antacids containing aluminum, calcium, or magnesium
Blood-thinning drugs such as warfarin (Coumadin)
Cimetidine (Tagamet)
Diabetes medications such as insulin and glyburide (Micronase)
Disulfiram (Antabuse)
Iron (including vitamins that contain iron)
Lithium (Lithonate)
Penicillin
Phenobarbital
Phenytoin (Dilantin)
Probenecid (Benemid)
Sodium bicarbonate (baking soda)
Sulfinpyrazone (Anturane)
Zinc (including vitamins that contain zinc)

Special information
if you are pregnant or breastfeeding
Do not undertake Helidac therapy during this period.

Recommended dosage

ADULTS

Take all 4 Helidac pills 4 times daily, with each meal and at bedtime.

Overdosage
An overdose of the bismuth subsalicylate part of Helidac can be fatal. The other components can have serious consequences as well.

- **Symptoms of Helidac overdose may include:**
  Confusion, coma, convulsions, coordination problems, diarrhea, fast heartbeat, high fever, lethargy, nausea, numbness or pain in the arms and legs, rapid breathing, ringing in the ears, severe heart and lung problems, vomiting

If you suspect an overdose, seek medical attention immediately.

Brand name:

HISMANAL

Pronounced: HISS-man-al
Generic name: Astemizole

Why is this drug prescribed?
Hismanal is an antihistamine prescribed to relieve hay fever and to treat chronic hives. Hismanal is for long-term use; it will not provide immediate relief.

Most important fact about this drug
Never take more than the prescribed dose of Hismanal in an attempt to speed its action. Higher doses have been known to cause dangerously irregular heartbeats.

How should you take this medication?
Hismanal should be taken on an empty stomach—for example, 1 hour before you eat or 2 hours after eating. Taking the drug with food may make it less effective.

■ *If you miss a dose...*
Take it as soon as you remember. If it is almost time for your next dose, skip the one you missed and go back to your regular schedule. Never take 2 doses at the same time.

■ *Storage instructions...*
Store at room temperature. Protect from moisture.

What side effects may occur?
Side effects cannot be anticipated. If any develop or change in intensity, inform your doctor as soon as possible. Only your doctor can determine if it is safe for you to continue taking Hismanal.

■ *More common side effects may include:*
Drowsiness, dry mouth, fatigue, headache, increase in appetite, weight gain

■ *Less common side effects may include:*
Asthma-like symptoms, burning, prickling, or tingling, depression, diarrhea, dizziness, fluid retention, hepatitis, inflammation of the eyelids, itching, joint pain, muscle pain, nausea, nervousness, nosebleed, palpitations, sensitivity to light, skin rash, sore throat, stomach and intestinal pain

■ *Rare side effects may include:*
Low blood pressure

Why should this drug not be prescribed?
Avoid Hismanal if you have a known allergy to it.

Special warnings about this medication
Rare—but serious—heart-related side effects have been reported when Hismanal is used with erythromycin (PCE, E-Mycin), ketoconazole (Nizoral), or itraconazole (Sporanox). If you are taking these medicines, do not take Hismanal. The same reaction can be caused by combining Hismanal with a large dose of quinine. However, the amount of quinine in tonic water is too small to cause the problem under ordinary circumstances.

If you are being treated for a lower respiratory tract disease such as asthma or for liver or kidney disease, consult with your doctor before taking Hismanal.

Possible food and drug interactions
when taking this medication

Taking this drug with food can decrease its effectiveness. Hismanal should not be taken with grapefruit juice.

If Hismanal is taken with certain other drugs the effects of either may be increased, decreased, or altered. It is especially important to check with your doctor before combining Hismanal with the following:

Alcohol
Antibiotics such as Flagyl
Antifungal drugs such as Diflucan, Nizoral, and Sporanox
Drugs that affect heart rhythms such as Vascor, Elavil, and Thorazine
"Macrolide" antibiotics such as Zithromax, Biaxin, E-Mycin, PCE, and Tao
Protease inhibitors (AIDS drugs) such as Crixivan, Fortovase, Norvir, and Viracept
Quinine
Serotonin-boosting drugs such as Luvox, Paxil, Prozac, Serzone, and Zoloft
Zyflo

See "Special warnings about this medication" for more information.

Special information
if you are pregnant or breastfeeding

The effects of Hismanal during pregnancy have not been adequately studied. Therefore, this medication should be prescribed only when the benefits of therapy outweigh any potential risk to the fetus. It is not known whether Hismanal appears in breast milk. If this medication is essential to your health, your doctor may advise you to stop nursing your baby until your treatment with this drug is finished.

Recommended dosage

ADULTS

The usual dose for adults and children 12 years and over is 10 milligrams (1 tablet) once daily.

CHILDREN

Safety and effectiveness in children under 12 have not been established.

Overdosage

Hismanal is generally safe; however, large amounts may cause serious symptoms. If you suspect an overdose, get medical help immediately.

■ *Symptoms of Hismanal overdose may include:*
Cardiac arrest, fainting, irregular heartbeat, seizures

Brand name:

HIVID

Pronounced: HIV-id
Generic name: Zalcitabine

Why is this drug prescribed?
Hivid is one of the drugs used against the human immunodeficiency virus (HIV)—the deadly cause of AIDS. HIV does its damage by slowly undermining the immune system, finally leaving the body without any defense against infection. Hivid staves off collapse of the immune system by interfering with the virus's ability to reproduce.

Hivid is often combined with one of the new protease inhibitors (Crixivan, Fortovase, and Norvir) as part of the "cocktail" of drugs that has proven so effective in halting or even reversing the progress of HIV. Hivid can also be combined with the HIV drug Retrovir, provided you have not already been taking Retrovir for more than 3 months. For people with advanced cases of HIV, Hivid is sometimes prescribed by itself when other drugs don't work or can't be tolerated.

Most important fact about this drug
Although Hivid can slow the progress of HIV, it is not a cure. You may continue to develop complications, including frequent infections. Even if you feel better, regular physical exams and blood counts by your doctor are highly advisable. Also be sure to notify your doctor immediately if you experience any changes in your general health.

How should you take this medication?
Hivid should be taken every 8 hours, exactly as prescribed. It is important to keep levels of the drug in your body as constant as possible, so be sure to take every scheduled dose. Never take more than the prescribed dose; nerve disorders could result.

■ *If you miss a dose...*
Take it as soon as you remember. If it is almost time for the next dose, skip the one you missed and go back to your regular schedule. Never take 2 doses at once.

■ *Storage instructions...*
Store at room temperature in a tightly closed bottle.

What side effects may occur?
Although side effects can never be predicted, they are more likely—and more apt to be severe—in people with an advanced case of HIV. If any side effects develop or change in intensity, inform your doctor as soon as possible. Only your doctor can determine if it is safe for you to continue using Hivid.

■ *More common side effects may include:*
Abdominal pain, fatigue, hives, itching, mouth sores and inflammation, nausea and vomiting, rash, tingling, burning, numbness, or pain in the hands and feet

■ *Less common side effects may include:*
Constipation, convulsions, diarrhea, fever, headache

There have been isolated reports of an extremely wide variety of additional problems occurring during Hivid therapy. Whether these problems were caused by the drug remains unclear. Nevertheless, it's wise to check with your doctor whenever any unexplained symptom develops.

Why should this drug not be prescribed?
If Hivid gives you an allergic reaction, you cannot use this medication.

Special warnings about this medication
If you have an advanced case of HIV, there is a one-in-three chance that Hivid will cause a serious nerve disorder called peripheral neuropathy. The first signs of this problem are numbness, tingling, and burning pain in the hands and feet. Check with your doctor as soon as any of these symptoms develop. If you continue to take Hivid, they will be followed by episodes of intense, sharp, shooting pain or severe, continuous, burning pain—and the condition could become irreversible. If Hivid is stopped promptly, the symptoms will gradually disappear.

Much more rarely, Hivid has been known to cause a dangerous inflammation of the pancreas (pancreatitis), especially in people who have previously had the problem. The chief signs are bouts of severe abdominal pain—usually lasting for days—accompanied by nausea and vomiting. If these symptoms develop, call your doctor without delay. Hivid therapy must be discontinued permanently.

Other rare but dangerous side effects to watch for include liver failure, weakening of the heart, and ulcers in the mouth and the canal to the stomach (esophagus). Kidney disease increases the risk of these side effects. If you've ever had kidney, liver, or heart problems, or tend to abuse alcohol, be sure your doctor is aware of the situation.

Remember that Hivid does not eliminate HIV from the body. The infection can still be passed to others through sexual contact or blood contamination.

Possible food and drug interactions
when taking this medication

A number of drugs can cause peripheral neuropathy and should not be taken with Hivid. The list includes:

Chloramphenicol (Chloromycetin)
Cisplatin (Platinol)
Dapsone
Disulfiram (Antabuse)
Ethionamide (Trecator-SC)
Glutethimide
Gold
Hydralazine (Ser-Ap-Es)
Iodoquinol (Yodoxin)
Isoniazid (Nydrazid)
Metronidazole (Flagyl)
Nitrofurantoin (Macrodantin)
Phenytoin (Dilantin)
Ribavirin (Virazole)
Vincristine (Oncovin)

Several other drugs should be either avoided or taken with caution while on Hivid therapy. Check with your doctor before taking the following:

Aminoglycosides such as Garamycin
Amphotericin B (Fungizone)
Antacids containing magnesium and aluminum, including Maalox and
    Mylanta
Cimetidine (Tagamet)
Didanosine (Videx)
Foscarnet (Foscavir)
Metoclopramide
Pentamidine (Pentam 300)
Probenecid (Benemid)

**Special information
if you are pregnant or breastfeeding**

The safety of Hivid during pregnancy has not been adequately studied. Take contraceptive measures while using Hivid. If you are pregnant or plan to become pregnant, notify your doctor immediately.

Do not breastfeed your baby. HIV can be passed to an infant through breast milk.

Recommended dosage

ADULTS

The usual dose, alone or in combination with Retrovir, is one 0.750 milligram tablet every 8 hours. Your doctor may adjust the dosage if you have kidney problems or are taking other HIV medications.

CHILDREN

Safety and effectiveness have not been established for children under 13.

Overdosage

Any medication taken in excess can have serious consequences. If you suspect an overdose, seek medical attention immediately.

■ *Symptoms of Hivid overdose may include:*
Drowsiness, vomiting, numbness, tingling, burning, and pain in the arms and legs

Brand name:

HUMULIN

See Insulin, page 639.

Brand name:

HYDERGINE

*Pronounced: HY-der-jeen
Generic name: Ergoloid mesylates*

Why is this drug prescribed?

Hydergine helps relieve symptoms of declining mental capacity, thought to be related to aging or dementia, seen in some people over age 60. The symptoms include reduced understanding and motivation, and a decline in self-care and interpersonal skills.

Most important fact about this drug

It may take several weeks or more for Hydergine to produce noticeable results. In fact, your doctor may need up to 6 months to determine whether the drug is right for you. Keep taking your regular doses even if you feel no effect.

How should you take this medication?

Take Hydergine exactly as prescribed.

■ *If you miss a dose...*
Skip the dose you missed and go back to your regular schedule. Do not take 2 doses at once. If you miss 2 or more doses in a row, consult your doctor.

■ *Storage instructions...*
Store at room temperature. Protect from heat and light. Do not freeze capsules or oral solution.

What side effects may occur?

Side effects cannot be anticipated. If any develop or change in intensity, notify your doctor as soon as possible. Only your doctor can determine whether it is safe to continue taking Hydergine.

■ *Side effects may include:*
Stomach upset, temporary nausea

Why should this drug not be prescribed?

Do not use Hydergine if you have ever had an allergic reaction to or are sensitive to the drug, or if you have a mental disorder.

Special warnings about this medication

Since the symptoms treated with Hydergine are of unknown origin and may change or evolve into a specific disease, your doctor will make a careful diagnosis before prescribing Hydergine and then watch closely for any changes in your condition.

Possible food and drug interactions
when taking this medication

No interactions have been reported.

Special information
if you are pregnant or breastfeeding
Hydergine is not intended for use by women of childbearing age.

Recommended dosage

ADULTS

The usual dose of Hydergine is 1 milligram, 3 times a day.

Overdosage
Any medication taken in excess can have serious consequences. If you
suspect an overdose of Hydergine, seek medical attention immediately.

Brand name:

HYDROCET

See Vicodin, page 1403.

Generic name:

HYDROCHLOROTHIAZIDE

See HydroDIURIL, page 601.

Generic name:

HYDROCHLOROTHIAZIDE WITH TRIAMTERENE

See Dyazide, page 443.

Generic name:

HYDROCODONE WITH ACETAMINOPHEN

See Vicodin, page 1403.

Generic name:

HYDROCODONE WITH CHLORPHENIRAMINE

See Tussionex, page 1356.

Generic name:

HYDROCODONE WITH IBUPROFEN

See Vicoprofen, page 1406.

Generic name:

HYDROCORTISONE SKIN PREPARATIONS

Pronounced: hi-droh-COURT-i-zone
Brand names: Cetacort, Dermacort, Hytone, Nutracort

Why is this drug prescribed?
Hydrocortisone creams and lotions contain a steroid medication that relieves a variety of itchy rashes and inflammatory skin conditions.

Most important fact about this drug
When you apply a hydrocortisone cream or lotion, you inevitably absorb some of the medication through your skin and into the bloodstream. Too much absorption can lead to unwanted side effects elsewhere in the body. To keep this problem to a minimum, avoid using large amounts of hydrocortisone over extensive areas, and do not cover it with airtight dressings such as plastic wrap or adhesive bandages unless specifically told to by your doctor.

How should you use this medication?
Use hydrocortisone exactly as directed, and only to treat the condition for which your doctor prescribed it.

Apply the medication directly to the affected area. Hydrocortisone cream and lotion are for use only on the skin. Be careful to keep them out of your eyes.

If you are using hydrocortisone for psoriasis or a condition that has been difficult to cure, your doctor may advise you to use a bandage or covering over the affected area. If an infection develops, remove the bandage and contact your doctor.

- *If you miss a dose...*
  Apply it as soon as you remember. If it is almost time for the next dose, skip the one you missed and go back to your regular schedule.

- *Storage instructions...*
  Keep the container tightly closed, and store it at room temperature, away from heat. Protect from freezing.

What side effects may occur?
Side effects cannot be anticipated. If any develop or change in intensity, inform your doctor as soon as possible. Only your doctor can determine if it is safe for you to continue using hydrocortisone.

■ *Side effects may include:*
Acne-like skin eruptions, burning, dryness, growth of excessive hair, inflammation of the hair follicles, inflammation around the mouth, irritation, itching, peeling skin, prickly heat, secondary infection, skin inflammation, skin softening, stretch marks, unusual lack of skin color

Why should this drug not be prescribed?
Do not use Hydrocortisone if it has ever given you an allergic reaction.

Special warnings about this medication
Avoid covering a treated area with waterproof diapers or plastic pants. They can increase unwanted absorption of hydrocortisone.

If you use this medication over large areas of skin for prolonged periods of time—or cover the treated area—the amount of the hormone absorbed into your bloodstream may eventually lead to Cushing's syndrome: a moon-faced appearance, fattened neck and trunk, and purplish streaks on the skin. You can also develop glandular problems or high blood sugar, or show sugar in your urine. Children, because of their relatively larger ratio of skin surface area to body weight, are particularly susceptible to overabsorption of hydrocortisone.

Long-term treatment of children with steroids such as hydrocortisone may interfere with growth and development.

If an irritation develops, stop using the medication and contact your doctor.

Possible food and drug interactions
when using this medication
No interactions have been reported.

Special information
if you are pregnant or breastfeeding
The effects of hydrocortisone during pregnancy have not been adequately studied. If you are pregnant or plan to become pregnant, inform your doctor immediately. It is not known whether this medication appears in breast milk in sufficient amounts to affect a nursing baby. To avoid any possible harm to your baby, use hydrocortisone sparingly, and only with your doctor's permission, when breastfeeding.

Recommended dosage

ADULTS

Apply hydrocortisone cream or lotion to the affected area 2 to 4 times a day, depending on the severity of the condition.

CHILDREN

Limit use to the least amount necessary, as directed by your doctor.

Overdosage

Extensive or long-term use can cause Cushing's syndrome (see "Special warnings about this medication"), glandular problems, higher than normal amounts of sugar in the blood, and high amounts of sugar in the urine. If you suspect an overdose of hydrocortisone, seek medical treatment immediately.

Brand name:

HYDRODIURIL

Pronounced: High-dro-DYE-your-il
Generic name: Hydrochlorothiazide
Other brand name: Esidrix

Why is this drug prescribed?

HydroDIURIL is used in the treatment of high blood pressure and other conditions that require the elimination of excess fluid (water) from the body. These conditions include congestive heart failure, cirrhosis of the liver, corticosteroid and estrogen therapy, and kidney disorders. When used for high blood pressure, HydroDIURIL can be used alone or with other high blood pressure medications. HydroDIURIL contains a form of thiazide, a diuretic that prompts your body to produce and eliminate more urine, which helps lower blood pressure.

Most important fact about this drug

If you have high blood pressure, you must take HydroDIURIL regularly for it to be effective. Since blood pressure declines gradually, it may be several weeks before you get the full benefit of HydroDIURIL; and you must continue taking it even if you are feeling well. HydroDIURIL does not cure high blood pressure; it merely keeps it under control.

How should you take this medication?

Take HydroDIURIL exactly as prescribed by your doctor.

■ *If you miss a dose...*
If you forget a dose, take it as soon as you remember. If it is almost time for your next dose, skip the one you missed and go back to your regular schedule. Never take 2 doses at the same time.

■ *Storage instructions...*
Keep container tightly closed. Protect from light, moisture, and freezing cold. Store at room temperature.

What side effects may occur?

Side effects cannot be anticipated. If any develop or change in intensity, inform your doctor as soon as possible. Only your doctor can determine if it is safe for you to continue taking HydroDIURIL.

■ *Side effects may include:*
Abdominal cramping, diarrhea, dizziness upon standing up, headache, loss of appetite, low blood pressure, low potassium (leading to symptoms such as dry mouth, excessive thirst, weak or irregular heartbeat, muscle pain or cramps), stomach irritation, stomach upset, weakness

■ *Less common or rare side effects may include:*
Anemia, blood disorders, changes in blood sugar, constipation, difficulty breathing, dizziness, fever, fluid in the lung, hair loss, high levels of sugar in the urine, hives, hypersensitivity reactions, impotence, inflammation of the lung, inflammation of the pancreas, inflammation of the salivary glands, kidney failure, muscle spasms, nausea, rash, reddish or purplish spots on the skin, restlessness, sensitivity to light, skin disorders including Stevens-Johnson syndrome (blisters in the mouth and eyes), skin peeling, tingling or pins and needles, vertigo, vision changes, vomiting, yellow eyes and skin

Why should this drug not be prescribed?

If you are unable to urinate, you should not take this medication.

If you are sensitive to or have ever had an allergic reaction to HydroDIURIL or similar drugs, or if you are sensitive to sulfa or other sulfonamide-derived drugs, you should not take this medication.

Special warnings about this medication

Diuretics can cause your body to lose too much potassium. Signs of an excessively low potassium level include muscle weakness and rapid or irregular heartbeat. To boost your potassium level, your doctor may recommend eating potassium-rich foods or taking a potassium supplement.

If you are taking HydroDIURIL, your kidney function should be given a complete assessment, and should continue to be monitored.

If you have liver disease, diabetes, gout, or lupus erythematosus (a form of rheumatism), HydroDIURIL should be used with caution.

If you have bronchial asthma or a history of allergies, you may be at greater risk for an allergic reaction to this medication.

Dehydration, excessive sweating, severe diarrhea or vomiting could deplete your body's fluids and cause your blood pressure to become too low. Be careful when exercising and in hot weather.

**Possible food and drug interactions
when taking this medication**

HydroDIURIL may increase the effects of alcohol. Do not drink alcohol while taking this medication.

If HydroDIURIL is taken with certain other drugs, the effects of either could be increased, decreased, or altered. It is especially important to check with your doctor before combining HydroDIURIL with the following:

  Barbiturates such as phenobarbital
  Cholestyramine (Questran)
  Colestipol (Colestid)
  Corticosteroids such as prednisone and ACTH
  Digoxin (Lanoxin)
  Drugs to treat diabetes such as insulin or Micronase
  Lithium (Lithonate)
  Narcotics such as Percocet
  Nonsteroidal anti-inflammatory drugs such as Naprosyn
  Norepinephrine (Levophed)
  Other high blood pressure medications such as Aldomet
  Skeletal muscle relaxants, such as tubocurarine

**Special information
if you are pregnant or breastfeeding**

The effects of HydroDIURIL during pregnancy have not been adequately studied. If you are pregnant or plan to become pregnant, inform your doctor immediately. HydroDIURIL appears in breast milk and could affect a nursing infant. If this medication is essential to your health, your doctor may advise you to discontinue breastfeeding until your treatment is finished.

Recommended dosage

Dosage should be adjusted to each individual's needs. The smallest dose that is effective should be used.

ADULTS

Water Retention

The usual dose is 25 milligrams to 100 milligrams per day. Your doctor may tell you to take the drug in a single dose or to divide the total amount into more than one dose. Your doctor may put you on a day on, day off schedule or some other alternate day schedule to suit your needs.

High Blood Pressure

The usual dose is 25 milligrams as a single dose. Your doctor may increase the dose to 50 milligrams, as a single dose or divided into 2 doses. Dosages should be adjusted when used with other high blood pressure medications.

CHILDREN

Dosages for children should be adjusted according to weight, generally 0.5 to 1 milligram per pound of body weight in 1 or 2 doses per day. Infants under 2 years should not receive more than 37.5 milligrams per day, and children aged 2 to 12 should not get more than 100 milligrams a day. Infants under 6 months may need 1.5 milligrams per pound per day in 2 doses.

Under 2 years

Based on age and body weight, the daily dosage is 12.5 milligrams to 37.5 milligrams per day.

2 to 12 years

The daily dosage, based on body weight, is 37.5 milligrams to 100 milligrams.

HydroDIURIL tablets come in strengths of 25, 50 and 100 milligrams.

Overdosage

Any medication taken in excess can cause symptoms of overdose. If you suspect an overdose, seek medical attention immediately.

■ *Symptoms of HydroDIURIL overdose may include:*
Dry mouth, excessive thirst, muscle pain or cramps, nausea and vomiting, weak or irregular heartbeat, weakness and dizziness

Generic name:

HYDROMORPHONE

See Dilaudid, page 404.

Generic name:

HYDROXYCHLOROQUINE

See Plaquenil, page 1007.

Generic name:

HYDROXYZINE

See Atarax, page 104.

Brand name:

HYGROTON

Pronounced: HIGH-grow-ton
Generic name: Chlorthalidone
Other brand name: Thalitone

Why is this drug prescribed?

Hygroton is a diuretic (water pill) used to treat high blood pressure and fluid retention associated with congestive heart failure, cirrhosis of the liver (a disease of the liver caused by damage to its cells), corticosteroid and estrogen therapy, and kidney disease. When used for high blood pressure, Hygroton may be used alone or in combination with other high blood pressure medications. Diuretics help your body produce and eliminate more urine, which helps lower blood pressure.

Most important fact about this drug

If you have high blood pressure, you must take Hygroton regularly for it to be effective. Since blood pressure declines gradually, it may be several weeks before you get the full benefit of Hygroton; and you must continue taking it even if you are feeling well. Hygroton does not cure high blood pressure; it merely keeps it under control.

How should you take this medication?

Diuretics such as Hygroton increase urination; therefore Hygroton should be taken in the morning.

Do not interchange Hygroton or generic chlorthalidone with Thalitone without consulting your doctor or pharmacist.

Hygroton may be taken with food. Take it exactly as prescribed.

■ *If you miss a dose...*
Take it as soon as you remember. If it is almost time for the next dose, skip the one you missed and go back to your regular schedule. Do not take 2 doses at the same time.

■ *Storage instructions...*
Store at room temperature.

What side effects may occur?
Side effects cannot be anticipated. If any side effects develop or change in intensity, tell your doctor immediately. Only your doctor can determine whether it is safe to continue taking Hygroton.

■ *Side effects may include:*
Allergic reaction, anemia, changes in blood sugar, changes in potassium levels (causing such symptoms as dry mouth, excessive thirst, weak or irregular heartbeat, and muscle pain or cramps), constipation, cramping, diarrhea, dizziness, dizziness upon standing up, flaky skin, headache, hives, impotence, inflammation of the pancreas, itching, loss of appetite, low blood pressure, muscle spasms, nausea, rash, restlessness, sensitivity to light, stomach irritation, tingling or pins and needles, vision changes, vomiting, weakness, yellow eyes and skin

Why should this drug not be prescribed?
If you are unable to urinate or if you have ever had an allergic reaction to or are sensitive to chlorthalidone or other sulfa drugs, do not take Hygroton.

Special warnings about this medication
Diuretics can cause your body to lose too much potassium. Signs of an excessively low potassium level include muscle weakness and rapid or irregular heartbeat. To boost your potassium level, your doctor may recommend eating potassium-rich foods or taking a potassium supplement.

Tell your doctor if you have ever had an allergic reaction to other diuretics or if you have asthma, kidney or liver disease, gout, or lupus.

If you have a history of bronchial asthma, you are more likely to have an allergic reaction to Hygroton.

Be careful in hot weather not to become dehydrated. Contact your doctor if you experience excessive thirst, tiredness, restlessness, muscle pains or cramps, nausea, vomiting, or increased heart rate or pulse.

This medication may aggravate lupus erythematosus, a disease of the connective tissue.

Avoid prolonged exposure to sunlight.

Possible food and drug interactions
when taking this medication
Drinking alcohol may increase the chance of dizziness. Do not drink alcohol while taking this medication.

If Hygroton is taken with certain other drugs, the effects of either could be increased, decreased, or altered. It is especially important to check with your doctor before combining Hygroton with the following:

Appetite-control medicines such as Tenuate
Cholestyramine (Questran)
Colestipol (Colestid)
Decongestants (medicines for colds, cough, hay fever, or sinus)
Digitalis (Lanoxin)
Insulin
Lithium (Lithonate)
Oral diabetes drugs such as Micronase
Other high blood pressure medications such as Catapres and Aldomet
Steroids such as prednisone

Special information
if you are pregnant or breastfeeding
Information is not available about the safety of Hygroton during pregnancy. If you are pregnant or plan to become pregnant, inform your doctor immediately. Hygroton may appear in breast milk and could affect a nursing infant. If Hygroton is essential to your health, your doctor may advise you to stop breastfeeding until your treatment is finished.

Recommended dosage
Your doctor will tailor your individual dose to the lowest possible amount that delivers a satisfactory response.

Once desired control of blood pressure or fluid retention has been achieved, your doctor may adjust your dose downward.

HIGH BLOOD PRESSURE

Hygroton
The usual initial dosage is a single dose of 25 milligrams. Your doctor may increase the dose to 100 milligrams once daily.

Thalitone
The usual initial dose is a single dose of 15 milligrams. Your doctor may increase the dose to 45 to 50 milligrams once daily.

FLUID RETENTION

Hygroton
The usual recommended initial dose is 50 to 100 milligrams daily or 100 milligrams every other day. Some people may require up to 150 to 200 milligrams at these intervals.

Thalitone
The usual initial dose is 30 to 60 milligrams daily or 60 milligrams on alternate days. Some people may require up to 90 to 120 milligrams at these intervals.

Overdosage
Any medication taken in excess can have serious consequences. If you suspect an overdose, seek medical treatment immediately.

■ *Symptoms of Hygroton overdose may include:*
Confusion, dizziness, nausea, weakness

Generic name:

HYOSCYAMINE

See Levsin, page 683.

Brand name:

HYTONE

See Hydrocortisone Skin Preparations, page 599.

Brand name:

HYTRIN

Pronounced: HIGH-trin
Generic name: Terazosin hydrochloride

Why is this drug prescribed?

Hytrin is prescribed to reduce high blood pressure. It may be used alone or in combination with other blood pressure lowering drugs, such as HydroDIURIL (a diuretic) or Inderal, a beta blocker.

Hytrin is also prescribed to relieve the symptoms of benign prostatic hyperplasia or BPH. BPH is an enlargement of the prostate gland that surrounds the urinary canal. It leads to the following symptoms:

- a weak or interrupted stream when urinating
- a feeling that you cannot empty your bladder completely
- a feeling of delay when you start to urinate
- a need to urinate often, especially at night
- a feeling that you must urinate right away

Hytrin relaxes the tightness of a certain type of muscle in the prostate and at the opening of the bladder. This can reduce the severity of the symptoms.

Most important fact about this drug

If you have high blood pressure, you must take Hytrin regularly for it to be effective. Since blood pressure declines gradually, it may be several weeks before you get the full benefit of Hytrin; and you must continue taking it even if you are feeling well. Hytrin does not cure high blood pressure; it merely keeps it under control.

How should you take this medication?

You may take Hytrin with or without food. Take your first dose at bedtime. Do not take more than the 1 milligram your doctor has prescribed.

- *If you miss a dose...*
  Take it as soon as you remember. If it is almost time for the next dose, skip the one you missed and go back to your regular schedule. Do not take 2 doses at the same time.

■ *Storage instructions...*
Store at room temperature in a cool, dry place. Protect from light.

What side effects may occur?
Side effects cannot be anticipated. If any develop or change in intensity, inform your doctor as soon as possible. Only your doctor can determine if it is safe for you to continue taking Hytrin.

■ *More common side effects may include:*
Difficult or labored breathing, dizziness, headache, heart palpitations, light-headedness upon standing, nausea, pain in the arms and legs, sleepiness, stuffy nose, swollen wrists and ankles, weakness

If these symptoms persist, tell your doctor. Your dosage of Hytrin may be higher than needed.

■ *Less common or rare side effects may include:*
Anxiety, back pain, blurred vision, bronchitis, conjunctivitis (inflamed eyes), constipation, decreased sex drive, depression, diarrhea, dimmed vision, dry mouth, facial swelling, fainting, fever, flu or cold symptoms (cough, sore throat, runny nose), fluid retention, frequent urination, gas, gout, impotence, inability to hold urine, increased heart rate, indigestion, inflamed sinuses, insomnia, irregular heartbeat, itching, joint pain and inflammation, low blood pressure, muscle aches, nasal inflammation, nervousness, nosebleed, numbness or tingling, painful lasting erection, pain in the abdomen, chest, neck, or shoulder, rash, ringing in the ears, severe allergic reaction, sweating, urinary tract infection, vertigo, vision changes, vomiting, weight gain

Why should this drug not be prescribed?
Do not take Hytrin if you are sensitive to it or have ever had an allergic reaction to it.

Special warnings about this medication
When your blood pressure falls in response to Hytrin, you may faint. Other less severe reactions include dizziness, heart palpitations, light-headedness, and drowsiness. You are also likely to feel dizzy or faint whenever you rise from a sitting or lying position; this should disappear as your body becomes accustomed to Hytrin. If your occupation is such that these symptoms might cause serious problems, make sure your doctor knows this from the start; he or she will increase your Hytrin dosage very cautiously.

Regardless of your occupation, avoid driving, climbing, and other hazardous tasks at the following times:

- For 12 hours after your first dose of Hytrin
- With each new dosage increase
- When you re-start Hytrin after any treatment interruption

If you are taking Hytrin for benign prostatic hyperplasia, remember that although Hytrin helps relieve the symptoms of BPH, it does NOT change the size of the prostate, which may continue to grow. You may still need surgery in the future. In addition, it *is* possible to have BPH and prostate cancer at the same time.

If you develop the side effect called priapism—a painful erection that lasts for hours—call your doctor without delay. The condition can lead to impotence if not treated immediately.

Possible food and drug interactions
when taking this medication

If Hytrin is taken with certain other drugs, the effects of either could be increased, decreased, or altered. It is especially important to check with your doctor before combining Hytrin with the following:

Nonsteroidal anti-inflammatory painkillers such as Motrin and Naprosyn
Other blood pressure medications, such as Dyazide, Vasotec, Calan, and
   Verelan

Special information
if you are pregnant or breastfeeding

The effects of Hytrin during pregnancy have not been adequately studied. If you are pregnant or plan to become pregnant, notify your doctor immediately. Hytrin is not recommended during pregnancy unless the benefit outweighs the potential risk to the unborn baby. It is not known whether Hytrin appears in breast milk. Because many drugs do appear in breast milk, your doctor may advise you to stop breastfeeding until your treatment with this drug is finished.

Recommended dosage

ADULTS

High Blood Pressure

The usual initial dose is 1 milligram at bedtime. Your doctor may slowly increase the dose until your blood pressure has been lowered sufficiently. The usual recommended dosage range is 1 milligram to 5 milligrams taken once a day; however, some people may benefit from doses as high as 20 milligrams per day.

Benign Prostatic Hyperplasia
The starting dose is 1 milligram at bedtime. Your doctor will gradually increase the dose to 10 milligrams, taken once a day, usually for at least 4 to 6 weeks. A few men have needed a dose of 20 milligrams a day.

If you stop taking Hytrin for several days or longer, your doctor will re-start your treatment with 1 milligram at bedtime.

CHILDREN

Safety and effectiveness of Hytrin in children have not been established.

Overdosage
If you take too much Hytrin, dizziness, light-headedness, and fainting may occur within 90 minutes. A large overdose may lead to shock. If you suspect an overdose of Hytrin, seek medical attention immediately.

Brand name:

HYZAAR

Pronounced: HIGH-zahr
Generic ingredients: Losartan potassium and
*   Hydrochlorothiazide*

Why is this drug prescribed?
Hyzaar is a combination medication used in the treatment of high blood pressure. One component, losartan, belongs to a new class of blood pressure medications that work by preventing the hormone angiotensin II from constricting the blood vessels, thus allowing blood to flow more freely and keeping the blood pressure down. The other component, hydrochlorothiazide, is a diuretic that increases the output of urine, removing excess fluid from the body and thus lowering blood pressure.

Most important fact about this drug
You must take Hyzaar regularly for it to be effective. Since blood pressure declines gradually, it may be several weeks before you get the full benefit of Hyzaar, and you must continue taking it even if you are feeling well. Hyzaar does not cure high blood pressure; it merely keeps it under control.

How should you take this medication?
Hyzaar may be taken with or without food. Take Hyzaar exactly as directed. Try to take it at the same time each day so that it is easier to remember.

■ *If you miss a dose...*
Take the forgotten dose as soon as you remember. If it is almost time for your next dose, skip the one you missed and go back to your regular schedule.

■ *Storage instructions...*
Keep in a tightly closed container at room temperature. Protect from light.

What side effects may occur?
Side effects cannot be anticipated. If any develop or change in intensity, inform your doctor as soon as possible. Only your doctor can determine if it is safe for you to continue taking Hyzaar.

■ *More common side effects include:*
Dizziness, upper respiratory infection

■ *Less common side effects include:*
Abdominal pain, back pain, cough, fluid retention and swelling, heart palpitations, sinus inflammation, skin rash

Why should this drug not be prescribed?
If you have ever had an allergic reaction to losartan, hydrochlorothiazide, or sulfa drugs, you should not take this medication. If you are unable to urinate, do not take Hyzaar.

Special warnings about this medication
If you are taking Hyzaar and have kidney disease, your doctor will watch your kidney function carefully.

Hyzaar can cause low blood pressure, especially if you are also taking another diuretic. You may feel light-headed or faint, especially during the first few days of therapy. If these symptoms occur, contact your doctor. Your dosage may need to be adjusted or discontinued. If you actually faint, stop taking the medication until you have talked to your doctor.

If you have liver or kidney disease, diabetes, gout, or lupus erythematosus, Hyzaar should be used with caution. This drug may bring out hidden diabetes. If you are already taking insulin or oral diabetes drugs, your medication may have to be adjusted. If you have bronchial asthma or a history of allergies, you may be at greater risk for an allergic reaction to this medication.

Excessive sweating, severe diarrhea or vomiting could deplete your body fluids and cause your blood pressure to drop too low. Be careful when exercising and in hot weather. Call your doctor if your mouth becomes dry, you feel weak or tired or sluggish, you are unusually thirsty, you feel restless or confused, you ache all over, your heart starts beating faster, or you are nauseated.

Possible food and drug interactions when taking this medication

Hyzaar may increase the effects of alcohol. Avoid alcohol while taking this medication.

If Hyzaar is taken with certain other drugs, the effects of either could be increased, decreased, or altered. It is especially important to check with your doctor before taking Hyzaar with the following:

Barbiturates such as phenobarbital and Seconal
Cholestyramine (Questran)
Colestipol (Colestid)
Corticosteroids (Prednisone)
Insulin
Ketoconazole (Nizoral)
Lithium (Eskalith, Lithobid)
Narcotic painkillers such as Demerol, Tylenol with Codeine, and Percocet
Nonsteroidal anti-inflammatory drugs such as Aleve, Anaprox, and Motrin
Other blood pressure-lowering drugs such as Procardia XL and Tenormin
Oral diabetes drugs such as Diabinese, DiaBeta, and Glucotrol
Potassium supplements such as Slow-K
Salt substitutes containing potassium
Sulfaphenazole
Troleandomycin (Tao)

Special Information if you are pregnant or breastfeeding

When used in the second or third trimester of pregnancy, Hyzaar can cause injury or even death to the unborn child. Stop taking Hyzaar as soon as you know you are pregnant. If you are pregnant or plan to become pregnant, tell your doctor immediately. Hyzaar appears in breast milk and can affect the nursing infant. If this medication is essential to your health, your doctor may advise you to stop breastfeeding while you are taking Hyzaar.

Recommended dosage

ADULTS

The usual starting dose of Hyzaar is 1 tablet once daily (losartan 50 milligrams/hydrochlorothiazide 12.5 milligrams).

If your blood pressure does not respond to this dose, after about 3 weeks the dose may be increased to 2 tablets once daily. Taking more than 2 tablets daily is not recommended.

CHILDREN

The safety and effectiveness of Hyzaar in children have not been studied.

Overdosage

Any medication taken in excess can have serious consequences. Information concerning Hyzaar overdosage is limited. However, extremely low blood pressure and abnormally rapid or slow heartbeat may be signs of an overdose. Other signs may include dryness and thirst, overall weakness and tiredness, restlessness and confusion, muscle pains, nausea, and vomiting.

If you suspect an overdose, seek medical attention immediately.

Generic name:

IBUPROFEN

See Motrin, page 830.

Brand name:

ILETIN

See Insulin, page 639.

Brand name:

ILOSONE

See Erythromycin, Oral, page 482.

Brand name:

IMDUR

Pronounced: IM-duhr
Generic name: Isosorbide mononitrate
Other brand names: Ismo, Monoket

Why is this drug prescribed?

Imdur is prescribed to prevent angina pectoris (crushing chest pain that results when partially clogged arteries restrict the flow of needed oxygen-rich blood to the heart muscle). This medication does not relieve angina attacks already underway.

Most important fact about this drug

Imdur may cause severe low blood pressure (possibly marked by dizziness or fainting), especially when you are standing or if you sit up quickly. People taking blood pressure medication or those who have low blood pressure should use Imdur with caution.

How should you take this medication?

To maintain this drug's protective effect, it is important that you take it exactly as prescribed.

Take Imdur once a day, when you get up in the morning. It may be taken with or without food. Imdur tablets should not be crushed or chewed. Swallow them with half a glass of liquid.

Do not switch to another brand of isosorbide mononitrate without consulting your doctor or pharmacist.

- *If you miss a dose...*
  Take it as soon as you remember. If it is almost time for your next dose, skip the one you missed and go back to your regular schedule. Do not take 2 doses at the same time.

- *Storage instructions...*
  Store at room temperature.

What side effects may occur?

Side effects cannot be anticipated. If any develop or change in intensity, tell your doctor as soon as possible. Only your doctor can determine if it is safe for you to continue taking Imdur.

Headache is the most common side effect; usually, aspirin or acetaminophen will relieve the pain. The headaches associated with Imdur usually subside within a short time after treatment with the drug begins. Check with your doctor if your headaches persist or become more intense. Another common side effect is dizziness.

- *Less common or rare side effects may include:*
  Abdominal pain, abnormal hair texture, abnormal heart sounds, abnormal or terrifying dreams, abnormal vision, acne, anemia, anxiety, back pain, bacterial infection, black stools, breast pain, bronchitis, chest pain, confusion, constipation, coughing, decreased sex drive, depression,

diarrhea, difficult or labored breathing, difficulty concentrating, diminished sense of touch, drooping eyelid, dry mouth, earache, excessive amount of urine, fatigue, fever, fluid retention and swelling, flu-like symptoms, flushing, frozen shoulder, gas, general feeling of illness, heart attack, heart failure, heart murmur, hemorrhoids, high blood pressure, hot flashes, impotence, inability to sleep, increased mucus from the lungs, increased sweating, indigestion, inflamed eyes, inflammation of the stomach, inflammation of the tongue, inflammation of the vagina, intolerance of light, irregular heartbeat, itching, joint pain, kidney stones, leg ulcer, loose stools, low blood pressure, migraine, muscle and/or bone pain, muscle weakness, nasal or sinus inflammation, nausea, nervousness, palpitations (throbbing or fluttering heartbeat), paralysis, perforated eardrum, pneumonia, purple or red spots on the skin, rapid heartbeat, rash, ringing in the ears, severe pain in calf muscles during walking, sleepiness, slow heartbeat, sore throat, stomach ulcer with or without bleeding, stuffy nose, tingling or pins and needles, tremor, twisted neck, urinary tract infection, varicose veins, vertigo, viral infection, vomiting, weakness, wheezing, worsening of angina pectoris, yeast infection

Why should this drug not be prescribed?

You should not take Imdur if you have had a previous allergic reaction to it or to other heart medications containing nitrates or nitrites. Your doctor will probably not prescribe Imdur if you have had a recent heart attack or congestive heart failure. If the doctor decides that this medication is essential, your heart function and blood pressure will need to be closely monitored to avoid potential side effects.

Special warnings about this medication

Do not abruptly stop taking this medication. Follow your doctor's plan for a gradual withdrawal.

Since Imdur can cause dizziness, you should be careful while driving, operating machinery, or performing other tasks that demand concentration.

Nitrate-type medications such as Imdur may aggravate angina caused by certain heart conditions.

Do not try to avoid a headache by changing your dose. If your headache stops, it may mean the drug has lost its effectiveness.

Be sure to tell your doctor about any medical conditions you have before starting Imdur therapy.

Possible food and drug interactions
when taking this medication

If Imdur is taken with certain other drugs, the effects of either could be increased, decreased, or altered. Extreme low blood pressure with dizziness and fainting upon standing up may occur if Imdur is taken with calcium-blocking blood pressure medications such as Calan, Cardizem, and Procardia.

Alcohol may interact with Imdur and cause a swift decrease in blood pressure, possibly resulting in light-headedness.

Special information
if you are pregnant or breastfeeding

The effects of Imdur during pregnancy have not been adequately studied. If you are pregnant or plan to become pregnant, tell your doctor immediately. Imdur should be used during pregnancy only if it is clearly needed.

It is not known whether Imdur appears in breast milk. If the drug is essential to your health, your doctor may advise you to stop nursing until your treatment is finished.

Recommended dosage

ADULTS

The usual starting dose is 30 milligrams (taken as a single 30-milligram tablet or as one-half of a 60-milligram tablet) or 60 milligrams once a day.

After several days, your doctor may increase the dose to 120 milligrams (a single 120-milligram tablet or two 60-milligram tablets) once daily.

Your doctor may further adjust the dosage according to your response to the medication.

CHILDREN

Safety and effectiveness of Imdur in children have not been established.

Overdosage

Any medication taken in excess can have serious consequences. Severe overdosage of Imdur can be fatal. If you suspect an overdose, seek medical help immediately.

- *Symptoms of Imdur overdose may include:*
  Air hunger, bloody diarrhea, coma, confusion, difficulty breathing, fainting, fever, nausea, palpitations, paralysis, pressure in the head, profuse sweating, seizures, skin either cold and clammy or flushed, slow heartbeat, throbbing headache, vertigo, visual disturbances, vomiting

Generic name:

IMIPRAMINE

See Tofranil, page 1315.

Brand name:

IMITREX

Pronounced: IM-i-trex
Generic name: Sumatriptan succinate

Why is this drug prescribed?
Imitrex is prescribed for the treatment of a migraine attack with or without the presence of an aura (visual disturbances, usually sensations of halos or flickering lights, which precede an attack). The injectable form is also used to relieve cluster headache attacks. (Cluster headaches come on in waves, then disappear for long periods of time. They are limited to one side of the head, and occur mainly in men.)

Imitrex cuts headaches short. It will not reduce the number of attacks you experience.

Most important fact about this drug
Imitrex should be used only to treat an acute, classic migraine attack or a cluster headache. It should not be used for certain unusual types of migraine.

How should you take this medication?
Imitrex should be taken as soon as your symptoms appear, but may be used at any time during an attack. It is available in three forms: injection, tablets, and nasal spray.

Imitrex injection is administered just below the skin with an autoinjector (self-injection device). Choose a site where the skin is thick enough to take the full length of the needle (1/4 inch). Avoid injecting Imitrex into a muscle or a vein. Your doctor should instruct you on how to use the autoinjector and how to dispose of the empty syringes. You should also read the instruction pamphlet that comes with the medication.

You can take a second injection if your headache returns; however, never take more than 2 injections within 24 hours, and be sure to wait 1 hour between doses.

Imitrex tablets should be swallowed whole, with liquid. If you have had no relief 2 hours after taking Imitrex Tablets, you may take a second dose of up to 100 milligrams, if your doctor advises it. If the headache returns, you may take additional doses at intervals of at least 2 hours. You should not take more than 300 milligrams in one day. If your headache returns after you have had an Imitrex injection, you may take single Imitrex Tablets, at intervals of at least 2 hours, up to a maximum of 200 milligrams in a day.

Imitrex nasal spray is packaged in single-dose bottles containing either 5 or 20 milligrams of the drug. The usual dosage is a single spray in one nostril. If the headache returns, you may repeat the dose once after 2 hours. Do not take more than 40 milligrams a day.

■ *If you miss a dose...*
Imitrex is *not* for regular use. Take it only during an attack.

■ *Storage instructions...*
Store Imitrex away from heat and light, at room temperature, in the case provided. If your medication has expired (the expiration date is printed on the treatment pack), throw it away as instructed, but keep the autoinjector. If your doctor decides to stop your treatment, do not keep any leftover medicine unless your doctor tells you to. Throw away your medicine as instructed.

What side effects may occur?
Side effects cannot be anticipated. If any develop or change in intensity, inform your doctor as soon as possible. Only your doctor can determine if it is safe for you to continue taking Imitrex.

■ *More common side effects may include:*
Burning sensation, dizziness or vertigo, feeling of heaviness, feeling of tightness, flushing, mouth and tongue discomfort, muscle weakness, nausea (nasal spray), neck pain and stiffness, numbness, pressure sensation, redness at the site of injection, sinus or nasal discomfort (nasal spray), sore throat, tingling, unusual taste (nasal spray), vomiting (nasal spray), warm/cold sensation

■ *Less common or rare side effects may include:*
Abdominal discomfort, agitation, allergic reactions (severe), anxiety, asthma, backache, backflow of stomach contents, bleeding between periods, bleeding in ears, nose or throat, breast tenderness, burning/numbness of tongue, changes in heart rhythm, chills, cold sensation, confusion, constipation, cough, depression, diarrhea, difficult or labored breathing, difficult or painful urination, difficulty concentrating, difficulty speaking, difficulty swallowing, drowsiness/calmness, dry mouth, ear infection, exaggerated feeling of well-being, eye irritation, facial pain,

fainting, fatigue, feeling strange, fever, general feeling of illness, headache, hearing loss, hearing disturbance, heavy feeling, hives, incoordination, increased urination, intolerance of noise or light, itching, jaw discomfort, joint problems, muscle cramps, muscle pain or tenderness, painful menstruation, pressure in chest, rapid and throbbing heartbeat, rash, ringing in the ears, rise or fall in blood pressure (temporary), sensation of lightness, sensitivity to noise or heat, shivering, shortness of breath, sinus inflammation, sinus or nasal discomfort, skin eruptions, skin redness or tenderness, sleep disturbances, smell disturbances, stomach problems, sweating, swelling, tearing, thirst, tight feeling in head, tightness in chest, tremors, vision changes

In addition to the above side effects, people taking Imitrex for cluster headache may experience nausea, a "pins and needles" sensation, vomiting, or wheezing.

Why should this drug not be prescribed?
If you are sensitive to or have had an allergic reaction to sumatriptan you should not use this drug again. Make sure your doctor is aware of any drug reactions you have experienced.

Imitrex should not be used if you have certain types of heart or blood vessel disease, including angina (crushing chest pain) or a history of heart attack, if you suffer from uncontrolled high blood pressure, or within 24 hours of taking a medication containing ergotamine (often used in other migraine medications) or drugs such as D.H.E. 45 Injection and Sansert.

Special warnings about this medication
Although the danger is minimal, Imitrex has triggered serious heart problems in people with heart disease. For that reason, the doctor may want you to take your first dose of Imitrex in the office, where you can be closely watched for ill effects. Be sure to tell the doctor if you have any conditions that increase your risk of heart disease, such as high blood pressure, high cholesterol, or diabetes. Also let him know if you smoke, have heart disease in the family, or have gone through menopause. If you develop pain or tightness in the chest, throat, or jaw after taking a dose of Imitrex, consult your doctor before taking any more.

If you develop severe chest pain, call the doctor immediately. Also seek immediate attention if you suffer sudden, severe abdominal pain after a dose of Imitrex. It could signal a blood vessel problem.

Be careful not to inject Imitrex into a vein. This can cause a serious heart irregularity.

If your fingers turn pale, then blue, after a dose of Imitrex, you may have a circulatory problem such as hardening of the arteries. Be sure to let your doctor know.

This medication should not be used for other types of migraine headache. If the first dose does not relieve your symptoms, your doctor will re-evaluate you; you may not have migraine or cluster headache.

If your headache does not feel like any you have been experiencing, do not take Imitrex.

Use Imitrex cautiously if you have liver or kidney disease. Also, if you have any trouble with your eyes, tell your doctor.

Imitrex has not been tested in children or adults over age 65.

Although very rare, severe and even fatal allergic reactions have occurred in people taking Imitrex. Such reactions are more likely in people who have several allergies. In rare cases, people have suffered seizures after taking Imitrex.

Possible food and drug interactions when taking this medication

If Imitrex is taken with certain other drugs, the effects of either may be increased, decreased, or altered. It is important to check with your doctor before combining Imitrex with the following:

Drugs classified as MAO inhibitors, including the antidepressants Nardil and Parnate
Ergot-containing drugs such as Cafergot and Ergostat
Fluoxetine (Prozac)
Fluvoxamine (Luvox)
Paroxetine (Paxil)
Sertraline (Zoloft)

Special information if you are pregnant or breastfeeding

The effects of Imitrex during pregnancy have not been adequately studied. If you are pregnant or plan to become pregnant, inform your doctor immediately. Imitrex does appear in breast milk and could affect a nursing infant. If this medication is essential to your health, your doctor may advise you to discontinue breastfeeding until your treatment with Imitrex is finished.

Recommended dosage

IMITREX INJECTION

The maximum single recommended adult dose is 6 milligrams injected under the skin.

The maximum recommended dose that may be given within 24 hours is two 6 milligram injections taken at least 1 hour apart.

IMITREX TABLETS

The usual adult dose is one 25-, 50-, or 100-milligram tablet taken with water or other liquid. The most you should take at one time is 100 milligrams, and the most you should take in 1 day is 200 milligrams. Doses should be spaced at least 2 hours apart.

If you have liver disease, you should not take more than 50 milligrams of Imitrex Tablets at one time.

IMITREX NASAL SPRAY

The recommended adult dose ranges from 5 to 20 milligrams taken when the attack begins and repeated once, if necessary, 2 hours later. Doses are usually taken as a single spray in one nostril, but if a 10-milligram dose works best for you, you can take it as a 5-milligram spray in each nostril. Do not use more than 20 milligrams at a time, or take more than 40 milligrams a day.

Overdosage

Any medication taken in excess can have serious consequences. If you suspect an overdose, seek medical attention immediately.

- *Symptoms of Imitrex overdose may include:*
  Bluish tinge to the skin, convulsions, dilated pupils, inactivity, lack of coordination, paralysis, redness in the arms and legs, skin changes at the site of injection, slow breathing, sluggishness, tremor

Brand name:

IMODIUM

Pronounced: i-MOH-dee-um
Generic name: Loperamide hydrochloride

Why is this drug prescribed?

Imodium is prescribed for the control and relief of symptoms of diarrhea not known to be caused by a specific germ, and for diarrhea associated with long-term inflammatory bowel disease. This drug is also prescribed for reducing the volume of discharge from an ileostomy (a surgical opening of the small intestine onto the abdominal wall for purposes of elimination).

Some doctors also prescribe Imodium, along with antibiotics such as Septra or Bactrim, to treat traveler's diarrhea.

Most important fact about this drug
If your diarrhea does not stop after a couple of days, if you have blood in your stools, or a fever develops, notify your doctor immediately.

How should you take this medication?
Do not take more than the prescribed dose of this medication.

Imodium may cause dryness of the mouth. Sucking on a hard candy or chewing gum can help relieve the problem.

- *If you miss a dose...*
  If you are taking Imodium on a regular schedule for chronic diarrhea and miss a dose, take it as soon as you remember then take the remaining doses for that day at evenly spaced intervals. However, if you are not having diarrhea, skip the missed dose completely.

- *Storage instructions...*
  Imodium should be stored at room temperature.

What side effects may occur?
Side effects reported from the use of Imodium are difficult to distinguish from symptoms associated with diarrhea. Those reported, however, were more commonly observed during the treatment of long-lasting diarrhea.

- *Side effects may include:*
  Abdominal distention, abdominal pain or discomfort, allergic reactions, including skin rash, constipation, dizziness, drowsiness, dry mouth, nausea and vomiting, tiredness

Why should this drug not be prescribed?
If you are sensitive to or have ever had an allergic reaction to Imodium, you should not take this medication. Make sure that your doctor is aware of any drug reactions that you have experienced.

Unless you are directed to do so by your doctor, do not take Imodium if constipation must be avoided.

Special warnings about this medication
Imodium may cause drowsiness and/or dizziness. You should exercise extra caution while driving or performing tasks requiring mental alertness.

Imodium is not good for all types of diarrhea. It is not prescribed for acute dysentery (an inflammation of the intestines characterized by abdominal pain, watery—sometimes bloody—stools, and fever, caused by bacteria, viruses, or parasites).

Dehydration can be a problem when you have diarrhea. It is important that you drink plenty of fluids while taking Imodium.

Use special caution when giving Imodium to a young child. Response to the drug can be unpredictable.

If you have a liver problem, your doctor should closely watch for signs of central nervous system reactions, such as drowsiness or convulsions.

If you have colitis and develop abdominal distention, constipation or an intestinal blockage, notify your doctor immediately. The use of Imodium should be discontinued.

**Possible food and drug interactions
when taking this medication**
There are no reported food or drug interactions.

**Special information
if you are pregnant or breastfeeding**
The effects of Imodium during pregnancy have not been adequately studied. If you are pregnant or plan to become pregnant, notify your doctor. It is not known whether Imodium appears in breast milk. If this medication is essential to your health, your doctor may advise you to discontinue breastfeeding until your treatment is finished.

Recommended dosage

ADULTS

Severe Diarrhea
The recommended starting dosage is 2 capsules (4 milligrams) followed by 1 capsule (2 milligrams) after each unformed stool. Daily dosage should not exceed 8 capsules (16 milligrams). Improvement should be observed within 48 hours.

Long-Lasting or Frequently Recurring Diarrhea
The recommended starting dosage is 2 capsules (4 milligrams) followed by 1 capsule (2 milligrams) after each unformed stool until diarrhea is controlled, after which the dosage of Imodium should be reduced by your doctor to meet your individual needs. When the ideal daily dosage has been established, this amount may then be given as a single dose or in divided doses. The average

maintenance dosage is 2 to 4 capsules per day, not to exceed 8 capsules. If improvement is not observed after treatment with 8 capsules (16 milligrams) per day for at least 10 days, notify your doctor.

CHILDREN

Imodium is not recommended in children under 2 years of age.

Severe Diarrhea

In children 2 to 5 years of age or 44 pounds or less, the nonprescription liquid medication (Imodium A-D) should be used. For children between the ages of 6 and 12, either Imodium capsules (2 milligrams per capsule) or Imodium A-D Liquid (1 milligram per teaspoonful) may be used.

For children 2 to 12 years of age, the following schedule for capsules or liquid will usually fulfill starting dosage requirements:

2 to 5 years (28-44 pounds):
1 milligram (1 teaspoonful of Imodium A-D liquid) taken 3 times a day (3 milligrams daily)

6 to 8 years (45-66 pounds):
2 milligrams taken 2 times a day (4 milligrams daily)

8 to 12 years (67 pounds and over):
2 milligrams taken 3 times a day (6 milligrams daily)

After the first day of treatment, additional Imodium doses (1 milligram per 22 pounds of body weight) should be given only after a loose stool. The total daily dosage should not exceed the recommended dosages for the first day.

Long-Lasting or Frequently Recurring Diarrhea

A dosage has not been established for children with long-lasting or frequently recurring diarrhea.

Overdosage

Any medication taken in excess can have serious consequences. If you suspect an Imodium overdose, seek medical attention immediately.

■ *Symptoms of an Imodium overdose may include:*
Constipation, drowsiness, lethargy and depression, nausea

Generic name:

INDAPAMIDE

See Lozol, page 738.

Brand name:

INDERAL

Pronounced: IN-der-al
Generic name: Propranolol hydrochloride
Other brand name: Inderal LA

Why is this drug prescribed?

Inderal, a type of medication known as a beta blocker, is used in the treatment of high blood pressure, angina pectoris (chest pain, usually caused by lack of oxygen to the heart due to clogged arteries), changes in heart rhythm, prevention of migraine headache, hereditary tremors, hypertrophic subaortic stenosis (a condition related to exertional angina), and tumors of the adrenal gland. It is also used to reduce the risk of death from recurring heart attack.

When used for the treatment of high blood pressure, it is effective alone or combined with other high blood pressure medications, particularly thiazide-type diuretics. Beta blockers decrease the force and rate of heart contractions, reducing the heart's demand for oxygen and lowering blood pressure.

Most important fact about this drug

If you have high blood pressure, you must take Inderal regularly for it to be effective. Since blood pressure declines gradually, it may be several weeks before you get the full benefit of Inderal; and you must continue taking it even if you are feeling well. Inderal does not cure high blood pressure; it merely keeps it under control.

How should you take this medication?

Inderal works best when taken before meals. Take it exactly as prescribed, even if your symptoms have disappeared.

Try not to miss any doses. If this medication is not taken regularly, your condition may worsen.

- *If you miss a dose...*
  Take it as soon as you remember. If it is within 8 hours of your next scheduled dose, skip the one you missed and go back to your regular schedule. Never take 2 doses at the same time.

- *Storage instructions...*
  Store at room temperature in a tightly closed, light-resistant container. Protect from freezing or excessive heat.

What side effects may occur?

Side effects cannot be anticipated. If any develop or change in intensity, inform your doctor as soon as possible. Only your doctor can determine if it is safe for you to continue taking Inderal.

■ *Side effects may include:*

Abdominal cramps, colitis, congestive heart failure, constipation, decreased sexual ability, depression, diarrhea, difficulty breathing, disorientation, dry eyes, fever with sore throat, hair loss, hallucinations, headache, light-headedness, low blood pressure, lupus erythematosus (a disease of the connective tissue), nausea, rash, reddish or purplish spots on the skin, short-term memory loss, slow heartbeat, tingling, prickling in hands, tiredness, trouble sleeping, upset stomach, visual changes, vivid dreams, vomiting, weakness, worsening of certain heartbeat irregularities

Why should this drug not be prescribed?

If you have inadequate blood supply to the circulatory system (cardiogenic shock), certain types of irregular heartbeat, a slow heartbeat, bronchial asthma, or severe congestive heart failure, you should not take this medication.

Special warnings about this medication

If you have a history of congestive heart failure, your doctor will prescribe Inderal cautiously.

Inderal should not be stopped suddenly. This can cause increased chest pain and heart attack. Dosage should be gradually reduced.

If you suffer from asthma or other bronchial conditions, coronary artery disease, or kidney or liver disease, this medication should be used with caution.

Ask your doctor if you should check your pulse while taking Inderal. This medication can cause your heartbeat to become too slow.

This medication may mask the symptoms of low blood sugar or alter blood sugar levels. If you are diabetic, discuss this with your doctor.

Notify your doctor or dentist that you are taking Inderal if you have a medical emergency, and before you have surgery or dental treatment.

Possible food and drug interactions
when taking this medication

If Inderal is taken with certain other drugs, the effects of either could be increased, decreased, or altered. It is especially important to check with your doctor before combining Inderal with the following:

Alcohol
Aluminum hydroxide gel (Amphojel)
Antipyrine (Auralgan)
Calcium-blocking blood pressure drugs such as Cardizem, Procardia, and
    Calan
Certain high blood pressure medications such as Diupres and Ser-Ap-Es
Chlorpromazine (Thorazine)
Cimetidine (Tagamet)
Epinephrine (EpiPen)
Haloperidol (Haldol)
Insulin
Lidocaine (Xylocaine)
Nonsteroidal anti-inflammatory drugs such as Motrin and Naprosyn
Oral diabetes drugs such as Micronase
Phenobarbitone
Phenytoin (Dilantin)
Rifampin (Rifadin)
Theophylline (Theo-Dur and others)
Thyroid medications such as Synthroid

Special information
if you are pregnant or breastfeeding

The effects of Inderal during pregnancy have not been adequately studied. If
you are pregnant or plan to become pregnant, inform your doctor immediately. Inderal appears in breast milk and could affect a nursing infant. If this
medication is essential to your health, your doctor may advise you to
discontinue breastfeeding until your treatment with this medication is
finished.

Recommended dosage

ADULTS

All dosages of Inderal, for any problem, must be tailored to the individual.
Your doctor will determine when and how often you should take this drug.
Remember to take it exactly as directed.

Hypertension

The usual starting dose is 40 milligrams 2 times a day. This dose may be in
combination with a diuretic. Dosages are gradually increased to between 120
milligrams and 240 milligrams per day for maintenance. In some cases, a
dose of 640 milligrams per day may be needed. Depending on the individual,
maximum effect of this drug may not be reached for a few days or even
several weeks. Some people may do better taking this medication 3 times a
day.

Angina Pectoris
The usual daily dosage is 80 milligrams to 320 milligrams, divided into 2, 3, or 4 smaller doses. When your treatment is being discontinued, your doctor will reduce the dosage gradually over a period of several weeks.

Irregular Heartbeat
The usual dose is 10 milligrams to 30 milligrams 3 or 4 times a day, before meals and at bedtime.

Heart Attack
The usual daily dosage is 180 milligrams to 240 milligrams divided into smaller doses. The usual maximum dose is 240 milligrams, although your doctor may increase the dose when treating heart attack with angina or high blood pressure.

Migraine
The usual starting dosage is 80 milligrams per day divided into smaller doses. Dosages can be increased gradually to between 160 milligrams and 240 milligrams per day. If this dose does not relieve your symptoms in 4 to 6 weeks, your doctor will slowly take you off the drug.

Tremors
The usual starting dose is 40 milligrams, 2 times per day. Symptoms will usually be relieved with a dose of 120 milligrams per day; however, on occasion, dosages of 240 milligrams to 320 milligrams per day may be necessary.

Hypertrophic Subaortic Stenosis
The usual dose is 20 milligrams to 40 milligrams, 3 to 4 times a day, before meals and at bedtime.

Before Adrenal Gland Surgery
The usual dose is 60 milligrams a day divided into smaller doses for 3 days before surgery in combination with an alpha-blocker drug.

Inderal may also be taken by people with inoperable tumors in doses of 30 milligrams a day, divided into smaller doses.

CHILDREN

Inderal will be carefully individualized for use in children and is used only for high blood pressure. Doses in children are calculated by body weight, and range from 2 milligrams to 4 milligrams per 2.2 pounds daily, divided into 2 equal doses. The maximum dose is 16 milligrams per 2.2 pounds per day.

If treatment is stopped, this drug must be gradually reduced over a 7- to 14-day period.

Inderal is also available in a sustained-release formulation, called Inderal LA, for once-a-day dosing.

Overdosage

No specific information on Inderal overdosage is available; however, overdose symptoms with other beta blockers include:

Extremely slow heartbeat, irregular heartbeat, low blood pressure, severe congestive heart failure, seizures, wheezing

Any medication taken in excess can have serious consequences. If you suspect an overdose, seek medical attention immediately.

Brand name:

INDERIDE

Pronounced: IN-deh-ride
Generic ingredients: Inderal (Propranolol hydrochloride),
Hydrochlorothiazide
Other brand name: Inderide LA

Why is this drug prescribed?

Inderide is used in the treatment of high blood pressure. It combines a beta blocker (Inderal) with a thiazide diuretic (hydrochlorothiazide). Beta blockers decrease the force and rate of heart contractions, thus lowering blood pressure. Diuretics help your body produce and eliminate more urine, which also helps lower blood pressure.

Most important fact about this drug

You must take Inderide regularly for it to be effective. Since blood pressure declines gradually, it may be several weeks before you get the full benefit of Inderide; and you must continue taking it even if you are feeling well. Inderide does not cure high blood pressure; it merely keeps it under control.

How should you take this medication?

Take Inderide exactly as prescribed, even if your symptoms have disappeared.

Try not to miss any doses. If this medication is not taken regularly, your condition may worsen.

■ *If you miss a dose...*
Take it as soon as you remember. If the next dose is within 8 hours, skip the one you missed and go back to your regular schedule. Do not take 2 doses at the same time.

■ *Storage instructions...*
Store at room temperature in a tightly closed container, protected from moisture, freezing, and excessive heat.

What side effects may occur?
Side effects cannot be anticipated. If any develop or change in intensity, inform your doctor as soon as possible. Only your doctor can determine if it is safe for you to continue taking Inderide.

■ *Side effects may include:*
Allergic reactions (including fever, rash, aching and sore throat), anemia, blood disorders, blurred vision, constipation, congestive heart failure, cramps, decreased mental clarity, depression, diarrhea, difficulty breathing, difficulty sleeping, disorientation, dizziness, dizziness when standing, dry eyes, emotional changeability, exhaustion, fatigue, hair loss, hallucinations, headache, high blood sugar, hives, increased skin sensitivity to sunlight, inflammation of the large intestine or the pancreas, inflammation of the salivary glands, light-headedness, loss of appetite, low blood pressure, lupus erythematosus (a connective tissue disease), male impotence, muscle spasms, nausea, restlessness, short-term memory loss, slow heartbeat, stomach irritation, sugar in the urine, tingling or pins and needles, upset stomach, vertigo, visual disturbances, vivid dreams, vomiting, weakness, wheezing, yellow eyes and skin

Why should this drug not be prescribed?
If you have inadequate blood supply to the circulatory system (cardiogenic shock), certain types of irregular heartbeat, slow heartbeat, bronchial asthma, or congestive heart failure, you should not take this medication.

Do not take Inderide if you are unable to urinate or if you are sensitive to or have ever had an allergic reaction to any of its ingredients or to sulfa drugs.

Special warnings about this medication
Inderide should not be stopped suddenly. This can cause chest pain and even heart attack. Dosage should be gradually reduced.

Diuretics can cause your body to lose too much potassium. Signs of an excessively low potassium level include muscle weakness and rapid or irregular heartbeat. To boost your potassium level, your doctor may recommend eating potassium-rich foods or taking a potassium supplement.

If you suffer from asthma, seasonal allergies or other bronchial conditions, or kidney or liver disease, your doctor will prescribe this medication with caution.

This medication may mask the symptoms of low blood sugar or alter blood sugar levels. If you are diabetic, discuss this with your doctor.

If you have a history of allergies or bronchial asthma, you are more likely to have an allergic reaction to Inderide.

Inderide may interfere with the screening test for glaucoma (excessive pressure in the eyes) and pressure within the eyes may increase when the medication is stopped.

Notify your doctor or dentist that you are taking Inderide if you have a medical emergency, and before you have surgery or dental treatment.

Possible food and drug interactions
when taking this medication

If Inderide is taken with certain other drugs, the effects of either could be increased, decreased, or altered. It is especially important to check with your doctor before combining Inderide with the following:

ACTH (adrenocorticotropic hormone)
Alcohol
Aluminum hydroxide gel (Amphojel)
Antipyrine (Auralgan)
Calcium-blocking blood pressure drugs such as Calan, Cardizem, and
    Procardia XL
Certain blood pressure medications such as Diupres and Ser-Ap-Es
Chlorpromazine (Thorazine)
Cimetidine (Tagamet)
Corticosteroids such as prednisone
Digitalis (Lanoxin)
Epinephrine (EpiPen)
Haloperidol (Haldol)
Insulin
Lidocaine (Xylocaine)
Nonsteroidal anti-inflammatory drugs such as Motrin
Norepinephrine (Levophed)

Oral diabetes drugs such as Micronase
Phenobarbitone
Phenytoin (Dilantin)
Rifampin (Rifadin)
Theophylline (Theo-Dur)
Thyroid medications such as Synthroid

Special information
if you are pregnant or breastfeeding

The effects of Inderide during pregnancy have not been adequately studied. If you are pregnant or plan to become pregnant, inform your doctor immediately. Inderide appears in breast milk and could affect a nursing infant. If Inderide is essential to your health, your doctor may advise you to discontinue breastfeeding until your treatment is finished.

Recommended dosage

ADULTS

Your doctor will tailor your dosage according to your response to Inderide's main ingredients.

The usual dose is one Inderide tablet, 2 times per day.

Your doctor may use this medication in combination with other high blood pressure drugs to achieve the desired effect.

This drug is also available in a sustained-release formulation, called Inderide LA, for once-a-day dosing.

CHILDREN

The safety and effectiveness of this drug in children have not been established.

OLDER ADULTS

Your doctor will adjust your dosage with extra caution.

Overdosage

Any medication taken in excess can have severe consequences. If you suspect an overdose, seek medical attention immediately.

■ *Symptoms of Inderide overdose may include:*
Coma, extremely slow heartbeat, heart failure, increased urination, irritation and overactivity of the stomach and intestines, low blood pressure, sluggishness, stupor, wheezing

Generic name:

INDINAVIR

See Crixivan, page 311.

Brand name:

INDOCIN

Pronounced: IN-doh-sin
Generic name: Indomethacin

Why is this drug prescribed?

Indocin, a nonsteroidal anti-inflammatory drug, is used to relieve the inflammation, swelling, stiffness and joint pain associated with moderate or severe rheumatoid arthritis and osteoarthritis (the most common form of arthritis), and ankylosing spondylitis (arthritis of the spine). It is also used to treat bursitis, tendinitis (acute painful shoulder), acute gouty arthritis, and other kinds of pain.

Most important fact about this drug

You should have frequent checkups with your doctor if you take Indocin regularly. Ulcers or internal bleeding can occur without warning.

How should you take this medication?

Indocin should be taken with food or an antacid, and with a full glass of water. Never take on an empty stomach.

Take this medication exactly as prescribed by your doctor.

If you are using Indocin for arthritis, it should be taken regularly.

If you are taking the liquid form of this medicine, shake the bottle well before each use.

Indocin SR capsules should be swallowed whole, not crushed or broken.

Do not lie down for about 20 to 30 minutes after taking Indocin. This helps prevent irritation that could lead to trouble in swallowing.

If you are using the suppository form of this medicine:

1. If the suppository is too soft to insert, hold it under cool water or chill it before removing the wrapper.
2. Remove the foil wrapper and moisten your rectal area with cool tap water.

3. Lie down on your side and use your finger to push the suppository well up into the rectum. Hold your buttocks together for a few seconds.
4. Indocin suppositories should be kept inside the rectum for at least 1 hour so that all of the medicine can be absorbed by your body.

■ *If you miss a dose...*
Take the forgotten dose as soon as you remember. If it is time for your next dose, skip the one you missed and return to your regular schedule. Never take a double dose.

■ *Storage instructions...*
The liquid and suppository forms of Indocin may be stored at room temperature. Keep both forms from extreme heat, and protect the liquid from freezing.

What side effects may occur?
Side effects cannot be anticipated. If any develop or change in intensity inform your doctor as soon as possible. Only your doctor can determine if it is safe for you to continue taking Indocin.

■ *More common side effects may include:*
Abdominal pain, constipation, depression, diarrhea, dizziness, fatigue, headache, heartburn, indigestion, nausea, ringing in the ears, sleepiness or excessive drowsiness, stomach pain, stomach upset, vertigo, vomiting

■ *Less common or rare side effects may include:*
Anemia, anxiety, asthma, behavior disturbances, bloating, blurred vision, breast changes, changes in heart rate, chest pain, coma, congestive heart failure, convulsions, decrease in white blood cells, fever, fluid in lungs, fluid retention, flushing, gas, hair loss, hepatitis, high or low blood pressure, hives, itching, increase in blood sugar, insomnia, kidney failure, labored breathing, light-headedness, loss of appetite, mental confusion, muscle weakness, nosebleed, peptic ulcer, problems in hearing, rash, rectal bleeding, Stevens-Johnson syndrome (skin peeling), stomach or intestinal bleeding, sweating, twitching, unusual redness of skin, vaginal bleeding, weight gain, worsening of epilepsy, yellow eyes and skin

Why should this drug not be prescribed?
If you are sensitive to or have ever had an allergic reaction to Indocin, aspirin, or similar drugs, or if you have had asthma attacks caused by aspirin or other drugs of this type, you should not take this medication. Make sure that your doctor is aware of any drug reactions that you have experienced.

Do not use Indocin suppositories if you have a history of rectal inflammation or recent rectal bleeding.

Special warnings about this medication

Indocin prolongs bleeding time. If you are taking blood-thinning medication, this drug should be taken with caution.

Your doctor should prescribe the lowest possible effective dose. The incidence of side effects increases as dosage increases.

Peptic ulcers and bleeding can occur without warning.

This drug should be used with caution if you have kidney or liver disease, and it can cause liver inflammation in some people.

Do not take aspirin or any other anti-inflammatory medications while taking Indocin, unless your doctor tells you to do so.

If you have heart disease or high blood pressure, this drug can increase water retention.

This drug can mask the symptoms of an existing infection.

Indocin may cause you to become drowsy or less alert; therefore, driving or operating dangerous machinery or participating in any hazardous activity that requires full mental alertness is not recommended.

Possible food and drug interactions
when taking this medication

If Indocin is taken with certain other drugs, the effects of either could be increased, decreased or altered. It is especially important to check with your doctor before combining Indocin with the following:

Aspirin
Beta-blockers such as the blood pressure medications Tenormin and
    Inderal
Blood-thinning medicines such as Coumadin
Captopril (Capoten)
Cyclosporine (Sandimmune)
Diflunisal (Dolobid)
Digoxin (Lanoxin)
Lithium (Eskalith)
Loop diuretics (Lasix)
Other nonsteroidal anti-inflammatory drugs such as Advil, Aleve, and
    Motrin
Potassium-sparing water pills such as Aldactone
Probenecid (Benemid, ColBENEMID)

The anticancer drug methotrexate
Thiazide-type water pills such as Diuril
Triamterene (Dyazide)

Special information
if you are pregnant or breastfeeding

The effects of Indocin during pregnancy have not been adequately studied. If you are pregnant or plan to become pregnant inform your doctor immediately. Indocin appears in breast milk and could affect a nursing infant. If this medication is essential to your health, your doctor may advise you to discontinue breastfeeding until your treatment with this medication is finished.

Recommended dosage

ADULTS

This medication is available in liquid, capsule, and suppository form. The following dosages are for the capsule form. If you prefer the liquid form, ask your doctor to make the proper substitution. Do not try to convert the medication or dosage yourself.

Moderate to Severe Rheumatoid Arthritis, Osteoarthritis, Ankylosing Spondylitis

The usual dose is 25 milligrams 2 or 3 times a day, increasing to a total daily dose of 150 to 200 milligrams. Your doctor should monitor you carefully for side effects when you are taking this drug.

Your doctor may prescribe a single daily 75-milligram capsule of Indocin SR in place of regular Indocin.

Bursitis or Tendinitis

The usual dose is 75 to 150 milligrams daily divided into 3 to 4 small doses for 1 to 2 weeks, until symptoms disappear.

Acute Gouty Arthritis

The usual dose is 50 milligrams 3 times a day until pain is reduced to a tolerable level (usually 3 to 5 days). Your doctor will advise you when to stop taking this drug for this condition. Keep him informed of its effects on your symptoms.

CHILDREN

The safety and effectiveness of Indocin have not been established in children under 14 years of age. However, your doctor may decide that the benefits of this medication outweigh any potential risks.

OLDER ADULTS

Your doctor will adjust the dosage as needed.

Overdosage

Any medication taken in excess can cause symptoms of overdose. If you suspect an overdose seek medical attention immediately.

■ *The symptoms of Indocin overdose may include:*
Convulsions, disorientation, dizziness, intense headache, lethargy, mental confusion, nausea, numbness, tingling or pins and needles, vomiting

Generic name:

INDOMETHACIN

See Indocin, page 635.

Generic name:

INSULIN

Pronounced: IN-suh-lin
Available formulations:
Insulin, Human:
Humulin
Insulin, Human Isophane Suspension:
Humulin N
Insulin, Human NPH:
Novolin N
Insulin, Human Regular:
Novolin R
Humulin BR & R
Velosulin BR
Insulin, Human Regular and Human NPH mixture:
Humulin 70/30
Novolin 70/30
Insulin, Human, Zinc Suspension:
Humulin L & U
Novolin L
Insulin, NPH:
NPH Iletin I (also II, Beef; II, Pork)
NPH Insulin
Insulin, Zinc Crystals:
NPH Iletin I

Insulin, Regular:
    Iletin I Regular (also II, Beef; II, Pork)
    Regular Insulin
Insulin, Zinc Suspension:
    Iletin I, Lente
    Protamine, Zinc and Iletin
    Iletin I, Semilente
    Iletin I
    Lente Insulin
    Ultralente Insulin

Why is this drug prescribed?

Insulin is prescribed for diabetes mellitus when this condition does not improve with oral medications or by modifying your diet. Insulin is a hormone produced by the pancreas, a large gland that lies near the stomach. This hormone is necessary for the body's correct use of food, especially sugar. Insulin apparently works by helping sugar penetrate the cell wall, where it is then utilized by the cell. In people with diabetes, the body either does not make enough insulin, or the insulin that is produced cannot be used properly.

There are actually two forms of diabetes: Type I insulin-dependent and Type II non-insulin-dependent. Type I usually requires insulin injection for life, while Type II diabetes can usually be treated by dietary changes and/or oral antidiabetic medications such as Diabinese and Glucotrol. Occasionally, Type II diabetics must take insulin injections on a temporary basis, especially during stressful periods or times of illness.

The various insulin brands above differ in several ways: in the source (animal, human, or genetically engineered), in the time requirements for the insulin to take effect, and in the length of time the insulin remains working.

Regular insulin is manufactured from beef and pork pancreas, begins working within 30 to 60 minutes, and lasts for 6 to 8 hours. Variations of insulin have been developed to satisfy the needs of individual patients. For example, zinc suspension insulin is an intermediate-acting insulin that starts working within 1 to 1½ hours and lasts approximately 24 hours. Insulin combined with zinc and protamine is a longer-acting insulin that takes effect within 4 to 6 hours and lasts up to 36 hours. The time and course of action may vary considerably in different individuals or at different times in the same individual. The genetically engineered insulin lispro injection works faster and for a shorter length of time than human regular insulin and should be used along with a longer-acting insulin. It is available only by prescription.

Animal-based insulin is a very safe product. However, some components may cause an allergic reaction (see "What side effects may occur?").

Therefore, genetically engineered human insulin has been developed to lessen the chance of an allergic reaction. It is structurally identical to the insulin produced by your body's pancreas. However, some human insulin may be produced in a semi-synthetic process that begins with animal-based ingredients, which may cause an allergic reaction.

Most important fact about this drug
Regardless of the type of insulin your doctor has prescribed, you should follow carefully the dietary and exercise guidelines he or she has recommended. Failure to follow these guidelines or to take your insulin as prescribed may result in serious and potentially life-threatening complications such as hypoglycemia (lowered blood sugar levels).

How should you take this medication?
Take your insulin exactly as prescribed, being careful to follow your doctor's dietary and exercise recommendations.

- *If you miss a dose...*
  Your doctor should tell you what to do if you miss an insulin injection or meal.

- *Storage instructions...*
  Store insulin in a refrigerator (but not in the freezer) or in another cool, dark place. Do not expose insulin to heat or direct sunlight.

Some brands of prefilled syringes can be kept at room temperature for a week or a month. The vial or cartridge of genetically engineered insulin lispro can be kept unrefrigerated for up to 28 days. Check your product's label. Never use insulin after the expiration date which is printed on the label and carton.

What side effects may occur?
While side effects from insulin use are rare, allergic reactions or low blood sugar (sometimes called "an insulin reaction") may pose significant health risks. Your doctor should be notified if any of the following occur:

- *Mild allergic reactions:*
  Swelling, itching or redness at the injection site (usually disappears within a few days or weeks)

- *More serious allergic reactions:*
  Fast pulse, low blood pressure, perspiration, rash over the entire body, shortness of breath, shallow breathing, or wheezing

Other side effects are virtually eliminated when the correct dose of insulin is matched with the proper diet and level of physical activity. Low blood sugar may develop in poorly controlled or unstable diabetes. Consuming sugar or a sugar-containing product will usually correct the condition, which can be brought about by taking too much insulin, missing or delaying meals, exercising or working more than usual, an infection or illness, a change in the body's need for insulin, drug interactions, or consuming alcohol.

■ *Symptoms of low blood sugar include:*
Abnormal behavior, anxiety, blurred vision, cold sweat, confusion, depressed mood, dizziness, drowsiness, fatigue, headache, hunger, inability to concentrate, light-headedness, nausea, nervousness, personality changes, rapid heartbeat, restlessness, sleep disturbances, slurred speech, sweating, tingling in the hands, feet, lips, or tongue, tremor, unsteady movement

Contact your physician if these symptoms persist.

■ *Symptoms of more severe low blood sugar include:*
Coma, disorientation

Remember, too, the symptoms associated with an under-supply of insulin, which can be brought on by taking too little of it, overeating, or fever and infection.

■ *Symptoms of insufficient insulin include:*
Drowsiness, flushing, fruity breath, heavy breathing, loss of appetite, rapid pulse, thirst

If you are ill, you should check your urine for ketones (acetone), and notify your doctor if the test is positive. This condition can be life-threatening.

Why should this drug not be prescribed?
Insulin should be used only to correct diabetic conditions.

Special warnings about this medication
Wear personal identification that states clearly that you are diabetic. Carry a sugar-containing product such as hard candy to offset any symptoms of low blood sugar.

Do not change the type of insulin or even the model and brand of syringe or needle you use without your physician's instruction. Failure to use the proper syringe may lead to improper dosage levels of insulin.

If you become ill from any cause, especially with nausea and vomiting or —

fever, your insulin requirements may change. It is important to eat as normally as possible. If you have trouble eating, drink fruit juices, soda, or clear soups, or eat small amounts of bland foods. Test your urine and/or blood sugar and tell your doctor at once. If you have severe and prolonged vomiting, seek emergency medical care.

If you are taking insulin, you should check your glucose levels with home blood and urine testing devices. If your blood tests consistently show above-normal sugar levels or your urine tests consistently show the presence of sugar, your diabetes is not properly controlled, and you should tell your doctor.

To avoid infection or contamination, use disposable needles and syringes or sterilize your reusable syringe and needle carefully.

Always keep handy an extra supply of insulin as well as a spare syringe and needle.

**Possible food and drug interactions
when taking this medication**
Follow your physician's dietary guidelines as closely as you can and inform your physician of any medication, either prescription or non-prescription, that you are taking. Specific medications, depending on the amount present, that affect insulin levels or its effectiveness include:

ACE inhibitors such as the blood pressure medications Capoten and
  Lotensin
Anabolic steroids such as Anadrol-50
Appetite suppressants such as Tenuate
Aspirin
Beta-blocking blood pressure medicines such as Tenormin and Lopressor
Diuretics such as Lasix and Dyazide
Epinephrine (EpiPen)
Estrogens such as Premarin
Isoniazid (Nydrazid)
Major tranquilizers such as Mellaril and Thorazine
MAO inhibitors (drugs such as the antidepressants Nardil and Parnate)
Niacin (Nicobid)
Octreotide (Sandostatin)
Oral contraceptives
Oral drugs for diabetes such as Diabinese and Orinase
Phenytoin (Dilantin)
Steroid medications such as prednisone
Sulfa antibiotics such as Bactrim and Septra
Thyroid medications such as Synthroid

Use alcohol carefully, since excessive alcohol consumption can cause low blood sugar. Don't drink unless your doctor has approved it.

Special information
if you are pregnant or breastfeeding

Insulin is considered safe for pregnant women, but pregnancy may make managing your diabetes more difficult.

Properly controlled diabetes is essential for the health of the mother and the developing baby; therefore, it is extremely important that pregnant women follow closely their physician's dietary and exercise guidelines and prescribing instructions.

Since insulin does not pass into breast milk, it is safe for nursing mothers. It is not known whether genetically engineered insulin lispro appears in breast milk.

Recommended dosage

Your doctor will specify which insulin to use, how much, when, and how often to inject it. Your dosage may be affected by changes in food, activity, illness, medication, pregnancy, exercise, travel, or your work schedule. Proper control of your diabetes requires close and constant cooperation with your doctor. Failure to use your insulin as prescribed may result in serious and potentially fatal complications.

Some insulins should be clear, and some have a cloudy precipitate. Find out what your insulin should look like and check it carefully before using.

Genetically engineered insulin lispro injection should not be used by children under age 12.

Overdosage

An overdose of insulin can cause low blood sugar (hypoglycemia). Symptoms include:

Depressed mood, dizziness, drowsiness, fatigue, headache, hunger, inability to concentrate, irritability, nausea, nervousness, personality changes, rapid heartbeat, restlessness, sleep disturbances, slurred speech, sweating, tingling, tremor, unsteady movements

■ *Symptoms of more severe low blood sugar include:*
  Coma, disorientation, pale skin, seizures

Your doctor should be contacted immediately if these symptoms of severe low blood sugar occur.

Eating sugar or a sugar-based product will often correct the condition. If you suspect an overdose, seek medical attention immediately.

Brand name:

INTAL

Pronounced: IN-tahl
Generic name: Cromolyn sodium
Other brand name: Nasalcrom

Why is this drug prescribed?
Intal contains the antiasthmatic/antiallergic medication cromolyn sodium.

Different forms of the drug are used to manage bronchial asthma, to prevent asthma attacks, and to prevent and treat seasonal and chronic allergies.

The drug works by preventing certain cells in the body from releasing substances that can cause allergic reactions or prompt too much bronchial activity. It also helps prevent bronchial constriction caused by exercise, aspirin, cold air, and certain environmental pollutants such as sulfur dioxide.

Most important fact about this drug
Intal does not help an acute asthma attack. When taken to prevent severe bronchial asthma, it can be 4 weeks before you feel its maximum benefit, though some people get relief sooner. Do not discontinue the inhalation capsules or nasal solution abruptly without the advice of your doctor.

How should you take this medication?
Intal capsules should not be swallowed. They are for inhalation using the Spinhaler turbo-inhaler. The contents of 1 capsule are usually inhaled 4 times daily at regular intervals. Wash the Spinhaler in warm water at least once a week; dry thoroughly. Replace the Spinhaler every 6 months.

Intal nebulizer solution should be inhaled using a power-operated nebulizer equipped with an appropriate face mask or mouthpiece. Hand-operated nebulizers are not suitable. It is important that the solution be inhaled at regular intervals, usually 4 times per day.

Intal aerosol spray can be used either for chronic asthma or to prevent an asthma attack. For chronic asthma, it must be inhaled at regular intervals, as directed by your doctor, usually 2 sprays inhaled 4 times daily. To prevent an asthma attack caused by exercise, cold air, or other irritants, the usual dose of 2 inhalation sprays should be taken between 10 and 60 minutes before exercising or exposure to cold or pollutants.

Nasalcrom nasal solution should be used with a metered nasal spray device, which should be replaced every 6 months. Blow your nose to clear your nasal passages before administering the spray. The nasal solution is used for nasal congestion due to seasonal or chronic allergies. For seasonal allergies, treatment is more effective if begun before the start of the allergy season. Treatment should then continue throughout the season. For year-round allergies, treatment may be required for up to 4 weeks before results are seen. Your doctor may find it necessary to add other allergy medications, such as antihistamines or decongestants, during initial treatment.

■ *If you miss a dose...*
Take it as soon as you remember. Then take the rest of that day's doses at equally spaced intervals. Do not take 2 doses at once.

■ *Storage instructions...*
Store at room temperature, away from light and heat. Keep the ampules in their foil pouch until you are ready to use them.

What side effects may occur?
Side effects cannot be anticipated. If any develop or change in intensity, inform your doctor as soon as possible. Only your doctor can determine if it is safe for you to continue taking Intal.

■ *More common side effects may include:*
Cough, nasal congestion or irritation, nausea, sneezing, throat irritation, wheezing

■ *Less common or rare side effects may include:*
Angioedema (swelling of face around lips, tongue, and throat, swollen arms and legs), bad taste in mouth, burning in chest, difficulty swallowing, dizziness, ear problems, headache, hives, joint swelling and pain, nosebleed, painful urination or frequent urination, postnasal drip, rash, severe allergic reaction, swollen glands, swollen throat, teary eyes, tightness in throat

Why should this drug not be prescribed?
If you are sensitive to or have ever had an allergic reaction to cromolyn sodium or lactose, you should not take this medication. Make sure your doctor is aware of any drug reactions you have experienced.

Special warnings about this medication

Asthma symptoms may recur if the recommended dosage of Intal is reduced or discontinued. Intal has no role in the treatment of an acute asthmatic attack once it has begun. Obtain medical help immediately if you experience a severe attack.

If you have liver or kidney problems, your doctor may have to reduce the dosage or even take you off the drug altogether.

When using the capsules, you may accidentally inhale some powder, which can irritate your throat or make you cough. Try rinsing your mouth or taking a drink of water immediately before and/or after using the Spinhaler.

If your heartbeat is ever irregular or if you have any other kind of heart trouble, be sure your doctor knows about it before you use Intal aerosol spray.

Intal aerosol spray may not help you if your attack has been brought on by exercise.

Possible food and drug interactions
when taking this medication

If you are taking other prescription or nonprescription drugs, discuss this with your doctor to determine if these drugs would interact with Intal.

Special information
if you are pregnant or breastfeeding

The effects of Intal during pregnancy have not been adequately studied. If you are pregnant or plan to become pregnant, inform your doctor immediately. It is not known whether Intal appears in breast milk. As with all medication, a nursing woman should use this drug only after careful consultation with her doctor.

Recommended dosage

INTAL CAPSULES FOR INHALATION
INTAL NEBULIZER SOLUTION

Adults and Children 2 Years Old and Over

For management of bronchial asthma, the usual dosage is 20 milligrams (1 capsule or ampule) inhaled 4 times daily at regular intervals, using the Spinhaler turbo-inhaler or power-operated nebulizer. If you have chronic asthma, this drug's effectiveness depends on your taking it regularly, as directed, and only after an attack has been controlled and you can inhale adequately.

For the prevention of an acute attack following exercise or exposure to cold, dry air or environmental irritants, the usual dose is 1 capsule or ampule inhaled shortly before exposure to the irritant. You may repeat the inhalation as needed for continued protection during prolonged exposure.

INTAL INHALER AEROSOL SPRAY

Adults and Children 5 Years Old and Over

For the management of bronchial asthma, the usual starting dose is 2 metered sprays taken at regular intervals, 4 times daily. This is the maximum dose that should be taken, and lower dosages may be effective in children. This drug should be used only after an asthma attack has been controlled and you can inhale adequately.

For the prevention of an acute asthma attack following exercise, exposure to cold air or environmental agents, the usual dose is inhalation of 2 metered sprays shortly (10 to 15 minutes but not more than 60 minutes) before exposure to the irritant.

NASALCROM NASAL SOLUTION

Adults and Children 6 Years Old and Over

For the prevention and treatment of allergies caused by exposure to certain irritants, the usual dosage is 1 spray in each nostril 3 to 4 times per day at regular intervals, using the metered spray device. Your doctor may have you use the spray 6 times a day if you need it.

Overdosage

Any medication taken in excess can have serious consequences. If you suspect an overdose, seek medical attention immediately.

■ *Symptoms of Intal overdose may include:*
 Difficulty breathing, heart failure, low blood pressure, slow heartbeat

Brand name:

IONAMIN

See Fastin, page 506.

Generic name:

IPRATROPIUM

See Atrovent, page 110.

Generic name:

IRBESARTAN

See Avapro, page 119.

Brand name:

ISMO

See Imdur, page 615.

Generic name:

ISOMETHEPTENE, DICHLORALPHENAZONE, AND ACETAMINOPHEN

See Midrin, page 798.

Brand name:

ISOPTIN

See Calan, page 181.

Brand name:

ISOPTO CARPINE

See Pilocar, page 1005.

Brand name:

ISORDIL

Pronounced: ICE-or-dill
Generic name: Isosorbide dinitrate
Other brand name: Sorbitrate

Why is this drug prescribed?

Isordil is prescribed to relieve or prevent angina pectoris (suffocating chest pain). Angina pectoris occurs when the arteries and veins become constricted and sufficient oxygen does not reach the heart. Isordil dilates the blood vessels by relaxing the muscles in their walls. Oxygen flow improves as the vessels relax, and chest pain subsides.

In swallowed capsules or tablets, Isordil helps to increase the amount of exercise you can do before chest pain begins.

In chewable or sublingual (held under the tongue) tablets, Isordil can help relieve chest pain that has already started or prevent pain expected from a strenuous activity such as walking up a hill or climbing stairs.

Most important fact about this drug
Isordil may cause severe low blood pressure (possibly marked by dizziness or fainting), especially when you stand or sit up quickly. People taking diuretic medication or those who have low blood pressure should use Isordil with caution.

How should you take this medication?
Swallowed capsules or tablets should be taken on an empty stomach. While regular tablets may be crushed for easier use, sustained- or prolonged-release products should not be chewed, crushed or altered.

Chewable tablets should be chewed thoroughly and held in the mouth for a couple of minutes. Do not eat, drink, smoke, or use chewing tobacco while a sublingual tablet is dissolving.

This drug's effectiveness is closely linked to the dose, so follow your doctor's instructions carefully.

■ *If you miss a dose...*
If you are taking this drug regularly, take the forgotten dose as soon as you remember. If your next dose is within 2 hours—or 6 hours for controlled-release tablets and capsules—skip the one you missed and go back to your regular schedule. Do not take 2 doses at once.

■ *Storage information...*
Store at room temperature in a tightly closed container, away from light.

What side effects may occur?
Side effects cannot be anticipated. If any develop or change in intensity, inform your doctor as soon as possible. Only your doctor can determine if it is safe for you to continue taking Isordil.

Headache is the most common side effect; usually, standard headache treatments with over-the-counter pain products will relieve the pain. The headaches associated with Isordil usually subside within 2 weeks after treatment with the drug begins. Do not change your dose to avoid the headache. At a dose that eliminates headaches, the drug may not be as effective against angina.

■ *Other common side effects may include:*
   Dizziness, light-headedness, low blood pressure, weakness

■ *Less common or rare side effects may include:*
   Collapse, fainting, flushed skin, high blood pressure, nausea, pallor, perspiration, rash, restlessness, skin inflammation and flaking, vomiting

Why should this drug not be prescribed?
You should not take Isordil if you have had a previous allergic reaction to it or to other nitrates or nitrites.

Special warnings about this medication
You should use Isordil with caution if you have anemia, the eye condition called glaucoma, a previous head injury or heart attack, heart disease, low blood pressure, or thyroid disease.

If you stop using Isordil, you should follow your doctor's plan for a gradual withdrawal schedule. Abruptly stopping this medication could result in additional chest pain.

Some people may develop a tolerance to Isordil, which causes its effects to be reduced over time. Tell your doctor if you think Isordil is starting to lose its effectiveness.

Possible food and drug interactions
when taking this medication
If Isordil is taken with certain other drugs, the effects of either could be increased, decreased, or altered.

Extreme low blood pressure (marked by dizziness, fainting, and numbness) may occur if you take Isordil with certain other high blood pressure drugs such as Cardizem and Procardia.

Alcohol may interact with Isordil and produce a swift decrease in blood pressure, possibly causing dizziness and fainting.

Special information
if you are pregnant or breastfeeding
The effects of Isordil in pregnancy have not been adequately studied. Isordil should be used only when the benefits of therapy clearly outweigh the potential risks to the developing baby. If you are pregnant or plan to become pregnant, inform your doctor immediately. It is not known if Isordil appears in breast milk; therefore, nursing mothers should use Isordil with caution.

Recommended dosage
Because you can develop a tolerance to this drug, your doctor may schedule a daily period of time when you do not take any drug.

ADULTS

The usual sublingual starting dose for the treatment of angina pectoris is 2.5 milligrams to 5 milligrams. Your doctor will increase this initial dose gradually until the pain subsides or side effects prove bothersome.

The usual sublingual starting dose for the prevention of an impending attack of angina pectoris is usually 5 or 10 milligrams every 2 to 3 hours.

To prevent chronic stable angina pectoris, the usual starting dose for swallowed, immediately released Isordil is 5 to 20 milligrams. Your doctor may increase this initial dose to 10 to 40 milligrams every 6 hours.

To prevent chronic stable angina pectoris with controlled-release Isordil, the usual initial dose is 40 milligrams. Your doctor may increase this dose from 40 to 80 milligrams given every 8 to 12 hours.

CHILDREN

The safety and effectiveness of Isordil have not been established for children.

Overdosage
Any medication taken in excess can have serious consequences. Severe overdosage of Isordil can be fatal. If you suspect an overdose, seek medical help immediately.

■ *Symptoms of Isordil overdose may include:*
Bloody diarrhea, coma, confusion, convulsions, fainting, fever, flushed and perspiring skin (later cold and blue), nausea, palpitations, paralysis, rapid decrease in blood pressure, rapid, then difficult and slow breathing, slow pulse, throbbing headache, vertigo, visual disturbances, vomiting

Generic name:

ISOSORBIDE DINITRATE

See Isordil, page 649.

Generic name:

ISOSORBIDE MONONITRATE

See Imdur, page 615.

Generic name:

ISOTRETINOIN

See Accutane, page 7.

Generic name:

ISRADIPINE

See DynaCirc, page 449.

Generic name:

ITRACONAZOLE

See Sporanox, page 1214.

Brand name:

KADIAN

See MS Contin, page 834.

Brand name:

KAON-CL

See Micro-K, page 791.

Brand name:

K-DUR

See Micro-K, page 791.

Brand name:

KEFLEX

Pronounced: KEF-lecks
Generic name: Cephalexin hydrochloride
Other brand name: Keftab

Why is this drug prescribed?

Keflex and Keftab are cephalosporin antibiotics. They are prescribed for bacterial infections of the respiratory tract including middle ear infection, bone, skin, and the reproductive and urinary systems. Because they are effective for only certain types of bacterial infections, before beginning treatment your doctor may perform tests to identify the organisms causing the infection.

Keflex is available in capsules and an oral suspension form for use in children. Keftab, available only in tablet form, is prescribed exclusively for adults.

Most important fact about this drug
If you are allergic to either penicillin or cephalosporin antibiotics in any form, consult your doctor *before taking Keflex*. There is a possibility that you are allergic to both types of medication and if a reaction occurs, it could be extremely severe. If you take the drug and feel signs of a reaction, seek medical attention immediately.

How should you take this medication?
Keflex may be taken with or without meals. However, if the drug upsets your stomach, you may want to take it after you have eaten.

Take Keflex at even intervals around the clock as prescribed by your doctor.

If you are taking the liquid form of Keflex, use the specially marked spoon to measure each dose accurately.

To obtain maximum benefit, it is important that you finish taking all of this medication, even if you are feeling better.

- *If you miss a dose...*
  Take it as soon as you remember. If it is almost time for the next dose, and you take 2 doses a day, take the one you missed and the next dose 5 to 6 hours later. If you take 3 or more doses a day, take the one you missed and the next dose 2 to 4 hours later, or double the next dose. Then go back to your regular schedule.

- *Storage instructions...*
  Store capsules and tablets at room temperature. Store the liquid suspension in a refrigerator; discard any unused medication after 14 days.

What side effects may occur?
Side effects cannot be anticipated. If any develop or change in intensity, inform your doctor as soon as possible. Only your doctor can determine if it is safe for you to continue taking Keflex.

■ *More common side effects may include:*
Diarrhea

■ *Less common or rare side effects may include:*
Abdominal pain, agitation, colitis (inflammation of the large intestine), confusion, dizziness, fatigue, fever, genital and rectal itching, hallucinations, headache, hepatitis, hives, indigestion, inflammation of joints, inflammation of the stomach, joint pain, nausea, rash, seizures, severe allergic reaction, skin peeling, skin redness, swelling due to fluid retention, vaginal discharge, vaginal inflammation, vomiting, yellowing of skin and whites of eyes

Why should this drug not be prescribed?
If you are sensitive to or have ever had an allergic reaction to the cephalosporin group of antibiotics, you should not use this medication. Make sure your doctor is aware of any drug reactions you have experienced.

Special warnings about this medication
If you have a history of stomach or intestinal disease, especially colitis, check with your doctor before taking Keflex.

If you have ever had an allergic reaction, particularly to drugs, be sure to tell your doctor.

If diarrhea occurs while taking cephalexin, check with your doctor before taking a remedy. Certain diarrhea medications (for instance, Lomotil) may increase your diarrhea or make it last longer.

Prolonged use of Keflex may result in an overgrowth of bacteria that do not respond to the medication, causing a secondary infection. Your doctor will monitor your use of this drug on a regular basis.

If you have a kidney disorder, check with your doctor before taking Keflex. You may need a reduced dose.

If you are diabetic, it is important to note that Keflex may cause false results in tests for urine sugar. Notify your doctor that you are taking this medication before being tested. Do not change your diet or dosage of diabetes medication without first consulting with your doctor.

If your symptoms do not improve within a few days, or if they get worse, notify your doctor immediately.

Do not give this medication to other people or use it for other infections before checking with your doctor.

Possible food and drug interactions
when taking this medication

If Keflex is taken with certain other drugs, the effects of either could be increased, decreased, or altered. It is especially important to check with your doctor before combining Keflex with the following:

Certain diarrhea medications such as Lomotil
Oral contraceptives

Special information
if you are pregnant or breastfeeding

The effects of Keflex during pregnancy have not been adequately studied. If you are pregnant or plan to become pregnant, notify your doctor immediately. Keflex appears in breast milk and could affect a nursing infant. If this medication is essential to your health, your doctor may advise you to discontinue breastfeeding until your treatment is finished.

Recommended dosage

ADULTS

Throat, Skin, and Urinary Tract Infections
The usual adult dosage is 500 milligrams taken every 12 hours. Cystitis (bladder infection) therapy should be continued for 7 to 14 days.

Other Infections
The usual recommended dosage is 250 milligrams taken every 6 hours. For more severe infections, larger doses may be needed, as determined by your doctor.

CHILDREN

Keflex
The usual dose is 25 to 50 milligrams for each 2.2 pounds of body weight per day, divided into smaller doses.

For strep throat in children over 1 year of age and for skin infections, the dose may be divided into 2 doses taken every 12 hours. For strep infections, the medication should be taken for at least 10 days. Your doctor may double the dose if your child has a severe infection.

For middle ear infection, the dose is 75 to 100 milligrams per 2.2 pounds per day, divided into 4 doses.

Keftab
Safety and effectiveness have not been established in children.

Overdosage
Any medication taken in excess can have serious consequences.

If you suspect an overdose, seek emergency medical treatment immediately.

- *Symptoms of Keflex overdose may include:*
  Blood in the urine, diarrhea, nausea, upper abdominal pain, vomiting

Brand name:

KEFTAB

See Keflex, page 653.

Generic name:

KETOCONAZOLE

See Nizoral, page 887.

Generic name:

KETOPROFEN

See Orudis, page 937.

Generic name:

KETOROLAC

See Toradol, page 1328.

Brand name:

KLONOPIN

Pronounced: KLON-uh-pin
Generic name: Clonazepam

Why is this drug prescribed?
Klonopin is used alone or along with other medications to treat convulsive
disorders such as epilepsy. It is also prescribed for panic disorder—

unexpected attacks of overwhelming panic accompanied by fear of recurrence. Klonopin belongs to a class of drugs known as benzodiazepines.

Most important fact about this drug
Klonopin works best when there is a constant amount in the bloodstream. To keep blood levels as constant as possible, take your doses at regularly spaced intervals and try not to miss any.

How should you take this medication?
Klonopin should be taken exactly as prescribed by your doctor.

Take Klonopin exactly as prescribed. If you are taking it for panic disorder and you find it makes you sleepy, your doctor may recommend a single dose at bedtime.

■ *If you miss a dose...*
If it is within an hour after the missed time, take the dose as soon as you remember. If you do not remember until later, skip the dose and go back to your regular schedule. Never take 2 doses at the same time.

■ *Storage instructions...*
Store at room temperature away from heat, light, and moisture.

What side effects may occur?
Side effects cannot be anticipated. If any develop or change in intensity, inform your doctor as soon as possible. Only your doctor can determine if it is safe for you to continue taking Klonopin.

■ *More common side effects in seizure disorders may include:*
Behavior problems, drowsiness, lack of muscular coordination

■ *Less common or rare side effects in seizure disorders may include:*
Abnormal eye movements, anemia, bed wetting, chest congestion, coated tongue, coma, confusion, constipation, dehydration, depression, diarrhea, double vision, dry mouth, excess hair, fever, fluttery or throbbing heartbeat, "glassy-eyed" appearance, hair loss, hallucinations, headache, inability to fall or stay asleep, inability to urinate, increased sex drive, involuntary rapid movement of the eyeballs, loss of or increased appetite, loss of voice, memory loss, muscle and bone pain, muscle weakness, nausea, nighttime urination, painful or difficult urination, partial paralysis, runny nose, shortness of breath, skin rash, slowed breathing, slurred

speech, sore gums, speech difficulties, stomach inflammation, swelling of ankles and face, tremor, uncontrolled body movement or twitching, vertigo, weight loss or gain

Klonopin can also cause aggressive behavior, agitation, anxiety, excitability, hostility, irritability, nervousness, nightmares, sleep disturbances, and vivid dreams.

- *Side effects due to rapid decrease or abrupt withdrawal from Klonopin may include:*
  Abdominal and muscle cramps, behavior disorders, convulsions, depressed feeling, hallucinations, restlessness, sleeping difficulties, tremors

- *More common side effects in panic disorder may include:*
  Allergic reaction, constipation, coordination problems, depression, dizziness, fatigue, inflamed sinuses or nasal passages, flu, memory problems, menstrual problems, nervousness, reduced thinking ability, respiratory infection, sleepiness, speech problems

- *Less common or rare side effects in panic disorder may include:*
  Abdominal pain/discomfort, abnormal hunger, acne, aggressive reaction, anxiety, apathy, asthma attack, bleeding from the skin, blood clots, bronchitis, burning sensation, changes in appetite, changes in sex drive, confusion, coughing, difficulty breathing, dizziness when standing, ear problems, emotional changeability, excessive dreaming, excitement, fever, flushing, fluttery or throbbing heartbeat, frequent bowel movements, gas, general feeling of illness, gout, hair loss, hemorrhoids, hoarseness, increased salivation, indigestion, infections, inflamed stomach and intestines, lack of attention, lack of sensation, leg cramps, loss of taste, male sexual problems, migraine, motion sickness, muscle pain/cramps, nightmares, nosebleed, overactivity, pain (anywhere in the body), paraylsis, pneumonia, shivering, skin problems, sleep problems, sneezing, sore throat, swelling with fluid retention, swollen knees, thick tongue, thirst, tingling/pins and needles, tooth problems, tremor, twitching, upset stomach, urinary problems, vertigo, vision problems, weight gain or loss, yawning

Why should this drug not be prescribed?
If you are sensitive to or have ever had an allergic reaction to Klonopin or similar drugs, such as Librium and Valium, you should not take this medication. Make sure your doctor is aware of any reactions you have experienced.

You should not take this medication if you have severe liver disease or the eye condition known as acute narrow angle glaucoma.

Special warnings about this medication

Klonopin may cause you to become drowsy or less alert; therefore, you should not drive or operate dangerous machinery or participate in any hazardous activity that requires full mental alertness until you know how this drug affects you.

If you have several types of seizures, this drug may increase the possibility of grand mal seizures (epilepsy). Inform your doctor if this occurs. Your doctor may wish to prescribe an additional anticonvulsant drug or increase your dose.

Klonopin can be habit-forming and can lose its effectiveness as you build up a tolerance to it. You may experience withdrawal symptoms—such as convulsions, hallucinations, tremor, and abdominal and muscle cramps—if you stop using this drug abruptly. Discontinue or change your dose only in consultation with your doctor.

Possible food and drug interactions
when taking this medication

Klonopin slows the nervous system and its effects may be intensified by alcohol. Do not drink while taking this medication.

If Klonopin is taken with certain other drugs, the effects of either could be increased, decreased, or altered. It is especially important to check with your doctor before combining Klonopin with the following:

Antianxiety drugs such as Valium
Antidepressant drugs such as Elavil, Nardil, Parnate, and Tofranil
Barbiturates such as phenobarbital
Carbamazepine (Tegretol)
Major tranquilizers such as Haldol, Navane, and Thorazine
Narcotic pain relievers such as Demerol and Percocet
Oral antifungal drugs such as Fungizone, Mycelex, Mycostatin
Other anticonvulsants such as Dilantin, Depakene, and Depakote
Sedatives such as Halcion

Special information
if you are pregnant or breastfeeding

Avoid Klonopin if at all possible during the first 3 months of pregnancy; there is a risk of birth defects. When taken later in pregnancy, the drug can cause other problems, such as withdrawal symptoms in the newborn. If you are pregnant or plan to become pregnant, inform your doctor immediately. Klonopin appears in breast milk and could affect a nursing infant. If this medication is essential to your health, you should not breastfeed until your treatment with this medication is finished.

Recommended dosage

SEIZURE DISORDERS

Adults
The starting dose should be no more than 1.5 milligrams per day, divided into 3 doses. Your doctor may increase your daily dosage by 0.5 to 1 milligram every 3 days until your seizures are controlled or the side effects become too bothersome. The most you should take in 1 day is 20 milligrams.

SEIZURE DISORDERS

Children
The starting dose for infants and children up to 10 years old or up to 66 pounds should be 0.01 to 0.03 milligram—no more than 0.05 milligram—per 2.2 pounds of body weight daily. The daily dosage should be given in 2 or 3 smaller doses. Your doctor may increase the dose by 0.25 to 0.5 milligram every 3 days until seizures are controlled or side effects become too bad. If the dose cannot be divided into 3 equal doses, the largest dose should be given at bedtime. The maximum maintenance dose is 0.1 to 0.2 milligram per 2.2 pounds daily.

PANIC DISORDER

Adults
The startng dose is 0.25 milligram twice a day. After 3 days, your doctor may increase the dose to 1 milligram daily. Some people need as much as 4 milligrams a day.

PANIC DISORDER

Children
For panic disorder, safety and effectiveness have not been established in children under age 18.

Overdosage

Any medication taken in excess can have serious consequences. If you suspect an overdose, seek medical attention immediately.

- *The symptoms of Klonopin overdose may include:*
  Coma, confusion, sleepiness, slowed reaction time

Brand name:

KLOR-CON

See Micro-K, page 791.

Brand name:

K-TAB

See Micro-K, page 791.

Brand name:

KWELL

Pronounced: QUELL
Generic name: Lindane

Why is this drug prescribed?

Kwell cream and lotion are used to treat scabies, a contagious skin disease caused by an almost invisible organism known as the "itch mite." Kwell shampoo is used to treat people with head lice and pubic (crab) lice and their eggs.

Most important fact about this drug

Use Kwell only as directed by your doctor. Using too much or applying it more often than directed can result in seizures or even death, particularly in the young. Read the "Instructions to Patients" information sheet accompanying the Kwell package before using. If you have any questions, call your doctor.

How should you use this medication?

CREAM AND LOTION

Shake the lotion well before using. Apply cream or lotion in a thin layer to dry skin, starting from the neck and working down, including the soles of your feet (unless otherwise directed by your doctor), and rub in thoroughly. Trim your nails and apply the medication under the nails with a toothbrush, then throw the toothbrush away. If you take a warm bath or shower before using Kwell, dry your skin thoroughly and let it cool completely before applying the medication. Leave the cream or lotion on for no less than 8 and no more than 12 hours (usually overnight), then take a shower or bath to wash it off thoroughly. Apply only once, and use only enough to cover the body in a thin layer.

SHAMPOO

Before applying Kwell shampoo, wash your hair with regular shampoo, without conditioners, then rinse it and dry it completely. Shake the shampoo well, then apply directly to dry hair, without adding water. Work thoroughly into your hair and leave it on for 4 minutes. After 4 minutes, add a little water until you have a good lather. Immediately rinse all the lather away. Do not let the lather touch any other part of the body any more than necessary. Towel-dry your hair. Remove nits (eggs) with a nit comb or tweezers. If you are using Kwell on another person, try to keep it off your skin as much as possible. If you are using Kwell on more than one person, wear rubber gloves (this applies especially to pregnant women and nursing mothers).

■ *If you miss a dose...*
Use Kwell only once per infection. Multiple applications are dangerous.

■ *Storage instructions...*
Store away from heat and direct light. Keep out of the reach of children.

What side effects may occur?
Side effects are extremely rare, but can be serious. If any develop, contact your doctor as soon as possible.

■ *Side effects may include:*
Convulsions, dizziness, seizures, skin eruptions, skin rash

Why should this drug not be prescribed?
If you are sensitive to or have ever had an allergic reaction to Kwell or any of its ingredients, do not use it again. Do not use Kwell on premature infants, their skin is more sensitive and more drug could be absorbed into the body. Do not use Kwell if you have any kind of seizure disorder; and do not use the cream or lotion for Norwegian scabies (an extremely contagious skin disease with a thin, flaky, rash).

Special warnings about this medication
Be careful to avoid contact with your eyes. If any Kwell does get in your eyes, immediately flush them with cold water; if they become irritated or you have an allergic reaction, call your doctor.

Do not swallow Kwell. If you accidentally swallow any, call your doctor or your local poison control center immediately. Do not allow your child to apply Kwell without close adult supervision.

Be sure to cover an infant's hands and feet during treatment with Kwell cream or lotion to prevent the child from sucking or licking the medication.

Do not use Kwell on open wounds such as cuts or sores unless directed by your doctor. After one application of Kwell cream or lotion, your itching may continue for several weeks. The itching is quite normal and does not require a reapplication of Kwell. You will not usually need a second treatment with Kwell shampoo, but if you find living lice in your hair 7 days after treatment, call your doctor. You may need retreatment.

Wash all recently worn clothing, underwear and pajamas, used sheets, pillow cases, and towels in very hot water or have them dry cleaned.

Use Kwell cream or lotion cautiously on young children and the elderly because their skin may absorb more of the medication. To avoid reinfection, make sure that any sexual partners are treated at the same time that you are. Kwell cannot be used to prevent scabies or lice, since no effects remain after it has been washed off.

Possible food and drug interactions
when taking this medication
Oils may cause more Kwell to be absorbed through the skin into the body, possibly causing serious side effects. Therefore, do not use oils, creams, or ointments at the same time you are using Kwell cream or lotion and do not use oil treatments or oil-based hair dressings or conditioners immediately before and after you apply Kwell shampoo.

Special information
if you are pregnant or breastfeeding
If you are pregnant, follow your doctor's directions carefully. Do not use more Kwell than your doctor recommends, and do not use it more than twice during your pregnancy.

If you are breastfeeding, be sure to check with your doctor before using Kwell. Small amounts pass into breast milk, so even though Kwell has not been found to cause problems in nursing infants, your doctor may have you give up breastfeeding for 4 days after using Kwell.

Recommended dosage

CREAM AND LOTION

Adults and children aged 6 and over
Use 1 to 2 ounces. Apply only once; and do not leave on for more than 12 hours.

Children under age 6
Use 1 ounce (half of a 2-ounce container). Apply only once.

SHAMPOO

Use 1 ounce (1/2 bottle) for short hair, 1 1/2 ounces (3/4 bottle) for medium-length hair, and 2 ounces (1 bottle) for long hair. Do not use more than 2 ounces.

Overdosage

Any medication used in excess can have serious consequences. If you suspect an overdose, seek medical attention immediately.

■ *Symptoms of Kwell overdose may include:*
Convulsions, dizziness

Generic name:

LABETALOL

See Normodyne, page 896.

Generic name:

LACTULOSE

See Chronulac Syrup, page 244.

Brand name:

LAMICTAL

Pronounced: LAM-ic-tal
Generic name: Lamotrigine

Why is this drug prescribed?

Lamictal is prescribed to control partial seizures in people with epilepsy. It is used in combination with other antiepileptic medications such as Tegretol and Depakene.

Most important fact about this drug

You may develop a rash during the first 2 to 8 weeks of Lamictal therapy, particularly if you are also taking Depakene. If this happens, notify your doctor immediately. The rash could become severe and even dangerous, particularly in children. A slight possibility of this problem remains for up to 6 months.

How should you take this medication?

Take Lamictal exactly as prescribed by your doctor. Taking more than the prescribed amount can increase your risk of developing a serious rash. Do not stop taking this medication without first discussing it with your doctor. An abrupt halt could increase your seizures. Your doctor can schedule a gradual reduction in dosage.

■ *If you miss a dose...*
Take it as soon as you remember. If it is almost time for your next dose, skip the one you missed and go back to your regular schedule. Do not take 2 doses at once.

■ *Storage instructions...*
Store in a tightly closed container at room temperature. Keep dry and protect from light.

What side effects may occur?

Side effects cannot be anticipated. If any develop or change in intensity, tell your doctor as soon as possible. Only your doctor can determine if it is safe for you to continue taking Lamictal.

■ *More common side effects may include:*
Blurred vision, dizziness, double vision, headache, nausea, rash, sleepiness, uncoordinated movements, vomiting

■ *Less common side effects may include:*
Abdominal pain, accidental injury, anxiety, constipation, depression, diarrhea, fever, "flu-like" symptoms, increased cough, inflammation of vagina, irritability, painful menstruation, sore throat, tremor

■ *Rare side effects may include:*
Absence of menstrual periods, chills, confusion, dry mouth, ear pain, emotional changes, heart palpitations, hot flashes, joint disorders, memory decrease, mind racing, muscle weakness, muscle spasm, poor concentration, ringing in ears, sleep disorder, speech disorder

Why should this drug not be prescribed?
If you are sensitive to or have ever had an allergic reaction to Lamictal, you should not take this medication. Make sure your doctor is aware of any drug reactions you have experienced.

Special warnings about this medication
Lamictal may cause some people to become drowsy, dizzy, or less alert. Do not drive or operate dangerous machinery or participate in any activity that requires full mental alertness until you are certain the drug does not have this kind of effect on you. Remember to be alert for development of any type of rash, especially during the first 2 to 8 weeks of treatment.

Be sure to tell your doctor about any medical problems you have before starting therapy with Lamictal. If you have kidney or liver disease, or heart problems, Lamictal should be used with caution.

Lamictal may cause vision problems. If any develop, notify your doctor immediately. Also be quick to call your doctor if you develop a fever or have any other signs of an allergic reaction. Notify your doctor, too, if your seizures get worse.

Possible food and drug interactions
when taking this medication
Lamictal is not used alone; it is combined with other medications used to treat epilepsy, including the following:

Carbamazepine (Tegretol)
Phenobarbital (Donnatal, Quadrinal, others)
Phenytoin (Dilantin)
Primidone (Mysoline)
Valproic acid (Depakene)

Be sure to check with your doctor before combining any other drugs with your seizure medications. Lamictal, in particular, may inhibit the action of sulfa drugs such as Bactrim, Proloprim, and Septra.

Special information
if you are pregnant or breastfeeding

The effects of Lamictal during pregnancy have not been adequately studied. If you are pregnant or plan to become pregnant, tell your doctor immediately. Lamictal should be used during pregnancy only if clearly needed. Lamictal appears in breast milk. Because the effects of Lamictal on an infant exposed to this medication are unknown, breastfeeding is not recommended.

Recommended dosage

ADULTS

Lamictal combined with Tegretol, Dilantin, Phenobarbital, and Mysoline:
One 50-milligram dose per day for 2 weeks, then two 50-milligram doses per day, for 2 weeks. After that, your doctor will have you take a total of 300 milligrams to 500 milligrams a day, divided into 2 doses.

Lamictal combined with Depakene and any of the above medications:
One 25-milligram dose every other day for 2 weeks, then 25 milligrams once a day for 2 weeks. After that, the doctor will prescribe a total of 100 milligrams to 150 milligrams a day, divided into 2 doses. You should not take more than 25 milligrams every other day because of the increased risk of rash with this combination of drugs.

CHILDREN

Safety and effectiveness of Lamictal in children below the age of 16 have not been established.

Overdosage

Any medication taken in excess can have serious consequences. If you suspect an overdose, seek medical treatment immediately. There has been little experience with Lamictal overdose. However, the following symptoms might be seen.

■ *Symptoms of Lamictal overdose may include:*
  Coma, dizziness, headache, sleepiness

Generic name:

LAMIVUDINE

See Epivir, page 479.

Generic name:

LAMOTRIGINE

See Lamictal, page 665.

Brand name:

LANOXIN

Pronounced: la-NOCKS-in
Generic name: Digoxin

Why is this drug prescribed?

Lanoxin is used in the treatment of congestive heart failure, certain types of irregular heartbeat, and other heart problems. It improves the strength and efficiency of your heart, which leads to better circulation of blood and reduction of the uncomfortable swelling that is common in people with congestive heart failure. Lanoxin is usually prescribed along with a water pill (to help relieve swelling) and a drug called an ACE inhibitor (to further improve circulation). It belongs to a class of drugs known as digitalis glycosides.

Most important fact about this drug

You should not stop taking Lanoxin without first consulting your doctor. A sudden absence of the drug could cause a serious change in your heart function. You will probably have to take Lanoxin for a long time—possibly for the rest of your life.

How should you take this medication?

Lanoxin usually is taken once daily. To help you remember your dose, try to take it at the same time every day, for instance when brushing your teeth in the morning or going to bed at night.

Lanoxin is available in tablet, capsule, liquid, and injectable forms. If you are taking the liquid form, use the specially marked dropper that comes with it.

It's best to take this medicine on an empty stomach. However, if this upsets your stomach, you can take Lanoxin with food.

Avoid taking this medicine with high-bran/high-fiber foods, such as certain breakfast cereals.

Do not change from one brand of this drug to another without first consulting your doctor or pharmacist.

Your doctor may ask you to check your pulse rate while taking Lanoxin.

Slowing or quickening of your pulse could mean you are developing side effects to your prescribed dose. The amount of Lanoxin needed to help most people is very close to the amount that could cause serious problems from overdose, so monitoring your pulse can be very important.

■ *If you miss a dose...*
If you remember within 12 hours, take it immediately. If you remember later, skip the dose you missed and go back to your regular schedule. Never take 2 doses at the same time. If you miss doses 2 or more days in a row, consult your doctor.

■ *Storage instructions...*
Store this medication at room temperature in the container it came in, tightly closed, and away from moist places and direct light. Keep out of reach of children. Digitalis-type drugs such as Lanoxin are a major cause of accidental poisoning in the young.

What side effects may occur?
Side effects cannot be anticipated. If any develop or change in intensity, inform your doctor as soon as possible. Only your doctor can determine if it is safe for you to continue taking Lanoxin.

■ *Side effects may include:*
Apathy, blurred vision, breast development in males, change in heartbeat, confusion, diarrhea, dizziness, headache, loss of appetite, lower stomach pain, nausea, psychosis, rash, vomiting, weakness, yellow vision

Why should this drug not be prescribed?
If you are sensitive to or have ever had an allergic reaction to Lanoxin or other digitalis preparations, you should not take this medication. Make sure your doctor is aware of any drug reactions you have experienced.

Lanoxin should not be taken by people with the heart irregularity known as ventricular fibrillation.

Lanoxin should not be used, alone or with other drugs, for weight reduction. It can cause irregular heartbeat and other dangerous, even fatal, reactions.

Special warnings about this medication
Your doctor will prescribe Lanoxin with caution—if at all—in the presence of certain heart disorders, including sinus node disease, AV block, certain disorders of the left ventricle, and "Wolff-Parkinson-White syndrome." Caution is also advised if you have poor kidneys, a thyroid disorder, or an imbalance in your calcium, potassium, or magnesium levels.

Tell the doctor that you are taking Lanoxin if you have a medical emergency and before you have surgery or dental treatment.

Even if you have no symptoms, do not change your dose or discontinue the use of Lanoxin before consulting with your doctor.

Possible food and drug interactions when taking this medication

In general, you should avoid nonprescription medicines, such as antacids; laxatives; cough, cold, and allergy remedies; and diet aids, except on professional advice.

If Lanoxin is taken with certain other drugs, the effects of either can be increased, decreased, or altered. It is especially important to check with your doctor before combining Lanoxin with the following:

Airway-opening drugs such as Proventil and Ventolin
Alprazolam (Xanax)
Amiloride (Midamor)
Amiodarone (Cordarone)
Antacids such as Maalox and Mylanta
Antibiotics such as neomycin, tetracycline, erythromycin, and
    clarithromycin
Beta-blocking blood pressure drugs such as Tenormin and Inderal
Calcium (injectable form)
Calcium-blocking blood pressure drugs such as Calan SR, Cardizem, and
    Procardia
Certain anticancer drugs such as Neosar
Cholestyramine (Questran)
Colestipol (Colestid)
Cyclosporine (Sandimmune)
Diphenoxylate (Lomotil)
Disopyramide (Norpace)
Heartbeat-regulating drugs such as Quinidex
Indomethacin (Indocin)
Itraconazole (Sporanox)
Kaolin-pectin
Metoclopramide (Reglan)
Propafenone (Rythmol)
Propantheline (Pro-Banthine)
Rifampin (Rifadin)
Spironolactone (Aldactone)
Steroids such as Decadron and Deltasone
Succinylcholine (Anectine)
Sucralfate (Carafate)

Sulfasalazine (Azulfidine)
Thyroid hormones such as Synthroid
Water pills such as Lasix

Special information
if you are pregnant or breastfeeding

The effects of Lanoxin during pregnancy have not been adequately studied. If you are pregnant or plan to become pregnant, inform your doctor immediately. Lanoxin appears in breast milk and could affect a nursing infant. If this medication is essential to your health, your doctor may advise you to discontinue breastfeeding.

Recommended dosage

Your doctor will determine your dosage based on several factors: (1) the disease being treated; (2) your body weight; (3) your kidney function; (4) your age; and (5) other diseases you have or drugs you are taking.

If you are receiving Lanoxin for the first time, you may be rapidly "digitalized" (a larger first dose may be taken, followed by smaller maintenance doses), or gradually "digitalized" (maintenance doses only), depending on your doctor's recommendation.

ADULTS

If your doctor feels you need rapid digitalization, your first few doses may be given intravenously. You'll then be switched to tablets or capsules for long-term maintenance. A typical maintenance dose might be a 0.125 milligram or 0.25 milligram tablet once daily, but individual requirements vary widely. The exact dose will be determined by your doctor, based on your needs.

CHILDREN

Infants and young children usually have their daily dose divided into smaller doses; children over age 10 need adult dosages in proportion to body weight as determined by your doctor.

Overdosage

Suspected overdoses of Lanoxin must be treated immediately; you should contact your doctor or emergency room without delay.

■ *Symptoms of Lanoxin overdose include:*
Abdominal pain, diarrhea, irregular heartbeat, loss of appetite, nausea, very slow pulse, vomiting

In infants and children, irregular heartbeat is the most common sign of overdose.

Generic name:

LANSOPRAZOLE

See Prevacid, page 1041.

Brand name:

LASIX

Pronounced: LAY-six
Generic name: Furosemide

Why is this drug prescribed?
Lasix is used in the treatment of high blood pressure and other conditions that require the elimination of excess fluid (water) from the body. These conditions include congestive heart failure, cirrhosis of the liver, and kidney disease. When used to treat high blood pressure, Lasix is effective alone or in combination with other high blood pressure medications. Diuretics help your body produce and eliminate more urine, which helps lower blood pressure. Lasix is classified as a "loop diuretic" because of its point of action in the kidneys.

Lasix is also used with other drugs in people with fluid accumulation in the lungs.

Most important fact about this drug
Lasix acts quickly, usually within 1 hour. However, since blood pressure declines gradually, it may be several weeks before you get the full benefit of Lasix; and you must continue taking it even if you are feeling well. Lasix does not cure high blood pressure; it merely keeps it under control.

How should you take this medication?
Take this medication exactly as prescribed by your doctor.

■ *If you miss a dose...*
  Take the forgotten dose as soon as you remember. If it is almost time for your next dose, skip the one you missed and go back to your regular schedule. Never take 2 doses at the same time.

■ *Storage instructions...*
  Keep this medication in the container it came in, tightly closed, and away from direct light. Store at room temperature.

What side effects may occur?

Side effects cannot be anticipated. If any develop or change in intensity, inform your doctor as soon as possible. Only your doctor can determine if it is safe for you to continue taking Lasix.

■ *Side effects may include:*

Anemia, blood disorders, blurred vision, constipation, cramping, diarrhea, dizziness, dizziness upon standing, fever, headache, hearing loss, high blood sugar, hives, itching, loss of appetite, low potassium (leading to symptoms like dry mouth, excessive thirst, weak or irregular heartbeat, muscle pain or cramps), muscle spasms, nausea, rash, reddish or purplish spots on the skin, restlessness, ringing in the ears, sensitivity to light, skin eruptions, skin inflammation and flaking, stomach or mouth irritation, tingling or pins and needles, vertigo, vision changes, vomiting, weakness, yellow eyes and skin

Why should this drug not be prescribed?

If you are sensitive to or have ever had an allergic reaction to Lasix or diuretics, or if you are unable to urinate, you should not take this medication.

Special warnings about this medication

Lasix can cause your body to lose too much potassium. Signs of an excessively low potassium level include muscle weakness and rapid or irregular heartbeat. To improve your potassium level, your doctor may prescribe a potassium supplement or recommend potassium-rich foods, such as bananas, raisins, and orange juice.

Make sure the doctor knows if you have kidney disease, liver disease, diabetes, gout, or the connective tissue disease, lupus erythematosus. Lasix should be used with caution.

If you are allergic to sulfa drugs, you may also be allergic to Lasix.

If you have high blood pressure, avoid over-the-counter medications that may increase blood pressure, including cold remedies and appetite suppressants.

Your skin may be more sensitive to the effects of sunlight.

Possible food and drug interactions
when taking this medication

If Lasix is taken with certain other drugs, the effects of either could be increased, decreased, or altered. It is especially important to consult with your doctor before taking Lasix with any of the following:

Aminoglycoside antibiotics such as Garamycin
Aspirin and other salicylates

Ethacrynic acid (Edecrin)
Indomethacin (Indocin)
Lithium (Lithonate)
Norepinephrine (Levophed)
Other high blood pressure medications such as Hytrin and Cardura
Sucralfate (Carafate)

**Special information
if you are pregnant or breastfeeding**
The effects of Lasix during pregnancy have not been adequately studied. If
you are pregnant or plan to become pregnant, inform your doctor immediately. Lasix appears in breast milk and could affect a nursing infant. If this
medication is essential to your health, your doctor may advise you to
discontinue breastfeeding until your treatment is finished.

Recommended dosage
Your doctor will adjust the dosages of this strong diuretic to meet your
specific needs.

ADULTS

Fluid Retention
You will probably be started at a single dose of 20 to 80 milligrams. If
needed, the same dose can be repeated 6 to 8 hours later, or the dose may
be increased. Your doctor may raise the dosage by 20 milligrams or 40
milligrams with each successive administration—each 6 to 8 hours after the
previous dose—until the desired effect is achieved. This dosage is then taken
once or twice daily thereafter. Your doctor should monitor you carefully using
laboratory tests. The maximum daily dose is 600 milligrams.

High Blood Pressure
The usual starting dose is 80 milligrams per day divided into 2 doses. Your
doctor will adjust the dosages and may add other high blood pressure
medications if Lasix is not enough.

CHILDREN

The usual initial dose is 2 milligrams per 2.2 pounds of body weight given in
a single oral dose. The doctor may increase subsequent doses by 1 to 2
milligrams per 2.2 pounds. Doses are spaced 6 to 8 hours apart. A child's
dosage will be adjusted to the lowest needed to achieve maximum effect,
and should not exceed 6 milligrams per 2.2 pounds.

Overdosage

Any medication taken in excess can have serious consequences. An overdose of Lasix can cause symptoms of severe dehydration. If you suspect an overdose, seek medical attention immediately.

- *Symptoms of Lasix overdose may include:*
  Dry mouth, excessive thirst, low blood pressure, muscle pain or cramps, nausea and vomiting, weak or irregular heartbeat, weakness or drowsiness

Generic name:

LATANOPROST

See Xalatan, page 1434.

Generic name:

LEFLUNOMIDE

See Arava, page 81.

Brand name:

LESCOL

Pronounced: LESS-cahl
Generic name: Fluvastatin sodium

Why is this drug prescribed?

Lescol reduces cholesterol levels in the blood, and can lower your chances of developing clogged arteries and heart disease. It is also prescribed to slow the accumulation of plaque in the arteries of people who already have coronary heart disease. Your doctor will prescribe the drug only if you have been unable to reduce your blood cholesterol level sufficiently with a low-fat, low-cholesterol diet alone.

Most important fact about this drug

Lescol is usually prescribed only if diet, exercise, and weight loss fail to bring your cholesterol levels under control. It's important to remember that Lescol is a supplement—not a substitute—for those other measures. To get the full benefit of the medication, you need to stick to the diet and exercise program prescribed by your doctor. All these efforts to keep your cholesterol levels normal are important because together they may lower your risk of heart disease.

How should you take this medication?

If you've been prescribed a small, single dose per day, take it at bedtime. A large dosage (80 milligrams) may be divided into 2 smaller doses and taken twice a day. You may take Lescol with or without food.

■ *If you miss a dose...*

If you miss a dose of this medication, take it as soon as you remember. However, if it is almost time for your next dose, skip the one you missed and go back to your regular schedule. Do not take 2 doses at the same time.

■ *Storage instructions...*

Store at room temperature. Protect from direct light and excessive heat. Keep out of reach of children.

What side effects may occur?

Side effects cannot be anticipated. If any develop or change in intensity, tell your doctor as soon as possible. Only your doctor can determine if it is safe for you to continue taking Lescol.

■ *More common side effects may include:*

Abdominal pain, accidental injury, back pain, constipation, diarrhea, flu-like symptoms, headache, indigestion, joint pain, muscle pain, nasal inflammation, nausea, sore throat, upper respiratory infection

■ *Less common side effects may include:*

Allergy, arthritis, constipation, coughing, dizziness, dental problems, fatigue, gas, inflamed sinuses, insomnia, rash

Why should this drug not be prescribed?

Do not take Lescol while pregnant or nursing. Also avoid Lescol if you are experiencing liver problems, or if you have ever been found to be excessively sensitive to it.

Special warnings about this medication

Because Lescol may damage the liver, your doctor may order a blood test to check your liver enzyme levels before you start taking this medication. Blood tests will probably be done 6 and 12 weeks after you start Lescol therapy and periodically after that. If your liver enzymes rise too high, your doctor may tell you to stop taking Lescol. Your doctor will monitor you especially closely if you have ever had liver disease or if you are, or have ever been, a heavy drinker.

Since Lescol may cause damage to muscle tissue, be sure to tell your doctor of any unexplained muscle pain, tenderness, or weakness right away, especially if you also have a fever or feel sick. Your doctor may want to do a blood test to check for signs of muscle damage. If your blood test shows signs of muscle damage, your doctor may suggest discontinuing this medication.

If your risk of muscle and/or kidney damage suddenly increases because of major surgery or injury, or conditions such as low blood pressure, severe infection, or seizures, your doctor may tell you to stop taking Lescol for a while.

Be sure to tell your doctor about any medical conditions you may have before starting therapy with Lescol.

Possible food and drug interactions when taking this medication

If you take Lescol with certain drugs, the effects of either could be increased, decreased, or altered. It is especially important to check with your doctor before combining Lescol with the following:

Cholestyramine (Questran)
Cimetidine (Tagamet)
Clofibrate (Atromid-S)
Cyclosporine (Sandimmune, Neoral)
Digoxin (Lanoxin, Lanoxicaps)
Erythromycin (E-Mycin, E.E.S.)
Gemfibrozil (Lopid)
Ketoconazole (Nizoral)
Omeprazole (Prilosec)
Ranitidine (Zantac)
Rifampin (Rifadin)

Special information if you are pregnant or breastfeeding

You must not become pregnant while taking Lescol. This medication lowers cholesterol, and cholesterol is needed for a baby to develop properly. Because of the possible risk of birth defects, your doctor will prescribe Lescol only if you are highly unlikely to get pregnant while taking this medication. If you do become pregnant while taking Lescol, stop taking the drug and notify your doctor right away.

Lescol does appear in breast milk. Therefore, Lescol could cause severe side effects in a nursing baby. Do not take Lescol while breastfeeding your baby.

Recommended dosage
Your doctor will put you on a cholesterol-lowering diet before starting treatment with Lescol. You should continue on this diet while you are taking Lescol.

ADULTS

The usual starting dose is 20 to 40 milligrams per day, taken as a single dose at bedtime. The usual range after that is 20 to 80 milligrams per day. At the 80-milligram level, the dosage will be split into two 40-milligram doses taken 2 times a day. After 4 weeks of therapy with Lescol, your doctor will check your cholesterol level and adjust your dosage if necessary.

Combined Drug Therapy
If you are taking Lescol with another cholesterol medication such as Questran, make sure you take the other drug at least 2 hours before your dose of Lescol.

CHILDREN

The safety and effectiveness of Lescol in children under 18 years old have not been established. Do not give Lescol to children under 18 years of age.

Overdosage
Although no specific information about Lescol overdose is available, any medication taken in excess can have serious consequences. If you suspect an overdose of Lescol, seek medical attention immediately.

Brand name:

LEVAQUIN

Pronounced: LEAV-ah-kwin
Generic name: Levofloxacin

Why is this drug prescribed?
Levaquin cures a variety of bacterial infections, including several types of sinus infection and pneumonia. It is also prescribed for flare-ups of chronic bronchitis, acute kidney infections, certain urinary infections, and mild to moderate skin infections. Levaquin is a member of the quinolone family of antibiotics.

Most important fact about this drug

Levaquin has been known to cause dangerous allergic reactions as soon as you take the first dose. Stop taking the drug and call your doctor immediately if you develop any of the following warning signs:

Skin rash, hives, or any other skin reaction
Rapid heartbeat
Difficulty swallowing or breathing
Swelling of the face, lips, tongue, or throat

How should you take this medication?

Take your complete prescription exactly as directed, even if you begin to feel better. If you stop taking Levaquin too soon, the infection may come back.

You may take Levaquin at mealtimes or in-between, but you should avoid taking it within 2 hours of the following:

Aluminum or magnesium antacids such as Maalox, Mylanta, or
  Gaviscon
Iron supplements such as Ferro-Sequels or Feosol
Any multivitamin preparation containing zinc
The ulcer medication Carafate

Be sure to drink plenty of fluid while taking Levaquin.

■ *If you miss a dose...*
Take it as soon as you remember. If it is almost time for your next dose, skip the one you missed and go back to your regular schedule. Do not take 2 doses at once.

■ *Storage instructions...*
Store at room temperature. Keep container tightly closed.

What side effects may occur?

Side effects cannot be anticipated. If any develop or change in intensity, tell your doctor as soon as possible. Only your doctor can determine if it is safe for you to continue taking Levaquin.

■ *Side effects may include:*
Abdominal pain, anxiety, bad taste, constipation, diarrhea, dizziness, fatigue, gas, general feeling of illness, headache, hives, indigestion, itching, lack of appetite, nausea, nervousness, rash, sleeplessness and sleep disorders, sweating, swelling, tremors, vaginal discharge, vaginal inflammation, vomiting, yeast infection

Why should this drug not be prescribed?

If any other quinolone antibiotic—such as Cipro, Floxin, Maxaquin, Noroxin, or Penetrex—has ever given you an allergic reaction, avoid Levaquin.

Special warnings about this medication

In rare cases, Levaquin has caused convulsions and other nervous disorders. If you develop any warning signs of a nervous reaction—ranging from restlessness and tremors to depression and hallucinations—stop taking this medication and call your doctor.

Hypersensitivity to quinolone antibiotics can, in rare instances, lead to severe illnesses ranging from blood disorders to liver or kidney failure. The first sign of a developing problem is often a rash; so you should stop taking Levaquin and check with your doctor when any type of skin disorder appears. Remember, too, that an immediate allergic reaction is also a possibility (see "Most important fact about this drug").

A case of diarrhea during Levaquin therapy could signal development of the potentially dangerous condition known as pseudomembranous colitis, an inflammation of the bowel. Call your doctor for treatment at the first sign of a problem.

Stop taking Levaquin, avoid exercise, and call your doctor if you develop pain, inflammation, or a rupture in a tendon. Quinolone antibiotics have been known to cause tendon rupture during and after therapy.

If you have a kidney condition, make sure the doctor is aware of it. Your dosage may need to be lowered.

Possible food and drug interactions
when taking this medication

Nonsteroidal anti-inflammatory drugs such as Advil, Motrin, and Naprosyn can increase the risk of a nervous reaction to Levaquin. Also, check with your doctor before combining Levaquin with an oral diabetes drug such as Glucotrol, Micronase, or Orinase; changes in blood sugar levels could result.

If you are taking the asthma drug, theophylline, or the blood-thinning drug, Coumadin, make sure the doctor is aware of it. Other quinolone antibiotics have been known to interact with these medications.

Special information
if you are pregnant or breastfeeding

The effects of this drug during pregnancy have not been adequately studied. If you are pregnant or plan to become pregnant, inform your doctor immediately. Levaquin is likely to appear in breast milk and could harm a nursing infant. If the drug is essential to your health, your doctor may advise you to stop nursing until your treatment is finished.

Recommended dosage

ADULTS

Respiratory and skin infections
The usual dose is 500 milligrams once a day.

Kidney and urinary infections
The usual dose is 250 milligrams once a day

CHILDREN

Not for children under 18. Levaquin might damage developing bones and joints.

Overdosage

Levaquin is not especially poisonous. However, an overdose could still be dangerous. If you suspect one, seek emergency treatment immediately.

■ *Symptoms of Levaquin overdose may include:*
Breathlessness, lack of movement, poor coordination, tremors, convulsions, collapse

Brand name:

LEVBID

See Levsin, page 683.

Brand name:

LEVLEN

See Oral Contraceptives, page 926.

Generic name:

LEVOBUNOLOL

See Betagan, page 158.

Generic name:

LEVODOPA

See Sinemet CR, page 1196.

Generic name:

LEVOFLOXACIN

See Levaquin, page 679.

Brand name:

LEVOTHROID

See Synthroid, page 1237.

Generic name:

LEVOTHYROXINE

See Synthroid, page 1237.

Brand name:

LEVOXYL

See Synthroid, page 1237.

Brand name:

LEVSIN

Pronounced: LEV-sin
Generic name: Hyoscyamine sulfate
Other brand names: Anaspaz, Levbid, Levsinex

Why is this drug prescribed?

Levsin is an antispasmodic medication given to help treat various stomach, intestinal, and urinary tract disorders that involve cramps, colic, or other painful muscle contractions. Because Levsin has a drying effect, it may also be used to dry a runny nose or to dry excess secretions before anesthesia is administered.

Together with morphine or other narcotics, Levsin is prescribed for the pain of gallstones or kidney stones. For inflammation of the pancreas, Levsin may be used to help control excess secretions and reduce pain. Levsin may also be taken in Parkinson's disease to help reduce muscle rigidity and tremors and to help control drooling and excess sweating.

Doctors also give Levsin as part of the preparation for certain diagnostic x-rays (for example, of the stomach, intestines, or kidneys).

Levsin comes in several forms, including regular tablets, tablets to be dissolved under the tongue, sustained-release capsules (Levsinex Timecaps) and sustained-release tablets (Levbid), liquid, drops, and an injectable solution.

Most important fact about this drug
Levsin may make you sweat less, causing your body temperature to increase and putting you at the risk of heatstroke. Try to stay inside as much as possible on hot days, and avoid warm places such as very hot baths and saunas.

How should you take this medication?
If you take Levsin for a stomach disorder, you may also need to take antacid medication. However, antacids make Levsin more difficult for the body to absorb. To minimize this problem, take Levsin before meals and the antacid after meals.

Take Levsin exactly as prescribed. Although the sublingual tablets (Levsin/SL) are designed to be dissolved under the tongue, they may also be chewed or swallowed. The regular tablets should be swallowed. Levbid extended-release tablets should not be crushed or chewed.

Levsin can cause dry mouth. For temporary relief, suck on a hard candy or chew gum.

- *If you miss a dose...*
  Take it as soon as you remember. If it is almost time for your next dose, skip the one you missed and go back to your regular schedule. Do not take 2 doses at once.

- *Storage instructions...*
  Store at room temperature.

What side effects may occur?
Side effects cannot be anticipated. If any side effects develop or change in intensity, tell your doctor immediately. Only your doctor can determine whether it is safe for you to continue taking Levsin.

■ *Side effects may include:*
Allergic reactions, bloating, blurred vision, confusion, constipation, decreased sweating, dilated pupils, dizziness, drowsiness, dry mouth, excitement, headache, hives, impotence, inability to urinate, insomnia, itching, heart palpitations, lack of coordination, loss of sense of taste, nausea, nervousness, rapid heartbeat, skin reactions, speech problems, vomiting, weakness

Why should this drug not be prescribed?
Do not take Levsin if you have ever had an allergic reaction to it or similar drugs such as scopolamine. Also, you should not be given Levsin if you have any of the following:

Bowel or digestive tract obstruction or paralysis
Glaucoma (excessive pressure in the eyes)
Myasthenia gravis (a disorder in which muscles become weak and tire easily)
Ulcerative colitis (severe bowel inflammation)
Urinary obstruction

Levsin is not appropriate if you have diarrhea, especially if you have a surgical opening to the bowels (an ileostomy or colostomy).

Special warnings about this medication
Be careful using Levsin if you have an overactive thyroid gland, heart disease, congestive heart failure, irregular heartbeats, high blood pressure, or kidney disease.

Because Levsin may make you dizzy or drowsy, or blur your vision, do not drive, operate other machinery, or do any other hazardous work while taking this medication.

While you are taking Levsin, you may experience confusion, disorientation, short-term memory loss, hallucinations, difficulty speaking, lack of coordination, coma, an exaggerated sense of well-being, decreased anxiety, fatigue, sleeplessness and agitation. These symptoms should disappear 12 to 48 hours after you stop taking the drug.

Possible food and drug interactions
when taking this medication
If Levsin is taken with certain other drugs, the effects of either drug could be increased, decreased, or altered. It is especially important to check with your doctor before combining Levsin with the following:

Amantadine (Symmetrel)
Antacids

Antidepressant drugs such as Elavil, Nardil, Parnate, and Tofranil
Antihistamines such as Benadryl
Major tranquilizers such as Thorazine and Haldol
Other antispasmodic drugs such as Bentyl
Potassium supplements such as Slow-K

Special information
if you are pregnant or breastfeeding

If you are pregnant or plan to become pregnant, inform your doctor immediately. Although it is not known whether Levsin can cause birth defects, pregnant women should avoid all drugs except those necessary to health.

Levsin appears in breast milk. Your doctor may ask you to forgo breastfeeding when taking this drug.

Recommended dosage

LEVSIN AND LEVSIN/SL TABLETS

Levsin tablets should be swallowed. Levsin/SL tablets may be placed under the tongue, swallowed, or chewed.

Adults and Children 12 Years of Age and Older

The usual dose is 1 to 2 tablets every 4 hours or as needed. Do not take more than 12 tablets in 24 hours.

Children 2 to Under 12 Years of Age

The usual dose is one-half to 1 tablet every 4 hours or as needed. Do not give a child more than 6 tablets in 24 hours.

LEVSIN ELIXIR

Adults and Children 12 Years of Age and Older

The recommended dosage is 1 to 2 teaspoonfuls every 4 hours or as needed, but no more than 12 teaspoonfuls in 24 hours.

Children 2 to 12 Years of Age

Dosage is by body weight. Doses may be given every 4 hours or as needed. Do not give a child more than 6 teaspoonfuls in 24 hours.

Weight	Dose
22 pounds	1/4 teaspoon
44 pounds	1/2 teaspoon
88 pounds	3/4 teaspoon
110 pounds	1 teaspoon

LEVSIN DROPS

Adults and Children 12 Years of Age and Older
The recommended dosage is 1 to 2 milliliters every 4 hours or as needed, but no more than 12 milliliters in 24 hours.

Children 2 to 12 Years of Age
The usual dosage is one-quarter to 1 milliliter every 4 hours or as needed. Do not give a child more than 6 milliliters in 24 hours.

Children under 2 Years of Age
Your doctor will determine the dosage based on body weight. The doses may be repeated every 4 hours or as needed.

Weight	Usual Dose	Do Not Exceed in 24 Hours
7.5 pounds	4 drops	24 drops
11 pounds	5 drops	30 drops
15 pounds	6 drops	36 drops
22 pounds	8 drops	48 drops

LEVSINEX TIMECAPS

Adults and Children 12 Years of Age and Older
The recommended dosage is 1 to 2 capsules every 12 hours. Your doctor may adjust the dosage to 1 capsule every 8 hours if needed. Do not take more than 4 capsules in 24 hours.

LEVBID EXTENDED-RELEASE TABLETS

Adults and Children 12 Years of Age and Older
The dosage is 1 to 2 tablets every 12 hours. The tablets are scored so that you can break them in half if your doctor wants you to. Do not crush or chew them. You should not take more than 4 tablets in 24 hours.

Overdosage

Any medication taken in excess can have serious consequences. If you suspect an overdose, seek medical attention immediately.

■ *Symptoms of Levsin overdose may include:*
Blurred vision, dilated pupils, dizziness, dry mouth, excitement, headache, hot dry skin, nausea, swallowing difficulty, vomiting

Brand name:

LEVSINEX

See Levsin, page 683.

Brand name:

LEXXEL

Pronounced: LECKS-ell
Generic ingredients: Enalapril maleate, Felodipine

Why is this drug prescribed?

Lexxel is used to treat high blood pressure. It combines two blood pressure drugs: an ACE inhibitor and a calcium channel blocker. The ACE inhibitor (enalapril) lowers blood pressure by preventing a chemical in your blood called angiotensin I from converting to a more potent form that narrows the blood vessels and increases salt and water retention. The calcium channel blocker (felodipine) also works to keep the blood vessels open, and eases the heart's workload by reducing the force and rate of your heartbeat.

Lexxel can be prescribed alone or in combination with other blood pressure medicines, especially water pills (diuretics) such as HydroDIURIL or Esidrix.

Most important fact about this drug

Doctors usually prescribe Lexxel for patients who have been taking one of its components—enalapril (Vasotec) or extended-release felodipine (Plendil)—without showing improvement. Like other blood pressure medications, Lexxel must be taken regularly for it to be effective. Since blood pressure declines gradually, it may be 1 or 2 weeks before you get the full benefit of Lexxel; and you must continue taking it even if you are feeling well. Lexxel does not cure high blood pressure; it merely keeps it under control.

How should you take this medication?

Lexxel can be taken with a light meal or without food. Remember, however, that a high-fat meal can reduce its effectiveness, and that grapefruit juice increases its impact.

Swallow Lexxel tablets whole. Do not crush, divide, or chew them.

■ *If you miss a dose...*
Take it as soon as you remember. If it is almost time for your next dose, skip the one you missed and go back to your regular schedule. Never take 2 doses at the same time.

■ *Storage instructions...*
Store at room temperature. Keep the container tightly closed and protect from light and humidity.

What side effects may occur?

Side effects cannot be anticipated. If any develop or change in intensity, inform your doctor as soon as possible. Only your doctor can determine if it is safe for you to continue taking Lexxel.

■ *More common side effects may include:*
Dizziness, headache, swelling

■ *Less common side effects may include:*
Cough, fatigue, flushing, lack of strength

■ *Rare side effects may include:*
Abdominal pain, agitation, breast enlargement, chest pain, constipation, diarrhea, difficulty breathing, drowsiness, dry mouth or throat, dry skin, facial swelling, fainting, gas, gout, hair loss, heartburn, hot flashes, impotence, increased pressure within the eyes, indigestion, insomnia, itching, joint swelling, nausea, neck pain, nervousness, poor coordination, rash, rectal pain, respiratory congestion, skin swelling, slow heartbeat, sore throat, tingling sensation, tremor, vomiting

Why should this drug not be prescribed?

Avoid Lexxel if you have ever had an allergic reaction to it, or have ever developed a swollen throat and difficulty swallowing (angioedema) while taking similar drugs such as Capoten, Vasotec, or Zestril. Make sure your doctor is aware of the incident.

Special warnings about this medication

Call your doctor immediately if you begin to suffer angioedema while taking Lexxel. Warning signs include swelling of the face, lips, tongue, or throat; swelling of the arms and legs; and difficulty swallowing or breathing.

Bee or wasp venom given to prevent an allergic reaction to stings may cause a severe allergic reaction to Lexxel. Kidney dialysis can also prompt an allergic reaction to the drug.

Lexxel sometimes causes a severe drop in blood pressure. The danger is especially great if you have been taking water pills (diuretics), or if you have heart disease, kidney disease, or a potassium or salt imbalance. Excessive sweating, severe diarrhea, and vomiting are also a threat. They can rob the body of water, causing a dangerous drop in blood pressure. If you feel light-headed or faint, have chest pain, or feel your heart racing, contact your doctor immediately.

Because another of the ACE inhibitors, Capoten, has been known to cause serious blood disorders, your doctor will check your blood regularly while you are taking Lexxel. If you develop signs of infection such as a sore throat or a fever, you should contact your doctor at once—an infection could be a signal of blood abnormalities.

Lexxel may also affect the liver; and your doctor will need to adjust your dosage with extra care if you are over 65 or have liver disease. Report these symptoms of liver problems to your doctor immediately: a generally run-down feeling, pain in the upper right abdomen, or yellowing of the skin or the whites of your eyes.

If you suffer from heart failure or kidney disease, make certain that your doctor knows about it. Lexxel should be used with caution under these circumstances.

Some people taking Lexxel develop a dry, nagging cough. This will go away when you stop taking the drug. Others are troubled by swollen gums. Good dental hygiene makes this less likely.

Possible food and drug interactions when taking this medication

If Lexxel is taken with certain other drugs, the effects of either could be increased, decreased, or altered. It is especially important to check with your doctor before combining Lexxel with the following:

Blood pressure medicines known as beta-blockers, including Lopressor, Inderal, and Tenormin
Cimetidine (Tagamet)

Diuretics such as Lasix or HydroDIURIL
Diuretics that leave potassium in the body, such as Aldactone,
    Midamor, and Dyrenium
Epilepsy medications such as Dilantin, phenobarbital, and Tegretol
Grapefruit juice
High-fat meals
Lithium (Eskalith, Lithobid)
Potassium supplements such as K-Lyte, K-Tabs, and Slow-K

Because Lexxel tends to increase your potassium level, avoid potassium-containing salt substitutes unless your doctor approves.

Special information
if you are pregnant or breastfeeding
Do not take Lexxel during pregnancy. When taken during the final 6 months, the ACE inhibitor in Lexxel can cause birth defects, prematurity, and death in the developing or newborn baby. If you are pregnant, inform your doctor immediately.

Lexxel may appear in breast milk and could affect a nursing infant. If this medication is essential to your health, your doctor may advise you to stop breastfeeding.

Recommended dosage

ADULTS

The usual starting dose is 1 tablet once a day. If there is no change in your blood pressure after 1 or 2 weeks, the doctor may increase your dose to 2 tablets daily.

CHILDREN

The safety and effectiveness of Lexxel in children have not been established.

OLDER ADULTS

If you are over 65, your doctor may have to monitor your blood pressure closely at the beginning of treatment, and adjust your dose with care.

Overdosage
Any medication taken in excess can have serious consequences. If you suspect an overdose, seek medical treatment immediately.

- *Symptoms of Lexxel overdose may include:*
  Low blood pressure, rapid heartbeat

Brand name:

LIBRAX

Pronounced: LIB-racks
Generic ingredients: Chlordiazepoxide hydrochloride,
*   Clidinium bromide*

Why is this drug prescribed?
Librax is used, in combination with other therapy, for the treatment of peptic ulcer, irritable bowel syndrome (spastic colon), and acute enterocolitis (inflammation of the colon and small intestine). Librax is a combination of a benzodiazepine (chlordiazepoxide) and an antispasmodic medication (clidinium).

Most important fact about this drug
Because of its sedative effects, you should not operate heavy machinery, drive, or engage in other hazardous tasks that require you to be mentally alert while you are taking Librax.

How should you take this medication?
Take Librax as directed by your doctor. Other therapy may be prescribed to be used at the same time.

Librax can make your mouth dry. For temporary relief, suck a hard candy or chew gum.

Take Librax before meals and at bedtime.

■ *If you miss a dose...*
   Take it as soon as you remember. If it is almost time for your next dose, skip the one you missed and go back to your regular schedule. Do not take 2 doses at once.

■ *Storage instructions...*
   Store away from heat, light, and moisture.

What side effects may occur?
Side effects cannot be anticipated. If any develop or change in intensity, inform your doctor as soon as possible. Only your doctor can determine if it is safe for you to continue taking Librax.

■ *Side effects may include:*
   Blurred vision, changes in sex drive, confusion, constipation, drowsiness, dry mouth, fainting, lack of coordination, liver problems, minor menstrual

irregularities, nausea, skin eruptions, swelling due to fluid retention, urinary difficulties, yellowing of skin and eyes

Why should this drug not be prescribed?

You should not take this drug if you have glaucoma (elevated pressure in the eye), prostatic hypertrophy (enlarged prostate), or a bladder obstruction. If you are sensitive to or have ever had an allergic reaction to Librax or any of its ingredients, you should not take this medication. Make sure your doctor is aware of any drug reactions you have experienced.

Special warnings about this medication

Librax can be habit-forming and has been associated with drug dependence and addiction. Be very careful taking this medication if you have ever had problems with alcohol or drug abuse. Never take more than the prescribed amount.

In addition, you should not stop taking Librax suddenly, because of the risk of withdrawal symptoms (convulsions, cramps, tremors, vomiting, sweating, feeling depressed, and insomnia). If you have been taking Librax over a long period of time, your doctor will have you taper off gradually.

The elderly are more likely to develop side effects such as confusion, excessive drowsiness, and uncoordinated movements when taking Librax. The doctor will probably prescribe a low dose.

Long-term treatment with Librax may call for periodic blood and liver function tests.

Possible food and drug interactions
when taking this medication

If Librax is taken with certain other drugs, the effects of either can be increased, decreased, or altered. It is especially important to check with your doctor before combining Librax with the following:

Antidepressant drugs known as MAO inhibitors, such as Nardil and
   Parnate
Blood-thinning drugs such as Coumadin
Certain diarrhea medications such as Donnagel and Kaopectate
Ketoconazole (Nizoral)
Major tranquilizers such as Stelazine and Thorazine
Potassium supplements such as Micro-K

In addition, you may experience excessive drowsiness and other potentially dangerous side effects if you combine Librax with alcohol or other drugs, such as Benadryl and Valium, that make you drowsy.

Special information
if you are pregnant or breastfeeding

Several studies have found an increased risk of birth defects if Librax is taken during the first 3 months of pregnancy. Therefore, Librax is rarely recommended for use by pregnant women. If you are pregnant, plan to become pregnant, or are breastfeeding, inform your doctor immediately.

Recommended dosage

ADULTS

The usual dose is 1 or 2 capsules, 3 or 4 times a day before meals and at bedtime.

OLDER ADULTS

Your doctor will have you take the lowest dose that is effective.

Overdosage

Any medication taken in excess can have serious consequences. A severe overdose of Librax can be fatal. If you suspect an overdose, seek medical help immediately.

■ *Symptoms of Librax overdose may include:*
  Blurred vision, coma, confusion, constipation, excessive sleepiness, excessively dry mouth, slow reflexes, urinary difficulties

Brand name:

LIBRIUM

Pronounced: LIB-ree-um
Generic name: Chlordiazepoxide

Why is this drug prescribed?

Librium is used in the treatment of anxiety disorders. It is also prescribed for short-term relief of the symptoms of anxiety, symptoms of withdrawal in acute alcoholism, and anxiety and apprehension before surgery. It belongs to a class of drugs known as benzodiazepines.

Most important fact about this drug

Librium is habit-forming and you can become dependent on it. You could experience withdrawal symptoms if you stopped taking it abruptly. (See "What side effects may occur?") Discontinue or change your dose only on advice of your doctor.

How should you take this medication?
Take this medication exactly as prescribed.

■ *If you miss a dose...*
Take it as soon as you remember if it is within an hour or so of your scheduled time. If you do not remember until later, skip the dose you missed and go back to your regular schedule. Do not take 2 doses at once.

■ *Storage instructions...*
Store away from heat, light, and moisture.

What side effects may occur?
Side effects cannot be anticipated. If any develop or change in intensity, inform your doctor as soon as possible. Only your doctor can determine if it is safe for you to continue taking Librium.

■ *Side effects may include:*
Confusion, constipation, drowsiness, fainting, increased or decreased sex drive, liver problems, lack of muscle coordination, minor menstrual irregularities, nausea, skin rash or eruptions, swelling due to fluid retention, yellow eyes and skin

■ *Side effects due to rapid decrease or abrupt withdrawal from Librium include:*
Abdominal and muscle cramps, convulsions, exaggerated feeling of depression, sleeplessness, sweating, tremors, vomiting

Why should this drug not be prescribed?
If you are sensitive to or have ever had an allergic reaction to Librium or similar tranquilizers, you should not take this medication.

Anxiety or tension related to everyday stress usually does not require treatment with Librium. Discuss your symptoms thoroughly with your doctor.

Special warnings about this medication
Librium may cause you to become drowsy or less alert; therefore, you should not drive or operate dangerous machinery or participate in any hazardous activity that requires full mental alertness until you know how you react to this drug.

If you are severely depressed or have suffered from severe depression, consult with your doctor before taking this medication.

This drug may cause children to become less alert.

If you have a hyperactive, aggressive child taking Librium, inform your doctor if you notice contrary reactions such as excitement, stimulation, or acute rage.

Consult with your doctor before taking Librium if you are being treated for porphyria (a rare metabolic disorder) or kidney or liver disease.

Possible food and drug interactions
when taking this medication

Librium is a central nervous system depressant and may intensify the effects of alcohol or have an additive effect. Do not drink alcohol while taking this medication.

If Librium is taken with certain other drugs, the effects of either can be increased, decreased, or altered. It is especially important to check with your doctor before combining Librium with the following:

Antacids such as Maalox and Mylanta
Antidepressant drugs known as MAO inhibitors, including Nardil and Parnate
Barbiturates such as phenobarbital
Blood-thinning drugs such as Coumadin
Cimetidine (Tagamet)
Disulfiram (Antabuse)
Levodopa (Larodopa)
Major tranquilizers such as Stelazine and Thorazine
Narcotic pain relievers such as Demerol and Percocet
Oral contraceptives

Special information
if you are pregnant or breastfeeding

Do not take Librium if you are pregnant or planning to become pregnant. There may be an increased risk of birth defects. This drug may appear in breast milk and could affect a nursing infant. If the medication is essential to your health, your doctor may advise you to discontinue breastfeeding until your treatment with the drug is finished.

Recommended dosage

ADULTS

Mild or Moderate Anxiety
The usual dose is 5 or 10 milligrams, 3 or 4 times a day.

Severe Anxiety
The usual dose is 20 to 25 milligrams, 3 or 4 times a day.

Apprehension and Anxiety before Surgery
On days preceding surgery, the usual dose is 5 to 10 milligrams, 3 or 4 times a day.

Withdrawal Symptoms of Acute Alcoholism
The usual starting oral dose is 50 to 100 milligrams; the doctor will repeat this dose, up to a maximum of 300 milligrams per day, until agitation is controlled. The dose will then be reduced as much as possible.

CHILDREN

The usual dose for children 6 years of age and older is 5 milligrams, 2 to 4 times per day. Some children may need to take 10 milligrams, 2 or 3 times per day. The drug is not recommended for children under 6.

OLDER ADULTS

Your doctor will limit the dose to the smallest effective amount in order to avoid oversedation or lack of coordination. The usual dose is 5 milligrams, 2 to 4 times per day.

Overdosage
Any medication taken in excess can cause symptoms of overdose. If you suspect an overdose, seek medical attention immediately.

- *The symptoms of Librium overdose may include:*
  Coma, confusion, sleepiness, slow reflexes

Brand name:

LIDEX

Pronounced: LYE-decks
Generic name: Fluocinonide

Why is this drug prescribed?
Lidex is a steroid medication that relieves the itching and inflammation of a wide variety of skin problems, including redness and swelling.

Most important fact about this drug
When you use Lidex, you inevitably absorb some of the medication through your skin and into the bloodstream. Too much absorption can lead to unwanted side effects elsewhere in the body. To keep this problem to a minimum, avoid using large amounts of Lidex over large areas, and do not cover it with airtight dressings such as plastic wrap or adhesive bandages unless specifically told to by your doctor.

How should you use this medication?
Lidex is for use only on the skin. Be careful to keep it out of your eyes. If the medication gets in your eyes and causes irritation, immediately flush your eyes with a large amount of water.

Apply Lidex as directed by your doctor. Do not use more of the medication than suggested by your doctor.

- *If you miss a dose...*
  Apply it as soon as you remember. If it is almost time for the next dose, skip the one you missed and go back to your regular schedule.

- *Storage instructions...*
  Store at room temperature. Avoid excessive heat.

What side effects may occur?
Side effects cannot be anticipated. If any develop or change in intensity, inform your doctor immediately. Only your doctor can determine if it is safe for you to continue using Lidex.

- *Side effects may include:*
  Acne-like eruptions, burning, dryness, excessive hair growth, infection of the skin, irritation, itching, lack of skin color, prickly heat, skin inflammation, skin loss or softening, stretch marks

Why should this drug not be prescribed?
You should not be using Lidex if you are allergic to any of its components.

Special warnings about this medication
Do not use Lidex more often or for a longer time than your doctor ordered. If enough of the drug is absorbed through the skin, it may produce unusual side effects, including increased sugar in your blood and urine and a group of symptoms called Cushing's syndrome, characterized by a moon-shaped face, emotional disturbances, high blood pressure, weight gain, and growth of body hair in women.

Some factors that may increase absorption include:

Using bandages over the area where the medication is applied;
Using the medication over a large area of skin or on broken skin; or
Using the medication for an extended period of time.

Children may absorb a proportionally greater amount of steroid drugs and may be more sensitive to the effects of these drugs. Avoid covering a treated area with waterproof diapers or plastic pants. They can increase absorption of Lidex.

■ *Effects experienced by children may include:*
Bulges on the head
Delayed weight gain
Headache
Slow growth

Lidex should be discontinued if irritation develops, and another treatment should be used.

Extended treatment time with any steroid product may cause skin to waste away. This may also occur with short-term use on the face, armpits, and skin creases.

Possible food and drug interactions
when taking this medication
No interactions have been reported with Lidex.

Special information
if you are pregnant or breastfeeding
Pregnant women should not use steroids on the skin in large amounts or for long periods of time. During pregnancy, these medications should be used only if the possible gains outweigh the possible risks to the baby.

Steroids do appear in breast milk. Women who breastfeed an infant should use them cautiously.

Recommended dosage
ADULTS

Lidex is applied to the affected areas in a thin film 2 to 4 times a day. If hair covers the infected area, part the hair so that the medication can be applied directly.

CHILDREN

Children should be given the smallest effective dose.

Overdosage

Lidex can be absorbed in amounts large enough to have temporary effects on the adrenal, hypothalamic, and pituitary glands.

- *Some effects of steroid drugs may include:*
  Abnormal sugar levels in urine, excessive blood sugar levels, symptoms of Cushing's syndrome

- *Symptoms of Cushing's syndrome may include:*
  Easily bruised skin, increased blood pressure, mood swings, water retention, weak muscles, weight gain

If you suspect a Lidex overdose, seek medical help immediately.

Generic name:

LINDANE

See Kwell, page 662.

Brand name:

LIPITOR

Pronounced: LIP-ih-tor
Generic name: Atorvastatin calcium

Why is this drug prescribed?

Lipitor is a cholesterol-lowering drug. Your doctor may prescribe it along with a special diet if your blood cholesterol or triglyceride level is high enough to put you in danger of heart disease, and you have been unable to lower your readings by diet alone.

The drug works by helping to clear harmful low density lipoprotein (LDL) cholesterol out of the blood and by limiting the body's ability to form new LDL cholesterol.

Most important fact about this drug

Lipitor is usually prescribed only if diet, exercise, and weight loss fail to bring your cholesterol levels under control. It's important to remember that Lipitor is a supplement—not a substitute—for those other measures. To get the full benefit of the medication, you need to stick to the diet and exercise program prescribed by your doctor. All these efforts to keep your cholesterol levels normal are important because they may lower your risk of heart disease.

How should you take this medication?

Lipitor should be taken once a day, with or without food. You can take it in the morning or the evening, but should hold to the same time each day. The drug generally begins working within 2 weeks.

For an even greater cholesterol-lowering effect, your doctor may prescribe Lipitor along with a different kind of lipid-lowering drug such as Questran or Colestid. It's important to avoid taking the two drugs at the same time of day. Take Lipitor at least 1 hour before or 4 hours after the other drug.

■ *If you miss a dose...*
Take the forgotten dose as soon as you remember. If it is almost time for your next dose, skip the one you missed and go back to your regular schedule. Do not take 2 doses at the same time.

■ *Storage instructions...*
Store at room temperature.

What side effects may occur?

Side effects cannot be anticipated. If any develop or change in intensity, inform your doctor as soon as possible. Only your doctor can determine if it is safe for you to continue taking Lipitor. The side effects of Lipitor—if any develop—are usually mild.

■ *Side effects may include:*
Abdominal pain, abnormal heart beats, accidental injury, acne, allergic reaction, amnesia, back pain, black stools, bleeding, breast enlargement, changes in eyesight, changes in taste sensation, chest pain, constipation, decreased sex drive, depression, diarrhea, difficulty swallowing, distorted facial muscles, dizziness, dry eyes, fatigue, fever, flu symptoms, fluid retention, gas, hair loss, headache, hearing difficulties, heartburn, increased muscle movement, increased sensations, indigestion, inflammation of sinus and nasal passages, insomnia, itching, joint pain, lack of coordination, leg cramps, muscle aching or weakness, purple or red spots on the skin, rash, respiratory problems, ringing in the ears, sensitivity to light, skin irritations, sore throat, strange dreams, sweating, tingling of extremities, unstable emotions, urinary problems, vomiting, weakness, weight gain, weight loss

Why should this drug not be prescribed?
Never take Lipitor during pregnancy or while breastfeeding. You should also avoid Lipitor if you have liver disease, or if the drug gives you an allergic reaction.

Special warnings about this medication
There is a slight chance of liver damage from Lipitor, so your doctor may order a blood test to check your liver function before you start taking the drug, again 6 weeks and 12 weeks after you begin therapy or your dosage is increased, and every 6 months thereafter. If the tests reveal a problem, you may have to stop using the drug.

Drugs like Lipitor have occasionally been known to damage muscle tissue, so be sure to tell your doctor immediately if you notice any unexplained muscle tenderness, weakness, or pain, especially if you also have a fever or feel sick. Your doctor may want to do a blood test to check for signs of muscle damage.

Possible food and drug interactions
when taking this medication
If you take Lipitor with certain other drugs, the effects of either could be increased, decreased, or altered. It is especially important to check with your doctor before combining Lipitor with any of the following:

Cyclosporine (Sandimmune, Neoral)
Digoxin (Lanoxin)
Erythromycin (E.E.S., Erythrocin, others)
Fluconazole (Diflucan)
Gemfibrozil (Lopid)
Itraconazole (Sporanox)
Ketoconazole (Nizoral)
Niacin (Nicobid, Nicolar)
Oral contraceptives

Special information
if you are pregnant or breastfeeding
Developing babies need plenty of cholesterol, so this cholesterol-lowering drug should never be used during pregnancy. In fact, your doctor is unlikely to prescribe Lipitor if there is even a chance that you may become pregnant. If you do conceive while taking this drug, notify your doctor right away. Lipitor does make its way into breast milk, so you should not take the drug while breastfeeding your baby.

Recommended dosage

You need to follow a standard cholesterol-lowering diet before starting Lipitor, and should continue following it throughout your therapy.

ADULTS

The usual starting dose is 10 milligrams once a day, with or without food. The doctor will check your cholesterol levels every 2 to 4 weeks and adjust the dose accordingly. The maximum recommended daily dose is 80 milligrams.

CHILDREN

Use in children is rare. The drug has never been prescribed for children under 9 years of age.

Overdosage

Although no specific information about Lipitor overdose is available, any medication taken in excess can have serious consequences. If you suspect an overdose of Lipitor, seek medical attention.

Generic name:

LISINOPRIL

See Zestril, page 1457.

Generic name:

LISINOPRIL WITH HYDROCHLOROTHIAZIDE

See Zestoretic, page 1452.

Generic name:

LITHIUM

See Lithonate, page 704.

Brand name:

LITHOBID

See Lithonate, page 704.

Brand name:

LITHONATE

Pronounced: LITH-oh-nate
Generic name: Lithium carbonate
Other brand names: Eskalith, Lithobid, Lithotabs

Why is this drug prescribed?

Lithonate is used to treat the manic episodes of manic-depressive illness, a condition in which a person's mood swings from depression to excessive excitement. A manic episode may involve some or all of the following symptoms:

Aggressiveness
Elation
Fast, urgent talking
Frenetic physical activity
Grandiose, unrealistic ideas
Hostility
Little need for sleep
Poor judgment

Once the mania subsides, Lithonate treatment may be continued over the long term, at a somewhat lower dosage, to prevent or reduce the intensity of future manic episodes.

Some doctors also prescribe lithium for premenstrual tension, eating disorders such as bulimia, certain movement disorders, and sexual addictions.

Most important fact about this drug

If the Lithonate dosage is too low, you will derive no benefit; if it is too high, you could suffer lithium poisoning. You and your doctor will need to work together to find the correct dosage. Initially, this means frequent blood tests to find out how much of the drug is actually circulating in your bloodstream. As long as you take Lithonate, you will need to watch for side effects. Signs of lithium poisoning include vomiting, unsteady walking, diarrhea, drowsiness, tremor, and weakness. Stop taking the drug and call your doctor if you have any of these symptoms.

How should you take this medication?

To avoid stomach upset, take Lithonate immediately after meals or with food or milk.

Do not change from one brand of lithium to another without consulting your doctor or pharmacist. Take the drug exactly as prescribed.

While taking Lithonate, you should drink 10 to 12 glasses of water or fluid a day. To minimize the risk of harmful side effects, eat a balanced diet that includes some salt and lots of liquids. If you have been sweating a great deal or have had diarrhea, make sure you get extra liquids and salt.

If you develop an infection with a fever, you may need to cut back on your Lithonate dosage or even quit taking it temporarily. While you are ill, keep in close touch with your doctor.

Long-acting forms of lithium, such as Eskalith CR or Lithobid, should be swallowed whole. Do not chew, crush, or break.

■ *If you miss a dose...*
Ask your doctor what to do; requirements vary for each individual. Do not take 2 doses at once.

■ *Storage instructions...*
Store at room temperature.

What side effects may occur?
The possibility of side effects varies with the level of lithium in your bloodstream. If you experience unfamiliar symptoms of any kind, inform your doctor as soon as possible.

■ *Side effects that may occur when you start taking lithium include:*
Discomfort, frequent urination, hand tremor, mild thirst, nausea

■ *Side effects that may occur at a high dosage include:*
Diarrhea, drowsiness, lack of coordination, muscular weakness, vomiting

Why should this drug not be prescribed?
Although your doctor will be cautious under certain conditions, lithium may be prescribed for anyone.

Special warnings about this medication
Lithonate may affect your judgment or coordination. Do not drive, climb, or perform hazardous tasks until you find out how this drug affects you.

Your doctor will prescribe Lithonate with extra caution if you have a heart or kidney problem, brain or spinal cord disease, or a weak, run-down, or dehydrated condition.

Also make sure your doctor is aware of any medical problems you may have, including diabetes, epilepsy, thyroid problems, Parkinson's disease, and difficulty urinating.

You should be careful in hot weather to avoid activities that cause you to sweat heavily. Also avoid drinking large amounts of coffee, tea, or cola, which can cause dehydration through increased urination. Do not make a major change in your eating habits or go on a weight loss diet without consulting your doctor. The loss of water and salt from your body could lead to lithium poisoning.

Possible food and drug interactions when taking this medication
If Lithonate is taken with certain other drugs, the effects of either could be increased, decreased, or altered. It is especially important to check with your doctor before combining Lithonate with the following:

ACE-inhibitor blood pressure drugs such as Capoten or Vasotec
Acetazolamide (Diamox)
Amphetamines such as Dexedrine
Antidepressant drugs that boost serotonin levels, including Paxil, Prozac, and Zoloft
Anti-inflammatory drugs such as Indocin and Feldene
Bicarbonate of soda
Caffeine (No-Doz)
Calcium-blocking blood pressure drugs such as Calan and Cardizem
Carbamazepine (Tegretol)
Diuretics such as Lasix or HydroDIURIL
Fluoxetine (Prozac)
Iodine-containing preparations such as potassium iodide (Quadrinal)
Major tranquilizers such as Haldol and Thorazine
Methyldopa (Aldomet)
Metronidazole (Flagyl)
Phenytoin (Dilantin)
Sodium bicarbonate
Tetracyclines such as Achromycin V and Sumycin
Theophylline (Theo-Dur, Quibron, others)

Special information if you are pregnant or breastfeeding
The use of Lithonate during pregnancy is usually not recommended because of the possibility that it might cause birth defects. If you are pregnant or plan to become pregnant, inform your doctor immediately.

Lithonate appears in breast milk and is considered potentially harmful to a nursing infant. If this medication is essential to your health, your doctor may advise you to discontinue breastfeeding while you are taking it.

Recommended dosage

ADULTS

Acute Episodes
The usual dosage is a total of 1,800 milligrams per day. Immediate-release forms are taken in 3 doses per day; long-acting forms are taken twice a day. The usual dose of syrup is 2 teaspoons, taken 3 times a day.

Your doctor will individualize your dosage according to the levels of the drug in your blood. Your blood levels will be checked at least twice a week when the drug is first prescribed and on a regular basis thereafter.

Long-term Control
Dosage will vary from one individual to another, but a total of 900 milligrams to 1,200 milligrams per day is typical. Immediate-release forms are taken in 3 or 4 doses per day; long-acting forms are taken two or three times a day. The usual dose of syrup is 1 teaspoon 3 or 4 times a day.

Blood levels in most cases should be checked every 2 months.

CHILDREN

Safety and effectiveness of Lithonate in children under 12 years of age have not been established.

OLDER ADULTS

Older people often need less Lithonate and may show signs of overdose at a dosage younger people can handle well.

Overdosage
Any medication taken in excess can have serious consequences. If you suspect symptoms of an overdose of Lithonate, seek medical attention immediately.

The harmful levels are close to those that will treat your condition. Watch for early signs of overdose, such as diarrhea, drowsiness, lack of coordination, vomiting, and weakness. If you develop any of these signs, stop taking the drug and call your doctor.

Brand name:

LITHOTABS

See Lithonate, page 704.

Brand name:

LODINE

Pronounced: LOW-deen
Generic name: Etodolac

Why is this drug prescribed?

Lodine, a nonsteroidal anti-inflammatory drug, is available in regular and extended-release forms (Lodine XL). Both forms are used to relieve the inflammation, swelling, stiffness, and joint pain of osteoarthritis (the most common form of arthritis) and rheumatoid arthritis. Regular Lodine is also used to relieve pain in other situations.

Most important fact about this drug

You should have frequent checkups with your doctor if you take Lodine regularly. Ulcers or internal bleeding can occur without warning.

How should you take this medication?

Your doctor may ask you to take Lodine with food or an antacid, and with a full glass of water. Never take it on an empty stomach.

Take this medication exactly as prescribed by your doctor.

You should see results in 1 to 2 weeks.

If you are using Lodine for arthritis, it should be taken regularly.

- *If you miss a dose...*
  Take the forgotten dose as soon as you remember. If it is almost time for the next dose, skip the one you missed and go back to your regular schedule. Never try to "catch up" by doubling the dose.

- *Storage instructions...*
  Store at room temperature. Protect capsules from moisture. Protect Lodine tablets from light; protect Lodine XL tablets from excessive heat and humidity.

What side effects may occur?
Side effects cannot be anticipated. If any develop or change in intensity, inform your doctor as soon as possible. Only your doctor can determine if it is safe for you to continue taking Lodine.

■ *More common side effects may include:*
Abdominal pain, black stools, blurred vision, chills, constipation, depression, diarrhea, dizziness, fever, gas, increased frequency of urination, indigestion, itching, nausea, nervousness, rash, ringing in ears, painful or difficult urination, vomiting, weakness

■ *Less common or rare side effects may include:*
Abdominal bleeding, abnormal intolerance of light, anemia, asthma, blood disorders, congestive heart failure, dry mouth, fainting, flushing, hepatitis and other liver problems, high blood pressure, high blood sugar in some diabetics, hives, inability to sleep, inflamed blood vessels, inflammation of mouth or upper intestine, kidney problems, including kidney failure, loss of appetite, peptic ulcer, rapid heartbeat, rash, severe allergic reactions, skin disorders including increased pigmentation, sleepiness, Stevens-Johnson syndrome (peeling skin), sweating, swelling (fluid retention), thirst, visual disturbances, yellowed skin and eyes

Why should this drug not be prescribed?
If you are sensitive to or have ever had an allergic reaction to Lodine, or if you have had asthma attacks, hives, or other allergic reactions caused by aspirin or other nonsteroidal anti-inflammatory drugs such as Motrin, you should not take this medication; it might cause a severe allergic reaction. Make sure your doctor is aware of any drug reactions you have experienced; and be careful about taking this drug if you have asthma—even if you've never had a drug reaction before. If you do suffer an allergic reaction, call for emergency help immediately.

Special warnings about this medication
Peptic ulcers and bleeding can occur without warning. You may have other problems with bleeding as well.

Call your doctor if you have any signs or symptoms of stomach or intestinal ulcers or bleeding, blurred vision or other eye problems, skin rash, weight gain, or fluid retention and swelling.

This drug should be used with caution if you have kidney or liver disease; and it can cause liver inflammation in some people.

Do not take aspirin or any other anti-inflammatory medications while taking Lodine, unless your doctor tells you to do so.

If you are taking Lodine over an extended period of time, your doctor should check your blood for anemia.

This drug can increase water retention. Use with caution if you have heart disease or high blood pressure.

Possible food and drug interactions
when taking this medication

If Lodine is taken with certain other drugs, the effects of either could be increased, decreased, or altered. It is especially important to check with your doctor before combining Lodine with the following:

    Aspirin
    Cyclosporine (Sandimmune, Neoral)
    Digoxin (Lanoxin)
    Lithium (Lithobid, others)
    Methotrexate
    Phenylbutazone (Butazolidin)
    The blood-thinning drug warfarin (Coumadin)

Special information
if you are pregnant or breastfeeding

The effects of Lodine during pregnancy have not been adequately studied. However, you should definitely not take it in late pregnancy. If you are pregnant or plan to become pregnant, inform your doctor immediately. Lodine may appear in breast milk and could affect a nursing infant. If this medication is essential to your health, your doctor may advise you to discontinue breastfeeding until your treatment with this medication is finished.

Recommended dosage

ADULTS

General Pain Relief
Take 200 to 400 milligrams every 6 to 8 hours as needed. Ordinarily, you should not take more than 1,000 milligrams a day, although your doctor may increase the dose to 1,200 milligrams a day if absolutely necessary.

Osteoarthritis and Rheumatoid Arthritis
The starting dose of Lodine is 300 milligrams 2 or 3 times a day, or 400 or 500 milligrams twice a day. The usual daily maximum ranges from 600 to

1,000 milligrams, although your doctor may prescribe as much as 1,200 milligrams a day if necessary.

The usual dose of Lodine XL is 400 to 1,000 milligrams taken once a day.

Your doctor will stick with the lowest dose that proves effective.

CHILDREN

The safety and effectiveness of Lodine have not been established in children.

Overdosage
Any medication taken in excess can cause symptoms of overdose. If you suspect an overdose, seek medical attention immediately.

- *Symptoms of Lodine overdose may include:*
  Drowsiness, lethargy, nausea, stomach pain, vomiting

Brand name:

LOESTRIN

See Oral Contraceptives, page 926.

Generic name:

LOMEFLOXACIN

See Maxaquin, page 758.

Brand name:

LOMOTIL

Pronounced: loe-MOE-till
Generic ingredients: Diphenoxylate hydrochloride, Atropine sulfate

Why is this drug prescribed?
Lomotil is used, along with other drugs, in the treatment of diarrhea.

Most important fact about this drug
Lomotil is not a harmless drug, so never exceed your recommended dosage. An overdose could be fatal.

How should you take this medication?
Lomotil can be habit-forming. Take it exactly as prescribed.

Be sure to drink plenty of liquids to replace lost body fluids. Eat bland foods, such as cooked cereals, breads and crackers.

Lomotil may cause dry mouth. Suck on a hard candy or chew gum to relieve this problem.

■ *If you miss a dose...*
Take it as soon as you remember. If it is almost time for your next dose, skip the one you missed and go back to your regular schedule. Do not take 2 doses at once.

■ *Storage instructions...*
Store away from heat, light, and moisture. Keep the liquid from freezing.

What side effects may occur?
Side effects cannot be anticipated. If any develop or change in intensity, inform your doctor as soon as possible. Only your doctor can determine if it is safe for you to continue taking Lomotil.

■ *Side effects may include:*
Abdominal discomfort, confusion, depression, difficulty urinating, dizziness, dry mouth and skin, exaggerated feeling of elation, fever, flushing, general feeling of not being well, headache, hives, intestinal blockage, itching, lack or loss of appetite, nausea, numbness of arms and legs, rapid heartbeat, restlessness, sedation/drowsiness, severe allergic reaction, sluggishness, swelling due to fluid retention, swollen gums, vomiting

Why should this drug not be prescribed?
If you are sensitive to or have ever had an allergic reaction to the ingredients of Lomotil, diphenoxylate or atropine, you should not take this medication. Make sure your doctor is aware of any drug reactions you have experienced.

Unless you are directed to do so by your doctor, do not take Lomotil if you have obstructive jaundice (a disease in which bile made in the liver does not reach the intestines because of a bile duct obstruction such as gallstones). Do not take Lomotil if you have diarrhea associated with pseudomembranous enterocolitis (inflammation of the intestines) or an infection with enterotoxin-producing bacteria (an enterotoxin is a poisonous substance that affects the stomach and intestines).

Special warnings about this medication
Certain antibiotics such as Ceclor, Cleocin, PCE and Achromycin V may cause diarrhea. Lomotil can make this type of diarrhea worse and longer-lasting. Check with your doctor before using Lomotil while taking an antibiotic.

Lomotil may cause drowsiness or dizziness. Therefore, you should not drive a car, operate dangerous machinery, or participate in any hazardous activity that requires full mental alertness until you know how this drug affects you.

Lomotil slows activity of the digestive system; this can result in a buildup of fluid in the intestine, which may worsen the dehydration and imbalance in normal body salts that usually occur with diarrhea.

If you have severe ulcerative colitis (an inflammation of the intestines), your doctor will want to monitor your condition while you are taking this drug. If your abdomen becomes distended, or enlarged, notify your doctor.

Use Lomotil with extreme caution if you have kidney and liver disease or if your liver is not functioning normally.

Lomotil should be used with caution in children, since side effects may occur even with recommended doses, especially in children with Down's syndrome (congenital mental retardation).

Since addiction to diphenoxylate hydrochloride is possible at high doses, you should never exceed the recommended dosage.

Possible food and drug interactions when taking this medication
Lomotil may intensify the effects of alcohol. It's better not to drink alcohol while taking this medication.

If Lomotil is taken with certain other drugs, the effects of either could be increased, decreased, or altered. It is especially important to check with your doctor before combining Lomotil with the following:

  Barbiturates (anticonvulsants and sedatives such as phenobarbital)
  MAO inhibitors (antidepressants such as Nardil and Parnate)
  Tranquilizers (such as Valium and Xanax)

Special information if you are pregnant or breastfeeding
The effects of Lomotil during pregnancy have not been adequately studied. If you are pregnant or plan to become pregnant, notify your doctor immediately.

Lomotil appears in breast milk and could affect a nursing infant. If this medication is essential to your health, your doctor may advise you to discontinue breastfeeding until your treatment is finished.

Recommended dosage

ADULTS

The recommended starting dosage is 2 tablets 4 times a day or 2 regular teaspoonfuls (10 milliliters) of liquid 4 times per day.

Once your diarrhea is under control, your doctor may reduce the dosage; you may need as little as 5 milligrams (2 tablets or 10 milliliters of liquid) per day.

You should see improvement within 48 hours. If your diarrhea persists after you have taken 20 milligrams a day for 10 days, the drug is not likely to work for you.

CHILDREN

Lomotil is not recommended for children under 2 years of age.

Your doctor will take into account your child's nutritional status and degree of dehydration before prescribing this drug.

In children under 13 years of age, use only Lomotil liquid and administer with the plastic dropper. The recommended starting dosage is 0.3 to 0.4 milligram per 2.2 pounds of body weight per day, divided into 4 equal doses. The following provides approximate starting dosage recommendations for children:

2 years (24-31 pounds):
    1.5-3.0 milligrams, 4 times daily
3 years (26-35 pounds):
    2.0-3.0 milligrams, 4 times daily
4 years (31-44 pounds):
    2.0-4.0 milligrams, 4 times daily
5 years (35-51 pounds):
    2.5-4.5 milligrams, 4 times daily
6-8 years (38-71 pounds):
    2.5-5.0 milligrams, 4 times daily
9-12 years (51-121 pounds):
    3.5-5.0 milligrams, 4 times daily

Your doctor may reduce the dosage as soon as symptoms are controlled. A maintenance dosage may be as low as one-quarter of the starting dose. If your child does not show improvement within 48 hours, Lomotil is unlikely to work.

Overdosage
An overdose of Lomotil can be dangerous and even fatal. If you suspect an overdose, seek medical attention immediately.

■ *Symptoms of Lomotil overdose may include:*
Coma, dry skin and mucous membranes, enlarged pupils of the eyes, extremely high body temperature, flushing, involuntary eyeball movement, lower than normal muscle tone, pinpoint pupils, rapid heartbeat, restlessness, sluggishness, suppressed breathing

Suppressed breathing may be seen as late as 30 hours after an overdose.

Brand name:

LO/OVRAL

See Oral Contraceptives, page 926.

Generic name:

LOPERAMIDE

See Imodium, page 623.

Brand name:

LOPID

Pronounced: LOH-pid
Generic name: Gemfibrozil

Why is this drug prescribed?
Lopid is prescribed, along with a special diet, for treatment of people with very high levels of serum triglycerides (a fatty substance in the blood) who are at risk of developing pancreatitis (inflammation of the pancreas) and who do not respond adequately to a strict diet.

This drug can also be used to reduce the risk of coronary heart disease in people who have failed to respond to weight loss, diet, exercise, and other triglyceride- or cholesterol-lowering drugs.

Most important fact about this drug
Lopid is usually prescribed only if diet, exercise, and weight-loss fail to bring your cholesterol levels under control. It's important to remember that Lopid is a supplement—not a substitute—for these other measures. To get the

full benefit of the medication, you need to stick to the diet and exercise program prescribed by your doctor. All these efforts to keep your cholesterol levels normal are important because together they may lower your risk of heart disease.

How should you take this medication?
Take this medication 30 minutes before the morning and evening meal, exactly as prescribed.

■ *If you miss a dose...*
Take it as soon as you remember. If it is almost time for the next dose, skip the one you missed and go back to your regular schedule. Do not take 2 doses at the same time.

■ *Storage instructions...*
Store at room temperature.

What side effects may occur?
Side effects cannot be anticipated. If any develop or change in intensity, inform your doctor as soon as possible. Only your doctor can determine if it is safe for you to continue taking Lopid.

■ *More common side effects may include:*
Abdominal pain, acute appendicitis, constipation, diarrhea, eczema, fatigue, headache, indigestion, nausea/vomiting, rash, vertigo

■ *Less common or rare side effects may include:*
Anemia, blood disorders, blurred vision, confusion, convulsions, decreased male fertility, decreased sex drive, depression, dizziness, fainting, hives, impotence, inflammation of the colon, irregular heartbeat, itching, joint pain, laryngeal swelling, muscle disease, muscle pain, muscle weakness, painful extremities, sleepiness, tingling sensation, weight loss, yellow eyes and skin

Why should this drug not be prescribed?
There is a slight possibility that Lopid may cause malignancy, gallbladder disease, abdominal pain leading to appendectomy, or other serious, possibly fatal, abdominal disorders. This drug should not be used by those who have only mildly elevated cholesterol levels, since the benefits do not outweigh the risk of these severe side effects.

If you are sensitive to or have ever had an allergic reaction to Lopid or similar drugs such as Atromid-S, you should not take this medication. Make sure your doctor is aware of any drug reactions you have experienced.

Unless you are directed to do so by your doctor, do not take this medication if you are being treated for severe kidney or liver disorders or gallbladder disease.

Special warnings about this medication

Excess body weight and excess alcohol intake may be important risk factors leading to unusually high levels of fats in the body. Your doctor will probably want you to lose weight and stop drinking before he or she tries to treat you with Lopid.

Your doctor will probably do periodic blood level tests during the first 12 months of therapy with Lopid because of blood diseases associated with the use of this medication.

Liver disorders have occurred with the use of this drug. Therefore, your doctor will probably test your liver function periodically.

If you are being treated for any disease that contributes to increased blood cholesterol, such as an overactive thyroid, diabetes, nephrotic syndrome (kidney and blood vessel disorder), dysproteinemia (excess of protein in the blood), or obstructive liver disease, consult with your doctor before taking Lopid.

Lopid should begin to reduce cholesterol levels during the first 3 months of therapy. If your cholesterol is not lowered sufficiently, this medication should be discontinued. Therefore, it is important that your doctor check your progress regularly.

The use of this medication may cause gallstones leading to possible gallbladder surgery. If you develop gallstones, your doctor will tell you to stop taking the drug.

The use of this drug may be associated with myositis, a muscle disease. If you have muscle pain, tenderness, or weakness, consult with your doctor. If myositis is suspected, your doctor will stop treating you with this drug.

Possible food and drug interactions
when taking this medication

If Lopid is taken with certain other drugs, the effects of either could be increased, decreased, or altered. It is especially important to check with your doctor before combining Lopid with the following:

Blood-thinning drugs such as Coumadin
Fluvastatin (Lescol)
Lovastatin (Mevacor)
Pravastatin (Pravachol)
Simvastatin (Zocor)

Special information
if you are pregnant or breastfeeding

The effects of Lopid during pregnancy have not been adequately studied. If you are pregnant or plan to become pregnant, inform your doctor immediately. This medication causes tumors in animals, and it could have an effect on nursing infants. If Lopid is essential to your health, your doctor may advise you to discontinue breastfeeding until your treatment with Lopid is finished.

Recommended dosage

ADULTS

The recommended dose is 1,200 milligrams divided into 2 doses, given 30 minutes before the morning and evening meals.

CHILDREN

Safety and effectiveness of Lopid have not been established for use in children.

OLDER ADULTS

This drug should be used with caution by older adults.

Overdosage

There have been no reported cases of overdose with Lopid. However, should you suspect a Lopid overdose, seek medical attention immediately.

Brand name:

LOPRESSOR

Pronounced: low-PRESS-or
Generic name: Metoprolol tartrate
Other brand name: Toprol-XL

Why is this drug prescribed?

Lopressor, a type of medication known as a beta blocker, is used in the treatment of high blood pressure, angina pectoris (chest pain, usually caused by lack of oxygen to the heart due to clogged arteries), and heart attack.

When prescribed for high blood pressure, it is effective when used alone or in combination with other high blood pressure medications. Beta blockers decrease the force and rate of heart contractions, thereby reducing the demand for oxygen and lowering blood pressure.

Occasionally doctors prescribe Lopressor for the treatment of aggressive behavior, prevention of migraine headache, and relief of temporary anxiety.

An extended-release form of this drug, called Toprol-XL, is also available.

Most important fact about this drug
If you have high blood pressure, you must take Lopressor regularly for it to be effective. Since blood pressure declines gradually, it may be several weeks before you get the full benefit of Lopressor; and you must continue taking it even if you are feeling well. Lopressor does not cure high blood pressure; it merely keeps it under control.

How should you take this medication?
Lopressor should be taken with food or immediately after you have eaten.

Take Lopressor exactly as prescribed, even if your symptoms have disappeared.

Try not to miss any doses. If this medication is not taken regularly, your condition may worsen.

- *If you miss a dose...*
  If it is within 4 hours of your next dose, skip the one you missed and go back to your regular schedule. Never take 2 doses at the same time.

- *Storage instructions...*
  Store at room temperature in a tightly closed container, away from light. Protect from moisture.

What side effects may occur?
Side effects cannot be anticipated. If any develop or change in intensity, inform your doctor as soon as possible. Only your doctor can determine if it is safe for you to continue taking Lopressor.

- *More common side effects may include:*
  Depression, diarrhea, dizziness, itching, rash, shortness of breath, slow heartbeat, tiredness

■ *Less common or rare side effects may include:*
Blurred vision, cold hands and feet, confusion, congestive heart failure, constipation, difficult or labored breathing, dry eyes, dry mouth, gas, hair loss, headache, heart attack, heartburn, low blood pressure, muscle pain, nausea, nightmares, rapid heartbeat, ringing in the ears, short-term memory loss, stomach pain, swelling due to fluid retention, trouble sleeping, wheezing, worsening of heart irregularities

Why should this drug not be prescribed?
If you have a slow heartbeat, certain heart irregularities, low blood pressure, inadequate output from the heart, or heart failure, you should not take this medication.

Special warnings about this medication
If you have a history of congestive heart failure, Lopressor should be used with caution.

Do not stop Lopressor abruptly. This can cause increased chest pain and heart attack. Dosage should be gradually reduced.

If you suffer from asthma, seasonal allergies or other bronchial conditions, or liver disease, this medication should be used with caution.

Ask your doctor if you should check your pulse while taking Lopressor. This medication can cause your heartbeat to become too slow.

This medication may mask some symptoms of low blood sugar in diabetics or alter blood sugar levels. If you are diabetic, discuss this with your doctor.

Lopressor may cause you to become drowsy or less alert; therefore, driving or operating dangerous machinery or participating in any hazardous activity that requires full mental alertness is not recommended until you know how you respond to this medication.

Notify your doctor or dentist that you are taking Lopressor if you have a medical emergency, or before you have surgery or dental treatment.

Notify your doctor if you have any difficulty in breathing.

Possible food and drug interactions
when taking this medication
If Lopressor is taken with certain other drugs, the effects of either could be increased, decreased, or altered. It is especially important to check with your doctor before combining Lopressor with certain high blood pressure drugs such as reserpine (Ser-Ap-Es).

- *Other medications that might interact with Lopressor include:*
  Albuterol (Proventil, Ventolin)
  Amiodarone (Cordarone)
  Barbiturates such as phenobarbital
  Calcium channel blockers such as Calan and Cardizem
  Cimetidine (Tagamet)
  Ciprofloxacin (Cipro)
  Clonidine (Catapres)
  Epinephrine (EpiPen)
  Hydralazine (Apresoline)
  Insulin
  Nonsteroidal anti-inflammatory drugs such as Motrin and Indocin
  Oral diabetes drugs such as Glucotrol and Micronase
  Prazosin (Minipress)
  Quinidine (Quinaglute)
  Ranitidine (Zantac)
  Rifampin (Rifadin)

Special information
if you are pregnant or breastfeeding

The effects of Lopressor during pregnancy have not been adequately studied. If you are pregnant or plan to become pregnant, inform your doctor immediately. Lopressor appears in breast milk and could affect a nursing infant. If this medication is essential to your health, your doctor may advise you to discontinue breastfeeding until your treatment with this medication is finished.

Recommended dosage

ADULTS

Dosages of Lopressor should be individualized by your doctor. It should be taken with or immediately following meals.

High Blood Pressure

The usual starting dosage of Lopressor is a total of 100 milligrams a day taken in 1 or 2 doses, whether taken alone or with a diuretic. The initial dosage of Toprol-XL ranges from 50 to 100 milligrams once a day. Your doctor may gradually increase the dosage up to 400 milligrams a day. Generally, the effectiveness of each dosage increase will be seen within a week.

Angina Pectoris

The usual starting dosage is a total of 100 milligrams a day taken in 2 doses of Lopressor or a single dose of Toprol-XL. Your doctor may gradually increase the dosage up to 400 milligrams a day.

Generally, the effectiveness of each dosage increase will be seen within a week. If treatment is to be discontinued, your doctor will withdraw the drug gradually over a period of 1 to 2 weeks.

Heart Attack

Lopressor can be used for treatment of heart attack both in the hospital during the early phases and after the individual's condition has stabilized. Your doctor will determine the dosage according to your needs.

CHILDREN

The safety and effectiveness of Lopressor have not been established in children.

Overdosage

Any medication taken in excess can cause symptoms of overdose. If you suspect an overdose, seek medical attention immediately.

■ *The symptoms of Lopressor overdose may include:*
Asthma-like symptoms, heart failure, low blood pressure, slow heartbeat

Brand name:

LOPROX

Pronounced: LOW-prox
Generic name: Ciclopirox olamine

Why is this drug prescribed?

Loprox is prescribed for the treatment of the following fungal skin infections:

Athlete's foot
Fungal infection of the groin (jock itch)
Fungal infection of non-hairy parts of the skin
Candidiasis (yeastlike fungal infection of the skin, nails, mouth, vagina, and lungs)
Tinea versicolor—infection of the skin that is characterized by brown or tan patches on the trunk.

Loprox is available in cream and lotion forms.

Most important fact about this drug
Loprox is for external treatment of skin infections. Do not use Loprox in the eyes.

How should you use this medication?
Use this medication for the full treatment time even if your symptoms have improved. Notify your doctor if there is no improvement after 4 weeks.

Shake Loprox lotion vigorously before each use.

- *If you miss a dose...*
  Apply the forgotten dose as soon as you remember. If it is almost time for your next dose, skip the one you missed and go back to your regular schedule.

- *Storage instructions...*
  Store at room temperature.

What side effects may occur?
Loprox rarely causes side effects. If any develop or change in intensity, inform your doctor as soon as possible. Only your doctor can determine if it is safe for you to continue using Loprox.

- *Rare side effects may include:*
  Burning, itching, worsening of infection symptoms

Why should this drug not be prescribed?
If you are sensitive to or have ever had an allergic reaction to ciclopirox olamine or any other ingredient in Loprox, you should not take this medication. Make sure your doctor is aware of any drug reactions you have experienced.

Special warnings about this medication
If the affected area of skin shows signs of increased irritation (redness, itching, burning, blistering, swelling, oozing), notify your doctor.

Avoid the use of airtight dressings or bandages.

Special information
if you are pregnant or breastfeeding
The effects of Loprox during pregnancy have not been adequately studied. If you are pregnant or plan to become pregnant, inform your doctor immediate-

ly. It is not known whether this drug appears in breast milk. If this medication is essential to your health, your doctor may advise you to discontinue breastfeeding your baby until your treatment is finished.

Recommended dosage

ADULTS

Gently massage Loprox into the affected and surrounding skin areas 2 times a day, in the morning and evening. For most infections, improvement usually occurs within the first week of treatment. People with tinea versicolor usually show signs of improvement after 2 weeks of treatment.

CHILDREN

Safety and effectiveness have not been established in children under 10 years of age.

Overdosage

Any medication taken in excess can have serious consequences. If you suspect an overdose, seek medical treatment immediately.

Brand name:

LORABID

Pronounced: LOR-a-bid
Generic name: Loracarbef

Why is this drug prescribed?

Lorabid is used to treat mild-to-moderate bacterial infections of the lungs, ears, throat, sinuses, skin, urinary tract, and kidneys.

Most important fact about this drug

If you have ever had an allergic reaction to Lorabid, penicillin, cephalosporins, or any other drug, be sure your doctor is aware of it before you take Lorabid. You may experience a severe reaction if you are sensitive to penicillin-type medications.

How should you take this medication?

Take Lorabid at least 1 hour before or 2 hours after eating. It is best to take your medication at evenly spaced intervals, day and night.

Do not stop taking your medication even if you begin to feel better after a few days. If you stop taking your medicine too soon, your symptoms may return. If you have a "strep" infection, you should take your medication for at least 10 days.

■ *If you miss a dose...*
Take it as soon as possible. This will help keep a constant amount of medicine in your system. If it is almost time for your next dose, skip the one you missed and go back to your regular schedule. Do not take 2 doses at once.

■ *Storage instructions...*
Lorabid can be stored at room temperature. The liquid form can be kept in the refrigerator, but not in the freezer. Discard any unused portion.

What side effects may occur?
Side effects cannot be anticipated. If any develop or change in intensity, tell your doctor as soon as possible. Only your doctor can determine if it is safe for you to continue taking Lorabid.

■ *More common side effects in children may include:*
Diarrhea, inflamed, runny nose, vomiting

■ *Less common or rare side effects in children may include:*
Headache, loss of appetite, rash, sleepiness

■ *More common side effects in adults may include:*
Diarrhea, headache

■ *Less common side effects in adults may include:*
Abdominal pain, nausea, rhinitis, skin rashes, vaginitis (inflammation of the vaginal tissues), vomiting, yeast infection

■ *Rare side effects may include:*
Blood disorders, dizziness, hives, insomnia, itching, loss of appetite, nervousness, red bumps on skin, sleepiness, vasodilation (widening of the blood vessels)

- *Side effects for other drugs of this class may include:*
  Allergic reactions (sometimes severe), anemia, blood disorders, hemorrhage, kidney problems, serum sickness (fever, skin rash, joint pain, swollen lymph nodes), skin peeling

Why should this drug not be prescribed?
If you are allergic to penicillin, cephalosporins, or other medications, you should not take Lorabid. Make sure you tell your doctor about any drug reactions you have experienced.

Special warnings about this medication
As with many antibiotics, Lorabid can cause colitis—an inflammation of the bowel. This condition can range from mild to life-threatening. If you develop diarrhea while taking Lorabid, notify your doctor, and do not take any diarrhea medication without your doctor's approval.

Prolonged use of Lorabid may result in development of bacteria that do not respond to the medication, leading to a second infection. Because of this danger, you should not use any left-over Lorabid for later infections, even if they have similar symptoms. Take Lorabid only when your doctor prescribes it for you.

If you have known or suspected kidney problems, your doctor will perform blood tests to check your urine and kidney function before and during Lorabid therapy.

Possible food and drug interactions
when taking this medication
If Lorabid is taken with certain other drugs, the effects of either could be increased, decreased, or altered. It is especially important to check with your doctor before combining Lorabid with the following:

Diuretics such as Lasix and Bumex
Probenecid (the gout medication Benemid)

Special information
if you are pregnant or breastfeeding
The effects of Lorabid during pregnancy have not been adequately studied. If you are pregnant or plan to become pregnant, tell your doctor immediately. Lorabid should be used during pregnancy only if clearly needed. It is not known whether Lorabid appears in human breast milk. Your doctor will determine whether it is safe for you to take Lorabid while breastfeeding.

Recommended dosage

ADULTS (13 YEARS AND OLDER)

Bronchitis
The usual dose is 200 to 400 milligrams every 12 hours for 7 days.

Pneumonia
The usual dose is 400 milligrams every 12 hours for 14 days.

Sinusitis
The usual dose is 400 milligrams every 12 hours for 10 days.

Skin and Soft Tissue Infections
The usual dose is 200 milligrams every 12 hours for 7 days.

Streptococcal Pharyngitis ("Strep Throat") and Tonsillitis
The usual dose is 200 milligrams every 12 hours for 10 days. For strep throat, take Lorabid for at least 10 days.

Bladder Infections
The usual dose is 200 milligrams every 24 hours for 7 days.

Kidney Infections
The usual dose is 400 milligrams every 12 hours for 14 days.

If you have impaired kidney function, your doctor will adjust the dosage according to your needs.

CHILDREN (6 MONTHS TO 12 YEARS OF AGE)

Otitis Media
This infection of the middle ear should be treated with the suspension. Do not use the pulvules.

The dose is based on body weight. The usual dose is 30 milligrams of liquid per 2.2 pounds of body weight per day in divided doses (half the dose every 12 hours), for 10 days.

Streptococcal Pharyngitis ("Strep Throat") and Tonsillitis
The dose is based on body weight. The usual dose is 15 milligrams per 2.2 pounds of body weight per day in divided doses (half the dose every 12 hours), for at least 10 days.

Impetigo (Skin Infection)
The dose is based on body weight. The usual dose is 15 milligrams of liquid per 2.2 pounds of body weight per day in divided doses (half the dose every 12 hours), for 7 days.

Overdosage
Any medication taken in excess can have serious consequences. If you suspect an overdose, seek medical attention immediately.

■ *Symptoms of Lorabid overdose may include:*
Diarrhea, nausea, stomach upset, vomiting

Generic name:

LORACARBEF

See Lorabid, page 724.

Generic name:

LORATADINE

See Claritin, page 251.

Generic name:

LORATADINE WITH PSEUDOEPHEDRINE

See Claritin-D, page 254.

Generic name:

LORAZEPAM

See Ativan, page 107.

Brand name:

LORCET

See Vicodin, page 1403.

Brand name:

LORTAB

See Vicodin, page 1403.

Generic name:

LOSARTAN

See Cozaar, page 308.

Generic name:

LOSARTAN WITH HYDROCHLOROTHIAZIDE

See Hyzaar, page 612.

Brand name:

LOTENSIN

Pronounced: Lo-TEN-sin
Generic name: Benazepril hydrochloride

Why is this drug prescribed?

Lotensin is used in the treatment of high blood pressure. It is effective when used alone or in combination with thiazide diuretics. Lotensin is in a family of drugs called ACE (angiotensin-converting enzyme) inhibitors. It works by preventing a chemical in your blood called angiotensin I from converting into a more potent form that increases salt and water retention in your body. Lotensin also enhances blood flow throughout your blood vessels.

Most important fact about this drug

You must take Lotensin regularly for it to be effective. Since blood pressure declines gradually, it may be several weeks before you get the full benefit of Lotensin; and you must continue taking it even if you are feeling well. Lotensin does not cure high blood pressure; it merely keeps it under control.

How should you take this medication?

Lotensin can be taken with or without food. Do not use salt substitutes containing potassium.

Take Lotensin exactly as prescribed. Suddenly stopping Lotensin could cause your blood pressure to increase.

■ *If you miss a dose...*
Take the forgotten dose as soon as you remember. If it is almost time for the next dose, skip the one you missed and go back to your regular schedule. Never try to "catch up" by doubling the dose.

■ *Storage instructions...*
Store at room temperature in a tightly closed container. Protect from light.

What side effects may occur?
Side effects cannot be anticipated. If any develop or change in intensity, inform your doctor as soon as possible. Only your doctor can determine if it is safe for you to continue taking Lotensin.

■ *More common side effects may include:*
Cough, dizziness, fatigue, headache, high potassium levels (dry mouth, excessive thirst, weak or irregular heartbeat, muscle pain or cramps), nausea

If you develop swelling of your face, around the lips, tongue, or throat; swelling of arms and legs; sore throat, fever, and chills; or difficulty swallowing, you should contact your doctor immediately. You may need emergency treatment.

■ *Less common or rare side effects may include:*
Allergic reactions, anxiety, arthritis, asthma, blisters, bronchitis, chest pain, constipation, dark tarry stool containing blood, decreased sex drive, difficulty sleeping, dizziness when standing, fainting, fluid retention, flushing, impotence, infection, inflammation or peeling of the skin, inflammation of the stomach or pancreas, itching, joint pain, low blood pressure, muscle pain, nervousness, pounding heartbeat, rash, sensitivity to light, shortness of breath, sinus inflammation, sweating, swelling of arms, legs, face, tingling or pins and needles, urinary infections, vomiting, weakness

Why should this drug not be prescribed?
If you are sensitive to or have ever had an allergic reaction to Lotensin or other angiotensin-converting enzyme (ACE) inhibitors, do not take this medication.

Special warnings about this medication
Your kidney function should be assessed when you start taking Lotensin and then monitored for the first few weeks. If you are on kidney dialysis, your doctor may need to use a different medication.

Lotensin can cause low blood pressure, especially if you are also taking a diuretic. You may feel light-headed or faint, especially during the first few days of therapy. If these symptoms occur, contact your doctor. Your dosage may need to be adjusted or discontinued.

If you have congestive heart failure, this drug should be used with caution.

Do not use potassium supplements or salt substitutes containing potassium without talking to your doctor first.

If you develop a sore throat or fever, you should contact your doctor immediately. It could indicate a more serious illness.

Excessive sweating, dehydration, severe diarrhea, or vomiting could make you lose too much water, causing your blood pressure to become too low.

Possible food and drug interactions
when taking this medication
If Lotensin is taken with certain other drugs, the effects of either could be increased, decreased, or altered. It is especially important to check with your doctor before combining Lotensin with the following:

Diuretics such as Lasix and HydroDIURIL
Lithium (Lithonate)
Potassium supplements such as Slow-K
Potassium-sparing diuretics such as Moduretic and Dyazide

Special information
if you are pregnant or breastfeeding
Lotensin can cause injury or death to developing and newborn babies, especially if taken during the second and third trimesters of pregnancy. If you are pregnant or plan to become pregnant and are taking Lotensin, contact your doctor immediately to discuss the potential hazard to your unborn child. Minimal amounts of Lotensin appear in breast milk. If this medication is essential to your health, your doctor may advise you to discontinue breastfeeding until your treatment with this medication is finished.

Recommended dosage

ADULTS

For people not taking a diuretic drug, the usual starting dose is 10 milligrams, once a day. Regular total dosages range from 20 to 40 milligrams per day either taken in a single dose or divided into 2 equal doses. The maximum dose is 80 milligrams per day. Your doctor will closely monitor the effect of this drug and adjust it according to your individual needs.

For people already taking a diuretic, the diuretic should be stopped, if possible, 2 to 3 days before taking Lotensin. This reduces the possibility of fainting or light-headedness. If blood pressure cannot be controlled by Lotensin alone, then diuretic use should begin again. If the diuretic cannot be discontinued, the starting dosage of Lotensin should be 5 milligrams.

For people with reduced kidney function, the dosages should be individualized according to the amount of reduced function. The usual starting dose in these instances is 5 milligrams per day, adjusted upwards to a maximum of 40 milligrams per day. If you are on kidney dialysis, your doctor may need to use a different medication.

CHILDREN

The safety and effectiveness of Lotensin have not been established in children.

Overdosage

Although there is no specific information available, a sudden drop in blood pressure would most likely be the primary symptom of Lotensin overdose. If you suspect a Lotensin overdose, seek medical attention immediately.

Brand name:

LOTREL

Pronounced: LOW-trel
Generic names: Amlodipine and Benazepril Hydrochloride

Why is this drug prescribed?

Lotrel is used in the treatment of high blood pressure. It is a combination medicine that is used when treatment with a single drug has not been successful or has caused side effects.

One component, amlodipine, is a calcium channel blocker. It eases the workload of the heart by slowing down the passage of nerve impulses and hence the contractions of the heart muscle. This improves blood flow through the heart and throughout the body and reduces blood pressure. The other component, benazepril, is an angiotensin-converting enzyme (ACE) inhibitor. It works by preventing the transformation of a hormone called angiotensin I into a more potent substance that increases salt and water retention in your body.

Most important fact about this drug

You must take Lotrel regularly for it to be effective. Since blood pressure declines gradually, it may take 1 to 2 weeks for the full effect of Lotrel to be seen. Even if you are feeling well, you must continue to take the medication. Lotrel does not cure high blood pressure; it merely keeps it under control.

How should you take this medication?

Take Lotrel exactly as prescribed by your doctor. Try to take your medication at the same time each day, such as before or after breakfast, so that it is easier to remember.

■ *If you miss a dose...*
Take it as soon as you remember. However, if it is almost time for your next dose, skip the one you missed and go back to your regular schedule. Do not take 2 doses at once.

■ *Storage instructions...*
Store at room temperature. Store away from moisture and light; avoid excessive heat.

What side effects may occur?

Side effects cannot be anticipated. If any develop or change in intensity, tell your doctor as soon as possible. Only your doctor can determine if it is safe for you to continue taking Lotrel.

If you develop swelling of your face, around the lips, tongue, or throat; swelling of arms and legs; or difficulty swallowing, you should contact your doctor immediately. You may need emergency treatment.

■ *More common side effects may include:*
Cough

■ *Less common side effects may include:*
Abdominal pain, anxiety, back pain, bloating and gas, constipation, cramps, decreased sex drive, diarrhea, dizziness, dry mouth, excessive urination, fluid retention and swelling, flushing, headache, hot flashes, impotence, insomnia, muscle and bone pain, muscle cramps, nausea, nervousness, rash, skin disorders, sore throat, tremor, weakness and fatigue

■ *Rare side effects may include:*
Anemia, blisters that leave dark spots on the skin, heart attack, pancreatitis (inflammation of the pancreas), worsening of angina pectoris (crushing chest pain)

Why should this drug not be prescribed?

If you are sensitive to or have ever had an allergic reaction to amlodipine, benazepril, or any angiotensin-converting enzyme (ACE) inhibitors, do not take this medication.

Special warnings about this medication

Your kidney function should be assessed when you start taking Lotrel, then monitored for the first few weeks.

Lotrel can cause low blood pressure, especially if you are taking high doses of diuretics. You may feel light-headed or faint, especially during the first few days of therapy. If these symptoms occur, contact your doctor. Your dosage may need to be adjusted or discontinued.

If you have congestive heart failure, use this drug with caution. If you have kidney disease or severe liver disease, diabetes, lupus erythematosus, or scleroderma (a rare disease affecting the blood vessels or connective tissue), use Lotrel with caution.

Excessive sweating, severe diarrhea, or vomiting could make you lose too much water, causing a severe drop in blood pressure. If you notice a yellow coloring to your skin or the whites of your eyes, stop taking the drug and notify your doctor immediately. You could be developing liver problems.

If you develop a persistent, dry cough, tell your doctor. It may be due to the medication and, if so, will disappear if you stop taking Lotrel. In a medical emergency and before you have surgery, notify your doctor or dentist that you are taking Lotrel.

Possible food and drug interactions
when taking this medication

If Lotrel is taken with certain other drugs, the effects of either could be increased, decreased, or altered. It is especially important to check with your doctor before combining Lotrel with the following:

Lithium (Eskalith, Lithobid)
Potassium supplements (Slow-K)
Potassium-sparing water pills such as Aldactazide, Moduretic, and
    Maxzide
Other water pills such as Diuril, Lasix, HydroDIURIL

Special information
if you are pregnant or breastfeeding

Lotrel can cause injury or death to developing and newborn babies, especially if taken during the second and third trimesters of pregnancy. If you are pregnant and are taking Lotrel, contact your doctor immediately to discuss the potential hazard to your unborn child. Minimal amounts of benazepril appear in breast milk. If this medication is essential to your health, your doctor may advise you to discontinue breastfeeding while you are taking Lotrel.

Recommended dosage

ADULTS

Your doctor will closely monitor the effects of this drug and adjust the dosage according to your blood pressure response. For small, older, frail, or liver-impaired individuals, the usual starting dose is a capsule containing 2.5 milligrams amlodipine and 10 milligrams benazepril.

CHILDREN

Safety and effectiveness in children have not been established.

Overdosage

Any medication taken in excess can have serious consequences. Although there is no specific information available, a sudden drop in blood pressure and rapid heartbeat would be the primary symptoms of a Lotrel overdose. If you suspect an overdose, seek medical attention immediately.

Brand name:

LOTRIMIN

See Gyne-Lotrimin, page 576.

Brand name:

LOTRISONE

Pronounced: LOE-trih-sone
Generic ingredients: Clotrimazole, Betamethasone
  dipropionate

Why is this drug prescribed?

Lotrisone, a combination of a steroid (betamethasone) and an antifungal drug (clotrimazole), is used to treat skin infections caused by fungus, such as athlete's foot, jock itch, and ringworm of the body.

Betamethasone treats symptoms (such as itching, redness, swelling, and inflammation) that result from fungus infections, while clotrimazole treats the cause of the infection by inhibiting the growth of certain yeast and fungus organisms.

Most important fact about this drug
When you use Lotrisone, you inevitably absorb some of the medication through your skin and into the bloodstream. Too much absorption can lead to unwanted side effects elsewhere in the body. To keep this problem to a minimum, avoid using large amounts of Lotrisone over wide areas, and do not cover it with airtight dressings such as plastic wrap or adhesive bandage unless specifically told to by your doctor.

How should you use this medication?
Wash your hands before and after applying Lotrisone. Gently massage it into the affected area and surrounding skin twice a day, in the morning and evening. Do not get it in your eyes.

Use Lotrisone for the full time prescribed, even if your condition has improved.

Lotrisone should be applied sparingly to the groin area, and it should not be used for longer than 2 weeks. Wear loose-fitting clothing.

■ *If you miss a dose...*
Apply it as soon as you remember. If it is almost time for your next dose, skip the one you missed and go back to your regular schedule.

■ *Storage instructions...*
Store at room temperature.

What side effects may occur?
Side effects cannot be anticipated. If any develop or change in intensity, inform your doctor as soon as possible. Only your doctor can determine if it is safe for you to continue using Lotrisone.

■ *More common side effects may include:*
Blistering, hives, infection, irritated skin, itching, peeling, reddened skin, skin eruptions and rash, stinging, swelling due to fluid retention, tingling sensation

■ *Less common side effects may include:*
Acne, burning, dryness, excessive hair growth, inflamed hair follicles, inflamed skin, irritated skin around mouth, loss of skin color, softening of the skin, streaks in the skin

Why should this drug not be prescribed?

You should not use Lotrisone if you are sensitive to clotrimazole or betamethasone or any of its other ingredients, or to similar steroid and antifungal medications.

Special warnings about this medication

Steroid drugs (such as betamethasone) can affect the functioning of the adrenal, hypothalamic, and pituitary glands and temporarily produce sugar in the urine, excessive blood sugar levels, and a disorder called Cushing's syndrome. Symptoms of Cushing's syndrome include easily bruised skin, increased blood pressure, low potassium levels, low sex hormone levels, mood swings, water retention, weak muscles, and weight gain.

Do not take Lotrisone internally and be sure to keep it away from your eyes.

If you are using Lotrisone to treat jock itch (tinea cruris) or a fungal infection of the skin, called tinea corporis, and there has been no improvement after 1 week, notify your doctor.

If you are using Lotrisone to treat athlete's foot (tinea pedis), notify your doctor if there is no improvement after 2 weeks of treatment.

Do not use Lotrisone for any condition other than the one for which it was prescribed, and do not use it for longer than 4 weeks.

Lotrisone is not for use on diaper rash.

Possible food and drug interactions
when taking this medication

No interactions have been reported.

Special information
if you are pregnant or breastfeeding

Pregnant women should not use steroid drugs in large amounts or for prolonged periods of time. The effects of Lotrisone during pregnancy have not been adequately studied. The medication should be used during pregnancy only if the potential benefits justify the potential risk to the developing baby. It is not known whether Lotrisone appears in breast milk. Nursing mothers should use Lotrisone with caution and only when clearly needed.

Recommended dosage

ADULTS AND CHILDREN OVER 12 YEARS OLD

*Jock Itch (Tinea Cruris) or Fungal Skin Infections
(Tinea Corporis)*
Gently massage Lotrisone into the affected and surrounding skin areas twice a day, in the morning and the evening, for 2 weeks. Lotrisone should be applied sparingly to the groin area. Notify your doctor if there has been no improvement after 1 week of treatment.

Athlete's Foot (Tinea Pedis)
Gently massage Lotrisone into the affected and surrounding skin areas twice a day, in the morning and the evening, for 4 weeks. Notify your doctor if there has been no improvement after 2 weeks of treatment.

CHILDREN

The safety and effectiveness of Lotrisone have not been established for children under 12 years of age. Children may absorb proportionally larger amounts of topical Lotrisone and be more sensitive to its effects than are adults.

Overdosage

Any medication used in excess can have serious consequences. A serious overdose of Lotrisone, which is applied to the skin, is unlikely. However, seek medical help immediately if you suspect an overdose.

Generic name:

LOVASTATIN

See Mevacor, page 781.

Brand name:

LOZOL

Pronounced: LOW-zoll
Generic name: Indapamide

Why is this drug prescribed?

Lozol is used in the treatment of high blood pressure, either alone or in combination with other high blood pressure medications. Lozol is also used to relieve salt and fluid retention. During pregnancy, your doctor may prescribe Lozol to relieve fluid retention caused by a specific condition or when fluid retention causes extreme discomfort that is not relieved by rest.

Most important fact about this drug
If you have high blood pressure, you must take Lozol regularly for it to be effective. Since blood pressure declines gradually, it may be several weeks before you get the full benefit of Lozol; and you must continue taking it even if you are feeling well. Lozol does not cure high blood pressure; it merely keeps it under control.

How should you take this medication?
Take Lozol exactly as prescribed by your doctor. Suddenly stopping Lozol could cause your condition to worsen.

Lozol is best taken in the morning.

- *If you miss a dose...*
  Take the forgotten dose as soon as you remember. If it is almost time for your next dose, skip the one you missed and go back to your regular schedule. Never take 2 doses at the same time.

- *Storage instructions...*
  Store Lozol at room temperature. Protect from excessive heat. Keep the container tightly closed.

What side effects may occur?
Side effects cannot be anticipated. If any side effects develop or change in intensity, tell your doctor immediately. Only your doctor can determine whether it is safe to continue taking Lozol. Most side effects are mild and temporary.

- *More common side effects may include:*
  Agitation, anxiety, back pain, dizziness, headache, infection, irritability, muscle cramps or spasms, nasal inflammation, nervousness, numbness in hands and feet, pain, tension, weakness, fatigue, loss of energy or tiredness

- *Less common or rare side effects may include:*
  Abdominal pain or cramps, blurred vision, chest pain, conjunctivitis, constipation, cough, depression, diarrhea, dizziness when standing up too quickly, drowsiness, dry mouth, excessive urination at night, fluid retention, flu-like symptoms, flushing, fluttering heartbeat, frequent urination, hives, impotence or reduced sex drive, indigestion, insomnia, irregular heartbeat, itching, light-headedness, loss of appetite, nausea, nervousness, premature heart contractions, production of large amounts of

pale urine, rash, runny nose, sore throat, stomach irritation, tingling in hands and feet, vertigo, vomiting, weakness, weak or irregular heartbeat, weight loss

Why should this drug not be prescribed?

Avoid using Lozol if you are unable to urinate or if you have ever had an allergic reaction or are sensitive to indapamide or other sulfa-containing drugs.

Special warnings about this medication

Diuretics such as Lozol can cause the body to lose too much salt and potassium, especially among elderly women. Signs of an excessively low potassium level include muscle weakness and rapid or irregular heartbeat. To boost your potassium level, your doctor may recommend eating potassium-rich foods or taking a potassium supplement.

The risk of potassium loss increases when larger doses are used, if you have cirrhosis, or if you are also using corticosteroids or ACTH. Your doctor should check your blood regularly, especially if you have an irregular heartbeat or are taking heart medications.

Lozol should be used with care if you have gout or high uric acid levels, liver disease, diabetes, or lupus erythematosus, a disease of the connective tissue.

This medication should be used with caution if you have severe kidney disease. Your kidney function should be given a complete assessment and should continue to be monitored.

In general, diuretics should not be taken if you are taking lithium, as they increase the risk of lithium poisoning.

Possible food and drug interactions
when taking this medication

If Lozol is taken with certain other drugs, the effects of either could be increased, decreased, or altered. It is especially important to check with your doctor before combining Lozol with the following:

Lithium (Eskalith)
Norepinephrine (a drug used to treat cardiac arrest and to maintain
  blood pressure)
Other high blood pressure medications such as Aldomet and Tenormin

Special information
if you are pregnant or breastfeeding

If you are pregnant or plan to become pregnant, tell your doctor immediately. No information is available about the safety of Lozol during pregnancy.

Lozol may appear in breast milk and could affect a nursing infant. If Lozol is essential to your health, your doctor may advise you to stop breastfeeding until your treatment is finished.

Recommended dosage

ADULTS

High Blood Pressure

The usual starting dose is 1.25 milligrams as a single daily dose taken in the morning. If Lozol does not seem to be working for you, your doctor may gradually increase your dosage up to 5 milligrams taken once a day.

Fluid Buildup in Congestive Heart Failure

The usual starting dose is 2.5 milligrams as a single daily dose taken in the morning. Your doctor may increase your dosage to 5 milligrams taken once daily.

Overdosage

Any medication taken in excess can have serious consequences. If you suspect an overdose, seek medical treatment immediately.

■ *Symptoms of Lozol overdose may include:*
Electrolyte imbalance (potassium or salt depletion due to too much fluid loss), nausea, stomach disorders, vomiting, weakness

Brand name:

LURIDE

Pronounced: LUHR-ide
Generic name: Sodium fluoride

Why is this drug prescribed?

Luride is prescribed to strengthen children's teeth against decay during the period when the teeth are still developing.

Studies have shown that children who live where the drinking water contains a certain level of fluoride have fewer cavities than others. Fluoride helps prevent cavities in three ways: by increasing the teeth's resistance to dissolving on contact with acid, by strengthening teeth, and by slowing down the growth of mouth bacteria.

Luride may be given to children who live where the water fluoride level is 0.6 parts per million or less.

Most important fact about this drug
Before Luride is prescribed, it is important for the doctor to know the fluoride content of the water your child drinks every day. Your water company, or a private laboratory, can tell you the level of fluoride in your water.

How should you take this medication?
Give your child Luride exactly as prescribed by your doctor. It is preferable to give the tablet at bedtime after the child's teeth have been brushed. The youngster may chew and swallow the tablet or simply suck on it until it dissolves. The liquid form of this medicine is to be taken by mouth only. It may be dropped directly into the mouth or mixed with water or fruit juice. Always store Luride drops in the original plastic dropper bottle.

■ *If you miss a dose...*
Give it as soon as you remember. If it is almost time for the next dose, skip the one you missed and go back to your regular schedule. Do not give 2 doses at once.

■ *Storage instructions...*
Store at room temperature away from heat, light, and moisture. Keep the liquid from freezing.

What side effects may occur?
Side effects cannot be anticipated. If any develop, tell your doctor immediately. Only your doctor can determine whether it is safe for your child to continue taking Luride.

In rare cases, Luride may cause an allergic rash or some other unexpected effect.

Why should this drug not be prescribed?
Your child should not take Luride if he or she is sensitive to it or has had an allergic reaction to sodium fluoride in the past.

Your child should not take the 1-milligram strength of Luride if the drinking water in your area contains 0.3 parts per million of fluoride or more. He or she should not take the other forms of Luride if the water contains 0.6 parts per million of fluoride or more.

Special warnings about this medication

Do not give full-strength tablets (1 milligram) to children under the age of 6. Do not give the half-strength tablets (0.5 milligram) to children under 3, or to children under 6 when your drinking water fluoride content is 0.3 parts per million or more. Do not give the quarter-strength tablets (0.25 milligrams) to children under 6 months, or to children under 3 years when fluoride content is 0.3 parts per million or more.

Possible food and drug interactions
when taking this medication

Avoid giving your child Luride with dairy products. The calcium in dairy products may interact with the fluoride to create calcium fluoride, which the body cannot absorb well.

Recommended dosage

Since this drug is used to supplement water with low fluoride content, consult your physician to determine the proper amount based on the local water content. Also check with your doctor if you move to a new area, change to bottled water, or begin using a water-filtering device. Dosages are determined by both age and the fluoride content of the water.

INFANTS AND CHILDREN

The following daily dosages are recommended for areas where the drinking water contains fluoride at less than 0.3 parts per million:

Children 6 Months to 3 Years of Age
1 quarter-strength (0.25 milligram) tablet or half a dropperful of liquid

3 to 6 Years of Age
1 half-strength (0.5 milligram) tablet or 1 dropperful of liquid

6 to 16 Years of Age
1 full-strength (1 milligram) tablet or 2 droppersful of liquid

For areas where the fluoride content of drinking water is between 0.3 and 0.6 parts per million, the recommended daily dosage of the tablets is one-half the above dosages. Dosage of the liquid should be reduced to half a dropperful for children ages 3 to 6 and 1 dropperful for children over 6.

Overdosage
Any medication taken in excess can have serious consequences. Taking too much fluoride for a long period of time may cause discoloration of the teeth. Notify your doctor or dentist if you notice white, brown, or black spots on the teeth.

Swallowing large amounts of fluoride can cause burning in the mouth and a sore tongue, followed by diarrhea, nausea, salivation, stomach cramping and pain, and vomiting sometimes with blood.

Brand name:

LUVOX

Pronounced: LOO-voks
Generic name: Fluvoxamine maleate

Why is this drug prescribed?
Luvox is prescribed for obsessive compulsive disorder. An obsession is marked by continual, unwanted thoughts that prevent proper functioning in everyday living. Compulsive behavior is typified by ritualistic actions such as repetitious washing, repeating certain phrases, completing steps in a process over and over, counting and recounting, checking and rechecking to make sure that something has not been forgotten, excessive neatness, and hoarding of useless items.

Most important fact about this drug
Before starting therapy with Luvox, be sure your doctor knows what medications you are taking—both prescription and over-the-counter—since combining Luvox with certain drugs may cause serious or even life-threatening effects. You should never take Luvox with the antihistamines Seldane and Hismanal or the heartburn medication Propulsid. You should also avoid taking Luvox within 14 days of taking any antidepressant drug classified as an MAO inhibitor, including Nardil and Parnate.

How should you take this medication?
Take this medication only as directed by your doctor.

Luvox may be taken with or without food.

■ *If you miss a dose...*
   If you are taking 1 dose a day, skip the missed dose and go back to your regular schedule. If you are taking 2 doses a day, take the missed dose as

soon as possible, then go back to your regular schedule. Never take 2 doses at the same time.

■ *Storage instructions...*
Store at room temperature and protect from humidity.

What side effects may occur?
Side effects cannot be anticipated. If any develop or change in intensity, tell your doctor immediately. Only your doctor can determine if it is safe for you to continue taking Luvox.

■ *More common side effects may include:*
Abnormal ejaculation, abnormal tooth decay and toothache, anxiety, blurred vision, constipation, decreased appetite, diarrhea, dizziness, dry mouth, feeling "hot or flushed," "flu-like" symptoms, frequent urination, gas and bloating, headache, heart palpitations, inability to fall asleep, indigestion, nausea, nervousness, sleepiness, sweating, taste alteration, tremor, unusual tiredness or weakness, upper respiratory infection, vomiting

■ *Less common side effects may include:*
Abnormal muscle tone, agitation, chills, decreased sex drive, depression, difficult or labored breathing, difficulty swallowing, extreme excitability, impotence, inability to urinate, lack of orgasm, yawning

Why should this drug not be prescribed?
If you are sensitive to or have ever had an allergic reaction to Luvox or similar drugs, such as Prozac and Zoloft, do not take this medication. Make sure your doctor is aware of any drug reactions you have experienced.

Never combine Luvox with Seldane, Hismanal, or Propulsid, or take it within 14 days of taking an MAO inhibitor such as Nardil or Parnate. (See "Most important fact about this drug.")

Special warnings about this medication
You should discuss all your medical problems with your doctor before starting therapy with Luvox, as certain physical conditions or diseases may affect your reaction to Luvox.

If you suffer from seizures, use this medication cautiously. If you experience a seizure while taking Luvox, stop taking the drug and call your doctor immediately.

If you have or have ever had suicidal thoughts, be sure to tell your doctor, as your dosage may need to be adjusted.

If you have a history of mania (excessively energetic, out-of-control behavior), use this medication cautiously.

If you have liver disease, your doctor will adjust the dosage.

Luvox may cause you to become drowsy or less alert and may affect your judgment. Therefore, avoid driving, operating dangerous machinery, or participating in any hazardous activity that requires full mental alertness until you know your reaction to this medication.

If you develop a rash or hives, or any other allergic-type reaction, notify your physician immediately.

Possible food and drug interactions when taking this medication

Do not drink alcohol while taking this medication. If you smoke, be sure to tell your doctor before starting Luvox therapy, as your dosage may need adjustment.

If Luvox is taken with certain other drugs, the effects of either could be increased, decreased, or altered. It is especially important to check with your doctor before combining Luvox with the following:

Anticoagulant drugs such as Coumadin
Antidepressant medications such as Anafranil, Elavil, and Tofranil, as
    well as the MAO inhibitors Nardil and Parnate
Blood pressure medications known as beta blockers, including Inderal
    and Lopressor
Carbamazepine (Tegretol)
Cisapride (Propulsid)
Clozapine (Clozaril)
Diazepam (Valium)
Diltiazem (Cardizem)
Lithium (Lithonate)
Methadone (Dolophine)
Phenytoin (Dilantin)
Quinidine (Quinidex)
Theophylline (Theo-Dur)
Tranquilizers and sedatives such as Halcion, Valium, Versed, and Xanax
Tryptophan

Special information
if you are pregnant or breastfeeding

The effects of Luvox in pregnancy have not been adequately studied. If you are pregnant or plan to become pregnant, consult your doctor immediately. Luvox passes into breast milk and may cause serious reactions in a nursing baby. If this medication is essential to your health, your doctor may advise you to discontinue breastfeeding until your treatment with Luvox is finished.

Recommended dosage

ADULTS

The usual starting dose is one 50-milligram tablet taken at bedtime.

Your doctor may increase your dose, depending upon your response. The maximum daily dose is 300 milligrams. If you take more than 100 milligrams a day, your doctor will divide the total amount into 2 doses; if the doses are not equal, you should take the larger dose at bedtime.

CHILDREN

The safety and effectiveness of Luvox have not been established in children under age 18.

Overdosage

Any medication taken in excess can have serious consequences. If you suspect an overdose, seek medical attention immediately.

■ *Symptoms of Luvox overdose may include:*
  Breathing difficulties, changes in pulse rate, coma, convulsions, diarrhea, dizziness, drowsiness, low blood pressure, liver problems, vomiting

Brand name:

MAALOX

See Antacids, page 75.

Brand name:

MACROBID

See Macrodantin, page 748.

Brand name:

MACRODANTIN

Pronounced: Mack-row-DAN-tin
Generic name: Nitrofurantoin
Other brand name: Macrobid

Why is this drug prescribed?
Nitrofurantoin, an antibacterial drug, is prescribed for the treatment of urinary tract infections caused by certain strains of bacteria.

Most important fact about this drug
Breathing disorders have occurred in people taking nitrofurantoin. The drug can cause inflammation of the lungs marked by coughing, difficulty breathing, and wheezing. It has also been known to cause pulmonary fibrosis (an abnormal increase in fibrous tissue of the lungs). This condition can develop gradually without symptoms and can be fatal. An allergic reaction to this drug is also possible and may occur without warning. Symptoms include a feeling of ill health and a persistent cough. However, all these reactions occur rarely and generally in those receiving nitrofurantoin therapy for 6 months or longer.

Sudden and severe lung reactions are characterized by fever, chills, cough, chest pain, and difficulty breathing. These acute reactions usually occur within the first week of treatment and subside when therapy with nitrofurantoin is stopped.

Your doctor should monitor your condition closely, especially if you are receiving long-term treatment with this medication.

How should you take this medication?
To improve absorption of the drug, nitrofurantoin should be taken with food.

Follow your doctor's instructions carefully. Take the full amount prescribed, even if you are feeling better.

This medication works best if your urine is acidic. Ask your doctor whether you should be taking special measures to assure its acidity.

Nitrofurantoin may turn the urine brown.

■ *If you miss a dose...*
  Take the forgotten dose as soon as you remember, then space out the rest of the day's doses at equal intervals.

■ *Storage instructions...*
Store at room temperature. Protect from light and keep the container tightly closed.

What side effects may occur?
Side effects cannot be anticipated. If any develop or change in intensity, inform your doctor as soon as possible. Only your doctor can determine if it is safe for you to continue taking nitrofurantoin.

■ *More common side effects may include:*
Lack or loss of appetite, nausea, vomiting

■ *Less common or rare side effects may include:*
Abdominal pain/discomfort, blue skin, chills, confusion, cough, chest pain, depression, diarrhea, difficulty breathing, dizziness, drowsiness, exaggerated sense of well-being, eye disorder, fever, hair loss, headache, hepatitis, hives, inflammation of the nerves causing symptoms of numbness, tingling, pain, or muscle weakness, intestinal inflammation, involuntary eye movement, irregular heartbeat, itching, itchy red skin patches, joint pain, muscle pain, peeling skin, psychotic reactions, rash, severe allergic reactions, skin inflammation with flaking, skin swelling or welts, vertigo, yellowing of the skin and whites of the eyes, weakness

Why should this drug not be prescribed?
If you are sensitive to or have ever had an allergic reaction to nitrofurantoin or other drugs of this type, such as Furoxone, you should not take this medication. Make sure that your doctor is aware of any drug reactions that you have experienced.

Unless you are directed to do so by your doctor, do not take this medication if you have poor kidneys, producing little or no urine.

Nitrofurantoin should not be taken at term of pregnancy or during labor and delivery; it should not be given to infants under 1 month of age.

Special warnings about this medication
Tell your doctor if you have any unusual symptoms while you are taking this drug.

Fatalities have been reported from hepatitis (liver disease) during treatment with nitrofurantoin. Long-lasting, active hepatitis can develop without symptoms; therefore, if you are receiving long-term treatment with this drug, your doctor should test your liver function periodically.

Fatalities from peripheral neuropathy—a disease of the nerves—have also been reported in people taking nitrofurantoin. Conditions such as a kidney disorder, anemia, diabetes mellitus, a debilitating disease, or a vitamin B deficiency make peripheral neuropathy more likely. If you develop symptoms such as muscle weakness or lack of sensation, check with your doctor immediately.

If you experience diarrhea, tell your doctor. It may be a sign of serious intestinal inflammation.

Hemolytic anemia (destruction of red blood cells) has occurred in people taking nitrofurantoin.

Continued or prolonged use of this drug may result in growth of bacteria that do not respond to it. This can cause a renewed infection, so it is important that your doctor monitor your condition on a regular basis.

Possible food and drug interactions
when taking this medication

If nitrofurantoin is taken with certain other drugs, the effects of either could be increased, decreased, or altered. It is especially important to check with your doctor before combining nitrofurantoin with the following:

Magnesium trisilicate (Gaviscon Antacid Tablets)
The gout drugs Benemid and Anturane, and other drugs that increase
    the amount of uric acid in the urine

Special information
if you are pregnant or breastfeeding

The safety of nitrofurantoin during pregnancy and breastfeeding has not been established. Nitrofurantoin does appear in human breast milk. If you are pregnant or breastfeeding or you plan to become pregnant or breastfeed, inform your doctor immediately.

Recommended dosage

Treatment with nitrofurantoin should be continued for 1 week or for at least 3 days after obtaining a urine specimen free of infection. If your infection has not cleared up, your doctor should re-evaluate your case.

ADULTS

The recommended dosage of Macrodantin is 50 to 100 milligrams taken 4 times a day. For long-term treatment, your doctor may reduce your dosage to 50 to 100 milligrams taken at bedtime.

The recommended dosage of Macrobid is one 100 milligram capsule every 12 hours for 7 days.

CHILDREN

This medication should not be prescribed for children under 1 month of age.

The recommended daily dosage of Macrodantin for infants and children over 1 month of age is 5 to 7 milligrams per 2.2 pounds of body weight, divided into 4 doses over 24 hours.

For the long-term treatment of children, the doctor may prescribe daily doses as low as 1 milligram per 2.2 pounds of body weight taken in 1 or 2 doses per day.

The dosage of Macrobid for children over 12 years of age is one 100 milligram capsule every 12 hours for 7 days. Safety and effectiveness have not been established for children under 12.

Overdosage
An overdose of nitrofurantoin does not cause any specific symptoms other than vomiting. If vomiting does not occur soon after an excessive dose, it should be induced.

If you suspect an overdose, seek emergency medical treatment immediately.

Brand name:

MATERNA

See Stuartnatal Plus, page 1223.

Brand name:

MAVIK

Pronounced: MA-vick
Generic name: Trandolapril

Why is this drug prescribed?
Mavik controls high blood pressure. It is effective when used alone or combined with other high blood pressure medications such as diuretics that help rid the body of excess water. Mavik is also used to treat heart failure or dysfunction following a heart attack.

Mavik is in a family of drugs known as ACE (angiotensin converting enzyme) inhibitors. It works by preventing a chemical in your blood called angiotensin I from converting into a more potent form that increases salt and water retention in your body. ACE inhibitors also expand your blood vessels, further reducing blood pressure.

Most important fact about this drug
You will get the full benefit of Mavik within a week; but you must continue taking it regularly to maintain the effect. Mavik does not cure high blood pressure, it merely keeps it under control.

How should you take this medication?
Mavik can be taken with or without food. Try to make Mavik part of your regular daily routine. If you take it at the same time each day—for example, right after breakfast—you will be less likely to forget a dose.

■ *If you miss a dose...*
Take it as soon as you remember. However, if it is almost time for your next dose, skip the one you missed and go back to your regular schedule.

■ *Storage instructions...*
Mavik may be stored at room temperature.

What side effects may occur?
Side effects cannot be anticipated. If any develop or change in intensity, tell your doctor as soon as possible. Only your doctor can determine if it is safe for you to continue taking Mavik.

■ *Side effects may include:*
Abdominal pain, anxiety, bloating, chest pain, constipation, cough, cramps, decreased sex drive, diarrhea, difficult or labored breathing, dizziness, drowsiness, fainting, flushing, fluid retention, gout, impotence, indigestion, insomnia, itching, low blood pressure, muscle cramps, nosebleed, pains in arms and legs, palpitations, pins and needles, rash, severe skin disease, slowed heartbeat, swelling of face and lips, swelling of tongue and throat, swelling of arms or legs, throat inflammation, upper respiratory infection, vertigo, vomiting, yellow eyes and skin

Why should this drug not be prescribed?
If you have ever had an allergic reaction to Mavik or similar drugs such as Capoten or Vasotec, you should not take this medication. Make sure your doctor is aware of any drug reactions you have experienced.

Special warnings about this medication

If you develop signs of an allergic reaction, such as swelling of the face, lips, tongue, or throat and difficulty swallowing (or swelling of the arms and legs), you should stop taking Mavik and contact your doctor immediately. You may need emergency treatment. Desensitization treatments with bee or wasp venom make an allergic reaction more likely. Kidney dialysis also increases the danger.

When prescribing Mavik, your doctor will perform a complete assessment of your kidney function and will continue to monitor your kidneys.

If you have congestive heart failure, your blood pressure may drop sharply after the first few doses of Mavik and you may feel light-headed for a time. Your doctor should monitor you closely when you start taking this medication and when your dosage is increased.

High doses of diuretics combined with Mavik may cause excessively low blood pressure. Your doctor may need to reduce your diuretic dose to avoid this problem.

Mavik sometimes affects the liver. If you notice a yellow coloring to your skin or the whites of your eyes, stop taking Mavik and notify your doctor immediately.

Dehydration may cause a drop in blood pressure. If you do not drink enough water, perspire a lot, or suffer vomiting or diarrhea, notify your doctor immediately.

Also contact your doctor promptly if you develop a sore throat or fever. It could indicate a more serious illness.

If you develop a persistent, dry cough, tell your doctor. It may be due to the medication and, if so, will disappear if Mavik is discontinued.

Heart and circulatory problems, diabetes, lupus erythematosus, and kidney disease are all reasons for using Mavik with care. Also be sure to tell your doctor or dentist that you are taking Mavik if you are planning any type of surgery.

Possible food and drug interactions
when taking this medication

If Mavik is taken with certain other drugs, the effects of either could be increased, decreased, or altered. It is especially important to check with your doctor before combining Mavik with the following:

Diuretics such as HydroDIURIL

Diuretics that spare the body's potassium, such as Aldactone, Dyazide, and Moduretic
Lithium (Lithonate)
Potassium preparations such as Micro-K and Slow-K

Also check with your doctor before using potassium-containing salt substitutes.

Special information
if you are pregnant or breastfeeding

ACE inhibitors such as Mavik can cause injury and even death to the developing baby when used during the last 6 months of pregnancy. At the first sign of pregnancy, stop taking Mavik and contact your doctor immediately.

Mavik may appear in breast milk and could affect a nursing infant. Do not take this medication while you are nursing.

Recommended dosage

ADULTS

The usual starting dose if you are not taking a diuretic is 1 milligram once a day; African-Americans should start on 2 milligrams once a day.

Depending on your blood pressure response, your doctor may increase your dosage at 1-week intervals, up to 2 to 4 milligrams once a day. If your blood pressure still does not respond, your dosage may be increased to 4 milligrams twice a day and the doctor may add a diuretic to your regimen.

If you are already taking a diuretic, your doctor will have you stop taking it 2 to 3 days before you start treatment with Mavik. If your diuretic should not be stopped, your starting dose of Mavik will be 0.5 milligram. A starting dose of 0.5 milligram daily is also recommended for people with liver or kidney disease.

CHILDREN

The safety and effectiveness of Mavik in children have not been established.

Overdosage

Any medication taken in excess can have serious consequences. The most likely effects of a Mavik overdose are light-headedness or dizziness due to a sudden drop in blood pressure. If you suspect an overdose, seek medical attention immediately.

Brand name:

MAXALT

Pronounced: MAX-alt
Generic name: Rizatriptan benzoate
Other brand name: Maxalt-MLT

Why is this drug prescribed?
Maxalt is prescribed for the treatment of a migraine attack with or without the presence of an aura (visual disturbances, usually sensations of halos or flickering lights, which precede an attack). It cuts headaches short, but won't prevent attacks.

Most important fact about this drug
Maxalt should be used only for typical migraine headaches. It is not recommended for any other type of headache, or for unusual types of migraine such as hemiplegic or basilar migraine.

How should you take this medication?
Take Maxalt as soon as your first symptoms appear. The drug is available in standard and orally disintegrating tablets (Maxalt-MLT). The standard tablets should be swallowed whole with liquid. No liquid is needed for Maxalt-MLT.

When using Maxalt-MLT, leave each individual blister pack in its foil pouch until needed. When ready, remove the pack from the pouch, peel it open with dry hands, and place the tablet on your tongue. The tablet will dissolve rapidly and can be swallowed with your saliva alone.

If your headache comes back, you may take a second dose as soon as 2 hours have elapsed. If the first dose provides no relief at all, check with your doctor before taking another.

Do not take more than 30 milligrams of Maxalt in a 24-hour period. Check with your doctor if you need to take the drug more than 4 times a month.

■ *If you miss a dose...*
Maxalt is not for regular use. Take it only during a migraine attack.

■ *Storage instructions...*
Maxalt and Maxalt-MLT may be stored at room temperature. Keep the Maxalt bottle tightly closed. Leave each Maxalt-MLT tablet in its pouch.

What side effects may occur?
Side effects cannot be anticipated. If any develop or change in intensity, inform your doctor as soon as possible. Only your doctor can determine if it is safe for you to continue taking Maxalt.

■ *More common side effects may include:*
Chest pain, dizziness, drowsiness, dry mouth, fatigue, nausea, pain, tingling skin, weakness

■ *Less common side effects may include:*
Clouded thinking, cold sensations, decreased sensitivity to pain, diarrhea, difficulty breathing, feeling of well-being, flushing, hot flashes, jaw tightness, headache, neck tightness, palpitations, throat tightness, tremor, vomiting, warm sensations

■ *Rare side effects may include:*
Acid indigestion, agitation, anxiety, blurred vision, bone pain, burning eyes, chills, cold hands and feet, confusion, constipation, dehydration, depression, disorientation, difficulty swallowing, dream abnormality, dry eyes, ear pain, eye irritation, eye pain, face swelling, fast or slow heartbeat, gas, hangover feeling, heat sensitivity, hives, increased blood pressure, increased urination, increased sensitivity to pain, indigestion, insomnia, irregular heartbeat, irritability, itching, joint pain, lack of coordination, loss of body fluids, memory impairment, menstruation disorder, muscle cramp, muscle pain, muscle spasm, muscle weakness, nasal congestion, nasal dryness, nasal irritation, nervousness, nose bleeds, rash, ringing in the ears, sinus problems, skin swelling, speech difficulties, stiffness, stomach bloating, sweating, tearing eyes, thirst, tongue swelling, throat irritation, throat dryness, upper respiratory infection, urinary frequency, walking abnormalities, vertigo, yawning

Why should this drug not be prescribed?
If Maxalt gives you an allergic reaction, you won't be able to use it. You should also avoid this drug if you have certain types of heart or blood vessel disease, including angina (crushing chest pain) or a history of heart attack. Do not use it if you have uncontrolled high blood pressure.

Never take Maxalt within 24 hours of using an ergotamine-type migraine medication such as Cafergot, D.H.E. 45 Injection, Migranal Nasal Spray, or Sansert, or a drug in the same family as Maxalt, such as Amerge, Imitrex, or Zomig. You should also refrain from using Maxalt within 2 weeks of taking an MAO inhibitor such as the antidepressants Marplan, Nardil, and Parnate.

Special warnings about this medication

Because some people with heart disease have suffered serious heart problems after taking Maxalt, your doctor may ask you to take the first dose in the office, where you can be monitored for cardiac side effects. High blood pressure, high cholesterol, diabetes, smoking, a history of heart disease in your family, and menopause all increase the odds of such side effects.

Maxalt can cause drowsiness and dizziness. Do not participate in any activities that require full alertness until you are certain of the drug's effect. Use Maxalt with caution if you have liver disease or need kidney dialysis. Also alert your doctor if you have an eye condition. There is a theoretical possibility that Maxalt could affect the eyes.

If your first dose of Maxalt has no effect on your symptoms, you may not be suffering from migraine. Ask your doctor for a re-evaluation.

If you have a condition called phenylketonuria, you should be aware that the Maxalt-MLT tablets contain phenylalanine.

Maxalt has not been tested in people under 18 years old and should not be used by this age group.

Possible food and drug interactions
when taking this medication

The following drugs may boost or add to the effect of Maxalt and should never be combined with it:

    Drugs classified as MAO inhibitors, including the antidepressants
        Marplan, Nardil, and Parnate
    Ergot-containing drugs such as Cafergot, D.H.E. Injection, Ergostat, and
        Migranal Nasal Spray
    Other drugs in the Maxalt family, including Amerge, Imitrex, and Zomig

Certain other drugs may also interact with Maxalt. Check with your doctor before combining it with the following:

    Fluoxetine (Prozac)
    Fluvoxamine (Luvox)
    Paroxetine (Paxil)
    Propranolol (Inderal)
    Sertraline (Zoloft)

Special information
if you are pregnant or breastfeeding

The effects of Maxalt during pregnancy have not been adequately studied. If you are pregnant or plan to become pregnant, inform your doctor immediately. It is not known whether Maxalt appears in breast milk, but because many drugs do, you should use Maxalt with caution while nursing an infant.

Recommended dosage

ADULTS

The usual dose of Maxalt and Maxalt-MLT is one 5- or 10-milligram tablet. Doses should be spaced at least 2 hours apart. Take no more than 30 milligrams a day.

Overdosage

Any medication taken in excess can have serious consequences. If you suspect an overdose, seek medical attention immediately.

■ *Symptoms of Maxalt overdose may include:*
Dizziness, fainting, heart and blood vessel problems, high blood pressure, loss of bowel and bladder control, slow heartbeat, vomiting

Brand name:

MAXAQUIN

Pronounced: MAX-ah-kwin
Generic name: Lomefloxacin hydrochloride

Why is this drug prescribed?

Maxaquin is a quinolone antibiotic used to treat lower respiratory infections, including chronic bronchitis, and urinary tract infections, including cystitis (inflammation of the inner lining of the bladder). Maxaquin is also given before bladder surgery and prostate biopsy to prevent the infections that sometimes follow these operations.

Most important fact about this drug

During and following treatment, Maxaquin causes sensitivity reactions in people exposed to sunlight or sunlamps. The reactions can occur despite use of sunscreens and sunblocks, and can be prompted by shaded or diffused light or exposure through glass. Avoid even indirect sunlight while taking Maxaquin and for several days following therapy.

How should you take this medication?

It is important to finish your prescription of Maxaquin completely. If you stop taking your medication too soon, your symptoms may return.

Maxaquin may be taken with or without food. Take it with a full 8-ounce glass of water; and be sure to drink plenty of fluids while on this medication.

You can reduce the risk of a reaction to sunlight by taking Maxaquin in the evening (at least 12 hours before you will be exposed to the sun).

■ *If you miss a dose...*
Take it as soon as you remember. If it is almost time for your next dose, skip the one you missed and go back to your regular schedule. Do not take 2 doses at the same time.

■ *Storage instructions...*
Store at room temperature.

What side effects may occur?
Side effects cannot be anticipated. If any develop or change in intensity, tell your doctor as soon as possible. Only your doctor can determine if it is safe for you to continue taking Maxaquin.

■ *More common side effects may include:*
Headache, nausea

■ *Less common side effects may include:*
Diarrhea, dizziness, sensitivity to light

■ *Rare side effects may include:*
Abdominal pain, abnormal or terrifying dreams, abnormal vision, agitation, allergic reaction, altered taste, angina pectoris (crushing chest pain), anxiety, back pain, bleeding between menstrual periods, bleeding in the stomach and intestines, blood clots in the lungs, blood in the urine, blue skin color, chest pain, chills, coma, confusion, conjunctivitis (pinkeye), constipation, convulsions, cough, decreased heat tolerance, depression, difficult or labored breathing, difficulty swallowing, dry mouth, earache, eye pain, facial swelling, fainting, fatigue, fluid retention and swelling, flu-like symptoms, flushing, gas, general feeling of illness, gout, harsh, high-pitched sound during breathing, heart attack, heart failure, high blood pressure, hives, inability to sleep, increased appetite, increased mucus from the lungs, increased sweating, indigestion, inflammation in the male genital area, inflammation of the stomach and intestines, inflammation of the vagina, irregular heartbeat, itching, joint pain, lack of urine, leg cramps, loss of appetite, loss of sense of identity, low blood pressure, low blood sugar, lung infection or other problems, muscle pain, nervousness,

nosebleed, overactivity, pain in the genital-rectal area, problems with urination, purple or red spots on the skin, rapid heartbeat, rash, ringing in the ears, skin disorders, skin eruptions or peeling, sleepiness, slow heartbeat, thirst, tingling or a "pins and needles" feeling, tongue discoloration, tremor, vaginal yeast infection, vertigo, vomiting, weakness, wheezing, white or yellow vaginal discharge

Why should this drug not be prescribed?
If you are sensitive to or have ever had an allergic reaction to Maxaquin or other quinolone antibiotics such as Cipro and Floxin, you should not take this medication. Make sure your doctor is aware of any drug reactions you have experienced.

Special warnings about this medication
Use Maxaquin cautiously if you have disorders such as epilepsy, severe hardening of the arteries in the brain, and other conditions that can lead to seizures. Maxaquin may cause convulsions.

In rare cases, people taking antibiotics similar to Maxaquin have experienced severe, even fatal reactions, sometimes after only one dose. These reactions may include confusion, convulsions, difficulty breathing, hallucinations, hives, itching, light-headedness, loss of consciousness, rash, restlessness, swelling in the face or throat, tingling, and tremors. If you develop any of these symptoms, stop taking Maxaquin immediately and seek medical help.

If other antibiotics have given you diarrhea, or it develops while you are taking Maxaquin, be sure to tell your doctor. Maxaquin may cause inflammation of the bowel, ranging from mild to life-threatening.

Maxaquin may cause dizziness or light-headedness and may impair your ability to drive a car or operate potentially dangerous machinery. Do not participate in any activities that require full alertness until you know how Maxaquin affects you.

Maxaquin can cause rupture of muscle tendons. If you notice any pain or inflammation, stop exercising the affected tendon until your doctor has examined you.

Possible food and drug interactions
when taking this medication
If Maxaquin is taken with certain other drugs, the effects of either could be increased, decreased, or altered. It is especially important to check with your doctor before combining Maxaquin with the following:

Antacids containing magnesium or aluminum, such as Maalox or
   Gaviscon
Caffeine (including coffee, tea, and some soft drinks)
Cimetidine (Tagamet)
Cyclosporine (Sandimmune and Neoral)
Probenecid (Benemid)
Sucralfate (Carafate)
Theophylline (Theo-Dur)
Warfarin (Coumadin)
Vitamins or products containing iron or zinc

Special information
if you are pregnant or breastfeeding
The effects of Maxaquin in pregnancy have not been adequately studied. If
you are pregnant or plan to become pregnant, notify your doctor immediately.
It is not known if Maxaquin appears in breast milk. Because many drugs do
make their way into breast milk, your doctor may have you stop nursing
while you are taking Maxaquin.

Recommended dosage

ADULTS

Chronic Bronchitis
The usual dosage is 400 milligrams once a day for 10 days.

Cystitis
The usual dosage is 400 milligrams once a day for 10 days.

Complicated Urinary Tract Infections
The dosage is 400 milligrams once a day for 14 days.

People With Impaired Renal Function or Cirrhosis
Your doctor will adjust the dosage according to your needs.

People on Dialysis
The recommended dosage for people on dialysis is 400 milligrams, followed
by daily maintenance doses of 200 milligrams (one half tablet) once a day for
the duration of treatment.

CHILDREN

Safety and efficacy have not been established for children under the age
of 18.

Overdosage
There is no information on overdosage with Maxaquin. However, any medication taken in excess can have serious consequences. If you suspect an overdose, seek medical help immediately.

Brand name:

MAXZIDE

See Dyazide, page 443.

Generic name:

MECLIZINE

See Antivert, page 79.

Brand name:

MEDROL

Pronounced: MED-rohl
Generic name: Methylprednisolone

Why is this drug prescribed?
Medrol, a corticosteroid drug, is used to reduce inflammation and improve symptoms in a variety of disorders, including rheumatoid arthritis, acute gouty arthritis, and severe cases of asthma. Medrol may be given to people to treat primary or secondary adrenal cortex insufficiency (inability of the adrenal gland to produce sufficient hormone). It is also given to help treat the following disorders:

Severe allergic conditions (including drug-induced allergic states)
Blood disorders (leukemia and various anemias)
Certain cancers (along with other drugs)
Skin diseases (including severe psoriasis)
Connective tissue diseases such as systemic lupus erythematosus
Digestive tract diseases such as ulcerative colitis
High serum levels of calcium associated with cancer
Fluid retention due to nephrotic syndrome (a condition in which damage to the kidney causes loss of protein in urine)
Various eye diseases
Lung diseases such as tuberculosis
Worsening of multiple sclerosis

Most important fact about this drug
Medrol lowers your resistance to infections and can make them harder to treat. Medrol may also mask some of the signs of an infection, making it difficult for your doctor to diagnose the actual problem.

How should you take this medication?
Take Medrol exactly as prescribed. It can be taken every day or every other day, depending on the condition being treated.

Do not abruptly stop taking Medrol without checking with your doctor. If you have been using Medrol for a long time, the dose should be reduced gradually.

Medrol may cause stomach upset. Take Medrol with meals or snacks.

■ *If you miss a dose...*
If you take your dose once a day, take it as soon as you remember. Then go back to your regular schedule. If you don't remember until the next day, skip the one you missed. Do not take 2 doses at once.

If you take it several times a day, take it as soon as you remember. Then go back to your regular schedule. If you don't remember until your next dose, double the dose you take.

If you take your dose every other day, and you remember it the same morning, take it as soon as you remember and go back to your regular schedule. If you don't remember until the afternoon, do not take it until the following morning, then skip a day and go back to your regular schedule.

■ *Storage instructions...*
Store at room temperature.

What side effects may occur?
Side effects cannot be anticipated. If any develop or change in intensity, tell your doctor immediately. Only your doctor can determine whether it is safe for you to continue taking Medrol.

■ *Side effects may include:*
Abdominal swelling, allergic reactions, bone fractures, bruising, cataracts, congestive heart failure, convulsions, Cushingoid symptoms (moon face, weight gain, high blood pressure, emotional disturbances, growth of facial hair in women), face redness, fluid and salt retention, headache, high blood pressure, increased eye pressure, increased sweating, increase in amounts of insulin or hypoglycemic medications needed, inflammation of the pancreas, irregular menstruation, muscle wasting and weakness,

osteoporosis, poor healing of wounds, protruding eyes, stomach ulcer, suppression of growth in children, symptoms of diabetes, thin, fragile skin, tiny red or purplish spots on the skin, vertigo

Why should this drug not be prescribed?

Medrol should not be used if you have a fungal infection or if you are sensitive to or allergic to steroids (corticosteroids).

Special warnings about this medication

The 24-milligram Medrol tablet contains FD&C Yellow No. 5 (tartrazine), which has caused allergic reactions (including asthma) in some people. Although this is rare, it is more common in people who are sensitive to aspirin.

Medrol can alter the way your body responds to unusual stress. If you are injured, need surgery, or develop an acute illness, inform your doctor. Your dosage may need to be increased.

You should avoid immunization shots with live or live, attenuated vaccines while taking high doses of Medrol, because Medrol can suppress the immune system. Immunization with killed or inactivated vaccines is safe, but may have diminished effect.

Long-term use of Medrol may cause cataracts, glaucoma (increased eye pressure), and eye infections.

Large doses of Medrol may cause high blood pressure, salt and water retention, and potassium and calcium loss. It may be necessary to restrict your salt intake and take a potassium supplement.

Medrol may reactivate dormant cases of tuberculosis. If you have inactive tuberculosis and must take Medrol for an extended period of time, your doctor will prescribe anti-TB medication as well.

Medrol should be used cautiously if you have an underactive thyroid, liver cirrhosis, or herpes simplex (virus) infection of the eye.

This medication may aggravate existing emotional problems or cause new ones. You may experience euphoria (an exaggerated sense of well-being) and difficulty sleeping, mood swings, or mental problems. If you have any changes in mood, contact your doctor.

People taking corticosteroids, such as Medrol, have developed Kaposi's sarcoma, a form of cancer.

Medrol should also be taken with caution if you have any of the following conditions:

Diverticulitis or other inflammatory conditions of the intestine
High blood pressure
Certain kidney diseases
Active or dormant peptic ulcer
Myasthenia gravis (a muscle weakness disorder)
Osteoporosis (brittle bones)
Threadworm
Ulcerative colitis with impending danger of infection

Long-term use of Medrol can slow the growth and development of infants and children.

Use aspirin cautiously with Medrol if you have a blood-clotting disorder.

Avoid exposure to chickenpox and measles.

Possible food and drug interactions
when taking this medication

If Medrol is taken with certain other drugs, the effects of either drug could be increased, decreased, or altered. It is especially important to check with your doctor before combining Medrol with the following:

Aspirin
Barbiturates such as phenobarbital
Blood thinners such as Coumadin
Carbamazepine (Tegretol)
Cyclosporine (Sandimmune, Neoral)
Estrogen medications such as Premarin
Insulin
Ketoconazole (Nizoral)
Nonsteroidal anti-inflammatory medications such as Indocin
Oral diabetes drugs such as Glucotrol
Phenytoin (Dilantin)
Rifampin (Rifadin)
Troleandomycin (Tao)
Water pills such as Lasix and HydroDIURIL

Special information
if you are pregnant or breastfeeding

If you are pregnant or plan to become pregnant, tell your doctor immediately. There is no information about the safety of Medrol during pregnancy. Babies born to mothers who have taken doses of Medrol (corticosteroids) during pregnancy should be carefully watched for adrenal problems. Medrol may appear in breast milk and could affect a nursing infant. If Medrol is essential to your health, your doctor may advise you to stop breastfeeding until your treatment with Medrol is finished.

Recommended dosage

The starting dose of Medrol tablets may vary from 4 milligrams to 48 milligrams per day, depending on the specific problem being treated.

Once you've shown a satisfactory response, the doctor will gradually lower the dosage to the smallest effective amount. If you are taking Medrol for an extended period, the doctor may instruct you to take the drug only every other day, at twice your daily dosage.

For a worsening of multiple sclerosis, the dosage is 160 milligrams a day for one week, then 64 milligrams every other day for a month.

Overdosage

Any medication taken in excess can have serious consequences. If you suspect an overdose of Medrol, seek medical treatment immediately.

Generic name:

MEDROXYPROGESTERONE

See Provera, page 1078.

Generic name:

MEFENAMIC ACID

See Ponstel, page 1019.

Brand name:

MELLARIL

Pronounced: MEL-ah-rill
Generic name: Thioridazine hydrochloride

Why is this drug prescribed?

Mellaril is used to reduce the symptoms of psychotic disorders such as schizophrenia, and to treat depression and anxiety in adults. Mellaril is also used in the treatment of agitation, fears, sleep disturbances, tension, depression, and anxiety in elderly people, and for certain behavior problems in children.

Most important fact about this drug

Mellaril may cause tardive dyskinesia—a condition marked by involuntary muscle spasms and twitches in the face and body. This condition may be permanent, and appears to be most common among the elderly, especially women. Ask your doctor for information about this possible risk.

How should you take this medication?

If you are taking Mellaril in a liquid concentrate form, you can dilute it with a liquid such as distilled water, soft tap water, or juice just before taking it.

Do not change from one brand of thioridazine to another without consulting your doctor.

■ *If you miss a dose...*
If you take 1 dose a day and remember later in the day, take the dose immediately. If you don't remember until the next day, skip the dose and go back to your regular schedule.

If you take more than 1 dose a day and remember the forgotten dose within an hour or so after its scheduled time, take it immediately. If you don't remember until later, skip the dose and go back to your regular schedule.

Never try to "catch up" by doubling a dose.

■ *Storage instructions...*
Store at room temperature, tightly closed, in the container the medication came in.

What side effects may occur?

Side effects cannot be anticipated. If any develop or change in intensity, inform your doctor as soon as possible. Only your doctor can determine if it is safe for you to continue taking Mellaril.

■ *Side effects may include:*
Abnormal and excessive secretion of milk, agitation, anemia, asthma, blurred vision, body spasm, breast development in males, changed mental state, changes in sex drive, chewing movements, confusion (especially at night), constipation, diarrhea, discolored eyes, drowsiness, dry mouth, excitement, eyeball rotation, fever, fluid accumulation and swelling, headache, inability to hold urine, inability to urinate, inhibition of ejaculation, intestinal blockage, involuntary movements, irregular blood pressure, pulse, and heartbeat, irregular or missed menstrual periods, jaw spasm, loss of appetite, loss of muscle movement, mouth puckering, muscle rigidity, nasal congestion, nausea, overactivity, painful muscle spasm, paleness, pinpoint pupils, protruding tongue, psychotic reactions,

puffing of cheeks, rapid heartbeat, redness of the skin, restlessness, rigid and masklike face, sensitivity to light, skin pigmentation and rash, sluggishness, stiff, twisted neck, strange dreams, sweating, swelling in the throat, swelling or filling of breasts, swollen glands, tremors, vomiting, weight gain, yellowing of the skin and whites of eyes

Why should this drug not be prescribed?
Never combine this drug with excessive amounts of central nervous system depressants such as alcohol, barbiturates, or narcotics. Do not take Mellaril if you have heart disease accompanied by severe high or low blood pressure.

Special warnings about this medication
This drug may impair your ability to drive a car or operate potentially dangerous machinery. Do not participate in any activities that require full alertness until you are certain the drug will not interfere.

If you have ever had breast cancer, make sure your doctor is aware of it.

Mellaril may cause false positive results in tests for pregnancy.

Possible food and drug interactions
when taking this medication
If Mellaril is taken with certain other drugs, the effects of either could be increased, decreased, or altered. It is especially important to check with your doctor before combining Mellaril with the following:

Epinephrine (EpiPen)
Phosphorus insecticides
Pindolol (Visken)
Propranolol (Inderal)

Extreme drowsiness and other potentially serious effects can result if Mellaril is combined with alcohol or other central nervous system depressants such as narcotics, painkillers, and sleeping medications.

Special information
if you are pregnant or breastfeeding
Pregnant women should use Mellaril only if clearly needed. If you are pregnant or plan to become pregnant, inform your doctor immediately.

Recommended dosage
Your doctor will tailor your dose to your needs, using the smallest effective amount.

ADULTS

Psychotic Disorders

The starting dose ranges from 150 to 300 milligrams a day, divided into 3 equal doses. Your doctor may increase your dosage to as much as 800 milligrams a day, taken in 2 to 4 small doses. Once your symptoms improve, your doctor will decrease the dosage to the lowest effective amount.

Depression and Anxiety

The initial dose is 75 milligrams a day, divided into 3 doses per day. Dosage may range from 20 to 200 milligrams a day, divided into 2 to 4 doses.

CHILDREN

Behavior Problems

Mellaril should not be given to children younger than 2 years old. For children 2 to 12 years old, doses are determined by body weight. Total daily doses range from 0.5 milligram to 3 milligrams for every 2.2 pounds of body weight.

The usual beginning dose for children with moderate disorders is from 20 to 30 milligrams a day, divided into 2 or 3 doses.

OLDER ADULTS

In general, older people take dosages of Mellaril in the lower range. Older people (especially older women) may be more susceptible to tardive dyskinesia—a possibly irreversible condition marked by involuntary muscle spasms and twitches in the face and body. Consult your doctor for information about these potential risks.

Depression, Anxiety and Sleep Disturbances

The starting dose is 75 milligrams a day, divided into 3 doses per day. The dosage may range from 20 to 200 milligrams a day, divided into 2 to 4 doses.

Overdosage

Any medication taken in excess can have serious consequences. An overdose of Mellaril can be fatal. If you suspect an overdose, seek medical help immediately.

- **Symptoms of Mellaril overdose may include:**
  Agitation, blurred vision, coma, confusion, constipation, difficulty breathing, dilated or constricted pupils, diminished flow of urine, dry mouth, dry skin, excessively high or low body temperature, extremely low blood

pressure, fluid in the lungs, heart abnormalities, inability to urinate, intestinal blockage, nasal congestion, restlessness, sedation, seizures, shock

Generic name:

MEPERIDINE

See Demerol, page 362.

Generic name:

MEPROBAMATE

See Miltown, page 804.

Brand name:

MERIDIA

Pronounced: mer-ID-dee-uh
Generic name: Sibutramine hydrochloride

Why is this drug prescribed?
Meridia helps the seriously overweight shed pounds and keep them off. It is especially recommended for those who in addition to being overweight have other health problems such as high blood pressure, diabetes, or high cholesterol. It is used in conjunction with a low-calorie diet.

Meridia works by boosting levels of certain chemical messengers in the nervous system, including serotonin, dopamine, and norepinephrine.

Most important fact about this drug
Make a point of keeping follow-up appointments with your doctor. Meridia can increase your blood pressure, so it's important to have your blood pressure and pulse monitored at the beginning of therapy and regularly thereafter.

How should you take this medication?
Meridia can be taken with or without food.

■ *If you miss a dose...*
Take it as soon as you remember. If it is almost time for your next dose, skip the one you missed and go back to your regular schedule. Do not take 2 doses at once.

- *Storage instructions...*
  Store at room temperature away from heat and moisture in a tight, light-resistant container.

What side effects may occur?
Side effects cannot be anticipated. If any develop or change in intensity, inform your doctor as soon as possible. Only your doctor can determine if it is safe for you to continue taking Meridia.

- *More common side effects may include:*
  Abdominal pain, acid indigestion, anxiety, back pain, constipation, cough increase, depression, dizziness, dry mouth, flu symptoms, headache, increased appetite, insomnia, joint pain, loss of appetite, loss of strength, nasal inflammation, nausea, nervousness, painful menstruation, rash, sinus inflammation, stomachache, sore throat

- *Less common side effects may include:*
  Acne, abnormal thinking, agitation, allergic reaction, arthritis, bronchitis, changes in taste, chest pain, dental problems, diarrhea, difficulty breathing, drowsiness, ear pain, ear problems, emotional changes, fever, gas, heavy uterine bleeding, herpes simplex virus, increased heart rate, increased blood pressure, itching, laryngitis, leg cramps, menstrual problems, migraine headache, muscle ache, neck pain, rectal problems, reduced vision, stimulation, stomach and intestinal inflammation, sweating, swelling, thirst, throbbing heartbeat, tingling skin sensation, urinary tract infection, vaginal yeast infection, vomiting

- *Rare side effects may include:*
  Bleeding problems, kidney problems, seizures

Why should this drug not be prescribed?
If Meridia gives you an allergic reaction, you won't be able to use it. You should also avoid Meridia (and certainly don't need it) if you suffer from the compulsive dieting disorder known as anorexia nervosa. Do not combine Meridia with other drugs used to suppress appetite, and do not use it within 2 weeks of taking a drug classified as an MAO inhibitor, including the antidepressant medications Marplan, Nardil, and Parnate.

Special warnings about this medication
Use Meridia with caution if you have uncontrolled high blood pressure; it could make the problem worse. Avoid Meridia completely if you've had a stroke or suffer from heart disease, heart failure, or irregular heartbeat. Also

avoid it if you have severe kidney or liver problems; the drug has not been tested under these conditions. Seizures are a rare, but possible, side effect. If you've had seizures in the past, use Meridia with caution. If you have a seizure while taking the drug, stop using it and call your doctor immediately.

Any drug that acts on the nervous system can theoretically impair judgment, thinking, and motor skills. Meridia does not seem to have this effect, but caution is still in order until you know how the drug affects you.

If you have narrow-angle glaucoma or thyroid problems, make sure the doctor knows; Meridia should be used with caution in these circumstances. If you are prone to gallstones, be aware that weight loss can cause more of them to form. Meridia has not been tested in people under 16 years old. It should be used with caution in those over 65. Although it has been classified as a controlled substance (potentially subject to abuse), the possibility of developing physical or psychological dependence is low.

Possible food and drug interactions when taking this medication

Remember that Meridia must never be taken within 2 weeks of using an MAO inhibitor such as Marplan, Nardil, or Parnate. The combination could lead to serious, even fatal, overstimulation.

Meridia may also interact with a wide variety of other prescription and over-the-counter drugs, especially weight-reducing agents, decongestants, antidepressants, allergy medications, and cough suppressants that contain ephedrine, phenylpropanolamine, or pseudoephedrine. Among the many drugs that pose a potential problem are the following:

Alcohol (excessive amounts)
Dextromethorphan (found in many over-the-counter cough preparations)
Dihydroergotamine (D.H.E. Injection, Migranal Nasal Spray)
Erythromycin (Eryc, Ery-Tab, PCE)
Fentanyl (Duragesic)
Fluoxetine (Prozac)
Fluvoxamine (Luvox)
Ketoconazole (Nizoral)
Lithium (Lithobid, Lithonate)
Meperidine (Demerol)
Naratriptan (Amerge)
Paroxetine (Paxil)
Pentazocine (Talwin NX, Talacen)
Sertraline (Zoloft)

Stimulants such as amphetamines, Dexedrine, Desoxyn, Adderall,
Didrex, and Ionamin
Sumatriptan (Imitrex)
Tryptophan (L-Tryptophan, Trofan)
Venlafaxine (Effexor)
Zolmitriptan (Zomig)

If you have any doubt about the safety of a combination, be sure to check with your doctor.

Special information
if you are pregnant or breastfeeding
The use of Meridia during pregnancy is not recommended. If you are in your child-bearing years, take reliable contraceptive measures while using this drug. If you do become pregnant, or plan on becoming pregnant, tell your doctor immediately. It is not known whether Meridia appears in breast milk; its use while breastfeeding is not recommended.

Recommended dosage

ADULTS

The starting dose is 10 milligrams once daily. If you have not lost at least 4 pounds after 4 weeks, the doctor may increase the dose to 15 milligrams daily. This is the maximum; if weight loss still fails to appear, Meridia will be discontinued.

For those who experience side effects at the 10-milligram level, a 5-milligram dose may prove sufficient.

Use of Meridia for longer than 1 year has not been studied.

Overdosage
Although doctors have had little experience with overdoses of Meridia, increased heart rate and blood pressure are possible results. Since any medication taken in excess can have serious consequences, seek medical attention immediately if you suspect an overdose.

Generic name:

MESALAMINE

See Rowasa, page 1152.

Brand name:

METAPREL

See Alupent, page 43.

Generic name:

METAPROTERENOL

See Alupent, page 43.

Generic name:

METFORMIN

See Glucophage, page 563.

Generic name:

METHAZOLAMIDE

See Neptazane, page 865.

Generic name:

METHENAMINE

See Urised, page 1380.

Brand name:

METHERGINE

Pronounced: METH-er-jin
Generic name: Methylergonovine maleate

Why is this drug prescribed?
Methergine, a blood-vessel constrictor, is given to prevent or control excessive bleeding following childbirth. It works by causing the uterine muscles to contract, thereby reducing the mother's blood loss.

Methergine comes in tablet and injectable forms.

Most important fact about this drug
Some blood-vessel disorders and certain infections make the use of Methergine dangerous. Make sure your doctor is aware of any medical conditions you may have.

How should you take this medication?
Take Methergine tablets exactly as prescribed.

■ *If you miss a dose...*
Do not take the missed dose at all and do not double the next one. Instead, go back to your regular schedule.

■ *Storage instructions...*
Store at room temperature in a tightly closed container, away from light.

What side effects may occur?
Side effects cannot be anticipated. If any develop or change in intensity, inform your doctor as soon as possible. Only your doctor can determine if it is safe for you to continue taking Methergine.

The most common side effect is high blood pressure, which may cause a headache or even a seizure. In some people, however, Methergine may cause low blood pressure.

■ *Less common or rare side effects may include:*
Bad taste, blood clots, blood in urine, chest pains (temporary), diarrhea, difficult or labored breathing, dizziness, edema, hallucinations, heart attack, leg cramps, nasal congestion, nausea, palpitations (throbbing heartbeat), ringing in the ears, sweating, vomiting

Why should this drug not be prescribed?
You should not take Methergine if you are allergic to it, if you are pregnant, or if you have high blood pressure or toxemia (poisons circulating in the blood).

Special warnings about this medication
It may be dangerous to take Methergine if you have an infection, certain blood vessel disorders, or a liver or kidney problem. Inform your doctor if you think you have any such condition.

Your doctor will use intravenous Methergine only when necessary, because of the possibility of a sudden rise in blood pressure or a stroke.

Possible food and drug interactions
when taking this medication

If Methergine is taken with certain other drugs, the effects of either may be increased, decreased, or altered. It is especially important to check with your doctor before combining Methergine with the following:

Other blood-vessel constrictors such as EpiPen
Other ergot-derived medications such as Ergotrate

Special information
if you are pregnant or breastfeeding

Methergine should not be taken during pregnancy. Methergine appears in breast milk. Although no specific information is available about possible effects of Methergine on a nursing baby, the general rule is that a mother who is breastfeeding should not take any drug unless it is clearly needed.

Recommended dosage

The usual dose is 1 tablet (0.2 milligram) 3 or 4 times daily after childbirth for a maximum of 1 week.

Overdosage

Any medication taken in excess can have serious consequences. If you suspect symptoms of a Methergine overdose, seek medical attention immediately.

■ *Symptoms of Methergine overdose may include:*
Abdominal pain, coma, convulsions, elevated blood pressure, hypothermia (drop in body temperature), lowered blood pressure, nausea, numbness, slowed breathing, tingling of the arms and legs, vomiting

Generic name:

METHOCARBAMOL

See Robaxin, page 1146.

Generic name:

METHOTREXATE

Pronounced: meth-oh-TREX-ate
Brand name: Rheumatrex

Why is this drug prescribed?

Methotrexate is an anticancer drug used in the treatment of lymphoma (cancer of the lymph nodes) and certain forms of leukemia. It is also given to treat some forms of cancers of the uterus, breast, lung, head, neck, and ovary. Methotrexate is also given to treat rheumatoid arthritis when other treatments have proved ineffective, and is sometimes used to treat very severe and disabling psoriasis (a skin disease characterized by thickened patches of red, inflamed skin often covered by silver scales).

Most important fact about this drug

Be certain to remember that in the treatment of psoriasis and rheumatoid arthritis, methotrexate is taken once a *week*, not once a day. Accidentally taking the recommended weekly dosage on a daily basis can lead to fatal overdosage. Be sure to read the patient instructions that come with the package.

How should you take this medication?

Take methotrexate exactly as prescribed, and promptly report to your doctor any new symptoms that may develop.

Methotrexate is given at a higher dosage for cancer than for psoriasis or rheumatoid arthritis. After high-dose methotrexate treatment, a drug called leucovorin may be given to limit the toxic effects.

■ *If you miss a dose...*
Skip it and go back to your regular schedule. Do not take 2 doses at once.

■ *Storage instructions...*
Store at room temperature, away from light.

What side effects may occur?

Side effects cannot be anticipated. If any develop or change in intensity, inform your doctor as soon as possible. Only your doctor can determine whether it is safe for you to continue taking methotrexate.

■ *More common side effects may include:*
Abdominal pain and upset, chills and fever, decreased resistance to infection, dizziness, fatigue, general feeling of illness, mouth ulcers, nausea

■ *Less common side effects may include:*
Abortion, acne, anemia, birth defects, black or tarry stool, boils, bruises, changes in skin coloration, convulsions, diarrhea, drowsiness, eye or vision problems, fatigue, hair loss, headaches, hives, inability to speak, infection

– of hair follicles, infertility, inflammation of the gums or mouth, intestinal inflammation, kidney failure, loss of appetite, lung disease, menstrual problems, partial or complete paralysis, rash or itching, red patches on skin, sensitivity to light, skin peeling or flaking, sore throat, stomach and intestinal ulcers and bleeding, stomach pain, vaginal discharge, vomiting, vomiting blood

■ *Rare side effects may include:*
Diabetes, impotence, infection, joint pain, loss of sexual desire, muscular pain, osteoporosis, ringing in the ears, severe allergic reaction, shortness of breath, sleepiness, sudden death, sweating

If you are taking methotrexate for psoriasis, you may also experience hair loss and/or sun sensitivity, and your patches of psoriasis may give a burning sensation.

Methotrexate can sometimes cause serious lung damage that makes it necessary to limit the treatment. If you experience a dry cough, fever, or breathing difficulties while taking methotrexate, be sure to tell your doctor right away.

During and immediately after treatment with methotrexate, fertility may be impaired. Men may have an abnormally low sperm count; women may have menstrual irregularities.

People on high doses of methotrexate may develop a brain condition signaled by confusion, partial paralysis, seizures, or coma.

Why should this drug not be prescribed?
Do not take this medication if you are sensitive to it or it has given you an allergic reaction.

Do not take this medication if you are pregnant.

Methotrexate treatment is not suitable for you if you suffer from psoriasis or rheumatoid arthritis and also have one of the following conditions:

- Abnormal blood cell count
  Alcoholic liver disease or other chronic liver disease
  Alcoholism
  Anemia
  Immune-system deficiency

Special warnings about this medication
Before you start taking methotrexate, your doctor will do a chest X-ray plus blood tests to determine your blood cell counts, liver enzyme levels, and the

efficiency of your kidney function. While you are taking methotrexate, the blood tests will be repeated at regular intervals; if you develop a cough or chest pain, the chest X-ray will be repeated.

If you are being treated for psoriasis or rheumatoid arthritis, your doctor will test your liver function at regular intervals. You should avoid alcoholic beverages while taking this drug.

You may develop an opportunistic infection—one that takes advantage of your altered body chemistry—while you are taking methotrexate. Before receiving an immunization or vaccination, be sure to inform health care workers that you are taking this drug.

Older or physically debilitated people are particularly vulnerable to toxic effects from methotrexate. Your doctor will prescribe methotrexate with great caution if you have any of the following:

Active infection
Liver disease
Peptic ulcer
Ulcerative colitis

Possible food and drug interactions
when taking this medication

If you are being given methotrexate for the treatment of cancer or psoriasis, you should not take aspirin or other nonsteroidal painkillers such as Advil or Naprosyn; this combination could increase the toxic effects of methotrexate. If you are taking methotrexate for rheumatoid arthritis, you may be able to continue taking aspirin or a nonsteroidal painkiller, but your doctor should monitor you carefully.

Other drugs that may increase the toxic effects of methotrexate include:

Cisplatin (Platinol)
Etretinate (Tegison)
Penicillins
Phenylbutazone
Phenytoin (Dilantin)
Probenecid (Benemid)
Sulfa drugs such as Bactrim and Gantrisin

Sulfa drugs may increase methotrexate's toxic effect on the bone marrow, where new blood cells are made.

Certain antibiotics, including tetracycline (Achromycin) and chloramphenicol (Chloromycetin), may reduce the effectiveness of methotrexate. This is also true of vitamin preparations that contain folic acid.

In addition, methotrexate can alter the effect of theophylline (Marax, Quibron).

Special information
if you are pregnant or breastfeeding

A woman should not start methotrexate therapy until the doctor is sure she is not pregnant. Because methotrexate causes birth defects and miscarriages, it must not be taken during pregnancy by women with psoriasis or rheumatoid arthritis. It should be taken by women being treated for cancer only if the potential benefit outweighs the risk to the developing baby. In fact, a couple should avoid pregnancy if either the man or the woman is taking methotrexate. After the end of methotrexate treatment, a man should wait at least 3 months, and a woman should wait for the completion of at least one menstrual cycle, before attempting to conceive a child.

Methotrexate should not be taken by a woman who is breastfeeding; it does pass into breast milk and may harm a nursing baby.

Recommended dosage

Treatment with methotrexate is highly individualized. Your doctor will carefully tailor your dosage of methotrexate in order to avoid serious side effects and possible under- or overdosing.

Overdosage

Taken in excess, methotrexate can cause serious and even fatal damage to the liver, kidneys, bone marrow, lungs, or other parts of the body. Symptoms of overdosage may include lung or breathing problems, mouth ulcers, or diarrhea. Initially, however, serious damage caused by methotrexate may be apparent only in the results of blood tests. For this reason, careful, regular monitoring by your doctor is necessary. If for any reason you suspect symptoms of an overdose of this drug, seek medical attention immediately.

Generic name:

METHYLDOPA

See Aldomet, page 32.

Generic name:

METHYLERGONOVINE

See Methergine, page 774.

Generic name:

METHYLPHENIDATE

See Ritalin, page 1142.

Generic name:

METHYLPREDNISOLONE

See Medrol, page 762.

Generic name:

METOCLOPRAMIDE

See Reglan, page 1099.

Generic name:

METOLAZONE

See Zaroxolyn, page 1446.

Generic name:

METOPROLOL

See Lopressor, page 718.

Generic name:

METRONIDAZOLE

See Flagyl, page 528.

Brand name:

MEVACOR

Pronounced: MEV-uh-core
Generic name: Lovastatin

Why is this drug prescribed?

Mevacor is used, along with diet, to lower cholesterol levels in the blood of people with primary hypercholesterolemia (too much cholesterol), a condition caused by a lack of the low-density lipoprotein (LDL) receptors that remove cholesterol from the bloodstream. However, Mevacor is usually prescribed only when a low-fat, low-cholesterol diet does not lower cholesterol levels enough. Mevacor is also used to slow down hardening of arteries in people with coronary heart disease.

Most important fact about this drug
Mevacor is usually prescribed only if diet, exercise, and weight-loss fail to bring your cholesterol levels under control. It's important to remember that Mevacor is a supplement—not a substitute—for these other measures. To get the full benefit of the medication, you need to stick to the diet and exercise program prescribed by your doctor. All these efforts to keep your cholesterol levels normal are important because together they may lower your risk of heart disease.

How should you take this medication?
Take Mevacor exactly as prescribed by your doctor.

Mevacor should be taken with meals.

- *If you miss a dose...*
  Take it as soon as you remember. If it is almost time for your next dose, skip the one you missed and go back to your regular schedule. Never take 2 doses at the same time.

- *Storage instructions...*
  Protect Mevacor from light. Store at room temperature. Keep container tightly closed.

What side effects may occur?
Mevacor is generally well tolerated. Any side effects that have occurred have usually been mild and short-lived. If any side effects develop or change in intensity, inform your doctor as soon as possible. Only your doctor can determine if it is safe for you to continue taking Mevacor.

- *Side effects may include:*
  Abdominal pain/cramps, altered sense of taste, blurred vision, constipation, diarrhea, dizziness, gas, headache, heartburn, indigestion, itching, muscle cramps, muscle pain, nausea, rash, weakness

Why should this drug not be prescribed?
If you are sensitive to or have ever had an allergic reaction to Mevacor or similar anticholesterol drugs, you should not take this medication. Make sure that your doctor is aware of any drug reactions that you have experienced.

Unless you are directed to do so by your doctor, do not take this medication if you are being treated for liver disease.

Do not take this drug if you are pregnant or nursing.

Special warnings about this medication
If you are being treated for any disease that contributes to increased blood cholesterol, such as hypothyroidism, diabetes, nephrotic syndrome (kidney and blood vessel disorder), dysproteinemia (an excess of protein in the blood), or liver disease, your doctor will closely monitor your reaction to Mevacor.

It is recommended that liver function tests be performed by your doctor before treatment with Mevacor begins, at 6 and 12 weeks after your treatment has started or your dosage has been raised, and periodically (about 6-month intervals) thereafter.

This drug should be used with caution if you consume substantial quantities of alcohol or have a past history of liver disease.

Possible food and drug interactions
when taking this medication
If Mevacor is taken with certain other drugs, the effects of either could be increased, decreased, or altered. It is especially important to check with your doctor before combining Mevacor with the following:

Blood-thinning drugs such as Coumadin
Clarithromycin (Biaxin)
Cyclosporine (Sandimmune, Neoral) and other immunosuppressive drugs
    (medications that lower the body's defense reaction to a foreign or
    invading substance)
Erythromycin (E.E.S., PCE, others)
Gemfibrozil (Lopid)
Itraconazole (Sporanox)
Ketoconazole (Nizoral)
Nefazodone (Serzone)
Nicotinic acid or niacin (Nicobid)

If you are taking Mevacor in combination with nicotinic acid, Lopid, or immunosuppressive drugs such as cyclosporine, alert your doctor immediately if you experience muscle pain, tenderness, or weakness, especially with fever or general bodily discomfort. This could be the first sign of impending kidney damage.

If you are taking cyclosporine and need to take Sporanox as well, the doctor will temporarily take you off Mevacor.

Special information
if you are pregnant or breastfeeding

You should take Mevacor only if pregnancy is highly unlikely. If you become pregnant while taking this drug, discontinue using it and notify your physician immediately. There may be a potential hazard to the developing baby. This medication may appear in breast milk and may have an effect on nursing infants. If this medication is essential to your health, you should discontinue breastfeeding until your treatment with this medication is finished.

Recommended dosage

ADULTS

The recommended starting dose is 20 milligrams once a day, taken with the evening meal. The maximum recommended dose is 80 milligrams per day, taken as a single dose or divided into smaller doses, as determined by your doctor. Adjustments to any dose, as determined by your doctor, should be made at intervals of 4 weeks or more.

If you are taking immunosuppressive drugs in combination with Mevacor, your dose of Mevacor should begin with 10 milligrams and should not exceed 20 milligrams per day.

Cholesterol levels should be monitored periodically by your doctor, who may decide to reduce the dose if your cholesterol level falls below the targeted range.

If you have reduced kidney function, your doctor will be cautious about increasing your dosage.

CHILDREN

The safety and effectiveness of this drug have not been established in children.

Overdosage

There have been no reported cases of overdose with Mevacor. However, if you suspect an overdose, seek medical attention immediately.

Generic name:

MEXILETINE

See Mexitil, below.

Brand name:

MEXITIL

Pronounced: MEX-ih-till
Generic name: Mexiletine hydrochloride

Why is this drug prescribed?
Mexitil is used to treat severe irregular heartbeat (arrhythmia). Irregular heart rhythms are generally divided into two main types: heartbeats that are faster than normal (tachycardia) and heartbeats that are slower than normal (bradycardia). Arrhythmias are often caused by drugs or disease but can occur in otherwise healthy people with no history of heart disease or other illness.

Most important fact about this drug
While you are taking Mexitil, your doctor should carefully monitor your heartbeat to make sure the drug is working properly.

How should you take this medication?
Take Mexitil with food or an antacid. Take it exactly as prescribed.

- *If you miss a dose...*
  If you remember within 4 hours, take it immediately. If more than 4 hours have passed, skip the missed dose and return to your regular schedule. Never take 2 doses at the same time.

- *Storage instructions...*
  Store at room temperature.

What side effects may occur?
Side effects cannot be anticipated. If any develop or change in intensity, inform your doctor as soon as possible. Only your doctor can determine if it is safe for you to continue taking Mexitil.

- *More common side effects may include:*
  Blurred vision, changes in sleep habits, chest pain, constipation, depression, diarrhea, difficult or labored breathing, dizziness, headache, heart-

burn, light-headedness, nausea, nervousness, numbness, poor coordination, rash, swelling due to fluid retention, throbbing heartbeat, tingling or pins and needles, tremors, upset stomach, vision changes, vomiting

■ *Less common or rare side effects may include:*
Abdominal pain/cramps, angina (crushing chest pain), appetite changes, behavior changes, bleeding from the stomach, confusion, congestive heart failure, decreased sex drive, depression, difficulty swallowing, difficulty urinating, dry mouth, dry skin, excessive perspiration, fainting, fatigue, fever, hallucinations, hair loss, hepatitis, hiccups, high blood pressure, hot flashes, impotence, joint pain, loss of consciousness, low blood pressure, peptic ulcer, ringing in the ears, seizures, short-term memory loss, skin inflammation and flaking, skin peeling, slow heartbeat, sore throat, speech difficulties, taste changes, vague feeling of bodily discomfort, weakness, worsening of irregular heartbeat

Why should this drug not be prescribed?
This drug should not be used if you have heart failure, a heartbeat irregularity called heart block that has not been corrected by a pacemaker, structural heart disease, or if you have recently had a heart attack.

Special warnings about this medication
If you have heart block and a pacemaker Mexitil may be prescribed, but you should be continuously monitored while taking it.

Mexitil can aggravate low blood pressure and severe congestive heart failure so will be prescribed cautiously for people with these conditions.

You should be monitored carefully if you have liver disease or abnormal liver function as a result of congestive heart failure.

Diets that change the pH (acid/alkaline content) of your urine can alter the excretion of Mexitil from your body. Talk to your doctor or pharmacist about proper diet.

Blood disorders have occurred with Mexitil use. Make sure your doctor performs periodic blood tests while you are using this medication.

If you have a seizure disorder, use Mexitil with caution.

Possible food and drug interactions when taking this medication
If Mexitil is taken with certain other drugs, the effects of either may be increased, decreased, or altered. It is especially important that you consult with your doctor before taking any of the following:

Antacids such as Maalox
Caffeine products such as No-Doz
Cimetidine (Tagamet)
Other antiarrhythmic drugs such as Norpace and Quinidex
Phenobarbital
Phenytoin (Dilantin)
Rifampin (Rifadin)
Theophylline products such as Theo-Dur

Special information
if you are pregnant or breastfeeding

The effects of Mexitil during pregnancy have not been adequately studied. If you are pregnant or plan to become pregnant, inform your doctor immediately. Mexitil appears in breast milk and could affect a nursing infant. If this medication is essential to your health, your doctor may advise you to discontinue breastfeeding until your treatment is finished.

Recommended dosage

Treatment is usually begun in the hospital.

ADULTS

The dosage of Mexitil will be adjusted to your individual needs on the basis of your response to the drug.

The usual starting dose is 200 milligrams every 8 hours when quick control of an irregular heartbeat is not necessary. Your doctor may adjust the dose by 50 or 100 milligrams up or down every 2 to 3 days.

Most people will do well on 200 to 300 milligrams taken every 8 hours with food or antacids. If you do not, your doctor may raise your dose to 400 milligrams every 8 hours. You should not take more than 1,200 milligrams in a day.

When fast relief is needed, your doctor may start you on 400 milligrams of Mexitil, followed by 200 milligrams in 8 hours. You should see the effects of this drug within 30 minutes to 2 hours.

In general, people with reduced kidney function are prescribed the usual doses of Mexitil, but those with severe liver disease may require lower doses and will be monitored closely.

Some people who handle this drug well may be transferred to a 12-hour dosage schedule that will make it easier and more convenient to take Mexitil. If you do well on a Mexitil dose of 300 milligrams or less every 8 hours, your doctor may decide to divide the daily total into 2 doses taken every 12 hours.

CHILDREN

The safety and efficacy of this drug have not been established in children.

OLDER ADULTS

Dosages will be adjusted according to the individual's needs.

Overdosage

Any medication taken in excess can have serious consequences. There have been deaths from Mexitil overdose. If you suspect an overdose, seek medical attention immediately.

■ *The symptoms of Mexitil overdose may include:*
Coma, low blood pressure, nausea, seizures, slow heartbeat or other heart problems, tingling or pins and needles

Brand name:

MIACALCIN

Pronounced: my-ah-CAL-sin
Generic name: Calcitonin-salmon
Other brand name: Calcimar

Why is this drug prescribed?

Miacalcin is a synthetic form of calcitonin, a naturally occurring hormone produced by the thyroid gland. Miacalcin reduces the rate of calcium loss from bones. Since less calcium passes from the bones to the blood, Miacalcin also helps control blood calcium levels.

Miacalcin Nasal Spray is used to treat postmenopausal osteoporosis (bone loss occurring after menopause) in women who cannot or will not take estrogen. Calcimar, an injectable form of the drug, is also used to treat Paget's disease (abnormal bone growth leading to deformities) and hypercalcemia (abnormally high calcium blood levels).

Most important fact about this drug

Although no allergic reactions have been reported with Miacalcin Nasal Spray, the injectable form, Calcimar, has been reported to cause serious allergic reactions (such as shock, difficulty breathing, wheezing, and swelling of the throat or tongue) in a few people. The possibility exists for such a reaction with the nasal spray. Your doctor may give you a skin test to see if you are allergic to calcitonin-salmon.

How should you take this medication?
Spray Miacalcin into one nostril one day, the other the next.

Follow the manufacturer's instructions for activating the pump before the first dose.

Keep your head upright. Put the nozzle into your nostril and depress the pump toward the bottle.

Be sure your diet provides enough calcium and vitamin D. Foods that are good sources of calcium include dairy products (such as milk and cheese) and fish. Good sources of vitamin D include fish (such as salmon, sardines, and tuna), liver, and dairy products. Sunlight is an indirect source of vitamin D.

- *If you miss a dose...*
  Take it as soon as you remember. Never take 2 doses at once.

- *Storage instructions...*
  Store the unopened medication in the refrigerator. Protect from freezing. Before you prime the pump and open a new bottle, let it come to room temperature. You can keep the bottle at room temperature for 30 days; be sure it stays upright.

What side effects may occur?
Side effects cannot be anticipated. If any develop or change in intensity, inform your doctor as soon as possible. Only your doctor can determine if it is safe for you to continue using Miacalcin Nasal Spray.

- *More common side effects may include:*
  Back pain, headache, joint pain, nasal inflammation, nasal symptoms (crusts, dryness, redness, sores, irritation, itching, thick feeling, soreness, paleness, infection, narrowing of passages, runny or blocked nose, small wounds, bleeding wound, uncomfortable feeling), nosebleed

- *Less common side effects may include:*
  Flushing, nausea, possible allergic reaction, respiratory tract irritation

Why should this drug not be prescribed?
You should not be using Miacalcin if you are allergic to calcitonin-salmon.

Special warnings about this medication
Your doctor will examine your nose before you use Miacalcin Nasal Spray and periodically while you are using it.

If your nose becomes very irritated, notify your doctor.

Miacalcin may cause small wounds or ulcers in your nose.

**Possible food and drug interactions
when taking this medication**
There are no interactions listed for this drug. However, people with Paget's disease who have taken certain drugs such as Didronel may find that Miacalcin Nasal Spray is not working as well as it should.

**Special information
if you are pregnant or breastfeeding**
The effects of calcitonin-salmon in pregnancy have not been adequately studied, but use of Miacalcin Nasal Spray if you are pregnant is not recommended.

It is not known whether Miacalcin appears in breast milk. Women are usually advised not to use Miacalcin while breastfeeding an infant.

Recommended dosage
The usual dose is 1 spray (200 I.U.) a day, sprayed into the nose. Alternate nostrils. Ask your doctor about taking supplemental vitamin D and calcium.

Miacalcin Nasal Spray should not be used by children.

Overdosage
Any medication taken in excess can have serious consequences. If you suspect an overdose, seek medical help immediately.

■ *Symptoms of Miacalcin overdose may include:*
  Spasms

Generic name:

MICONAZOLE

See Monistat, page 821.

Brand name:

MICRO-K

Pronounced: MY-kroe kay
Generic name: Potassium chloride
Other brand names: Klor-Con, K-Dur, K-Tab, Kaon-CL,
  Slow-K

Why is this drug prescribed?
Micro-K is used to treat or prevent low potassium levels in people who may face potassium loss caused by digitalis (Lanoxin), non-potassium-sparing diuretics (such as Diuril and Dyazide), and certain diseases.

Potassium plays an essential role in the proper functioning of a wide range of systems in the body, including the kidneys, muscles, and nerves. As a result, a potassium deficiency may have a wide range of effects, including dry mouth, thirst, reduced urination, weakness, fatigue, drowsiness, low blood pressure, restlessness, muscle cramps, abnormal heart rate, nausea, and vomiting.

Micro-K and the other products discussed here are slow-release potassium formulations.

Most important fact about this drug
There have been reports of intestinal and gastric ulcers and bleeding associated with use of slow-release potassium chloride medications. Micro-K should be used only by people who cannot take potassium chloride in liquid or effervescent forms.

Do not change from one brand of potassium chloride to another without consulting your doctor or pharmacist.

How should you take this medication?
Take Micro-K with meals and with a full glass of water or some other liquid.

Tell your doctor if you have difficulty swallowing Micro-K. You may sprinkle the contents of the capsule onto a spoonful of soft food. Capsules and tablets should not be crushed, chewed, or sucked.

■ *If you miss a dose...*
If it is within 2 hours of the scheduled time, take it as soon as you remember. If you do not remember until later, skip the dose you missed and go back to your regular schedule. Do not take 2 doses at once.

■ *Storage instructions...*
Store at room temperature in a tightly closed container.

What side effects may occur?
Side effects cannot be anticipated. If any develop or change in intensity, inform your doctor as soon as possible. Only your doctor can determine if it is safe for you to continue taking Micro-K.

■ *Side effects may include:*
Abdominal pain or discomfort, diarrhea, gas, nausea, stomach and intestinal ulcers and bleeding, blockage, or perforation, vomiting

Why should this drug not be prescribed?
You should not be using Micro-K in a solid form if you are taking any drug or have any condition that could stop or slow Micro-K as it goes through the gastrointestinal tract.

If you have high potassium levels, you should not use Micro-K.

You should not use these products if you are allergic to any of their ingredients.

People with certain heart conditions should not use slow-release forms of potassium.

Special warnings about this medication
Before taking Micro-K, tell your doctor if you have ever had acute dehydration, heat cramps, adrenal insufficiency, diabetes, heart disease, kidney disease, liver disease, ulcers, or severe burns.

Tell your doctor immediately if you notice that your stools are black or tarry.

Possible food and drug interactions
when taking this medication
If Micro-K is taken with certain other drugs, the effects of either could be increased, decreased, or altered. It is important to check with your doctor before combining Micro-K with the following:

Antispasmodic drugs such as Bentyl
Blood pressure medications classified as ACE inhibitors, such as Vasotec and Capoten

Digitalis (Lanoxin)
Potassium-sparing diuretics such as Midamor and Aldactone

Also tell your doctor if you use salt substitutes.

Special information
if you are pregnant or breastfeeding
Micro-K is generally considered safe for pregnant women or women who breastfeed their babies.

Recommended dosage
Dosages must be adjusted for each individual. Safety and effectiveness in children have not been established. The following are typical dosages for Micro-K and other leading slow-release potassium supplements.

TO TREAT LOW POTASSIUM LEVELS

Micro-K, Klor-Con 8, Slow-K
The usual dosage is 5 to 12 tablets or capsules per day.

Micro-K 10, Klor-Con 10, K-Dur 10, K-Tab, Kaon-CL 10
The usual dose is 4 to 10 tablets or capsules per day.

K-DUR 20
The usual dose is 2 to 5 tablets per day.

TO PREVENT LOW POTASSIUM LEVELS

Micro-K, Klor-Con 8, Slow-K, K-Dur 10, Kaon-CL 10
The usual dosage is 2 or 3 tablets or capsules per day.

K-Tab, Micro-K 10, Klor-Con 10
The usual dose is 2 tablets or capsules per day.

If you are taking more than 2 tablets or capsules per day, your total daily dose will be divided into smaller doses.

Overdosage
Any medication taken in excess can have serious consequences. Overdoses of these supplements can result in potentially fatal levels of potassium. Overdose symptoms may not be noticeable in their early stages. Therefore, if you have any reason to suspect an overdose, seek medical help immediately.

■ *Symptoms of potassium overdose may include:*
Blood in stools, cardiac arrest, irregular heartbeat, muscle paralysis, muscle weakness

Brand name:

MICRONASE

Pronounced: MIKE-roh-naze
Generic name: Glyburide
Other brand names: DiaBeta, Glynase

Why is this drug prescribed?
Micronase is an oral antidiabetic medication used to treat Type 2 diabetes, the kind that occurs when the body either does not make enough insulin or fails to use insulin properly. Insulin transfers sugar from the bloodstream to the body's cells, where it is then used for energy.

There are two forms of diabetes: Type 1 and Type 2. Type 1 diabetes results from a complete shutdown of normal insulin production and usually requires insulin injections for life, while Type 2 diabetes can usually be treated by dietary changes, exercise, and/or oral antidiabetic medications such as Micronase. This medication controls diabetes by stimulating the pancreas to produce more insulin and by helping insulin to work better. Type 2 diabetics may need insulin injections, sometimes only temporarily during stressful periods such as illness, or on a long-term basis if an oral antidiabetic medication fails to control blood sugar.

Micronase can be used alone or along with a drug called metformin (Glucophage) if diet plus either drug alone fails to control sugar levels.

Most important fact about this drug
Always remember that Micronase is an aid to, not a substitute for, good diet and exercise. Failure to follow a sound diet and exercise plan can lead to serious complications, such as dangerously high or low blood sugar levels. Remember, too, that Micronase is *not* an oral form of insulin, and cannot be used in place of insulin.

How should you take this medication?
In general, Micronase should be taken with breakfast or the first main meal of the day.

■ *If you miss a dose...*
Take it as soon as you remember. If it is almost time for your next dose, skip the one you missed and go back to your regular schedule. Never take 2 doses at the same time.

■ *Storage instructions...*
Keep this medication in the container it came in, tightly closed. Store it at room temperature.

What side effects may occur?
Side effects cannot be anticipated. If any develop or change in intensity, inform your doctor as soon as possible. Only your doctor can determine if it is safe for you to continue taking Micronase.

Many side effects from Micronase are rare and seldom require discontinuation of the medication.

■ *More common side effects may include:*
Bloating, heartburn, nausea

■ *Less common or rare side effects may include:*
Anemia and other blood disorders, blurred vision, changes in taste, headache, hives, itching, joint pain, liver problems, muscle pain, reddening of the skin, skin eruptions, skin rash, yellowing of the skin

Micronase, like all oral antidiabetics, may cause hypoglycemia (low blood sugar) especially in elderly, weak, and undernourished people, and those with kidney, liver, adrenal, or pituitary gland problems. The risk of hypoglycemia can be increased by missed meals, alcohol, other medications, fever, trauma, infection, surgery, or excessive exercise. To avoid hypoglycemia, you should closely follow the dietary and exercise plan suggested by your physician.

■ *Symptoms of mild hypoglycemia may include:*
Cold sweat, drowsiness, fast heartbeat, headache, nausea, nervousness

■ *Symptoms of more severe hypoglycemia may include:*
Coma, pale skin, seizures, shallow breathing

Eating sugar or a sugar-based product will often correct mild hypoglycemia.

Severe hypoglycemia should be considered a medical emergency, and prompt medical attention is essential.

Why should this drug not be prescribed?

You should not take Micronase if you have had an allergic reaction to it or to similar drugs such as Glucotrol or Diabinese.

Micronase should not be taken if you are suffering from diabetic ketoacidosis (a life-threatening medical emergency caused by insufficient insulin and marked by excessive thirst, nausea, fatigue, pain below the breastbone, and fruity breath).

Special warnings about this medication

It's possible that drugs such as Micronase may lead to more heart problems than diet treatment alone, or diet plus insulin. If you have a heart condition, you may want to discuss this with your doctor.

If you are taking Micronase, you should check your blood or urine periodically for abnormal sugar (glucose) levels.

It is important that you closely follow the diet and exercise plan recommended by your doctor.

The effectiveness of any oral antidiabetic, including Micronase, may decrease with time. This may occur either because of a diminished responsiveness to the medication or a worsening of the diabetes.

Possible food and drug interactions
when taking this medication

If Micronase is taken with certain other drugs, the effects of either could be increased, decreased, or altered. It is especially important to check with your doctor before combining Micronase with the following:

Airway-opening drugs such as Proventil and Ventolin
Anabolic steroids such as testosterone and Danazol
Antacids such as Mylanta
Aspirin
Beta blockers such as the blood pressure medications Inderal and
  Tenormin
Blood thinners such as Coumadin
Calcium channel blockers such as the blood pressure medications
  Cardizem and Procardia
Certain antibiotics such as Cipro
Chloramphenicol (Chloromycetin)
Cimetidine (Tagamet)
Clofibrate (Atromid-S)
Estrogens such as Premarin

Fluconazole (Diflucan)
Furosemide (Lasix)
Gemfibrozil (Lopid)
Isoniazid (a drug used for tuberculosis)
Itraconazole (Sporanox)
Major tranquilizers such as Stelazine and Mellaril
MAO inhibitors such as the antidepressants Nardil and Parnate
Metformin (Glucophage)
Niacin (Nicolar, Nicobid)
Nonsteroidal anti-inflammatory drugs such as Advil, Motrin, Naprosyn, and Voltaren
Oral contraceptives
Phenytoin (Dilantin)
Probenecid (Benemid, ColBENEMID)
Steroids such as prednisone
Sulfa drugs such as Gantanol
Thiazide diuretics such as the water pills Diuril and HydroDIURIL
Thyroid medications such as Synthroid

Be careful about drinking alcohol, since excessive alcohol consumption can cause low blood sugar.

Special information
if you are pregnant or breastfeeding

The effects of Micronase during pregnancy have not been adequately studied in humans. This drug should be used during pregnancy only if the benefit outweighs the potential risk to the unborn baby. Since studies suggest the importance of maintaining normal blood sugar (glucose) levels during pregnancy, your physician may prescribe insulin injections during pregnancy.

While it is not known if Micronase appears in breast milk, other oral diabetes medications do. Therefore, women should discuss with their doctors whether to discontinue the medication or to stop breastfeeding. If the medication is discontinued, and if diet alone does not control glucose levels, then your doctor may consider insulin injections.

Recommended dosage
Your doctor will tailor your dosage to your individual needs.

ADULTS

Usually the doctor will prescribe an initial daily dose of 2.5 to 5 milligrams. Maintenance therapy usually ranges from 1.25 to 20 milligrams daily. Daily doses greater than 20 milligrams are not recommended. In most cases,

Micronase is taken once a day; however, people taking more than 10 milligrams a day may respond better to twice-a-day dosing.

CHILDREN

The safety and effectiveness of Micronase have not been established in children.

OLDER ADULTS

Older, malnourished or debilitated individuals, or those with impaired kidney and liver function, usually receive lower initial and maintenance doses to minimize the risk of low blood sugar (hypoglycemia).

Overdosage

An overdose of Micronase can cause low blood sugar (hypoglycemia).

- *Symptoms of severe hypoglycemia include:*
  Coma, pale skin, seizure, shallow breathing

If you suspect a Micronase overdose, seek medical attention immediately.

Brand name:

MICRONOR

See Oral Contraceptives, page 926.

Brand name:

MIDRIN

Pronounced: MID-rin
Generic ingredients: Isometheptene mucate,
  Dichloralphenazone, Acetaminophen

Why is this drug prescribed?

Midrin is prescribed for the treatment of tension headaches. It is also used to treat vascular headaches such as migraine.

Most important fact about this drug

Midrin can be used only after the headache starts. It does not prevent headaches.

How should you take this medication?

You should start taking Midrin at the first sign of a migraine attack.

Do not take more than the maximum dose of Midrin.

Take this medication exactly as prescribed by your doctor.

■ *If you miss a dose...*
Take this medication only as needed.

■ *Storage instructions...*
Store at room temperature in a dry place.

What side effects may occur?
Side effects cannot be anticipated. If any develop or change in intensity, tell your doctor immediately. Only your doctor can determine whether it is safe for you to continue taking Midrin.

■ *Side effects may include:*
Short periods of dizziness, skin rash

Why should this drug not be prescribed?
Unless directed to do so by your doctor, do not take Midrin if you have the eye condition called glaucoma or severe kidney disease, high blood pressure, a physical defect of the heart, or liver disease, or if you are currently taking antidepressant drugs known as MAO inhibitors, including Nardil and Parnate.

Special warnings about this medication
Take Midrin cautiously if you have high blood pressure or any abnormal condition of the blood vessels outside of the heart, or have recently had a cardiovascular attack such as a heart attack or stroke.

Possible food and drug interactions
when taking this medication
Avoid alcoholic beverages.

If Midrin is taken with certain other drugs, the effects of either drug could be increased, decreased, or altered. It is especially important to check with your doctor before combining Midrin with the following:

Acetaminophen-containing pain relievers such as Tylenol
Antidepressants classified as MAO inhibitors, including Nardil and
   Parnate
Antihistamines such as Benadryl
Central nervous system depressants such as Halcion, Valium and Xanax

Special information
if you are pregnant or breastfeeding
If you are pregnant, plan to become pregnant, or are breastfeeding your baby, check with your doctor before taking Midrin.

Recommended dosage

ADULTS

Relief of Migraine Headache
The usual dosage is 2 capsules at once, followed by 1 capsule every hour until the headache is relieved; do not take more than 5 capsules within a 12-hour period.

Relief of Tension Headache
The usual dosage is 1 or 2 capsules every 4 hours up to a maximum of 8 capsules a day.

Overdosage
Any medication taken in excess can have serious consequences. If you suspect a Midrin overdose, seek emergency medical treatment immediately.

Brand name:

MIGRANAL

Pronounced: MY-grah-nal
Generic name: Dihydroergotamine mesylate

Why is this drug prescribed?
Migranal Nasal Spray is used for relief of migraine headache attacks, whether or not preceded by an aura (visual disturbances, usually including sensations of halos or flickering lights).

This nasally administered remedy contains the same active ingredient as D.H.E. 45, an injectable form of the drug. It constricts the blood vessels, and may defeat migraine through this action.

Most important fact about this drug
Migranal Nasal Spray is for use only during a genuine attack of classic migraine. Do not attempt to prevent migraines with this drug, and do not use it for tension headaches, cluster headaches, or unusual types of migraine such as hemiplegic or basilar migraine.

How should you take this medication?

Migranal comes in single-dose ampuls, each with an accompanying nasal sprayer. Do not open an ampul until needed. Once opened, the drug must be used within 8 hours to be fully effective.

Take this medication at the first sign of a developing migraine. Assemble the ampul and sprayer according to package directions, pump the sprayer 4 times to prime it with medication, then spray once in each nostril. While spraying, do NOT tilt your head back or inhale through your nose. Wait 15 minutes, then spray once in each nostril again. After the second spray, discard the sprayer and the ampul's cap. To be prepared for the next attack, remember to load a new ampul and sprayer into the assembly case that comes with the medication.

Migranal will be effective even if you have a stuffy nose, a cold, or allergies.

■ *If you miss a dose...*
Migranal Nasal Spray is not for regular use. Use it only during a migraine attack.

■ *Storage instructions...*
Store at room temperature away from heat and light. Do not refrigerate or freeze.

What side effects may occur?
Side effects cannot be anticipated. If any develop or change in intensity, inform your doctor as soon as possible. Only your doctor can determine if it is safe for you to continue using Migranal Nasal Spray.

■ *More common side effects may include:*
Altered sense of taste, dizziness, drowsiness, nasal inflammation, nausea, sore throat, vomiting

■ *Less common side effects may include:*
Diarrhea, dry mouth, fatigue, hot flushes, loss of strength, sinus inflammation, stiffness, tingling sensation

■ *Rare side effects may include:*
Abdominal pain, altered sense of smell, cold clammy skin, confusion, conjunctivitis (pinkeye), cramps, decreased sensation, difficulty breathing, difficulty swallowing, earache, ear ringing, excessive muscle tone, feeling cold or ill, feeling of well-being, fever, hiccups, increased urination, increased sweating, impaired concentration, indigestion, insomnia, intoler-

ance to light, itching, lack of muscle tone, loss of voice, muscle aches, muscle weakness, nervousness, rapid or throbbing heartbeat, rash, red/purple blotches on the skin, respiratory tract infection, swelling, tearing abnormalities, tremor, vision abnormalities, yawning

Why should this drug not be prescribed?

Do not take Migranal if you have ever had an allergic reaction to an ergotamine-based drug such as the migraine remedies Cafergot, Ergostat, and D.H.E. 45 Injection, or the senility drug Hydergine.

You should avoid Migranal if you have certain types of heart or blood vessel disease, including angina (crushing chest pain) or a history of heart attack, or if you suffer from uncontrolled high blood pressure, severe kidney or liver disease, or a severe blood infection. Avoid it, too, if you have recently had blood vessel surgery.

Do not use Migranal within 24 hours of taking another ergotamine-based drug, another migraine remedy such as Amerge, Imitrex, Maxalt, or Zomig, or the migraine-preventing drug Sansert. Also avoid combining Migranal with other drugs that constrict the blood vessels, such as the decongestants pseudoephedrine and phenylpropanolamine found in many over-the-counter cold products.

Do not use Migranal Nasal Spray while pregnant or nursing.

Special warnings about this medication

If you have heart disease, Migranal could trigger a serious problem. Risk factors for this disorder include high blood pressure, high cholesterol, diabetes, a family history of heart disease, smoking, and passing menopause. Your doctor will probably want to observe your reaction to the first dose of Migranal if any of these factors apply.

Because Migranal constricts blood vessels, you should use it with caution if you have circulation problems in your arms, legs, fingers, or toes. Use it cautiously, too, if you are being treated for high blood pressure; it occasionally aggravates the problem.

Alert your doctor immediately if you have any of the following side effects: pain in the arms and legs, numbness or tingling in your fingers or toes, coldness, pallor, weakness in the legs, chest pain, temporary speeding or slowing of the heart rate, swelling, itching, or a bluish color in your fingers and toes.

Possible food and drug interactions
when taking this medication

If Migranal is taken with certain other drugs, the effects of either can be increased, decreased, or altered. Completely avoid other migraine remedies and ergotamine-based drugs, and check with your doctor before combining Migranal with the following:

Azithromycin (Zithromax)
Clarithromycin (Biaxin)
Erythromycin (Ery-Tab, Eryc)
Nicotine (from any source, including cigarettes, patches, or inhalers)
Phenylpropanolamine (Propagest)
Propranolol (Inderal)
Pseudoephedrine (Afrin, Sudafed)
Troleandomycin (Tao)

Special information
if you are pregnant or breastfeeding

Migranal can harm a developing baby; do not use it during pregnancy. Also avoid while breastfeeding. It appears in breast milk and may cause diarrhea, vomiting, weak pulse, and unstable blood pressure in a nursing infant.

Recommended dosage

ADULTS

Use one spray (0.5 milligram) in each nostril followed by another spray in each nostril 15 minutes later for a total of 4 sprays (2 milligrams).

Do not use more than 3 milligrams (6 sprays) in 24 hours or 4 milligrams (8 sprays) in 7 days.

Overdosage

Any medication taken in excess can have serious consequences. If you suspect an overdose, seek medical attention immediately.

■ *Symptoms of Migranal overdose may include:*
Abdominal pain, abnormal speech, coma, confusion, convulsions, hallucinations, increase and/or decrease in blood pressure, nausea, numbness, tingling, pain, and a bluish color of your fingers and toes, slowed breathing, vomiting

Brand name:

MILTOWN

Pronounced: MILL-town
Generic name: Meprobamate
Other brand name: Equanil

Why is this drug prescribed?
Miltown is a tranquilizer used in the treatment of anxiety disorders and for short-term relief of the symptoms of anxiety.

Most important fact about this drug
Miltown can be habit forming. You can develop tolerance and dependence, and you may experience withdrawal symptoms if you stop using this drug abruptly. Discontinue this drug or change your dose only on your doctor's advice.

How should you take this medication?
Take Miltown exactly as prescribed.

■ *If you miss a dose...*
Take it as soon as you remember if it is within an hour of your scheduled time. If you do not remember until later, skip the dose you missed and go back to your regular schedule. Never take 2 doses at the same time.

■ *Storage instructions...*
Store at room temperature in a tightly closed container.

What side effects may occur?
Side effects cannot be anticipated. If any develop or change in intensity, inform your doctor as soon as possible. Only your doctor can determine if it is safe for you to continue taking Miltown.

■ *More common side effects may include:*
Allergic reactions, blood disorders, bruises, diarrhea, dizziness, drowsiness, exaggerated feeling of well-being, fainting, fast throbbing heartbeat, fever, headache, inappropriate excitement, itchy rash, loss of muscle coordination, nausea, rapid or irregular heartbeat, skin eruptions, slurred speech, small, purplish spots on the skin, sudden severe drop in blood

pressure, swelling due to fluid retention, tingling sensation or numbness, vertigo, vision problems, vomiting, weakness

■ *Less common or rare side effects may include:*
Breathing difficulty, chills, high fever, inflammation of mouth, inflammation of the rectum, little or no urine, redness and swelling of skin, severe allergic reaction, skin inflammation and flaking, Stevens-Johnson syndrome (peeling skin)

■ *Side effects due to rapid decrease in dose or abrupt withdrawal from Miltown:*
Anxiety, confusion, convulsions, hallucinations, inability to fall or stay asleep, loss of appetite, loss of coordination, muscle twitching, tremors, vomiting

Withdrawal symptoms usually become apparent within 12 to 48 hours after discontinuation of this medication and should disappear in another 12 to 48 hours.

Why should this drug not be prescribed?
If you are sensitive to or have ever had an allergic reaction to Miltown or related drugs such as carisoprodol (Soma), you should not take this medication.

You should not take Miltown if you have acute intermittent porphyria, an inherited disease of the body's metabolism. It can make your symptoms worse.

Anxiety or tension related to everyday stress usually does not require treatment with Miltown. Discuss your symptoms thoroughly with your doctor.

Special warnings about this medication
If you develop a skin rash, sore throat, fever, or shortness of breath, contact your doctor immediately. You may be having an allergic reaction to the drug.

Miltown may cause you to become drowsy or less alert; therefore, you should not drive or operate dangerous machinery, or participate in any hazardous activity that requires full mental alertness until you know how this drug affects you.

Long-term use of this drug should be evaluated by your doctor periodically for its usefulness.

If you have liver or kidney disorders, make sure your doctor is aware of these conditions before you begin using this medication.

If you have epilepsy, use of this drug may bring on seizures. Consult your doctor before taking it.

**Possible food and drug interactions
when taking this medication**

Miltown may intensify the effects of alcohol. Do not drink alcohol while taking this medication.

If Miltown is taken with certain other drugs, the effects of either could be increased, decreased, or altered. It is especially important to check with your doctor before combining Miltown with mood-altering drugs and central nervous system depressants such as the following:

  Antidepressant drugs such as Elavil, Nardil, and Tofranil
  Barbiturates such as Seconal and phenobarbital
  Major tranquilizers such as Thorazine and Mellaril
  Narcotics such as Percocet or Demerol
  Tranquilizers such as Halcion, Restoril, and Valium

**Special information
if you are pregnant or breastfeeding**

Do not take Miltown if you are pregnant or planning to become pregnant. There is an increased risk of birth defects. Miltown appears in breast milk and could affect a nursing infant. If this medication is essential to your health, your doctor may advise you to discontinue breastfeeding until your treatment is finished.

Recommended dosage

ADULTS

The usual dosage is 1,200 milligrams to 1,600 milligrams per day divided into 3 or 4 doses. You should not take more than 2,400 milligrams a day.

CHILDREN

The usual dose for children 6 to 12 years of age is 200 to 600 milligrams per day divided into 2 or 3 doses.

Miltown is not recommended for children under age 6.

OLDER ADULTS

Your doctor will limit your dose to the smallest effective amount to avoid oversedation.

Overdosage
Any medication taken in excess can cause symptoms of overdose. If you suspect an overdose, seek emergency medical attention immediately.

■ *The symptoms of Miltown overdose may include:*
Coma, drowsiness, loss of muscle control, severely impaired breathing, shock, sluggishness, and unresponsiveness

Brand name:

MINIPRESS

Pronounced: MIN-ee-press
Generic name: Prazosin hydrochloride

Why is this drug prescribed?
Minipress is used to treat high blood pressure. It is effective used alone or with other high blood pressure medications such as diuretics or beta-blocking medications (drugs that ease heart contractions) such as Tenormin.

Minipress is also prescribed for the treatment of benign prostatic hyperplasia (BPH), an abnormal enlargement of the prostate gland.

Most important fact about this drug
If you have high blood pressure, you must take Minipress regularly for it to be effective. Since blood pressure declines gradually, it may be several weeks before you get the full benefit of Minipress; and you must continue taking it even if you are feeling well. Minipress does not cure high blood pressure; it merely keeps it under control.

How should you take this medication?
Minipress can be taken with or without food.

This medication should be taken exactly as prescribed by your doctor even if your symptoms have disappeared. Try not to miss any doses. If this medication is not taken regularly, your blood pressure will increase.

■ *If you miss a dose...*
Take it as soon as you remember. If it is almost time for your next dose, skip the one you missed and go back to your regular schedule. Never take 2 doses at the same time.

■ *Storage instructions...*
Protect from heat, light, and moisture.

What side effects may occur?

Side effects cannot be anticipated. If any develop or change in intensity, inform your doctor as soon as possible. Only your doctor can determine if it is safe for you to continue taking Minipress.

■ *More common side effects may include:*
Dizziness, drowsiness, headache, lack of energy, nausea, palpitations (pounding heartbeat), weakness

■ *Less common side effects may include:*
Blurred vision, constipation, depression, diarrhea, dizziness on standing up, dry mouth, fainting, fluid retention, frequent urination, nasal congestion, nervousness, nosebleeds, rash, red eyes, shortness of breath, vertigo, vomiting

■ *Rare side effects may include:*
Abdominal discomfort/pain, excessive perspiration, fever, hair loss, hallucinations, impotence, inability to hold urine, inflammation of the pancreas, itching, itchy purple spots on wrists, forearms, and thighs, joint pain, persistent, painful erection, rapid heartbeat, ringing in ears, tingling or pins and needles

Why should this drug not be prescribed?

There are no known reasons to avoid this drug.

Special warnings about this medication

Minipress can cause low blood pressure, especially when you first start taking the medication. This can cause you to become faint, dizzy, or light-headed, particularly on standing up. You should avoid driving or any hazardous tasks where injury could occur for 24 hours after taking the first dose or after your dose has been increased. Dizziness, fainting, or light-headedness may also occur in hot weather, when exercising, or when standing for long periods of time. Ask your doctor what precautions you should take.

Possible food and drug interactions
when taking this medication

Minipress can intensify the effects of alcohol. Be careful of the amount you drink.

If Minipress is taken with certain other drugs, the effects of either could be increased, decreased, or altered. It is especially important that you check with your doctor before combining Minipress with the following:

Beta blockers such as Inderal
Dextroamphetamine (Dexedrine)
Diuretics such as Dyazide
Ibuprofen (Motrin, Advil, others)
Other high blood pressure medications
Verapamil (Calan, Verelan)

Special information
if you are pregnant or breastfeeding

The effects of Minipress during pregnancy have not been adequately studied. If you are pregnant or plan to become pregnant, notify your doctor immediately. Minipress appears in breast milk and can affect a nursing infant. If this medication is essential to your health, your doctor may advise you to discontinue breastfeeding until your treatment is finished.

Recommended dosage

ADULTS

Dosages of this drug should be adjusted by your doctor according to your response.

The usual starting dose is 1 milligram, 2 or 3 times per day.

To determine your regular dose, your doctor may slowly increase this medication to as much as 20 milligrams per day, divided into smaller doses. The commonly prescribed daily dose is 6 milligrams to 15 milligrams per day, divided into smaller doses. Although doses higher than 20 milligrams per day have not been found to be effective, there are some people who may benefit from a daily dose of 40 milligrams, divided into smaller doses.

If Minipress is used with a diuretic or other high blood pressure drug, the dose can be reduced to 1 to 2 milligrams, 3 times a day.

CHILDREN

Safety and effectiveness of this drug have not been established in children.

Overdosage

Any medication taken in excess can have serious consequences. If you suspect a Minipress overdose, seek medical treatment immediately.

- *The symptoms of Minipress overdose may include:*
  Extreme drowsiness, low blood pressure

Brand name:

MINOCIN

Pronounced: MIN-o-sin
Generic name: Minocycline hydrochloride
Other brand name: Dynacin

Why is this drug prescribed?
Minocin is a form of the antibiotic tetracycline.

It is given to help treat many different kinds of infection, including:

Acne
Amebic dysentery
Anthrax (a rare skin infection)
Cholera
Gonorrhea (when penicillin cannot be given)
Plague
Respiratory infections such as pneumonia
Rocky Mountain spotted fever
Syphilis (when penicillin cannot be given)
Urinary tract infections caused by certain microbes

Most important fact about this drug
To help clear up your infection completely, keep taking Minocin for the full time of treatment, even if you begin to feel better after a few days. Minocin, like other antibiotics, works best when there is a constant amount in the body. To help keep the level constant, take the doses at evenly spaced times around the clock.

How should you take this medication?
You may take Minocin with or without food. Take Minocin exactly as directed. Your doctor will prescribe it for a specific number of days according to the type of infection being treated; keep taking the medication until you have used it all up.

To reduce the risk of throat irritation, take the capsule form of Minocin with plenty of fluids.

You should avoid use of antacids that contain aluminum, calcium, or magnesium, such as Maalox and Mylanta, and iron preparations such as Feosol. If you must take these medicines, take them 2 to 3 hours before or after taking Minocin.

- *If you miss a dose...*
  Take it as soon as you remember, then space out evenly any remaining doses for that day. Never take 2 doses at the same time.

- *Storage instructions...*
  Store capsules and liquid at room temperature. Keep capsules away from moist places and direct light. Do not freeze the liquid.

What side effects may occur?
Side effects cannot be anticipated. If any develop or change in intensity, inform your doctor as soon as possible. Only your doctor can determine if it is safe for you to continue taking Minocin.

- *Side effects may include:*
  Aching, inflamed joints, anal or genital sores with fungus infection, anaphylaxis (life-threatening allergic reaction), anemia, appetite loss, blurry vision, bulging of soft spots in infants' heads, decreased hearing, diarrhea, difficulty swallowing, discoloration of children's teeth, fever, fluid retention, headache, hepatitis, hives, inflammation of the penis, inflammation of the intestines, inflammation of the tongue, joint pain, kidney or liver failure, nausea, rash, sensitivity to light, skin coloration, skin eruptions, skin inflammation and peeling, throat irritation, thyroid gland problems, vomiting

Why should this drug not be prescribed?
Do not take Minocin if you have ever had an allergic reaction to it or to any other tetracycline antibiotic.

Although Minocin may be given to kill meningococcal (spinal) bacteria in people who are carriers, it should not be given to treat actual meningococcal meningitis (inflammation in the spinal canal).

Minocin is not a first-choice drug for treating any staphylococcal ("staph") infection.

Special warnings about this medication
If you have a kidney problem, a normal dose of Minocin may amount to an overdose for you. It is likely that you will need a lower-than-average dosage; if you need to take Minocin for an extended period of time, your doctor may order frequent blood tests to make sure you are not getting too much of the drug.

Because Minocin may make you dizzy or light-headed or cause a whirling feeling, do not drive, climb, or perform hazardous tasks until you know how the medication affects you.

Minocin should not be given to children 8 years old or younger, since it may cause discoloration of the teeth. Occasionally, Minocin has also caused tooth discoloration in adults.

Like other tetracycline antibiotics, Minocin may cause a sensitivity to light, and you may sunburn very easily. Be careful in sun and under sunlamps. If your skin turns red and hot, stop taking Minocin immediately.

While taking Minocin you may be especially susceptible to infections, including fungus infections such as vaginal yeast infection. If you do get an infection, check with your doctor immediately.

If you get a headache and blurry vision while taking Minocin, or if an infant receiving Minocin develops bulging of the "soft spots" (fontanels) on the head, this could mean that the drug is causing a buildup of fluid within the skull. It is important to stop taking Minocin and see a doctor immediately.

Minocin liquid contains a sulfite that can cause severe allergic reactions in susceptible people.

Possible food and drug interactions
when taking this medication

If Minocin is taken with certain other drugs, the effects of either could be increased, decreased, or altered. It is especially important to check with your doctor before combining Minocin with the following:

Antacids containing aluminum, calcium, or magnesium, such as Mylanta
Blood thinners such as Coumadin
Iron-containing preparations such as Feosol
Oral contraceptives
Penicillin (Pen-Vee K)

Special information
if you are pregnant or breastfeeding

If you are pregnant or plan to become pregnant, inform your doctor immediately. If you take Minocin during the second half of pregnancy, it may cause permanent yellow, gray, or brown discoloration of your baby's teeth.

There is reason to believe that taking Minocin during pregnancy could also harm the baby in other ways. Therefore, Minocin should be taken during pregnancy only if an antibiotic is clearly needed and only if a non-tetracycline antibiotic cannot be used instead. Because Minocin appears in breast milk and could harm the baby, it should not be taken by a woman who is breastfeeding. If this drug is essential to your health, your doctor may advise you to discontinue breastfeeding until treatment is finished.

Recommended dosage

ADULTS

The usual dosage of Minocin is 200 milligrams to start with, followed by 100 milligrams every 12 hours. If you need to take more frequent doses, your doctor may prescribe two or four 50-milligram capsules initially, and then one 50-milligram capsule 4 times daily.

The dosage and the length of time you take the drug can vary according to your condition and the specific infection.

CHILDREN ABOVE 8 YEARS OF AGE

The usual dosage of Minocin is 4 milligrams per 2.2 pounds of body weight to start, followed by 2 milligrams per 2.2 pounds every 12 hours.

Overdosage

Although no specific information is available, any medication taken in excess can have serious consequences. If you suspect symptoms of an overdose of Minocin, seek medical attention immediately.

Generic name:

MINOCYCLINE

See Minocin, page 810.

Brand name:

MIRAPEX

Pronounced: MERE-a-pecks
Generic name: Pramipexole dihydrochloride

Why is this drug prescribed?

Although it is not a cure, Mirapex eases the symptoms of Parkinson's disease—a progressive disorder marked by muscle rigidity, weakness, shaking, tremor, and eventually difficulty with walking and talking. Parkinson's disease results from a shortage of the chemical messenger dopamine in certain areas of the brain. Mirapex is believed to work by boosting the action of whatever dopamine is available. The drug can be used with other Parkinson's medications such as Eldepryl, Sinemet, and Larodopa.

Most important fact about this drug

If you are taking Sinemet or Larodopa, Mirapex may allow a reduction in your dosage. And if you suffer from the "on-off" effect that often develops during

Parkinson's therapy (symptom-free periods alternating with severe attacks), Mirapex may extend the good "on" times and shorten your "off" periods.

How should you take this medication?
Take Mirapex exactly as prescribed. If it makes you nauseous, try taking it with food.

When discontinuing Mirapex therapy, it's best to do it gradually. Your doctor will tell you how to taper your dose over a week's time.

■ *If you miss a dose...*
Take it as soon as you remember. If it is almost time for your next dose, skip the one you missed and go back to your regular schedule. Do not take 2 doses at the same time.

■ *Storage instructions...*
Store at room temperature; protect from light.

What side effects may occur?
Side effects cannot be anticipated. If any develop or change in intensity, inform your doctor as soon as possible. Only your doctor can determine if it is safe for you to continue taking Mirapex.

■ *More common side effects may include:*
Abnormal dreams, arthritis, chest pain, confusion, constipation, decreased sensitivity to touch, difficulty breathing, difficulty walking, dizziness, dizziness upon standing, drowsiness, dry mouth, hallucinations, increased muscle tone, increased urination, insomnia, involuntary movement (jerky motions), lack of appetite, memory loss, nasal inflammation, nausea, swelling, urinary tract infections, vision abnormalities, weakness

■ *Less common side effects may include:*
Decreased sex drive, delusions, difficulty swallowing, fever, general feeling of illness, impotence, inability to hold urine, muscle spasms or twitching, pneumonia, skin disorders, thinking abnormalities, uncontrollable restlessness, weight loss

■ *Rare side effects may include:*
Abnormal ejaculation, abnormal heartbeat, agitation, blood clots, blood in urine, blood circulation problems, convulsions, difficult or painful urination, enlarged abdomen, eye disorders, heart attack, heart problems, joint problems, lung problems, mental illness, muscular problems, prostate problems, severe chest pain (angina), thirst

Why should this drug not be prescribed?
If Mirapex gives you an allergic reaction, you'll be unable to use it.

Special warnings about this drug
Mirapex can cause your blood pressure to drop when you first stand up, resulting in symptoms such as dizziness, nausea, fainting, blackouts, and, sometimes, sweating. To avoid or reduce these symptoms, try to stand up slowly, especially at the beginning of treatment with Mirapex.

Mirapex can cause drowsiness and may trigger hallucinations, especially if you are over 65 or have an advanced case of Parkinson's. Do not drive a car or operate complex machinery until you know how Mirapex affects your performance. Be especially cautious when taking other drugs that cause sleepiness.

If you have a kidney condition, make sure the doctor is aware of it. You'll probably need regular blood tests to check your kidney function, and your dosage of Mirapex may have to be reduced.

In very rare cases, Mirapex may cause muscle wasting. If you develop muscle aches or soreness after you start Mirapex, be sure to tell your doctor. Also alert your doctor if you notice any changes in your eyesight.

Possible food and drug interactions
when taking this medication
If Mirapex is taken with certain other drugs, the effects of either could be increased, decreased, or altered. It is especially important to check with your doctor before combining Mirapex with the following:

Carbidopa/Levodopa (Sinemet)
Cimetidine (Tagamet)
Diltiazem (Cardizem, Dilacor XR)
Major tranquilizers such as Compazine, Haldol, Mellaril, Navane, Prolixin, Stelazine, and Thorazine
Metoclopramide (Reglan)
Quinidine (Quinidex, Quinaglute)
Quinine
Ranitidine (Zantac)
Sedatives and tranquilizers such as chloral hydrate, codeine products, Dalmane, Halcion, and phenobarbital
Triamterene (Dyrenium)
Verapamil (Calan, Isoptin)

Combining Mirapex with Sinemet or Larodopa sometimes triggers twitching and jerky movements. If this happens, tell your doctor. A reduction in your dose of Sinemet or Larodopa may solve the problem.

Special information
if you are pregnant or breastfeeding

The effects of Mirapex during pregnancy have not been adequately studied, so it's best to avoid it if you're expecting. If you are pregnant or plan to become pregnant, inform your doctor immediately.

It is not known whether Mirapex appears in breast milk. If the drug is considered essential to your health, your doctor may advise you to stop breastfeeding while taking the medication.

Recommended dosage

ADULTS

The usual starting dose is 0.125 milligrams 3 times a day. If necessary, your doctor may increase the dose every 5 to 7 days until the maximum dose of 4.5 milligrams a day is reached. Dosage is usually increased gradually to minimize the drug's potential side effects. If you have kidney disease, the doctor will keep the dosage quite low.

CHILDREN

The safety and effectiveness of this drug in children have not been established.

Overdosage

Researchers have had no experience with a massive overdose of Mirapex. However, any medication taken in excess can have dangerous consequences. If you suspect an overdose, seek medical attention immediately.

Generic name:

MIRTAZAPINE

See Remeron, page 1105.

Generic name:

MISOPROSTOL

See Cytotec, page 325.

Brand name:

MODICON

See Oral Contraceptives, page 926.

Brand name:

MODURETIC

Pronounced: mod-your-ET-ik
Generic ingredients: Amiloride, Hydrochlorothiazide

Why is this drug prescribed?

Moduretic is a diuretic combination used in the treatment of high blood pressure and congestive heart failure, conditions which require the elimination of excess fluid (water) from the body. When used for high blood pressure, Moduretic can be used alone or with other high blood pressure medications. Diuretics help your body produce and eliminate more urine, which helps lower blood pressure. Amiloride, one of the ingredients, helps minimize the potassium loss that can be caused by the other component, hydrochlorothiazide.

Most important fact about this drug

If you have high blood pressure, you must take Moduretic regularly for it to be effective. Since blood pressure declines gradually, it may be several weeks before you get the full benefit of Moduretic; and you must continue taking it even if you are feeling well. Moduretic does not cure high blood pressure; it merely keeps it under control.

How should you take this medication?

Take this medication with food.

Take Moduretic exactly as prescribed by your doctor. Stopping Moduretic suddenly could cause your condition to worsen.

■ *If you miss a dose...*
Take the forgotten dose as soon as you remember. If it is almost time for your next dose, skip the one you missed and go back to your regular schedule. Never take a double dose.

■ *Storage instructions...*
Store at room temperature. Keep this medication in the container it came in, tightly closed, and protected from moisture, light, and freezing.

What side effects may occur?
Side effects cannot be anticipated. If any develop or change in intensity, inform your doctor as soon as possible. Only your doctor can determine if it is safe for you to continue taking Moduretic.

■ *More common side effects may include:*
Diarrhea, dizziness, elevated potassium levels, fatigue, headache, irregular heartbeat, itching, leg pain, loss of appetite, nausea, rash, shortness of breath, stomach and intestinal pain, weakness

■ *Less common or rare side effects may include:*
Anemia, appetite changes, back pain, bad taste, breast development in males, changes in liver function, changes in potassium levels leading to symptoms such as dry mouth, excessive thirst, weak or irregular heartbeat, muscle pain or cramps, chest pain, constipation, cough, decreased sex drive, dehydration, depression, dermatitis, dizziness on standing up, dry mouth, excessive perspiration, excessive urination at night, fainting, fever, fluid in lungs, flushing, frequent urination, fullness in abdomen, gas, gout, hair loss, heartburn, hiccups, hives, impotence, incontinence, indigestion, insomnia, itching, joint pain, mental confusion, muscle cramps, nasal congestion, neck and shoulder ache, nervousness, numbness, painful or difficult urination, rapid heartbeat, ringing in ears, sensitivity to light, sleepiness, Stevens-Johnson syndrome (severe blisters), stomach and intestinal bleeding, stupor, sugar in blood or urine, thirst, tingling or pins and needles, tremors, vague feeling of bodily discomfort, vertigo, vision changes, vomiting, yellow eyes and skin

Why should this drug not be prescribed?
If you are unable to urinate or have serious kidney disease, or if you have high potassium levels in your blood, you should not take this medication.

If you are sensitive to or have ever had an allergic reaction to amiloride, hydrochlorothiazide or similar drugs, or if you are sensitive to other sulfonamide-derived drugs, you should not take this medication. Make sure your doctor is aware of any drug reactions you may have experienced.

Special warnings about this medication
Potassium supplements, potassium-containing salt substitutes, and other diuretics (such as Dyazide) that minimize loss of potassium should not be used while you are taking Moduretic unless your doctor specifically says

otherwise. You should also limit your consumption of potassium-rich foods such as bananas, prunes, raisins, orange juice, and whole and skim milk. Ask your doctor for advice on how much of these foods to consume.

If you are taking Moduretic, a complete assessment of your kidney function should be done; kidney function should continue to be monitored.

If you are taking an ACE-inhibitor type of blood pressure medication such as Vasotec, this drug should be used with extreme caution.

If you have liver disease, diabetes, gout, or collagen vascular disease (lupus erythematosus), Moduretic should be used with caution.

If you have bronchial asthma or a history of allergies, you may be at risk for an allergic reaction to this medication.

Dehydration, excessive sweating, severe diarrhea or vomiting could deplete your fluids and cause your blood pressure to become too low. Be careful when exercising and in hot weather.

Notify your doctor or dentist that you are taking Moduretic if you have a medical emergency or before you have surgery.

Possible food and drug interactions
when taking this medication
Moduretic may increase the effects of alcohol. Avoid alcohol while taking this medication.

If Moduretic is taken with certain other drugs, the effects of either could be increased, decreased, or altered. It is especially important to check with your doctor before combining Moduretic with the following:

ACE inhibitors such as Vasotec
Barbiturates such as phenobarbital
Cholestyramine (Questran)
Colestipol (Colestid)
Corticosteroids such as prednisone
Insulin
Lithium (Lithonate)
Muscle relaxants such as tubocurarine
Narcotics such as Percocet
Nonsteroidal anti-inflammatory drugs such as Naprosyn
Norepinephrine (Levophed)
Oral drugs for treating diabetes such as Micronase, DiaBeta
Other high blood pressure medications

Special information
if you are pregnant or breastfeeding

The effects of Moduretic during pregnancy have not been adequately studied. If you are pregnant or plan to become pregnant, inform your doctor immediately. Moduretic appears in breast milk and could affect a nursing infant. If this medication is essential to your health, your doctor may advise you to discontinue breastfeeding until your treatment is finished.

Recommended dosage

Your doctor will tailor the dosage to meet your individual requirements, taking into consideration other medical conditions you may have and other medications you may be taking.

ADULTS

The usual starting dose is 1 tablet per day, which may be increased to 2 tablets per day taken at the same time or separately.

CHILDREN

The safety and effectiveness of Moduretic have not been established in children.

Overdosage

Any medication taken in excess can cause symptoms of overdose. If you suspect an overdose, seek medical attention immediately.

No specific information on symptoms of Moduretic overdose is available, but dehydration might be expected.

Generic name:

MOEXIPRIL

See Univasc, page 1377.

Generic name:

MOEXIPRIL WITH HYDROCHLOROTHIAZIDE

See Uniretic, page 1372.

Generic name:

MOMETASONE

See Elocon, page 467.

Brand name:

MONISTAT

Pronounced: MON-ih-stat
Generic name: Miconazole nitrate

Why is this drug prescribed?
Monistat is available in several formulations, including Monistat 3 vaginal suppositories, Monistat 7 vaginal cream and suppositories, and Monistat-Derm skin cream. Monistat's active ingredient, Miconazole, fights fungal infections.

Monistat 3 and Monistat 7 are used for vaginal yeast infections. Monistat-Derm is used for skin infections such as athlete's foot, ringworm, jock itch, yeast infection on the skin (cutaneous candidiasis), and tinea versicolor (a common skin condition that produces patches of white, tan, or brown finely flaking skin over the neck and trunk).

Most important fact about this drug
Keep using this medicine regularly for the full time of the treatment, even if the infection seems to have disappeared. If you stop too soon, the infections could return. You should continue using the vaginal forms of the medicine even during your menstrual period.

How should you use this medication?
Use this medication exactly as prescribed.

Keep all forms of this medicine away from your eyes.

Before applying Monistat-Derm to your skin, be sure to wash your hands. Massage the medication gently into the affected area and the surrounding skin.

If you are using the vaginal cream or suppository, follow these steps:

1. Load the applicator to the fill line with cream, or unwrap a tablet, wet it with warm water, and place it in the applicator as shown in the instructions you received with the product.
2. Lie on your back with your knees drawn up.
3. Gently insert the application high into the vagina and push the plunger.
4. Withdraw the applicator and discard it if disposable, or wash with soap and water.

To keep the vaginal medication from getting on your clothing, wear a sanitary napkin. Do not use tampons because they will absorb the medicine. Wear cotton underwear—avoid synthetic fabrics such as rayon or nylon. Do not douche unless your doctor tells you to do so.

Dry the genital area thoroughly after a shower, bath, or swim. Change out of a wet bathing suit or damp workout clothes as soon as possible. Yeast is less likely to flourish in a dry environment.

Do not scratch if you can help it. Scratching can cause more irritation and can spread the infection.

■ *If you miss a dose...*
Make up for it as soon as you remember. However, if it is almost time for your next dose, skip the one you missed and go back to your regular schedule.

■ *Storage instructions...*
Store at room temperature.

What side effects may occur?
Side effects cannot be anticipated. If any develop or change in intensity, inform your doctor. Only your doctor can determine whether it is safe for you to continue taking Monistat.

■ *Side effects may include:*
Burning sensation, cramping, headaches, hives, irritation, rash, vulval or vaginal itching

Why should this drug not be prescribed?
If you have ever had an allergic reaction to or are sensitive to miconazole nitrate, you should not use this medication. Make sure your doctor is aware of any drug reactions you have experienced.

Special warnings about this medication
If symptoms persist, or if an irritation or allergic reaction develops while you are using Monistat, notify your doctor.

The hydrogenated vegetable oil base of Monistat 3 may interact with the latex in vaginal diaphragms, so concurrent use of these two products is not recommended.

Your doctor may recommend Monistat 7 Vaginal Cream if you are using a diaphragm. However, you should be aware that the mineral oil in the vaginal cream can weaken the latex in condoms and diaphragms, making them less reliable for prevention of pregnancy or sexually transmitted disease.

If you are using Monistat 3 or Monistat 7 suppositories, you should either avoid sexual intercourse or make sure your partner uses a condom.

Do not give Monistat 7 to girls less than 12 years of age. Also avoid using Monistat 7 if you have any of the following symptoms:

Fever above 100°F orally
Foul-smelling vaginal discharge
Pain in the lower abdomen, back, or either shoulder

If these symptoms develop while you are using Monistat 7, stop treatment and contact your doctor right away. You may have a more serious infection.

If the infection fails to improve or worsens within 3 days, or you do not obtain complete relief within 7 days, or symptoms return within two months, you may have something other than a yeast infection.

**Possible food and drug interactions
when taking this medication**
No interactions have been reported.

**Special information
if you are pregnant or breastfeeding**
Unless you are directed to do so by your doctor, do not use Monistat during the first trimester (three months) of pregnancy because it is absorbed in small amounts from the vagina. It is not known whether miconazole appears in breast milk. If Monistat is essential to your health, your doctor may advise you to discontinue breastfeeding until your treatment with this medication is finished.

Recommended dosage

MONISTAT-7 VAGINAL CREAM

The usual daily dose is 1 applicatorful inserted into the vagina at bedtime for 7 consecutive days.

MONISTAT-7 VAGINAL SUPPOSITORIES

The usual daily dose is 1 suppository inserted into the vagina at bedtime for 7 consecutive days.

MONISTAT-DERM

For jock itch, ringworm, athlete's foot, or yeast infection of the skin, apply a thin layer of Monistat-Derm over the affected area morning and night. For tinea versicolor, apply a thin layer over the affected area once daily.

Overdosage
Overdose of Monistat has not been reported. However, any medication used in excess can have serious consequences. If you suspect an overdose, seek medical attention immediately.

Brand name:

MONOKET

See Imdur, page 615.

Brand name:

MONOPRIL

Pronounced: MON-oh-prill
Generic name: Fosinopril sodium

Why is this drug prescribed?
Monopril is a high blood pressure medication known as an ACE inhibitor. It is effective when used alone or in combination with other medications for the treatment of high blood pressure. Monopril is also prescribed for heart failure.

Monopril works by preventing the conversion of a chemical in your blood called angiotensin I into a more potent substance that increases salt and water retention in your body. Monopril also enhances blood flow in your circulatory system.

Most important fact about this drug
You must take Monopril regularly for it to be effective. Since blood pressure declines gradually, it may be several weeks before you get the full benefit of Monopril; and you must continue taking it even if you are feeling well. Monopril does not cure high blood pressure; it merely keeps it under control.

How should you take this medication?
Monopril is best taken 1 hour before meals; but it can be taken with food if it upsets your stomach.

Take this medication exactly as prescribed by your doctor.

■ *If you miss a dose...*
Suddenly stopping Monopril could cause your blood pressure to increase. If you forget to take a dose, take it as soon as you remember. If it is almost time for your next dose, skip the one you missed and go back to your regular schedule. Never take 2 doses at the same time.

■ *Storage instructions...*
Store Monopril at room temperature in a tightly closed container to protect the medication from moisture.

What side effects may occur?
Side effects cannot be anticipated. If any develop or change in intensity, inform your doctor as soon as possible. Only your doctor can determine if it is safe for you to continue taking Monopril.

WHEN TAKEN FOR HIGH BLOOD PRESSURE

■ *More common side effects may include:*
Cough, dizziness, nausea, vomiting

■ *Less common or rare side effects may include:*
Abdominal pain, anaphylaxis (severe allergic reaction), changes in appetite and weight, changes in sexual performance, confusion, constipation, decreased sex drive, diarrhea, drowsiness, dry mouth, excessive sweating, eye irritation, fatigue, gas, headache, heartburn, itching, kidney failure, liver failure, muscle cramps, rash, ringing in ears, skin sensitivity to sunlight, sleep disturbances, tremors, vertigo, vision disturbances, weakness, yellow eyes and skin

WHEN TAKEN FOR HEART FAILURE

■ *More common side effects may include:*
Cough, dizziness, low blood pressure, muscle and bone pain

■ *Less common or rare side effects may include:*
Abnormal breathing, arm or leg weakness, behavior change, bronchitis, chest pain, constipation, decreased appetite, depression, diarrhea, distended abdomen, dry mouth, excessive sweating, fainting, fever, flu, fluid retention/swelling, gas, gout, heart rhythm disturbances, high blood pressure, itching, kidney pain, light-headedness on standing up, muscle ache, nasal inflammation, nausea, numbness, pain, pins and needles, rapid or slow heartbeat, sensation of cold, sexual problems, shock, sinus problems, speaking abnormality, stoppage of breathing/heart, stroke, swelling in legs or arms, taste disturbance, tremor, upper respiratory infection, urinary problems, vertigo, vision problems, vomiting, weakness, weight gain

Why should this drug not be prescribed?
If you are sensitive to or have ever had an allergic reaction to Monopril or other ACE inhibitors such as Capoten, you should not take this medication. Make sure that your doctor is aware of any drug reactions that you have experienced.

Special warnings about this medication
If you develop a sore throat or fever, you should contact your doctor immediately. It could indicate a more serious illness.

If you develop swelling of your face, lips, tongue or throat, or arms and legs, or have difficulty swallowing, you should contact your doctor immediately. You may need emergency treatment.

Make sure your doctor knows about any kidney or liver problems you may have. If you notice your skin or the whites of your eyes turning yellow, stop taking Monopril and contact your doctor immediately.

Your kidney function should be monitored while you are taking Monopril for either high blood pressure or heart failure. If you have heart failure and your kidneys are not functioning properly, you may develop low blood pressure. Also, certain blood tests may be needed if you have a disease of the connective tissue.

If you are taking high doses of a diuretic along with Monopril, you may develop excessively low blood pressure.

You may experience light-headedness while taking Monopril, especially during the first few days of therapy. If this occurs, notify your doctor. If you actually faint, discontinue the use of this medication and notify your doctor immediately.

Do not use potassium-containing salt substitutes without consulting your doctor.

If you have heart failure, this drug should be started under close medical supervision. Your doctor should continue to monitor your progress for the first 2 weeks of treatment and whenever your dosage is increased.

Excessive sweating, dehydration, severe diarrhea, or vomiting could lead to excessive loss of water and cause your blood pressure to drop dangerously. Take precautions to avoid excessive water loss while exercising.

This drug should be used with caution if you are on dialysis. There have been reports of extreme allergic reactions during dialysis in people taking ACE inhibitors such as Monopril. There have also been reports of severe allergic reactions in people given bee or wasp venom to protect against stings.

Possible food and drug interactions
when taking this medication

If Monopril is taken with certain other drugs, the effects of either could be increased, decreased, or altered. It is especially important to check with your doctor before combining Monopril with the following:

Antacids such as Mylanta and Maalox
Lithium (Eskalith, Lithonate)
Potassium preparations such as K+10 and K-Lyte
Potassium-sparing diuretics such as Moduretic and Aldactone
Thiazide diuretics such as Esidrix and Diuril

Special information
if you are pregnant or breastfeeding

ACE inhibitors such as Monopril have been shown to cause injury and even death in the developing baby when used in pregnancy during the second or third trimesters. If you are pregnant your doctor should discontinue the use of this medication as soon as possible. If you plan to become pregnant and are taking Monopril, contact your doctor immediately to discuss the potential hazard to your unborn child. Monopril appears in breast milk and could affect a nursing infant. If this medication is essential to your health, your doctor may advise you to discontinue breastfeeding until your treatment with this medication is finished.

Recommended dosage

ADULTS

High Blood Pressure
The usual initial dose is 10 milligrams, taken once a day, either alone or when added to a diuretic. Dosage, after blood pressure is adjusted, should be

20 to 40 milligrams a day in a single dose. For some patients, the doctor may divide the daily total into several smaller doses.

Diuretic use should, if possible, be stopped before using Monopril. If not, your physician may give an initial dose of 10 milligrams under supervision before any further medication is prescribed.

Heart Failure

The usual starting dose is 10 milligrams once a day, with diuretics and possibly digitalis. Your doctor will gradually increase the dose to one that works for you—usually between 20 milligrams daily and the maximum dose of 40 milligrams per day. If your kidneys are impaired you will probably start with a dose of 5 milligrams.

CHILDREN

The safety and effectiveness of Monopril have not been established in children.

Overdosage

Any medication taken in excess can have serious consequences. If you suspect an overdose, seek medical attention immediately.

The primary effect of a Monopril overdose is likely to be a sudden drop in blood pressure.

Generic name:

MONTELUKAST

See Singulair, page 1204.

Brand name:

MONUROL

Pronounced: MON-your-all
Generic name: Fosfomycin tromethamine

Why is this drug prescribed?

Monurol is an antibiotic used to treat bladder infections (cystitis) in women.

Most important fact about this drug
You need take only one dose of Monurol. Additional doses won't speed a cure, but will make side effects more likely. If your symptoms do not improve in 2 to 3 days, contact your physician.

How should you take this medication?
Monurol is packaged in a sachet, which contains granules of the drug. Open the sachet and pour the contents in 3 or 4 ounces (half a cup) of cold water, stir to dissolve, and drink immediately. Do not use hot water. Do not take the drug in its dry form. The solution can be taken with or without food.

■ *If you miss a dose...*
Only one dose is needed.

■ *Storage instructions...*
Store at room temperature.

What side effects may occur?
Side effects cannot be anticipated. If any develop or change in intensity, inform your doctor as soon as possible. Only your doctor can determine if it is safe for you to continue taking Monurol.

■ *More common side effects may include:*
Diarrhea, headache, nausea, vaginal inflammation

■ *Less common side effects may include:*
Dizziness, indigestion, weakness

Why should this drug not be prescribed?
If you have an allergic reaction to Monurol, avoid it in the future. It is used only for bladder infections, not for infections of the kidney (pyelonephritis).

Special warnings about this medication
Call your doctor if symptoms fail to improve within 2 to 3 days. You may need a different prescription.

**Possible food and drug interactions
when taking this medication**
Check with your doctor before combining Monurol with Reglan, a drug that speeds digestion. Reglan and similar drugs will reduce Monurol's effectiveness.

Special information
if you are pregnant or breastfeeding
There have been no adequate studies in pregnant women; and it is not known whether Monurol appears in breast milk. If you are pregnant or plan to become pregnant, make sure the doctor is aware of it.

Recommended dosage

ADULTS
The usual dose for women 18 years and older is 1 sachet (3 grams) dissolved in water.

CHILDREN
Safety and effectiveness have not been established in children 12 and under.

Overdosage
No Monurol overdoses have been reported. However, any medication taken in excess can have serious consequences. If you suspect an overdose, seek medical treatment immediately.

Generic name:

MORPHINE

See MS Contin, page 834.

Brand name:

MOTRIN

Generic name: Ibuprofen
Other brand name: Advil

Why is this drug prescribed?
Motrin is a nonsteroidal anti-inflammatory drug available in both prescription and nonprescription forms. Prescription Motrin is used in adults for relief of the symptoms of rheumatoid arthritis and osteoarthritis, treatment of menstrual pain, and relief of mild to moderate pain. In children aged 6 months and older it can be given to reduce fever and relieve mild to moderate pain. It is also used to relieve the symptoms of juvenile arthritis.

Motrin IB tablets, caplets, and gelcaps; Children's Motrin Suspension; and Advil tablets and caplets are available without a prescription. Check the packages for uses, dosage, and other information on these products.

Most important fact about this drug
You should have frequent checkups with your doctor if you take Motrin regularly. Ulcers or internal bleeding can occur without warning.

How should you take this medication?
Your doctor may ask you to take Motrin with food or an antacid to avoid stomach upset. The suspension can be given with meals or milk if it upsets the stomach.

A drink of water or other fluid after taking a chewable tablet can help your body absorb the drug.

If you are using Motrin for arthritis, you should take it regularly, exactly as prescribed.

■ *If you miss a dose...*
  Take it as soon as you remember. If it is almost time for your next dose, skip the one you missed and go back to your regular schedule. Never take 2 doses at the same time.

■ *Storage information...*
  Store at room temperature.

What side effects may occur?
Side effects cannot be anticipated. If any develop or change in intensity, inform your doctor as soon as possible. Only your doctor can determine if it is safe for you to continue taking Motrin.

■ *More common side effects may include:*
  Abdominal cramps or pain, abdominal discomfort, bloating and gas, constipation, diarrhea, dizziness, fluid retention and swelling, headache, heartburn, indigestion, itching, loss of appetite, nausea, nervousness, rash, ringing in ears, stomach pain, vomiting

■ *Less common or rare side effects may include:*
  Abdominal bleeding, anemia, black stool, blood in urine, blurred vision, changes in heartbeat, chills, confusion, congestive heart failure, depression, dry eyes and mouth, emotional volatility, fever, hair loss, hearing loss, hepatitis, high or low blood pressure, hives, inability to sleep, inflammation of nose, inflammation of the pancreas or stomach, kidney or liver failure, severe allergic reactions, shortness of breath, skin eruptions or peeling, sleepiness, stomach or upper intestinal ulcer, ulcer of gums, vision loss, vomiting blood, wheezing, yellow eyes and skin

Why should this drug not be prescribed?
If you are sensitive to or have ever had an allergic reaction to ibuprofen, aspirin, or similar drugs, such as Aleve and Naprosyn, or if you have had asthma attacks caused by aspirin or other drugs of this type, or if you have angioedema, a condition whose symptoms are skin eruptions, you should not take this medication.

Make sure that your doctor is aware of any drug reactions that you have experienced.

Special warnings about this medication
Peptic ulcers and bleeding can occur without warning. Tell your doctor if you have bleeding or any other problems.

This drug should be used with caution if you have kidney or liver disease, or are severely dehydrated; it can cause liver or kidney inflammation or other problems in some people.

Do not take aspirin or any other anti-inflammatory medications while taking Motrin unless your doctor tells you to do so.

If you have a severe allergic reaction, seek medical help immediately.

Motrin may cause vision problems. If you experience any changes in your vision, inform your doctor.

Motrin may prolong bleeding time. If you are taking blood-thinning medication, this drug should be taken with caution.

This drug can cause water retention. It should be used with caution if you have high blood pressure or poor heart function.

Avoid the use of alcohol while taking this medication.

Motrin may mask the usual signs of infection or other diseases. Use with care in the presence of an existing infection.

If you have diabetes, remember that the suspension contains 1.5 grams of sucrose and 8 calories per teaspoonful.

Motrin chewable tablets contain phenylalanine. If you have a hereditary disease called phenylketonuria, you should be aware of this.

**Possible food and drug interactions
when taking this medication**
If Motrin is taken with certain other drugs, the effects of either could be increased, decreased, or altered. It is especially important to check with your doctor before combining Motrin with the following:

Aspirin

Blood pressure medications known as ACE inhibitors, including Vasotec and Capoten

Blood-thinning drugs such as Coumadin

Diuretics such as Lasix and HydroDIURIL

Lithium (Lithonate)

Methotrexate (Rheumatrex)

Special information
if you are pregnant or breastfeeding

The effects of ibuprofen during pregnancy have not been adequately studied. If you are pregnant or plan to become pregnant, inform your doctor immediately. Ibuprofen may appear in breast milk and could affect a nursing infant. If this medication is essential to your health, your doctor may advise you to discontinue breastfeeding until your treatment with this medication is finished.

Recommended dosage

ADULTS

Rheumatoid Arthritis and Osteoarthritis

The usual dosage is 1,200 to 3,200 milligrams per day divided into 3 or 4 doses. Your doctor will tailor the dose to your individual needs. Symptoms should be reduced within 2 weeks. Daily dosage should not be greater than 3,200 milligrams.

Mild to Moderate Pain

The usual dose is 400 milligrams every 4 to 6 hours as necessary.

Menstrual Pain

The usual dose is 400 milligrams every 4 hours as necessary. Begin treatment when symptoms first appear.

CHILDREN 6 MONTHS TO 12 YEARS OF AGE

Fever reduction

The recommended dose is 5 milligrams per 2.2 pounds of body weight if temperature is less than 102.5°F or 10 milligrams per 2.2 pounds of body weight if temperature is 102.5°F or greater. The fever should go down for 6 to 8 hours. Do not give the child more than 40 milligrams per 2.2 pounds of body weight in one day.

Mild to Moderate Pain

The usual dose is 10 milligrams per 2.2 pounds of body weight every 6 to 8 hours. Do not give the child more than 4 such doses per day.

Juvenile Arthritis
The usual dose is 30 to 40 milligrams daily per 2.2 pounds of body weight, divided into 3 or 4 doses. Some children may need only 20 milligrams daily per 2.2 pounds.

Overdosage
Any medication taken in excess can have serious consequences. An overdose of Motrin can be fatal. If you suspect an overdose, seek medical attention immediately.

■ *Symptoms of Motrin overdose may include:*
 Abdominal pain, breathing difficulties, coma, drowsiness, headache, irregular heartbeat, kidney failure, low blood pressure, nausea, ringing in the ears, seizures, sluggishness, vomiting

Brand name:

MS CONTIN

Pronounced: em-ess KON-tin
Generic name: Morphine sulfate
Other brand name: Kadian

Why is this drug prescribed?
MS Contin, a controlled-release tablet containing morphine, is used to relieve moderate to severe pain. While regular morphine is usually given every 4 hours, MS Contin is typically taken every 12 hours—only twice a day. The Kadian brand may be taken once or twice a day. The drugs are intended for people who need a morphine painkiller for more than just a few days.

Most important fact about this drug
Like other narcotics, MS Contin is potentially addictive. If you take MS Contin for some time and then stop abruptly, you could experience withdrawal symptoms. For this reason, do not make dosage changes on your own; always consult your doctor.

How should you take this medication?
Take MS Contin exactly as prescribed by your doctor—typically one tablet every 12 hours. Swallow the tablets whole. If you crush or chew the tablets, a dangerously large amount of morphine could enter your bloodstream all at once.

Kadian capsules and the pellets they contain should not be dissolved, or mixed with food, either.

Do not increase the dose or take the drug more frequently than prescribed. It will take a little time for the drug to begin working.

Do not drink alcoholic beverages while using MS Contin.

■ *If you miss a dose...*
Take the forgotten dose as soon as you remember. If it is almost time for your next dose, skip the one you missed and go back to your regular schedule. Do not take 2 doses at once.

■ *Storage instructions...*
Store at room temperature in a tightly closed container, away from light and moisture.

What side effects may occur?
Side effects cannot be anticipated. If any develop or change in intensity, tell your doctor immediately. Only your doctor can determine whether it is safe for you to continue taking MS Contin.

As with other narcotics, the most hazardous potential side effect of MS Contin is respiratory depression (dangerously slow breathing). If you are older or in a weakened condition, you are particularly vulnerable to respiratory depression; you may be at special risk at any age if you have a lung or breathing problem.

■ *More common side effects may include:*
Anxiety, constipation, depressed or irritable mood, dizziness, drowsiness, exaggerated sense of well-being, light-headedness, nausea, sedation, sweating, vomiting

You may be able to lessen some of these side effects by lying down.

■ *Less common side effects may include:*
Agitation, appetite loss, apprehension, blurred vision, chills, constipation, cramps, depression, diarrhea, difficult urination, disorientation, double vision, dreams, dry mouth, facial flushing, fainting, faintness, floating feeling, hallucinations, headache, high blood pressure, hives, inability to urinate, insomnia, involuntary movement of the eyeball, itching, low blood pressure, mood changes, nervousness, "pinpoint" pupils, rapid heartbeat, rash, rigid muscles, seizure, sexual drive or performance problems, slow heartbeat, sweating, swelling due to fluid retention, taste alterations, throbbing heartbeat, tingling or pins and needles, tremor, uncoordinated muscle movements, vision disturbances, weakness

■ *Other side effects reported during trials of Kadian include:*

Abdominal pain, abnormal thinking, accidental injury, anemia, apathy, asthma, back pain, bedsores, blood disorders, bone pain, breast development in males, chest pain, confusion, conjunctivitis (pinkeye), difficulty swallowing, feeling of illness, fever, fluid in the lungs, flushing, flu symptoms, heartburn, hiccups, inability to concentrate, indigestion, irregular heartbeat, joint pain, lack of menstrual period, lack of sensation, memory loss, nasal inflammation, pain, pallor, sluggishness, slurred speech, vertigo, voice changes

If you stop taking MS Contin after a long period of use, you will probably experience some degree of narcotic withdrawal syndrome. During the first 24 hours, you may have: dilated pupils, goose bumps, restlessness, restless sleep, runny nose, sweating, tearing, or yawning.

Over the next 72 hours, the following may be added:

Abdominal and leg pains, abdominal and muscle cramps, anxiety, diarrhea, hot and cold flashes, inability to fall or stay asleep, increase in body temperature, blood pressure, and breathing and heart rate, kicking movements, loss of appetite, nasal discharge, nausea, severe backache, sneezing, twitching and spasm of muscles, vomiting, weakness

Even without treatment, your withdrawal symptoms will probably disappear within a week or two. However, you could experience a second phase of withdrawal, involving aching muscles, irritability, and insomnia, which might last for 2 to 6 months.

Why should this drug not be prescribed?
Do not take MS Contin if you have ever had an allergic reaction to morphine or are sensitive to it, or if you have bronchial asthma.

If your breathing is abnormally slow, you should not take MS Contin unless there is resuscitation equipment nearby.

MS Contin should not be prescribed if you are suffering an intestinal blockage.

Special warnings about this medication
MS Contin should not be used by anyone who might have a brain injury, or the beginnings of an abdominal problem requiring surgery; the drug could mask the symptoms, making correct diagnosis difficult or impossible. For people facing biliary tract surgery, there is a chance that the drug could make their condition worse. Your doctor will also prescribe MS Contin with extreme caution if you have any of the following conditions:

Alcoholism
Coma
Curvature of the spine
Delirium tremens (severe alcohol withdrawal)
Drug-related psychosis
Enlarged prostate or constricted urinary canal
Kidney disorder
Liver disorder
Low adrenaline levels
Low thyroid levels
Lung disorder
Swallowing difficulty

If taken by an epileptic person, MS Contin could increase the likelihood of a seizure.

Since MS Contin can impair judgment and coordination, do not drive, climb, or operate hazardous equipment while taking this drug. If you become overly calm or lethargic, call your doctor.

MS Contin can lower blood pressure; you may feel dizzy or light-headed, especially when you first stand up.

Possible food and drug interactions
when taking this medication
If MS Contin is taken with certain other drugs, the effects of either could be increased, decreased, or altered. It is especially important to check with your doctor before combining MS Contin with the following:

Alcohol
Certain analgesics such as Talwin, Nubain, Stadol, and Buprenex
Drugs that control vomiting, such as Compazine and Tigan
Drugs classified as MAO inhibitors, such as the antidepressants Nardil and Parnate
Major tranquilizers such as Thorazine and Haldol
Muscle relaxants such as Flexeril and Valium
Sedatives such as Dalmane and Halcion
Tranquilizers such as Librium and Xanax
Water pills such as Diuril and Lasix

Special information
if you are pregnant or breastfeeding
If you are pregnant or plan to become pregnant, inform your doctor immediately. Although there is no evidence so far that a pregnant woman's

short-term use of MS Contin can harm her unborn baby, this drug should be taken during pregnancy only if the benefit to the mother outweighs a possible risk to the child.

MS Contin is not recommended for use as a painkiller during childbirth. If a woman takes this drug shortly before giving birth, her baby may have trouble breathing. Babies born to mothers who use morphine chronically may suffer from drug withdrawal symptoms.

Since some of the morphine from MS Contin appears in breast milk, do not take this medication while breastfeeding. If you do nurse while using MS Contin, your baby could experience withdrawal symptoms once you stop taking this medication.

Recommended dosage

ADULTS

Because MS Contin and Kadian are so potent, the doctor will set the dosage schedule and amount to meet your individual needs.

Overdosage

Any medication taken in excess can have serious consequences. An overdose of MS Contin can be fatal. If you suspect an overdose, seek medical attention immediately.

■ *Symptoms of MS Contin overdose may include:*
Cold, clammy skin, flaccid muscles, fluid in the lungs, lowered blood pressure, "pinpoint" or dilated pupils, sleepiness leading to stupor and coma, slowed breathing, slow pulse rate

Category:

MULTIVITAMINS

Brand names: Centrum, Theragran, Vi-Daylin

Why is this supplement prescribed?

Multivitamins are nutritional supplements for people whose diet may be deficient in certain vitamins and minerals. You may need a supplement if you are on a special diet, or don't eat the right foods. A supplement may also be necessary if you are a strict vegetarian, take medications that prevent the body from using certain nutrients, or have an illness that affects your appetite. In addition, special formulas are available for use during pregnancy.

Vitamin/mineral supplements come in a wide range of formulations. Three of the most widely used are Centrum, Theragran, and Vi-Daylin. Each of these brands offers a variety of formulas tailored to the needs of different groups.

Centrum is a multivitamin/multimineral supplement that includes all antioxidants, the vitamins that strengthen the body's natural defenses against cell damage. *Centrum Silver* contains higher strengths of the vitamins that people 50 years of age or older need the most. *Centrum, Jr.*, formulations are geared to children's needs.

Theragran is a multivitamin supplement. *Theragran-M* adds minerals to the formulation. *Theragran Stress Formula* contains higher strengths of the B vitamins that may be needed for people under stress, plus extra vitamin C.

Vi-Daylin is a multivitamin supplement; *Vi-Daylin + Iron* is a multivitamin plus iron, which may be needed by women who have heavy menstrual periods. Some Vi-Daylin formulations also contain fluoride. *Vi-Daylin drops* are given to infants and young children.

Most important fact about this supplement
Do not use supplements as a replacement for a diet rich in essential vitamins and minerals. Food contains many important ingredients not available in supplements.

How should you take this supplement?
Follow the dosing instructions on the bottle, or use as directed by your doctor.

Do not take more than suggested.

- *If you miss a dose...*
  If you forget to take your multivitamin for a day, don't be concerned. Resume your regular schedule the following day.

- *Storage instructions...*
  Keep out of the reach of children. Store at room temperature, and keep tightly closed.

Why should this supplement not be used?
If you have any serious chronic medical conditions check with your doctor before starting on a multivitamin supplement. You may have special requirements.

If your multivitamin supplement contains fluoride, check with your doctor. You should not use it if your drinking water contains more than 0.7 parts per million of fluoride.

Special warnings about this supplement

Do not take more of a multivitamin supplement than suggested on the packaging, or directed by your doctor. Very high doses of some vitamins and minerals can be harmful or even dangerous.

Possible food and drug interactions
when taking this supplement

When taken as suggested on the packaging, there are no known supplement interactions.

Special information
if you are pregnant or breastfeeding

Ask your doctor whether you should take a multivitamin supplement while you are pregnant or breastfeeding. Taking too much of any supplement may be harmful to you or your unborn child.

Recommended dosage

ADULTS

The usual dose is 1 tablet, teaspoonful, or tablespoonful daily according to package instructions, or as directed by your doctor.

CHILDREN

The usual dose of children's formulations is 1 tablet, teaspoonful, or dropperful daily or as directed by your doctor. Younger children may require only half this dose. Check the instructions on the package.

Overdosage

Megadoses of some vitamins and minerals can be harmful when taken for extended periods. If you have unexplained symptoms and suspect an overdose, check with your doctor.

Generic name:

MUPIROCIN

See Bactroban, page 139.

Brand name:

MUSE

See Caverject, page 217.

Brand name:

MYCELEX

See Gyne-Lotrimin, page 576.

Brand name:

MYCOLOG-II

Pronounced: MY-koe-log too
Generic ingredients: Nystatin, Triamcinolone acetonide
Other brand names: Myco-Triacet II, Mytrex

Why is this drug prescribed?
Mycolog-II Cream and Ointment are prescribed for the treatment of candidiasis (a yeast-like fungal infection) of the skin. The combination of an antifungal (nystatin) and a steroid (triamcinolone acetonide) provides greater benefit than nystatin alone during the first few days of treatment. Nystatin kills the fungus or prevents its growth; triamcinolone helps relieve the redness, swelling, itching, and other discomfort that can accompany a skin infection.

Most important fact about this drug
Absorption of this drug through the skin can affect the whole body instead of just the surface of the skin being treated. Although unusual, it is possible that you could experience symptoms of steroid excess such as weight gain, reddening and rounding of the face and neck, growth of excess body and facial hair, high blood pressure, emotional disturbances, increased blood sugar, and urinary excretion of glucose (marked by an increase in frequency of urination).

Use of this medication over large surface areas, for prolonged periods, or with airtight dressings or bandages, could cause these problems. Your doctor will watch your condition and periodically check for symptoms.

How should you use this medication?
Use this medicine for the full course of treatment, even if your symptoms are gone. Apply a thin layer to the affected area and gently rub it in. Do not

bandage or wrap the area being treated, unless your doctor tells you to. Keep the area cool and dry.

Use this medication exactly as prescribed by your doctor. Do not use it more often or for a longer time. It is for external use only. Avoid contact with the eyes.

■ *If you miss a dose...*
Apply it as soon as you remember. If it is almost time for your next dose, skip the one you missed and go back to your regular schedule.

■ *Storage instructions...*
Store away from heat and light. Do not freeze.

What side effects may occur?
Side effects cannot be anticipated. If any develop or change in intensity, inform your doctor as soon as possible. Only your doctor can determine if it is safe for you to continue taking Mycolog-II.

■ *Side effects may include:*
Blistering, burning, dryness, eruptions resembling acne, excessive discoloring of the skin, excessive growth of hair (especially on the face), hair loss (especially on the scalp), inflammation around the mouth, inflammation of hair follicles, irritation, itching, peeling, prickly heat, reddish purple lines on skin, secondary infection, severe inflammation of the skin, softening of the skin, stretch marks, stretching or thinning of the skin

Why should this drug not be prescribed?
If you are sensitive to or have ever had an allergic reaction to nystatin, triamcinolone acetonide, or other antifungals or steroids, you should not take this medication. Make sure your doctor is aware of any drug reactions you have experienced.

Special warnings about this medication
Do not use this drug for any disorder other than the one for which it was prescribed.

Remember to avoid wrapping or bandaging the affected area. The use of tight-fitting diapers or plastic pants is not recommended for a child being treated in the diaper area with Mycolog-II. These garments may act in the same way as airtight dressings or bandages.

If an irritation or allergic reaction develops while using Mycolog-II, notify your doctor.

If used in the groin area, apply Mycolog-II sparingly and wear loose-fitting clothing.

If your condition does not show improvement after 2 to 3 weeks, or if it gets worse, consult your doctor.

**Possible food and drug interactions
when taking this medication**
No interactions have been reported.

**Special information
if you are pregnant or breastfeeding**
The effects of Mycolog-II in pregnancy have not been adequately studied. If you are pregnant or plan to become pregnant, inform your doctor before using Mycolog-II.

It is not known whether this medication appears in breast milk. If this drug is essential to your health, your doctor may advise you to discontinue breastfeeding until your treatment with this medication is finished.

Recommended dosage

ADULTS

Mycolog-II Cream
Mycolog-II Cream is usually applied to the affected areas 2 times a day, in the morning and evening, by gently and thoroughly massaging the preparation into the skin. Your doctor will have you stop using the cream if your symptoms persist after 25 days of treatment.

Mycolog-II Ointment
A thin film of Mycolog-II Ointment is usually applied to the affected areas 2 times a day, in the morning and the evening. Your doctor will have you stop using the ointment if your symptoms persist after 25 days of treatment.

CHILDREN

Your doctor will limit use of Mycolog-II for children to the least amount that is effective. Long-term treatment may interfere with the growth and development of children.

Overdosage
An acute overdosage is unlikely with the use of Mycolog-II; however, long-term or prolonged use can produce reactions throughout the body. See "Most important fact about this drug."

Brand name:

MYCO-TRIACET II

See Mycolog-II, page 841.

Brand name:

MYKROX

See Zaroxolyn, page 1446.

Brand name:

MYLANTA

See Antacids, page 75.

Brand name:

MYSOLINE

Pronounced: MY-soh-leen
Generic name: Primidone

Why is this drug prescribed?
Mysoline is used to treat epileptic and other seizures. It can be used alone or with other anticonvulsant drugs. It is chemically similar to barbiturates.

Most important fact about this drug
Mysoline should not be stopped suddenly; this could cause you to have seizures. If you no longer need the medication, your doctor will reduce the dosage gradually.

How should you take this medication?
Take Mysoline exactly as prescribed. Do not change from one manufacturer's product to another without consulting your doctor.

If using Mysoline Suspension, shake well before using.

■ *If you miss a dose...*
  Take it as soon as you remember. If it is within an hour of your next dose, skip the one you missed and go back to your regular schedule. Never take 2 doses at the same time.

■ *Storage instructions...*
Store at room temperature in a tightly closed container, away from light.

What side effects may occur?
Side effects cannot be anticipated. If any develop or change in intensity, inform your doctor as soon as possible. Only your doctor can determine if it is safe for you to continue taking Mysoline.

■ *More common side effects may include:*
Lack of muscle coordination, vertigo or severe dizziness

■ *Less common side effects may include:*
Double vision, drowsiness, emotional disturbances, excessive irritability, fatigue, impotence, loss of appetite, nausea, skin eruptions that resemble measles, uncontrolled movement of the eyeballs, vomiting

Why should this drug not be prescribed?
You should not take Mysoline if you have porphyria (an inherited metabolic disorder) or if you are allergic to phenobarbital.

Special warnings about this medication
Remember that you must not stop taking Mysoline suddenly.

It can take several weeks for the full effectiveness of Mysoline to be seen.

Since Mysoline is generally given for long periods of time, your doctor will check your blood count every 6 months.

**Possible food and drug interactions
when taking this medication**
If Mysoline is taken with certain other drugs, the effects of either could be increased, decreased, or altered. It is especially important to check with your doctor before combining Mysoline with the following:

Antidepressants called MAO inhibitors, such as Parnate and Nardil
Blood-thinning drugs such as Coumadin
Doxycycline (Doryx, Vibramycin)
Estrogen-containing oral contraceptives such as Ortho-Novum and
     Triphasil
Griseofulvin (Fulvicin-U/F, Grifulvin V)
Steroid drugs such as Decadron

Avoid alcoholic beverages while you are taking Mysoline.

Special information
if you are pregnant or breastfeeding

Although the effects of Mysoline in pregnancy and nursing infants are not known, recent studies show an increase in birth defects in infants born to epileptic women taking anticonvulsant medications (particularly Dilantin and phenobarbital). Although most pregnant women taking anticonvulsant medication give birth to normal, healthy babies, this possibility may also exist with Mysoline. If you are pregnant or plan to become pregnant, inform your doctor immediately. Mysoline appears in breast milk and can affect a nursing infant, causing excessive sleepiness and drowsiness. If this medication is essential to your health, your doctor may advise you to stop breastfeeding.

Recommended dosage

ADULTS

For people 8 years of age and older who have not been treated before, the doctor will start Mysoline as follows, using either 50-milligram or scored 250-milligram Mysoline tablets:

Days 1 to 3: 100 to 125 milligrams at bedtime

Days 4 to 6: 100 to 125 milligrams 2 times a day

Days 7 to 9: 100 to 125 milligrams 3 times a day

Day 10 to maintenance: 250 milligrams 3 times a day

For most adults and children 8 years of age and over, the usual maintenance dosage is 250 milligrams 3 or 4 times a day. If you need more, your doctor may increase the dose to five or six 250-milligram tablets. You should not take more than 500 milligrams 4 times a day (2000 milligrams or 2 grams).

In patients already receiving other anticonvulsants, the usual starting dose of Mysoline is 100 to 125 milligrams at bedtime; your doctor will gradually increase this dose to a maintenance level as the other drug is gradually decreased. Your doctor will either find a working level for the combination or withdraw the other medication completely. When Mysoline is to be used as a single drug, it will take at least 2 weeks to make the transition from two drugs to one.

CHILDREN UNDER AGE 8

Days 1 to 3: 50 milligrams at bedtime

Days 4 to 6: 50 milligrams 2 times a day

Days 7 to 9: 100 milligrams 2 times a day

Day 10 to maintenance: 125 milligrams 3 times a day to 250 milligrams 3 times a day

The usual maintenance dosage is 125 to 250 milligrams 3 times daily or 10 to 25 milligrams per 2.2 pounds of body weight per day, divided into smaller doses.

Overdosage
Any medication taken in excess can have serious consequences. If you suspect a Mysoline overdose, seek medical attention immediately.

Brand name:

MYTREX

See Mycolog-II, page 841.

Generic name:

NABUMETONE

See Relafen, page 1102.

Generic name:

NADOLOL

See Corgard, page 294.

Generic name:

NADOLOL WITH BENDROFLUMETHIAZIDE

See Corzide, page 300.

Generic name:

NALTREXONE

See ReVia, page 1122.

Generic name:

NAPHAZOLINE WITH PHENIRAMINE

See Naphcon-A, page 848.

Brand name:

NAPHCON-A

Pronounced: NAFF-kon ay
Generic ingredients: Naphazoline hydrochloride,
  Pheniramine maleate
Other brand name: Opcon-A

Why is this drug prescribed?
Naphcon-A, an eyedrop containing both a decongestant and an antihistamine, is used to relieve itchy, red eyes caused by ragweed, pollen, and animal hair.

Most important fact about this drug
If this medication causes changes in your vision, be careful when driving or performing other tasks that could be hazardous.

How should you use this medication?
Remove contact lenses before administering this medication. Do not use the solution if it becomes cloudy or changes color.

To administer the eyedrops, follow these steps:
1. Wash your hands thoroughly.
2. Gently pull your lower eyelid down to form a pocket between your eye and the lid.
3. Hold the eyedrop bottle on your forehead or the bridge of your nose.
4. Do not touch the applicator tip to your eye or any other surface.
5. Tilt your head back and squeeze the medication into your eye.
6. Close your eyes gently and keep them closed for a minute or two.
7. Do not rinse the dropper.

■ *If you miss a dose...*
  Use this medication only as needed.

■ *Storage instructions...*
  Store at room temperature in a tightly closed bottle. Protect from light.

What side effects may occur?
Naphcon is unlikely to cause side effects. However, overuse can cause reddening of the eyes.

Why should this drug not be prescribed?

Do not take Naphcon-A if you have ever had an allergic reaction to it or are sensitive to any of its ingredients.

Do not use Naphcon-A if you have heart disease, high blood pressure, or trouble urinating because of enlargement of the prostate gland.

Do not use this medication if you have glaucoma.

Special warnings about this medication

Contact your doctor before giving Naphcon-A to infants or children under 6 years of age. Swallowing this medication can cause stupor or coma and a serious drop in body temperature in an infant or child.

If your eyes hurt or continue to be red or irritated, if you experience changes in vision, if your eyes get worse, or if the itching and redness last more than 72 hours, stop using Naphcon-A and call your doctor.

Recommended dosage

ADULTS

Place 1 or 2 drops in the affected eyes, up to 4 times a day.

Overdosage

Overdose from accidental oral use can have serious consequences, especially in young children. If you suspect an overdose, seek medical attention immediately.

Brand name:

NAPRELAN

See Anaprox, page 66.

Brand name:

NAPROSYN

Pronounced: NA-proh-sinn
Generic name: Naproxen
Other brand name: EC-Naprosyn

Why is this drug prescribed?

Naprosyn, a nonsteroidal anti-inflammatory drug, is used to relieve the inflammation, swelling, stiffness, and joint pain associated with rheumatoid arthritis, osteoarthritis (the most common form of arthritis), juvenile arthritis, ankylosing spondylitis (spinal arthritis), tendinitis, bursitis, and acute gout; it is also used to relieve menstrual cramps and other types of mild to moderate pain.

Most important fact about this drug
You should have frequent checkups with your doctor if you take Naprosyn regularly. Ulcers or internal bleeding can occur without warning.

How should you take this medication?
Naprosyn may be taken with food or an antacid, and with a full glass of water to avoid stomach upset. Avoid taking it on an empty stomach.

If you are using Naprosyn for arthritis, it should be taken regularly; take it exactly as prescribed.

Do not break, crush, or chew an EC-Naprosyn tablet.

- *If you miss a dose...*
  And you take the drug on a regular schedule, take the dose as soon as you remember. If it is almost time for your next dose, skip the one you missed and go back to your regular schedule. Do not take 2 doses at once.

- *Storage instructions...*
  Store at room temperature in a well-closed container. Protect from light and extreme heat.

What side effects may occur?
Side effects cannot be anticipated. If any develop or change in intensity, inform your doctor as soon as possible. Only your doctor can determine if it is safe for you to continue taking Naprosyn.

- *More common side effects may include:*
  Abdominal pain, bruising, constipation, difficult or labored breathing, dizziness, drowsiness, headache, heartburn, indigestion, itching, nausea, ringing in ears, skin eruptions, swelling due to fluid retention

- *Less common or rare side effects may include:*
  Abdominal bleeding, black stools, blood in the urine, changes in liver function, chills and fever, colitis, congestive heart failure, depression, diarrhea, dream abnormalities, general feeling of illness, hair loss, hearing disturbances or loss, inability to concentrate, inability to sleep, inflammation of the lungs, inflammation of the mouth, kidney disease or failure, light-headedness, menstrual disorders, muscle pain and weakness, peptic ulcer, red or purple spots on the skin, severe allergic reaction, skin

inflammation due to sensitivity to light, skin rashes and hives, sweating, thirst, throbbing heartbeat, vertigo, visual disturbances, vomiting, vomiting of blood, yellow skin and eyes

Why should this drug not be prescribed?

If you are sensitive to or have ever had an allergic reaction to Naprosyn, EC-Naprosyn, Anaprox, Anaprox DS, or Aleve, you should not take this drug. Also, if aspirin or other nonsteroidal anti-inflammatory drugs have ever given you asthma or nasal inflammation or tumors, you should not take this medication. Make sure your doctor is aware of any drug reactions you have experienced.

Special warnings about this medication

Remember that peptic ulcers and bleeding can occur without warning. Call your doctor immediately if you suspect a problem.

Use this drug with caution if you have kidney or liver disease; it can cause liver or kidney problems in some people.

Naprosyn may prolong bleeding time. If you are taking blood-thinning medication, your doctor will prescribe Naprosyn with caution.

By reducing fever and inflammation, Naprosyn may hide an underlying condition.

This medication may cause vision problems. If you experience any changes in your vision, inform your doctor.

This drug can increase water retention. It will be prescribed with caution if you have heart disease or high blood pressure. Naprosyn suspension contains a significant amount of sodium. If you are on a low-sodium diet, discuss this with your doctor.

Naprosyn may cause you to become drowsy or less alert; therefore, avoid driving, operating dangerous machinery, or participating in any hazardous activity that requires full mental alertness until you are sure of the drug's effect on you.

Possible food and drug interactions
when taking this medication

If Naprosyn is taken with certain other drugs, the effects of either could be increased, decreased, or altered. It is especially important to check with your doctor before combining Naprosyn with the following:

ACE inhibitors such as the blood-pressure drug Capoten
Aspirin
Beta blockers such as the blood-pressure drug Tenormin

Blood-thinning drugs such as Coumadin
Furosemide (Lasix)
Lithium (Lithonate)
Methotrexate
Naproxen sodium (Aleve, Anaprox)
Oral diabetes drugs such as Diabinese and Micronase
Phenytoin (Dilantin)
Probenecid (Benemid)
Sulfa drugs such as the antibiotics Bactrim and Septra

EC-Naprosyn should not be used with antacids, H_2 blockers such as Tagamet, or sucralfate (Carafate).

Special information
if you are pregnant or breastfeeding
The effects of Naprosyn during pregnancy have not been adequately studied. If you are pregnant or plan to become pregnant, inform your doctor immediately. Naprosyn appears in breast milk and could affect a nursing infant. If this medication is essential to your health, your doctor may advise you to discontinue breastfeeding until your treatment with this medication is finished.

Recommended dosage
Naprosyn is available in tablet and liquid form. When taking the liquid, use a teaspoon or the measuring cup, marked in one-half teaspoon and 2.5 milliliter increments, that comes with Naprosyn suspension.

ADULTS

Rheumatoid Arthritis, Osteoarthritis, and Ankylosing Spondylitis
The usual dose of Naprosyn is 250 milligrams (10 milliliters or 2 teaspoons of suspension), 375 milligrams (15 milliliters or 3 teaspoons), or 500 milligrams (20 milliliters or 4 teaspoons) 2 times a day (morning and evening). EC-Naprosyn is taken in doses of 375 or 500 milligrams twice a day. Your dose may be adjusted by your doctor over your period of treatment. Improvement of symptoms should be seen in 2 to 4 weeks.

Acute Gout
Starting dose of Naprosyn is 750 milligrams (30 milliliters or 6 teaspoons), followed by 250 milligrams (10 milliliters or 2 teaspoons) every 8 hours until the symptoms are relieved. EC-Naprosyn should not be used to treat gout.

Mild to Moderate Pain, Menstrual Cramps, Acute Tendinitis and Bursitis

Starting dose is 500 milligrams (20 milliliters or 4 teaspoons of suspension), followed by 250 milligrams (10 milliliters or 2 teaspoons) every 6 to 8 hours as needed. The most you should take in a day is 1,250 milligrams (50 milliliters or 10 teaspoons). Do not take EC-Naprosyn for these problems.

CHILDREN

Juvenile Arthritis

The usual daily dose is 10 milligrams per 2.2 pounds of body weight, divided into 2 doses. Follow your doctor's directions carefully when giving a child this medicine.

The safety and effectiveness of Naprosyn have not been established in children under 2 years of age.

OLDER ADULTS

Your doctor will probably have you take a reduced dose.

Overdosage

Any medication taken in excess can have serious consequences. If you suspect an overdose, seek medical attention immediately.

■ *Symptoms of Naprosyn overdose may include:*
   Drowsiness, heartburn, indigestion, nausea, vomiting

Generic name:

NAPROXEN

See Naprosyn, page 849.

Generic name:

NAPROXEN SODIUM

See Anaprox, page 66.

Generic name:

NARATRIPTAN

See Amerge, page 54.

Brand name:

NARDIL

Pronounced: NAHR-dill
Generic name: Phenelzine sulfate

Why is this drug prescribed?

Nardil is a monoamine oxidase (MAO) inhibitor used to treat depression as well as anxiety or phobias mixed with depression. MAO is an enzyme responsible for breaking down certain neurotransmitters (chemical messengers) in the brain. By inhibiting MAO, Nardil helps restore more normal mood states. Unfortunately, MAO inhibitors such as Nardil also block MAO activity throughout the body, an action that can have serious, even fatal, side effects—especially if MAO inhibitors are combined with other foods or drugs containing a substance called tyramine.

Most important fact about this drug

Avoid the following foods, beverages, and medications while taking Nardil and for 2 weeks thereafter:

Beer (including alcohol-free or reduced-alcohol beer)
Caffeine (in excessive amounts)
Cheese (except for cottage cheese and cream cheese)
Chocolate (in excessive amounts)
Dry sausage (including Genoa salami, hard salami, pepperoni, and
    Lebanon bologna)
Fava bean pods
Liver
Meat extract
Pickled herring
Pickled, fermented, aged, or smoked meat, fish, or dairy products
Sauerkraut
Spoiled or improperly stored meat, fish, or dairy products
Wine (including alcohol-free or reduced-alcohol wine)
Yeast extract (including large amounts of brewer's yeast)
Yogurt

■ *Medications to avoid:*
Amphetamines
Antidepressants and related medications such as Prozac, Effexor,
    Luvox, Paxil, Remeron, Serzone, Wellbutrin, Zoloft, Elavil, Triavil,
    Tegretol, and Flexeril

Appetite suppressants such as Redux and Tenuate

Asthma inhalants such as Proventil and Ventolin

Cold and cough preparations including those with dextromethorphan, such as Robitussin DM

Hay fever medications such as Contac and Dristan

L-tryptophan-containing products

Nasal decongestants in tablet, drop, or spray form such as Sudafed

Sinus medications such as Sinutab

Taking Nardil with any of the above foods, beverages, or medications can cause serious, potentially fatal, high blood pressure. Therefore, when taking Nardil you should immediately report the occurrence of a headache, heart palpitations, or any other unusual symptom. In addition, make certain that you inform any other physician or dentist you see that you are currently taking Nardil or have taken Nardil within the last 2 weeks.

How should you take this medication?

Nardil may be taken with or without food. Take it exactly as prescribed. It can take up to 4 weeks for the drug to begin working.

Use of Nardil may complicate other medical treatment. Always carry a card that says you take Nardil, or wear a Medic Alert bracelet.

■ *If you miss a dose...*

Take it as soon as you remember. If it is within 2 hours of your next dose, skip the one you missed and go back to your regular schedule. Do not take 2 doses at once.

■ *Storage instructions...*

Store at room temperature.

What side effects may occur?

Side effects cannot be anticipated. If any develop or change in intensity, inform your doctor as soon as possible. Only your doctor can determine if it is safe for you to continue taking Nardil.

■ *More common side effects may include:*

Constipation, disorders of the stomach and intestines, dizziness, drowsiness, dry mouth, excessive sleeping, fatigue, headache, insomnia, itching, low blood pressure (especially when rising quickly from lying down or sitting up), muscle spasms, sexual difficulties, strong reflexes, swelling due to fluid retention, tremors, twitching, weakness, weight gain

■ *Less common or rare side effects may include:*
Anxiety, blurred vision, coma, convulsions, delirium, exaggerated feeling of well-being, fever, glaucoma, inability to urinate, involuntary eyeball movements, jitteriness, lack of coordination, liver damage, mania, muscular rigidity, onset of the mental disorder schizophrenia, rapid breathing, rapid heart rate, repetitious use of words and phrases, skin rash or lupus-like disease, sweating, swelling in the throat, tingling sensation, yellowed skin and whites of eyes

Why should this drug not be prescribed?
You should not take this drug if you have pheochromocytoma (a tumor of the adrenal gland), congestive heart failure, or a history of liver disease, or if you have had an allergic reaction to it.

You should not take Nardil if you are taking medications that may increase blood pressure (such as amphetamines, cocaine, allergy and cold medications, or Ritalin), other MAO inhibitors, L-dopa, methyldopa (Aldomet), phenylalanine, L-tryptophan, L-tyrosine, fluoxetine (Prozac), buspirone (BuSpar), bupropion (Wellbutrin), guanethidine (Ismelin), meperidine (Demerol), dextromethorphan, or substances that slow the central nervous system such as alcohol and narcotics; or if you must consume the foods, beverages, or medications listed in the "Most important fact about this drug" section.

Special warnings about this medication
You must follow the food and drug limitations established by your physician; failure to do so may lead to potentially fatal side effects. While taking Nardil, you should promptly report the occurrence of a headache or any other unusual symptoms.

If you are diabetic, your doctor will prescribe Nardil with caution, since it is not clear how MAO inhibitors affect blood sugar levels.

If you are taking Nardil, talk to your doctor before you decide to have elective surgery.

If you stop taking Nardil abruptly, you may have withdrawal symptoms. They may include nightmares, agitation, strange behavior, and convulsions.

Possible food and drug interactions
when taking this medication
If Nardil is taken with certain other drugs, the effects of either could be increased, decreased, or altered. It is important that you closely follow your doctor's dietary and medication limitations when taking Nardil. Consult the "Most important fact about this drug" and "Why should this drug not be

prescribed?" sections for lists of the foods, beverages, and medications that should be avoided while taking Nardil.

In addition, you should use blood pressure medications (including water pills and beta blockers) with caution when taking Nardil, since excessively low blood pressure may result. Symptoms of low blood pressure include dizziness when rising from a lying or sitting position, fainting, and tingling in the hands or feet.

Special information
if you are pregnant or breastfeeding

The effects of Nardil during pregnancy have not been adequately studied. Nardil should be used during pregnancy only if the benefits of therapy clearly outweigh the potential risks to the fetus. If you are pregnant or plan to become pregnant, inform your doctor immediately. Nursing mothers should use Nardil only after consulting their physician, since it is not known whether Nardil appears in human milk.

Recommended dosage

ADULTS

The usual starting dose is 15 milligrams (1 tablet) 3 times a day. Your doctor may increase the dosage to 90 milligrams per day.

It may be 4 weeks before the drug starts to work.

Once you have had good results, your doctor may gradually reduce the dose, possibly to as low as 15 milligrams daily or every 2 days.

CHILDREN

Nardil is not recommended, since safety and efficacy for children under the age of 16 have not been determined.

Overdosage

Any medication taken in excess can have serious consequences. An overdose of Nardil can be fatal. If you suspect an overdose, seek medical help immediately.

- *Symptoms of overdose may include:*
  Agitation, backward arching of the head, neck, and back, cool, clammy skin, coma, convulsions, difficult breathing, dizziness, drowsiness, faint-ness, hallucinations, high blood pressure, high fever, hyperactivity, irritability, jaw muscle spasms, low blood pressure, pain in the heart area, rapid and irregular pulse, rigidity, severe headache, sweating

Brand name:

NASACORT

See Azmacort, page 126.

Brand name:

NASALCROM

See Intal, page 645.

Brand name:

NASALIDE

See AeroBid, page 21.

Brand name:

NATALINS RX

See Stuartnatal Plus, page 1223.

Brand name:

NAVANE

Pronounced: NA-vain
Generic name: Thiothixene

Why is this drug prescribed?
Navane is used to treat psychotic disorders (a severe sense of distorted reality). Researchers theorize that antipsychotic medications such as Navane work by lowering levels of dopamine, a neurotransmitter (or chemical messenger) in the brain. Excessive levels of dopamine are believed to be related to psychotic behavior.

Most important fact about this drug
Navane may cause tardive dyskinesia—a condition marked by involuntary muscle spasms and twitches in the face and body. This condition can be permanent and appears to be most common among the elderly, especially women. Ask your doctor for information about this possible risk.

How should you take this medication?
Navane may be taken in liquid or capsule form. In liquid form, a dropper is supplied.

■ *If you miss a dose...*
Take it as soon as you remember. If it is within 2 hours of your next dose, skip the one you missed and go back to your regular schedule. Do not take 2 doses at once.

■ *Storage instructions...*
Store at room temperature away from heat, light, and moisture. Keep the liquid form from freezing.

What side effects may occur?
Side effects cannot be anticipated. If any develop or change in intensity, inform your doctor as soon as possible. Only your doctor can determine if it is safe for you to continue taking Navane.

■ *Side effects may include:*
Abnormal muscle rigidity, abnormal secretion of milk, abnormalities in movements and posture, agitation, anemia, blurred vision, breast development in males, chewing movements, constipation, diarrhea, dizziness, drowsiness, dry mouth, excessive thirst, eyeball rotation or state of fixed gaze, fainting, fatigue, fluid accumulation and swelling, headache, high fever, high or low blood sugar, hives, impotence, insomnia, intestinal blockage, involuntary movements of the arms and legs, irregular menstrual periods, itching, light-headedness, loss or increase of appetite, low blood pressure, narrow or dilated pupils of the eye, nasal congestion, nausea, painful muscle spasm, protruding tongue, puckering of mouth, puffing of cheeks, rapid heartbeat, rash, restlessness, salivation, sedation, seizures, sensitivity to light, severe allergic reaction, skin inflammation and peeling, strong reflexes, sweating, swelling of breasts, tremors, twitching in the body, neck, shoulders, and face, visual problems, vomiting, weakness, weight increase, worsening of psychotic symptoms

Why should this drug not be prescribed?
Do not give Navane to comatose individuals. Do not take Navane if you are known to be hypersensitive to it. Also, you should not be using Navane if the activity of your central nervous system is slowed down for any reason—for example, by a sleeping medication, if you have had circulatory system collapse, or if you have an abnormal bone marrow or blood condition.

Special warnings about this medication
Navane may hide symptoms of brain tumor and intestinal obstruction. Your doctor will prescribe Navane cautiously if you have or have ever had a brain tumor, breast cancer, convulsive disorders, the eye condition called glaucoma, intestinal blockage, or heart disease; or if you are exposed to extreme heat or are recovering from alcohol addiction.

This drug may impair your ability to drive a car or operate potentially dangerous machinery. Do not participate in any activities that require full alertness if you are unsure of your ability.

**Possible food and drug interactions
when taking this medication**
If Navane is taken with certain other drugs, the effects of either could be increased, decreased, or altered. It is especially important to check with your doctor before combining Navane with the following:

    Antihistamines such as Benadryl
    Barbiturates such as phenobarbital
    Drugs that contain atropine, such as Donnatal

Extreme drowsiness and other potentially serious effects can result if Navane is combined with alcohol or other central nervous system depressants such as painkillers, narcotics, or sleeping medications.

**Special information
if you are pregnant or breastfeeding**
If you are pregnant or plan to become pregnant, inform your doctor immediately; pregnant women should use Navane only if clearly needed. Consult your doctor if you are breastfeeding; he or she may have you stop while you are taking Navane.

Recommended dosage
Dosages of Navane are tailored to the individual. Usually treatment begins with a small dose, which is increased if needed.

ADULTS

For Milder Conditions
The usual starting dosage is a daily total of 6 milligrams, divided into doses of 2 milligrams and taken 3 times a day. Your doctor may increase the dose to a total of 15 milligrams a day.

For More Severe Conditions
The usual starting dosage is a daily total of 10 milligrams, taken in 2 doses of 5 milligrams each. Your doctor may increase this dose to a total of 60 milligrams a day.

Taking more than 60 milligrams a day rarely increases the benefits of Navane.

Some people are able to take Navane once a day. Check with your doctor to see whether you can follow this schedule.

CHILDREN

Navane is not recommended for children younger than 12 years old.

OLDER ADULTS

In general, older adults are prescribed dosages of Navane in the lower ranges. Because older adults may develop low blood pressure while taking Navane, their doctors will monitor them closely. Older adults (especially women) may be more susceptible to such side effects as involuntary muscle spasms and twitches in the face and body. Check with your doctor for more information about these potential risks.

Overdosage
Any medication taken in excess can have serious consequences. If you suspect an overdose, seek medical help immediately.

■ *Symptoms of Navane overdose may include:*
Central nervous system depression, coma, difficulty swallowing, dizziness, drowsiness, head tilted to the side, low blood pressure, muscle twitching, rigid muscles, salivation, tremors, walking disturbances, weakness

Generic name:

NEDOCROMIL

See Tilade, page 1306.

Generic name:

NEFAZODONE

See Serzone, page 1190.

Generic name:

NELFINAVIR

See Viracept, page 1413.

Brand name:

NEODECADRON OPHTHALMIC OINTMENT AND SOLUTION

Pronounced: Nee-oh-DECK-uh-drohn
Generic ingredients: Dexamethasone sodium phosphate,
  Neomycin sulfate

Why is this drug prescribed?

Neodecadron is a steroid and antibiotic combination that is used to treat inflammatory eye conditions in which there is also a bacterial infection or the possibility of a bacterial infection. Dexamethasone (the steroid) decreases inflammation. Neomycin, the antibiotic, kills some of the more common bacteria.

Most important fact about this drug

Prolonged use of Neodecadron may increase the possibility of developing additional eye infections. It could also cause vision problems, raise the pressure inside your eyes, and even lead to glaucoma and cataracts. If you take this medication for 10 days or longer, your doctor will routinely check your eye pressure.

How should you use this medication?

Neodecadron Ophthalmic Solution

1. Wash your hands thoroughly before use.
2. Tilt your head backward or lie down and gaze upward.
3. Gently pull the lower eyelid away from the eye to form a pouch.
4. Drop the medicine in the pouch and gently close your eyes. Try not to blink.
5. Keep your eye closed for a couple of minutes. Do not rub the eye.
6. Do not touch the applicator tip or dropper to any surface, including the eye.

Neodecadron Ophthalmic Ointment

1. Wash your hands thoroughly before use.
2. Hold the ointment tube in your hand for a few minutes to warm the ointment and make it flow more smoothly.

3. Tilt your head backward or lie down and gaze upward.
4. Gently pull the lower eyelid away from the eye to form a pouch.
5. Squeeze the tube gently, and with a sweeping motion along the inside of the lower lid, apply 0.25 to 0.5 inch of ointment.
6. Close your eyes for a couple of minutes and roll them in all directions.

■ *If you miss a dose...*
Take the forgotten dose as soon as you remember. If it is almost time for the next dose, skip the one you missed and go back to your regular schedule. Never try to "catch up" by doubling the dose.

■ *Storage instructions...*
Store at room temperature. Protect solution from light.

What side effects may occur?
Side effects cannot be anticipated. If any develop or change in intensity, notify your doctor as soon as possible. Only your doctor can determine whether it is safe to continue using Neodecadron.

■ *Side effects may include:*
Allergic skin reactions, cataracts, delay in healing of wounds, development of additional eye infections, increased eye pressure with possible glaucoma and optic nerve damage

Why should this drug not be prescribed?
Neodecadron should be avoided if you have an inflammation of the cornea (the transparent surface of the eye); chickenpox; or other bacterial, fungal, or viral eye infections. Do not use Neodecadron if you have ever had an allergic reaction or are sensitive to any of its ingredients.

Neodecadron solution contains a sulfite that can cause an allergic reaction in susceptible people.

Special warnings about this medication
Neodecadron is absorbed into your bloodstream when applied to your eye. Its steroid component can lower your resistance to infection and it can prolong or worsen the severity of many viral infections of the eye. Diseases such as measles and chickenpox can be serious and even fatal in adults. If you are using Neodecadron and are exposed to chickenpox or measles, notify your doctor immediately.

Remember that using Neodecadron for a long time may result in increased pressure in the eye, including glaucoma, as well as vision changes and cataracts. Long-term use also increases the chances of developing an additional eye infection. If you use Neodecadron for 10 days or longer, your doctor should check your eye pressure regularly.

If you undergo eye surgery, sustain an eye injury, or develop an eye infection, check with your doctor immediately.

Eye medications can become contaminated if they are not used properly, causing dangerous infections. Do not let the tip of the container touch anything. If your eyes continue to be red, irritated, swollen, or painful, or if they get worse, notify your doctor immediately.

A preservative in Neodecadron solution can be absorbed by soft contact lenses. If you wear contacts, wait at least 15 minutes after using the solution before you insert your lenses.

If you develop a skin rash or any other allergic reaction, stop using the medication and contact your doctor.

If you have had cataract surgery, Neodecadron may delay healing.

Neodecadron may cause temporary blurring of vision or stinging.

This prescription should not be renewed unless your doctor has re-examined your eyes.

If your signs and symptoms have not improved after two days, your doctor will reconsider your treatment.

**Possible food and drug interactions
when taking this medication**
No interactions have been reported.

**Special information
if you are pregnant or breastfeeding**
Neodecadron has not been adequately studied during pregnancy. If you are pregnant or plan to become pregnant, inform your doctor immediately. Steroids can appear in breast milk. Your doctor may advise you not to breastfeed while you are using Neodecadron.

Recommended dosage
The length of treatment varies with the type of condition being treated. Treatment can take a few days or several weeks.

NEODECADRON OPHTHALMIC OINTMENT

Apply a thin coating of Neodecadron Ophthalmic Ointment 3 or 4 times a day. When the condition gets better, daily applications should be reduced to 2 and later to 1 if a maintenance dose is required to control the symptoms.

NEODECADRON OPHTHALMIC SOLUTION

The recommended initial dose is to place 1 or 2 drops into the conjunctival sac every hour during the day and every 2 hours during the night. When your condition improves, the doctor will lower the dose to 1 drop every 4 hours, and then to 1 drop 3 or 4 times a day.

Overdosage

Any medication taken in excess can have serious consequences. If you suspect a Neodecadron overdose, seek medical treatment immediately.

Brand name:

NEORAL

See Sandimmune, page 1164.

Brand name:

NEPTAZANE

Pronounced: NEP-tuh-zayne
Generic name: Methazolamide

Why is this drug prescribed?

Neptazane anhydrase is used to treat the eye condition called chronic open-angle glaucoma. This type of glaucoma is caused by a gradual blockage of the outflow of fluid in the front compartment of the eye over a period of years, causing a slow rise in pressure. It rarely occurs before the age of 40. Neptazane is also used in the type called acute angle-closure glaucoma when pressure within the eye must be lowered before surgery.

Most important fact about this drug

This medication is related to sulfa drugs and can cause allergic reactions, including fever, rash, redness and peeling of the skin, hives, difficulty breathing, serious skin and blood disorders, and even death. Make sure your doctor is aware of any drug reactions you have experienced. He or she should monitor your blood while you are taking this drug. Call your doctor immediately if you experience any allergic symptoms.

How should you take this medication?

Take Neptazane exactly as prescribed. Your doctor may have you use it with other eye medications.

■ *If you miss a dose...*
Take it as soon as you remember. If it is almost time for your next dose, skip the one you missed and go back to your regular schedule. Do not take 2 doses at once.

■ *Storage instructions...*
Store at room temperature.

What side effects may occur?
Side effects cannot be anticipated. If any occur or change in intensity, inform your doctor as soon as possible. Only your doctor can determine if it is safe for you to continue taking Neptazane. Most reactions to Neptazane have been mild and disappear when the medication is stopped or the dosage is adjusted.

■ *More common side effects may include:*
Confusion, depression, diarrhea, dizziness, drowsiness, excessive urination, fatigue, fever, general feeling of not being well, headache, hearing problems, loss of appetite, nausea and vomiting, rash, ringing in the ears, severe allergic reaction, taste changes, temporary nearsightedness, tingling in fingers, toes, hands, or feet

■ *Rare side effects may include:*
Black, tarry stools, blood in the urine, convulsions, hives, increased sensitivity to light, kidney stones, paralysis

Why should this drug not be prescribed?
Neptazane is not for use against all types of glaucoma—only the ones mentioned in "Why is this drug prescribed?" Also, you should not use Neptazane if you have kidney or liver disease, adrenal gland disorders, or low sodium or potassium levels.

Special warnings about this medication
Neptazane can aggravate acidosis, a condition in which the blood is too acidic.

If you have emphysema or a lung blockage, this drug will be prescribed cautiously.

Possible food and drug interactions
when taking this medication
If Neptazane is taken with certain other drugs, the effects of either could be increased, decreased, or altered.

Neptazane and high-dose aspirin taken at the same time can cause loss of appetite, rapid breathing, lethargy, coma, and even death.

Use of Neptazane with steroids may lower your potassium level.

Special information
if you are pregnant or breastfeeding
The effects of Neptazane in pregnancy have not been adequately studied. Neptazane should be used by a pregnant woman only if the potential benefit outweighs the potential risk to the developing baby. If you are pregnant or plan to become pregnant, inform your doctor immediately. Neptazane may appear in breast milk and could affect a nursing infant. If this medication is essential to your health, your doctor may advise you to stop breastfeeding until your treatment with Neptazane is finished.

Recommended dosage

ADULTS

The usual dosage is 50 milligrams to 100 milligrams taken 2 to 3 times a day.

Overdosage
Any drug taken in excess can have serious consequences. If you suspect an overdose of Neptazane, seek medical attention immediately.

Brand name:

NEURONTIN

Pronounced: NUHR-on-tin
Generic name: Gabapentin

Why is this drug prescribed?
Neurontin, an epilepsy medication, is used with other medications to treat certain types of difficult to manage seizures, including elementary partial seizures (brief and no loss of consciousness) and complex partial seizures (consciousness impaired), with and without secondary generalization (grand mal epilepsy with loss of consciousness).

Most important fact about this drug
Take Neurontin exactly as directed by your doctor. To effectively control your seizures, it is important that you take Neurontin 3 times a day, approximately every 8 hours. You should not go longer than 12 hours without a dose of medication.

How should you take this medication?

Do not increase or decrease dosage of this medication without your doctor's approval; and do not suddenly stop taking it, as this may cause an increase in the frequency of your seizures. If you are taking an antacid such as Maalox, take Neurontin at least 2 hours after the antacid.

You may take Neurontin with or without food.

- ■ *If you miss a dose...*
  Try not to allow more than 12 hours to pass between doses. Do not double doses.

- ■ *Storage instructions...*
  Store at room temperature.

What side effects may occur?

Side effects cannot be anticipated. If any develop or change in intensity, inform your doctor as soon as possible. Because Neurontin is used with other antiseizure drugs, it may not be possible to determine whether a side effect is due to Neurontin alone. Only your doctor can determine if it is safe for you to continue taking Neurontin.

- ■ *More common side effects may include:*
  Blurred, dimmed, or double vision, dizziness, drowsiness, fatigue, involuntary eye movement, itchy, runny nose, lack of muscular coordination, nausea, tremor, vomiting

- ■ *Less common or rare side effects may include:*
  Abnormal coordination, abnormal dreams, abnormal thinking, agitation, allergy, altered reflexes, anemia, angina pectoris (crushing chest pain), anxiety, apathy, arthritis, back pain, behavioral or psychological problems, bladder problems, bleeding gums, bloody stools, bruising, cataracts, chill, conjunctivitis (pinkeye), constipation, cough, cysts, decreased sensitivity to touch, depression, difficult or labored breathing, dry eyes, dry mouth or throat, dry or scaly skin, ear problems, exaggerated feeling of well-being, excessive body hair, eye pain or disorder, fainting, feeling "high," "fever" blisters on lips and mouth, fluid retention, fracture, gas, general feeling of illness, hair loss, hallucination, heart murmur, heartburn, hemorrhoids, high blood pressure, hostility, hyperactivity, increased appetite, increased salivation, increased sweating, indigestion, inflammation of the mouth, gums, or tongue, inflammation of the stomach and intestinal lining, irregular heartbeat, itching, joint pain, stiffness, or swelling, liver enlargement, loss of appetite, loss of bowel control, loss of memory, low

blood pressure, menstrual problems, migraines, mouth sores, muscle pain or weakness, nervousness, nosebleeds, paralysis, pneumonia, sexual problems, shortness of breath, skin disorders, sore throat, speech difficulties, stupor, swelling of the face, taste loss, tendinitis, thirst, tingling or pins and needles, twitching, vaginal hemorrhage, vertigo, weight increase or decrease

Why should this drug not be prescribed?

You should not take Neurontin if you have ever had an allergic reaction to it.

Special warnings about this medication

Neurontin causes some people to become drowsy and less alert. Do not drive or operate dangerous machinery or participate in any hazardous activity that requires full mental alertness until you are certain Neurontin does not have this effect on you.

Be sure to tell your doctor if you have any kidney problems or are on hemodialysis, as your doctor will need to adjust your dosage of Neurontin.

Tell your doctor about any medications you are taking, including over-the-counter drugs.

Possible food and drug interactions
when taking this medication

If Neurontin is taken with certain other drugs, the effects of either can be increased, decreased, or altered. It is especially important to check with your doctor before combining Neurontin with the following:

Antacids such as Maalox

Special information
if you are pregnant or breastfeeding

The effects of Neurontin on pregnant women have not been adequately studied, although birth defects have occurred in babies whose mothers took an antiepileptic drug while they were pregnant. It should be used during pregnancy only if clearly needed. If you are pregnant or plan to become pregnant, tell your doctor immediately. This medication may appear in breast milk and could affect a nursing infant. Check with your doctor if you plan to breastfeed your baby.

Recommended dosage

ADULTS AND CHILDREN 12 YEARS AND OVER

Your doctor will probably start your therapy with one 300-milligram dose at bedtime on the first day, two 300-milligram doses the second day, and three

300-milligram doses the third day. After that, the usual daily dosage ranges from 900 to 1,800 milligrams divided into 3 doses, using 300-milligram or 400-milligram capsules.

If Neurontin is discontinued or another drug added to therapy, your doctor will do this gradually, over a 1-week period.

Overdosage
Any medication taken in excess can have serious consequences. If you suspect an overdose, seek medical treatment immediately.

■ *Symptoms of Neurontin overdose may include:*
Diarrhea, double vision, drowsiness, lethargy, slurred speech

Generic name:

NEVIRAPINE

See Viramune, page 1417.

Generic name:

NICARDIPINE

See Cardene, page 198.

Brand name:

NICODERM CQ

See Nicotine Patches, below.

Generic name:

NICOTINE INHALATION SYSTEM

See Nicotrol Inhaler, 875.

Category:

NICOTINE PATCHES

Brand names: Habitrol, Nicoderm, Nicotrol, ProStep

Why is this drug prescribed?

Nicotine patches, which are available under several brand names, are designed to help you quit smoking by reducing your craving for tobacco. Each adhesive patch contains a specific amount of nicotine embedded in a pad or gel.

Nicotine, the habit-forming ingredient in tobacco, is a stimulant and a mood lifter. When you give up smoking, lack of nicotine makes you crave cigarettes and may also cause anger, anxiety, concentration problems, irritability, frustration, or restlessness.

When you wear a nicotine patch, a specific amount of nicotine steadily travels out of the patch, through your skin, and into your bloodstream, keeping a constant low level of nicotine in your body. Although the resulting level of nicotine is less than you would get from smoking, it may be enough to keep you from craving cigarettes or experiencing other withdrawal symptoms.

Habitrol patches are round and come in three strengths: 21, 14, or 7 milligrams of nicotine per patch. You wear a Habitrol patch 24 hours a day.

Nicoderm patches are rectangular and come in three strengths: 21, 14, or 7 milligrams of nicotine per patch. You wear a Nicoderm patch 24 hours a day.

Nicotrol patches are rectangular and deliver 15 milligrams of nicotine per patch. You put on a Nicotrol patch in the morning, wear it all day, and remove it at bedtime. You do not use it when you sleep. Nicotrol is available over-the-counter.

ProStep patches are round and come in two strengths: 22 or 11 milligrams of nicotine per patch. You wear a ProStep patch 24 hours a day.

Most important fact about this drug

Nicotine patch therapy should be part of an overall stop-smoking program that also includes behavior modification, counseling, and support. The goal of the therapy should be complete cessation of smoking, not just "cutting down."

How should you use this medication?

Use nicotine patches exactly as prescribed. The general procedure is as follows:

- Take a fresh patch out of its packaging and remove the protective liner from the adhesive. Save the wrapper for later disposal of the used patch.
- Stick the patch onto your outer upper arm or any clean, non-hairy part of your trunk.
- Press the patch firmly onto your skin for about 10 seconds, making sure that the edges are sticking well.

- Wash your hands. Any nicotine sticking to your hands could get into your eyes or nose, causing irritation.
- After 16 or 24 hours (depending on the brand), remove that patch and apply a fresh patch to a different spot on your body. To reduce the chances of irritation, do not return to a previously used spot for at least a week.
- Fold the used patch in half, place it back in its own wrapper, and throw it in a trash container that cannot be reached by children or pets.

Water will not harm the nicotine patch. You may keep wearing your patch while bathing, showering, swimming, or using a hot tub.

If your patch does fall off, dispose of it carefully and apply a new patch.

As a memory aid, pick a specific time of day and always apply a fresh patch at that time. You may change the schedule if you need to. Just remember not to wear any single patch for more than the recommended time (16 or 24 hours), since after that time the patch will begin to lose strength and may begin to irritate your skin.

Do not change brands without consulting your doctor, and do not attempt to adjust your dosage by cutting a patch in pieces.

If you are unable to stop smoking after 4 to 6 weeks of wearing nicotine patches, it is likely that patch treatment will not work for you.

- *If you miss a dose...*
  Apply the patch as soon as you remember. Never use 2 patches at once.

- *Storage instructions...*
  Do not remove a patch from its wrapping until you are ready to use it. Store your supply of patches at temperatures no higher than 86 degrees Fahrenheit; remember that in warm weather the inside of a car can get much hotter than this.

What side effects may occur?
Side effects cannot be anticipated. If any develop or change in intensity, inform your doctor as soon as possible. Only your doctor can determine if it is safe for you to continue using nicotine patches.

- *Most common side effects may include:*
  Dizziness, high blood pressure, itching and burning at the application site, nausea, redness of the skin

- *Less common side effects may include:*
  Abnormal dreaming, allergic reactions, back pain, chest pain, constipation, cough, diarrhea, drowsiness, dry mouth, headache, impaired concentra-

tion, indigestion, inflammation of sinuses, menstrual irregularities, numbness, pain, pins and needles sensation, rash, sleeplessness, sore throat, stomach pain, sweating, taste changes, tingling, vomiting, weakness

Why should this drug not be prescribed?
Do not take this medication if you are sensitive to or have ever had an allergic reaction to nicotine. Be cautious if you have ever had a bad reaction to a different brand of nicotine patch or to adhesive tape or other adhesive material.

Special warnings about this medication
Do not smoke, chew, or sniff any form of tobacco while wearing a patch; doing so could give you an overdose of nicotine. Be aware that for several hours after you remove a patch, nicotine from the patch is still in your skin and passing into your bloodstream, so you should not smoke even when the patch is off.

The use of nicotine patches may aggravate certain medical conditions. Before you use any brand of nicotine patch, make sure your doctor knows if you have, or have ever had, any of the following conditions:

Allergies to drugs, adhesive tape, or bandages
Chest pain from a heart condition (angina)
Diabetes requiring insulin injections
Heart attack or heart disease
High blood pressure (severe)
Irregular heartbeat (heart arrhythmia)
Kidney disease
Liver disease
Overactive thyroid
Skin disease
Stomach ulcer

Nicotine, from any source, can be toxic and addictive. Do not use nicotine patches any longer than your doctor prescribes or the product instructions recommend. Thoroughly discuss with your doctor the benefits and risks of nicotine replacement therapy.

If your heartbeat becomes irregular or you have heart palpitations, stop using the patch and call your doctor. Do the same if redness caused by the patch doesn't go away in 4 days or if your skin swells or develops a rash.

Do not use a patch if its pouch is unsealed.

The safety and effectiveness of nicotine patches have not been tested in children. Over-the-counter Nicotrol is not for use by children under age 18.

Because a used nicotine patch still contains enough nicotine to poison a child or a pet, you must dispose of used patches with special care. Wrap each patch in the opened pouch or aluminum foil in which it came and throw it in a trash receptacle that is out of the reach of youngsters and animals.

Possible food and drug interactions
when taking this medication
If nicotine patches are used with certain other drugs, the effects of either could be increased, decreased, or altered. It is especially important to check with your doctor before combining nicotine patches with the following:

   Acetaminophen-containing drugs such as Tylenol
   Caffeine-containing drugs such as No Doz
   Certain airway-opening drugs such as Isuprel, Dristan, and Neo-
      Synephrine
   Certain blood pressure medicines such as Minipress, Trandate, and
      Normodyne
   Cimetidine (Tagamet)
   Haloperidol (Haldol)
   Imipramine (Tofranil)
   Insulin
   Lithium (Lithonate)
   Oxazepam (Serax)
   Pentazocine (Talwin)
   Propranolol (Inderal)
   Theophylline (Theo-Dur)

Special information
if you are pregnant or breastfeeding
If you are pregnant or plan to become pregnant, inform your doctor immediately. Ideally, a pregnant woman should not take nicotine in any form. Do your best to quit smoking with the aid of counseling and support and without drug therapy. If you are unable to quit, you and your doctor should discuss which is more likely to harm your unborn baby: continued smoking or use of nicotine patches to help you quit smoking. Because nicotine passes very readily into breast milk, ideally it should not be taken in any form during breastfeeding. If you are breastfeeding and are unable to quit smoking, discuss with your doctor the pros and cons of using nicotine patches.

Remember that if you smoke while wearing a patch, you are giving your body a "double dose" of nicotine; if you are pregnant or breastfeeding, your baby will get the "double dose," too.

Recommended dosage

Nicotine patches come in one, two, or three strengths, depending on the brand; larger patches contain higher doses of nicotine. The usual starting dose is 1 high-strength patch per day. If you weigh less than 100 pounds, however, or if you smoke less than half a pack of cigarettes a day or have heart disease, your doctor may start you on a lower-dose patch.

Your doctor will work closely with you to determine the best product and the most effective cessation program.

Overdosage

Any medication used in excess, including nicotine patches, can have serious consequences. If you suspect symptoms of an overdose of nicotine, either from a patch or from smoking while wearing a patch, seek medical attention immediately.

■ *Symptoms of nicotine overdose may include:*
Abdominal pain, blurred vision, breathing abnormalities, cold sweat, confusion, diarrhea, dizziness, drooling, fainting, hearing difficulties, heart palpitations, low blood pressure, nausea, pallor, rapid heartbeat, salivation, severe headaches, sweating, tremor, upset stomach, vision problems, vomiting, weakness

Brand name:

NICOTROL

See Nicotine Patches, page 870.

Brand name:

NICOTROL INHALER

Pronounced: NICK-o-trole
Generic name: Nicotine inhalation system

Why is this drug prescribed?

A quit-smoking aid, the Nicotrol Inhaler provides a substitute source of nicotine when you first give up cigarettes. A sudden decline in nicotine levels can cause such withdrawal symptoms as nervousness, restlessness, irritability, anxiety, depression, dizziness, drowsiness, concentration problems, sleep disturbances, increased appetite, weight gain, headache, constipation, fatigue, muscle aches, and a craving for tobacco. Nicotrol Inhaler prevents these symptoms and, through a familiar hand-to-mouth ritual, acts as a replacement for cigarettes. (Most of the nicotine in the product is, however, deposited in the mouth instead of the lungs.)

Most important fact about this drug

To get the most from this system, you must be genuinely committed to quitting, and should give up smoking completely before you begin using the inhaler. It should be employed as part of an overall stop-smoking program that includes behavior modification, counseling, and support. The goal is to become a total non-smoker. If you find that you are still smoking after 4 weeks with the inhaler, you should probably stop treatment and try again when you are really ready to quit.

How should you take this medication?

Each Nicotrol Inhaler package includes a mouthpiece and 42 cartridges of nicotine. Treatment takes place in two stages. During the first stage (up to 12 weeks) you should use as many Nicotrol cartridges as needed (at least 6, but no more than 16 daily) to quell the craving for cigarettes. During the second stage (6 to 12 weeks) you should gradually reduce your daily consumption until you are nicotine-free.

For best effect, puff frequently on each cartridge for about 20 minutes. Remember to clean the mouthpiece regularly with soap and water.

■ *If you miss a dose...*
Use the inhaler no more than needed to control the urge to smoke.

■ *Storage instructions...*
Store at room temperature away from light. Keep the mouthpiece in its plastic storage case.

What side effects may occur?

Side effects cannot be anticipated. If any develop or change in intensity, inform your doctor as soon as possible. Only your doctor can determine if it is safe for you to continue using the Nicotrol Inhaler.

■ *Side effects may include:*
Acid indigestion, allergies, back pain, coughing, diarrhea, fever, flu-like symptoms, gas, headache, hiccups, jaw and neck pain, mouth and throat

irritation, nasal inflammation, nausea, pain, sinus inflammation, taste
disturbances, tingling skin sensation, tooth disorders

Why should this drug not be prescribed?
Nicotrol Inhaler should not be used by anyone allergic to nicotine or menthol.

Special warnings about this medication
Nicotine from any source can be toxic and addictive, and you can become
dependent on the Nicotrol Inhaler. To minimize this risk, it's important to
gradually cut back on use of the inhaler after the first 3 months. Its use for
more than 6 months is not recommended.

Do not smoke while using the inhaler. The added nicotine will increase your
risk of developing nicotine toxicity.

Nicotrol Inhaler may not be your best quit-smoking option if you have angina,
heartbeat irregularities, Raynaud's phenomenon (periodic loss of circulation
in the fingers), Buerger's disease (a dangerous decline in circulation in the
hands and feet) or a history of heart attack. If you develop an irregular
heartbeat or palpitations, stop using the product and call your doctor
immediately.

Nicotrol Inhaler should also be used with caution if you have a respiratory
disease, an overactive thyroid, pheochromocytoma (adrenal tumors), insulin-
dependent diabetes, an ulcer, severe high blood pressure, or advanced kidney
disease.

The nicotine in Nicotrol cartridges can be fatal if inhaled or swallowed by
children or pets. Keep used and unused cartridges in a safe place.

Possible food and drug interactions
when taking this medication
If you have been taking certain medications regularly, their effects may
increase, decrease, or change when you stop smoking. It is especially
important to check with your doctor if you have been taking the following
drugs:

Antidepressants such as Anafranil
Elavil
Norpramin
Pamelor
Sinequan, and Tofranil
Theophylline (Theo-Dur, Theo-24, Slo-bid)

Special information
if you are pregnant or breastfeeding

Cigarette smoking during pregnancy is associated with low birth weight, an increased risk of stillbirth, and a greater chance of miscarriage, so it's extremely important to quit. The Nicotrol Inhaler system may be less harmful than cigarettes, since it does not contain the hydrogen cyanide and carbon monoxide present in cigarette smoke. Nevertheless, nicotine alone can cause fetal harm in lab animals, and your best course is to avoid nicotine in any form. Quitting with the aid of a nicotine-replacement system such as Nicotrol Inhaler should be considered only if all other quit-smoking strategies fail. Discuss the problem thoroughly with your doctor.

Nicotine passes into breast milk and ideally should not be taken in any form during breastfeeding. However, use of the Nicotrol Inhaler system could be preferable to smoking, since it may reduce the level of nicotine in your system. If you are breastfeeding, discuss with your doctor the relative pros and cons of quitting with the Nicotrol Inhaler.

Recommended dosage

ADULTS

Dosage varies with the stage of treatment.

Initial Treatment (Up to 12 Weeks):
Use at least 6 cartridges a day for the first 3 to 6 weeks. Additional doses may be needed to control the urge to smoke, up to a maximum of 16 cartridges a day. The average number of doses falls between these extremes.

Gradual Reduction of Dose (Up to 12 Weeks):
Start using Nicotrol Inhaler less frequently. You may find it helpful to keep a tally of daily usage, set a steadily diminishing target, or plan a fixed quit date. Some people find that they can stop abruptly with success.

Overdosage

Excessive doses of nicotine can cause severe symptoms, and may even be fatal. If you suspect an overdose, seek medical attention immediately.

■ *Symptoms of nicotine overdose may include:*
Abdominal pain, breathing abnormalities, cold sweat, confusion, diarrhea, dizziness, exhaustion, headaches, hearing difficulties, increased salivation, low blood pressure, nausea, pallor, tremor, vision problems, vomiting, weakness

Generic name:

NIFEDIPINE

See Procardia, page 1055.

Brand name:

NILANDRON

Pronounced: nigh-LAND-ron
Generic name: Nilutamide

Why is this drug prescribed?

Nilandron is used for advanced prostate cancer—cancer that has begun to spread beyond the prostate gland. An "antiandrogen" drug, it blocks the effects of the male hormone testosterone, which is known to encourage prostate cancer. The drug is part of a treatment program that begins with removal of the testes, a major—but not the only—source of testosterone.

Most important fact about this drug

Nilandron treatment must begin on the same day as, or on the day after, surgical removal of the testes. You should not interrupt the doses or stop taking Nilandron without consulting your doctor.

How should you take this medication?

Take Nilandron exactly as prescribed. You may take Nilandron with or without food.

- *If you miss a dose...*
  Take the forgotten dose as soon as you remember. If it is almost time for your next dose, skip the one you missed and go back to your regular schedule. Never take 2 doses at the same time.

- *Storage instructions...*
  Store at room temperature away from light.

What side effects may occur?

Side effects cannot be anticipated. If any develop or change in intensity, inform your doctor immediately. Only your doctor can determine if it is safe for you to continue taking Nilandron.

■ *More common side effects may include:*
Abnormal vision, alcohol intolerance, constipation, decreased sex drive, difficulty breathing, dizziness, heart failure, hot flashes, impotence, increase in blood pressure, lung problems, nausea, poor adaptation to the dark, tingling feeling, urinary tract infection

■ *Less common side effects may include:*
Abdominal bleeding or discomfort, angina (chest pain), arthritis, cataracts, coughing, diarrhea, dry mouth, fainting, general feeling of discomfort, high sensitivity to light, inflammation of the nasal passages, itching, nervousness, swelling, tarry stools, weight loss

Why should this drug not be prescribed?
Do not take Nilandron if you have ever had an allergic reaction to it or to any of its ingredients. If you have severe liver disease or severe breathing problems, you should not take this medication. Make sure your doctor is aware of these conditions.

Special warnings about this medication
Nilandron occasionally causes inflammation of the lungs; and if a problem does develop, you may have to stop taking the drug. Report any symptoms that might suggest a lung problem to your doctor right away. Warning signs include difficulty breathing upon exertion or worsening of a pre-existing problem, cough, chest pain, and fever. This lung condition almost always goes away when Nilandron treatment is stopped.

Nilandron may also cause liver damage in some people. Your doctor will do blood tests to check your liver function before you start treatment and every 3 months thereafter. If a liver problem does develop, you may have to stop taking Nilandron. Report any symptoms of liver damage to your doctor immediately. Warning signs include dark urine, jaundice (a yellowing of the skin and eyes), fatigue, abdominal pain, nausea, or vomiting.

While taking Nilandron, you may also find that your eyes are slow to adapt to the dark when you leave a lighted area. Be careful when driving at night or through tunnels. Tinted glasses will help this problem.

**Possible food and drug interactions
when taking this medication**
Nilandron can cause a reaction to alcohol. If you develop a facial flush, flu-like symptoms, and a decrease in blood pressure after drinking alcohol, you'll need to give up alcoholic beverages while taking this drug.

If Nilandron is taken with certain drugs, the effects of either could be increased, decreased, or altered. It is especially important to check with your doctor before combining Nilandron with the following:

Phenytoin (Dilantin)
Theophylline (Theo-Dur)
Vitamin K antagonists (Coumadin)

If you are already taking Coumadin, you will need to be monitored especially closely after treatment with Nilandron begins. Your doctor may need to lower your dosage of Coumadin.

**Special information
if you are pregnant or breastfeeding**
Nilandron is for use only by men.

Recommended dosage
The recommended adult dosage is 6 tablets once a day for 30 days. The dosage is then reduced to 3 tablets once a day.

Overdosage
Any medication taken in excess can have serious consequences. If you suspect an overdose, seek medical attention immediately.

■ *Symptoms of Nilandron overdose may include:*
Dizziness, general discomfort, headache, nausea, vomiting

Generic name:

NILUTAMIDE

See Nilandron, page 879.

Generic name:

NISOLDIPINE

See Sular, page 1224.

Brand name:

NITRO-BID

See Nitroglycerin, page 882.

Brand name:

NITRO-DUR

See Nitroglycerin, below.

Generic name:

NITROFURANTOIN

See Macrodantin, page 748.

Generic name:

NITROGLYCERIN

Pronounced: NIGHT-row-GLISS-err-in
Brand names: Nitro-Bid, Nitro-Dur, Nitrolingual Spray,
  Nitrostat Tablets, Transderm-Nitro

Why is this drug prescribed?
Nitroglycerin is prescribed to prevent and treat angina pectoris (suffocating chest pain). This condition occurs when the coronary arteries become constricted and are not able to carry sufficient oxygen to the heart muscle. Nitroglycerin is thought to improve oxygen flow by relaxing the walls of arteries and veins, thus allowing them to dilate.

Nitroglycerin is used in different forms. As a patch or ointment, nitroglycerin may be applied to the skin. The patch and the ointment are for *prevention* of chest pain.

Swallowing nitroglycerin in capsule or tablet form also helps to *prevent* chest pain from occurring.

In the form of sublingual (held under the tongue) or buccal (held in the cheek) tablets, or in oral spray (sprayed on or under the tongue), nitroglycerin helps relieve chest pain that has *already occurred*. The spray can also prevent anginal pain. The type of nitroglycerin you use will depend on your condition.

Most important fact about this drug
Nitroglycerin may cause severe low blood pressure (possibly marked by dizziness or light-headedness), especially if you are in an upright position or have just gotten up from sitting or lying down. You may also find your heart rate slowing and your chest pain increasing. People taking diuretic

medication, or who have low systolic blood pressure (less than 90 mm Hg) should use nitroglycerin with caution.

How should you take this medication?
Since nitroglycerin is available in many forms, it is crucial for you to follow your doctor's directions for taking the type of nitroglycerin prescribed for you. Never interchange brands.

Ideally, you should take nitroglycerin while sitting down—especially if you feel dizzy or light-headed—so as to avoid a fall.

■ *If you miss a dose...*
If you are using a skin patch or ointment:

Apply it as soon as you remember. If it is almost time for your regular dose, skip the one you missed and go back to your regular schedule. Never apply 2 skin patches at the same time.

If you are taking oral tablets or capsules:

Take the forgotten dose as soon as you remember. However, if it is within 2 hours of your next dose, skip the one you missed and go back to your regular schedule. Never take 2 doses at the same time.

■ *Storage instructions...*
Keep this medication in the container it came in, tightly closed. Store it at room temperature. Do not refrigerate.

Avoid puncturing the spray container and keep it away from excess heat.

Do not open the container of sublingual tablets until you need a dose. Close the container tightly immediately after each use. Do not put other medications, a cotton plug, or anything else in the container. Keep the sublingual tablets handy at all times. Keep the patches in the protective pouches they come in until use.

What side effects may occur?
Side effects cannot be anticipated. If any develop or change in intensity, inform your doctor as soon as possible. Only your doctor can determine if it is safe for you to continue taking nitroglycerin.

■ *More common side effects may include:*
Dizziness, flushed skin (neck and face), headache, light-headedness, worsened angina pain

■ *Less common or rare side effects may include:*
Diarrhea, fainting, heart pounding, low blood pressure, nausea, numbness, pallor, restlessness, severe allergic reactions, skin rashes and eruptions, sweating, vertigo, vomiting, weakness

Why should this drug not be prescribed?

You should not be using nitroglycerin if you are allergic to it or to the adhesive in the patch, if you have a head injury, or if you have any condition caused by increased fluid pressure in your head. Nitroglycerin should not be taken if you have severe anemia or if you recently had a heart attack. The capsule form should not be used if you have closed-angle glaucoma (pressure in the eye) or suffer from postural hypotension (dizziness upon standing up).

Special warnings about this medication

If your vision becomes blurry or your mouth becomes dry while taking nitroglycerin, it should be discontinued. Contact your doctor immediately if these symptoms develop.

You may develop acute headaches if you take nitroglycerin excessively. Also, some people may develop a tolerance to nitroglycerin, and it may become less beneficial over time, especially if used in excess.

If you are taking sublingual nitroglycerin, you may notice a burning or tingling sensation. This does not necessarily mean the tablets are still good.

Take no more than the smallest possible amount needed to relieve pain.

Daily headaches may be an indicator of the drug's activity. Do not change your dose to avoid the headache, because you may reduce the drug's effectiveness at the same time.

Before taking nitroglycerin, tell your doctor if you have had a recent heart attack, head injury, or stroke; or if you have anemia, glaucoma (pressure in the eye), or heart, kidney, liver, or thyroid disease.

If you use a patch, dispose of it carefully. There is enough drug left in a used patch to be harmful to children and pets.

Since nitroglycerin can cause dizziness, you should observe caution while driving, operating machinery, or performing other tasks that demand concentration.

The benefits of applying nitroglycerin to the skin of people experiencing heart attacks or congestive heart failure have not been established. If you are using the medication for these conditions, your doctor will monitor you to prevent low blood pressure and pounding heartbeat.

Possible food and drug interactions when taking this medication

If nitroglycerin is taken with certain other drugs, the effects of either could be increased, decreased, or altered.

Taken with many high blood pressure drugs, nitroglycerin may cause extreme low blood pressure (dizziness, fainting, numbness). Take particular care with calcium channel blockers such as Calan and Procardia XL, as well as isosorbide dinitrate (Sorbitrate, Isordil, others), isosorbide mononitrate (Ismo, others), blood vessel dilators such as Loniten, and beta-blocker medications such as Tenormin.

Aspirin can increase the effects of nitroglycerin.

Alcohol may interact with nitroglycerin and cause a swift decrease in blood pressure, possibly causing dizziness and fainting.

Also be alert for an interaction with dihydroergotamine (D.H.E.). Check with your doctor if you are uncertain about any combination you plan to take.

Special information if you are pregnant or breastfeeding

It has not been determined whether nitroglycerin might harm a fetus or a pregnant woman. As a result, nitroglycerin should be used only when the benefits of therapy clearly outweigh the potential risks to the fetus and woman. It is not known if nitroglycerin appears in breast milk; therefore, a nursing mother should use nitroglycerin only on advice of her doctor.

Recommended dosage

The following section is intended to provide guidelines for taking nitroglycerin. Follow your doctor's instructions carefully for using nitroglycerin in the form prescribed for you.

ADULTS

Sublingual or Buccal Tablets

At the first sign of chest pain, 1 tablet should be dissolved under the tongue or inside the cheek. You may repeat the dose every 5 minutes until the pain is relieved. If your pain continues after you have taken 3 tablets in a 15-minute period, notify your doctor or seek medical attention immediately.

You may take sublingual or buccal nitroglycerin from 5 to 10 minutes before starting activities that may cause chest pain.

Patch Form
A patch is applied to the skin for 12 to 14 hours. After this time, the patch is removed; it is not applied again for 10 to 12 hours (a "patch-off" period). Apply the patch as soon as you remove it from its protective pouch.

Spray Form
At the first sign of chest pain, spray 1 or 2 premeasured doses onto or under the tongue. You should not use more than 3 doses within a 15-minute period. If your chest pain continues, you should contact your doctor or seek medical attention immediately.

The spray can be used 5 to 10 minutes before activity that might precipitate an attack.

Ointment Form
Your initial dose may be a daily total of 1 inch of ointment. Apply one-half inch on rising in the morning, and the remaining one-half inch 6 hours later. If needed, follow your doctor's instructions for increasing your dosage. Apply in a thin, uniform layer, regardless of the amount of your dosage. There should be a daily period where no ointment is applied. Usually, the "ointment-off" period will last from 10 to 12 hours.

Absorption varies with site of application—more is absorbed through the chest.

Sustained-Release Capsules or Tablets
The smallest effective amount should be taken 2 or 3 times a day at 8- to 12-hour intervals.

CHILDREN

The safety and effectiveness of nitroglycerin have not been established for children.

OLDER ADULTS

In general, dosages less than the above adult dosages are recommended, since the elderly may be more susceptible to low blood pressure and headaches.

Overdosage
Any medication taken in excess can have serious consequences. Severe overdosage of nitroglycerin may result in death. If you suspect an overdose, seek medical attention immediately.

■ *Symptoms of overdose may include:*
Bluish skin, clammy skin, colic, coma, confusion, diarrhea (may be bloody), difficult and/or slow breathing, dizziness, fainting, fever, flushed skin, headache (persistent, throbbing), increased pressure within the skull, irregular pulse, loss of appetite, nausea, palpitations (an abnormally rapid throbbing or fluttering of the heart), paralysis, rapid decrease in blood pressure, seizures, slow or fast pulse/heartbeat, sweating, vertigo, visual disturbances, vomiting

Brand name:

NITROLINGUAL SPRAY

See Nitroglycerin, page 882.

Brand name:

NITROSTAT TABLETS

See Nitroglycerin, page 882.

Generic name:

NIZATIDINE

See Axid, page 121.

Brand name:

NIZORAL

Pronounced: NYE-zore-al
Generic name: Ketoconazole

Why is this drug prescribed?
Nizoral, a broad-spectrum antifungal drug available in tablet form, may be given to treat several fungal infections within the body, including oral thrush and candidiasis.

It may also be given to treat severe, hard-to-treat fungal skin infections that have not cleared up after treatment with creams or ointments, or the oral drug griseofulvin (Fulvicin, Grisactin).

Most important fact about this drug
In some people, Nizoral may cause serious or even fatal damage to the liver. Before starting to take Nizoral, and at frequent intervals while you are taking

it, you should have blood tests to evaluate your liver function. Tell your doctor immediately if you experience any signs or symptoms that could mean liver damage: these include unusual fatigue, loss of appetite, nausea or vomiting, jaundice, dark urine, or pale stools.

How should you take this medication?
Take Nizoral exactly as prescribed.

You should keep taking the drug until tests show that your fungal infection has subsided. If you stop too soon, the infection might return.

You may want to take Nizoral Tablets with meals to avoid stomach upset.

Avoid alcohol and do not take with antacids. If antacids are necessary, you should wait 2 to 3 hours before taking them.

■ *If you miss a dose...*
Take the forgotten dose as soon as you remember. This will help to keep the proper amount of medicine in the body. However, if it is almost time for your next dose, skip the one you missed and go back to your regular schedule. Do not take double doses.

■ *Storage instructions...*
Nizoral should be stored at room temperature.

What side effects may occur?
Side effects from Nizoral cannot be anticipated. If any develop or change in intensity, inform your doctor as soon as possible. Only your doctor can determine if it is safe for you to continue taking Nizoral.

■ *More common side effects may include:*
Nausea, vomiting

■ *Less common side effects may include:*
Abdominal pain, itching

■ *Rare side effects may include:*
Breast swelling (in men), depression, diarrhea, dizziness, drowsiness, fever and chills, headache, hives, impotence, light-sensitivity, rash

Why should this drug not be prescribed?
Do not take Nizoral if you are sensitive to it or have ever had an allergic reaction to it. Never take Nizoral together with Seldane, Hismanal, Halcion,

or Propulsid. Rare, but sometimes fatal reactions have been reported when these drugs are combined.

Special warnings about this medication

In rare cases, people have had anaphylaxis (a life-threatening allergic reaction) after taking their first dose of Nizoral.

Observe caution when driving or performing other tasks requiring alertness, due to potential side effects of headache, dizziness, and drowsiness.

Possible food and drug interactions
when taking this medication

If Nizoral is taken with certain other drugs, the effects of either could be increased, decreased, or altered. It is especially important to check with your doctor before combining Nizoral with the following:

Alcoholic beverages
Antacids such as Di-Gel, Maalox, Mylanta, and others
Anticoagulants such as Coumadin, Dicumarol, and others
Anti-ulcer medications such as Axid, Pepcid, Tagamet, and Zantac
Astemizole (Hismanal)
Cisapride (Propulsid)
Cyclosporine (Sandimmune, Neoral)
Digoxin (Lanoxin)
Drugs that relieve spasms, such as Donnatal
Isoniazid (Nydrazid)
Methylprednisolone (Medrol)
Midazolam (Versed)
Oral diabetes drugs such as Diabinese and Micronase
Phenytoin (Dilantin)
Rifampin (Rifadin, Rifamate, and Rimactane)
Tacrolimus (Prograf)
Terfenadine (Seldane)
Theophyllines (Slo-Phyllin, Theo-Dur, others)
Triazolam (Halcion)

Special information
if you are pregnant or breastfeeding

If you are pregnant or plan to become pregnant, inform your doctor immediately. Nizoral should be taken during pregnancy only if the benefit outweighs the possible harm to your unborn child.

Since Nizoral can probably make its way into breast milk, it should not be taken during breastfeeding. If you are a new mother, check with your doctor. You may need to stop breastfeeding while you are taking Nizoral.

Recommended dosage

ADULTS

The recommended starting dose of Nizoral is a single daily dose of 200 milligrams (1 tablet).

In very serious infections, or if the problem does not clear up within the expected time, the dose of Nizoral may be increased to 400 milligrams (2 tablets) once daily. Treatment lasts at least 1 to 2 weeks, and for some infections much longer.

CHILDREN

In small numbers of children over 2 years of age, a single daily dose of 3.3 to 6.6 milligrams per 2.2 pounds of body weight has been used.

Nizoral has not been studied in children under 2 years of age.

Overdosage

Although no specific information is available, any medication taken in excess can have serious consequences. If you suspect an overdose of Nizoral, seek medical attention immediately.

Brand name:

NOLVADEX

Pronounced: NOLL-vah-decks
Generic name: Tamoxifen citrate

Why is this drug prescribed?

Nolvadex, an anticancer drug, may be given to treat breast cancer. It also has proved effective when cancer has spread to other parts of the body. Nolvadex is most effective in stopping the kind of breast cancer that thrives on estrogen.

Most important fact about this drug

Women taking Nolvadex should have routine gynecological examinations and report any abnormal vaginal bleeding, changes in menstrual periods, change in vaginal discharge, or pelvic pain or pressure to the doctor immediately. Even after Nolvadex therapy has stopped, any abnormal vaginal bleeding should be reported at once.

How should you take this medication?
Take Nolvadex exactly as prescribed. Do not stop taking this medication without first consulting your doctor. It may be necessary to continue taking the drug for several years.

■ *If you miss a dose...*
Do not try to make it up. Go back to your regular schedule with the next dose.

■ *Storage instructions...*
Nolvadex may be stored at room temperature.

What side effects may occur?
Side effects from Nolvadex are usually mild and rarely require the drug to be stopped. If any develop or change in intensity, inform your doctor as soon as possible. Only your doctor can determine if it is safe for you to continue taking Nolvadex.

■ *More common side effects may include:*
Hot flashes, nausea, vomiting

■ *Less common side effects may include:*
Bone pain, diarrhea, menstrual irregularities, skin rash, tumor pain, vaginal bleeding, vaginal discharge

■ *Rare side effects may include:*
Blood clots, depression, distaste for food, dizziness, hair thinning or partial loss, headache, light-headedness, liver disorders, swelling of arms or legs, vaginal itching or dryness, visual problems

Why should this drug not be prescribed?
Do not take Nolvadex if you are sensitive to it or have ever had an allergic reaction to it.

Special warnings about this medication
If you experience visual problems while taking Nolvadex, notify your doctor immediately.

In a few women Nolvadex may raise the level of cholesterol and other fats in the blood. Your doctor may periodically do blood tests to check your cholesterol and triglyceride levels.

Nolvadex may produce an abnormally high level of calcium in the blood.

Symptoms include muscle pain and weakness, loss of appetite, and, if severe, kidney failure. If you experience any of these symptoms, notify your doctor as soon as possible.

If tests show that your blood contains too few white blood cells or platelets while you are taking Nolvadex, your doctor should monitor you with special care. These problems have sometimes been found in women taking Nolvadex; whether the drug caused the blood-cell abnormalities is uncertain.

Possible food and drug interactions
when taking this medication

If Nolvadex is taken with certain other drugs, the effects of either could be increased, decreased, or altered. It is especially important to check with your doctor before combining Nolvadex with the following:

Blood-thinning drugs such as Coumadin
Bromocriptine (Parlodel)
Cancer drugs such as Hydrea
Phenobarbital

Special information
if you are pregnant or breastfeeding

It is important to avoid pregnancy while taking Nolvadex, because the drug could harm the unborn child. Since Nolvadex is an anti-estrogen drug, you will need to use a non-hormonal form of contraception, such as a condom and/or diaphragm, and not birth control pills. If you accidentally become pregnant while taking Nolvadex, or within 2 months after you have stopped taking it, discuss this with your doctor immediately.

Because Nolvadex might cause serious harm to a nursing infant, you should not breastfeed your baby while taking this drug. If this medication is essential to your health, your doctor may advise you to discontinue breastfeeding until your treatment is finished.

Recommended dosage

ADULTS

The daily dosage ranges from 20 to 40 milligrams. If you are taking more than 20 milligrams a day, your doctor will have you divide the total into 2 smaller doses taken in the morning and evening. Nolvadex comes in 10- and 20-milligram tablets.

CHILDREN

Safety and efficacy in children have not been established.

Overdosage

Any medication taken in excess can have serious consequences. If you suspect an overdose of Nolvadex, seek medical attention immediately.

■ *Symptoms of Nolvadex overdose may include:*
Dizziness, overactive reflexes, tremor, unsteady gait

Brand name:

NORDETTE

See Oral Contraceptives, page 926.

Brand name:

NORETHIN

See Oral Contraceptives, page 926.

Generic name:

NORFLOXACIN

See Noroxin, page 899.

Brand name:

NORGESIC

Pronounced: nor-JEE-zic
Generic ingredients: Orphenadrine citrate, Aspirin, Caffeine
Other brand name: Norgesic Forte

Why is this drug prescribed?

Norgesic is prescribed, along with rest, physical therapy, and other measures, for the relief of mild to moderate pain of severe muscle disorders.

Most important fact about this drug

Norgesic may impair your ability to drive a car or operate dangerous machinery. Do not participate in potentially hazardous activities until you know how you react to this medication.

How should you take this medication?

If aspirin upsets your stomach, you may take Norgesic with food. Take it exactly as prescribed.

■ *If you miss a dose...*
If it is within an hour of your scheduled time, take it as soon as you remember. If you do not remember until later, skip the dose you missed and go back to your regular schedule. Do not take 2 doses at once.

■ *Storage instructions...*
Store at room temperature.

What side effects may occur?

Side effects cannot be anticipated. If any develop or change in intensity, inform your doctor as soon as possible. Only your doctor can determine if it is safe for you to continue taking Norgesic.

■ *Side effects may include:*
Blurred vision, confusion (in the elderly), constipation, difficulty in urinating, dilation of the pupils, dizziness, drowsiness, dry mouth, fainting, hallucinations, headache, hives, light-headedness, nausea, palpitations, rapid heart rate, skin diseases, stomach and intestinal bleeding, vomiting, weakness

Why should this drug not be prescribed?

If you are sensitive to or have ever had an allergic reaction to the ingredients of Norgesic—orphenadrine, aspirin, and caffeine—you should not take this medication. Make sure your doctor is aware of any drug reactions you have experienced.

You should not be taking Norgesic if you have the eye condition called glaucoma, a stomach or intestinal blockage, an enlarged prostate gland, a bladder obstruction, achalasia (failure of stomach or intestinal muscles to relax), or myasthenia gravis (muscle weakness and fatigue).

Because taking aspirin while you have chickenpox or flu may cause a rare but serious condition called Reye's syndrome, do not give Norgesic to anyone with these diseases. Call your doctor if fever or swelling develops.

Special warnings about this medication

Because the safety of continuous, long-term therapy with Norgesic has not been established, your doctor should monitor your blood, urine, and liver function if you use this drug for a prolonged period of time.

Because Norgesic contains aspirin, you should be careful taking it if you have a peptic ulcer or problems with blood clotting.

Possible food and drug interactions
when taking this medication
If Norgesic is taken with certain other drugs, the effects of either could be increased, decreased, or altered. It is especially important to check with your doctor before combining Norgesic with propoxyphene (Darvon). The combination can cause confusion, anxiety, and tremors.

Special information
if you are pregnant or breastfeeding
The effects of Norgesic during pregnancy have not been adequately studied. If you are pregnant or plan to become pregnant, inform your doctor immediately. This drug may appear in breast milk and could affect a nursing infant. If this medication is essential to your health, your doctor may advise you to discontinue breastfeeding until your treatment is finished.

Recommended dosage

ADULTS

The usual dose of Norgesic is 1 to 2 tablets taken 3 or 4 times a day.

The usual dosage of Norgesic Forte, which is exactly twice the strength of Norgesic, is one-half to 1 tablet, taken 3 or 4 times per day.

CHILDREN

The safety and effectiveness of Norgesic have not been established in children.

OLDER ADULTS

Some older adults have experienced confusion when taking this drug. Your doctor may adjust the dosage accordingly.

Overdosage
Any medication taken in excess can have serious consequences. If you suspect an overdose of Norgesic, seek emergency medical treatment immediately.

Brand name:

NORINYL

See Oral Contraceptives, page 926.

Brand name:

NORMODYNE

Pronounced: NORM-oh-dine
Generic name: Labetalol hydrochloride
Other brand name: Trandate

Why is this drug prescribed?

Normodyne is used in the treatment of high blood pressure. It is effective when used alone or in combination with other high blood pressure medications, especially thiazide diuretics such as HydroDIURIL and "loop" diuretics such as Lasix.

Most important fact about this drug

You must take Normodyne regularly for it to be effective. Since blood pressure declines gradually, it may be several weeks before you get the full benefit of Normodyne; and you must continue taking it even if you are feeling well. Normodyne does not cure high blood pressure; it merely keeps it under control.

How should you take this medication?

Normodyne can be taken with or without food. The amount of Normodyne absorbed into your bloodstream is actually increased by food.

This medication should be taken exactly as prescribed by your doctor, even if your symptoms have disappeared.

Try not to miss any doses. If Normodyne is not taken regularly, your condition may worsen.

■ *If you miss a dose...*
Take it as soon as you remember. If it is almost time for your next dose, skip the one you missed and go back to your regular schedule. Never take 2 doses at the same time.

■ *Storage instructions...*
Store at room temperature.

What side effects may occur?

Side effects cannot be anticipated. If any develop or change in intensity, inform your doctor as soon as possible. Only your doctor can determine if it is safe for you to continue taking Normodyne.

- *More common side effects may include:*
  Dizziness, fatigue, indigestion, nausea, stuffy nose

- *Less common or rare side effects may include:*
  Anaphylaxis (severe allergic reaction), angioedema (swelling of the face, lips, tongue and throat, difficulty swallowing), changes in taste, depression, diarrhea, difficulty urinating, dizziness upon standing up (especially among the elderly), drowsiness, dry eyes, ejaculation failure, fainting, fluid retention, hair loss, headache, heart block (conduction disorder), hives, impotence, increased sweating, itching, low blood pressure, lupus erythematosus (fever, arthritis, skin eruptions), muscle cramps, rash, shortness of breath, slow heartbeat, tingling or pins and needles, tingling scalp, vertigo, vision changes, weakness, wheezing or asthma-like symptoms, vomiting, yellow eyes and skin

Why should this drug not be prescribed?

You should not take Normodyne if you are currently suffering from bronchial asthma, congestive heart failure, heart block (a heart irregularity), inadequate blood supply to the circulatory system (cardiogenic shock), a severely slow heartbeat, or any other condition that causes severe and continued low blood pressure.

If you are sensitive to or have ever had an allergic reaction to Normodyne or any of its ingredients you should not take this medication.

Special warnings about this medication

Normodyne has caused severe liver damage in some people. Although this is a rare occurrence, if you develop any symptoms of abnormal liver function—itching, dark urine, continuing loss of appetite, yellow eyes and skin, or unexplained "flu-like" symptoms—contact your doctor immediately.

If you have a history of congestive heart failure, or kidney or liver disease, Normodyne should be used with caution.

Normodyne should not be stopped suddenly. This can cause chest pain and heart attack. Dosage should be gradually reduced.

If you suffer from asthma, chronic bronchitis, emphysema, or other bronchial diseases, Normodyne should be used cautiously.

This medication may mask the symptoms of low blood sugar or alter blood sugar levels. If you are diabetic, discuss this with your doctor.

Notify your doctor or dentist that you are taking Normodyne if you have a medical emergency, and before you have surgery or dental treatment.

Possible food and drug interactions
when taking this medication

If Normodyne is taken with certain other drugs, the effects of either could be increased, decreased, or altered. It is especially important to check with your doctor before taking Normodyne with the following:

Airway opening drugs such as Proventil and Ventolin
Antidepressant medications such as Elavil
Cimetidine (Tagamet)
Diabetes drugs such as Micronase
Epinephrine (EpiPen)
Insulin
Nitroglycerin products such as Transderm-Nitro
Nonsteroidal anti-inflammatory drugs such as Advil and Motrin
Ritodrine (Yutopar)
Verapamil (Calan)

Special information
if you are pregnant or breastfeeding

The effects of Normodyne during pregnancy have not been adequately studied. If you are pregnant or plan to become pregnant, inform your doctor immediately. Normodyne appears in breast milk and could affect a nursing infant. If this medication is essential to your health, your doctor may advise you to discontinue breastfeeding until your treatment is finished.

Recommended dosage

ADULTS

Your doctor will adjust the dosages to fit your needs. Your doctor may observe the drug's effect in his or her office over a 1- to 3-hour period after you begin taking it, and then check your pressure again at regular office visits (12 hours after a dose) to make sure that the medicine is effective.

The usual starting dose is 100 milligrams, 2 times per day, alone or with a diuretic drug. After 2 to 3 days of checking your blood pressure, your doctor may begin increasing your dose by 100 milligrams, 2 times per day, at intervals of 2 to 3 days.

The regular dose ranges from 200 to 400 milligrams, 2 times per day. Some people may require total daily dosage of as much as 1,200 to 2,400 milligrams, either alone or with a thiazide diuretic. In these cases, your doctor will observe the drug's effect and adjust your dose accordingly.

CHILDREN

The safety and effectiveness of this drug in children have not been established.

OLDER ADULTS

The usual starting dose is the same as younger people's—100 milligrams twice a day. Your doctor may increase the dose, but usually to no more than 200 milligrams twice a day.

Overdosage

Any medication taken in excess can have serious consequences. If you suspect an overdose, seek medical treatment immediately.

■ *Symptoms of Normodyne overdose may include:*
Dizziness when standing up, severely low blood pressure, severely slow heartbeat

Brand name:

NOROXIN

Pronounced: Nor-OX-in
Generic name: Norfloxacin

Why is this drug prescribed?

Noroxin is an antibacterial medication used to treat infections of the urinary tract, including cystitis (inflammation of the inner lining of the bladder caused by a bacterial infection), prostatitis (inflammation of the prostate gland), and certain sexually transmitted diseases, such as gonorrhea.

Most important fact about this drug

Noroxin is not given for the treatment of syphilis. When used in high doses for a short period of time to treat gonorrhea, it may actually mask or delay the symptoms of syphilis. Your doctor may perform certain tests for syphilis at the time of diagnosing gonorrhea, and after treatment with Noroxin.

How should you take this medication?

Noroxin should be taken with a glass of water, either 1 hour *before* or 2 hours *after* eating a meal or drinking milk. Do not take more than the dosage prescribed by your doctor.

It is important to drink plenty of fluids while taking Noroxin.

Take all the Noroxin your doctor prescribes. If you stop taking the medicine too soon, you may have a relapse.

■ *If you miss a dose...*
Be sure to take it as soon as possible. This will help to keep a constant amount of Noroxin in your body. However, if it is almost time for your next dose, skip the one you missed and go back to your regular schedule. Do not take two doses at the same time.

■ *Storage instructions...*
Store at room temperature. Keep container tightly closed. Store out of reach of children.

What side effects may occur?
Side effects cannot be anticipated. If any develop or change in intensity, inform your doctor as soon as possible. Only your doctor can determine whether it is safe for you to continue taking Noroxin.

■ *More common side effects may include:*
Abdominal cramping, dizziness, headache, nausea, weakness

■ *Other side effects may include:*
Abdominal pain or swelling, allergies, anal itching, anal/rectal pain, anxiety, arthritis, back pain, bitter taste, blood abnormalities, blurred vision, bursitis, chest pain, chills, confusion, constipation, depression, diarrhea, difficult breathing, double vision, dry mouth, extreme sleepiness, fever, fluid retention and swelling, gas, heart attack, heartburn, heart palpitations, hives, indigestion, insomnia, intestinal inflammation, itching, joint pain, kidney failure (symptoms may include reduced amount of urine, drowsiness, nausea, vomiting, and coma), lack of coordination, loose stools, loss of appetite, menstrual disorders, mouth ulcer, muscle pain, peeling skin, rash, reddened skin, ringing in the ears, severe skin reaction to light, stomach pain, sweating, swelling of feet or hands, temporary hearing loss, tendon inflammation or tearing, tingling in fingers, vision problems, vomiting, yellow eyes and skin

Why should this drug not be prescribed?
You should not be using Noroxin if you are sensitive to it or to other drugs of the same type, such as Cipro, or if you have suffered tendon inflammation or tearing due to the use of such drugs. See "Special Warnings" section.

Special warnings about this medication

Noroxin is not recommended for:

Children (under the age of 18)
Nursing mothers
Pregnant women

People with disorders such as epilepsy, severe cerebral arteriosclerosis, and other conditions that might lead to seizures should use Noroxin cautiously. There have been reports of convulsions in some people taking Noroxin.

If you develop diarrhea, tell your doctor. It could be a symptom of a potentially serious intestinal inflammation.

Some people taking drugs chemically similar to Noroxin have experienced severe, sometimes fatal reactions, occasionally after only one dose. These reactions may include: Confusion, convulsions, difficulty breathing, hallucinations, heart collapse, hives, increased pressure in the head, itching, light-headedness, loss of consciousness, psychosis, rash, restlessness, shock, swelling in the face or throat, tingling, tremors.

If you experience any of these reactions you should immediately stop taking Noroxin and seek medical help.

There is a small chance that Noroxin may weaken the muscle tendons in your shoulder, hand, or heel, causing them to tear. Should this happen, surgery or at least a long period of disability would be in store. If you feel any pain, inflammation, or tearing, stop taking this drug immediately and call your doctor. Rest and avoid exercise until the doctor is certain the tendons are intact.

Some people find needle-shaped crystals in their urine after taking Noroxin. Drink plenty of fluids while taking Noroxin. This will increase urine output and reduce crystallization.

Noroxin may cause dizziness or light-headedness and might impair your ability to drive a car or operate potentially dangerous machinery. Use caution when undertaking any activities that require full alertness if you are unsure of your ability.

You should avoid excessive exposure to direct sunlight while taking Noroxin. Stop taking Noroxin and contact your doctor immediately if you have a severe reaction to sunlight, such as a skin rash.

**Possible food and drug interactions
when taking this medication**
If Noroxin is taken with certain other drugs, the effects of either could be
increased, decreased, or altered. It is especially important to check with your
doctor before combining Noroxin with the following:

Antacids such as Maalox and Tums
Caffeine (including coffee, tea, and some soft drinks)
Calcium supplements
Cyclosporine (Sandimmune, Neoral)
Multivitamins and other products containing iron or zinc
Nitrofurantoin (Macrodantin, Macrobid)
Oral blood thinners such as warfarin (Coumadin)
Probenecid (Benemid)
Sucralfate (Carafate)
Theophylline (Theo-Dur)

**Special information
if you are pregnant or breastfeeding**
The effects of Noroxin during pregnancy have not been adequately studied.
Inform your doctor if you are pregnant or planning a pregnancy.

Do not take Noroxin while breastfeeding. There is a possibility of harm to the
infant.

Recommended dosage
Take Noroxin with a full glass of water 1 hour before, or 2 hours after,
eating a meal or drinking milk. Drink plenty of liquids while taking Noroxin.

Uncomplicated Urinary Tract Infections
The suggested dose is 800 milligrams per day; 400 milligrams should be
taken twice a day for 3 to 10 days, depending upon the kind of bacteria
causing the infection. People with impaired kidney function may take 400
milligrams once a day for 3 to 10 days.

Complicated Urinary Tract Infections
The suggested dose is 800 milligrams per day; 400 milligrams should be
taken twice a day for 10 to 21 days.

Prostatitis
The usual daily dose is 800 milligrams, divided into 2 doses of 400
milligrams each, taken for 28 days.

Sexually Transmitted Diseases (Gonorrhea)
The usual recommended dose is one single dose of 800 milligrams for 1 day.

The total daily dosage of Noroxin should not be more than 800 milligrams.

Overdosage
The symptoms of overdose with Noroxin are not known. However, any medication taken in excess can have serious consequences. If you suspect a Noroxin overdose, seek medical help immediately.

Brand name:

NORPACE

Pronounced: NOR-pace
Generic name: Disopyramide phosphate
Other brand name: Norpace CR

Why is this drug prescribed?
Norpace is used to treat severe irregular heartbeat. It relaxes an overactive heart and improves the efficiency of the heart's pumping action.

Most important fact about this drug
Do not stop taking Norpace without first consulting your doctor. Stopping suddenly can cause serious changes in heart function.

How should you take this medication?
Be sure to take this medication exactly as prescribed.

Norpace may cause dry mouth. For temporary relief suck on a hard candy, chew gum, or melt ice chips in your mouth.

■ *If you miss a dose...*
Take it as soon as you remember, if the next dose is 4 or more hours away. If you do not remember until later, skip the dose you missed and go back to your regular schedule. Do not take 2 doses at once.

■ *Storage instructions...*
Store at room temperature.

What side effects may occur?
Side effects cannot be anticipated. If any develop or change in intensity, inform your doctor as soon as possible. Only your doctor can determine if it is safe for you to continue taking Norpace.

- *More common side effects may include:*
  Abdominal pain, aches and pains, bloating and gas, blurred vision, constipation, dizziness, dry eyes, nose, and throat, dry mouth, fatigue, headache, inability to urinate, increased urinary frequency and urgency, muscle weakness, nausea, vague feeling of bodily discomfort

- *Less common or rare side effects may include:*
  Breast development in males, chest pain, congestive heart failure, depression, diarrhea, difficulty breathing, difficulty sleeping, fainting, fever, impotence, itching, low blood pressure, low blood sugar (hypoglycemia), nervousness, numbness or tingling, painful urination, rash, psychosis, shortness of breath, skin diseases, swelling due to fluid retention, vomiting, weight gain, yellow eyes and skin

Why should this drug not be prescribed?
This drug should not be used if the output of your heart is inadequate (cardiogenic shock) or if you are sensitive to or have ever had an allergic reaction to Norpace.

Norpace can be used for only certain types of irregular heartbeat, and must not be used for others.

Special warnings about this medication
If you have structural heart disease, inflammation of the heart muscle, or other heart disorders, use this medication with extreme caution.

Norpace may cause or worsen congestive heart failure and can cause severe low blood pressure. If you have a history of heart failure, your doctor will carefully monitor your heart function while you are taking this medication.

Norpace can cause low blood sugar (hypoglycemia), especially if you have congestive heart failure; poor nutrition; or kidney, liver, or other diseases; or if you are taking beta-blocking blood pressure drugs such as Tenormin or drinking alcohol.

Your doctor will prescribe Norpace along with other heart-regulating drugs, such as quinidine, procainamide, encainide, flecainide, propafenone, and propranolol, only if the irregular rhythm is considered life-threatening and other antiarrhythmic medication has not worked.

If you have the eye condition called glaucoma, myasthenia gravis, or difficulty urinating (particularly if you have a prostate condition), use this drug cautiously.

You will take lower dosages if you have liver or kidney disease.

Your doctor should check your potassium levels before starting you on

Norpace. Low potassium levels may make this drug ineffective; high levels may increase its toxic effects.

Possible food and drug interactions
when taking this medication
Avoid alcoholic beverages while taking Norpace.

If Norpace is taken with certain other drugs, the effects of either could be increased, decreased, or altered. It is especially important to check with your doctor before combining Norpace with the following:

Drugs that inhibit the breakdown of other drugs by the liver, including Tagamet
Erythromycin (Eryc, Ery-Tab, PCE)
Other heart-regulating drugs such as quinidine (Quinidex), procainamide (Procan SR), lidocaine (Xylocaine), propranolol (Inderal), Verapamil (Calan)
Phenytoin (Dilantin)

Special information
if you are pregnant or breastfeeding
The effects of Norpace during pregnancy have not been adequately studied. If you are pregnant or plan to become pregnant, inform your doctor immediately. Norpace appears in breast milk and may affect a nursing infant. If this medication is essential to your health, your doctor may advise you to discontinue breastfeeding until your treatment with this medication is finished.

Recommended dosage
Treatment with Norpace should be started in the hospital.

ADULTS

Your doctor will adjust your dosage according to your own response to, and tolerance of, Norpace or Norpace CR.

The usual dosage range of Norpace and Norpace CR is 400 milligrams to 800 milligrams per day, divided into smaller doses.

The recommended dosage for most adults is 600 milligrams per day, divided into smaller doses (either 150 milligrams every 6 hours for immediate-release Norpace or 300 milligrams every 12 hours for Norpace CR).

For those who weigh less than 110 pounds, the recommended dosage is 400 milligrams per day, divided into smaller doses (either 100 milligrams every 6 hours for immediate-release Norpace or 200 milligrams every 12 hours for Norpace CR.

For people with severe heart disease, the starting dose will be 100 milligrams of immediate-release Norpace every 6 to 8 hours. Your doctor will adjust the dosage gradually and watch you closely for any signs of low blood pressure or heart failure.

For people with moderately reduced kidney or liver function, the dosage is 400 milligrams per day, divided into smaller doses (either 100 milligrams every 6 hours for immediate-release Norpace or 200 milligrams every 12 hours for Norpace CR).

For those who have severe kidney impairment, the dosage of immediate-release Norpace is 100 milligrams; the times will vary with the individual as determined by your doctor.

Norpace CR is not recommended for people with severe kidney disease.

CHILDREN

Dosage in children to age 18 is based on body weight. The total daily dosage should be divided into equal doses taken orally every 6 hours or at intervals that are best for the individual.

Overdosage

Any medication taken in excess can have serious consequences. An overdose of Norpace can be fatal. If you suspect an overdose, seek medical treatment immediately.

■ *The symptoms of Norpace overdose may include:*
Cessation of breathing, irregular heartbeat, loss of consciousness, low blood pressure, slow heartbeat, worsening of congestive heart failure

Brand name:

NORPRAMIN

Pronounced: NOR-pram-in
Generic name: Desipramine hydrochloride

Why is this drug prescribed?

Norpramin is used in the treatment of depression. It is one of a family of drugs called tricyclic antidepressants. Drugs in this class are thought to work by affecting the levels of the brain's natural chemical messengers (called neurotransmitters), and adjusting the brain's response to them.

Norpramin has also been used to treat bulimia and attention deficit disorders, and to help with cocaine withdrawal.

Most important fact about this drug
Serious, sometimes fatal, reactions have been known to occur when drugs such as Norpramin are taken with another type of antidepressant called an MAO inhibitor. Drugs in this category include Nardil and Parnate. Do not take Norpramin within two weeks of taking one of these drugs. Make sure your doctor and pharmacist know of all the medications you are taking.

How should you take this medication?
Norpramin should be taken exactly as prescribed.

Do not stop taking Norpramin if you feel no immediate effect. It can take up to 2 or 3 weeks for improvement to begin.

Norpramin can cause dry mouth. Sucking hard candy or chewing gum can help this problem.

■ *If you miss a dose...*
If you take several doses per day, take the forgotten dose as soon as you remember, then take any remaining doses for the day at evenly spaced intervals. If you take Norpramin once a day at bedtime and don't remember until morning, skip the missed dose. Never try to "catch up" by doubling the dose.

■ *Storage instructions...*
Norpramin can be stored at room temperature. Protect it from excessive heat.

What side effects may occur?
Side effects cannot be anticipated. If any develop or change in intensity, inform your doctor as soon as possible. Only your doctor can determine if it is safe for you to continue taking Norpramin.

■ *Side effects may include:*
Abdominal cramps, agitation, anxiety, black tongue, black, red, or blue spots on skin, blurred vision, breast development in males, breast enlargement in females, confusion, constipation, delusions, diarrhea, dilated pupils, disorientation, dizziness, drowsiness, dry mouth, excessive or spontaneous flow of milk, fatigue, fever, flushing, frequent urination or difficulty or delay in urinating, hallucinations, headache, heart attack,

heartbeat irregularities, hepatitis, high or low blood pressure, high or low blood sugar, hives, impotence, increased or decreased sex drive, inflammation of the mouth, insomnia, intestinal blockage, lack of coordination, light-headedness (especially when rising from lying down), loss of appetite, loss of hair, mild elation, nausea, nightmares, odd taste in mouth, painful ejaculation, palpitations, purplish spots on the skin, rapid heartbeat, restlessness, ringing in the ears, seizures, sensitivity to light, skin itching and rash, sore throat, stomach pain, stroke, sweating, swelling due to fluid retention (especially in face or tongue), swelling of testicles, swollen glands, tingling, numbness and pins and needles in hands and feet, tremors, urinating at night, visual problems, vomiting, weakness, weight gain or loss, worsening of psychosis, yellowed skin and whites of eyes

Why should this drug not be prescribed?
Norpramin should not be used if you are known to be hypersensitive to it, or if you have had a recent heart attack.

People who take antidepressant drugs known as MAO inhibitors (including Nardil and Parnate) should not take Norpramin.

Special warnings about this medication
Before using Norpramin, tell your doctor if you have heart or thyroid disease, a seizure disorder, a history of being unable to urinate, or glaucoma.

Nausea, headache, and uneasiness can result if you suddenly stop taking Norpramin. Consult your doctor and follow instructions closely when discontinuing Norpramin.

This drug may impair your ability to drive a car or operate potentially dangerous machinery. Do not participate in any activities that require full alertness if you are unsure about your ability.

Norpramin may increase your skin's sensitivity to sunlight. Overexposure could cause rash, itching, redness, or sunburn. Avoid direct sunlight or wear protective clothing.

If you are planning to have elective surgery, make sure that your doctor is aware that you are taking Norpramin. It should be discontinued as soon as possible prior to surgery.

Tell your doctor if you develop a fever and sore throat while you are taking Norpramin. He may want to do some blood tests.

**Possible food and drug interactions
when taking this medication**
People who take antidepressant drugs known as MAO inhibitors (including
Nardil and Parnate) should not take Norpramin.

If Norpramin is taken with certain other drugs, the effects of either could be
increased, decreased, or altered. It is especially important to check with your
doctor before combining Norpramin with the following:

  Cimetidine (Tagamet)
  Drugs that improve breathing, such as Proventil
  Drugs that relax certain muscles, such as Bentyl
  Fluoxetine (Prozac)
  Guanethidine (Ismelin)
  Paroxetine (Paxil)
  Sedatives/hypnotics (Halcion, Valium)
  Sertraline (Zoloft)
  Thyroid medications (Synthroid)

Extreme drowsiness and other potentially serious effects can result if
Norpramin is combined with alcohol or other depressants, including narcotic
painkillers such as Percocet and Demerol, sleeping medications such as
Halcion and Nembutal, and tranquilizers such as Valium and Xanax.

**Special information
if you are pregnant or breastfeeding**
Pregnant women or mothers who are nursing an infant should use Norpramin
only when the potential benefits clearly outweigh the potential risks. If you
are pregnant or planning to become pregnant, inform your doctor immediately.

Recommended dosage
Your doctor will tailor the dose to your individual needs.

ADULTS

The usual dose ranges from 100 to 200 milligrams per day, taken in 1 dose
or divided into smaller doses. If needed, dosages may gradually be increased
to 300 milligrams a day. Dosages above 300 milligrams per day are not
recommended.

CHILDREN

Norpramin is not recommended for children.

OLDER ADULTS AND ADOLESCENTS

The usual dose ranges from 25 to 100 milligrams per day. If needed, dosages may gradually be increased to 150 milligrams a day. Doses above 150 milligrams per day are not recommended.

Overdosage

Any medication taken in excess can have serious consequences. An overdosage of Norpramin can be fatal. If you suspect an overdose, seek medical help immediately.

- *Symptoms of overdose may include:*
  Agitation, coma, confusion, convulsions, dilated pupils, disturbed concentration, drowsiness, extremely low blood pressure, hallucinations, high fever, irregular heart rate, low body temperature, overactive reflexes, rigid muscles, stupor, vomiting

Generic name:

NORTRIPTYLINE

See Pamelor, page 943.

Brand name:

NORVASC

Pronounced: NOR-vask
Generic name: Amlodipine besylate

Why is this drug prescribed?

Norvasc is prescribed for angina, a condition characterized by episodes of crushing chest pain that usually results from a lack of oxygen in the heart muscle due to clogged arteries. Norvasc is also prescribed for high blood pressure. It is a type of medication called a calcium channel blocker. These drugs dilate blood vessels and slow the heart to reduce blood pressure and the pain of angina.

Most important fact about this drug

If you have high blood pressure, you must take Norvasc regularly for it to be effective. Since blood pressure declines gradually, it may be several weeks before you get the full benefit of Norvasc; and you must continue taking it even if you are feeling well. Norvasc does not cure high blood pressure; it merely keeps it under control.

How should you take this medication?

Norvasc may be taken with or without food. A once-a-day medication, Norvasc may be used alone or in combination with other drugs for high blood pressure or angina.

You should take this medication exactly as prescribed, even if your symptoms have disappeared. You will begin to see a drop in your blood pressure 24 hours after you start the medication.

■ *If you miss a dose...*
   If you forget to take a dose, take it as soon as you remember. If it is almost time for your next dose, skip the one you missed and go back to your regular schedule. Never take 2 doses at the same time.

■ *Storage instructions...*
   Store at room temperature in a tightly closed container, away from light.

What side effects may occur?

Side effects cannot be anticipated. If any develop or change in intensity, tell your doctor as soon as possible. Only your doctor can determine if it is safe for you to continue taking Norvasc.

■ *More common side effects may include:*
   Dizziness, fatigue, flushing, fluid retention and swelling, headache, palpitations (fluttery or throbbing heartbeat)

■ *Less common side effects may include:*
   Abdominal pain, nausea, sleepiness

■ *Rare side effects may include:*
   Abnormal dreams, agitation, altered sense of smell or taste, anxiety, apathy, back pain, chest pain, cold and clammy skin, conjunctivitis (pinkeye), constipation, coughing, depression, diarrhea, difficult or labored breathing, difficult or painful urination, difficulty swallowing, dizziness or light-headedness when standing, double vision, dry mouth, dry skin, excessive urination, eye pain, fainting, frequent urination, gas, general feeling of illness, hair loss, heart failure, hives, hot flashes, inability to sleep, increased appetite, increased sweating, indigestion, irregular heartbeat, irregular pulse, itching, joint pain or problems, lack of coordination, lack of sensation, loose stools, loss of appetite, loss of memory, loss of sense of identity, low blood pressure, migraine, muscle cramps or pain, muscle weakness, nasal inflammation, nervousness, nosebleed, pain, purple or red spots on the skin, rapid heartbeat, rash, ringing in the ears, sexual problems, skin discoloration, skin inflammation,

slow heartbeat, stomach inflammation, thirst, tingling or "pins and needles," tremor, twitching, urinating at night, urinating problems, vertigo, vision problems, vomiting, weakness, weight gain

Why should this drug not be prescribed?

If you are sensitive to or have ever had an allergic reaction to Norvasc, do not take this medication.

Special warnings about this medication

Check with your doctor before you stop taking Norvasc, as a slow reduction in the dose may be needed.

Your doctor will prescribe Norvasc with caution if you have certain heart conditions or liver disease. Make sure the doctor is aware of all your medical problems before you start therapy with Norvasc.

Although very rare, if you have severe heart disease, you may experience an increase in frequency and duration of angina attacks, or even have a heart attack, when you are starting on Norvasc or your dosage is increased.

Safety and effectiveness in children have not been established.

Possible food and drug interactions

There are no known food or drug interactions with this medication.

Special information
if you are pregnant or breastfeeding

The effects of Norvasc during pregnancy have not been adequately studied. If you are pregnant or planning to become pregnant, tell your doctor immediately. Norvasc should be used during pregnancy only if clearly needed. Norvasc may appear in breast milk. If this medication is essential to your health, your doctor may tell you to discontinue breastfeeding your baby until your treatment with Norvasc is finished.

Recommended dosage

HIGH BLOOD PRESSURE

Adults

The usual starting dose is 5 milligrams taken once a day. The most you should take in a day is 10 milligrams. If your doctor is adding Norvasc to other high blood pressure medications, the dose is 2.5 milligrams once daily. The lower 2.5-milligram starting dose also applies if you have liver disease.

Older Adults

You will be prescribed a lower starting dose of 2.5 milligrams.

ANGINA

Adults

The usual starting dose is 5 to 10 milligrams once daily. If you have liver disease, the lower 5-milligram dose will be used at the start.

Older Adults

The usual starting dose is 5 milligrams. Your doctor may adjust the dose based on your response to the drug.

Overdosage

Experience with Norvasc is limited; but if you suspect an overdose, seek medical attention immediately. The most likely symptoms are a drop in blood pressure and a faster heartbeat.

Brand name:

NORVIR

Pronounced: NOR-veer
Generic name: Ritonavir

Why is this drug prescribed?

Norvir is prescribed to slow the progress of HIV (human immunodeficiency virus) infection. HIV causes the immune system to break down so that it can no longer respond effectively to infection, leading to the fatal disease known as acquired immune deficiency syndrome (AIDS). Without treatment, HIV takes over certain human cells, especially white blood cells, and uses the inner workings of the infected cell to make additional copies of itself. Norvir belongs to a new class of HIV drugs, called protease inhibitors, which work by interfering with an important step in this process. Although Norvir cannot get rid of HIV already present in the body, it can reduce the amount of virus available to infect other cells.

Norvir is used alone or in combination with other HIV drugs called nucleoside analogues (Retrovir, Hivid, and others). Because these two types of drugs act against HIV in different ways, your doctor may prescribe a combination of Norvir and Retrovir or Hivid.

Most important fact about this drug
Do not take Norvir with the following medications. The combination could cause serious, even life-threatening, effects.

Amiodarone (Cordarone), astemizole (Hismanal), bepridil (Vascor), bupropion (Wellbutrin), cisapride (Propulsid), clozapine (Clozaril), encainide (Enkaid), flecainide (Tambocor), meperidine (Demerol), piroxicam (Feldene), propafenone (Rythmol), propoxyphene (Darvon), quinidine (Quinidex), rifabutin (Mycobutin), terfenadine (Seldane)

Norvir may also increase the effects of certain sedative and sleeping medications, leading to extreme sedation and difficulty breathing. Never combine Norvir with the following:

Alprazolam (Xanax), clorazepate (Tranxene), diazepam (Valium), estazolam (ProSom), flurazepam (Dalmane), midazolam (Versed), triazolam (Halcion), zolpidem (Ambien)

Be sure to tell your doctor and pharmacist what medications you are taking, both prescription and over-the-counter, and let them know when you *stop* taking any medication.

How should you take this medication?
Take Norvir every day, exactly as prescribed by your doctor. Do not share this medication with anyone and do not take more than your recommended dosage.

Take Norvir with food, if possible, or the medication may not work properly.

If you are taking Norvir oral solution and want to improve the taste, you can mix the liquid with chocolate milk or a liquid nutritional product (Ensure or Advera) within 1 hour of taking the dose. Use a measuring cup or spoon to measure each dose of the oral solution accurately. A household teaspoon may not hold the correct amount of oral solution.

■ *If you miss a dose...*
Take it as soon as possible. If it is almost time for the next dose, skip the one you missed and go back to your regular schedule. Never double the dose.

■ *Storage instructions...*
Capsules should be refrigerated and protected from light. The oral solution is best kept in the refrigerator, although it does not require refrigeration if used within 30 days and stored below 77°F. Avoid exposure to extreme heat and keep the cap tightly closed. Keep the oral solution in its original container.

What side effects may occur?
Side effects cannot be anticipated. If any develop or change in intensity, tell your doctor as soon as possible. Only your doctor can determine if it is safe for you to continue taking Norvir.

■ *Possible side effects may include:*
Abdominal pain, bodily weakness, constipation, diarrhea, disturbed thoughts, dizziness, drowsiness, fever, gas, general feeling of illness, headache, indigestion, insomnia, loss of appetite, muscle aches, nausea, numbness or tingling sensation around the face or mouth, "pins and needles" sensation in the arms and legs, rash, sore or irritated throat, sweating, taste alteration, vomiting

Why should this drug not be prescribed?
If you have ever had an allergic reaction to Norvir or any of its ingredients, do not take the drug. Never combine Norvir with the drugs listed under "Most important fact about this drug."

Special warnings about this medication
Norvir is very new and has been studied for only a limited period of time. Its long-term effects are still unknown.

Norvir is not a cure for AIDS or HIV infection. You may continue to experience symptoms and develop complications, including opportunistic infections (rare diseases that attack when the immune system falters, such as certain types of pneumonia, tuberculosis, and fungal infections).

Norvir does not reduce the danger of transmission of HIV to others through sexual contact or blood contamination. Therefore, you should continue to avoid practices that could give HIV to others. If you have liver disease, you should take this medication with caution.

**Possible food and drug interactions
when taking this medication**
Combining Norvir with certain drugs (see "Most important fact about this drug") may cause serious or life-threatening effects. Other drugs may cause less dangerous—but still worrisome—effects. It is especially important to check with your doctor before combining Norvir with the following:

Clarithromycin (Biaxin)
Desipramine (Norpramin)
Disulfiram (Antabuse)
Metronidazole (Flagyl)
Oral contraceptives

Saquinavir (Invirase)
Theophylline (Theo-Dur)

Less significant interactions may occur with many other drugs. Your wisest course is to check with your doctor before combining *any* drug with Norvir.

Tobacco use decreases the effects of Norvir. The effects of antacids taken with Norvir have not been studied.

Special information
if you are pregnant or breastfeeding

The effects of Norvir during pregnancy have not been adequately studied. If you are pregnant or plan to become pregnant, tell your doctor immediately. This drug may appear in breast milk and could affect a nursing infant. To avoid transmitting HIV to a newborn baby, HIV-positive women should not breastfeed.

Recommended dosage

ADULTS AND ADOLESCENTS OVER 12 YEARS OF AGE

The recommended dose of Norvir is 600 milligrams twice a day with food.

Should you experience nausea when first starting on Norvir, your doctor may lower your starting dosage to 300 milligrams twice a day for 1 day, 400 milligrams twice a day for 2 days, 500 milligrams twice a day for 1 day, and then 600 milligrams twice a day thereafter.

If Norvir is to be used in combination with other HIV drugs, your doctor may suggest taking Norvir alone at first and adding the second drug later in the first 2 weeks of therapy. This approach may cause fewer stomach problems.

CHILDREN

The safety and effectiveness of Norvir in children below the age of 12 have not been established at this time.

Overdosage

Information on acute overdose with Norvir is limited. However, any medication taken in excess can have serious consequences. If you suspect an overdose, seek emergency medical treatment immediately.

■ *Symptoms of Norvir overdose may include:*
  Numbness, tingling, or a "pins and needles" sensation, particularly in the arms and legs

Brand name:

NOVOLIN

See Insulin, page 639.

Brand name:

NUTRACORT

See Hydrocortisone Skin Preparations, page 599.

Generic name:

NYSTATIN WITH TRIAMCINOLONE

See Mycolog-II, page 841.

Brand name:

OBY-CAP

See Fastin, page 506.

Generic name:

OFLOXACIN

See Floxin, page 537.

Brand name:

OGEN

Pronounced: OH-jen
Generic name: Estropipate
Other brand name: Ortho-Est

Why is this drug prescribed?

Ogen and Ortho-Est are estrogen replacement drugs. The tablets are used to reduce symptoms of menopause, including feelings of warmth in face, neck, and chest, and the sudden intense episodes of heat and sweating known as "hot flashes." They also may be prescribed for teenagers who fail to mature at the usual rate.

In addition, either the tablets or Ogen vaginal cream can be used for other conditions caused by lack of estrogen, such as dry, itchy external genitals and vaginal irritation.

Along with diet, calcium supplements, and exercise, Ogen and Ortho-Est tablets are also prescribed to prevent osteoporosis, a condition in which the bones become brittle and easily broken.

Some doctors also prescribe these drugs to treat breast cancer and cancer of the prostate.

Most important fact about this drug
Because estrogens have been linked with increased risk of endometrial cancer (cancer in the lining of the uterus) in women who have had their menopause, it is essential to have regular checkups and to report any unusual vaginal bleeding to your doctor immediately.

How should you take this medication?
Be careful to follow the cycle of administration your doctor establishes for you. Take the medication exactly as prescribed.

When using Ogen Vaginal Cream, follow the instructions printed on the carton. It is for short-term use only. Remove the cap from the tube and make sure the plunger of the applicator is all the way into the barrel. Screw the nozzle of the applicator onto the tube and squeeze the cream into the applicator. The number on the plunger, which indicates the dose you should take, should be level with the top of the barrel. Unscrew the applicator and replace the cap on the tube. Insert the applicator into the vagina and push the plunger all the way down. Between uses, take the plunger out of the barrel and wash the applicator with warm, soapy water. Never use hot or boiling water.

■ *If you miss a dose...*
  Take the forgotten dose as soon as you remember. If it is almost time for the next dose, skip the one you missed and go back to your regular schedule. Never try to "catch up" by doubling the dose.

■ *Storage instructions...*
  Store at room temperature.

What side effects may occur?
Side effects cannot be anticipated. If any develop or change in intensity, notify your doctor as soon as possible. Only your doctor can determine if it is safe for you to continue taking estrogen.

■ *Side effects may include:*

Abdominal cramps, bloating, breakthrough bleeding, breast enlargement, breast tenderness and secretions, change in amount of cervical secretion, changes in sex drive, changes in vaginal bleeding patterns, chorea (irregular, rapid, jerky movements, usually affecting the face and limbs), depression, dizziness, enlargement of benign tumors (fibroids), excessive hairiness, fluid retention, hair loss, headache, inability to use contact lenses, menstrual changes, migraine, nausea, reduced ability to tolerate carbohydrates, spotting, spotty darkening of the skin, especially around the face, skin eruptions (especially on the legs and arms) with bleeding, skin irritation, skin redness and scaling, vaginal yeast infection, vision problems, vomiting, weight gain or loss, yellow eyes and skin

Why should this drug not be prescribed?

Estrogens should not be used if you know or suspect you have breast cancer or other cancers promoted by estrogen. Do not use estrogen if you are pregnant or think you may be pregnant. Also avoid estrogen if you have abnormal, undiagnosed genital bleeding, or if you have blood clots or a blood clotting disorder or a history of blood clotting disorders associated with previous estrogen use.

Ogen Vaginal Cream should not be used if you are sensitive to or have ever had an allergic reaction to any of its components.

Special warnings about this medication

The risk of cancer of the uterus increases when estrogen is used for a long time or taken in large doses. There also may be increased risk of breast cancer in women who take estrogen for an extended period of time.

Women who take estrogen after menopause are more likely to develop gallbladder disease.

Ogen also increases the risk of blood clots. These blood clots can cause stroke, heart attack, or other serious disorders.

Your doctor will check your blood pressure regularly. It could go up or down.

While taking estrogen, get in touch with your doctor right away if you notice any of the following:

Abdominal pain, tenderness, or swelling
Abnormal bleeding from the vagina
Breast lumps
Coughing up blood
Pain in your chest or calves
Severe headache, dizziness, or faintness

Speech changes
Sudden shortness of breath
Vision changes
Vomiting
Weakness or numbness in an arm or leg
Yellowing of the skin

Ogen may cause fluid retention in some people. If you have asthma, epilepsy, migraine, or heart or kidney disease, use this medication with care.

Estrogen therapy may cause uterine bleeding or breast pain.

Possible food and drug interactions
when taking this medication
If Ogen is taken with certain other drugs, the effects of either could be increased, decreased, or altered. It is especially important to check with your doctor before combining Ogen with the following:

Barbiturates such as phenobarbital
Blood thinners such as Coumadin
Epilepsy drugs (Tegretol, Dilantin, others)
Insulin
Rifampin (Rifadin)
Tricyclic antidepressants (Elavil, Tofranil, others)

Special information
if you are pregnant or breastfeeding
Estrogens should not be used during pregnancy. If you are pregnant or plan to become pregnant, notify your doctor immediately. These drugs may appear in breast milk and could affect a nursing infant. If this medication is essential to your health, your doctor may advise you to discontinue breastfeeding until your treatment is finished.

Recommended dosage

HOT FLASHES AND NIGHT SWEATS

Ogen Tablets:
The usual dose ranges from one .625 tablet to two 2.5 tablets per day. Tablets should be taken in cycles, according to your doctor's instructions.

Ortho-Est Tablets:
The usual dose ranges from half a tablet to 4 tablets per day of Ortho-Est 1.25 or 1 to 8 tablets of Ortho-Est .625. Tablets should be taken in cycles, according to your doctor's instructions.

VAGINAL INFLAMMATION AND DRYNESS

Ogen Tablets:
The usual dose ranges from one .625 tablet to two 2.5 tablets per day. Tablets should be taken in cycles, according to your doctor's instructions.

Ortho-Est Tablets:
The usual dose ranges from half a tablet to 4 tablets per day of Ortho-Est 1.25 or 1 to 8 tablets of Ortho-Est .625. Tablets should be taken in cycles, according to your doctor's instructions.

Ogen Vaginal Cream:
The usual dose is 2 to 4 grams daily. Cream should be used in cycles, and only for limited periods of time.

ESTROGEN HORMONE DEFICIENCY

Ogen Tablets:
The usual dose ranges from one 1.25 tablet to three 2.5 tablets per day, taken for 3 weeks, followed by a rest period of 8 to 10 days.

Ortho-Est Tablets:
The usual dose ranges from 1 to 6 tablets per day of Ortho-Est 1.25 or 2 to 12 tablets of Ortho-Est .625, given for 3 weeks, followed by a rest period of 8 to 10 days.

OVARIAN FAILURE

Ogen Tablets:
The usual dose ranges from one 1.25 tablet to three 2.5 tablets per day for 3 weeks, followed by a rest period of 8 to 10 days. Your doctor may increase or decrease your dosage according to your response.

Ortho-Est Tablets:
The usual dose ranges from 1 to 6 tablets per day of Ortho-Est 1.25 or 2 to 12 tablets of Ortho-Est .625 for 3 weeks, followed by a rest period of 8 to 10 days. Your doctor may increase or decrease your dosage according to your response.

PREVENTION OF OSTEOPOROSIS

Ogen and Ortho-Est Tablets:
The usual dose is one .625 tablet per day for 25 days of a 31-day monthly cycle.

Overdosage
Any medication taken in excess can have serious consequences. If you suspect an overdose, seek emergency medical treatment immediately.

■ *Symptoms of Ogen overdose may include:*
Nausea, vomiting, withdrawal bleeding

Generic name:

OLANZAPINE

See Zyprexa, page 1491.

Generic name:

OLSALAZINE

See Dipentum, page 413.

Generic name:

OMEPRAZOLE

See Prilosec, page 1047.

Brand name:

OMNIPEN

Pronounced: AHM-nee-pen
Generic name: Ampicillin
Other brands: Principen, Totacillin

Why is this drug prescribed?
Omnipen is a penicillin-like antibiotic prescribed for a wide variety of infections, including gonorrhea and other genital and urinary infections, respiratory infections, and gastrointestinal infections, as well as meningitis (inflamed membranes of the spinal cord or brain).

Most important fact about this drug
If you are allergic to either penicillin or cephalosporin antibiotics in any form, consult your doctor *before taking Omnipen*. There is a possibility that you are allergic to both types of medication; and if a reaction occurs, it could be extremely severe. If you take the drug and develop a skin reaction, diarrhea, shortness of breath, wheezing, sore throat, or fever, seek medical attention immediately.

How should you use this medication?

Take Omnipen Capsules with a full glass of water, a half hour before or 2 hours after a meal.

Omnipen Oral Suspension should be shaken well before using.

Take Omnipen exactly as prescribed. It works best when there is a constant amount in the body. Take your doses at evenly spaced times around the clock, and try not to miss a dose.

■ *If you miss a dose...*
Take it as soon as you remember. If it is almost time for the next dose, and you take 2 doses a day, take the one you missed and the next dose 5 to 6 hours later. If you take 3 or more doses a day, take the one you missed and the next dose 2 to 4 hours later. Then go back to your regular schedule. Do not take 2 doses at once.

■ *Storage information...*
Store Omnipen Capsules at room temperature in a tightly closed container.

Keep Omnipen Oral Suspension in the refrigerator, in a tightly closed container. Discard the unused portion after 14 days.

What side effects may occur?

Side effects cannot be anticipated. If any develop or change in intensity, inform your doctor as soon as possible. Only your doctor can determine whether it is safe for you to continue taking Omnipen.

■ *Side effects may include:*
Colitis (inflammation of the bowel), diarrhea, fever, itching, nausea, rash or other skin problems, sore tongue or mouth, vomiting

Why should this drug not be prescribed?

You should not take Omnipen if you are allergic to penicillin or cephalosporin antibiotics.

Special warnings about this medication

If you have an allergic reaction, stop taking Omnipen and contact your doctor immediately.

After you have taken Omnipen for a long time, you may get a new infection (called a superinfection) due to an organism this medication cannot treat. Consult your doctor if your symptoms do not improve or seem to get worse.

Omnipen sometimes causes diarrhea. Some diarrhea medications can make the diarrhea worse. Check with your doctor before taking any diarrhea remedy.

Oral contraceptives may not work properly while you are taking Omnipen. For greater certainty, use other measures while taking Omnipen.

If you are diabetic, be aware that Omnipen may cause a *false positive* in certain urine glucose tests. You should talk to your doctor about the right tests to use while you are taking Omnipen.

For infections such as strep throat, it is important to take Omnipen for the entire amount of time your doctor has prescribed. Even if you feel better, you need to continue taking the medication.

Possible food and drug interactions
when taking this medication
If Omnipen is taken with certain other drugs the effects of either could be increased, decreased, or altered. It is especially important to check with your doctor before combining Omnipen with any of the following:

Allopurinol (Zyloprim)
Atenolol (Tenormin)
Chloroquine (Aralen)
Mefloquine (Lariam)
Oral contraceptives

Special information
if you are pregnant or breastfeeding
The effects of Omnipen during pregnancy have not been adequately studied. If you are pregnant or plan to become pregnant, inform your doctor immediately. Omnipen should be used during pregnancy only if the potential benefit justifies the potential risk to the developing baby.

Omnipen appears in breast milk and could affect a nursing infant. If this medication is essential to your health, your doctor may advise you to stop breastfeeding until your treatment with Omnipen is finished.

Recommended dosage
Unless you are being treated for gonorrhea, your doctor will have you continue taking Omnipen for 2 to 3 days after your symptoms have disappeared. Dosages are for capsules and oral suspension.

ADULTS

Infections of the Genital, Urinary, or Gastrointestinal Tracts
The usual dose is 500 milligrams, taken every 6 hours.

Gonorrhea
The usual dose is 3.5 grams in a single oral dose along with 1 gram of probenecid.

Respiratory Tract Infections
The usual dose is 250 milligrams, taken every 6 hours.

CHILDREN

Children weighing over 44 pounds should follow the adult dose schedule.

Children weighing 44 pounds or less should have their dosage determined by their weight.

Infections of the Genital, Urinary, or Gastrointestinal Tracts
The usual dose is 100 milligrams for each 2.2 pounds of body weight daily, divided into 4 doses for the capsules, and 3 to 4 doses for the suspension.

Respiratory Tract Infections
The usual dose is 50 milligrams for each 2.2 pounds of body weight daily, divided into 3 to 4 doses.

Overdosage
Although no specific symptoms have been reported, any medication taken in excess can have serious consequences. If you suspect an overdose of Omnipen, seek medical attention immediately.

Generic name:

ONDANSETRON

See Zofran, page 1467.

Brand name:

OPCON-A

See Naphcon-A, page 848.

Category:

ORAL CONTRACEPTIVES

Brand names: Brevicon, Demulen, Desogen, Genora, Levlen, Loestrin, Lo/Ovral, Micronor, Modicon, Nordette, Norethin, Norinyl, Ortho-Cept, Ortho-Cyclen, Ortho-Novum, Ortho Tri-Cyclen, Ovcon, Ovral, Triphasil

Why is this drug prescribed?

Oral contraceptives (also known as "The Pill") are highly effective means of preventing pregnancy. Oral contraceptives consist of synthetic forms of two hormones produced naturally in the body: either progestin alone or estrogen and progestin. Estrogen and progestin regulate a woman's menstrual cycle, and the fluctuating levels of these hormones play an essential role in fertility.

To reduce side effects, oral contraceptives are available in a wide range of estrogen and progestin concentrations. Progestin-only products (such as Micronor) are usually prescribed for women who should avoid estrogens; however, they may not be as effective as estrogen/progestin contraceptives.

One variety of the Pill—the Ortho Tri-Cyclen 28-day Dial pak—is also used in the treatment of moderate acne in women aged 15 and older. It is taken just as it would be for contraception.

Most important fact about this drug

Cigarette smoking increases the risk of serious heart-related side effects (stroke, heart attack, blood clots, etc.) in women who use oral contraceptives. This risk increases with heavy smoking (15 or more cigarettes per day) and with age. There is an especially significant increase in heart disease risk in women over 35 years old who smoke and use oral contraceptives.

How should you take this medication?

Oral contraceptives should be taken daily, no more than 24 hours apart, for the duration of the prescribed cycle of 21 or 28 days. Ideally, you should take your pill at the same time every day to reduce the chance of forgetting a dose; with progestin-only contraceptives, taking the pill at the same time each day is essential.

■ *If you miss a dose...*

If you neglect to take only one estrogen/progestin pill, take it as soon as you remember, take the next pill at your regular time, and continue taking the rest of the medication cycle. The risk of pregnancy is small if you miss only one combination pill per cycle. If you miss more than one tablet, check your product's patient information for instructions.

Missing a single progestin-only tablet increases the chance of pregnancy. Consult your doctor immediately if you miss a single dose or if you take it 3 or more hours late, and use another method of birth control until your next period begins or pregnancy is ruled out.

■ *Storage instructions...*
To help keep track of your doses, use the original container. Store at room temperature.

What side effects may occur?
Side effects cannot be anticipated. If any develop or change in intensity, inform your doctor as soon as possible. Only your doctor can determine if it is safe for you to continue taking an oral contraceptive.

■ *Side effects may include:*
Abdominal cramps, acne, appetite changes, bladder infection, bleeding in spots during a menstrual period, bloating, blood clots, breast tenderness or enlargement, cataracts, chest pain, contact lens discomfort, decreased flow of milk when given immediately after birth, depression, difficulty breathing, dizziness, fluid retention, gallbladder disease, growth of face, back, chest, or stomach hair, hair loss, headache, heart attack, high blood pressure, inflammation of the large intestine, kidney trouble, lack of menstrual periods, liver tumors, lumps in the breast, menstrual pattern changes, migraine, muscle, joint, or leg pain, nausea, nervousness, premenstrual syndrome (PMS), secretion of milk, sex drive changes, skin infection, skin rash or discoloration, stomach cramps, stroke, swelling, temporary infertility, unexplained bleeding in the vagina, vaginal discharge, vaginal infections (and/or burning and itching), visual disturbances, vomiting, weight gain or loss, yellow skin or whites of eyes

Why should this drug not be prescribed?
You should not take oral contraceptives if you have had an allergic reaction to them or if you are pregnant (or think you might be).

If you have ever had breast cancer or cancer in the reproductive organs or liver tumors, you should not take oral contraceptives.

If you have or have ever had a stroke, heart disease, liver disease, angina (severe chest pain), or blood clots, you should not take oral contraceptives. Women who have had pregnancy-related jaundice or jaundice stemming from previous use of oral contraceptives should not take them.

If you have undiagnosed and/or unexplained abnormal vaginal bleeding, do not take oral contraceptives.

Special warnings about this medication

Oral contraceptives should be used with caution if you are over 40 years old; smoke tobacco; have liver, heart, gallbladder, kidney, or thyroid disease; have high blood pressure, high cholesterol, diabetes, epilepsy, asthma, or porphyria (a blood disorder); or tend to be seriously overweight. Caution is also advised if you have blood circulation problems or have had a heart attack or stroke in the past. Be cautious, too, if you have problems with depression, migraine or other headaches, irregular menstrual periods, or visual disturbances.

If you have a family history of breast cancer or other cancers, you might want to consider using a progestin-only product. The estrogen in combination oral contraceptives has been linked with a slight increase in the risk of breast cancer. If you do use a combination, chose one with a relatively low amount of estrogen. Take high-estrogen pills (0.05 milligrams of estrogen) only if your doctor feels it's necessary.

Since the blood's clotting ability may be affected by oral contraceptives, your doctor may take you off them prior to surgery. If bleeding lasts more than 8 days while you are on a progestin-only oral contraceptive, or if you have no period at all, be sure to let your doctor know. The risk of blood clots is greater with oral contraceptives that contain desogestrel, such as Ortho-Cept.

Oral contraceptives do not protect against HIV infection (AIDS) or any other sexually transmitted disease. If there is a danger of infection, use a latex condom and spermicide in addition to the pill.

If you develop a migraine or severe headache that does not let up or keeps recurring while you are taking a progestin-only oral contraceptive, check with your doctor. You may need to switch to a different type of pill.

If you miss a menstrual period but have taken your pills regularly, contact your doctor but do not stop taking your pills. If you miss a period and have not taken your pills regularly, or if you miss two consecutive periods, you may be pregnant; stop taking your pills and check with your doctor immediately to see if you are pregnant. Use another form of birth control while you are not taking your pills.

If you are taking a progestin-only oral contraceptive and you have sudden or severe abdominal pain, call your doctor immediately. There is a higher risk of ectopic (outside the womb) pregnancy or ovarian cysts with this type of contraceptive.

You should also be aware that oral contraceptives have been know to cause rare cases of noncancerous—but dangerous—liver tumors.

Possible food and drug interactions when taking this medication

If oral contraceptives are taken with certain other drugs, the effects of either could be increased, decreased, or altered. It is especially important to check with your doctor before combining oral contraceptives with the following:

Amitriptyline (Elavil, Endep)
Ampicillin (Principen, Totacillin)
Barbiturates (phenobarbital, Seconal)
Carbamazepine (Tegretol)
Chloramphenicol (Chloromycetin)
Clomipramine (Anafranil)
Diazepam (Valium)
Doxepin (Sinequan)
Glipizide (Glucotrol)
Griseofulvin (Fulvicin, Grisactin)
Imipramine (Tofranil)
Lorazepam (Ativan)
Metoprolol (Lopressor)
Oxazepam (Serax)
Penicillin (Veetids, Pen-Vee K)
Phenylbutazone (Butazolidin)
Phenytoin (Dilantin)
Prednisolone (Prelone, Pediapred)
Prednisone (Deltasone)
Primidone (Mysoline)
Propranolol (Inderal)
Rifampin (Rifadin, Rimactane)
Sulfonamides (Bactrim, Septra)
Tetracycline (Achromycin V, Sumycin)
Theophylline (Theo-Dur, Slo-bid)
Warfarin (Coumadin, Panwarfin)

In addition, oral contraceptives may affect tests for blood sugar levels and thyroid function and may cause an increase in blood cholesterol levels.

**Special information
if you are pregnant or breastfeeding**

If you are pregnant (or think you might be), you should not use oral contraceptives, since they are not safe during pregnancy. In addition, wait at least 4 weeks after delivery before starting an oral contraceptive.

Nursing mothers should not use most oral contraceptives, since these drugs can appear in breast milk and may cause jaundice and enlarged breasts in nursing infants. In this situation, your doctor may advise you to use a different form of contraception while you are nursing your baby. Progestin-only oral contraceptives should not affect your milk or your baby's health.

Recommended dosage

If you have any questions about how you should take oral contraceptives, consult your doctor or the patient instructions that come in the drug package. The following is a partial list of instructions for taking oral contraceptives; it should not be used as a substitute for consultation with your doctor.

Some brands can be started on the first day of your menstrual cycle or on the first Sunday afterwards. Others must be started on the fifth day of the cycle or the first Sunday afterwards. The instructions below are for the first-Sunday schedule.

Oral contraceptives are supplied in 21-day and 28-day packages.

FOR A 21-DAY SCHEDULE

Oral contraceptives are taken every day for a 3-week period, followed by 1 week of no oral contraceptives; this cycle is repeated each month.

1) Starting on the first Sunday after the beginning of your menstrual period, take one tablet daily (at the same time each day) for the next 21 days. Note: If your period begins on Sunday, take the first tablet that day.

2) Wait 1 week before taking any tablets. Your menstrual period should occur during this time.

3) Following this 1-week waiting time, begin taking a daily tablet again for the next 21 days.

FOR A 28-DAY SCHEDULE

Starting on the first Sunday after the beginning of your menstrual period, take one tablet daily (at the same time each day) for the next 28 days. Continue taking the oral contraceptives according to your physician's instructions. Note: If your period begins on Sunday, take the first tablet that day.

FOR BOTH 21- AND 28-DAY REGIMENS

When following a regimen with a Sunday or Day 5 start, use an additional method of birth control for the first 7 days of the cycle.

Progestin-only tablets should be taken at the same time of day every day of the year.

Overdosage
While any medication taken in excess can cause overdose, the risk associated with oral contraceptives is minimal. Even young children who have taken large amounts of oral contraceptives have not experienced serious adverse effects. However, if you suspect an overdose, seek medical help immediately.

- *Symptoms of overdose may include:*
  Nausea, withdrawal bleeding in females

Brand name:

ORASONE

See Deltasone, page 357.

Brand name:

ORINASE

Pronounced: OR-in-aze
Generic name: Tolbutamide

Why is this drug prescribed?
Orinase is an oral antidiabetic medication used to treat Type II (non-insulin-dependent) diabetes. Diabetes occurs when the body does not make enough insulin, or when the insulin that is produced no longer works properly. Insulin works by helping sugar get inside the body's cells, where it is then used for energy.

There are two forms of diabetes: Type I (insulin-dependent) and Type II (non-insulin-dependent). Type I diabetes usually requires taking insulin injections for life, while Type II diabetes can usually be treated by dietary changes, exercise, and/or oral antidiabetic medications such as Orinase. Orinase controls diabetes by stimulating the pancreas to secrete more insulin and by helping insulin work better.

Occasionally, Type II diabetics must take insulin injections temporarily during stressful periods or times of illness. When diet, exercise, and an oral antidiabetic medication fail to reduce symptoms and/or blood sugar levels, a person with Type II diabetes may require long-term insulin injections.

Most important fact about this drug

Always remember that Orinase is an aid to, not a substitute for, good diet and exercise. Failure to follow a sound diet and exercise plan can lead to serious complications, such as dangerously high or low blood sugar levels. Remember, too, that Orinase is *not* an oral form of insulin, and cannot be used in place of insulin.

How should you take this medication?

In general, Orinase should be taken 30 minutes before a meal to achieve the best control over blood sugar levels. However, the exact dosing schedule, as well as the dosage amount, must be determined by your physician. Ask your doctor when it is best for you to take this medication.

To help prevent low blood sugar levels (hypoglycemia) you should:

Understand the symptoms of hypoglycemia.
Know how exercise affects your blood sugar levels.
Maintain an adequate diet.
Keep a product containing quick-acting sugar with you at all times.
Limit alcohol intake. If you drink alcohol, it may cause breathlessness and facial flushing.

■ *If you miss a dose...*
Take it as soon as you remember. If it is almost time for the next dose, skip the one you missed and go back to your regular schedule. Do not take 2 doses at the same time.

■ *Storage instructions...*
Store at room temperature.

What side effects may occur?

Side effects cannot be anticipated. If any develop or change in intensity, inform your doctor as soon as possible. Only your doctor can determine if it is safe for you to continue taking Orinase.

Side effects from Orinase are rare and seldom require discontinuation of the medication.

- *More common side effects may include:*
  Bloating, heartburn, nausea

- *Less common or rare side effects may include:*
  Anemia and other blood disorders, blistering, changes in taste, headache, hepatic porphyria (a condition frequently characterized by sensitivity to light, stomach pain, and nerve damage, caused by excessive levels of a substance called porphyrin in the liver), hives, itching, redness of the skin, skin eruptions, skin rash

Orinase, like all oral antidiabetics, may cause hypoglycemia (low blood sugar). The risk of hypoglycemia can be increased by missed meals, alcohol, other medications, fever, trauma, infection, surgery, or excessive exercise. To avoid hypoglycemia, you should closely follow the dietary and exercise plan suggested by your physician.

- *Symptoms of mild hypoglycemia may include:*
  Cold sweat, drowsiness, fast heartbeat, headache, nausea, nervousness

- *Symptoms of more severe hypoglycemia may include:*
  Coma, pale skin, seizures, shallow breathing

Contact your doctor immediately if these symptoms of severe low blood sugar occur.

Ask your doctor what you should do if you experience mild hypoglycemia. Severe hypoglycemia should be considered a medical emergency, and prompt medical attention is essential.

Why should this drug not be prescribed?
You should not take Orinase if you have had an allergic reaction to it.

Orinase should not be taken if you are suffering from diabetic ketoacidosis (a life-threatening medical emergency caused by insufficient insulin and marked by excessive thirst, nausea, fatigue, pain below the breastbone, and fruity breath).

In addition, Orinase should not be used as the sole therapy in treating Type I (insulin-dependent) diabetes.

Special warnings about this medication
It's possible that drugs such as Orinase may lead to more heart problems than diet treatment alone, or diet plus insulin. If you have a heart condition, you may want to discuss this with your doctor.

If you are taking Orinase, you should check your blood or urine periodically for abnormal sugar (glucose) levels.

It is important that you closely follow the diet and exercise plan recommended by your doctor.

Even people with well-controlled diabetes may find that stress, illness, surgery, or fever results in a loss of control over their diabetes. In these cases, your physician may recommend that you temporarily stop taking Orinase and use injected insulin instead.

In addition, the effectiveness of any oral antidiabetic, including Orinase, may decrease with time. This may occur because of either a diminished responsiveness to the medication or a worsening of the diabetes.

Like other antidiabetic drugs, Orinase may produce severe low blood sugar if the dosage is wrong. While taking Orinase, you are particularly susceptible to episodes of low blood sugar if:

You suffer from a kidney or liver problem;

You have a lack of adrenal or pituitary hormone;

You are elderly, run-down, malnourished, hungry, exercising heavily, drinking alcohol, or using more than one glucose-lowering drug.

Possible food and drug interactions when taking this medication

If Orinase is taken with certain other drugs, the effects of either could be increased, decreased, or altered. It is especially important to check with your doctor before combining Orinase with the following:

Adrenal corticosteroids such as prednisone (Deltasone) and cortisone (Cortone)
Airway-opening drugs such as Proventil and Ventolin
Anabolic steroids such as testosterone
Barbiturates such as Amytal, Seconal, and phenobarbital
Beta blockers such as Inderal and Tenormin
Blood-thinning drugs such as Coumadin
Calcium channel blockers such as Cardizem and Procardia
Chloramphenicol (Chloromycetin)
Cimetidine (Tagamet)
Clofibrate (Atromid-S)
Colestipol (Colestid)
Epinephrine (EpiPen)
Estrogens (Premarin)
Fluconazole (Diflucan)
Furosemide (Lasix)

Isoniazid (Laniazid, Rifamate)

Itraconazole (Sporanox)

Major tranquilizers such as Stelazine and Mellaril

MAO inhibitors such as Nardil and Parnate

Methyldopa (Aldomet)

Miconazole (Monistat)

Niacin (Nicobid, Nicolar)

Nonsteroidal anti-inflammatory agents such as Advil, aspirin, Motrin, Naprosyn, and Voltaren

Oral contraceptives

Phenytoin (Dilantin)

Probenecid (Benemid)

Rifampin (Rifadin)

Sulfa drugs such as Bactrim and Septra

Thiazide and other diuretics such as Diuril and HydroDIURIL

Thyroid medications such as Synthroid

Be cautious about drinking alcohol, since excessive alcohol can cause low blood sugar.

Special information
if you are pregnant or breastfeeding

The effects of Orinase during pregnancy have not been adequately established in humans. Since Orinase has caused birth defects in rats, it is not recommended for use by pregnant women. Therefore, if you are pregnant or planning to become pregnant, you should take Orinase only on the advice of your physician. Since studies suggest the importance of maintaining normal blood sugar (glucose) levels during pregnancy, your physician may prescribe injected insulin during your pregnancy. While it is not known if Orinase enters breast milk, other similar medications do. Therefore, you should discuss with your doctor whether to discontinue the medication or to stop breastfeeding. If the medication is discontinued, and if diet alone does not control glucose levels, your doctor will consider giving you insulin injections.

Recommended dosage

Dosage levels are based on individual needs.

ADULTS

Usually an initial daily dose of 1 to 2 grams is recommended. Maintenance therapy usually ranges from 0.25 to 3 grams daily. Daily doses greater than 3 grams are not recommended.

CHILDREN

Safety and effectiveness have not been established in children.

OLDER ADULTS

Older, malnourished, or debilitated people, or those with impaired kidney or liver function, are usually prescribed lower initial and maintenance doses to minimize the risk of low blood sugar (hypoglycemia).

Overdosage

Any medication taken in excess can have serious consequences. An overdose of Orinase can cause low blood sugar (see "Special warnings about this medication"). Eating sugar or a sugar-based product will often correct mild hypoglycemia. If you suspect an overdose, seek medical attention immediately.

Generic name:

ORPHENADRINE, ASPIRIN, AND CAFFEINE

See Norgesic, page 893.

Brand name:

ORTHO-CEPT

See Oral Contraceptives, page 926.

Brand name:

ORTHO-CYCLEN

See Oral Contraceptives, page 926.

Brand name:

ORTHO-EST

See Ogen, page 917.

Brand name:

ORTHO-NOVUM

See Oral Contraceptives, page 926.

Brand name:

ORTHO TRI-CYCLEN

See Oral Contraceptives, page 926.

Brand name:

ORUDIS

Pronounced: Oh-ROO-dis
Generic name: Ketoprofen
Other brand names: Actron, Orudis KT, Oruvail

Why is this drug prescribed?
Orudis, a nonsteroidal anti-inflammatory drug, is used to relieve the inflammation, swelling, stiffness, and joint pain associated with rheumatoid arthritis and osteoarthritis (the most common form of arthritis). It is also used to relieve mild to moderate pain, as well as menstrual pain.

Oruvail, an extended-release form of the drug, is used to treat the signs and symptoms of rheumatoid arthritis and osteoarthritis over the long term, not severe attacks that come on suddenly.

Actron and Orudis KT are over-the-counter forms of the drug. They are used to relieve minor aches and pains associated with the common cold, headache, toothache, muscle aches, backache, minor arthritis, and menstrual cramps. They are also used to reduce fever.

Most important fact about this drug
You should have frequent check-ups with your doctor if you take Orudis regularly. Ulcers or internal bleeding can occur without warning.

How should you take this medication?
To minimize side effects, your doctor may recommend that you take Orudis with food, an antacid, or milk.

If you are using Orudis for arthritis, it should be taken regularly.

Orudis and Oruvail should not be taken together.

Actron and Orudis KT should be taken with a full glass of water or other fluid. Do not use them for more than 3 days for fever or 10 days for pain.

■ *If you miss a dose...*
If you take Orudis on a regular schedule, take the forgotten dose as soon as you remember. If it is almost time for your next dose, skip the one you missed and go back to your regular schedule. Do not take 2 doses at once.

■ *Storage instructions...*
Store at room temperature in a tightly closed container. Protect Oruvail capsules from direct light and excessive heat and humidity.

What side effects may occur?
Side effects cannot be anticipated. If any develop or change in intensity, inform your doctor as soon as possible. Only your doctor can determine if it is safe for you to continue taking Orudis.

■ *More common side effects may include:*
Abdominal pain, changes in kidney function, constipation, diarrhea, dreams, fluid retention, gas, headache, inability to sleep, indigestion, nausea, nervousness

■ *Less common or rare side effects may include:*
Allergic reaction, amnesia, anemia, asthma, belching, blood in the urine, bloody or black stools, change in taste, chills, confusion, congestive heart failure, coughing up blood, conjunctivitis (pinkeye), depression, difficult or labored breathing, dizziness, dry mouth, eye pain, facial swelling due to fluid retention, general feeling of illness, hair loss, hepatitis, high blood pressure, hives, impaired hearing, impotence, increase in appetite, increased salivation, infection, inflammation of the mouth, irregular or excessive menstrual bleeding, itching, jaundice (yellowing of the eyes and skin), kidney failure, liver problems, loosening of fingernails, loss of appetite, migraine, muscle pain, nasal inflammation, nosebleed, pain, peptic or intestinal ulcer, rapid heartbeat, rash, rectal bleeding, red or purple spots on the skin, ringing in the ears, sensitivity to light, skin discoloration, skin eruptions, skin inflammation and flaking, sleepiness, sore throat, stomach inflammation, sweating, swelling of the throat, thirst, throbbing heartbeat, tingling or pins and needles, vertigo, visual disturbances, vomiting, vomiting blood, weight gain or loss

Why should this drug not be prescribed?
If you are sensitive to or have ever had an allergic reaction to Orudis, or if you have had asthma attacks, hives, or other allergic reactions caused by aspirin or other nonsteroidal anti-inflammatory drugs, you should not take this medication. Make sure your doctor is aware of any drug reactions you have experienced.

Special warnings about this medication
Remember that stomach ulcers and bleeding can occur without warning.

This drug should be used with caution if you have kidney or liver disease.

If you are taking Orudis for an extended period of time, your doctor will check your blood for anemia.

This drug can increase water retention. Use with caution if you have heart disease or high blood pressure.

Make sure your doctor knows what other conditions you have and what other drugs you are taking.

Check with your doctor before taking Actron if the painful area is red or swollen. Also check with your doctor if, after you have started taking Actron, your symptoms continue or get worse, new symptoms appear, or you have stomach pain.

Possible food and drug interactions
when taking this medication
If Orudis is taken with certain other drugs, the effects of either could be increased, decreased, or altered. It is especially important to check with your doctor before combining Orudis with the following:

Aspirin
Blood thinners such as Coumadin
Diuretics such as hydrochlorothiazide (HydroDIURIL)
Lithium (Lithonate)
Methotrexate
Probenecid (the gout medication Benemid)

Orudis can prolong bleeding time. If you are taking blood-thinning medication, use this drug cautiously.

Do not combine pain relievers without asking your doctor.

If you usually have 3 or more alcoholic drinks a day, ask your doctor about taking pain relievers.

Special information
if you are pregnant or breastfeeding
The effects of Orudis during pregnancy have not been adequately studied. If you are pregnant or plan to become pregnant, inform your doctor immediately. It is particularly important not to use this product during the last 3 months of pregnancy unless your doctor has told you to; its use may cause problems in your baby or during delivery. Orudis may appear in breast milk

and could affect a nursing infant. If this medication is essential to your health, your doctor may advise you to discontinue breastfeeding until your treatment with this medication is finished.

Recommended dosage

ADULTS

Rheumatoid Arthritis and Osteoarthritis
The starting dose of Orudis is 75 milligrams 3 times a day or 50 milligrams 4 times a day; for Oruvail, 200 milligrams taken once a day. The most you should take in a day is 300 milligrams of Orudis or 200 milligrams of Oruvail. Some side effects, such as headache or upset stomach, increase in severity as the dose gets higher.

Mild to Moderate Pain and Menstrual Pain
The usual dose of Orudis is 25 to 50 milligrams every 6 to 8 hours as needed.

Smaller people, older people, and those with kidney or liver disease need smaller doses of Orudis. Doses above 75 milligrams have no additional effect.

The usual dose of Actron or Orudis KT is 1 tablet or caplet (12.5 milligrams) every 4 to 6 hours. If you get no relief in 1 hour, you may take another tablet or caplet. Do not take more than 2 tablets or caplets in a 4 to 6-hour period. Do not take more than 6 tablets or caplets each 24 hours.

CHILDREN

Not for use in children under 16 years of age, unless recommended by a doctor.

OLDER ADULTS

Dosage may be lower.

Overdosage
Any medication taken in excess can have serious consequences. If you suspect an overdose of Orudis, seek medical attention immediately.

- *Symptoms of Orudis overdose may include:*
  Breathing difficulty, coma, convulsions, drowsiness, high blood pressure, kidney failure, low blood pressure, nausea, sluggishness, stomach and intestinal bleeding, stomach pain, vomiting

Brand name:

ORUVAIL

See Orudis, page 937.

Brand name:

OVCON

See Oral Contraceptives, page 926.

Brand name:

OVRAL

See Oral Contraceptives, page 926.

Generic name:

OXAPROZIN

See Daypro, page 338.

Generic name:

OXAZEPAM

See Serax, page 1180.

Generic name:

OXICONAZOLE

See Oxistat, below.

Brand name:

OXISTAT

Pronounced: OX-ee-stat
Generic name: Oxiconazole nitrate

Why is this drug prescribed?
Oxistat is used to treat fungal skin diseases commonly called ringworm (tinea). Oxistat is prescribed for athlete's foot (tinea pedis), jock itch (tinea

cruris), ringworm of the entire body (tinea corporis), and tinea versicolor, which appears as patches on the skin. It is available as a cream or lotion.

Most important fact about this drug
Oxistat should not be used in, on, or near the eyes, or applied to the vagina.

How should you use this medication?
Use Oxistat exactly as prescribed.

Wash and dry the area to be treated before applying Oxistat and then apply the cream or lotion so that it covers the entire affected area and the area right around it.

Be careful when applying to raw, blistered, or oozing skin.

■ *If you miss a dose...*
Apply the cream or lotion when you remember, then return to your regular schedule.

■ *Storage instructions...*
Store Oxistat at room temperature.

What side effects may occur?
Side effects cannot be anticipated. If any develop or change in intensity, notify your doctor as soon as possible. Only your doctor can determine whether it is safe for you to continue using Oxistat.

■ *Side effects may include:*
Allergic skin inflammation, burning, cracks in the skin, eczema, irritation, itching, pain, rash, scaling, skin redness, skin softening, small, firm, raised skin eruptions similar to those of chickenpox, stinging, tingling

Why should this drug not be prescribed?
Do not use Oxistat if you have ever had an allergic reaction or are sensitive to oxiconazole or any other ingredients in the cream.

Special warnings about this medication
If you develop an irritation or sensitivity to the medication, notify your doctor.

Possible food and drug interactions
when taking this medication
No interactions have been reported.

Special information
if you are pregnant or breastfeeding
Oxistat has not been proved safe during pregnancy. If you are pregnant or plan to become pregnant, inform your doctor immediately.

Oxistat appears in breast milk and could affect a nursing infant. If Oxistat is essential to your health, your doctor may advise you to stop breastfeeding until your treatment is finished.

Recommended dosage

ADULTS AND CHILDREN
For athlete's foot, jock itch, or ringworm of the body, use Oxistat cream or lotion once or twice a day. Athlete's foot is treated for 1 month. Jock itch and ringworm of the body are treated for 2 weeks.

For tinea versicolor, apply Oxistat cream once a day for 2 weeks.

Overdosage
Overdose of Oxistat has not been reported. However, if you suspect an overdose, seek medical attention immediately.

Generic name:

OXYBUTYNIN

See Ditropan, page 421.

Brand name:

PAMELOR

Pronounced: PAM-eh-lore
Generic name: Nortriptyline hydrochloride
Other brand name: Aventyl

Why is this drug prescribed?
Pamelor is prescribed for the relief of symptoms of depression. It is one of the drugs known as tricyclic antidepressants.

Some doctors also prescribe Pamelor to treat chronic hives, premenstrual depression, attention deficit hyperactivity disorder in children, and bedwetting.

Most important fact about this drug
Pamelor must be taken regularly to be effective and it may be several weeks before you begin to feel better. Do not skip doses, even if they seem to make no difference.

How should you take this medication?
Take Pamelor exactly as prescribed. Pamelor may make your mouth dry. Sucking on hard candy, chewing gum, or melting ice chips in your mouth can provide relief.

■ *If you miss a dose...*
Take it as soon as you remember. If it is almost time for the next dose, skip the one you missed and go back to your regular schedule. If you take Pamelor once a day at bedtime and you miss a dose, do not take it in the morning, since disturbing side effects could occur. Never take 2 doses at once.

■ *Storage instructions...*
Keep Pamelor in the container it came in, tightly closed and away from light. Be sure to keep this drug out of reach of children; an overdose is particularly dangerous in the young. Store at room temperature.

What side effects may occur?
Side effects cannot be anticipated. If any develop or change in intensity, inform your doctor as soon as possible. Only your doctor can determine if it is safe for you to continue taking Pamelor.

■ *Side effects may include:*
Abdominal cramps, agitation, anxiety, black tongue, blurred vision, breast development in males, breast enlargement, confusion, constipation, delusions, diarrhea, dilation of pupils, disorientation, dizziness, drowsiness, dry mouth, excessive or spontaneous flow of milk, excessive urination at night, fatigue, fever, fluid retention, flushing, frequent urination, hair loss, hallucinations, headache, heart attack, high or low blood pressure, high or low blood sugar, hives, impotence, inability to sleep, inability to urinate, increased or decreased sex drive, inflammation of the mouth, intestinal blockage, itching, loss of appetite, loss of coordination, nausea, nightmares, numbness, panic, perspiration, pins and needles in the arms and legs, rapid, fluttery, or irregular heartbeat, rash, reddish or purplish spots on skin, restlessness, ringing in the ears, seizures, sensitivity to light, stomach upset, strange taste, stroke, swelling of the testicles, swollen glands, tingling, tremors, vision problems, vomiting, weakness, weight gain or loss, yellow eyes and skin

- *Side effects due to rapid decrease or abrupt withdrawal from Pamelor after a long term of treatment include:*
  Headache, nausea, vague feeling of bodily discomfort

These side effects do not indicate addiction to this drug.

Why should this drug not be prescribed?
If you are sensitive to or have ever had an allergic reaction to Pamelor or similar drugs, you should not take this medication. Make sure your doctor is aware of any drug reactions you have experienced.

Do not take Pamelor if you are taking—or have taken within the past 14 days—a drug classified as an MAO inhibitor. Drugs in this category include the antidepressants Nardil and Parnate. Combining these drugs with Pamelor can cause fever and convulsions, and could even be fatal.

Unless you are directed to do so by your doctor, do not take this medication if you are recovering from a heart attack or are taking any other antidepressant drugs.

If you have been taking Prozac, you may have to wait at least 5 weeks before beginning therapy with Pamelor. A drug interaction could result.

Special warnings about this medication
Pamelor may cause you to become drowsy or less alert; therefore, you should not drive or operate dangerous machinery or participate in any hazardous activity that requires full mental alertness until you know how this drug affects you.

Use Pamelor with caution if you have a history of seizures, difficulty urinating, diabetes, or chronic eye conditions such as glaucoma. Be careful, also, if you have heart disease, high blood pressure, or an overactive thyroid, or are receiving thyroid medication. You should discuss all of your medical problems with your doctor before taking this medication.

If you are being treated for a severe mental disorder (schizophrenia or manic depression), tell your doctor before taking Pamelor.

Pamelor may make your skin more sensitive to sunlight. Try to stay out of the sun, wear protective clothing, and apply a sun block.

Before having surgery, dental treatment, or any diagnostic procedure, tell your doctor that you are taking Pamelor. Certain drugs used during these procedures, such as anesthetics and muscle relaxants, may interact with Pamelor.

Possible food and drug interactions
when taking this medication
Combining Pamelor and MAO inhibitors can be fatal.

Pamelor may intensify the effects of alcohol. Do not drink alcohol while taking this medication.

If Pamelor is taken with certain other drugs, the effects of either can be increased, decreased, or altered. It is especially important to check with your doctor before combining Pamelor with the following:

Airway-opening drugs such as Ventolin and Proventil
Antidepressants such as Wellbutrin and Desyrel
Antidepressants that act on serotonin, such as Prozac, Paxil, and Zoloft
Blood pressure medications such as Catapres and Esimil
Chlorpropamide (Diabinese)
Cimetidine (Tagamet)
Drugs for heart irregularities, such as Tambocor and Rythmol
Drugs that control spasms, such as Donnatal and Bentyl
Levodopa (Larodopa)
Major tranquilizers such as Thorazine and Mellaril
Quinidine (Quinidex)
Reserpine (Diupres)
Stimulants such as Dexedrine
Thyroid medication such as Synthroid
Warfarin (Coumadin)

Special information
if you are pregnant or breastfeeding

The effects of Pamelor during pregnancy have not been adequately studied. If you are pregnant or planning to become pregnant, inform your doctor immediately. Also consult your doctor before breastfeeding.

Recommended dosage

This medication is available in tablet and liquid form. Only tablet dosages are listed. Consult your doctor if you cannot take the tablet form of this medication.

ADULTS

Your doctor will monitor your response to this medication carefully and will gradually increase or decrease the dose to suit your needs.

The usual starting dosage is 25 milligrams, 3 or 4 times per day.

Alternatively, your doctor may prescribe that the total daily dose be taken once a day.

Doses above 150 milligrams per day are not recommended.

Your doctor may want to perform a blood test to help in deciding the best dose you should receive.

CHILDREN

The safety and effectiveness of Pamelor have not been established for children and its use is not recommended. However, adolescents may be given 30 to 50 milligrams per day, either in a single dose or divided into smaller doses, as determined by your doctor.

OLDER ADULTS

The usual dose is 30 to 50 milligrams taken in a single dose or divided into smaller doses, as determined by your doctor.

Overdosage

An overdose of this type of antidepressant can be fatal. If you suspect an overdose, seek medical help immediately.

■ *Symptoms of Pamelor overdose may include:*
Agitation, coma, confusion, congestive heart failure, convulsions, dilated pupils, disturbed concentration, drowsiness, excessive reflexes, extremely high fever, fluid in the lungs, hallucinations, irregular heartbeat, low body temperature, restlessness, rigid muscles, severely low blood pressure, shock, stupor, vomiting

Brand name:

PANADOL

See Tylenol, page 1362.

Brand name:

PANCREASE

Pronounced: PAN-kree-ace
Generic name: Pancrelipase
Other brand names: Creon, Pancrease MT, Viokase,
 Ultrase

Why is this drug prescribed?

Pancrease is used to treat pancreatic enzyme deficiency. It is often prescribed for people with cystic fibrosis, chronic inflammation of the pancreas, or blockages of the pancreas or common bile duct caused by cancer. It is also taken by people who have had their pancreas removed or who have had gastrointestinal bypass surgery. Pancrease is taken to help with digestion of proteins, starches, and fats.

Most important fact about this drug
Pancrease capsules should not be chewed or crushed.

How should you take this medication?
Take this medication exactly as prescribed. If you are taking Pancrease for cystic fibrosis, your doctor may also prescribe a special diet for you. Be sure to follow the diet closely, as well as taking Pancrease.

Do not change brands or dosage forms of this medication without first checking with your doctor.

If swallowing the Pancrease capsule is difficult, open the capsule and shake the contents (microspheres) onto a small amount of soft food, such as applesauce or gelatin, that does not require chewing, then swallow immediately. Avoid mixing it with alkaline foods, such as ice cream or milk. They can reduce the medication's effect.

Pancrease should be taken with meals and snacks. Drink plenty of fluids while you are taking Pancrease.

■ *If you miss a dose...*
Resume taking the medication with your next meal or snack.

■ *Storage instructions...*
Store at room temperature in a tightly closed container away from moisture. Do not refrigerate.

What side effects may occur?
Side effects cannot be anticipated. If any develop or change in intensity, inform your doctor as soon as possible. Only your doctor can determine if it is safe for you to continue taking Pancrease.

■ *More common side effects may include:*
Stomach and intestinal upset

■ *Less common or rare side effects may include:*
Allergic-type reactions

Why should this drug not be prescribed?
Pancrease should not be used if you are sensitive to or have ever had an allergic reaction to pork protein, if you have a recently inflamed pancreas, or if you have a disease of the pancreas that gets worse.

Special warnings about this medication
If you develop an allergic reaction to Pancrease, stop taking the medication and inform your doctor immediately. If you have cystic fibrosis and develop any signs of an intestinal blockage, call your doctor.

Possible food and drug interactions
when taking this medication
If Pancrease is taken with certain other drugs, the effects of either can be increased, decreased, or altered. It is especially important that you check with your doctor before combining Pancrease with the following:

Certain antacids such as Tums and Milk of Magnesia
Certain acid-blocking ulcer medications, such as Pepcid and Zantac

Special information
if you are pregnant or breastfeeding
The effects of Pancrease during pregnancy have not been adequately studied. If you are pregnant or plan to become pregnant, inform your doctor immediately.

It is not known whether Pancrease appears in breast milk. Your doctor may advise you not to nurse while you are taking this drug.

Recommended dosage

ADULTS

Doses range from 4,000 units to 20,000 units (more if necessary) with each meal and with snacks. The dosage will be adjusted based on your response. Any increase in dosage should be made slowly. People with cystic fibrosis may require less.

CHILDREN

Your doctor will determine the best dosage of Pancrease based on the child's individual needs.

Overdosage
Although no specific information is available, any medication taken in excess can have serious consequences. If you suspect an overdose of Pancrease, seek medical treatment immediately.

Generic name:

PANCRELIPASE

See Pancrease, page 947.

Brand name:

PARAFON FORTE DSC

Pronounced: PAIR-a-fahn FOR-tay DEE-ESS-SEE
Generic name: Chlorzoxazone

Why is this drug prescribed?

Parafon Forte DSC is prescribed, along with rest and physical therapy, for the relief of discomfort associated with severe, painful muscle spasms.

Most important fact about this drug

Although rare, serious, sometimes fatal liver problems have been reported in people using Parafon Forte DSC. You should stop taking this medication and notify your doctor immediately if you develop any of the following signs of liver toxicity: fever, rash, loss of appetite, nausea, vomiting, fatigue, pain in the upper right part of your abdomen, dark urine, or yellow skin or eyes.

How should you take this medication?

Take Parafon Forte DSC exactly as prescribed by your doctor. Do not increase the dose or take it more often than prescribed.

Parafon Forte DSC occasionally discolors urine orange or purple red.

- *If you miss a dose...*
  Take it as soon as you remember, if it is within an hour or so of the missed time. Otherwise, skip the dose and go back to your regular schedule. Do not take 2 doses at once.

- *Storage instructions...*
  Store at room temperature in a tightly closed container.

What side effects may occur?

Parafon Forte DSC rarely produces undesirable side effects. However, if any develop or change in intensity, inform your doctor as soon as possible. Only your doctor can determine if it is safe for you to continue taking Parafon Forte DSC.

■ *Uncommon and rare side effects may include:*
Bruises, dizziness, drowsiness, feeling of illness, fluid retention, light-headedness, overstimulation, red or purple spots on the skin, severe allergic reaction, skin rashes, stomach or intestinal bleeding, urine discoloration

Why should this drug not be prescribed?
If you have had any reaction to this drug, notify your doctor. Make sure he or she is aware of any drug reactions you have experienced.

Special warnings about this medication
Be careful using this drug if you have allergies or have ever had an allergic reaction to a drug. If you have a sensitivity reaction such as hives, redness, or itching of skin while you are taking Parafon Forte DSC, notify your doctor immediately.

Possible food and drug interactions
when taking this medication
Parafon Forte DSC may intensify the effects of alcohol. Be cautious about drinking alcohol while taking this medication.

If Parafon Forte DSC is taken with certain other drugs, the effects of either could be increased, decreased, or altered. It is especially important to check with your doctor before combining Parafon Forte DSC with drugs that slow the action of the central nervous system, such as Percocet, Valium, and Xanax.

Special information
if you are pregnant or breastfeeding
The effects of Parafon Forte DSC during pregnancy have not been adequately studied. If you are pregnant or plan to become pregnant, inform your doctor immediately. This drug may appear in breast milk and could affect a nursing infant. If this medication is essential to your health, your doctor may advise you to discontinue breastfeeding until your treatment is finished.

Recommended dosage

ADULTS

The usual dosage of Parafon Forte DSC is 1 caplet taken 3 or 4 times per day. If you do not respond to this dosage, your doctor may increase it to one and a half caplets (750 milligrams) taken 3 or 4 times per day.

Overdosage

Any medication taken in excess can have serious consequences. If you suspect an overdose, seek medical treatment immediately.

- *Symptoms of Parafon Forte DSC overdose may include:*
  Diarrhea, dizziness, drowsiness, headache, light-headedness, nausea, vomiting

- *Symptoms that may develop after a period of time include:*
  Feeling of illness, loss of muscle strength, lowered blood pressure, sluggishness, troubled or rapid breathing

Brand name:

PARLODEL

Pronounced: PAR-luh-del
Generic name: Bromocriptine mesylate

Why is this drug prescribed?

Parlodel inhibits the secretion of the hormone prolactin from the pituitary gland. It also mimics the action of dopamine, a chemical lacking in the brain of someone with Parkinson's disease. It is used to treat a variety of medical conditions, including:

- Infertility in some women
- Menstrual problems such as the abnormal stoppage or absence of flow, with or without excessive production of milk
- Growth hormone overproduction leading to acromegaly, a condition characterized by an abnormally large skull, jaw, hands, and feet
- Parkinson's disease
- Pituitary gland tumors

Some doctors also prescribe Parlodel to treat cocaine addiction, the eye condition known as glaucoma, erection problems in certain men, restless leg syndrome, and a dangerous reaction to major tranquilizers called neuroleptic malignant syndrome.

Most important fact about this drug

Notify your doctor immediately if you develop a severe headache that does not let up or continues to get worse. It could be a warning of the possibility of other dangerous reactions, including seizure, stroke, or heart attack.

How should you take this medication?
Parlodel should be taken with food. Take the first dose while lying down. You may faint or become dizzy due to lower blood pressure, especially following the first dose.

You may not feel the full effect of this medication for a few weeks. Do not stop taking Parlodel without first checking with your doctor.

- *If you miss a dose...*
  Take it as soon as you remember if it is within 4 hours of the scheduled time. Otherwise, skip the dose you missed and go back to your regular schedule. Do not take 2 doses at once.

- *Storage information...*
  Store at room temperature in a tightly closed, light-resistant container.

What side effects may occur?
The number and severity of side effects depend on many factors, including the condition being treated, dosage, and duration of treatment. Side effects cannot be anticipated. If any develop or change in intensity, inform your doctor as soon as possible. Only your doctor can determine if it is safe for you to continue taking Parlodel.

- *More common side effects may include:*
  Abdominal cramps or discomfort, confusion, constipation, depression, diarrhea, dizziness, drop in blood pressure, drowsiness, dry mouth, fainting, fatigue, hallucinations (particularly in Parkinson's patients), headache, inability to sleep, indigestion, light-headedness, loss of appetite, loss of coordination, nasal congestion, nausea, shortness of breath, uncontrolled body movement, vertigo, visual disturbance, vomiting, weakness

- *Less common side effects may include:*
  Abdominal bleeding, anxiety, difficulty swallowing, frequent urination, heart attack, inability to hold urine, inability to urinate, nervousness, nightmares, rash, seizures, splotchy skin, stroke, swelling in feet and ankles, twitching of eyelids

Some of the above side effects are also symptoms of Parkinson's disease.

- *Rare side effects may include:*
  Abnormal heart rhythm, blurred vision or temporary blindness, cold feet, fast or slow heartbeat, hair loss, heavy-headedness, increase in blood

pressure, lower back pain, muscle cramps, muscle cramps in feet and legs, numbness, pale face, paranoia, prickling or tingling, reduced tolerance to cold, severe or continuous headache, shortness of breath, sluggishness, tingling of ears or fingers

Why should this drug not be prescribed?

You should not be using Parlodel if you have high blood pressure that is not under control or if you are pregnant (unless your doctor finds it medically necessary). You should also not take Parlodel if you are allergic to it or to any other drugs containing ergot alkaloids, such as Bellergal-S and Cafergot.

Women who have severe heart conditions should not use Parlodel after they have had a baby unless it is medically necessary.

Special warnings about this medication

Your doctor will check your pituitary gland thoroughly before you are treated with Parlodel.

Since Parlodel can restore fertility and pregnancy can result, women who do not want to become pregnant should use a "barrier" method of contraception during treatment with this medication. Do not use the "Pill" or oral contraceptives, as they may prevent Parlodel from working properly.

Notify your doctor immediately if you become pregnant while you are being treated with Parlodel.

If you have kidney or liver disease, consult your doctor before taking Parlodel.

If you are being treated with Parlodel for endocrine problems related to a tumor and stop taking this medication, the tumor may grow back rapidly.

Use Parlodel with caution if you have had mental problems, any disease of the heart and circulatory system, peptic ulcer, or bleeding in the stomach and intestines.

If you are being treated for Parkinson's disease, the use of Parlodel alone or Parlodel with levodopa may cause hallucinations, confusion, and low blood pressure. If this happens, notify your doctor immediately.

If you have an abnormal heartbeat rhythm caused by a previous heart attack, consult your doctor before taking Parlodel.

If you experience a persistent watery nasal discharge while taking Parlodel, notify your doctor.

This drug may impair your ability to drive a car or operate potentially dangerous machinery. Do not participate in any activities that require full alertness if you are unsure about your ability to do so.

Your first dose of Parlodel may cause dizziness. If so, check with your doctor.

Possible food and drug interactions
when taking this medication
Combining alcohol with Parlodel can cause blurred vision, chest pain, pounding heartbeat, throbbing headache, confusion, and other problems. Do not drink alcoholic beverages while taking this medication.

Certain drugs used for psychotic conditions, including Thorazine and Haldol, inhibit the action of Parlodel. It is important that you consult your doctor before taking these drugs while on Parlodel therapy.

- *Other drugs that may interact with Parlodel include:*
  Blood pressure-lowering drugs such as Aldomet and Catapres
  Metoclopramide (Reglan)
  Oral contraceptives
  Other ergot derivatives such as Hydergine
  Pimozide (Orap)

Special information
if you are pregnant or breastfeeding
The use of Parlodel during pregnancy should be discussed thoroughly with your doctor. If Parlodel is essential to your treatment, your doctor will carefully monitor you throughout your pregnancy.

You should not take Parlodel while breastfeeding.

Recommended dosage

ADULTS

Parlodel is available as 2.5-milligram tablets and 5-milligram capsules. Dosage information given is for 2.5-milligram tablets.

Excess Prolactin Hormone
If you are being treated for conditions associated with excess prolactin, such as menstrual problems, with or without excessive milk production, infertility, or pituitary gland tumors, the usual starting dose is one-half to 1 tablet daily. Your doctor may add a tablet every 3 to 7 days, until the treatment works. The usual longer term dose is 5 to 7.5 milligrams per day and ranges from 2.5 to 15 milligrams per day.

Growth Hormone Overproduction

Treatment for the overproduction of growth hormones is usually one-half to 1 tablet with food at bedtime for 3 days. Your doctor may add one-half to 1 tablet every 3 to 7 days. The usual treatment dose varies from 20 to 30 milligrams per day. The dose should not exceed 100 milligrams per day. Your doctor will do a monthly re-evaluation.

Parkinson's Disease

Parlodel taken in combination with levodopa may provide additional treatment benefits if you are currently taking high doses of levodopa, are beginning to develop a tolerance to levodopa, or are experiencing "end of dose failure" on levodopa therapy.

The usual starting dose of Parlodel is one-half tablet twice a day with meals. Your dose will be monitored by your doctor at 2-week intervals. If necessary, your doctor may increase the dose every 14 to 28 days by 1 tablet per day.

CHILDREN

The safety and effectiveness of Parlodel have not been established in children.

Overdosage

Any medication taken in excess can have serious consequences. If you suspect an overdose of Parlodel, contact your doctor immediately or seek other medical attention.

■ *Symptoms of Parlodel overdose may include:*
  Confusion, constipation, delusions, dizziness, drowsiness, feeling unwell, hallucinations, lethargy, nausea, pallor, severely low blood pressure, sweating, vomiting, yawning repeatedly

Generic name:

PAROXETINE

See Paxil, below.

Brand name:

PAXIL

Pronounced: PACKS-ill
Generic name: Paroxetine hydrochloride

Why is this drug prescribed?

Paxil is prescribed for a serious, continuing depression that interferes with your ability to function. Symptoms of this type of depression often include changes in appetite and sleep patterns, a persistent low mood, loss of interest in people and activities, decreased sex drive, feelings of guilt or worthlessness, suicidal thoughts, difficulty concentrating, and slowed thinking.

Paxil is also used to treat obsessive-compulsive disorder (OCD), a disease marked by unwanted, but stubbornly persistent thoughts, or unreasonable rituals you feel compelled to repeat. In addition, Paxil is described for panic disorder, a crippling emotional problem characterized by sudden attacks of at least four of the following symptoms: palpitations, sweating, shaking, numbness, chills or hot flashes, shortness of breath, a feeling of choking, chest pain, nausea or abdominal distress, dizziness or faintness, feelings of unreality or detachment, fear of losing control, or fear of dying.

Most important fact about this drug

Your depression may seem to improve within 1 to 4 weeks after beginning treatment with Paxil. Even if you feel better, continue to take the medication as long as your doctor tells you to do so.

How should you take this medication?

Paxil is taken once a day, usually in the morning. Inform your doctor if you are taking or plan to take any prescription or over-the-counter drugs, since they may interact unfavorably with Paxil.

Shake the oral suspension well before using.

- *If you miss a dose...*
  Skip the forgotten dose and go back to your regular schedule with the next dose. Do not take a double dose to make up for the one you missed.

- *Storage instructions...*
  Paxil tablets and suspension can be stored at room temperature.

What side effects may occur?

Side effects cannot be anticipated. If any develop or change in intensity, inform your doctor as soon as possible. Only your doctor can determine whether it is safe for you to continue taking this medication.

Over a 4 to 6 week period, you may find some side effects less troublesome (nausea and dizziness, for example) than others (dry mouth, drowsiness, and weakness).

■ *More common side effects may include:*
Constipation, decreased appetite, diarrhea, dizziness, drowsiness, dry mouth, gas, male genital disorders, nausea, nervousness, sleeplessness, sweating, tremor, weakness

■ *Less common side effects may include:*
Agitation, altered taste sensation, blurred vision, burning or tingling sensation, decreased sex drive, drugged feeling, increased appetite, muscle tenderness or weakness, pounding heartbeat, rash, tightness in throat, twitching, upset stomach, urinary disorders, vomiting, yawning

Why should this drug not be prescribed?
Do not take Paxil if you are also taking an MAO inhibitor antidepressant or within 14 days after you discontinue treatment with this type of medication.

Special warnings about this medication
Paxil should be used cautiously by people with a history of manic disorders.

If you have a history of seizures, make sure your doctor knows about it. Paxil should be used with caution in this situation. If you develop seizures once therapy has begun, the drug should be discontinued.

If you have a disease or condition that affects your metabolism or blood circulation, make sure your doctor is aware of it. Paxil should be used cautiously in this situation.

Paxil may impair your judgment, thinking, or motor skills. Do not drive, operate dangerous machinery, or participate in any hazardous activity that requires full mental alertness until you are sure the medication is not affecting you in this way.

Possible food and drug interactions
when taking this medication
Do not drink alcohol during your treatment with Paxil.

If Paxil is taken with certain other drugs, the effects of either could be increased, decreased, or altered. It is especially important to check with your doctor before combining Paxil with any of the following:

Antidepressants such as Elavil, Tofranil, Norpramin, Pamelor, Prozac, Nardil, and Parnate
Cimetidine (Tagamet)
Diazepam (Valium)
Digoxin (Lanoxin)
Flecainide (Tambocor)

Lithium (Lithonate)
Phenobarbital
Phenytoin (Dilantin)
Procyclidine (Kemadrin)
Propafenone (Rythmol)
Propranolol (Inderal, Inderide)
Quinidine (Quinaglute)
Sumatriptan (Imitrex)
Thioridazine (Mellaril)
Tryptophan
Warfarin (Coumadin)

Special information
if you are pregnant or breastfeeding

The effects of Paxil during pregnancy have not been adequately studied. If you are pregnant or plan to become pregnant, inform your doctor immediately. Paxil appears in breast milk and could affect a nursing infant. If this medication is essential to your health, your doctor may advise you to discontinue breastfeeding until your treatment with Paxil is finished.

Recommended dosage

DEPRESSION

The usual starting dose is 20 milligrams a day, taken as a single dose, usually in the morning. At intervals of at least 1 week, your physician may increase your dosage by 10 milligrams a day, up to a maximum of 50 milligrams a day.

OBSESSIVE-COMPULSIVE DISORDER

The usual starting dose is 20 milligrams a day, typically taken in the morning. At intervals of at least 1 week, your doctor may increase the dosage by 10 milligrams a day. The recommended long-term dosage is 40 milligrams daily. The maximum is 60 milligrams a day.

PANIC DISORDER

The usual starting dose is 10 milligrams a day, taken in the morning. At intervals of 1 week or more, the doctor may increase the dose by 10 milligrams a day. The target dose is 40 milligrams daily; dosage should never exceed 60 milligrams.

For older adults, the weak, and those with severe kidney or liver disease, starting doses are reduced to 10 milligrams daily, and later doses are limited to no more than 40 milligrams a day. Safety and effectiveness in children have not been established.

Overdosage

Any medication taken in excess can have serious consequences. If you suspect an overdose, seek medical attention immediately.

■ *The symptoms of Paxil overdose may include:*
Dizziness, drowsiness, facial flushing, nausea, sweating, vomiting

Brand name:

PCE

See Erythromycin, Oral, page 482.

Brand name:

PEDIAPRED

Pronounced: PEE-dee-uh-pred
Generic name: Prednisolone sodium phosphate

Why is this drug prescribed?

Pediapred, a steroid drug, is used to reduce inflammation and improve symptoms in a variety of disorders, including rheumatoid arthritis, acute gouty arthritis, and severe cases of asthma. It may be given to people to treat primary or secondary adrenal cortex insufficiency (lack of or insufficient adrenal cortical hormone in the body). It is also given to help treat the following disorders:

Blood disorders such as leukemia and various anemias
Certain cancers (along with other drugs)
Connective tissue diseases such as systemic lupus erythematosus
Digestive tract diseases such as ulcerative colitis
Eye diseases of various kinds
Fluid retention due to nephrotic syndrome (a condition in which damage
    to the kidneys causes a loss of protein in the urine)
High blood levels of calcium associated with cancer
Lung diseases such as tuberculosis
Severe allergic conditions such as drug-induced allergic reactions
Skin diseases such as severe psoriasis

Studies have shown that high doses of Pediapred are effective in controlling severe symptoms of multiple sclerosis, although they do not affect the ultimate outcome or natural history of the disease.

Most important fact about this drug
Pediapred decreases your resistance to infection. It may also mask some of the signs and symptoms of an infection, which makes it difficult for a doctor to diagnose the actual problem.

How should you take this medication?
Pediapred may cause stomach upset and should be taken with food. Take this medication exactly as prescribed.

■ *If you miss a dose...*
Take it as soon as you remember. If it is almost time for your next dose, skip the one you missed and go back to your regular schedule. Never take 2 doses at the same time.

■ *Storage instructions...*
Store Pediapred in a cool place, and keep the bottle tightly closed. This medication may be refrigerated.

What side effects may occur?
Side effects cannot be anticipated. If any develop or change in intensity, inform your doctor as soon as possible. Only your doctor can determine if it is safe for you to continue taking Pediapred.

■ *Side effects may include:*
Abnormal loss of bony tissue causing fragile bones, abnormal redness of the face, backbone break that collapses the spinal column, bruising, cataracts, convulsions, dizziness, fluid retention (edema), fracture of long bones, glaucoma (increased eye pressure), headache, high blood pressure, increased sweating, loss of muscle mass, menstrual irregularities, mental capacity changes, muscle disease, muscle weakness, peptic ulcer (stomach ulcer with possible bleeding), protrusion of eyeball, salt retention, slow growth in children, slow wound healing, sugar diabetes, swelling of the abdomen, thinning of the skin, vertigo

Why should this drug not be prescribed?
This drug should not be used for fungal infections within the body.

Special warnings about this medication
You should not be vaccinated against smallpox while being treated with Pediapred. Avoid other immunizations as well, especially if you are taking

Pediapred in high doses, because of the possible hazards of nervous system complications and a lack of natural immune response.

Because Pediapred reduces resistance to infection, people who have never had measles or chickenpox—or been vaccinated against them—should be careful to avoid exposure. These diseases can be severe, or even fatal, in people with lowered resistance.

Likewise, an ordinary case of threadworm can grow into a grave emergency when the immune system is weak. Symptoms of threadworm include stomach pain, vomiting, and diarrhea. If you suspect an infection, call your doctor immediately.

If you are taking Pediapred and are subjected to unusual stress, notify your doctor. The drug reduces the function of your adrenal glands, and they may be unable to cope. Your doctor may therefore increase your dosage of this rapidly acting steroid before, during, and after the stressful situation.

Prolonged use of steroids may produce posterior subcapsular cataracts (a disorder under the envelope-like structure at the back of the eye that causes the lens to become less transparent) or the eye disease glaucoma, and may intensify additional eye infections due to fungi or viruses.

Average and high doses of this medication may cause an increase in blood pressure, salt and water retention, and an increased loss of potassium. Your doctor may have you decrease your salt intake and increase your potassium intake.

The effects of Pediapred may be intensified if you have an underactive thyroid or long-term liver disease.

If you have ocular herpes simplex (painful blisters of the eye), you should be careful using this drug because of the possibility of corneal perforation (puncture of the outer, transparent part of the eye).

The use of Pediapred may cause mood swings, feelings of elation, insomnia, personality changes, severe depression, or even severe mental disorders.

If you are being treated for a blood clotting factor deficiency, use aspirin with caution when taking Pediapred. Do not use this drug for any disorder other than that for which it was prescribed.

Your doctor will prescribe this medication very cautiously if you have ulcerative colitis (inflammation of the colon and rectum) where there is a possibility of a puncture, abscess, or other infection; diverticulitis (inflammation of a sac formed at weak points of the colon); recent intestinal anastomoses (a surgical connection between two separate parts of the colon); active or inactive peptic (stomach) ulcers; unsatisfactory kidney function; high blood pressure; osteoporosis (brittle bones that may fracture); and myasthenia gravis (a long-term disease characterized by abnormal fatigue and weakness of certain muscles).

Do not discontinue the use of Pediapred abruptly or without medical supervision.

If you should develop a fever or other signs of infection while taking Pediapred, notify your doctor immediately.

Possible food and drug interactions
when taking this medication

If Pediapred is taken with certain other drugs, the effects of either could be increased, decreased, or altered. It is especially important to check with your doctor before combining Pediapred with the following:

Amphotericin B
Aspirin
Barbiturates such as phenobarbital and Seconal
Carbamazepine (Tegretol)
Cyclosporine (Sandimmune and Neoral)
Diabetes drugs such as Glucotrol
Estrogens such as Premarin
Isoniazid (Nydrazid)
Ketoconazole (Nizoral)
Nonsteroidal anti-inflammatory drugs such as Motrin
Oral contraceptives
Phenytoin (Dilantin)
Rifampin (Rifadin)
Water pills such as Lasix

Special information
if you are pregnant or breastfeeding

The effects of Pediapred during pregnancy have not been adequately studied. If you are pregnant or plan to become pregnant, inform your doctor immediately. This medication may appear in breast milk and could affect a nursing infant. If this drug is essential to your health, your doctor may advise you to discontinue breastfeeding until your treatment is finished.

Recommended dosage

The starting dosage of Pediapred may vary from 5 milliliters to 60 milliliters, depending on the specific disease being treated.

Your doctor will adjust the dose until the results are satisfactory. If your condition does not improve after a reasonable period of time, the doctor may switch you to another medication.

Once you've shown a favorable response, your doctor will gradually decrease the dosage to the minimum that maintains the effect.

If you stop taking Pediapred after long-term therapy, your doctor will have you withdraw slowly, rather than abruptly.

For acute flare-ups of multiple sclerosis (MS), the usual dose is 200 milligrams per day of Pediapred for one week followed by 80 milligrams every other day or 4 to 8 milligrams of dexamethasone every other day for 1 month.

Overdosage
Although no specific information is available, any medication taken in excess can have serious consequences. If you suspect an overdose of Pediapred, seek medical treatment immediately.

Brand name:

PEDIAZOLE

Pronounced: PEE-dee-uh-zole
Generic ingredients: Erythromycin ethylsuccinate, Sulfisoxazole acetyl
Other brand name: Eryzole

Why is this drug prescribed?
Pediazole is prescribed for the treatment of severe middle ear infections in children.

Most important fact about this drug
Sulfisoxazole is one of a group of drugs called sulfonamides, which prevent the growth of certain bacteria in the body. However, sulfonamides have been known to cause rare but sometimes fatal reactions such as Stevens-Johnson syndrome (a skin condition characterized by severe blisters and bleeding in the mucous membranes of the lips, mouth, nose, and eyes), sudden and severe liver damage, a severe blood disorder (agranulocytosis), and a lack of red and white blood cells because of a bone marrow disorder.

Notify your doctor at the first sign of a side effect such as skin rash, sore throat, fever, abnormal skin paleness, reddish or purplish skin spots, or yellowing of the skin or whites of the eyes.

How should you take this medication?

Be sure to keep giving Pediazole for the full time prescribed, even if your child begins to feel better after the first few days. Keep to a regular schedule; the medication works best when there is a constant amount in the blood.

Pediazole can be given with or without food. However, you should not give this medication with or immediately after carbonated beverages, fruit juice, or tea. If the child develops an upset stomach, give the medicine with crackers or a light snack.

To prevent sediment in the urine and the formation of stones, make sure that the child drinks plenty of fluids during treatment with Pediazole.

This medication increases the skin's sensitivity to sunlight. Overexposure can cause a rash, itching, redness, or sunburn. Keep the child out of direct sunlight, or provide protective clothing.

Shake well before using.

■ *If you miss a dose...*
Give the forgotten dose as soon as you remember, then give the rest of the day's doses at evenly spaced intervals.

■ *Storage instructions...*
Store Pediazole in the refrigerator. Keep tightly closed. Do not allow it to freeze. Use within 14 days; discard unused portion.

What side effects may occur?

Side effects cannot be anticipated. If any develop or change in intensity, inform your doctor as soon as possible. Only your doctor can determine if it is safe to continue giving Pediazole.

■ *More common side effects may include:*
Abdominal pain and discomfort, diarrhea, lack or loss of appetite, nausea, vomiting

■ *Less common or rare side effects may include:*
Anxiety, blood disorders, blood or stone formation in the urine, bluish discoloration of skin, chills, colitis, convulsions, cough, dark, tarry stools, depression, difficulty in urinating or inability to urinate, disorientation, dizziness, drowsiness, exhaustion, fainting, fatigue, fluid retention, flushing, fever, gas, hallucinations, headache, hepatitis, hives, inability to fall or stay asleep (insomnia), increased urine, inflammation of the mouth, irregular heartbeat, itching, lack of muscle coordination, low blood sugar,

palpitations, rapid heartbeat, redness and swelling of the tongue, ringing in the ears, scaling of dead skin due to inflammation, sensitivity to light, severe allergic reactions, severe skin welts or swelling, shortness of breath, skin eruptions, skin rash, Stevens-Johnson syndrome, stomach or intestinal bleeding, swelling around the eye, temporary hearing loss, tingling or pins and needles, vertigo, weakness, yellow eyes and skin

Why should this drug not be prescribed?

If your child is sensitive to or has ever had an allergic reaction to erythromycin, sulfonamides, or other drugs of this type, do not use this medication. Make sure that your doctor is aware of any drug reactions that your child has experienced.

Pediazole should not be used if the child is taking Seldane or Hismanal.

This medication should not be prescribed for infants under 2 months of age.

Pediazole should not be taken by pregnant women at the end of their pregnancy or by mothers nursing infants under 2 months of age.

Special warnings about this medication

If your child has impaired kidney or liver function or a history of severe allergies or bronchial asthma, Pediazole may not be the best drug to use. Check with your doctor.

Prolonged or repeated use of Pediazole may cause new infections. If your child develops a new infection (called a superinfection), talk to your doctor. A different antibiotic may be needed.

If your child develops a cough or becomes short of breath, call your doctor. Also seek care immediately if the child develops diarrhea; it could signal a serious intestinal disorder.

If your child has the muscle-weakening disorder myasthenia gravis, Pediazole could make the condition worse.

Your doctor may recommend frequent urine tests while your child is taking Pediazole.

Possible food and drug interactions when taking this medication

If Pediazole is taken with certain other drugs, the effects of either could be increased, decreased, or altered. It is especially important to check with your doctor before combining Pediazole with the following:

Astemizole (Hismanal)
Blood thinners such as warfarin (Coumadin)

Bromocriptine (Parlodel)
Carbamazepine (Tegretol)
Cyclosporine (Sandimmune)
Digoxin (Lanoxin)
Disopyramide (Norpace)
Ergotamine (Cafergot, Ergostat)
Lovastatin (Mevacor)
Methotrexate (Rheumatrex)
Oral antidiabetic drugs such as Micronase
Phenytoin (Dilantin)
Terfenadine (Seldane)
Theophylline (Theo-Dur)
Triazolam (Halcion)

Special information
if you are pregnant or breastfeeding

This drug is not prescribed for adults, and should never be taken at term of
pregnancy or when breastfeeding.

Recommended dosage

CHILDREN

The recommended dose for children 2 months of age or older is determined
by weight. The total daily amount is divided into several smaller doses given
3 or 4 times a day for 10 days.

Four-times-a-day schedule
   Less than 18 pounds: Determined by doctor
   18 pounds: ½ teaspoonful
   35 pounds: 1 teaspoonful
   53 pounds: 1½ teaspoonfuls
   Over 70 pounds: 2 teaspoonfuls

Three-times-a-day schedule
   Less than 13 pounds: Determined by doctor
   13 pounds: ½ teaspoonful
   26 pounds: 1 teaspoonful
   40 pounds: 1½ teaspoonfuls
   53 pounds: 2 teaspoonfuls
   Over 66 pounds: 2½ teaspoonfuls

Overdosage

Any medication taken in excess can have serious consequences. If you suspect an overdose, seek medical treatment immediately.

■ *Symptoms of Pediazole overdose may include:*
Blood in the urine, colic, dizziness, drowsiness, fever, headache, loss of appetite, nausea, unconsciousness, vomiting, yellowed eyes and skin

Generic name:

PEMOLINE

See Cylert, page 320.

Generic name:

PENCICLOVIR

See Denavir, page 365.

Brand name:

PENETREX

Pronounced: PEN-eh-trecks
Generic name: Enoxacin

Why is this drug prescribed?

Penetrex is used to treat urinary tract infections, including cystitis (inflammation of the inner lining of the bladder caused by bacterial infection), and certain sexually transmitted diseases such as gonorrhea. It is a quinolone antibiotic.

Most important fact about this drug

Penetrex, like other antibiotics, works best when there is a constant amount in the blood and urine. To help keep the level constant try not to miss any doses, and take them at evenly spaced intervals around the clock.

How should you take this medication?

Penetrex should be taken with a full glass of water, either 1 hour before or 2 hours after a meal. Do not take more than the prescribed dosage. Use up all the medicine. If you stop taking Penetrex too soon, your symptoms may return.

Be sure to drink plenty of fluids while taking Penetrex.

- *If you miss a dose...*
  Take it as soon as you remember. If it is almost time for your next dose, skip the one you missed and go back to your regular schedule. Do not take 2 doses at the same time.

- *Storage instructions...*
  Store at room temperature.

What side effects may occur?
Side effects cannot be anticipated. If any develop or change in intensity, tell your doctor as soon as possible. Only your doctor can determine whether it is safe for you to continue taking this medication.

- *More common side effects may include:*
  Nausea, vomiting

- *Less common or rare side effects may include:*
  Abdominal pain, agitation, back pain, bloody stools, chest pain, chills, confusion, constipation, convulsions, cough, depression, diarrhea, difficult or labored breathing, dizziness, dry mouth and throat, emotional change-ability, excessive sweating, fainting, fatigue, fever, fluid retention and swelling, fungal infection, gas, general feeling of illness, hallucinations, headache, hives, inability to hold urine, indigestion, inflammation of the large intestine, inflammation of the mouth, inflammation of the stomach, inflammation of the vagina, inflamed eyes, joint pain, kidney failure, lack of coordination, loss of appetite, loss of feeling of identity, loss of memory, mental disorders, muscle pain, nosebleed, overactivity, pounding heart-beat, purple or red spots on the skin, rapid heartbeat, ringing in the ears, sensitivity to light, skin eruptions, skin peeling, sleepiness, tingling or pins and needles, tremor, twitching, vaginal yeast infection, vision distur-bances, weakness

Why should this drug not be prescribed?
You should not take Penetrex if you are sensitive to this medication or to other quinolone antibiotics such as Cipro and Floxin, or if you have ever had inflamed or torn tendons due to the use of such drugs.

Special warnings about this medication
Penetrex may cause convulsions. Use Penetrex cautiously if you have problems such as epilepsy, kidney disorder, severe hardening of the arteries in the brain, and other conditions that might lead to seizures, or if you are taking any drugs that could make you seizure-prone.

In rare cases, other drugs in this class have caused severe, even fatal reactions, sometimes after a single dose. These reactions may include confusion, convulsions, depression, difficulty breathing, hallucinations, hives, insomnia, itching, light-headedness, loss of consciousness, nervousness or anxiety, nightmares, paranoia, rash, restlessness or agitation, swelling in the face or throat, thoughts of suicide (rare), tingling, and tremors. If you develop any of these symptoms, you should immediately stop taking Penetrex and seek medical help.

If you have experienced diarrhea when taking other antibacterial medications or develop it after you start taking Penetrex, be sure to tell your doctor. Penetrex may cause an inflammation of the bowel, ranging from mild to life-threatening.

Tell your doctor if you experience pain, inflammation, or rupture of a tendon. If you do, stop taking the drug, stop any exercise, and rest until you have seen your doctor.

Penetrex may cause dizziness or light-headedness and could impair your ability to drive a car or operate potentially dangerous machinery. Do not participate in any activities that require full alertness if you are unsure about the drug's effect on you.

You should avoid excessive exposure to direct sunlight while taking Penetrex. Stop taking Penetrex immediately if you have a severe reaction to sunlight, such as a skin rash.

Possible food and drug interactions
when taking this medication

If Penetrex is taken with certain other drugs, the effects of either could be increased, decreased, or altered. It is especially important to check with your doctor before combining Penetrex with the following:

Antacids containing calcium, magnesium, or aluminum, such as Maalox and Tums
Bismuth subsalicylate (Pepto-Bismol)
Caffeine (including certain drugs, coffee, tea, chocolate, and some soft drinks)
Cyclosporine (Sandimmune)
Digoxin (Lanoxin)
Ranitidine (Zantac)
Sucralfate (Carafate)
Theophylline (Theo-Dur)
Vitamins or products containing iron or zinc
Warfarin (Coumadin)

Special information
if you are pregnant or breastfeeding
The effects of Penetrex during pregnancy have not been adequately studied. If you are pregnant or plan to become pregnant, notify your doctor. Penetrex may appear in breast milk and may affect a nursing infant. Your doctor may have you stop nursing while you are taking this medication.

Recommended dosage

ADULTS

Uncomplicated Urinary Tract Infections
The usual dose is 200 milligrams every 12 hours for 7 days.

Other Urinary Tract Infections
The usual dose is 400 milligrams every 12 hours for 14 days.

Sexually Transmitted Disease (Gonorrhea)
The usual dose is 400 milligrams taken in a single dose.

CHILDREN

Safety and efficacy of Penetrex have not been established for children under 18 years of age.

Overdosage
There is no information on overdosage with Penetrex. However, any medication taken in excess can have serious consequences. If you suspect a Penetrex overdose, seek medical help immediately.

Generic name:

PENICILLIN V POTASSIUM

Brand names: Beepen-VK, Pen-Vee K, V-cillin K, Veetids

Why is this drug prescribed?
Penicillin V potassium is used to treat infections, including:

Dental infection, infections in the heart, middle ear infections, rheumatic fever, scarlet fever, skin infections, upper and lower respiratory tract infections

Penicillin V works against only certain types of bacteria—it is ineffective against fungi, viruses, and parasites.

Most important fact about this drug
If you are allergic to either penicillin or cephalosporin antibiotics in any form, consult your doctor before taking penicillin V. There is a possibility that you are allergic to both types of medication; and if a reaction occurs, it could be extremely severe. If you take the drug and feel signs of a reaction, seek medical attention immediately.

How should you take this medication?
Penicillin V may be taken on a full or empty stomach, though it is better absorbed when the stomach is empty. Be sure to take it for the full time of treatment.

Doses of the oral solution of penicillin V should be measured with a calibrated measuring spoon. Shake the solution well before using.

■ *If you miss a dose...*
Take it as soon as you remember. If it is almost time for the next dose, and you take 2 doses a day, take the one you missed and the next dose 5 to 6 hours later. If you take 3 or more doses a day, take the one you missed and the next dose 2 to 4 hours later, or double the next dose. Then go back to your regular schedule.

■ *Storage instructions...*
Store in a tightly closed container. The reconstituted oral solution must be refrigerated; discard any unused solution after 14 days.

Tablets and powder for oral solution may be stored at room temperature.

What side effects may occur?
Side effects cannot be anticipated. If any develop or change in intensity, inform your doctor as soon as possible. Only your doctor can determine if it is safe for you to continue taking this medication.

■ *Side effects may include:*
Anemia, black, hairy tongue, diarrhea, fever, hives, nausea, skin eruptions, stomach upset or pain, swelling in throat, vomiting

Why should this drug not be prescribed?
You should not be using penicillin V if you have had an allergic reaction to penicillin or cephalosporin antibiotics.

Special warnings about this medication

If any allergic reactions occur, stop taking penicillin V and contact your doctor immediately.

If new infections (called superinfections) occur, consult your doctor.

If you have ever had allergic reactions such as rashes, hives, or hay fever, consult with your doctor before taking penicillin V.

Before taking penicillin V, tell your doctor if you have ever had asthma, colitis (inflammatory bowel disease), diabetes, or kidney or liver disease.

For infections such as strep throat, it is important to take penicillin V for the entire amount of time your doctor has prescribed. Even if you feel better, you need to continue taking this medication. If you stop taking this medication before your treatment time is complete, your infection may recur.

**Possible food and drug interactions
when taking this medication**

If penicillin V is taken with certain other drugs, the effects of either could be increased, decreased, or altered. It is especially important to check with your doctor before combining penicillin V with the following:

Chloramphenicol (Chloromycetin)
Oral contraceptives
Tetracyclines such as Achromycin V and Sumycin

**Special information
if you are pregnant or breastfeeding**

The effects of penicillin V in pregnancy have not been adequately studied. If you are pregnant or planning to become pregnant, inform your doctor immediately. Penicillin V should be used during pregnancy only if your doctor determines that the potential benefit justifies the potential risk to the fetus. Since penicillin V appears in breast milk, you should consult with your doctor if you plan to breastfeed your baby. If this medication is essential to your health, your doctor may advise you to discontinue breastfeeding until your treatment is finished.

Recommended dosage

ADULTS AND CHILDREN 12 YEARS OLD AND OVER

Continue taking penicillin V for the full time of treatment, even if you begin to feel better after a few days. Failure to take a full course of therapy may prevent complete elimination of the infection. It is best to take the doses at evenly spaced times, around the clock.

For Mild to Moderately Severe Strep Infections of the Upper Respiratory Tract and Skin, and Scarlet Fever
The usual dosage is 125 to 250 milligrams every 6 to 8 hours for 10 days.

For Mild to Moderately Severe Pneumococcal Infections of the Respiratory Tract, Including Middle Ear Infections
The usual dosage is 250 milligrams to 500 milligrams every 6 hours until you have been without a fever for at least 2 days.

For Mild Staph Infections of Skin
The usual dosage is 250 milligrams to 500 milligrams every 6 to 8 hours.

For Mild to Moderately Severe Gum Infections Known as Vincent's Gingivitis
The usual dosage is 250 milligrams to 500 milligrams every 6 to 8 hours.

To Prevent Recurring Rheumatic Fever and/or Chorea (Infective Disorder of the Nervous System)
The usual dosage is 125 milligrams to 250 milligrams 2 times a day on a continuing basis.

Prevention of Bacterial Endocarditis (Inflammation of the Heart Membrane) in People with Heart Disease Who Are Undergoing Dental or Surgical Procedures
For oral therapy, the usual dose is 2 grams of penicillin V ½ to 1 hour before the procedure, then 1 gram 6 hours later.

Overdosage
Any medication taken in excess can have serious consequences. If you suspect an overdose, seek medical attention immediately.

■ *Symptoms of penicillin V overdose may include:*
  Diarrhea, nausea, vomiting

Brand name:

PENTASA

See Rowasa, page 1152.

Generic name:

PENTAZOCINE WITH ASPIRIN

See Talwin Compound, page 1245.

Generic name:

PENTOXIFYLLINE

See Trental, page 1336.

Brand name:

PEN-VEE K

See Penicillin V Potassium, page 971.

Brand name:

PEPCID

Pronounced: PEP-sid
Generic name: Famotidine
Other brand name: Pepcid AC

Why is this drug prescribed?
Pepcid is prescribed for the short-term treatment of active duodenal ulcer (in the upper intestine) for 4 to 8 weeks and for active, benign gastric ulcer (in the stomach) for 6 to 8 weeks. It is prescribed for maintenance therapy, at reduced dosage, after a duodenal ulcer has healed. It is also used for short-term treatment of GERD, a condition in which the acid contents of the stomach flow back into the food canal (esophagus), and for resulting inflammation of the esophagus. And it is prescribed for certain diseases that cause the stomach to produce excessive quantities of acid, such as Zollinger-Ellison syndrome. Pepcid belongs to a class of drugs known as histamine H_2 blockers.

An over-the-counter formulation, Pepcid AC, is used to relieve and prevent heartburn, acid indigestion, and sour stomach.

Most important fact about this drug
To cure your ulcer, you need to take Pepcid for the full time of treatment your doctor prescribes. Keep taking the drug even if you begin to feel better.

How should you take this medication?

It may take several days for Pepcid to begin relieving stomach pain. You can use antacids for the pain at the same time you take Pepcid.

If you are taking Pepcid suspension, shake it vigorously for 5 to 10 seconds before use.

If you are taking Pepcid orally disintegrating tablets, leave each tablet in its unopened blister until just before use, then open the blister with dry hands and place the tablet on your tongue. The tablet will dissolve immediately and can be swallowed with saliva. No water is needed.

Take Pepcid AC with water. To prevent symptoms take it 1 hour before a meal you expect will cause trouble.

■ *If you miss a dose...*
Take it as soon as you remember. If it is almost time for your next dose, skip the one you missed and go back to your regular schedule. Do not take 2 doses at once.

■ *Storage instructions...*
Store at room temperature in a dry place. Protect the suspension from freezing, and discard any unused portion after 30 days.

What side effects may occur?

Side effects cannot be anticipated. If any develop or change in intensity, inform your doctor as soon as possible. Only your doctor can determine if it is safe for you to continue taking Pepcid.

The most common side effect is headache.

■ *Less common or rare side effects may include:*
Abdominal discomfort, acne, agitation, altered taste, anxiety, breast development in males, changes in behavior, confusion, constipation, decreased sex drive, depression, diarrhea, difficulty sleeping, dizziness, dry mouth, dry skin, facial swelling due to fluid retention, fatigue, fever, flushing, grand mal seizures, hair loss, hallucinations, hives, impotence, irregular heartbeat, itching, loss of appetite, muscle, bone, or joint pain, nausea, pounding heartbeat, prickling, tingling, or pins and needles, rash, ringing in ears, severe allergic reaction, sleepiness, vomiting, weakness, wheezing, yellow eyes and skin

Why should this drug not be prescribed?

If you are sensitive to or have ever had an allergic reaction to Pepcid, you should not take this medication. Make sure your doctor is aware of any drug reactions you have experienced.

Special warnings about this medication

If you have stomach cancer, Pepcid may relieve the symptoms without curing the disease. Your doctor will be careful to rule out this possibility.

Use Pepcid with caution if you have severe kidney disease.

Although heartburn and acid indigestion are common, see your doctor if you have trouble swallowing or abdominal pain that does not let up.

If you have a condition known as phenylkentonuria, be aware that Pepcid orally disintegrating tablets contain phenylalanine.

Do not take 2 tablets of Pepcid AC a day continuously for more than 2 weeks unless your doctor tells you to.

You can help avoid heartburn and acid indigestion by:

Not lying down soon after eating
Keeping your weight down
Stopping smoking, or at least cutting down
Avoiding or limiting caffeine, chocolate, fatty foods, and alcohol
Not eating just before bedtime

Possible food and drug interactions
when taking this medication

If Pepcid is taken with certain other drugs, the effects of either can be increased, decreased, or altered. It is especially important that you check with your doctor before combining Pepcid with the following:

Itraconazole (Sporanox)
Ketoconazole (Nizoral)

Special information
if you are pregnant or breastfeeding

The effects of Pepcid during pregnancy have not been adequately studied. If you are pregnant or plan to become pregnant, inform your doctor immediately. Pepcid may appear in breast milk and could affect a nursing infant. If this medication is essential to your health, your doctor may advise you to discontinue breastfeeding until your treatment with this medication is finished.

Recommended dosage

ADULTS

For Duodenal Ulcer

The usual starting dose is 40 milligrams or 5 milliliters (1 teaspoonful) once a day at bedtime. Results should be seen within 4 weeks, and this medication should not be used at full dosage longer than 6 to 8 weeks. Your doctor may have you take 20 milligrams or 2.5 milliliters (half a teaspoonful) twice a day. The normal maintenance dose after your ulcer has healed is 20 milligrams or 2.5 milliliters (half a teaspoonful) once a day at bedtime.

Benign Gastric Ulcer

The usual dose is 40 milligrams or 5 milliliters (1 teaspoonful) once a day at bedtime.

Gastroesophageal Reflux Disease (GERD)

The usual dose is 20 milligrams or 2.5 milliliters (1/2 teaspoonful) twice a day for up to 6 weeks. For inflammation of the esophagus due to GERD, the dose is 20 or 40 milligrams or 2.5 to 5 milliliters twice a day for up to 12 weeks.

Excess Acid Conditions (such as Zollinger-Ellison Syndrome)

The usual starting dose is 20 milligrams every 6 hours, although some people need a higher dose. Doses of up to 160 milligrams every 6 hours have been given in severe cases.

If your kidneys are not functioning properly, your doctor will adjust the dosage.

CHILDREN

Pepcid can be given to children 1 to 16 years old. Safety and effectiveness have not been established in infants of less than 1 year.

Peptic Ulcer

The usual dose is 0.5 milligrams per 2.2 pounds of body weight. The entire dose may be given at bedtime, or divided and given in 2 smaller doses. Do not give more than 40 milligrams per day.

Gastroesophageal Reflux Disease (GERD)

The usual daily dose is 1 milligram per 2.2 pounds of body weight, divided and given in 2 smaller doses. Do not exceed 40 milligrams daily.

PEPCID AC

Pepcid AC should not be given to children under age 12. Take no more than 2 tablets per day.

Relief
Swallow 1 tablet with water.

Prevention
Take 1 tablet 1 hour before a meal that could cause symptoms.

Overdosage
Any medication taken in excess can have serious consequences. If you suspect an overdose, seek medical attention immediately.

Brand name:

PERCOCET

Pronounced: PERK-o-set
Generic ingredients: Acetaminophen, Oxycodone hydrochloride
Other brand names: Roxicet, Tylox

Why is this drug prescribed?

Percocet, a narcotic analgesic, is used to treat moderate to moderately severe pain. It contains two drugs—acetaminophen and oxycodone. Acetaminophen is used to reduce both pain and fever. Oxycodone, a narcotic analgesic, is used for its calming effect and for pain.

Most important fact about this drug

Percocet contains a narcotic and, even if taken only in prescribed amounts, can cause physical and psychological dependence when taken for a long time.

How should you take this medication?

Percocet may be taken with meals or with milk.

▪ *If you miss a dose...*
If you take Percocet on a regular schedule, take it as soon as you remember. If it is almost time for the next dose, skip the one you missed and go back to your regular schedule. Never take 2 doses at once.

■ *Storage instructions...*
Store at room temperature.

What side effects may occur?
Side effects cannot be anticipated. If any develop or change in intensity, inform your doctor as soon as possible. Only your doctor can determine if it is safe for you to continue taking Percocet.

■ *More common side effects may include:*
Dizziness, light-headedness, nausea, sedation, vomiting

You may be able to alleviate some of these side effects by lying down.

■ *Less common or rare side effects may include:*
Constipation, depressed feeling, exaggerated feeling of well-being, itchy skin, skin rash, slowed breathing (at higher doses)

Why should this drug not be prescribed?
You should not use Percocet if you are sensitive to either acetaminophen or oxycodone.

Special warnings about this medication
You should take Percocet cautiously and according to your doctor's instructions, as you would take any medication containing a narcotic. If you have ever had a problem with alcohol addiction, make sure your doctor is aware of it.

If you have experienced a head injury, consult your doctor before taking Percocet. The effects of Percocet may be stronger for people with head injuries, and using it may delay recovery.

If you have stomach problems, such as an ulcer, check with your doctor before taking Percocet. Percocet may hide the symptoms of stomach problems, making them difficult to diagnose and treat.

If you have ever had liver, kidney, thyroid gland, or Addison's disease (a disease of the adrenal glands), difficulty urinating, or an enlarged prostate, consult your doctor before taking Percocet.

Elderly people or those in a weakened condition should take Percocet cautiously.

This drug may impair your ability to drive a car or operate potentially dangerous machinery. Do not participate in any activities that require full alertness if you are unsure about the drug's effect on you.

Possible food and drug interactions when taking this medication

Alcohol may increase the sedative effects of Percocet. You should not take Percocet with alcohol.

If Percocet is taken with certain other drugs, the effects of either could be increased, decreased, or altered. It is especially important to check with your doctor before combining Percocet with the following:

Antidepressants such as Elavil, Nardil, Pamelor, and Parnate
Antispasmodic drugs such as Cogentin, Bentyl, and Donnatal
Major tranquilizers such as Thorazine and Mellaril
Other narcotic painkillers such as Darvon and Demerol
Sedatives such as phenobarbital and Seconal
Tranquilizers such as Xanax and Valium

Special information if you are pregnant or breastfeeding

It is not known whether Percocet can injure a developing baby or affect a woman's reproductive capacity. Using any medication that contains a narcotic during pregnancy may cause physical addiction for your newborn baby. If you are pregnant or plan to become pregnant, inform your doctor immediately. As with other narcotic painkillers, taking Percocet shortly before delivery (especially at higher dosages) may cause some degree of impaired breathing in the mother and newborn. It is not known whether Percocet appears in breast milk, possibly harming a nursing infant. If you are breastfeeding use Percocet only under a doctor's directions.

Recommended dosage

ADULTS

The usual dose is 1 tablet every 6 hours as needed.

CHILDREN

The safety and effectiveness of Percocet have not been established in children.

Overdosage

A severe overdose of Percocet can be fatal. If you suspect an overdose, seek medical help immediately.

■ *Symptoms of Percocet overdose may include:*
Bluish skin, eyes or skin with yellow tone, cold and clammy skin, decreased or irregular breathing (ceasing in severe overdose), extreme

sleepiness progressing to stupor or coma, heart attack, low blood pressure, muscle weakness, nausea, slow heartbeat, sweating, vague bodily discomfort, vomiting

Brand name:

PERIACTIN

Pronounced: pair-ee-AK-tin
Generic name: Cyproheptadine hydrochloride

Why is this drug prescribed?
Periactin is an antihistamine given to help relieve cold- and allergy-related symptoms such as hay fever, nasal inflammation, stuffy nose, red and inflamed eyes, hives, and swelling. Periactin may also be given after epinephrine to help treat anaphylaxis, a life-threatening allergic reaction.

Some doctors prescribe Periactin to treat cluster headache and to stimulate appetite in underweight people.

Most important fact about this drug
Like other antihistamines, Periactin may make you feel sleepy and sluggish. However, some people, particularly children, may have the opposite reaction and become excited.

How should you take this medication?
Take Periactin exactly as prescribed by your doctor.

■ *If you miss a dose...*
Take it as soon as you remember. If it is almost time for your next dose, skip the one you missed and go back to your regular schedule. Do not take 2 doses at once.

■ *Storage instructions...*
Store at room temperature in a tightly closed container.

What side effects may occur?
Side effects cannot be anticipated. If any develop or change in intensity, tell your doctor immediately. Only your doctor can determine whether it is safe for you to continue taking Periactin.

■ *Side effects may include:*
Anaphylaxis (life-threatening allergic reaction), anemia, appetite loss, chest congestion or tightness, chills, confusion, constipation, convulsions,

diarrhea, difficulty urinating, dizziness, dry mouth, nose, or throat, earlier-than-expected menstrual period, exaggerated feeling of well-being, excessive perspiration, excitement, faintness, fatigue, fluttery or throbbing heartbeat, frequent urination, hallucinations, headache, hives, hysteria, inability to urinate, increased appetite and weight gain, insomnia, irritability, lack of coordination, light sensitivity, low blood pressure, nausea, nervousness, rapid heartbeat, rash and swelling, restlessness, ringing in the ears, sleepiness, stomach pain, stuffy nose, tingling or pins and needles, tremor, vertigo, vision problems (double vision, blurred vision), vomiting, weight gain, wheezing, yellow eyes and skin

Older people, in particular, are likely to become dizzy or drowsy, or develop low blood pressure in response to Periactin.

Why should this drug not be prescribed?
Do not take Periactin if you are sensitive to it, or have ever had an allergic reaction to it or to a similar antihistamine.

Do not take Periactin if you are taking an antidepressant drug known as an MAO inhibitor. Drugs in this category include Nardil and Parnate.

Do not take Periactin if you have the eye condition called angle-closure glaucoma, a peptic ulcer, an enlarged prostate, obstruction of the neck of the bladder, or obstruction of the outlet of the stomach.

Newborn or premature infants should not be given this drug, nor should it be used by women who are breastfeeding an infant.

The elderly and those in a weakened condition should not take this drug.

Special warnings about this medication
Like other antihistamines, Periactin may make you drowsy or impair your coordination. Be very careful about driving, climbing, or operating machinery, or doing hazardous tasks until you know how you react to this medication.

Be cautious about taking Periactin if you have bronchial asthma, the eye condition called glaucoma, an overactive thyroid gland, high blood pressure, heart disease, or circulatory problems.

Possible food and drug interactions
when taking this medication
Avoid alcoholic beverages while taking Periactin.

If Periactin is taken with certain other drugs, the effects of either could be increased, decreased, or altered. It is especially important to check with your doctor before combining Periactin with the following:

Antidepressant drugs classified as MAO inhibitors, including Nardil and
    Parnate
Sedatives such as Nembutal and Seconal
Tranquilizers such as Librium and Valium

Special information
if you are pregnant or breastfeeding

Because of possible harm to the unborn baby, Periactin should not be used
during pregnancy unless it is clearly needed. Periactin should not be taken by
a woman who is breastfeeding. If you have just given birth, you will need to
choose between breastfeeding and taking Periactin.

Recommended dosage

ADULTS

The usual initial dose is 4 milligrams (1 tablet or 2 teaspoonfuls) 3 times
daily. Dosage may range from 4 to 20 milligrams a day, but most people will
take between 12 and 16 milligrams. Some may need as much as 32
milligrams a day.

CHILDREN

Ages 2 to 6 Years
The usual dose is 2 milligrams (one-half tablet or 1 teaspoon) 2 or 3 times a
day; your doctor may adjust the dose if necessary. A child this age should
not take more than 12 milligrams a day.

Ages 7 to 14 Years
The usual dose is 4 milligrams (1 tablet or 2 teaspoons) 2 or 3 times a day;
your doctor may adjust the dose if needed. A child this age should not take
more than 16 milligrams a day.

Overdosage

Any drug taken in excess may have serious consequences. An overdose of
Periactin can be fatal. If you suspect an overdose, seek medical attention
immediately.

■ *Symptoms of Periactin overdose may include:*
  Dilated pupils, dry mouth, extreme excitement and agitation, fever,
  flushing, stomach or bowel distress, stupor or coma

Overdosage in children may produce hallucinations and convulsions.

Brand name:

PERIDEX

Pronounced: PAIR-i-decks
Generic name: Chlorhexidine gluconate

Why is this drug prescribed?
Peridex is an oral rinse used to treat gingivitis, a condition in which the gums become red and swollen. Peridex is also used to control gum bleeding caused by gingivitis.

Most important fact about this drug
Peridex may stain front-tooth fillings, especially those with a rough surface. These stains have no adverse effect on the gums, and usually can be removed by a professional cleaning.

How should you take this medication?
You should get a thorough dental cleaning and examination before beginning treatment with Peridex.

After brushing, thoroughly rinsing, and flossing your teeth, rinse with Peridex by swishing one-half fluid ounce (marked in the cap) around in your mouth for 30 seconds, then spit it out. Do not dilute Peridex and do not rinse with water or mouthwash, eat, brush your teeth, or drink immediately after using this medication.

■ *If you miss a dose...*
Resume your regular schedule the next time you brush.

■ *Storage instructions...*
Protect from freezing.

What side effects may occur?
Side effects cannot be anticipated. If any develop or change in intensity, inform your doctor as soon as possible. Only your doctor can determine if it is safe for you to continue using Peridex.

■ *More common side effects may include:*
Change in taste, increase in plaque, staining of teeth, mouth, tooth fillings, dentures, or other appliances in the mouth

■ *Less common or rare side effects may include:*
Allergic symptoms, coated tongue, inflamed gums, irritation of the mouth, redness, scaling of the lining of the mouth, ulcers in the mouth

Why should this drug not be prescribed?
Unless you are directed to do so by your doctor, do not use Peridex if you have shown a sensitivity to or are allergic to Peridex.

Special warnings about this medication
If you have both gingivitis and periodontitis (disease of the tissue that supports and attaches the teeth), remember that Peridex is used only for gingivitis. Periodontitis may require additional treatment by your doctor or dentist.

The use of Peridex may leave a bitter after-taste. Rinsing your mouth with or drinking water after using Peridex may increase the bitterness.

In addition to staining, Peridex can also cause an excess of tartar build-up on your teeth. It is recommended that you have your teeth cleaned at least every 6 months.

Foods may taste different to you for several hours after rinsing with Peridex. In most cases, this effect becomes less noticeable after continued use. Taste should return to normal when treatment with Peridex is finished.

Possible food and drug interactions
when taking this medication
No interactions with other drugs have been reported.

Special information
if you are pregnant or breastfeeding
The effects of Peridex during pregnancy have not been adequately studied. If you are pregnant or plan to become pregnant, inform your doctor immediately. It is not known whether this medication appears in breast milk. If it is essential for you to use Peridex, your doctor may advise you to stop breastfeeding until your treatment is finished.

Recommended dosage

ADULTS

The usual dose of undiluted Peridex is one-half fluid ounce. Rinse for 30 seconds twice a day, morning and evening, after brushing. Peridex should be spit out after rinsing and never swallowed.

CHILDREN

The effectiveness and safety of Peridex have not been established in children under 18 years of age.

Overdosage

If you suspect that a child of 22 pounds or less has swallowed 4 or more ounces of Peridex, seek medical attention immediately.

Also seek immediate medical attention if any child shows signs of alcohol intoxication such as slurred speech, staggering, or sleepiness, and you suspect he or she has swallowed Peridex.

If a small child swallows 1 or 2 ounces of Peridex, he or she may have an upset stomach and nausea.

Brand name:

PERSANTINE

Pronounced: per-SAN-teen
Generic name: Dipyridamole

Why is this drug prescribed?

Persantine helps reduce the formation of blood clots in people who have had heart valve surgery. It is used in combination with blood thinners such as Coumadin.

Some doctors also prescribe Persantine in combination with other drugs, such as aspirin, to reduce the damage from a heart attack and prevent a recurrence, to treat angina, and to prevent complications during heart bypass surgery.

Most important fact about this drug

Persantine is sometimes used with aspirin to provide better protection against the formation of blood clots. However, the risk of bleeding may also be increased. To reduce this risk, take *only* the amount of aspirin prescribed by the *same* doctor who directed you to take Persantine. If you need a medication for pain or a fever, do not take extra aspirin without first consulting your doctor.

How should you take this medication?

Persantine must be taken exactly as your doctor prescribes, at regularly scheduled times.

It is best to take Persantine on an empty stomach, with a full glass of water.

However, if this upsets your stomach, you can take the drug with food or milk.

Do not change from one brand of dipyridamole to another without consulting your doctor or pharmacist. Products manufactured by different companies may not be equally effective.

■ *If you miss a dose...*
Take it as soon as you remember. If it is within 4 hours of your next scheduled dose, skip the dose you missed and go back to your regular schedule. Never take 2 doses at the same time.

■ *Storage instructions...*
Store at room temperature. Protect from excessive heat.

What side effects may occur?
Side effects cannot be anticipated. If any develop or change in intensity, inform your doctor as soon as possible. Only your doctor can determine if it is safe for you to continue taking Persantine.

■ *More common side effects may include:*
Abdominal distress, dizziness

■ *Less common or rare side effects may include:*
Angina pectoris (crushing chest pain), diarrhea, feeling flushed, headache, itching, liver problems, skin rash, vomiting

Why should this drug not be prescribed?
There is no known reason to avoid this drug.

Special warnings about this medication
Use this medication carefully if you have low blood pressure.

Tell the doctor that you are taking Persantine if you have a medical emergency, and before you have surgery or dental treatment.

Possible food and drug interactions
when taking this medication
If Persantine is taken with certain other drugs, the effects of either could be increased, decreased, or altered. It is especially important to check with your doctor before combining Persantine with the following:

Aspirin
Blood thinners such as Coumadin

Indomethacin (Indocin)
Ticlopidine (Ticlid)
Valproic acid (Depakene)

Special information
if you are pregnant or breastfeeding

The effects of Persantine during pregnancy have not been adequately studied. If you are pregnant or plan to become pregnant, inform your doctor immediately. This drug appears in breast milk and may affect a nursing infant. If this medication is essential to your health, your doctor may advise you to discontinue breastfeeding until your treatment with this medication is finished.

Recommended dosage

ADULTS

The usual recommended dose is 75 milligrams to 100 milligrams, 4 times a day.

CHILDREN

The safety and effectiveness of this medication have not been established in children under 12 years of age.

Overdosage

Low blood pressure is the most common symptom of overdose and usually lasts for a short period of time. If this occurs, contact your doctor or emergency room immediately.

Brand name:

PHENAPHEN WITH CODEINE

See Tylenol with Codeine, page 1365.

Generic name:

PHENAZOPYRIDINE

See Pyridium, page 1088.

Generic name:

PHENELZINE

See Nardil, page 854.

Brand name:

PHENERGAN

Pronounced: FEN-er-gan
Generic name: Promethazine hydrochloride

Why is this drug prescribed?
Phenergan is an antihistamine that relieves nasal stuffiness and inflammation and red, inflamed eyes caused by hay fever and other allergies. It is also used to treat itching, swelling, and redness from hives and other rashes; allergic reactions to blood transfusions; and, with other medications, anaphylactic shock (severe allergic reaction).

Phenergan is also used as a sedative and sleep aid for both children and adults, and is prescribed to prevent and control nausea and vomiting before and after surgery and to prevent and treat motion sickness. It is also used, with other medications, for pain after surgery.

Antihistamines work by decreasing the effects of histamine, a chemical the body releases in response to certain irritants. Histamine narrows air passages in the lungs and contributes to inflammation. Antihistamines reduce itching and swelling and dry up secretions from the nose, eyes, and throat.

Most important fact about this drug
Phenergan may cause considerable drowsiness. You should not drive or operate dangerous machinery or participate in any hazardous activity that requires full mental alertness until you know how you react to Phenergan. Children should be carefully supervised while they are bike-riding, roller-skating, or playing until the drug's effect on them is established.

How should you take this medication?
Take Phenergan exactly as prescribed.

■ *If you miss a dose...*
  If you are taking Phenergan on a regular schedule, take the forgotten dose as soon as you remember. If it is almost time for your next dose, skip the

one you missed and go back to your regular schedule. Never take 2 doses at once.

■ *Storage instructions...*
Tablets should be stored at room temperature, away from light. Suppositories should be stored in the refrigerator, in a tightly closed container.

What side effects may occur?
Side effects cannot be anticipated. If any develop or change in intensity, inform your doctor as soon as possible. Only your doctor can determine if it is safe for you to continue taking Phenergan.

■ *More common side effects may include:*
Blurred vision, dizziness, dry mouth, increased/decreased blood pressure, nausea, rash, sedation (extreme calm), sleepiness, vomiting

■ *Rare side effects may include:*
Abnormal eye movements, blood disorders, confusion, disorientation, protruding tongue, sensitivity to light, stiff neck

Why should this drug not be prescribed?
Phenergan should not be used to treat asthma or other breathing difficulties or if you are sensitive to or have ever had an allergic reaction to it or to related medications, such as Thorazine, Mellaril, Stelazine, or Prolixin.

Special warnings about this medication
If you are taking other medications that cause sedation, your doctor may reduce the dosage of these medications or eliminate them while you are using Phenergan.

If you have a seizure disorder, Phenergan may cause your seizures to occur more often.

Avoid this medication if you have sleep apnea (periods during sleep when breathing stops).

Use Phenergan cautiously if you have heart disease, high blood pressure or circulatory problems, liver problems, the eye condition called narrow-angle glaucoma, peptic ulcer or other abdominal obstructions, or urinary bladder obstruction due to an enlarged prostate.

Phenergan may affect the results of pregnancy tests and can raise your blood sugar.

Some people have developed jaundice (yellow eyes and skin) while on this medication.

Tell your doctor if you have any uncontrolled movements or seem to be unusually sensitive to sunlight.

Remember that Phenergan can cause drowsiness.

Possible food and drug interactions
when taking this medication
Phenergan may increase the effects of alcohol. Do not drink alcohol, or at least substantially reduce the amount you drink, while taking this medication.

If Phenergan is taken with certain other drugs, the effects of either could be increased, decreased, or altered. It is especially important to check with your doctor before combining Phenergan with the following:

Certain antidepressant drugs, including Elavil and Tofranil
Narcotic pain relievers such as Demerol and Dilaudid
Sedatives such as Halcion, Dalmane, and Seconal
Tranquilizers such as Xanax and Valium

Special information
if you are pregnant or breastfeeding
The effects of Phenergan during pregnancy have not been adequately studied. If you are pregnant or plan to become pregnant, inform your doctor immediately. Phenergan may appear in breast milk and may affect a nursing infant. If this medication is essential to your health, your doctor may advise you to discontinue breastfeeding until your treatment is finished.

Recommended dosage
Phenergan is available in tablet, syrup, and suppository form. Phenergan tablets and suppositories are not recommended for children under 2 years of age.

ALLERGY

Adults
The average oral dose is 25 milligrams taken before bed; however, your doctor may have you take 12.5 milligrams before meals and before bed.

Children
The usual dose is a single 25-milligram dose at bedtime, or 6.25 to 12.5 milligrams 3 times daily.

MOTION SICKNESS

Adults

The average adult dose is 25 milligrams taken twice daily. The first dose should be taken one-half to 1 hour before you plan to travel, and the second dose 8 to 12 hours later, if necessary. On travel days after that, the recommended dose is 25 milligrams when you get up and again before the evening meal.

Children

The usual dose of Phenergan tablets, syrup, or rectal suppositories is 12.5 to 25 milligrams taken twice a day.

NAUSEA AND VOMITING

The average dose of Phenergan for nausea and vomiting in children or adults is 25 milligrams. When oral medication cannot be tolerated, use the rectal suppository. Your doctor may have you take 12.5 to 25 milligrams every 4 to 6 hours, if necessary.

For nausea and vomiting in children, the dose is usually calculated at 0.5 milligram per pound of body weight and will also be based on the age of the child and the severity of the condition being treated.

INSOMNIA

Adults

The usual dose is 25 to 50 milligrams for nighttime sedation.

Children

The usual dose is 12.5 to 25 milligrams by tablets or rectal suppository at bedtime.

Overdosage

Any medication taken in excess can have serious consequences. If you suspect an overdose, seek medical treatment immediately.

■ *Symptoms of Phenergan overdose may include:*
Difficulty breathing, dry mouth, fixed, dilated pupils, flushing, loss of consciousness, slowdown in brain activity, slowed heartbeat, stomach and intestinal problems, very low blood pressure

Children may become overstimulated and have nightmares; rarely, they may have convulsions. The elderly may also become overstimulated.

Brand name:

PHENERGAN WITH CODEINE

Pronounced: FEN-er-gan
*Generic ingredients: Promethazine hydrochloride, Codeine
    phosphate*

Why is this drug prescribed?

Phenergan with Codeine is used to relieve coughs and other symptoms of allergies and the common cold. Promethazine, an antihistamine, helps reduce itching and swelling and dries up secretions from the nose, eyes, and throat. It also has sedative effects and helps control nausea and vomiting. Codeine, a narcotic analgesic, helps relieve pain and stops coughing.

Most important fact about this drug

Phenergan with Codeine may cause considerable drowsiness. You should not drive or operate dangerous machinery or participate in any hazardous activity that requires full mental alertness until you know how you react to this medication. Children should be carefully supervised while they are bike-riding, roller-skating, or playing until the drug's effect on them is established.

How should you take this medication?

Take this medication exactly as prescribed.

- *If you miss a dose...*
  If you take Phenergan with Codeine on a regular schedule, take the forgotten dose as soon as you remember. If it is almost time for your next dose, skip the one you missed and go back to your regular schedule. Never take 2 doses at once.

- *Storage instructions...*
  Store at room temperature, away from light.

What side effects may occur?

Side effects cannot be anticipated. If any develop or change in intensity, inform your doctor as soon as possible. Only your doctor can determine if it is safe for you to continue taking Phenergan with Codeine.

- *Side effects may include:*
  Blurred vision, constipation, convulsions, decreased amount of urine, depressed feeling, difficulty breathing, disorientation, dizziness, dizziness on standing, dry mouth, exaggerated sense of well-being, fainting,

faintness, fast, fluttery heartbeat, feeling of anxiety, restlessness, flushing, headache, hives, inability to urinate, increased/decreased blood pressure, itching, light-headedness, nausea, passing hallucinations, rapid heartbeat, rash, sedation (extreme calm), sleepiness, slow heartbeat, sweating, swelling due to fluid retention (including the throat), vision changes, vomiting, weakness, yellowed skin or whites of eyes

■ *Side effects seen rarely include:*
Abnormal eye movements, blood disorders, confusion, protruding tongue, skin sensitivity to light, stiff neck

Why should this drug not be prescribed?
Phenergan with Codeine should not be used if you have asthma or other breathing difficulties or if you are sensitive to or have ever had an allergic reaction to codeine, promethazine, or related medications, such as Thorazine, Mellaril, Stelazine, or Prolixin.

Special warnings about this medication
It is possible to develop psychological and physical dependence on codeine. Although the likelihood of this is quite low with oral codeine, be cautious if you have a history of drug abuse or dependence.

Never take more cough syrup than has been prescribed. If your cough does not seem better within 5 days, check back with your doctor.

Codeine can cause or worsen constipation.

Phenergan with Codeine should be used with extreme caution in young children.

Use this medication very carefully if you have a head injury, the eye condition called narrow-angle glaucoma, peptic ulcer or other abdominal obstruction, urinary bladder obstruction due to an enlarged prostate, heart disease, high blood pressure or circulatory problems, liver or kidney disease, fever, seizures, an underactive thyroid gland, intestinal inflammation, or Addison's disease (a disorder of the adrenal glands). Be cautious, too, if you have had recent stomach/intestinal or urinary tract surgery. The very young, the elderly, and people in a weakened condition may have problems taking Phenergan with Codeine.

This medication may make you dizzy when you first stand up. Getting up slowly can help prevent this problem.

If you are taking other medications with sedative effects, your doctor may reduce their dosage or eliminate them altogether while you are using Phenergan with Codeine.

If you have a seizure disorder, this medication may cause your seizures to occur more often.

Avoid using Phenergan with Codeine if you have sleep apnea (periods during sleep when breathing stops).

Phenergan with Codeine may affect the results of pregnancy tests; and it can raise your blood sugar.

Tell your doctor if you have any involuntary muscle movements or seem to be unusually sensitive to sunlight.

Possible food and drug interactions when taking this medication

Phenergan with Codeine may increase the effects of alcohol. Do not drink alcohol, or at least substantially reduce the amount you drink, while taking this medication.

If Phenergan with Codeine is taken with certain other drugs, the effects of either could be increased, decreased, or altered. It is especially important to check with your doctor before combining Phenergan with Codeine with the following:

    All antidepressant drugs, including Marplan, Nardil, Elavil and Prozac
    Narcotic pain relievers such as Demerol and Dilaudid
    Sedatives such as Seconal, Halcion and Dalmane
    Tranquilizers such as Xanax and Valium

Special information if you are pregnant or breastfeeding

The effects of Phenergan with Codeine during pregnancy have not been adequately studied. If you are pregnant or plan to become pregnant, inform your doctor immediately. Phenergan with Codeine may appear in breast milk and may affect a nursing infant. If this medication is essential to your health, your doctor may advise you to discontinue breastfeeding until your treatment is finished.

Recommended dosage

ADULTS

The usual dosage is 1 teaspoon (5 milliliters) every 4 to 6 hours, not to exceed 6 teaspoons, or 30 milliliters, in 24 hours.

CHILDREN 6 YEARS TO UNDER 12 YEARS

The usual dose is one-half to 1 teaspoon (2.5 to 5 milliliters) every 4 to 6 hours, not to exceed 6 teaspoons, or 30 milliliters, in 24 hours.

CHILDREN UNDER 6 YEARS

The usual dose is one-quarter to one-half teaspoon (1.25 to 2.5 milliliters) every 4 to 6 hours. The total daily dose should not exceed 9 milliliters for children weighing 40 pounds, 8 milliliters for 35 pounds, 7 milliliters for 30 pounds, and 6 milliliters for 25 pounds.

Phenergan with Codeine is not recommended for children under 2 years of age.

Overdosage

Any medication taken in excess can have serious consequences. An overdose of codeine can be fatal. If you suspect an overdose, seek medical treatment immediately.

■ *Symptoms of an overdose of Phenergan with Codeine may include:*
Bluish skin, cold, clammy skin, coma, convulsions, difficulty breathing, dilated pupils, dry mouth, extreme sleepiness, flushing, low blood pressure, muscle softness, nightmares, overexcitability, slow heartbeat, small pupils, stomach and intestinal problems, stupor, unconsciousness

Generic name:

PHENOBARBITAL

Pronounced: fee-noe-BAR-bi-tal

Why is this drug prescribed?

Phenobarbital, a barbiturate, is used as a sleep aid and in the treatment of certain types of epilepsy, including generalized or grand mal seizures and partial seizures.

Most important fact about this drug

Phenobarbital can be habit-forming. You may become tolerant (needing more and more of the drug to achieve the same effect) and physically and psychologically dependent with continued use. Never increase the amount of phenobarbital you take without checking with your doctor.

How should you take this medication?
Take this medication exactly as prescribed.

If you are taking phenobarbital for seizures, do not discontinue it abruptly.

- *If you miss a dose...*
  Take it as soon as you remember. If it is almost time for your next dose, skip the one you missed and go back to your regular schedule. Never take 2 doses at once.

- *Storage instructions...*
  Store at room temperature in a tightly closed container.

What side effects may occur?
Side effects cannot be anticipated. If any develop or change in intensity, notify your doctor as soon as possible. Only your doctor can determine whether it is safe for you to continue taking phenobarbital.

- *Side effects may include:*
  Abnormal thinking, aggravation of existing emotional disturbances and phobias, agitation, anemia, angioedema (swelling of face around lips, tongue, and throat, swollen arms and legs, difficulty breathing), allergic reactions (localized swelling, especially of the eyelids, cheeks, or lips, skin redness and inflammation), anxiety, confusion, constipation, decreased breathing, delirium, difficulty sleeping, dizziness, drowsiness, excitement, fainting, fever, hallucinations, headache, increased physical activity and muscle movement, irritability and hyperactivity in children, lack of muscle coordination, low blood pressure, muscle, nerve, or joint pain, especially in people with insomnia, nausea, nervousness, nightmares, psychiatric disturbances, rash, residual drowsiness, restlessness, excitement, and delirium when taken for pain, shallow breathing, sleepiness, slow heartbeat, slowdown of the nervous system, sluggishness, softening of bones, temporary cessation of breathing, vertigo, vomiting

Why should this drug not be prescribed?
Phenobarbital should not be used if you suffer from porphyria (an inherited metabolic disorder), liver disease, or a lung disease that causes blockages or breathing difficulties, or if you have ever had an allergic reaction to or are sensitive to phenobarbital or other barbiturates.

Special warnings about this medication
Remember that phenobarbital may be habit-forming. Make sure you take the medication exactly as prescribed.

Phenobarbital should be used with extreme caution, or not at all, by people who are depressed, or have a history of drug abuse.

Be sure to tell your doctor if you are in pain, or if you have constant pain, before you take phenobarbital.

Phenobarbital may cause excitement, depression, or confusion in elderly or weakened individuals, and excitement in children.

If you have been diagnosed with liver disease or your adrenal glands are not functioning properly, make sure the doctor knows about it. Phenobarbital should be prescribed with caution.

Barbiturates such as phenobarbital may cause you to become tired or less alert. Be careful driving, operating machinery, or doing any activity that requires full mental alertness until you know how you react to this medication.

Possible food and drug interactions
when taking this medication
Phenobarbital may increase the effects of alcohol. Avoid alcoholic beverages while taking phenobarbital.

If phenobarbital is taken with certain other drugs, the effects of either could be increased, decreased, or altered. It is especially important to check with your doctor before combining phenobarbital with the following:

Antidepressant drugs known as MAO inhibitors, including Nardil and
    Parnate
Antihistamines such as Benadryl
Blood-thinning medications such as Coumadin
Doxycycline (Doryx, Vibramycin)
Griseofulvin (Fulvicin-P/G, Grifulvin V)
Narcotic pain relievers such as Percocet
Oral contraceptives
Other epilepsy drugs such as Dilantin, Depakene, and Depakote
Other sedatives such as Nembutal and Seconal
Steroids such as Medrol and Deltasone
Tranquilizers such as Xanax and Valium

Special information
if you are pregnant or breastfeeding
Barbiturates such as phenobarbital may cause damage to the developing baby during pregnancy. Withdrawal symptoms may occur in an infant whose mother took barbiturates during the last 3 months of pregnancy. If you are pregnant or plan to become pregnant, inform your doctor immediately.

Phenobarbital appears in breast milk and could affect a nursing infant. If phenobarbital is essential to your health, your doctor may advise you to stop breastfeeding until your treatment is finished.

Recommended dosage

ADULTS

Sedation
The usual initial dose of phenobarbital is a single dose of 30 to 120 milligrams. Your doctor may repeat this dose at intervals, depending on how you respond to this medication.

You should not take more than 400 milligrams during a 24-hour period.

Daytime Sedation
The usual dose is 30 to 120 milligrams a day, divided into 2 to 3 doses.

To Induce Sleep
The usual dose is 100 to 200 milligrams.

Anticonvulsant Use
Phenobarbital dosage must be individualized on the basis of specific laboratory tests. Your doctor will determine the exact dose best for you. The usual dose is 60 to 200 milligrams daily.

CHILDREN

Anticonvulsant Use
The phenobarbital dosage must be individualized on the basis of specific laboratory tests. Your doctor will determine the exact dose best for your child.

The usual dose is 3 to 6 milligrams per 2.2 pounds of body weight per day.

OLDER ADULTS

If you are old or debilitated, your dose may be lower than the regular adult dose. People who have liver or kidney disease may also require a lower dose of phenobarbital.

Overdosage

Barbiturate overdose can be fatal. If you suspect an overdose, seek medical treatment immediately.

■ *Symptoms of phenobarbital overdose may include:*
Congestive heart failure, diminished breathing, extremely low body temperature, fluid in lungs, involuntary eyeball movements, irregular heartbeat, kidney failure, lack of muscle coordination, low blood pressure, poor reflexes, skin reddening or bloody blisters, slowdown of the central nervous system

Generic name:

PHENOBARBITAL, HYOSCYAMINE, ATROPINE, AND SCOPOLAMINE

See Donnatal, page 431.

Generic name:

PHENTERMINE

See Fastin, page 506.

Generic name:

PHENYLEPHRINE, CHLORPHENIRAMINE, AND PYRILAMINE

See Rynatan, page 1158.

Generic name:

PHENYTOIN

See Dilantin, page 399.

Brand name:

PHOSPHOLINE IODIDE

Pronounced: FOS-foh-lin I-o-dide
Generic name: Echothiophate iodide

Why is this drug prescribed?

Phospholine Iodide is used to treat chronic open-angle glaucoma, a partial loss of vision or blindness resulting from a gradual increase in pressure of fluid in the eye. Because the vision loss occurs slowly, people often do not experience any symptoms and do not realize that their vision has declined. By the time the loss is noticed, it may be irreversible. Phospholine Iodide helps by reducing fluid pressure in the eye.

Phospholine Iodide is also used to treat secondary glaucoma (such as glaucoma following surgery to remove cataracts), for subacute or chronic angle-closure glaucoma after iridectomy (surgical removal of a portion of the iris) or when someone cannot have surgery or refuses it. The drug is also prescribed for children with accommodative esotropia ("cross-eye").

Most important fact about this drug
Avoid exposure to certain pesticides or insecticides such as Sevin and Trolene. They can boost the side effects of Phospholine Iodide. If you work with these chemicals, wear a mask over your nose and mouth, wash and change your clothing frequently, and wash your hands often.

How should you use this medication?

To use Phospholine Iodide:
1. To minimize drainage of Phospholine Iodide into your nose, your doctor may instruct you to apply pressure with the middle finger to the inside corner of the eye for 1 to 2 minutes after placing the drops in your eyes.
2. Wipe off any excess Phospholine Iodide around the eye with a tissue.
3. Wash off any Phospholine Iodide that may get onto your hands.

■ *If you miss a dose...*
If you use 1 dose every other day: Apply the dose you missed as soon as you remember, if it is still the scheduled day. If you do not remember until the next day, apply it as soon as you remember, then skip a day and start your schedule again.

If you use 1 dose a day: Apply the dose you missed as soon as you remember. If you do not remember until the next day, skip the dose you missed and go back to your regular schedule.

If you use 2 doses a day: Apply the dose you missed as soon as you remember. If it is almost time for your next dose, skip the one you missed and go back to your regular schedule.

Never apply 2 doses at once.

■ *Storage instructions...*
You may keep the eye drops at room temperature for up to 4 weeks.

What side effects may occur?
Side effects cannot be anticipated. If any develop or change in intensity, tell your doctor immediately. Only your doctor can determine whether it is safe to continue taking Phospholine Iodide.

■ *Side effects may include:*
Ache above the eyes, blurred vision, burning, clouded eye lens, cyst formation, decreased pupil size, decreased visual sharpness, excess tears, eye pain, heart irregularities, increased eye pressure, inflamed iris, lid muscle twitching, nearsightedness, red eyes, stinging

Why should this drug not be prescribed?
You should not use Phospholine Iodide if you have an inflammation in the eye.

Most people with angle-closure glaucoma (a condition in which there is a sudden increase in pressure of fluid in the eye) should not use Phospholine Iodide.

If you have ever had an allergic reaction to or are sensitive to Phospholine Iodide or any of its ingredients, you should not use this medication.

Special warnings about this medication
Drugs such as Phospholine Iodide should be used cautiously (if at all) if you have or have ever had:

Bronchial asthma
Detached retina
Epilepsy
Extreme low blood pressure
Parkinson's disease
Peptic ulcer
Recent heart attack
Slow heartbeat
Stomach or intestinal problems

If you notice any problems with your heart, notify your doctor immediately.

Stop taking the drug and notify your doctor immediately if you experience any of the following: breathing difficulties, diarrhea, inability to hold urine, muscle weakness, profuse sweating, or salivation.

If you will be using Phospholine Iodide for a long time, your doctor should schedule regular examinations to make sure that Phospholine Iodide is not causing unwanted effects.

Phospholine Iodide may cause vision problems. Be careful when driving at night or performing tasks in dim or poor light.

Possible food and drug interactions when taking this medication

If Phospholine Iodide is taken with certain other drugs, the effects of either could be increased, decreased, or altered. It is especially important to check with your doctor before combining this medication with drugs such as Enlon, Mestinon, or Tensilon, used to treat myasthenia gravis, a condition of muscle weakness that usually affects muscles in the eyes, face, limbs, and throat.

Special information if you are pregnant or breastfeeding

If you are pregnant or plan to become pregnant, inform your doctor immediately. No information is available about the safety of Phospholine Iodide during pregnancy.

Phospholine Iodide should not be used by women who are breastfeeding.

Recommended dosage

ADULTS

For Glaucoma

A dose of 0.03 percent should be used 2 times a day, in the morning and at bedtime. Your doctor may increase the dose if necessary. Your doctor may have you take 1 dose a day or 1 dose every other day, instead.

CHILDREN

For Accommodative Esotropia

Place 1 drop of 0.125 percent solution in both eyes at bedtime for 2 or 3 weeks to diagnose the condition.

Your doctor may then change the schedule to 0.125 percent every other day or reduce the dose to 0.06 percent every day.

The maximum dose usually recommended is 0.125 percent solution once daily.

If the eye drops are slowly withdrawn after a year or two of treatment, and the eye problem returns, your doctor may want you to consider surgery.

Overdosage

Any medication used in excess can have serious consequences. If you suspect an overdose of Phospholine Iodide, seek medical help immediately.

Brand name:

PILOCAR

Pronounced: PYE-low-car
Generic name: Pilocarpine hydrochloride
Other brand names: Isopto Carpine, Pilopine HS Gel

Why is this drug prescribed?

Pilocar causes constriction of the pupils (miosis) and reduces pressure within the eye. It is used to treat the increased pressure of open-angle glaucoma and to lower eye pressure before surgery for acute angle-closure glaucoma. It can be used alone or in combination with other medications. Glaucoma, one of the leading causes of blindness in the United States, is characterized by increased pressure in the eye that can damage the optic nerve and cause loss of vision.

Most important fact about this drug

There is no cure for glaucoma. Pilocar and similar drugs can keep ocular pressure under control, but only as long as you take them. You will probably need to continue treatment for life; and you must be sure to take the medication regularly.

How should you use this medication?

Follow these steps to administer Pilocar:

1. Wash your hands thoroughly.
2. Gently pull your lower eyelid down to form a pocket next to your eye.
3. Brace the eyedrop bottle on the bridge of your nose or your forehead.
4. Tilt your head back and squeeze the medication into your eye.
5. Close your eyes gently. Keep them closed for 1 to 2 minutes.
6. Do not rinse the dropper.
7. Wait for 5 to 10 minutes before using a second eye medication.

To avoid contaminating the dropper and solution, do not touch the eyelids or surrounding areas with the tip of the dropper.

Do not use if the solution is discolored.

■ *If you miss a dose...*
 Apply it as soon as you remember. If it is almost time for your next dose, skip the one you missed and go back to your regular schedule. Do not take 2 doses at once.

■ *Storage instructions...*
Store away from heat and light. Do not freeze.

Keep the bottle tightly closed when it is not being used.

What side effects may occur?
Side effects cannot be anticipated. If any develop or change in intensity, inform your doctor as soon as possible. Only your doctor can determine if it is safe for you to continue using Pilocar.

■ *More common side effects may include:*
Cloudy vision, detached retina, headache over your eye, nearsightedness, reduced vision in poor light, spasms of the eyelids, tearing eyes

■ *Rare side effects may include:*
Breathing difficulty, diarrhea, excessive salivation, fluid in lungs, high blood pressure, nausea, rapid heartbeat, sweating, vomiting

Why should this drug not be prescribed?
Pilocar should not be used if you are sensitive to or have ever had an allergic reaction to any of the components of this solution. Your doctor will not prescribe it for you if you have an eye condition in which your pupils should not be constricted.

Special warnings about this medication
Pilocar may make it difficult for you to see in the dark. Be careful driving at night, or doing any hazardous activity in dim light.

Possible food and drug interactions
when using this medication
No interactions have been reported.

Special information
if you are pregnant or breastfeeding
The effects of Pilocar during pregnancy have not been adequately studied. If you are pregnant or plan to become pregnant, inform your doctor immediately. Pilocar may appear in breast milk and could affect a nursing infant. If this medication is essential to your health, your doctor may advise you to stop breastfeeding until your treatment with Pilocar is finished.

Recommended dosage

ADULTS

The usual starting dose is 1 or 2 drops up to 6 times a day, depending on the severity of the glaucoma and your response. During a severe attack, your doctor will tell you to put drops into the unaffected eye as well.

Overdosage
Any medication taken in excess can have serious consequences. If you suspect an overdose seek medical attention immediately.

Generic name:

PILOCARPINE

See Pilocar, page 1005.

Brand name:

PILOPINE HS GEL

See Pilocar, page 1005.

Generic name:

PINDOLOL

See Visken, page 1420.

Generic name:

PIROXICAM

See Feldene, page 512.

Brand name:

PLAQUENIL

Pronounced: PLAK-en-ill
Generic name: Hydroxychloroquine sulfate

Why is this drug prescribed?
Plaquenil is prescribed for the prevention and treatment of certain forms of malaria.

Plaquenil is also used to treat the symptoms of rheumatoid arthritis such as swelling, inflammation, stiffness, and joint pain. It is also prescribed for lupus erythematosus, a chronic inflammation of the connective tissue.

Most important fact about this drug

Children are especially sensitive to Plaquenil. Relatively small doses of this medication have caused fatalities. Keep this drug in a child-proof container and out of the reach of children.

How should you take this medication?

Take Plaquenil exactly as prescribed for the full course of therapy.

If you have been prescribed Plaquenil for rheumatoid arthritis, it will take several weeks for beneficial effects to appear. Take each dose with a meal or a glass of milk.

■ *If you miss a dose...*
   And you take 1 dose every 7 days, take it as soon as you remember, then go back to your regular schedule.

   If you take 1 dose a day and you miss your dose, take it as soon as you remember. If you do not remember until the next day, skip the one you missed and go back to your regular schedule.

   If you take more than one dose a day, take it as soon as you remember if it is within an hour or so of the missed time. If you do not remember until later on, skip the missed dose and go back to your regular schedule. Do not take 2 doses at once.

■ *Storage information...*
   Store at room temperature, away from heat, light, and moisture.

What side effects may occur?

Side effects cannot be anticipated. If any develop or change in intensity, inform your doctor as soon as possible. Only your doctor can determine if it is safe for you to continue taking Plaquenil.

■ *Side effects of treatment for an acute malarial attack may include:*
   Abdominal cramps, diarrhea, dizziness, lack or loss of appetite, mild headache, nausea, vomiting

■ *Side effects of treatment for lupus erythematosus and rheumatoid arthritis may include:*
   Abdominal cramps, abnormal eye pigmentation, anemia, bleaching of hair, blind spots, blood disorders, blurred vision, convulsions, decreased vision, diarrhea, difficulty focusing the eyes, dizziness, emotional changes, excessive coloring of the skin, eye muscle paralysis, "foggy vision," halos around lights, headache, hearing loss, hives, involuntary eyeball move-

ment, irritability, itching, lack of muscle coordination, light flashes and streaks, light intolerance, loss of hair, loss or lack of appetite, muscle weakness, nausea, nervousness, nightmares, psoriasis (dry, scaly, red skin patches), reading difficulties, ringing in the ears, skin eruptions, skin inflammation and scaling, skin rash, vertigo, vomiting, weariness, weight loss

Why should this drug not be prescribed?

If you are sensitive to or have ever had an allergic reaction to Plaquenil or similar drugs such as Aralen and Chloroquine, you should not take this medication. Make sure your doctor is aware of any drug reactions you have experienced.

Plaquenil should not be prescribed if you have suffered partial or complete loss of vision in small areas while taking this medication or similar drugs. Notify your doctor of any past or present visual changes you have experienced.

This drug should not be used for long-term therapy in children.

Special warnings about this medication

Unless you are directed to do so by your doctor, do not take this medication if you have psoriasis (a recurrent skin disorder characterized by patches of red, dry, scaly skin) or porphyria (an inherited metabolic disorder affecting the liver or bone marrow). The use of Plaquenil may cause a severe attack of psoriasis and may increase the severity of porphyria.

Disorders of the retina causing impairment or loss of vision may be related to the length of time and the dose of Plaquenil given for lupus and rheumatoid arthritis. Problems have occurred several months to several years after beginning daily therapy. When you are on prolonged therapy your doctor will perform eye examinations at the beginning of treatment and every 3 months after that. Visual disturbances may progress, even after you have stopped taking this drug. If you have any problem with your vision or your eyes, notify your doctor immediately.

All people on long-term therapy with this drug should have a physical examination periodically, including testing of knee and ankle reflexes, to detect any evidence of muscular weakness.

Consult your doctor if you experience ringing in the ears, or other hearing problems.

If you are being treated for rheumatoid arthritis and have shown no improvement (such as reduced joint swelling or increased mobility) within 6 months, your doctor may decide to discontinue this drug.

Plaquenil should be used with caution by alcoholics and those who have liver disease or kidney problems.

Your doctor should conduct periodic blood cell counts if you are on prolonged therapy with this medication. If any severe blood disorder develops that is not attributed to the disease you are being treated for, your doctor may discontinue use of this drug.

Consult your doctor if you are taking a drug that has a tendency to produce dermatitis (inflammation of the skin), because you may have some skin reactions while taking Plaquenil.

Possible food and drug interactions when taking this medication

If Plaquenil is taken with certain other drugs, the effects of either could be increased, decreased, or altered. It is especially important to check with your doctor before combining Plaquenil with the following:

Any medication that may cause liver damage
Aurothioglucose (Solganal)
Cimetidine (Tagamet)
Digoxin (Lanoxin)

Special information if you are pregnant or breastfeeding

Use of this drug during pregnancy should be avoided except in the suppression or treatment of malaria when, in the judgment of your doctor, the benefit outweighs the possible hazard. This drug may appear in breast milk and could affect a nursing infant. If this medication is essential to your health, your doctor may advise you to discontinue breastfeeding until your treatment is finished.

Recommended dosage

ADULTS

Restraint or Prevention of Malaria

The usual dose is 400 milligrams taken once every 7 days on exactly the same day of each week. If circumstances permit, preventive therapy should begin 2 weeks prior to exposure. If this is not possible, your doctor will have you take a starting dose of 800 milligrams, which may be divided into 2 doses taken 6 hours apart. You should continue this suppressive therapy for 8 weeks after leaving the area where malaria occurs.

Acute Attack of Malaria

The usual starting dose is 800 milligrams, to be followed by 400 milligrams in 6 to 8 hours and 400 milligrams on each of 2 consecutive days.

Alternatively, your doctor may prescribe a single dose of 800 milligrams.

Lupus Erythematosus

The usual starting dose for adults is 400 milligrams once or twice daily. You will continue to take this dose for several weeks or months, depending on your response. For longer-term maintenance therapy, your doctor may reduce the dose to 200 to 400 milligrams per day.

Rheumatoid Arthritis

The usual starting dose for adults is 400 to 600 milligrams a day taken with a meal or a glass of milk. If your condition improves, usually within 4 to 12 weeks, your doctor will reduce the dose to a maintenance level of 200 to 400 milligrams daily.

CHILDREN

For the treatment of malaria, your doctor will calculate the dosage on the basis of your child's weight.

This drug has not been proved safe for treatment of juvenile arthritis.

Overdosage

Any medication taken in excess can have serious consequences. If you suspect an overdose, seek emergency medical treatment immediately.

■ *Symptoms of an overdose of Plaquenil may occur within 30 minutes. They include:*
Convulsions, drowsiness, headache, heart problems and failure, inability to breathe, visual problems

Brand name:

PLAVIX

Pronounced: PLA-vicks
Generic name: Clopidogrel bisulfate

Why is this drug prescribed?

Plavix keeps blood platelets slippery and discourages formation of clots, thereby improving blood flow to your heart, brain, and body. The drug is prescribed to reduce the risk of heart attack, stroke, and circulation problems in people with hardening of the arteries.

Most important fact about this drug

Because Plavix slows clotting, it will take longer than usual to stop bleeding. Be sure to report any unusual bleeding to your doctor immediately, and tell any doctor or dentist planning a procedure that you have been taking Plavix. You should discontinue the drug 7 days before any kind of surgery.

How should you take this medication?

Plavix can be taken with or without food.

■ *If you miss a dose...*

Take it as soon as you remember. If it is almost time for your next dose, skip the one you missed and go back to your regular schedule. Do not take 2 doses at the same time.

■ *Storage instructions...*

Store at room temperature.

What side effects may occur?

Side effects cannot be anticipated. If any develop or change in intensity, inform your doctor as soon as possible. Only your doctor can determine if it is safe for you to continue using Plavix.

■ *More common side effects may include:*

Abdominal pain, back pain, bronchitis, chest pain, coughing, depression, diarrhea, difficulty breathing, dizziness, fatigue, fluid retention and swelling, flu symptoms, headache, high blood pressure, high cholesterol, indigestion, inflammation of the nasal passages, itching, joint pain, nausea, pain, purple discoloration of skin, rash, upper respiratory tract infection, urinary tract infection

■ *Less common side effects may include:*

Anemia, anxiety, arthritis, bruising and bleeding under the skin, cataracts, constipation, fainting, gout, heart problems, hernia, increased heart rate, insomnia, irregular heartbeat, joint disease, leg cramps, loss of sensitivity to touch, nosebleed, pinkeye, pneumonia, skin problems, stomach and intestinal bleeding, sinus inflammation, skin tingling, vomiting, weakness

■ *Rare side effects may include:*
Allergic reactions, decreased circulation in the skin, decreased white blood cell counts, excessive menstrual flow, liver problems, stomach ulcers, unusual or excessive bleeding

Why should this drug not be prescribed?
Do not take Plavix if you have a bleeding stomach ulcer or bleeding in the area around the brain. Also avoid this medication if it gives you an allergic reaction.

Special warnings about this medication
If you've ever had a stomach ulcer or bleeding in the digestive tract, make sure the doctor is aware of it; Plavix should be used with caution. The drug should also be used carefully if you have bleeding problems due to severe liver disease, or expect to be at risk of bleeding from any other cause.

If you develop a fever or any other signs of an infection while you are taking Plavix, tell your doctor immediately.

Possible food and drug interactions
when taking this medication
If Plavix is taken with certain other drugs, the effects of either could be increased, decreased, or altered. Ask your doctor before starting any new drug; and be doubly careful before combining Plavix with the following:

Aspirin
Fluvastatin (Lescol)
Heparin
Nonsteroidal anti-inflammatory drugs such as Advil, Aleve, Motrin, and Naprosyn
Phenytoin (Dilantin)
Tamoxifen (Nolvadex)
Tolbutamide (Orinase)
Torsemide (Demadex)
Warfarin (Coumadin)

Special information
if you are pregnant or breastfeeding
The effects of Plavix during pregnancy have not been adequately studied. If you are pregnant or plan to become pregnant, inform your doctor immediately. Use Plavix during pregnancy only if absolutely necessary. Do not breastfeed while taking Plavix, since the drug may appear in breast milk.

Recommended dosage

ADULTS

The usual dose is 75 milligrams once a day.

CHILDREN

The safety and effectiveness of Plavix have not been established in children.

Overdosage

Any medication taken in excess can have serious consequences. If you suspect an overdose of Plavix, seek medical attention immediately.

■ *Potential symptoms of Plavix overdose may include:*
Difficulty breathing, exhaustion, stomach or intestinal bleeding, vomiting

Brand name:

PLENDIL

Pronounced: PLEN-dill
Generic name: Felodipine

Why is this drug prescribed?

Plendil is prescribed for the treatment of high blood pressure. It is effective alone or in combination with other high blood pressure medications. A type of medication called a calcium channel blocker, Plendil eases the workload of the heart by slowing down its muscle contractions and the passage of nerve impulses through it. This improves blood flow through the heart and throughout the body, reduces blood pressure, and helps prevent angina pain (chest pain, often accompanied by a feeling of choking, usually caused by lack of oxygen in the heart due to clogged arteries).

Most important fact about this drug

If you have high blood pressure, you must take Plendil regularly for it to be effective. Since blood pressure declines gradually, it may be several weeks before you get the full benefit of Plendil; you must continue taking it even if you are feeling well. Plendil does not cure high blood pressure; it merely keeps it under control.

How should you take this medication?

Plendil can be taken with a light meal or without food. The tablets should be swallowed whole, not crushed or chewed.

Try not to miss any doses. If Plendil is not taken regularly, your blood pressure may increase.

■ *If you miss a dose...*
Take the forgotten dose as soon as you remember. If it is almost time for the next dose, skip the one you missed and go back to your regular schedule. Never try to "catch up" by doubling the dose.

■ *Storage instructions...*
Store at room temperature. Protect from light.

What side effects may occur?
Side effects cannot be anticipated. If any develop or change in intensity, inform your doctor as soon as possible. Only your doctor can determine if it is safe for you to continue taking Plendil.

■ *More common side effects may include:*
Flushing, headache, swelling of the legs and feet

■ *Less common or rare side effects may include:*
Anemia, angina pectoris (chest pain), ankle pain, anxiety disorders, arm pain, arthritis, back pain, blurred vision, breast enlargement, bronchitis, bruising, constipation, cough, diarrhea, dizziness, decreased sex drive, depression, difficulty sleeping, dry mouth, enlarged gums, excessive nighttime urination, excessive perspiration, facial swelling, fainting, fatigue, flu, foot pain, frequent urination, gas, muscle pain, heart attack, hip pain, hives, impotence, inflammation of the nose, irregular heartbeat, irritability, itching, joint pain, knee pain, leg pain, low blood pressure, nausea, neck pain, nervousness, nosebleeds, painful or difficult urination, rapid heartbeat, rash, respiratory infections, ringing in the ears, shortness of breath, shoulder pain, sinus inflammation, sleepiness, sneezing, sore throat, stomach and intestinal pain, tingling sensation, tremor, urgent urination, vomiting, warm sensation, weakness

Why should this drug not be prescribed?
If you are sensitive to or have ever had an allergic reaction to Plendil or other calcium channel blockers, such as Calan and Procardia, you should not take this medication. Make sure your doctor is aware of any drug reactions you have experienced.

Special warnings about this medication
Plendil can cause your blood pressure to become too low. If you feel light-headed or faint, or if you feel your heart racing or you experience chest pain, contact your doctor immediately.

If you have congestive heart failure, Plendil should be used with caution, especially if you are also taking one of the "beta-blocker" family of drugs, such as Inderal or Tenormin.

Your legs and feet may swell when you start taking Plendil, usually within the first 2 to 3 weeks of treatment.

If you have liver disease or are over age 65, your doctor should monitor your blood pressure carefully while adjusting your dosage of Plendil.

Your gums may become swollen and sore while you are taking Plendil. Good dental hygiene will help control this problem.

Possible food and drug interactions
when taking this medication
If Plendil is taken with certain other drugs, the effects of either could be increased, decreased, or altered. It is especially important to check with your doctor before combining Plendil with the following:

Beta-blocking blood pressure medicines such as Lopressor, Inderal, and
    Tenormin
Cimetidine (Tagamet)
Digoxin (Lanoxin)
Epilepsy medications such as Tegretol and Dilantin
Erythromycin (PCE, ERYC, others)
Phenobarbital
Theophylline (Theo-Dur)

Taking Plendil with grapefruit juice can more than double the effect of the drug.

Special information
if you are pregnant or breastfeeding
Although the effects of Plendil during pregnancy have not been adequately studied in humans, birth defects have occurred in animal studies. If you are pregnant or plan to become pregnant, inform your doctor immediately. Plendil may appear in breast milk and may affect a nursing infant. If this medication is essential to your health, your doctor may advise you to discontinue breastfeeding until your treatment is finished.

Recommended dosage

ADULTS

Your doctor will adjust the dosage according to your response to the drug.

The usual starting dose is 5 milligrams once a day; your doctor will adjust the dose at intervals of not less than 2 weeks.

The usual dosage range is 2.5 to 10 milligrams once daily.

CHILDREN

The safety and effectiveness of Plendil in children have not been established.

OLDER ADULTS

If you are over 65 years of age, your doctor will monitor your blood pressure closely during dosage adjustment. In general, you should not take more than 10 milligrams a day.

Overdosage

Any medication taken in excess can have serious consequences. If you suspect an overdose, seek medical treatment immediately.

■ *Symptoms of Plendil overdose may include:*
  Severely low blood pressure, slow heartbeat

Generic name:

POLYMYXIN B, NEOMYCIN, AND HYDROCORTISONE

See Cortisporin Ophthalmic Suspension, page 297.

Brand name:

POLY-VI-FLOR

Pronounced: pol-ee-VIE-floor
Generic ingredients: Vitamins, Fluoride

Why is this drug prescribed?
Poly-Vi-Flor is a multivitamin and fluoride supplement. The drops have 9 essential vitamins; the chewable tablets have 10. Poly-Vi-Flor is prescribed for children aged 2 and older to provide fluoride where the drinking water

contains less than the amount recommended by the American Dental Association to build strong teeth and prevent cavities. Poly-Vi-Flor also supplies significant amounts of vitamins to help prevent deficiencies. The American Academy of Pediatrics recommends that children up to age 16 take a fluoride supplement if they live in areas where the drinking water contains less than the recommended amount of fluoride.

Most important fact about this drug
Do not give your child more than the recommended dose. Too much fluoride can cause discoloration and pitting of teeth.

How should you take this medication?
Do not give your child more than your doctor prescribes.

Poly-Vi-Flor chewable tablets should be chewed or crushed before swallowing. You can put Poly-Vi-Flor drops directly into a child's mouth with the dropper provided or mix them into cereal, juice, or other food.

■ *If you miss a dose...*
Give it as soon as you remember. If it is almost time for the next dose, skip the one you missed and go back to your regular schedule. Do not give 2 doses at once.

■ *Storage instructions...*
Store away from heat, light, and moisture.

What side effects may occur?
Rarely, an allergic rash has occurred.

Why should this drug not be prescribed?
Children should not take Poly-Vi-Flor if they are getting significant amounts of fluoride from other medications or sources.

Special warnings about this medication
Do not give your child more than the recommended dosage. Your child's teeth should be checked periodically for discoloration or pitting. Notify your doctor if white, brown, or black spots appear on your child's teeth.

The fluoride level of your drinking water should be determined before Poly-Vi-Flor is prescribed.

Let your doctor know if you change drinking water or filtering systems.

Fluoride does not replace proper dental habits, such as brushing, flossing, and having dental checkups.

Recommended dosage

The usual dose is 1 tablet or 1 milliliter every day as prescribed by the doctor; your doctor will choose the strength according to your child's age and the amount of fluoride in the drinking water.

Overdosage

Although overdose is unlikely, any medication taken in excess can have serious consequences. If you suspect an overdose, seek medical treatment immediately.

Brand name:

PONSTEL

Pronounced: PON-stel
Generic name: Mefenamic acid

Why is this drug prescribed?

Ponstel, a nonsteroidal anti-inflammatory drug, is used for the relief of moderate pain (when treatment will not last for more than 7 days) and for the treatment of menstrual pain.

Most important fact about this drug

You should have frequent checkups with your doctor if you take Ponstel regularly. Ulcers or internal bleeding can occur without warning.

How should you take this medication?

Take Ponstel with food if possible. If it upsets your stomach, be sure to take it with food or an antacid or with a full glass of milk.

Take Ponstel exactly as prescribed by your doctor.

■ *If you miss a dose...*
If you take Ponstel on a regular schedule, take the forgotten dose as soon as you remember. If it is almost time for your next dose, skip the one you missed and go back to your regular schedule. Do not take 2 doses at once.

■ *Storage instructions...*
Store away from heat, light, and moisture.

What side effects may occur?

Side effects cannot be anticipated. If any develop or change in intensity, inform your doctor as soon as possible. Only your doctor can determine if it is safe for you to continue taking Ponstel.

- *More common side effects may include:*
  Abdominal pain, diarrhea, nausea, stomach and intestinal upset, vomiting

- *Less common or rare side effects may include:*
  Anemia, blood in the urine, blurred vision, changes in liver function, constipation, difficult or painful urination, dizziness, drowsiness, ear pain, eye irritation, facial swelling due to fluid retention, fluttery or throbbing heartbeat, gas, headache, heartburn, hives, inability to sleep, increased need for insulin in a diabetic, kidney failure, labored breathing, loss of appetite, loss of color vision, nervousness, rash, red or purple spots on the skin, sweating, ulcers and internal bleeding

Why should this drug not be prescribed?
Do not take Ponstel if you are sensitive to or have ever had an allergic reaction to it. You should not take it, either, if you have had asthma attacks, hay fever, or hives caused by aspirin or other nonsteroidal anti-inflammatory drugs, such as Motrin and Nuprin. Make sure your doctor is aware of any drug reactions you have experienced.

Do not take Ponstel if you have ulcerations or frequently recurring inflammation of your stomach or intestines.

Avoid this drug if you have serious kidney disease.

Special warnings about this medication
If you develop a rash, diarrhea, or other stomach problems, stop taking this medication and contact your doctor.

Ponstel should be used with caution if you have kidney disease, heart failure, or liver disease; it can cause liver inflammation in some people.

This drug may prolong bleeding time. If you are taking blood-thinning medication, take Ponstel with caution.

Possible food and drug interactions when taking this medication
If Ponstel is taken with certain other drugs, the effects of either can be increased, decreased, or altered. It is especially important to check with your doctor before combining Ponstel with the following:

Aspirin
Blood-thinning medications such as Coumadin
Diuretics such as Lasix and HydroDIURIL
Lithium (Lithonate)
Methotrexate

Special information
if you are pregnant or breastfeeding

The effects of Ponstel during pregnancy have not been adequately studied. If you are pregnant or plan to become pregnant, inform your doctor immediately. You should not use Ponstel in late pregnancy because nonsteroidal anti-inflammatory drugs affect the heart and blood vessels of the developing baby. Ponstel may appear in breast milk and could affect a nursing infant. If this medication is essential to your health, your doctor may advise you to discontinue breastfeeding until your treatment is finished.

Recommended dosage

ADULTS AND CHILDREN OVER 14

Moderate Pain
The usual starting dose is 500 milligrams, followed by 250 milligrams every 6 hours, if needed, for 1 week.

Menstrual Pain
The usual starting dose, once symptoms appear, is 500 milligrams, followed by 250 milligrams every 6 hours for 2 to 3 days.

CHILDREN

The safety and effectiveness of Ponstel have not been established in children under 14.

Overdosage
Although there is no information available on overdosage with Ponstel, any medication taken in excess can have serious consequences. If you suspect an overdose of Ponstel, seek medical attention immediately.

Generic name:

POTASSIUM CHLORIDE

See Micro-K, page 791.

Generic name:

PRAMIPEXOLE

See Mirapex, page 813.

Brand name:

PRANDIN

Pronounced: PRAN-din
Generic name: Repaglinide

Why is this drug prescribed?
Prandin is used to reduce blood sugar levels in people with Type 2 diabetes (the kind that does not require insulin shots). It's prescribed when diet and exercise alone fail to correct the problem. A combination of Prandin and a second diabetes drug called Glucophage can be prescribed if either drug alone proves insufficient.

Most important fact about this drug
Chronically high glucose levels have been implicated in the kidney failure, blindness, and loss of sensation that plague many people with long-standing diabetes. A low-calorie diet, weight loss, and exercise are your first line of defense against these problems. Medications such as Prandin are prescribed only as a back-up when these other measures still leave sugar too high. If diet, exercise, and a combination of Prandin and Glucophage all fail to do the job, your doctor may have to start you on insulin.

How should you take this medication?
Prandin should be taken shortly before each meal. You can take it 30 minutes ahead of time or wait until just before starting; a 15-minute period is typical. You can take Prandin 2, 3, or 4 times a day, depending on the number of meals you have. If you skip a meal (or add an extra meal), skip (or add) a dose accordingly.

- *If you miss a dose...*
  Wait until your next meal, then take your regular dose. Do not take 2 doses at once.

- *Storage instructions...*
  Store at room temperature away from moisture in a tightly closed container.

What side effects may occur?
Side effects cannot be anticipated. If any develop or change in intensity, inform your doctor as soon as possible. Only your doctor can determine if it is safe for you to continue taking Prandin.

■ *More common side effects may include:*
Back pain, bronchitis, chest pain, constipation, diarrhea, headache, indigestion, joint pain, low blood sugar, nasal inflammation, nausea, sinus inflammation, skin tingling, upper respiratory tract infection, urinary tract infection, vomiting

■ *Less common and rare side effects may include:*
Allergic reactions, angina (chest pain), tooth problems

Why should this drug not be prescribed?
If you have Type 1 (insulin-dependent) diabetes, you cannot use Prandin. The drug also cannot be used for diabetic ketoacidosis (a life-threatening emergency first signaled by excessive thirst, nausea, fatigue, and fruity-smelling breath). This condition must be treated with insulin.

If you find that Prandin gives you an allergic reaction, you'll be unable to continue using it.

Special warnings about this medication
While taking Prandin, you should check your blood sugar regularly. Your doctor will also watch it; and to measure long-term glucose control, he will probably give you a glycosylated hemoglobin (HbA1C) test as well.

Too much Prandin can cause low blood sugar (hypoglycemia), marked by shaking, sweating, and cold-clammy skin. If you develop these symptoms, take some orange juice or suck on a hard candy. The problem is more likely to surface if you are elderly, debilitated, or malnourished, have liver problems, or suffer from poor adrenal or pituitary function.

You should be aware that another oral diabetes drug, tolbutamide, has been blamed for a slight increase in heart-related deaths among people on long-term therapy. This finding is controversial, and Prandin itself has never been implicated. However, the authorities recommend approaching all oral diabetes drugs with caution.

Possible food and drug interactions
when taking this medication
If Prandin is taken with certain other drugs, the effects of either could be increased, decreased, or altered. It is especially important to check with your doctor before combining Prandin with the following:

Airway-opening medications such as Alupent, Proventil, and Ventolin
Alcohol (excessive amounts can cause low blood sugar)
Aspirin
Barbiturates such as the sedatives Seconal and Nembutal

Beta blockers such as the blood pressure medications Inderal and Tenormin

Blood thinners such as Dicumarol and Miradon

Calcium channel blockers such as the blood pressure medications Cardizem and Procardia

Carbamazepine (Tegretol)

Chloramphenicol (Chloromycetin)

Erythromycin (Eryc, Ery-Tab, PCE)

Estrogens such as Premarin

Ketoconazole (Nizoral)

Furosemide (Lasix)

Glucose lowering agents such as Glucotrol and Micronase

Isoniazid

Major tranquilizers such as Mellaril and Stelazine

MAO inhibitors such as the antidepressants Marplan, Nardil, and Parnate

Niacin (Nicobid)

Nonsteroidal anti-inflammatory drugs such as Advil, Motrin, Naprosyn, and Voltaren

Oral contraceptives

Phenytoin (Dilantin)

Probenecid (Benemid, ColBENEMID)

Rifampin (Rifadin, Rimactane)

Steroids such as prednisone

Sulfa drugs such as Gantanol

Thyroid medications such as Synthroid

Troglitazone (Rezulin)

Water pills such as the thiazide diuretics Dyazide and HydroDIURIL

Special information
if you are pregnant or breastfeeding

Because abnormal blood sugar during pregnancy can cause fetal defects, your doctor will probably prescribe insulin injections until the baby is born. The effects of Prandin during pregnancy have not been adequately studied.

It is not known whether Prandin appears in breast milk. Discuss with your doctor whether to discontinue breastfeeding or give up Prandin. If the medication is discontinued, and diet alone does not control your blood sugar levels, your doctor may recommend insulin injections.

Recommended dosage

ADULTS

Take Prandin before each meal. The recommended dose ranges from 0.5 milligram to 4 milligrams. If you have never taken a glucose-lowering medication before, you should start with the 0.5-milligram dose. If you have taken these drugs in the past, the starting dose is 1 or 2 milligrams. Take no more than 16 milligrams a day.

Dose Adjustment
Your dose of Prandin will be adjusted according to your fasting blood sugar levels. Your doctor will wait at least a week after each change in dose to check your response.

Switching to Prandin
When Prandin replaces another oral glucose-lowering medicine, you should start taking it the day after your final dose or the previous drug. Be alert for signs of low blood sugar; effects of the drugs may overlap.

Combination Therapy:
If Prandin is being added to Glucophage therapy, you should begin with a 0.5-milligram dose. Dosage will then be adjusted according to your blood glucose levels.

Overdosage
An overdose of Prandin taken without food can cause low blood sugar (hypoglycemia).

■ *Symptoms of mild hypoglycemia may include:*
   Cold sweat, confusion, depression, dizziness, drowsiness, fatigue, headache, hunger, nausea, nervousness, rapid heartbeat, shaking

■ *Symptoms of severe hypoglycemia may include:*
   Coma, pale skin, seizure, shallow breathing

Consuming some sugar will usually correct the problem. If symptoms persist or worsen, contact your doctor.

Brand name:

PRAVACHOL

Pronounced: PRAV-a-coll
Generic name: Pravastatin sodium

Why is this drug prescribed?
Pravachol is a cholesterol-lowering drug. Your doctor may prescribe it along with a cholesterol-lowering diet if your blood cholesterol level is dangerously high and you have not been able to lower it by diet alone.

High cholesterol can lead to heart problems. By lowering your cholesterol, Pravachol improves your chances of avoiding a heart attack, heart surgery, and death from heart disease. In people who already have hardening of the arteries, it slows progression of the disease and cuts the risk of acute attacks.

The drug works by helping to clear harmful low-density lipoprotein (LDL) cholesterol out of the blood and by limiting the body's ability to form new LDL cholesterol.

Most important fact about this drug

Pravachol is usually prescribed only if diet, exercise, and weight-loss fail to bring your cholesterol levels under control. It's important to remember that Pravachol is a supplement—not a substitute—for those other measures. To get the full benefit of the medication, you need to stick to the diet and exercise program prescribed by your doctor. All these efforts to keep your cholesterol levels normal are important because together they may lower your risk of heart disease.

How should you take this medication?

For an even greater cholesterol-lowering effect, your doctor may prescribe Pravachol along with a different kind of lipid-lowering drug such as Questran or Colestid. However, you must not take Pravachol at the same time of day as the other cholesterol-lowering drug. Take Pravachol at least 1 hour before or 4 hours after taking the other drug.

Pravachol should be taken once daily at bedtime. You may take it with or without food.

Your doctor will probably do blood tests for cholesterol levels every 4 weeks to determine the effectiveness of the dose.

■ *If you miss a dose...*
Take the forgotten dose as soon as you remember. If it is almost time for your next dose, skip the one you missed and go back to your regular schedule. Do not take a double dose.

■ *Storage instructions...*
Store at room temperature, in a tightly closed container, away from moisture and light.

What side effects may occur?
Side effects from Pravachol cannot be anticipated. If any develop or change in intensity, inform your doctor as soon as possible. Only your doctor can determine if it is safe for you to continue taking Pravachol.

■ *Side effects may include:*
Abdominal pain, chest pain, cold, constipation, cough, diarrhea, dizziness, fatigue, flu, gas, headache, heartburn, inflammation of nasal passages, muscle aching or weakness, nausea, rash, urinary problems, vomiting

Why should this drug not be prescribed?
Do not take Pravachol if you are sensitive or have ever had an allergic reaction to it.

Do not take Pravachol if you have liver disease.

Special warnings about this medication
Pravachol should not be used to try to lower high cholesterol that stems from a medical condition such as alcoholism, poorly controlled diabetes, an underactive thyroid gland, or a kidney or liver problem.

Because Pravachol may cause damage to the liver, your doctor will do blood tests regularly. Your doctor should monitor you especially closely if you have ever had liver disease or if you are or have ever been a heavy drinker.

Since Pravachol may cause damage to muscle tissue, promptly report to your doctor any unexplained muscle pain, tenderness, or weakness, especially if you also have a fever or you just generally do not feel well.

**Possible food and drug interactions
when taking this medication**
If Pravachol is taken with certain other drugs, the effects of either could be increased, decreased, or altered. It is especially important to check with your doctor before combining Pravachol with the following:

Cholestyramine (Questran)
Cimetidine (Tagamet)
Colestipol (Colestid)
Drugs that suppress the immune system, such as Sandimmune and Neoral
Erythromycin (E.E.S., Erythrocin, others)
Gemfibrozil (Lopid)
Niacin (Nicobid, Nicolar)
Warfarin (Coumadin)

Special information
if you are pregnant or breastfeeding
You must not become pregnant while taking Pravachol. Because this drug lowers cholesterol, and cholesterol is necessary for the proper development of an unborn baby, there is some suspicion that Pravachol might cause birth defects. Your doctor will prescribe Pravachol only if you are highly unlikely to become pregnant while taking the drug. If you do become pregnant while taking Pravachol, inform your doctor immediately.

Because Pravachol appears in breast milk, and because its cholesterol-lowering effects might prove harmful to a nursing baby, you should not take Pravachol while you are breastfeeding.

Recommended dosage

ADULTS

The usual starting dose is 10 to 20 milligrams once a day at bedtime.

For ongoing therapy, the recommended dose is 10 to 40 milligrams, once a day at bedtime.

OLDER ADULTS

The usual starting dose is 10 milligrams a day at bedtime; for ongoing therapy, the dose is 20 milligrams per day or less.

Overdosage
Although no specific information is available, any medication taken in excess can have serious consequences. If you suspect an overdose of Pravachol, seek medical attention immediately.

Generic name:

PRAVASTATIN

See Pravachol, page 1025.

Generic name:

PRAZOSIN

See Minipress, page 807.

Brand name:

PRECOSE

Pronounced: PREE-cohs
Generic name: Acarbose

Why is this drug prescribed?

Precose is an oral medication used to treat Type II (noninsulin-dependent) diabetes when high blood sugar levels cannot be controlled by diet alone. Precose works by slowing the body's digestion of carbohydrates so that blood sugar levels won't surge upward after a meal. Precose may be taken alone or in combination with certain other diabetes medications such as Diabinese, Micronase, Glucophage, and Insulin.

Most important fact about this drug

Always remember that Precose is an aid to, not a substitute for, good diet and exercise. Failure to follow the diet and exercise plan recommended by your doctor can lead to serious complications such as dangerously high or low blood sugar levels. If you are overweight, losing pounds and exercising are critically important in controlling your diabetes. Remember, too, that Precose is not an oral form of insulin and cannot be used in place of insulin.

How should you take this medication?

Do not take more or less of this medication than directed by your doctor. Precose is usually taken 3 times a day with the first bite of each main meal.

■ *If you miss a dose...*
Take it as soon as you remember. If it is almost time for your next dose, skip the one you missed and go back to your regular schedule. Never take 2 doses at the same time. Taking Precose with your 3 main meals will help you to remember your medication schedule.

■ *Storage instructions...*
Keep the container tightly closed. Protect from temperatures above 77°F. Store away from moisture.

What side effects may occur?

Side effects cannot be anticipated. If any develop or change in intensity, tell your doctor as soon as possible. Only your doctor can determine if it is safe for you to continue taking Precose.

If side effects do occur, they usually appear during the first few weeks of therapy and generally become less intense and less frequent over time. They are rarely severe.

■ *More common side effects may include:*
Abdominal pain, diarrhea, gas

Why should this drug not be prescribed?
Do not take Precose when suffering diabetic ketoacidosis (a life-threatening medical emergency caused by insufficient insulin and marked by mental confusion, excessive thirst, nausea, vomiting, headache, fatigue, and a sweet fruity smell to the breath).

You should not take Precose if you have cirrhosis (chronic degenerative liver disease). Also avoid Precose therapy if you have inflammatory bowel disease, ulcers in the colon, any intestinal obstruction or chronic intestinal disease associated with digestion, or any condition that could become worse as a result of gas in the intestine.

Special warnings about this medication
Every 3 months during your first year of treatment, your doctor will give you a blood test to check your liver and see how it is reacting to Precose. While you are taking Precose, you should check your blood and urine periodically for the presence of abnormal sugar (glucose) levels.

Even people with well-controlled diabetes may find that stress such as injury, infection, surgery, or fever results in a loss of control over their blood sugar. If this happens to you, your doctor may recommend that Precose be discontinued temporarily and injected insulin used instead.

When taken alone, Precose does not cause hypoglycemia (low blood sugar), but when you take it in combination with other medications such as Diabinese or Glucotrol, or with insulin, your blood sugar may fall too low. If you have any questions about combining Precose with other medications, be sure to discuss them with your doctor.

If you are taking Precose along with other diabetes medications, be sure to have some source of glucose, such as Glutose tablets, available in case you experience any symptoms of mild or moderate low blood sugar. (Table sugar won't work because Precose inhibits its absorption.)

■ *Symptoms of mild hypoglycemia may include:*
Cold sweat, fast heartbeat, fatigue, headache, nausea, and nervousness

■ *Symptoms of more severe hypoglycemia may include:*
Coma, pale skin, and shallow breathing

Severe hypoglycemia is an emergency. Contact your doctor immediately if the symptoms occur.

Possible food and drug interactions
when taking this medication

When you take Precose with certain other drugs, the effects of either could be increased, decreased, or altered. It is especially important to check with your doctor before taking Precose with the following:

Airway-opening drugs such as Sudafed and Proventil
Calcium channel blockers (heart and blood pressure medications such as Cardizem and Procardia)
Charcoal tablets
Digestive enzyme preparations such as Creon 20 and Donnazyme
Estrogens such as Premarin
Isoniazid (Rifamate)
Major tranquilizers such as Compazine and Mellaril
Nicotinic acid (Nicobid, Nicolar)
Oral contraceptives
Phenytoin (Dilantin)
Steroid medications such as Deltasone and Prelone
Thyroid medications such as Synthroid and Thyrolar
Water pills (diuretics) such as HydroDIURIL, Enduron, Moduretic

Special information
if you are pregnant or breastfeeding

The effects of Precose during pregnancy have not been adequately studied. If you are pregnant or plan to become pregnant, tell your doctor immediately. Since studies suggest the importance of maintaining normal blood sugar levels during pregnancy, your doctor may prescribe injected insulin. It is not known whether Precose appears in breast milk. Because many drugs do appear in breast milk, you should not take Precose while breastfeeding.

Recommended dosage

ADULTS

The recommended starting dose of Precose is 25 milligrams (half of a 50-milligram tablet) 3 times a day, taken with the first bite of each main meal.

Some people need to work up to this dose gradually and start with 25 milligrams only once a day. Your doctor will adjust your dosage at 4- to 8-week intervals, based on blood tests and your individual response to Precose. The doctor may increase the medication to 50 milligrams 3 times a day or, if needed, 100 milligrams 3 times a day. You should not take more than this amount. If you weigh less than 132 pounds, the maximum dosage is 50 milligrams 3 times a day.

If you are also taking another oral antidiabetic medication and you show signs of low blood sugar, your doctor will adjust the dosage of both medications.

CHILDREN

Safety and effectiveness of Precose in children have not been established.

Overdosage

An overdose of Precose alone will not cause low blood sugar. However, it may cause a temporary increase in gas, diarrhea, and abdominal discomfort. The symptoms will disappear quickly.

Brand name:

PRED FORTE

Pronounced: PRED FORT
Generic name: Prednisolone acetate

Why is this drug prescribed?

Pred Forte contains a steroid medication that eases redness, irritation, and swelling due to inflammation of the eye.

Most important fact about this drug

Do not use Pred Forte more often or for a longer period than your doctor orders. Overuse can increase the risk of side effects and can lead to eye damage. If your eye problems return, do not use any leftover Pred Forte without first consulting your doctor.

How should you use this medication?

Keep using Pred Forte for the full time prescribed.

To avoid spreading infection, do not let anyone else use your prescription.

Pred Forte may increase the chance of infection from contact lenses. Your doctor may advise you to stop wearing your contacts while using this medication.

Follow these steps to administer Pred Forte:
1. Wash your hands thoroughly.
2. Vigorously shake the dropper bottle.
3. Gently pull your lower eyelid down to form a pocket next to your eye.
4. Do not touch the applicator tip to any surface including your eye.
5. Brace the bottle against the bridge of your nose or your forehead.
6. Tilt your head back and squeeze the medication into your eye.
7. Close your eyes gently. Keep them closed for 1 to 2 minutes.
8. Do not rinse the dropper.
9. Wait for 5 to 10 minutes before using a second eye medication.

■ *If you miss a dose...*
Apply it as soon as you remember. If it is almost time for your next dose, skip the one you missed and go back to your regular schedule.

■ *Storage instructions...*
Store away from heat and direct light. Keep the bottle tightly closed and protect from freezing.

What side effects may occur?
Side effects cannot be anticipated. If any develop or change in intensity, inform your doctor as soon as possible. Only your doctor can determine if it is safe for you to continue taking Pred Forte.

■ *Side effects may include:*
Allergic reactions, blurred vision, burning/stinging, cataract formation, delayed wound healing, dilated pupils, drooping eyelid, increased pressure inside the eyeball, inflamed eyes, perforation of the eyeball, secondary infection, ulcers of the cornea

Since many of these developments could affect your vision temporarily or permanently, it is important to keep in close contact with your doctor while using Pred Forte eyedrops, and to use the drops only as directed.

Occasionally, long-term use of Pred Forte eyedrops may cause bodywide side effects due to an overload of steroid hormone. Such side effects may include a "moon-faced" appearance, obese trunk, humped upper back, wasted limbs, and purple stretch marks on the skin. These effects are likely to disappear once the medication is withdrawn. If bodywide side effects occur, you will need to stop using the eyedrops gradually rather than all at once.

Why should this drug not be prescribed?
You should not take Pred Forte if you have herpes or other viral diseases of the eye, or certain bacterial or fungal diseases of the eye.

Do not use Pred Forte if you are allergic to prednisolone or other steroids.

Special warnings about this medication
You must stay in close touch with your doctor while using this medication, for the following reasons:

If you use Pred Forte eyedrops extensively and/or for an extended period of time, you may be at increased risk for cataracts or vision problems. Prolonged use also increases the risk of another infection.

If you have had cataract surgery, this medication can delay healing.

Some eye diseases, together with long-term use of steroids, can cause thinning of the cornea; you may be at increased risk for perforation of the eyeball.

If you have a persistent ulceration of the cornea of your eye while using Pred Forte eyedrops, the problem may be a secondary fungus infection which Pred Forte cannot cure. An eye doctor should evaluate this possibility.

If you use Pred Forte eyedrops for 10 days or longer, an eye doctor should check your intraocular pressure (pressure inside the eyeball) frequently, since prolonged use of steroids may increase this pressure. If you already have glaucoma, use this medication cautiously. If increased pressure is allowed to continue, it may cause loss of vision.

Corticosteroids can mask, or worsen, pus-forming eye infections. If your eye inflammation or pain lasts longer than 48 hours or becomes worse, stop using Pred Forte and call your doctor.

Pred Forte contains sodium bisulfite, which can cause allergic-type reactions, including severe or even life-threatening asthma attacks. You are more likely to be sensitive to sulfites if you suffer from asthma.

**Possible food and drug interactions
when using this medication**
Prednisolone acetate, the active ingredient in Pred Forte eyedrops, is also available in tablet and injectable forms for the treatment of other disorders. It's known that when these other forms of prednisolone acetate are taken with certain drugs, the effects of either medication can be increased, decreased, or altered. Therefore, it's wise to check with your doctor before combining Pred Forte eyedrops with other medications.

Special information
if you are pregnant or breastfeeding

If you are pregnant or plan to become pregnant, inform your doctor immediately. Pred Forte eyedrops should be used during pregnancy only if the potential benefit outweighs the potential risk to the developing baby.

It is not known whether the hormone in Pred Forte eyedrops appears in breast milk. If it does, the small quantity involved would be unlikely to harm a breastfeeding baby. Nevertheless, caution is advised when using Pred Forte eyedrops while breastfeeding.

Recommended dosage

ADULTS

Put 1 to 2 drops under the eyelid 2 to 4 times daily. During the first 24 to 48 hours, your doctor may want you to use more frequent doses.

Overdosage

A one-time accidental overdose of Pred Forte eyedrops ordinarily will not cause acute problems. Over time, however, overdosage may have serious consequences (see "What side effects may occur?"). If you suspect symptoms of a chronic overdose with Pred Forte eyedrops, seek medical attention immediately.

If you accidentally swallow Pred Forte eyedrops, drink fluids to dilute the medication. Call your local poison center or your doctor for assistance.

Generic name:

PREDNISOLONE ACETATE

See Pred Forte, page 1032.

Generic name:

PREDNISOLONE SODIUM PHOSPHATE

See Pediapred, page 960.

Generic name:

PREDNISONE

See Deltasone, page 357.

Brand name:

PREMARIN

Pronounced: PREM-uh-rin
Generic name: Conjugated estrogens
Other brand names: Premphase, Prempro

Why is this drug prescribed?

Premarin is an estrogen replacement drug. The tablets are used to reduce symptoms of menopause, including feelings of warmth in face, neck, and chest, and the sudden intense episodes of heat and sweating known as "hot flashes." They also may be prescribed for teenagers who fail to mature at the usual rate, and to relieve the symptoms of certain types of cancer, including some forms of breast and prostate cancer.

In addition, either the tablets or Premarin vaginal cream can be used for other conditions caused by lack of estrogen, such as dry, itchy external genitals and vaginal irritation.

Along with diet, calcium supplements, and exercise, Premarin tablets are also prescribed to prevent osteoporosis, a condition in which the bones become brittle and easily broken.

The addition of progesterone to estrogen-replacement therapy has been shown to reduce the risk of uterine cancer. Prempro combines estrogen and progesterone in a single tablet taken once daily. Premphase is a 28-day supply of tablets. The first 14 contain only estrogen. The second 14 supply both estrogen and progesterone. Both Prempro and Premphase are prescribed to reduce the symptoms of menopause, including vaginal problems, and to prevent osteoporosis.

Most important fact about this drug

Because estrogens have been linked with increased risk of endometrial cancer (cancer in the lining of the uterus), it is essential to have regular checkups and to report any unusual vaginal bleeding to your doctor immediately.

How should you take this medication?

Take Premarin exactly as prescribed. Do not share it with anyone else.

If you are taking calcium supplements as a part of the treatment to help prevent brittle bones, check with your doctor about how much to take.

You should take a few moments to read the patient package insert provided with your prescription.

If you are using Premarin vaginal cream, apply it as follows:

1. Remove cap from tube.
2. Screw nozzle end of applicator onto tube.
3. Gently squeeze tube from the bottom to force sufficient cream into the barrel to provide the prescribed dose. Use the marked stopping points on the applicator as a guide.
4. Unscrew applicator from tube.
5. Lie on back with knees drawn up. Gently insert applicator deeply into the vagina and press plunger downward to its original position.

To cleanse the applicator, pull the plunger to remove it from the barrel, then wash with mild soap and warm water. Do not boil or use hot water.

■ *If you miss a dose...*
Take the forgotten dose as soon as you remember. If it is almost time for the next dose, skip the one you missed and go back to your regular schedule. Never try to "catch up" by doubling the dose.

■ *Storage instructions...*
Store at room temperature.

What side effects may occur?
Side effects cannot be anticipated. If any develop or change in intensity, inform your doctor immediately. Only your doctor can determine whether it is safe to continue taking Premarin.

■ *Side effects may include:*
Abdominal cramps, abnormal vaginal bleeding, bloating, blood clots, breast swelling and tenderness, depression, dizziness, enlargement of benign tumors in the uterus, fluid retention, gallbladder disease, hair loss from the scalp, increased body hair, inflammation of the pancreas, intolerance to contact lenses, migraine headache, nausea, vomiting, sex-drive changes, skin darkening, especially on the face, skin rash or redness, swelling of wrists and ankles, vaginal yeast infection, vomiting, weight gain or loss, yellow eyes and skin

■ *Other possible side effects of Premphase and Prempro:*
Appetite changes, backache, changes in blood pressure, excessive flow of breast milk, eye disorders, fatigue, fever, headache, nervousness, sleep disturbances, twitching

Why should this drug not be prescribed?
Do not take Premarin if you have ever had a bad reaction to it, or have undiagnosed abnormal vaginal bleeding.

Except in certain special circumstances, you should not be given Premarin if you have breast cancer or any other "estrogen-dependent" cancer.

Do not take Premarin if you have had any heart or circulation problem including a tendency for abnormal blood clotting.

Special warnings about this medication
The risk of cancer of the uterus increases when estrogen is used for a long time or taken in large doses.

There may be an increased risk of breast cancer in women who take estrogen for a long time. If you have a family history of breast cancer or have ever had an abnormal mammogram, you need to have more frequent breast examinations.

Women who take Premarin after menopause are more likely to develop gallbladder disease.

Premarin also increases the risk of blood clots. These blood clots can cause stroke, heart attack, or other serious disorders.

While taking Premarin, get in touch with your doctor right away if you notice any of the following:

Abdominal pain, tenderness, or swelling
Abnormal bleeding from the vagina
Breast lumps
Coughing up blood
Pain in your chest or calves
Severe headache, dizziness, or faintness
Sudden shortness of breath
Vision changes
Yellowing of the skin

If you have high levels of fat in your blood, specifically a high triglyceride level, conjugated estrogens are likely to cause side effects in the pancreas.

Possible food and drug interactions
when taking this medication
If Premarin is taken with certain other drugs, the effects of either could be increased, decreased, or altered. It is especially important to check with your doctor before combining Premarin with the following:

Barbiturates such as phenobarbital
Blood thinners such as Coumadin
Drugs used for epilepsy, such as Dilantin
Major tranquilizers such as Thorazine
Oral diabetes drugs such as Micronase
Rifampin (Rifadin)
Steroid medications such as Deltasone
Thyroid preparations such as Synthroid
Tricyclic antidepressants such as Elavil and Tofranil
Vitamin C

Special information
if you are pregnant or breastfeeding

If you are pregnant or plan to become pregnant, notify your doctor immediately. Premarin should not be taken during pregnancy because of the possibility of harm to the unborn child. Premarin cannot prevent a miscarriage. Estrogens can decrease the quantity and quality of breast milk, and progestins appear in breast milk. Your doctor may advise you not to breastfeed while you are taking this drug.

Recommended dosage

Your doctor will start therapy with this medication at a low dose. He or she will want to check you periodically at 3- to 6-month intervals to determine the need for continued therapy.

PREMARIN TABLETS

Hot Flashes Associated with Menopause

The usual dosage is 0.3 to 1.25 milligrams daily. If you are still having periods, the doctor will start the Premarin on the fifth day of your cycle, have you take it for 3 weeks, then give you 1 week off.

Tissue Degeneration in the Vagina

The usual dosage is 0.3 to 1.25 milligrams or more daily. The drug is taken cyclically (3 weeks on and 1 week off).

Low Estrogen Levels Due to Reduced Ovary Function

The usual dosage is 2.5 to 7.5 milligrams daily, taken in several small doses, for 20 days, followed by a 10-day rest period. If you do not have your period by the end of this time, the same dosage schedule is repeated.

If you start to bleed before the end of the 10-day period your doctor will start you on another 20-day cycle, with an oral progestin added during the last 5 days. If you start to bleed before the second cycle is over, stop taking the medication and tell your doctor.

Ovary Removal or Ovarian Failure
The usual dosage is 1.25 milligrams daily, cyclically (3 weeks on and 1 week off). Your doctor will adjust the dosage according to the severity of your symptoms and your response to treatment.

Prevention of Osteoporosis (Loss of Bone Mass)
The usual dosage is 0.625 milligram daily, taken cyclically (3 weeks on and 1 week off).

Advanced Androgen-Dependent Cancer of the Prostate, for Relief of Symptoms Only
The usual dosage is 1.25 to 2.5 milligrams 3 times daily.

Breast Cancer (for Relief of Symptoms Only) in Appropriately Selected Women and Men with Metastatic Disease
The suggested dosage is 10 milligrams 3 times daily for a period of at least 3 months. Tell your doctor if you have any unusual bleeding.

PREMARIN VAGINAL CREAM

Given cyclically for short-term use only.

Degeneration of Genital Tissue or Severe Itching in the Genital Area
The recommended dosage is one-half to 2 grams daily, inserted into the vagina, depending on the severity of the condition. You will use the cream for 3 weeks, then stop for 1 week. Tell your doctor if you notice any unusual bleeding.

PREMPHASE TABLETS

Follow a 28-day cycle. Take 1 maroon Premarin tablet every day for the first 14 days; on the 15th day, begin taking 1 light-blue tablet daily.

PREMPRO TABLETS

The usual starting dose is one 0.625-milligram/2.5-milligram tablet once a day. If this dose proves insufficient, your doctor may increase the dose to one 0.625-milligram/5-milligram tablet once a day.

Overdosage

Any medication taken in excess can have serious consequences. If you suspect an overdose of Premarin, seek medical attention immediately.

■ *Symptoms of Premphase/Prempro overdose may include:*
Nausea, vomiting, withdrawal bleeding

Brand name:

PREMPHASE

See Premarin, page 1036.

Brand name:

PREMPRO

See Premarin, page 1036.

Generic name:

PRENATAL VITAMINS AND MINERALS

See Stuartnatal Plus, page 1223.

Brand name:

PREVACID

Pronounced: PREH-va-sid
Generic name: Lansoprazole

Why is this drug prescribed?

Prevacid blocks the production of stomach acid. It is prescribed for the short-term treatment (up to 4 weeks) of duodenal ulcers (ulcers near the exit from the stomach). It is also used for up to 8 weeks in the treatment of stomach ulcers and a condition called erosive esophagitis (a severe inflammation of the passage to the stomach). Once a duodenal ulcer or case of esophagitis has cleared up, the doctor may continue prescribing Prevacid to prevent a relapse. The drug is also used for long-term treatment of certain diseases marked by excessive acid production, such as Zollinger-Ellison syndrome.

Prevacid is also prescribed as part of a combination treatment to eliminate the *H. pylori* bacterium that causes most cases of duodenal ulcer.

Most important fact about this drug
To relieve your symptoms and to heal your ulcer, you need to take Prevacid for the full time of treatment your doctor prescribes. Keep taking the drug even if you begin to feel better, and be sure to keep your appointments with your doctor.

How should you take this medication?
Prevacid should be taken before meals. If you have trouble swallowing the capsules, open them and sprinkle the granules on a tablespoon of applesauce; swallow immediately. Do not chew or crush the granules.

If you are taking antacids for pain, you may continue to do so. You also may continue to take sucralfate (Carafate), but take your dose of Prevacid at least 30 minutes prior to the Carafate.

■ *If you miss a dose...*
Take it as soon as you remember. If it is almost time for your next dose, skip the one you missed and go back to your regular schedule. Do not take 2 doses at once.

■ *Storage instructions...*
Store at room temperature in a tightly closed container. Keep away from moisture.

What side effects may occur?
Side effects cannot be anticipated. If any develop or change in intensity, tell your doctor as soon as possible. Only your doctor can determine if it is safe for you to continue taking Prevacid.

■ *More common side effects may include:*
Diarrhea

■ *Less common side effects may include:*
Abdominal pain, nausea

■ *Rare side effects may include:*
Abnormal thinking, acne, aggravation of hostility, agitation, anemia, anxiety, apathy, arthritis, asthma, bad breath, belching, black or discolored stools, blood in the urine, breast development in males, breast enlargement, breast tenderness, bronchitis, chest pain (including severe pain), colitis, confusion, constipation, cough, coughing up blood, deafness, decreased sex drive, depression, diabetes, difficult or labored breathing, difficulty swallowing, dizziness, dry mouth, ear infection, eye pain, fainting, fever, fluid retention, "flu-like" symptoms, flushing, gallstones,

gas, general feeling of illness, gout, hair loss, hallucinations, heart attack, hiccups, high blood pressure, high or low blood sugar, hives, impotence, increased appetite, increased salivation, indigestion, infection, inflammation of the esophagus or mouth, inflammation of the stomach lining, itching, kidney problems, kidney stones, loss of appetite, low blood pressure, memory loss, menstrual problems, muscle, bone, or joint pain, nervousness, nosebleeds, paralysis, pneumonia, prickling, tingling, or pins and needles, rash, rectal hemorrhage, rectal and bladder spasms, ringing in ears, shock, sore throat, stomach and intestinal hemorrhage, stroke, taste alteration, thirst, throbbing heartbeat, thyroid problems, visual disturbances, vomiting blood, weakness, weight gain or loss, wheezing, yeast infection

Why should this drug not be prescribed?
Avoid Prevacid if you have ever had an allergic reaction to it.

Special warnings about this medication
Do not take Prevacid any longer than your doctor has prescribed; this medication should not be used for long-term therapy of duodenal ulcer or erosive esophagitis.

If you have liver disease, be sure your doctor knows about it. Prevacid should be used cautiously.

If you do not begin to feel better on Prevacid therapy, or if your symptoms become worse, be sure to call your doctor.

Prevacid has no effect on stomach cancer. It could be present even if Prevacid relieves your symptoms.

Possible food and drug interactions
when taking this medication
If Prevacid is taken with certain other drugs, the effects of either could be increased, decreased, or altered. It is especially important to check with your doctor before combining Prevacid with the following:

Ampicillin
Digoxin (Lanoxin)
Iron salts (Ferro-Sequels, Ferro-Sulfate)
Ketoconazole (Nizoral)
Sucralfate (Carafate)
Theophylline (Theo-Dur)

Special information
if you are pregnant or breastfeeding

The effects of Prevacid in pregnant women have not been adequately studied. If you are pregnant or plan to become pregnant, tell your doctor. It is not known whether Prevacid appears in human breast milk. If this medication is essential to your health, your doctor may have you stop breastfeeding your baby while you are taking it.

Recommended dosage

ADULTS

For treatment of duodenal ulcer

The usual dose is 15 milligrams once daily, before eating, for 4 weeks.

To prevent relapse of duodenal ulcer

Take 15 milligrams once a day.

To eradicate ulcer-causing bacteria

To eliminate the *H. pylori* bacteria that cause most duodenal ulcers, Prevacid is taken with amoxicillin alone or amoxicillin and Biaxin. When combined with amoxicillin only, the usual dosage is 30 milligrams of Prevacid and 1 gram of amoxicillin 3 times daily for 14 days. If all three drugs are used, the usual dosage is 30 milligrams of Prevacid, 1 gram of amoxicillin, and 500 milligrams of Biaxin twice daily for 10 to 14 days.

For treatment of stomach ulcer

The usual dose is 30 milligrams once a day for up to 8 weeks.

For treatment of erosive esophagitis

The usual dose is 30 milligrams daily, before eating, for up to 8 weeks. Depending on your response to the medication your doctor may suggest another 8-week treatment regimen.

Other excess acid conditions (such as Zollinger-Ellison syndrome)

The usual starting dose is 60 milligrams once daily. This dose can be adjusted upward by your doctor, depending on your response. Dosages totalling more than 120 milligrams a day should be divided into smaller doses. If you have severe liver disease, your doctor will tailor your dosage to fit your needs.

CHILDREN

The safety and effectiveness of Prevacid have not been established in children.

Overdosage

Overdoses of Prevacid are not known to cause any problems. Nevertheless, no medication should be taken in excess. If you suspect an overdose, seek medical attention immediately.

Brand name:

PREVPAC

Pronounced: PREV-pack
Generic name: Amoxicillin, Clarithromycin, and
*   Lansoprazole*

Why is this drug prescribed?

Prevpac is a prepackaged combination of drugs designed to cure duodenal ulcers caused by *H. pylori* bacteria, the most common source of ulcers. With two antibiotics and an acid-blocking agent, Prevpac will eradicate the *H. pylori* infection and improve your odds of remaining ulcer-free. This type of therapy is usually reserved for people with an active ulcer and those who've had one for at least a year.

Most important fact about this drug

Prevpac will work only if you take all the medications as prescribed and finish your entire course of therapy. If you stop too soon, the ulcer may not heal completely and your symptoms may return.

How should you take this medication?

Each pack contains a full day's supply of medication, consisting of two 30-milligram capsules of lansoprazole (Prevacid), four 500-milligram capsules of amoxicillin, and two 500-milligram tablets of clarithromycin (Biaxin). Take half the supply before breakfast and the remainder before dinner. Swallow each pill whole; do not crush or chew.

■ *If you miss a dose...*
Take it as soon as you remember. If it is almost time for your next dose, skip the one you missed and go back to your regular schedule. Do not take 2 doses at the same time.

■ *Storage instructions...*
Store at room temperature, away from light and moisture.

What side effects may occur?
Side effects cannot be anticipated. If any develop or change in intensity, inform your doctor as soon as possible. Only your doctor can determine if it is safe for you to continue taking Prevpac.

■ *More common side effects may include:*
Diarrhea, headache, taste disturbances

■ *Less common and rare side effects may include:*
Abdominal pain, confusion, dark stools, dizziness, dry mouth, mouth infection, mouth sores, muscle aches, rectal itching, nausea, respiratory problems, skin reactions, thirst, tongue swelling or discoloration, vaginal infections, vaginal inflammation, vomiting

Why should this drug not be prescribed?
You cannot use Prevpac if you've ever had an allergic reaction to antibiotics such as amoxicillin, erythromycin, penicillin, or Biaxin. Also avoid Prevpac if you've had a reaction to a cephalosporin-type antibiotic such as Ceclor, Duricef, and Keflex.

While on Prevpac therapy, be sure to avoid taking Seldane, Propulsid, and Orap. Combining any of these drugs with Prevpac could cause serious heart irregularities.

Special warnings about this medication
If you develop severe diarrhea after taking Prevpac, call your doctor. Prevpac therapy is not recommended if you have severe kidney disease. Use Prevpac with caution if you are over 65 years old.

**Possible food and drug interactions
when taking this medication**
If Prevpac is taken with certain other drugs, the effects of either could be increased, decreased, or altered. It is especially important to check with your doctor before combining Prevpac with the following:

Ampicillin
Astemizole (Hismanal)
Blood-thinning pills such as Warfarin (Coumadin)
Bromocriptine (Parlodel)
Carbamazepine (Tegretol)
Cisapride (Propulsid)
Cyclosporine (Neoral, Sandimmune)
Digoxin (Lanoxin)
Disopyramide (Norpace)

Ergotamine-based drugs for migraine such as Cafergot, D.H.E. 45
  Injection, Ergostat, and Migranal Nasal Spray
Ketoconazole (Nizoral)
Iron supplements
Lovastatin (Mevacor)
Phenytoin (Dilantin)
Pimozide (Orap)
Sucralfate (Carafate)
Tacrolimus (Prograf)
Terfenadine (Seldane)
Theophylline (Theo-Dur, Theolair)
Triazolam (Halcion)

Special information
if you are pregnant or breastfeeding
Do not use Prevpac during pregnancy. The Biaxin component can harm the
developing baby. You should also avoid Prevpac while breastfeeding.

Recommended dosage

ADULTS

The recommended dosage is 1 capsule of lansoprazole (Prevacid), 2 capsules
of amoxicillin, and 1 tablet of clarithromycin (Biaxin) taken together twice a
day (morning and evening) for 14 days.

Your doctor will adjust your dose if you have kidney problems.

Overdosage
Any medication taken in excess can have serious consequences. If you
suspect an overdose of Prevpac, seek medical attention immediately.

Brand name:

PRILOSEC

Pronounced: PRILL-oh-sek
Generic name: Omeprazole

Why is this drug prescribed?
Prilosec is prescribed for the short-term treatment (4 to 8 weeks) of
stomach ulcer, duodenal ulcer (near the exit from the stomach), and erosive
esophagitis (inflammation of the esophagus), and for the treatment of
heartburn and other symptoms of gastroesophageal reflux disease (backflow
of acid stomach contents into the canal leading to the stomach). It is also
used to maintain healing of erosive esophagitis and for the long-term

treatment of conditions in which too much stomach acid is secreted, including Zollinger-Ellison syndrome, multiple endocrine adenomas (benign tumors), and systemic mastocytosis (cancerous cells).

Combined with the antibiotic clarithromycin (Biaxin), Prilosec is also used to cure patients whose ulcers are caused by infection with the germ *H. pylori*.

Most important fact about this drug
Prilosec's healing effect can mask the signs of stomach cancer. Your doctor should be careful to rule out this possibility.

How should you take this medication?
Prilosec works best when taken before meals. It can be taken with an antacid.

The capsule should be swallowed whole. It should not be opened, chewed, or crushed.

Avoid excessive amounts of caffeine while taking this drug.

It may take several days for Prilosec to begin relieving stomach pain. Be sure to continue taking the drug exactly as prescribed even if it seems to have no effect.

■ *If you miss a dose...*
Take it as soon as you remember. If it is almost time for your next dose, skip the one you missed and go back to your regular schedule. Do not take 2 doses at once.

■ *Storage information...*
Store at room temperature in a tightly closed container, away from light and moisture.

What side effects may occur?
Side effects cannot be anticipated. If any develop or change in intensity, inform your doctor as soon as possible. Only your doctor can determine if it is safe for you to continue taking Prilosec.

■ *More common side effects may include:*
Abdominal pain, diarrhea, headache, nausea, vomiting

■ *Less common or rare side effects may include:*
Abdominal swelling, abnormal dreams, aggression, anemia, anxiety, apathy, back pain, blood in urine, breast development in males, changes in liver function, chest pain, confusion, constipation, cough, depression, difficulty sleeping, discolored feces, dizziness, dry mouth, dry skin, fatigue, fever, fluid retention and swelling, fluttery heartbeat, frequent urination, gas, general

feeling of illness, hair loss, hallucinations, hepatitis, high blood pressure, hives, irritable colon, itching, joint and leg pain, loss of appetite, low blood sugar, muscle cramps and pain, nervousness, nosebleeds, pain, pain in testicles, rapid heartbeat, rash, ringing in ears, skin inflammation, sleepiness, slow heartbeat, stomach tumors, taste distortion, throat pain, tingling or pins and needles, tremors, upper respiratory infection, urinary tract infection, vertigo, weakness, weight gain, yellow eyes and skin

■ *When taken with Biaxin, side effects also may include:*
Flu symptoms, nasal inflammation, sore throat, taste alteration, tongue discoloration

Why should this drug not be prescribed?

If you are sensitive to or have ever had an allergic reaction to Prilosec or any of its ingredients, you should not take this medication. Make sure your doctor is aware of any drug reactions you have experienced.

You should avoid the Prilosec/Biaxin combination treatment if you are allergic to certain antibiotics called macrolides or if you are taking Orap, Propulsid, or Seldane.

Special warnings about this medication

Long-term use of this drug can cause severe stomach inflammation.

Possible food and drug interactions
when taking this medication

If Prilosec is taken with certain other drugs, the effects of either could be increased, decreased, or altered. It is especially important to check with your doctor before combining Prilosec with the following:

Ampicillin-containing drugs such as Unasyn
Cyclosporine (Sandimmune, Neoral)
Diazepam (Valium)
Disulfiram (Antabuse)
Iron
Ketoconazole (Nizoral)
Phenytoin (Dilantin)
Warfarin (Coumadin)

When taking the Prilosec/Biaxin combination treatment, it's best to avoid the hay-fever remedy Hismanal.

Special information
if you are pregnant or breastfeeding

The effects of Prilosec during pregnancy have not been adequately studied. If you are pregnant or plan to become pregnant, inform your doctor immediately. Avoid combined therapy with Biaxin unless there is no alternative. Prilosec (and Biaxin) may appear in breast milk and could affect a nursing infant. If this medication is essential to your health, your doctor may advise you to discontinue breastfeeding until your treatment with this medication is finished.

Recommended dosage

ADULTS

Short-term Treatment of Active Duodenal Ulcer
The usual dose is 20 milligrams once a day. Most people heal within 4 weeks.

Prevention of Duodenal Ulcers Caused by H. Pylori
The usual dosage is 40 milligrams of Prilosec every morning and 500 milligrams of clarithromycin 3 times a day, for 14 days, followed by 20 milligrams of Prilosec daily for an additional 14 days.

Gastric Ulcer
The usual dose is 40 milligrams once a day for 4 to 8 weeks.

Gastroesophageal Reflux Disease (GERD)
The usual dose for people with symptoms of GERD is 20 milligrams daily for up to 4 weeks. For erosive esophagitis accompanied by GERD symptoms, the usual dose is 20 milligrams a day for 4 to 8 weeks. The dose may be continued to maintain healing.

Pathological Hypersecretory Conditions
The usual starting dose is 60 milligrams once a day. If you take more than 80 milligrams a day, your doctor will divide the total into smaller doses. The dosing will be based on your needs.

CHILDREN

The safety and effectiveness of Prilosec in children have not been established.

Overdosage

Overdose with Prilosec has been rare, but any medication taken in excess can have serious consequences. If you suspect an overdose, seek medical attention immediately.

■ *Symptoms of Prilosec overdose may include:*
Blurred vision, confusion, drowsiness, dry mouth, flushing, headache, nausea, rapid heartbeat, sweating

Generic name:

PRIMIDONE

See Mysoline, page 844.

Brand name:

PRINCIPEN

See Omnipen, page 922.

Brand name:

PRINIVIL

See Zestril, page 1457.

Brand name:

PRINZIDE

See Zestoretic, page 1452.

Generic name:

PROCAINAMIDE

See Procan SR, below.

Brand name:

PROCANBID

See Procan SR, below.

Brand name:

PROCAN SR

Pronounced: PROH-can
Generic name: Procainamide hydrochloride
Other brand names: Procanbid, Pronestyl-SR

Why is this drug prescribed?
Procan SR is used to treat severe irregular heartbeats (arrhythmias). Arrhythmias are generally divided into two main types: heartbeats that are faster than normal (tachycardia), and heartbeats that are slower than normal

(bradycardia). Irregular heartbeats are often caused by drugs or disease but can occur in otherwise healthy people with no history of heart disease or other illness.

Most important fact about this drug

Procan SR can cause serious blood disorders, especially during the first 3 months of treatment. Be sure to notify your doctor if you notice any of the following: joint or muscle pain, dark urine, yellowing of skin or eyes, muscular weakness, chest or abdominal pain, appetite loss, diarrhea, hallucinations, dizziness, depression, wheezing, cough, easy bruising or bleeding, tremors, palpitations, rash, soreness or ulcers in the mouth, sore throat, fever, and chills.

How should you take this medication?

Take only your prescribed doses of Procan SR; never take more.

Procan SR should be swallowed whole. Do not break or chew the tablet. You may see the tablet matrix of Procan SR in your stool, since it does not disintegrate following release of procainamide.

Try not to miss any doses. Skipping doses, changing the intervals between doses, or "making up" missed doses by doubling up later may cause your condition to worsen and could be dangerous.

■ *If you miss a dose...*
Take it as soon as you remember if it is within 4 hours of your scheduled time. If you do not remember until later, skip the dose you missed and go back to your regular schedule. Never take 2 doses at the same time.

■ *Storage instructions...*
Store at room temperature in a tightly closed container, away from heat, light, and moisture.

What side effects may occur?

Side effects cannot be anticipated. If any develop or change in intensity, inform your doctor as soon as possible. Only your doctor can determine if it is safe for you to continue taking Procan SR.

■ *More common side effects may include:*
Abdominal pain, bitter taste, diarrhea, loss of appetite, nausea, symptoms similar to those of lupus erythematosus, an inflammatory disease of the

connective tissue (joint pain or inflammation, abdominal or chest pain, fever, chills, muscle pain, skin lesions), vomiting

■ *Less common side effects may include:*
Depression, dizziness, fluid retention, flushing, giddiness, hallucinations, hives, itching, rash, weakness

■ *Rare side effects may include:*
Anemia, changes in blood counts, low blood pressure

Why should this drug not be prescribed?
Procan SR should not be taken if you have the heart irregularity known as complete heart block or incomplete heart block without a pacemaker, or if you have ever had an allergic reaction to procaine or similar local anesthetics.

Your doctor will not prescribe this drug if you have been diagnosed with the connective-tissue disease lupus erythematosus or the heartbeat irregularity known as torsade de pointes.

Special warnings about this medication
To check for the serious blood disorders that can develop during Procan SR therapy, your doctor will do a complete blood count weekly for the first 12 weeks and will continue to monitor your blood count carefully after that.

If you develop a fever, chills, sore throat or mouth, bruising or bleeding, infections, chest or abdominal pain, loss of appetite, weakness, muscle or joint pain, skin rash, nausea, fluttery heartbeat, vomiting, diarrhea, hallucinations, dizziness, depression, wheezing, yellow eyes and skin, or dark urine, contact your doctor immediately. It could indicate a serious illness.

Use Procan SR cautiously if you have ever had congestive heart failure or other types of heart disease.

Your doctor will prescribe Procan SR along with other antiarrhythmic drugs, such as quinidine or disopyramide, only if they have been tried and have not worked when used alone.

If you have ever had kidney disease, liver disease, or myasthenia gravis (a disease that causes muscle weakness, especially in the face and neck), your doctor will watch you carefully while you are taking Procan SR.

Make sure your doctor is aware of any drug reactions you have experienced, especially to procaine, other local anesthetics, or aspirin.

Possible food and drug interactions
when taking this medication

If Procan SR is taken with certain other drugs, the effects of either could be increased, decreased, or altered. It is especially important to check with your doctor before combining Procan SR with the following:

Alcohol

Amiodarone (Cordarone)

Antiarrhythmic drugs such as quinidine (Quinidex), propranolol (Inderal), and mexiletine (Mexitil)

Cimetidine (Tagamet)

Drugs that ease muscle spasms, such as Cogentin and Artane

Lidocaine

Ranitidine (Zantac)

Trimethoprim (Proloprim)

Special information
if you are pregnant or breastfeeding

The effects of Procan SR during pregnancy have not been adequately studied. If you are pregnant or plan to become pregnant, inform your doctor immediately. Procan SR appears in breast milk and may affect a nursing infant. If this medication is essential to your health, your doctor may advise you to discontinue breastfeeding until your treatment is finished.

Recommended dosage

ADULTS

Dosages and intervals between doses will be adjusted for you, based on your doctor's assessment of the degree of underlying heart disease, your age, and the way your kidneys are functioning.

Younger people with normal kidney function will start with a total daily oral dose of up to 50 milligrams per 2.2 pounds of body weight, divided into smaller doses and taken every 6 hours (Procan SR) or divided into 2 doses and taken every 12 hours (Procanbid).

Older people, especially those over 50 years of age, or those with reduced kidney, liver, or heart function will get lower doses or wait a longer time between doses; this may decrease the probability of side effects that are related to the size of the dose.

CHILDREN

The safety and effectiveness of this drug have not been established in children.

Overdosage

Any medication taken in excess can have serious consequences. If you suspect an overdose, seek medical treatment immediately.

- *Symptoms of Procan SR overdose may include:*
  Changes in heart function and heartbeat

Brand name:

PROCARDIA

Pronounced: pro-CAR-dee-uh
Generic name: Nifedipine
Other brand names: Procardia XL, Adalat, Adalat CC

Why is this drug prescribed?

Procardia and Procardia XL are used to treat angina (chest pain caused by lack of oxygen to the heart due to clogged arteries or spasm of the arteries). Procardia XL is also used to treat high blood pressure. Procardia and Procardia XL are calcium channel blockers. They ease the workload of the heart by relaxing the muscles in the walls of the arteries, allowing them to dilate. This improves blood flow through the heart and throughout the body, reduces blood pressure, and helps prevent angina. Procardia XL is taken once a day and provides a steady rate of medication over a 24-hour period.

Most important fact about this drug

If you have high blood pressure, you must take Procardia XL regularly for it to be effective. Since blood pressure declines gradually, it may be several weeks before you get the full benefit of Procardia XL; and you must continue taking it even if you are feeling well. Procardia XL does not cure high blood pressure; it merely keeps it under control.

How should you take this medication?

Procardia and Procardia XL should be taken exactly as prescribed by your doctor, even if your symptoms have disappeared.

Procardia XL tablets are specially designed to release the medication into your bloodstream slowly. As a result, something that looks like a tablet may occasionally appear in your stool. This is normal and simply means that the medication has been released, and the shell that contained the medication has been eliminated from your body.

Procardia and Procardia XL tablets should be swallowed whole. Do not break, crush, or chew.

Procardia and Procardia XL can be taken with or without food.

Do not substitute another brand of nifedipine for Procardia or Procardia XL unless your doctor directs.

Procardia XL should be taken once a day. You can take it in the morning or evening, but should hold to the same time each day.

■ *If you miss a dose...*
Take the forgotten dose as soon as you remember. If it is almost time for your next dose, skip the one you missed. Never take 2 doses at the same time.

■ *Storage instructions...*
Procardia and Procardia XL can be stored at room temperature. Protect from moisture, light, humidity, and excessive heat.

What side effects may occur?
Side effects cannot be anticipated. If any develop or change in intensity, inform your doctor as soon as possible. Only your doctor can determine whether it is safe for you to continue taking Procardia or Procardia XL.

■ *More common side effects may include:*
Constipation, cough, dizziness, fatigue, flushing, giddiness, headache, heartburn, heat sensation, light-headedness, mood changes, muscle cramps, nasal congestion, nausea, sore throat, swelling of arms, legs, hands, and feet, tremors, wheezing

■ *Less common side effects may include:*
Abdominal pain, blurred vision, chest congestion, chills, cramps, diarrhea, difficult or labored breathing, difficulty in balance, difficulty sleeping, drowsiness, dry cough, dry mouth, excessive sweating, fever, fluttering heartbeat, gas, general chest pain, hives, impotence, indigestion, itching, jitteriness, joint pain, leg cramps, muscle and bone inflammation, nervousness, pain, production of large amounts of pale urine, rash, sexual difficulties, shakiness, shortness of breath, skin inflammation, sleep disturbances, sleepiness, stiff joints, tingling or pins and needles, weakness

■ *Rare side effects may include:*
Abnormal or terrifying dreams, anemia, anxiety, arthritis, back pain, belching, blood in the urine, breast development in males, breast pain,

breathing disorders, dark stools containing blood, decreased sex drive, depression, distorted taste, dulled sense of touch, excessive urination at night, facial swelling, fainting, fever, gout, gum overgrowth, hair loss, hepatitis, hives, hot flashes, increased angina, increased sweating, inflammation of the sinuses, inflamed and peeling skin and other skin disorders, irregular heartbeat, migraine, muscle incoordination, muscle pain, muscle tension, nosebleeds, painful or difficult urination, paranoia, rapid heartbeat, reddish or purplish spots under the skin, ringing in the ears, sensitivity to light, swelling around the eyes or mouth and throat with breathing difficulty, tearing eyes, temporary blindness, upper respiratory tract infection, vague feeling of illness, vertigo, vision changes, vomiting, weight gain

Why should this drug not be prescribed?

Procardia should not be used if you have ever had an allergic reaction to it or are sensitive to it or other calcium channel blockers (Adalat, Calan, others). Make sure your doctor is aware of any drug reactions you have experienced.

Special warnings about this medication

Procardia and Procardia XL may cause your blood pressure to become too low, which may make you feel light-headed or faint. This is more likely to happen when you start taking the medication and when the amount you take is increased. It is also more likely to occur if you are also taking a beta-blocker heart medication such as Tenormin or Inderal. Your doctor should check your blood pressure when you start taking Procardia or Procardia XL and continue monitoring it while your dosage is being adjusted.

Procardia XL can be used for high blood pressure; plain Procardia should be used only for angina—NOT for high blood pressure.

Do not take Procardia for the first week or two following a heart attack, or if you are in danger of a heart attack.

There is a remote possibility of experiencing increased angina when you start taking Procardia or Procardia XL, or when your dosage is increased. If this happens, contact your doctor immediately.

You may have angina pain if you suddenly stop taking beta blockers when beginning Procardia therapy. Your doctor will taper you off the other drug.

If you have tight aortic stenosis (a narrowing of the aortic valve that obstructs blood flow from the heart to the body) and have been taking a beta blocker, your doctor will monitor you carefully while you are taking Procardia or Procardia XL.

If you develop swelling of the arms, hands, legs, and feet, your doctor can prescribe a diuretic (water pill) to relieve the problem.

Procardia XL should be used cautiously if you have any stomach or intestinal narrowing.

Notify your doctor or dentist that you are taking Procardia if you have a medical emergency, and before you have surgery or dental treatment.

This drug is not recommended for use in children.

Possible food and drug interactions
when taking this medication

If Procardia or Procardia XL is taken with certain other drugs, the effects of either could be increased, decreased, or altered. It is especially important to check with your doctor before combining Procardia or Procardia XL with the following:

Cimetidine (Tagamet)
Digoxin (Lanoxin)
Quinidine (Quinaglute, Quinidex)

Taking Procardia with double-concentrated grapefruit juice can dramatically increase the effect of the drug.

Special information
if you are pregnant or breastfeeding

The effects of Procardia and Procardia XL during pregnancy have not been adequately studied, although new animal research points to possible birth defects in humans. If you are pregnant or plan to become pregnant, inform your doctor immediately. It is not known whether Procardia or Procardia XL appears in breast milk and can affect a nursing infant. If this medication is essential to your health, your doctor may advise you to discontinue breastfeeding until your treatment is finished.

Recommended dosage

ADULTS

The usual starting dose of Procardia is one 10-milligram capsule, 3 times a day. The usual range is 10 to 20 milligrams 3 times a day. Some people may need 20 to 30 milligrams, 3 or 4 times a day. Usually you will not take more than 120 milligrams in a day and should take no more than 180 milligrams.

The starting dose of Procardia XL is usually a 30- or 60-milligram tablet, taken once daily. Your doctor may increase the dose over 1 to 2 weeks if not satisfied with the way the drug is working. Doses above 120 milligrams per day are not recommended.

Although no serious side effects have been reported when Procardia XL is stopped, your doctor will probably have you lower the dose gradually under close supervision.

Overdosage

Any medication taken in excess can have serious consequences. If you suspect an overdose, seek medical treatment immediately.

- *Symptoms of Procardia overdose may include:*
  Dizziness, drowsiness, nausea, severe drop in blood pressure, slurred speech, weakness

Generic name:

PROCHLORPERAZINE

See Compazine, page 286.

Generic name:

PROMETHAZINE

See Phenergan, page 990.

Generic name:

PROMETHAZINE WITH CODEINE

See Phenergan with Codeine, page 994.

Brand name:

PRONESTYL-SR

See Procan SR, page 1051.

Generic name:

PROPAFENONE

See Rythmol, page 1161.

Brand name:

PROPECIA

Pronounced: pro-PEE-she-ah
Generic name: Finasteride

Why is this drug prescribed?

Propecia is a remedy for baldness in men with mild to moderate hair loss on the top of the head and the front of the mid-scalp area. It increases hair growth, improves hair regrowth, and slows down hair loss. It works only on scalp hair and does not affect hair on other parts of the body.

You may begin to see improvement as early as 3 months after you begin taking Propecia, but for many men it takes longer. The improvement lasts only as long as you take the drug; if you stop, new hair growth will cease and hair loss will resume.

Propecia is a low-dose form of Proscar, a drug prescribed for prostate enlargement.

Most important fact about this drug

Propecia is NOT for use by women. If taken during pregnancy, it can cause abnormal development of a male baby's genital organs.

How should you take this medication?

For maximum benefit, take Propecia regularly once a day. It can be taken with or without food.

- *If you miss a dose...*
  Take it as soon as you remember. If it is almost time for your next dose, skip the one you missed and go back to your regular schedule. Do not take 2 doses at the same time.

- *Storage instructions...*
  Store at room temperature in a closed container away from moisture.

What side effects may occur?

Propecia's side effects are primarily sexual, and relatively uncommon—they strike one or two men in a hundred. If any side effects develop or change in intensity, inform your doctor as soon as possible. Only your doctor can determine if it is safe for you to continue taking Propecia.

■ *Side effects may include:*
Decreased amount of semen per ejaculation, decreased sex drive, impotence

Why should this drug not be prescribed?
Due to the drug's effect on male babies, women should avoid Propecia if there is any chance that they may be pregnant.

Do not use Propecia if it gives you an allergic reaction, or if you've ever had an allergic reaction to its chemical twin, Proscar.

Special warnings about this medication
If there's even a possibility that they're pregnant, women should avoid handling a crushed or broken Propecia tablet for fear of absorbing some of the active ingredient through the skin. Whole tablets are safe to handle thanks to a protective outer coating.

Use Propecia with caution if you have liver problems.

Propecia lowers readings of the PSA screening test for prostate cancer. If you're scheduled to have your PSA level checked, make sure the doctor knows you're taking Propecia.

Possible food and drug interactions
when taking this medication
No significant drug interactions have been reported.

Special information
if you are pregnant or breastfeeding
Avoid even touching the active ingredient in Propecia if there's a chance that you're pregnant.

Recommended dosage

ADULT MEN
The recommended dosage, for men only, is 1 tablet daily.

Overdosage
Although no specific information is available on Propecia overdose, any medication taken in excess can have serious consequences. If you suspect an overdose, seek medical attention immediately.

Brand name:

PROPINE

Pronounced: PROH-peen
Generic name: Dipivefrin hydrochloride

Why is this drug prescribed?
Propine is used to treat chronic open-angle glaucoma, the most common form of the disease. In glaucoma, the fluid inside the eyeball is under abnormally high pressure, a condition which can cause vision problems or even blindness.

Propine belongs to a class of medication called "prodrugs," drugs that generally are not active by themselves, but are converted in the body to an active form. This makes for better absorption, stability, and comfort and reduces side effects.

Most important fact about this drug
There is no cure for glaucoma. Propine and similar drugs can keep ocular pressure under control, but only as long as you take them. You will probably need to continue treatment for life; and you must be sure to take the medication regularly.

How should you use this medication?
Use this medication exactly as prescribed. If you use too much, or use it too often, Propine may cause side effects.

Wash your hands before and after you use the eyedrops. Once the drops are in your eye, keep your eye closed for 1 to 2 minutes, applying pressure to the inside corner of your eye, so the medicine can be properly absorbed.

To keep the medication free of contamination, do not touch the applicator tip to your eye or any other surface.

A number appears on the cap of the dropper bottle to tell you what dose you are taking. When you are ready to take the first dose, make sure the number 1 appears in the window. After each dose, replace the cap and rotate it to the next number. Turn until you hear a click.

■ *If you miss a dose...*
   Apply it as soon as you remember. If it is almost time for your next dose, skip the one you missed and go back to your regular schedule. Never apply more than 1 dose at a time.

■ *Storage instructions...*
Keep Propine in the plastic dropper bottle it came in.

What side effects may occur?
Side effects cannot be anticipated. If any develop or change in intensity, inform your doctor as soon as possible. Only your doctor can determine if it is safe for you to continue taking Propine.

■ *More common side effects may include:*
Burning and stinging, red eye

■ *Less common or rare side effects may include:*
Allergic reactions, change in heart rhythm, conjunctivitis, extreme dilation of pupils, increased heart rate or blood pressure, increased sensitivity to light

Why should this drug not be prescribed?
If you are sensitive to or have ever had an allergic reaction to Propine or any of its ingredients, you should not use this medication. Make sure your doctor is aware of any drug reactions you have experienced.

Unless you are directed to do so by your doctor, do not use this medication if you have narrow-angle glaucoma.

Special warnings about this medication
Propine may cause vision problems, including blurry vision, for a short time after the eyedrops are applied. If this occurs, make sure you do not drive, use machinery, or participate in any hazardous activity that requires clear vision.

Possible food and drug interactions
when taking this medication
No significant interactions have been reported.

Special information
if you are pregnant or breastfeeding
The effects of Propine during pregnancy have not been adequately studied. If you are pregnant or plan to become pregnant, inform your doctor immediately. Propine may appear in breast milk and could affect a nursing infant. If this medication is essential to your health, your doctor may advise you to discontinue breastfeeding your baby until your treatment is finished.

Recommended dosage

ADULTS

The usual dose is 1 drop in the eye(s) every 12 hours. It usually takes about 30 minutes for Propine to start working. You should feel the maximum effects of the drug within 1 hour.

CHILDREN

The safety and effectiveness of Propine have not been established in children.

Overdosage

Any medication taken in excess can have serious consequences. If you suspect an overdose of Propine, seek medical attention immediately.

Generic name:

PROPOXYPHENE NAPSYLATE WITH ACETAMINOPHEN

See Darvocet-N, page 334.

Generic name:

PROPRANOLOL

See Inderal, page 627.

Generic name:

PROPRANOLOL WITH HYDROCHLOROTHIAZIDE

See Inderide, page 631.

Brand name:

PROPULSID

Pronounced: pro-PUHL-sid
Generic name: Cisapride

Why is this drug prescribed?

Propulsid is prescribed to treat nighttime heartburn caused by gastroesophageal reflux disease, a condition in which the valve between the esophagus and the stomach opens or leaks, allowing stomach acid to back up and cause burning or "heartburn."

Most important fact about this drug
There have been rare reports of dangerous heartbeat irregularities developing when Propulsid is combined with certain drugs. If you are taking any other medications, be sure to check "Why should this drug not be prescribed?" below.

How should you take this medication?
Take your medication 15 minutes before meals and at bedtime. Take Propulsid exactly as prescribed, even if your symptoms disappear.

■ *If you miss a dose...*
  Take the forgotten dose as soon as you remember. If it is almost time for your next dose, skip the one you missed and go back to your regular schedule. Do not take 2 doses at once.

■ *Storage instructions...*
  Store at room temperature. Protect from moisture.

What side effects may occur?
Side effects cannot be anticipated. If any develop or change in intensity, tell your doctor as soon as possible. Only your doctor can determine if it is safe for you to continue taking Propulsid.

■ *More common side effects may include:*
  Abdominal pain, bloating/gas, constipation, diarrhea, headache, inflamed nasal passages and sinuses, nausea, pain, upper respiratory and viral infections

■ *Less common side effects may include:*
  Abnormal vision, anxiety, back pain, chest pain, coughing, dehydration, depression, dizziness, fatigue, fever, frequent urination, indigestion, inflammation of the vagina, insomnia, itching, joint pain, muscle pain, nervousness, rash, sore throat, urinary tract infection, vomiting

Why should this drug not be prescribed?
You should not use Propulsid if you have bleeding, blockage, or leakage in the stomach or intestines. Do not use this drug if you are taking Nizoral, Sporanox, Monistat IV, Tao, Biaxin, erythromycin, or Diflucan. Also avoid

Propulsid if you are sensitive to or have ever had an allergic reaction to it.

Special warnings about this medication

Propulsid is used only for nighttime heartburn. It has not been shown to be effective for daytime heartburn.

Because irregular heartbeats have occurred in a few people taking Propulsid, be sure to tell your doctor if you have had any heart trouble.

Propulsid by itself rarely causes drowsiness. However, it may increase the effects of alcoholic beverages and tranquilizers.

Possible food and drug interactions
when taking this medication

If Propulsid is taken with certain other drugs, the effects of either could be increased, decreased, or altered. It is especially important to check with your doctor before combining Propulsid with the following:

Cimetidine (Tagamet)
Clarithromycin (Biaxin)
Drugs that control spasms, such as Bentyl and Cogentin
Erythromycin (E-Mycin, Eryc)
Fluconazole (Diflucan)
Itraconazole (Sporanox)
Ketoconazole (Nizoral)
Miconazole (Monistat IV)
Ranitidine (Zantac)
Tranquilizers such as Librium, Valium, and Xanax
Troleandomycin (TAO)
Warfarin (Coumadin)

Remember that Propulsid may increase the effects of alcohol. If you are taking oral blood thinners (warfarin), your doctor will give you a blood test 1 week after you start on Propulsid and after your therapy is completed. Your blood-thinning medication may need to be adjusted.

Special information
if you are pregnant or breastfeeding

The effects of Propulsid during pregnancy have not been adequately studied. If you are pregnant or plan to become pregnant, tell your doctor immediately. The drug appears in breast milk and could affect a nursing infant. If this medication is essential to your health, your doctor may advise you to discontinue breastfeeding until your treatment is finished.

Recommended dosage

ADULTS

The usual starting dose is one 10-milligram tablet or 10 milliliters of suspension 4 times daily, taken at least 15 minutes before meals and at bedtime.

Your doctor may need to adjust your dosage to 20 milligrams 4 times daily, depending on how well the drug works for you.

CHILDREN

The safety and effectiveness of Propulsid in children have not been established.

Overdosage

Any medication taken in excess can have serious consequences. If you suspect an overdose, seek medical attention immediately.

- *Symptoms of Propulsid overdose may include:*
  Frequent urination or bowel movements, gas, gurgling and rumbling in the stomach, retching

Brand name:

PROSCAR

Pronounced: PRAHS-car
Generic name: Finasteride

Why is this drug prescribed?

Proscar is prescribed to help shrink an enlarged prostate.

The prostate, a chestnut-shaped gland present in males, produces a liquid that forms part of the semen. This gland completely encloses the upper part of the urethra, the tube through which urine flows out of the bladder. Many men over age 50 suffer from a benign (noncancerous) enlargement of the prostate. The enlarged gland squeezes the urethra, obstructing the normal flow of urine. Resulting problems may include difficulty in starting urination, weak flow of urine, and the need to urinate urgently or frequently. Sometimes surgical removal of the prostate is necessary.

By shrinking the enlarged prostate, Proscar may alleviate the various associated urinary problems, making surgery unnecessary.

Some doctors are also prescribing Proscar for baldness and as a preventive measure against prostate cancer.

Most important fact about this drug
Different men have different responses to Proscar:

- You may experience early relief from your urinary problems.
- You may need to take the drug for 6 months or even a year before noticing any improvement.
- Or you may find that, even after a year of treatment, Proscar simply has not helped you.

How should you take this medication?
You may take Proscar either with a meal or between meals.

- *If you miss a dose...*
  Take it as soon as you remember. If it is almost time for your next dose, skip the one you missed and go back to your regular schedule. Never take 2 doses at the same time.

- *Storage instructions...*
  Store at room temperature in a tightly closed container. Protect from light.

What side effects may occur?
Side effects cannot be anticipated. If any develop or change in intensity, inform your doctor as soon as possible. Only your doctor can determine if it is safe for you to continue taking Proscar.

- *Side effects may include:*
  Decreased amount of semen per ejaculation, decreased sex drive, impotence

Why should this drug not be prescribed?
Proscar should never be taken by a woman or a child.

Do not take Proscar if you are sensitive to it or have ever had an allergic reaction to it.

Special warnings about this medication
Benign enlargement of the prostate is not the only condition that can cause male urinary inefficiency and discomfort. Other possibilities include infection, obstruction, cancer of the prostate, and bladder disorders. Before prescribing

Proscar, your doctor will want to do various tests to determine the cause of your urinary problems.

Even if Proscar does relieve your urinary symptoms, periodic checkups are necessary to test for possible development of cancer of the prostate. Proscar is not an effective treatment for prostate cancer.

Check the patient information that comes in the Proscar package for new information every time you renew your prescription.

**Possible food and drug interactions
when taking this medication**
No significant drug interactions have been reported.

**Special information
if you are pregnant or breastfeeding**
If accidentally absorbed by a pregnant woman who is carrying a male fetus, Proscar may cause abnormal development of the unborn baby's genital organs. Any woman who is pregnant or who may become pregnant should therefore never even touch a crushed Proscar tablet.

Recommended dosage

ADULTS

The recommended dosage, for men only, is one 5-milligram tablet per day.

Overdosage
Although no specific information is available, any medication taken in excess can have serious consequences. If you suspect an overdose of Proscar, seek medical attention immediately.

Brand name:

PROSOM

Pronounced: PROE-som
Generic name: Estazolam

Why is this drug prescribed?
ProSom, a sleeping pill, is given for the short-term treatment of insomnia. Insomnia may involve difficulty falling asleep, frequent awakenings during the night, or too-early morning awakening.

Most important fact about this drug
As a chemical cousin of Valium and similar tranquilizers, ProSom is potentially addictive; thus, you should plan on taking this drug only as a temporary sleeping aid. Even after relatively short-term use of ProSom, you may experience some withdrawal symptoms when you stop taking the medication.

How should you take this medication?
Take ProSom exactly as prescribed by your doctor. A typical schedule is 1 tablet every night at bedtime. For small, physically run-down, or older people, one-half a tablet may be a safer starting dose.

Avoid drinking alcoholic beverages while taking ProSom.

If you have ever had seizures, do not abruptly stop taking ProSom, even if you are taking antiseizure medication. Instead, taper off from ProSom under your doctor's supervision.

Even if you have never had seizures, it is better to taper off from ProSom than to stop taking the medication abruptly. Experience suggests that tapering off can help prevent drug withdrawal symptoms.

Typically, the only withdrawal symptoms caused by ProSom are mild and temporary insomnia or irritability. Occasionally, however, withdrawal can involve considerable discomfort or even danger, with symptoms such as abdominal and muscle cramps, convulsions, sweating, tremors, and vomiting.

■ *If you miss a dose...*
   Take at bedtime only as needed. It is not necessary to make up a missed dose.

■ *Storage instructions...*
   Store at room temperature.

What side effects may occur?
Side effects cannot be anticipated. If any develop or change in intensity, inform your doctor as soon as possible. Only your doctor can determine whether it is safe for you to continue taking ProSom.

■ *More common side effects may include:*
   Abnormal coordination, cold symptoms, decreased movement or activity, dizziness, general feeling of illness, hangover, headache, leg and foot pain, nausea, nervousness, sleepiness, weakness

■ *Less common or rare side effects may include:*
Abdominal pain, abnormal dreaming, abnormal thinking, abnormal vision, acne, agitation, allergic reaction, altered taste, anxiety, apathy, arm and hand pain, arthritis, asthma, back pain, black stools, body pain, chest pain, chills, confusion, constant, involuntary eye movement, constipation, cough, decreased appetite, decreased hearing, decreased reflexes, depression, difficult/labored breathing, double vision, dry mouth, dry skin, ear pain, emotional changeability, fainting, fever, flushing, frequent urination, gas, hallucinations, hostility, inability to hold urine, inability to urinate, increased appetite, indigestion, inflamed sinuses, itching, lack of coordination, little or no urine flow, loss of memory, menstrual cramps, muscle stiffness, nasal inflammation, neck pain, nighttime urination, nosebleed, numbness or tingling around the mouth, purple or reddish spots on the skin, rapid, heavy breathing, rash, ringing in the ears, seizure, sleep problems, sore throat, stupor, swollen breast, thirst, throbbing or fluttering heartbeat, tingling or "pins and needles," tremor, twitch, urgent need to urinate, vaginal discharge/itching, vomiting, weight gain or loss

Why should this drug not be prescribed?
Do not take ProSom if you are sensitive or allergic to it, or if you have ever had an adverse reaction to another Valium-type medication.

Do not take ProSom if you are pregnant or planning to become pregnant. Drugs in this class may cause damage to the unborn child.

Special warnings about this medication
Since ProSom may cloud your thinking, impair your judgment, or interfere with your normal physical coordination, do not drive, climb, or perform hazardous tasks until you know your reaction to this medication. It is important to remember that the tablet you took in the evening may continue to affect you well into the following day.

If you are older or physically run-down, or if you have liver or kidney damage or breathing problems, you will be particularly vulnerable to side effects from ProSom, and you should use this medication with special caution.

Possible food and drug interactions
when taking this medication
Do not drink alcohol while you are taking ProSom; this combination could make you comatose or dangerously slow your breathing.

For the same reason, do not combine ProSom with any other medication that might calm or slow the functioning of your central nervous system. Among such drugs are:

Antihistamines such as Benadryl and Chlor-Trimeton
Antiseizure drugs such as Dilantin, Tegretol, and Depakene
Barbiturates such as phenobarbital
Major tranquilizers such as Haldol and Mellaril
MAO inhibitors such as the antidepressants Nardil and Parnate
Narcotics such as Percodan and Tylox
Tranquilizers such as Valium and Xanax

If you smoke, you will tend to process and eliminate ProSom fairly quickly compared with a nonsmoker.

Special information
if you are pregnant or breastfeeding

If you are pregnant, you must not take ProSom; it could cause birth defects in your child.

When a pregnant woman takes ProSom or a similar medication shortly before giving birth, her baby is likely to have poor muscle tone (flaccidity) and/or experience drug withdrawal symptoms.

Because ProSom is thought to pass into breast milk, you should not take this medication while breastfeeding.

Recommended dosage

ADULTS

The recommended initial dose is 1 milligram at bedtime; however, some people may need a 2-milligram dose.

CHILDREN

There is no information on the safety and effectiveness of ProSom in people under age 18.

OLDER ADULTS

The recommended usual dosage for older adults is 1 milligram. However, some people may require only 0.5 milligram.

Overdosage

Any medication taken in excess can have serious consequences. If you suspect an overdose, seek medical attention immediately.

■ *Symptoms of a ProSom overdose may include:*
Confusion, depressed breathing, drowsiness and eventually coma, lack of coordination, slurred speech

Brand name:

PROSTEP

See Nicotine Patches, page 870.

Brand name:

PROTOSTAT

See Flagyl, page 528.

Brand name:

PROVENTIL

Pronounced: Proh-VEN-till
Generic name: Albuterol sulfate
Other brand names: Proventil HFA, Ventolin, Volmax
  Extended-Release Tablets

Why is this drug prescribed?

Drugs containing albuterol are prescribed for the prevention and relief of bronchial spasms that narrow the airway. This especially applies to the treatment of asthma. Some brands of this medication are also used for the prevention of bronchial spasm due to exercise.

Most important fact about this drug

Do not take albuterol more frequently than your doctor recommends. Increasing the number of doses can be dangerous and may actually make symptoms of asthma worse.

If the dose your doctor recommends does not provide relief of your symptoms, or if your symptoms become worse, consult your doctor immediately.

How should you take this medication?

If you are taking extended-release tablets, swallow them whole with some liquid—never chew or crush them.

Shake the inhalation aerosol canister well before using. Test spray the device before using it for the first time, and after long periods of disuse. Use only the adapter that comes with the product; do not use this adapter with any other product.

If you are using an inhalation solution, be sure to protect it from contamination. Keep the tip of the dropper away from the lip of the bottle or any other surface. Do not use the solution if it changes color or becomes cloudy.

■ *If you miss a dose...*
Take the forgotten dose as soon as you remember; then take any remaining doses for that day at equally spaced intervals. Never take a double dose.

■ *Storage instructions...*
This medication can be kept in the refrigerator or at room temperature. The aerosol should be at room temperature before use. Ventolin nebules must be used within 2 weeks of being removed from the refrigerator.

What side effects may occur?
Side effects cannot be anticipated. If any develop or change in intensity, inform your doctor as soon as possible. Only your doctor can determine if it is safe for you to continue taking albuterol.

■ *More common side effects may include:*
Aggression, agitation, cough, diarrhea, dizziness, excitement, general bodily discomfort, headache, heartburn, increased appetite, increased blood pressure, increased difficulty breathing, indigestion, irritability, labored breathing, light-headedness, muscle cramps, nausea, nervousness, nightmares, nosebleed, overactivity, palpitations, rapid heartbeat, rash, ringing in the ears, shakiness, sleeplessness, stomachache, stuffy nose, throat irritation, tooth discoloration, tremors, vomiting, wheezing

■ *Proventil HFA may also cause the following:*
Allergic reaction, back pain, fever, inhalation site sensation, nasal inflammation, respiratory infection or disorder, taste sensation on inhalation, urinary problems

■ *Less common side effects may include:*
Chest pain (sometimes crushing) or discomfort, difficulty urinating, drowsiness, dry mouth and throat, flushing, high blood pressure, muscle spasm, restlessness, sweating, unusual taste, vertigo, weakness

■ *Proventil HFA may also cause the following:*
Anxiety, belching, chills and fever, coordination problems, depression, difficulty speaking, diabetes, dizziness, fluid retention and swelling, gas, heart palpitations, leg cramps, overactivity, ringing in the ears, sleepiness

- *Rare side effects following the use of inhaled albuterol include:*
  Hoarseness, increased breathing or wheezing, rapid heartbeat, skin rash or hives, unusual and unexpected swelling of mouth and throat

Why should this drug not be prescribed?
If you are sensitive to or have ever had an allergic reaction to albuterol or other bronchodilators, you should not take this medication. Make sure that your doctor is aware of any drug reactions that you have experienced.

Special warnings about this medication
When taking albuterol inhalation aerosol, you should not use other inhaled medications before checking with your doctor.

Make sure the doctor is aware of it if you have a heart condition, seizure disorder, high blood pressure, abnormal heartbeat, overactive thyroid gland, or diabetes. Call your doctor immediately if you notice any change in heartbeat or pulse while taking this medication.

You may have an immediate, serious allergic reaction to the first dose of albuterol. The drug has been known to cause life-threatening bronchial spasms, especially with the first dose from a new canister or vial. There have also been rare reports of skin reddening and peeling in children taking albuterol syrup.

Do not exceed your doctor's recommended dose of albuterol. If you need more than usual, check with your doctor. Your asthma may be getting unstable, and you may need another medication. Do not, however, change brands without first consulting your doctor or pharmacist.

Possible food and drug interactions
when taking this medication
Albuterol inhalation aerosol should not be used with other aerosol bronchodilators.

If albuterol is taken with certain other drugs, the effects of either could be increased, decreased, or altered. It is especially important to check with your doctor before combining albuterol with the following:

Antidepressants such as Elavil and Nardil
Beta blockers (heart and blood pressure drugs such as Inderal, Tenormin, and Sectral)
Digoxin (Lanoxin)
Drugs similar to albuterol, such as Alupent, Brethaire, Isuprel, and epinephrine

Drugs that lower potassium levels (water pills such as Lasix or HydroDIURIL)

Special information
if you are pregnant or breastfeeding

The effects of albuterol during pregnancy have not been adequately studied. If you are pregnant or plan to become pregnant, inform your doctor immediately. It is not known whether albuterol appears in breast milk. If this drug is essential to your health, your doctor may advise you to stop nursing your baby until your treatment is finished.

Recommended dosage

ADULTS

Inhalation Aerosol

Patient instructions are available with both products.

If you are being treated for a sudden or severe bronchial spasm or the prevention of asthma symptoms, the usual dosage of albuterol inhalation aerosol for adults and children aged 4 and over (Ventolin) or 12 and over (Proventil, Proventil HFA) is 2 inhalations repeated every 4 to 6 hours. More frequent use is not recommended. In some individuals, 1 inhalation every 4 hours may be sufficient.

The recommended dose of Proventil Inhalation Aerosol for prevention of recurring symptoms is 2 inhalations, 4 times a day.

For exercise-induced bronchial spasm, the usual dosage for adults and children 12 years and older is 2 inhalations, 15 minutes prior to exercise.

Tablets

The usual starting dose for adults and children 12 years of age and older is 2 or 4 milligrams 3 to 4 times a day. The daily dose should not exceed 32 milligrams per day.

Syrup

The usual starting dose for adults and children over 14 years of age is 1 or 2 teaspoonfuls 3 or 4 times a day.

Ventolin Rotacaps for Inhalation

The usual dosage for adults and children 4 years and older is the contents of one 200-microgram capsule inhaled every 4 to 6 hours using a Rotahaler inhalation device. Some people may require two 200-microgram capsules every 4 to 6 hours.

For exercise-induced bronchial spasm, the usual dosage for adults and children 4 years of age and older is the contents of one 200-microgram capsule inhaled 15 minutes before exercise.

Inhalation Solution

The usual dosage for adults and children 12 years of age and older is 2.5 milligrams administered 3 to 4 times daily by nebulization. Do not use more often or in higher doses. To administer 2.5 milligrams, dilute 0.5 milliliter of the 0.5 percent solution for inhalation with 2.5 milliliters of sterile normal saline solution.

Ventolin Nebules Inhalation Solution

The usual dosage for adults and children 2 years and older, and weighing at least 33 pounds, is 2.5 milligrams of Ventolin taken 3 to 4 times a day by nebulization. Children weighing less than 33 pounds should use inhalation solution instead of Ventolin Nebules.

Proventil Repetabs and Volmax Extended-Release Tablets

The usual recommended dosage for adults and children 12 years of age and older is 8 milligrams every 12 hours. In some people, 4 milligrams every 12 hours may be sufficient. If the desired effect is not achieved with the standard dosage, your doctor may increase doses to a maximum of 32 milligrams per day, divided into two 16-milligram doses spaced 12 hours apart. Those taking Ventolin Tablets or Ventolin Syrup can switch to Volmax Extended-Release Tablets. One Volmax tablet every 12 hours is equivalent to one 2-milligram Ventolin Tablet every 6 hours.

CHILDREN

Inhalation Aerosol

Safety and effectiveness in children below the age of 12 (Proventil, Proventil HFA, Volmax) and below the age of 4 (Ventolin) have not been established. For dosage in children above these ages, see adult section.

Tablets

The usual starting dose for children 6 to 12 years of age is 2 milligrams 3 or 4 times a day. The dose can be increased with caution but should not exceed 24 milligrams per day. Safety and effectiveness in children under 6 have not been established.

Syrup

The usual starting dose for children 6 to 14 years of age is 1 teaspoonful 3 to 4 times a day. For children 2 to 6 years of age, the starting dose is 0.1

milligram per 2.2 pounds of body weight, to a maximum of 4 milligrams, 3 times a day.

Proventil Repetabs
The usual starting dosage for children 6 to 11 years of age is 4 milligrams every 12 hours. The dosage can be increased with caution but should not exceed 24 milligrams per day.

Inhalation Solution
The starting dosage for children 2 to 12 years of age is based on body weight but should not exceed 2.5 milligrams 3 or 4 times daily.

OLDER ADULTS

Oral Dosage
The usual starting dose of tablets or syrup is 2 milligrams 3 or 4 times a day. If needed, the dosage may be increased gradually to as much as 8 milligrams 3 or 4 times a day.

Overdosage

■ *Symptoms of albuterol overdose may include:*
Fatigue, general feeling of illness, high or low blood pressure, insomnia, radiating chest pain, rapid or irregular heartbeat, seizures

Heart attack and even death have been associated with abuse of albuterol inhalation. Exaggerated side effects may also be a sign of an overdose. If you suspect an overdose, seek medical attention immediately.

Brand name:

PROVERA

Pronounced: pro-VAIR-uh
Generic name: Medroxyprogesterone acetate
Other brand name: Cycrin

Why is this drug prescribed?
Provera is derived from the female hormone progesterone. You may be given Provera if your menstrual periods have stopped or a female hormone imbalance is causing your uterus to bleed abnormally.

Other forms of medroxyprogesterone, such as Depo-Provera, are used as a contraceptive injection and prescribed in the treatment of endometrial cancer.

Some doctors prescribe Provera to treat endometriosis, menopausal symptoms, premenstrual tension, sexually aggressive behavior in men, and sleep apnea (temporary failure to breathe while sleeping).

Most important fact about this drug
You should never take Provera during the first 4 months of pregnancy. During this formative period, even a few days of treatment with Provera might put your unborn baby at increased risk for birth defects. If you take Provera and later discover that you were pregnant when you took it, discuss this with your doctor right away.

How should you take this medication?
Provera may be taken with or between meals.

Do not change from one brand to another without consulting your doctor or pharmacist.

Your doctor will probably have you take Provera for 5 to 10 days and then stop; you should have your period within 3 to 7 days after the last dose.

If you are being treated for lack of regular menstrual periods, your doctor may have you start taking Provera at any time. If you are being treated for abnormal uterine bleeding due to a female-hormone imbalance, your doctor will probably have you start taking Provera on day 16 or 21 of your menstrual cycle (i.e., 16 or 21 days after the start of your last period). You should have your period within 3 to 7 days after the last dose.

- *If you miss a dose...*
  Take it as soon as you remember. If it is almost time for your next dose, skip the one you missed and go back to your regular schedule. Never take 2 doses at the same time.

- *Storage instructions...*
  Store at room temperature.

What side effects may occur?
Side effects cannot be anticipated. If any develop or change in intensity, inform your doctor as soon as possible. Only your doctor can determine if it is safe for you to continue taking Provera.

- *Side effects may include:*
  Acne, anaphylaxis (life-threatening allergic reaction), blood clot in a vein, lungs, or brain, breakthrough bleeding (between menstrual periods), breast tenderness or sudden or excessive flow of milk, cervical erosion or changes in secretions, depression, excessive growth of hair, fever, fluid

retention, hair loss, headache, hives, insomnia, itching, lack of menstruation, menstrual flow changes, spotting, nausea, rash, skin discoloration,
sleepiness, weight gain or loss, yellowed eyes and skin

Why should this drug not be prescribed?

Do not take Provera if you are sensitive to it or have ever had an allergic
reaction to it.

If you suspect you may have become pregnant, do not take Provera as a test
for pregnancy. Doctors once prescribed Provera for this purpose, but no
longer do so for 2 reasons:

- Quicker, safer pregnancy tests are now available.
- If you are in fact pregnant, Provera might injure the baby.

Do not take Provera during your first 4 months of pregnancy. In the past,
Provera was sometimes given to try to prevent miscarriage. However,
doctors now believe that this treatment is not only ineffective but also
potentially harmful to the baby.

Do not take Provera if you have:

- Cancer of the breast or genital organs
- Liver disease or a liver condition
- A dead fetus still in the uterus
- Undiagnosed bleeding from the vagina

Do not take Provera if you have, or have ever developed, blood clots.

Special warnings about this medication

Before you start to take Provera, your doctor will give you a complete
physical exam, including examination of your breasts and pelvic organs. You
should also have a cervical smear (Pap test).

Provera may cause some degree of fluid retention. If you have a medical
condition that could be made worse by fluid retention—such as epilepsy,
migraine, asthma, or a heart or kidney problem—make sure your doctor
knows about it.

Provera may mask the onset of menopause. In other words, while taking
Provera you may continue to experience regular menstrual bleeding even if
your menopause has started.

Provera may make you depressed, especially if you have suffered from
depression in the past. If you become seriously depressed, tell your doctor;
you should probably stop taking Provera.

If you are diabetic, Provera could make your diabetes worse; your doctor will want to watch you closely while you are taking this drug.

There is some concern that Provera, like birth control pills, may increase your risk for a blood clot in a vein. If you experience any symptoms that might suggest the onset of such a condition—pain with swelling, warmth, and redness in a leg vein, coughing or shortness of breath, vision problems, migraine, or weakness or numbness in an arm or leg—see your doctor immediately.

Tell your doctor right away if you lose some or all of your vision or you start seeing double. You may have to stop taking the medication.

Possible food and drug interactions
when taking this medication
If Provera is taken with certain other drugs, the effects of either may be increased, decreased, or altered. It is especially important to check with your doctor before combining Provera with aminoglutethimide (Cytadren).

Special information
if you are pregnant or breastfeeding
You should not take Provera during pregnancy. If you are pregnant or plan to become pregnant, inform your doctor immediately.

Provera appears in breast milk. If you are a new mother, you may need to choose between taking Provera and breastfeeding your baby.

Recommended dosage

ADULTS

To Restore Menstrual Periods
Provera Tablets are taken in dosages of 5 to 10 milligrams daily for 5 to 10 days. Make sure you discuss what effect this will have on your menstrual cycle with your doctor. You should have bleeding 3 to 7 days after you stop taking Provera.

Abnormal Uterine Bleeding Due to Hormonal Imbalance
Beginning on the 16th or 21st day of your menstrual cycle, you will take 5 to 10 milligrams daily for 5 to 10 days. Make sure you discuss what effect this will have on your menstrual cycle with your doctor. You should have bleeding 3 to 7 days after you stop taking Provera.

Overdosage
Although no specific information is available, any medication taken in excess can have serious consequences. If you suspect an overdose of Provera, seek medical attention immediately.

Brand name:

PROZAC

Pronounced: PRO-zak
Generic name: Fluoxetine hydrochloride

Why is this drug prescribed?
Prozac is prescribed for the treatment of depression—that is, a continuing depression that interferes with daily functioning. The symptoms of major depression often include changes in appetite, sleep habits, and mind/body coordination; decreased sex drive; increased fatigue; feelings of guilt or worthlessness; difficulty concentrating; slowed thinking; and suicidal thoughts.

Prozac is also prescribed to treat obsessive-compulsive disorder. An obsession is a thought that won't go away; a compulsion is an action done over and over to relieve anxiety. The drug is also used in the treatment of bulimia (binge-eating followed by deliberate vomiting).

Prozac is thought to work by adjusting the balance of the brain's natural chemical messengers. It has also been used to treat obesity and eating disorders.

Most important fact about this drug
Serious, sometimes fatal, reactions have been known to occur when Prozac is used in combination with other antidepressant drugs known as MAO inhibitors, including Nardil and Parnate; and when Prozac is discontinued and an MAO inhibitor is started. Never take Prozac with one of these drugs or within at least 14 days of discontinuing therapy with one of them; and allow 5 weeks or more between stopping Prozac and starting an MAO inhibitor. Be especially cautious if you have been taking Prozac in high doses or for a long time.

If you are taking any prescription or nonprescription drugs, notify your doctor before taking Prozac.

How should you take this medication?
Prozac should be taken exactly as prescribed by your doctor.

Prozac usually is taken once or twice a day. To be effective, it should be taken regularly. Make a habit of taking it at the same time you do some other daily activity.

It may be 4 weeks before you feel any relief from your depression, but the drug's effects should last about 9 months after a 3-month treatment regimen. For obsessive-compulsive disorder, the full effect may take 5 weeks to appear.

- *If you miss a dose...*
  Take the forgotten dose as soon as you remember. If several hours have passed, skip the dose. Never try to "catch up" by doubling the dose.

- *Storage instructions...*
  Store at room temperature.

What side effects may occur?
Side effects cannot be anticipated. If any develop or change in intensity, inform your doctor as soon as possible. Only your doctor can determine if it is safe for you to continue taking Prozac.

- *More common side effects may include:*
  Abnormal dreams, abnormal ejaculation, agitation, amnesia, anxiety, bronchitis, changeable emotions, chills, confusion, conjunctivitis (pinkeye), cough, decreased sex drive, diarrhea, dilated pupils, dizziness, drowsiness and fatigue, dry eyes, dry mouth, ear pain, flu symptoms, frequent urination, gas, headache, hemorrhage, high blood pressure, impotence, inability to fall or stay asleep, increased appetite, indigestion, intolerance of light, itching, lack or loss of appetite, nausea, nervousness, rash, ringing in the ears, sinus or nasal inflammation, sore throat, sweating, taste alterations, tremors, vision problems, vomiting, weakness, weight gain, yawning

- *Less common side effects may include:*
  Abnormal gait, abnormal stoppage of menstrual flow, acne, apathy, arthritis, asthma, bone pain, breast pain, brief loss of consciousness, bursitis, chills and fever, convulsions, dark, tarry stool, difficulty in swallowing, exaggerated feeling of well-being, facial swelling due to fluid retention, fever, fluid retention, hair loss, hallucinations, hiccups, hives, hostility, infection, inflammation of the esophagus, inflammation of the stomach lining, inflammation of the tongue, involuntary movement, irrational ideas, irregular heartbeat, lack of muscle coordination, low blood pressure upon standing, migraine headache, mouth inflammation, muscle spasm, nosebleed, paranoid reaction, pelvic pain, rapid breathing, rapid or throbbing heartbeat, sensitivity to light, severe chest pain, skin inflamma-

tion, skin rash, thirst, tooth problems, twitching, uncoordinated movements, urinary disorders, vague feeling of bodily discomfort, vertigo, vision disturbances, vomiting, weight loss

■ *Rare side effects may include:*
Antisocial behavior, belching, bleeding gums, blood clots, blood in urine, bloody diarrhea, breast enlargement, bruising, coma, deafness, decreased reflexes, dehydration, delusions, diabetes, double vision, duodenal ulcer, enlargement of liver, enlargement or increased activity of thyroid gland, excess growth of coarse hair on face, chest, etc., excess uterine or vaginal bleeding, eye bleeding, female milk production, fluid buildup in larynx and lungs, gallstones, glaucoma, gout, heart attack, heart failure, hepatitis, high blood sugar, inability to control bowel movements, increased salivation, inflammation of eyes and eyelids, inflammation of fallopian tubes, inflammation of the intestines, inflammation of tissue below skin, irregular heartbeat, kidney disorders, leg cramps, low blood pressure, menstrual disorders, miscarriage, mouth sores, muscle inflammation, muscle spasms, weakness, or disease, psoriasis, rashes, reddish or purplish spots on the skin, reduction of body temperature, rheumatoid arthritis, salivation, seborrhea, shingles, skin discoloration, skin inflammation and disorders, slowing of heart rate, slurred speech, spitting blood, stomach and intestinal hemorrhage, stomach ulcer, stroke, stupor, suicidal thoughts, taste loss, temporary cessation of breathing, tingling sensation around the mouth, tongue swelling, urinary tract disorders, vomiting blood

Why should this drug not be prescribed?

If you are sensitive to or have ever had an allergic reaction to Prozac or similar drugs such as Paxil and Zoloft, you should not take this medication. Make sure that your doctor is aware of any drug reactions that you have experienced.

Do not take this drug while using an MAO inhibitor. (See "Most important fact about this drug.")

Special warnings about this medication

Unless you are directed to do so by your doctor, do not take this medication if you are recovering from a heart attack or if you have liver disease or diabetes.

Prozac may cause you to become drowsy or less alert and may affect your judgment. Therefore, driving or operating dangerous machinery or participating in any hazardous activity that requires full mental alertness is not recommended.

While taking this medication, you may feel dizzy or light-headed or actually faint when getting up from a lying or sitting position. If getting up slowly doesn't help or if this problem continues, notify your doctor.

If you develop a skin rash or hives while taking Prozac, discontinue use of the medication and notify your doctor immediately.

Prozac should be used with caution if you have a history of seizures. You should discuss all of your medical conditions with your doctor before taking this medication.

The safety and effectiveness of Prozac have not been established in children.

Possible food and drug interactions
when taking this medication
Combining Prozac with MAO inhibitors is dangerous.

Do not drink alcohol while taking this medication.

If Prozac is taken with certain other drugs, the effects of either could be increased, decreased, or altered. It is especially important to check with your doctor before combining Prozac with the following:

    Alprazolam (Xanax)
    Carbamazepine (Tegretol)
    Clozapine (Clozaril)
    Diazepam (Valium)
    Digitoxin (Crystodigin)
    Drugs that impair brain function, such as Xanax
    Flecainide (Tambocor)
    Haloperidol (Haldol)
    Lithium (Eskalith)
    Other antidepressants (Elavil)
    Phenytoin (Dilantin)
    Pimozide (Orap)
    Tryptophan
    Vinblastine (Velban)
    Warfarin (Coumadin)

Special information
if you are pregnant or breastfeeding
The effects of Prozac during pregnancy have not been adequately studied. If you are pregnant or plan to become pregnant, inform your doctor immediately. This medication appears in breast milk, and breastfeeding is not recommended while you are taking Prozac.

Recommended dosage

ADULTS

The usual starting dose is 20 milligrams per day, taken in the morning. Your doctor may increase your dose after several weeks if no improvement is observed. People with kidney or liver disease, the elderly, and those taking other drugs may have their dosages adjusted by their doctor.

Dosages above 20 milligrams daily should be taken once a day in the morning or in 2 smaller doses taken in the morning and at noon.

The usual daily dose for depression ranges from 20 to 60 milligrams. For obsessive-compulsive disorder the customary range is 20 to 60 milligrams per day, though a maximum of 80 milligrams is sometimes prescribed. For bulimia nervosa, the usual dose is 60 milligrams, taken in the morning. Your doctor may have you start with less and build up to this dosage.

Overdosage

Any medication taken in excess can have serious consequences. In addition, combining Prozac with certain other drugs can cause symptoms of overdose. If you suspect an overdose, seek medical attention immediately.

- *Symptoms of Prozac overdose include:*
  Agitation, nausea, restlessness, vomiting

Brand name:

PSORCON

Pronounced: SORE-kon
Generic name: Diflorasone diacetate

Why is this drug prescribed?
Psorcon is prescribed for the relief of the inflammatory and itching symptoms of skin disorders that respond to the topical application (applied directly to the skin) of steroids (hormones produced by the body that have potent anti-inflammatory effects).

Most important fact about this drug
When you use Psorcon, you inevitably absorb some of the medication through your skin and into the bloodstream. Too much absorption can lead to unwanted side effects elsewhere in the body. To keep this problem to a minimum, avoid using large amounts of Psorcon over large areas, and do not cover it with airtight dressings such as plastic wrap or adhesive bandages unless specifically told to by your doctor.

How should you use this medication?
Use this medication exactly as prescribed.

Psorcon is for use only on the skin. Be careful to keep it out of your eyes.

■ *If you miss a dose...*
   Apply it as soon as you remember. If it is almost time for the next dose, skip the one you missed and go back to your regular schedule.

■ *Storage instructions...*
   Store at room temperature.

What side effects may occur?
Side effects cannot be anticipated. If any develop or change in intensity, inform your doctor as soon as possible. Only your doctor can determine if it is safe for you to continue taking Psorcon.

■ *Side effects may include:*
   Burning, dryness, eruptions resembling acne, excessive discoloring of the skin, excessive growth of hair, inflammation of hair follicles, inflammation around the mouth, irritation, itching, prickly heat, secondary infection, severe inflammation of the skin, softening of the skin, stretch marks, stretching or thinning of the skin

Why should this drug not be prescribed?
If you are sensitive to or have ever had an allergic reaction to diflorasone diacetate or other drugs of this type (antifungals, steroids), you should not take this medication. Make sure your doctor is aware of any drug reactions you have experienced.

Special warnings about this medication
Remember that absorption of Psorcon through the skin can affect the whole body. Although it's unusual (most common if Psorcon is spread over large areas of the skin), you could develop symptoms of steroid excess such as weight gain, reddening and rounding of the face and neck, growth of excess body and facial hair, high blood pressure, emotional disturbances, loss of energy due to high blood sugar, and increase in frequency of urination.

Do not use this drug for any disorder other than the one for which it was prescribed.

The treated skin area should not be bandaged, covered, or wrapped unless otherwise directed by your doctor. Avoid covering a treated area with waterproof diapers or plastic pants. They can cause unwanted absorption of Psorcon.

If an irritation or allergic reaction develops while you are using Psorcon, notify your doctor.

Possible food and drug interactions
when taking this medication
No interactions with food or other drugs have been reported.

Special information
if you are pregnant or breastfeeding
If you are pregnant or plan to become pregnant, inform your doctor before using Psorcon. In general, women who are pregnant should not use steroids extensively, in large amounts, or over long periods of time. It is not known whether this medication appears in breast milk. If this drug is essential to your health, your doctor may advise you to discontinue breastfeeding until treatment with this medication is finished.

Recommended dosage

ADULTS

Psorcon ointment should be applied as a thin film over the affected area from 1 to 3 times a day, depending on the severity or resistant nature of the condition. Psorcon cream should be applied twice a day.

Your doctor may recommend airtight bandages for the management of psoriasis (a chronic skin disorder) or other stubborn skin conditions. If an infection develops, you should stop using airtight dressings.

CHILDREN

Your doctor will limit the use of Psorcon for your child to the least amount that is effective. Long-term treatment may interfere with the growth and development of children.

Overdosage
An acute overdosage is unlikely with the use of Psorcon; however, long-term or prolonged use can produce side effects throughout your body. If you suspect an overdose, seek medical attention immediately.

Brand name:

PYRIDIUM

Pronounced: pie-RI-di-um
Generic name: Phenazopyridine hydrochloride

Why is this drug prescribed?

Pyridium is a urinary tract analgesic that helps relieve the pain, burning, urgency, frequency, and irritation caused by infection, trauma, catheters, or various surgical procedures in the lower urinary tract. Pyridium is indicated for short-term use and can only relieve symptoms; it is not a treatment for the underlying cause of the symptoms.

Most important fact about this drug

Pyridium produces an orange to red color in urine, and may stain fabric. Staining of contact lenses has also been reported.

How should you take this medication?

Take Pyridium after meals, exactly as prescribed.

- *If you miss a dose...*
  Take it as soon as you remember. If it is almost time for your next dose, skip the one you missed and go back to your regular schedule. Never take 2 doses at the same time.

- *Storage instructions...*
  Store at room temperature.

What side effects may occur?

Side effects cannot be anticipated. If any occur or change in intensity, inform your doctor as soon as possible. Only your doctor can determine if it is safe for you to continue taking Pyridium.

- *Side effects may include:*
  Headache, itching, rash, severe allergic reaction (rash, difficulty breathing, fever, rapid heartbeat, convulsions), upset stomach

Why should this drug not be prescribed?

Pyridium should be avoided if you have kidney disease, or if you are sensitive to or have ever had an allergic reaction to it.

Special warnings about this medication

If your skin or the whites of your eyes develop a yellowish tone, it may indicate that your kidneys are not eliminating the medication as they should. Notify your doctor immediately. If you are older, your doctor will watch you more closely, since the kidneys work less effectively as we age.

**Possible food and drug interactions
when taking this medication**
No interactions have been reported.

**Special information
if you are pregnant or breastfeeding**
The effects of Pyridium during pregnancy have not been adequately studied.
If you are pregnant or plan to become pregnant, inform your doctor
immediately. To date, there is no information on whether Pyridium appears in
breast milk. If this medication is essential to your health, your doctor may
advise you to stop breastfeeding until your treatment with Pyridium is
finished.

Recommended dosage

ADULTS

The usual dose is two 100-milligram tablets or one 200-milligram tablet 3
times a day after meals.

You should not take Pyridium for more than 2 days if you are also taking an
antibiotic for the treatment of a urinary tract infection.

Overdosage
Any medication taken in excess can have serious consequences. If you
suspect an overdose, seek emergency medical treatment immediately.

■ *Symptoms of Pyridium overdose may include:*
  Blood disorders, bluish skin color, impaired kidney and liver function

Generic name:

QUAZEPAM

See Doral, page 434.

Brand name:

QUESTRAN

*Pronounced: KWEST-ran
Generic name: Cholestyramine
Other brand name: Questran Light*

Why is this drug prescribed?

Questran is used to lower cholesterol levels in the blood of people with primary hypercholesterolemia (too much LDL cholesterol). Hypercholesterolemia is a genetic condition characterized by a lack of the LDL receptors that remove cholesterol from the bloodstream.

This drug can be used to lower cholesterol levels in people who also have hypertriglyceridemia, a condition in which an excess of fat is stored in the body.

This drug may also be prescribed to relieve itching associated with gallbladder obstruction.

It is available in two forms: Questran and Questran Light. The same instructions apply to both.

Most important fact about this drug

It's important to remember that Questran is a supplement to—not a substitute for—diet, exercise, and weight loss. To get the full benefit of the medication, you need to stick to the diet and exercise program prescribed by your doctor. All these efforts to keep your cholesterol levels normal are important because together they may lower your risk of heart disease.

How should you take this medication?

Never take Questran in its dry form. Always mix it with water or other liquids *before* taking it. For Questran, use 2 to 6 ounces of liquid per packet or level scoopful; for Questran Light, use 2 to 3 ounces. Soups or fruits with a high moisture content, such as applesauce or crushed pineapple, can be used in place of beverages.

■ *If you miss a dose...*
Take the forgotten dose as soon as you remember. If it is almost time for the next dose, skip the one you missed and go back to your regular schedule. Never try to "catch up" by doubling the dose.

■ *Storage instructions...*
Store at room temperature. Protect from moisture and high humidity.

What side effects may occur?

Side effects cannot be anticipated. If any develop or change in intensity, inform your doctor as soon as possible. Only your doctor can determine if it is safe for you to continue taking Questran.

The most common side effect of Questran is constipation.

■ *Less common or rare side effects may include:*
Abdominal discomfort, anemia, anxiety, arthritis, asthma, backache, belching, black stools, bleeding around the teeth, blood in the urine, brittle bones, burnt odor to urine, dental cavities, diarrhea, difficulty swallowing, dizziness, drowsiness, fainting, fatigue, fluid retention, gas, headache, heartburn, hiccups, hives, increased sex drive, increased tendency to bleed due to vitamin K deficiency, inflammation of the eye, inflammation of the pancreas, irritation around the anal area, irritation of the skin and tongue, joint pain, lack or loss of appetite, muscle pain, nausea, night blindness due to vitamin A deficiency, painful or difficult urination, rash, rectal bleeding and/or pain, ringing in the ears, shortness of breath, sour taste, swollen glands, tingling sensation, ulcer attack, vertigo, vitamin D deficiency, vomiting, weight gain or loss, wheezing

Why should this drug not be prescribed?
If you are sensitive to or have ever had an allergic reaction to Questran or similar drugs such as Colestid, you should not take this medication. Make sure that your doctor is aware of any drug reactions that you have experienced.

Unless you are directed to do so by your doctor, do not take this medication if you are being treated for gallbladder obstruction.

Special warnings about this medication
If you have phenylketonuria, a genetic disorder, check with your doctor before taking Questran Light because this product contains phenylalanine.

If you are being treated for any disease that contributes to increased blood cholesterol, such as hypothyroidism (reduced thyroid function), diabetes, nephrotic syndrome (kidney and blood vessel disorder), dysproteinemia, obstructive liver disease, or alcoholism, or if you are taking any drugs that may raise cholesterol levels, consult your doctor before taking this medication. Caution is also in order if your kidney function is poor.

Questran should begin to reduce cholesterol levels during the first month of therapy. If adequate reduction of cholesterol is not obtained, your doctor may increase the dosage or add other cholesterol-lowering drugs. Therefore, it is important that your doctor check your progress regularly.

Questran does not cure the tendency to have high cholesterol levels; it merely helps control it. To maintain healthy levels, you therefore must continue taking the drug as directed.

The use of this medication may produce or worsen constipation and aggravate hemorrhoids. If this happens, inform your doctor. To prevent constipation, the doctor may increase your dosage very slowly, and ask you to drink more fluids, take more fiber, or take a stool softener. If severe constipation develops anyway, the doctor may switch to a different drug.

The prolonged use of Questran may change acidity in the bloodstream, especially in younger and smaller individuals in whom the doses are relatively higher. Again, it is important that you or your child be checked by your doctor on a regular basis.

Sipping Questran or holding it in your mouth for a long period can lead to tooth discoloration, enamel erosion, or decay. Be sure to brush and floss regularly.

Possible food and drug interactions when taking this medication

If Questran is taken with certain other drugs, the effects of either could be increased, decreased, or altered. It is especially important to check with your doctor before taking Questran with the following:

Digitalis (Lanoxin, Crystodigin)
Estrogens and progestins (hormones)
Oral diabetes drugs such as DiaBeta and Diabinese
Penicillin G (Pentids, others)
Phenobarbital
Phenylbutazone (Butazolidin)
Propranolol (Inderal)
Spironolactone (Aldactazide, Aldactone)
Tetracycline (Achromycin V)
Thiazide-type water pills such as Diuril
Thyroid medication such as Synthroid
Warfarin (Coumadin)

Your doctor may recommend that you take other medications at least 1 hour before or 4 to 6 hours after you take Questran.

If you are taking a drug such as digitalis (Lanoxin), stopping Questran could be hazardous, since you might experience exaggerated effects of the other drug. Consult your doctor before discontinuing Questran.

This drug may interfere with normal digestion and absorption of fats, including fat-soluble vitamins such as A, D, E, and K. If supplements of vitamins A, D, E, and K are essential to your health, your doctor may prescribe an alternative form of these vitamins.

There are no special considerations regarding alcohol use with this medication.

Special information
if you are pregnant or breastfeeding

The effects of Questran during pregnancy have not been adequately studied. If you are pregnant or plan to become pregnant, inform your doctor immediately. Because this medication can interfere with vitamin absorption, you may need to increase your vitamin intake before the baby is born and while nursing an infant.

Recommended dosage

ADULTS

The recommended starting dose is 1 single-dose packet or 1 level scoopful, 1 to 2 times daily. The usual maintenance dosage is a total of 2 to 4 packets or scoopfuls daily divided into 2 doses preferably at mealtime (usually before meals). The maximum daily dose is 6 packets or scoopfuls. Although the recommended dosing schedule is 2 times daily, your doctor may ask you to take Questran in up to 6 smaller doses per day.

CHILDREN

Experience with the use of Questran in infants and children is limited. If this medication is essential to your child's health, follow your doctor's recommended dosing schedule.

Overdosage

No ill effects from an overdose have been reported. The main potential harm of an overdose would be obstruction of the stomach and intestines. If you suspect an overdose, seek medical attention immediately.

Generic name:

QUETIAPINE

See Seroquel, page 1187.

Brand name:

QUIBRON-T/SR

See Theo-Dur, page 1293.

Generic name:

QUINAPRIL

See Accupril, page 3.

Brand name:

QUINIDEX EXTENTABS

Pronounced: KWIN-i-deks Eks-TEN-tabs
Generic name: Quinidine sulfate

Why is this drug prescribed?
Quinidex Extentabs are used to correct certain types of irregular heart rhythms and to slow an abnormally fast heartbeat.

Most important fact about this ~~drug~~
It is important to take only the prescribed amount of this medication—no more and no less. Try to keep your doses at regularly spaced intervals, and be sure not to miss any.

How should you take this medication?
Take Quinidex exactly as prescribed.

- *If you miss a dose...*
  Take it as soon as you remember, if it is within 2 hours of your scheduled time. If you do not remember until later, skip the dose you missed and go back to your regular schedule. Do not take 2 doses at once.

- *Storage instructions...*
  Store at room temperature in a tightly closed container, away from light.

What side effects may occur?
Side effects cannot be anticipated. If any develop or change in intensity, inform your doctor as soon as possible. Only your doctor can determine if it is safe for you to continue taking Quinidex Extentabs.

- *More common side effects include:*
  Abdominal pain, diarrhea, hepatitis, inflammation of the esophagus (gullet), loss of appetite, nausea, vomiting

- *Less common or rare side effects may include:*
  Allergic reaction (symptoms include: swelling of face, lips, tongue, throat, arms, and legs, sore throat, fever and chills, difficulty swallowing, chest pain), anemia, apprehension, asthma attack, blind spots, blood clots, blurred vision, changes in skin pigmentation, confusion, delirium, depression, dilated pupils, disturbed color perception, double vision, eczema, excitement, fainting, fever, fluid retention, flushing, headache, hearing

changes, hepatitis, hives, inability to breathe, intense itching, intolerance to light, irregular heartbeats, joint pain, lack of coordination, low blood pressure, lupus erythematosus (inflammation of connective tissue), mental decline, muscle pain, night blindness, psoriasis, rash, reddish or purplish spots below the skin, skin eruptions and scaling, skin sensitivity to light, vertigo, vision changes, wheezing

Another possible side effect is a sensitivity reaction called cinchonism. Symptoms include blurred or double vision, confusion, delirium, diarrhea, headache, intolerance to light, loss of hearing, ringing in the ears, vertigo, and vomiting.

Why should this drug not be prescribed?
Do not take this medication if you have ever had an allergic reaction to quinidine. Also avoid this medication if quinine or quinidine causes you to bruise easily.

Quinidex is prescribed only for certain specific types of heart irregularity, and should be avoided when other irregularities are present. It could also prove harmful if you have myasthenia gravis (abnormal muscle weakness) or a similar condition.

Special warnings about this medication
Quinidex is reserved for certain kinds of dangerously rapid heart irregularities. It works well for some people, providing them with significant symptomatic relief. However, you should know that—on average for all cases—it has not been shown to improve chances of long-term survival, and could actually lower the odds.

Remember, too, that under certain conditions (slow heart rate, low potassium or magnesium levels) Quinidex can *cause* certain types of heart irregularity. It can also cause the condition known as heart block, and should be used with caution if you have partial heart block.

Also use Quinidex Extentabs cautiously if you have kidney or liver disease. Your doctor will check your blood count and liver and kidney function periodically during long-term therapy.

There have been rare cases of severe allergic reaction to quinidine, especially during the first few weeks of therapy. Discuss any allergic reactions you have experienced with your doctor.

Do not confuse Quinidex with quinine, which, although related, is used to treat malaria.

**Possible food and drug interactions
when taking this medication**

Concentrations of digoxin (Lanoxin) in your blood may increase or even double when this drug is taken with Quinidex Extentabs. Your doctor may need to reduce the amount of digoxin you take.

If Quinidex Extentabs are taken with certain other drugs, the effects of either could be increased, decreased, or altered. It is especially important to check with your doctor before combining Quinidex Extentabs with the following:

Amiodarone (Cordarone)
Antacids containing magnesium, such as Maalox and Mylanta
Antispasmodic drugs such as Bentyl
Aspirin
Beta-blocking blood pressure medications such as Inderal and Tenormin
Blood thinners such as Coumadin
Certain antidepressants such as Elavil and Tofranil
Certain diuretic drugs such as Diamox and Daranide
Cimetidine (Tagamet)
Codeine
Decamethonium
Digitoxin (Crystodigin)
Disopyramide (Norpace)
Felodipine (Plendil)
Haloperidol (Haldol)
Hydrocodone (Vicodin)
Ketoconazole (Nizoral)
Major tranquilizers such as Stelazine and Thorazine
Mexiletine (Mexitil)
Nicardipine (Cardene)
Nifedipine (Procardia)
Nimodipine (Nimotop)
Phenobarbital
Phenytoin (Dilantin)
Physostigmine (Antilirium)
Procainamide (Procanbid)
Reserpine (Diupres)
Rifampin (Rifadin)
Sodium bicarbonate
Sucralfate (Carafate)
Thiazide diuretics such as Dyazide and HydroDIURIL
Verapamil (Calan)

Special information
if you are pregnant or breastfeeding
The effects of Quinidex Extentabs during pregnancy have not been adequately studied. If you are pregnant or plan to become pregnant, inform your doctor immediately. Quinidex appears in breast milk and can affect a nursing infant. If this medication is essential to your health, your doctor may advise you to discontinue breastfeeding until your treatment is finished.

Recommended dosage

ADULTS

The usual dosage is 1 Quinidex Extentab every 8 to 12 hours.

Overdosage
Any medication taken in excess can have serious consequences. If you suspect an overdose, seek medical treatment immediately.

■ *The symptoms of Quinidex Extentabs overdose may include:*
Abnormal heart rhythms, blurred or double vision, confusion, delirium, diarrhea, headache, intolerance to light, loss of hearing, low blood pressure, ringing in the ears, vertigo, vomiting

Generic name:

QUINIDINE POLYGALACTURONATE

See Cardioquin, page 202.

Generic name:

QUINIDINE SULFATE

See Quinidex Extentabs, page 1095.

Generic name:

RALOXIFENE

See Evista, page 500.

Generic name:

RAMIPRIL

See Altace, page 39.

Generic name:

RANITIDINE

See Zantac, page 1443.

Generic name:

RANITIDINE BISMUTH CITRATE

See Tritec, page 1353.

Brand name:

REGLAN

Pronounced: REG-lan
Generic name: Metoclopramide hydrochloride

Why is this drug prescribed?
Reglan increases the contractions of the stomach and small intestine, helping the passage of food. It is given to treat the symptoms of diabetic gastroparesis, a condition in which the stomach does not contract. These symptoms include vomiting, nausea, heartburn, feeling of indigestion, persistent fullness after meals, and appetite loss. Reglan is also used, for short periods, to treat heartburn in people with gastroesophageal reflux disorder (backflow of stomach contents into the esophagus). In addition, it is also given to prevent nausea and vomiting caused by cancer chemotherapy and surgery.

Most important fact about this drug
Reglan may cause mild to severe depression. If you have suffered from depression in the past, make sure your doctor is aware of it. Reglan may not be the best drug for you.

How should you take this medication?
Reglan is usually taken 30 minutes before a meal. If you suffer from heartburn that occurs only intermittently or only at certain times of day, your doctor may want you to schedule your Reglan therapy around those times.

You will probably take Reglan for only 4 to 12 weeks. Continuous treatment beyond 12 weeks is not recommended.

If you have diabetic "lazy stomach" (gastric stasis) that tends to recur, your doctor may want you to take Reglan at the first sign of a recurrence.

■ *If you miss a dose...*
Take it as soon as you remember. If it is almost time for your next dose, skip the one you missed and go back to your regular schedule. Do not take 2 doses at once.

■ *Storage instructions...*
Store at room temperature.

What side effects may occur?
Side effects cannot be anticipated. If any develop or change in intensity, inform your doctor as soon as possible. Only your doctor can determine if it is safe for you to continue taking Reglan.

■ *More common side effects may include:*
Drowsiness, fatigue, restlessness

■ *Less common or rare side effects may include:*
Breast development in males, confusion, continual discharge of milk from the breasts, depression, diarrhea, dizziness, fluid retention, frequent urination, hallucinations, headache, high or low blood pressure, high fever, hives, impotence, inability to hold urine, insomnia, menstrual irregularities, nausea, rapid or slow heartbeat, rash, rigid muscles, slow movement, swollen tongue or throat, tremor, vision problems, wheezing, yellowed eyes and skin

In addition, Reglan may cause symptoms similar to those of Parkinson's disease, such as slow movements, rigidity, tremor, or a mask-like facial appearance.

Reglan may produce tardive dyskinesia, a syndrome of jerky or writhing involuntary movements, particularly of the tongue, face, mouth, or jaw. Reglan may also cause involuntary movements of the arms and legs, and sometimes loud or labored breathing.

Reglan may cause intense restlessness with associated symptoms such as anxiety, agitation, foot-tapping, pacing, inability to sit still, jitteriness, and insomnia. These symptoms may disappear as your body gets used to Reglan, or if your dosage is reduced.

Why should this drug not be prescribed?
Do not take Reglan if you are sensitive to it or have ever had an allergic reaction to it.

You should not take Reglan if you have a condition such as obstruction, perforation, or hemorrhage of the stomach or small bowel that might be aggravated by increased stomach and small-bowel movement.

If you have pheochromocytoma (a nonmalignant tumor that causes hypertension), do not take Reglan; it could trigger a dangerous jump in blood pressure.

Do not take Reglan if you have epilepsy; it could increase the frequency and severity of seizures.

If you are taking a drug that is likely to cause side effects such as tremors, jerks, grimaces, or writhing movements, do not take Reglan; it could make such symptoms more severe.

Reglan is not recommended for patients under 18 years of age.

Special warnings about this medication

If you have Parkinson's disease, you should be given Reglan cautiously or not at all, since the drug may make your Parkinson's symptoms worse.

Because Reglan may make you drowsy and impair your coordination, you should not drive, climb, or perform hazardous tasks until you know how the medication affects you.

Use Reglan with caution if you have high blood pressure.

Possible food and drug interactions
when taking this medication

If Reglan is taken with certain other drugs, the effects of either could be increased, decreased, or altered. It is especially important to check with your doctor before combining Reglan with the following:

Acetaminophen (Tylenol)
Alcoholic beverages
Antispasmodic drugs such as Bentyl and Pro-Banthine
Cimetidine (Tagamet)
Cyclosporine (Sandimmune)
Digoxin (Lanoxin)
Insulin
MAO inhibitor antidepressants such as Nardil and Parnate
Levodopa (Dopar, Sinemet)
Narcotic painkillers such as Percocet and Demerol
Sleeping pills such as Dalmane, Halcion, and Restoril
Tetracycline (Achromycin, Sumycin, others)
Tranquilizers such as Valium and Xanax

If you take insulin for diabetes, your insulin dosage or dosing schedule may have to be adjusted while you are taking Reglan.

Special information
if you are pregnant or breastfeeding
The effects of Reglan during pregnancy have not been adequately studied. If you are pregnant or plan to become pregnant, inform your doctor immediately. Reglan should be used during pregnancy only if it is clearly needed. Reglan appears in breast milk. Your doctor may recommend that you discontinue Reglan while you are breastfeeding your baby.

Recommended dosage

ADULTS

Symptoms of Gastroesophageal Reflux
The usual dose is 10 milligrams to 15 milligrams of Reglan, up to 4 times a day, 30 minutes before each meal and at bedtime, depending upon the symptoms being treated and the effectiveness of the dose. Treatment usually lasts no longer than 12 weeks.

If symptoms occur only intermittently or at specific times of the day, your doctor may give you a single dose of up to 20 milligrams as a preventive measure.

Symptoms Associated with Diabetic Gastroparesis or Gastric Stasis
The usual dose is 10 milligrams 30 minutes before each meal and at bedtime for 2 to 8 weeks.

OLDER ADULTS

Relief of Symptomatic Gastroesophageal Reflux
Older adults may need only 5 milligrams per dose.

Overdosage
Any medication taken in excess can have serious consequences. If you suspect an overdose, seek medical attention immediately.

■ *Symptoms of Reglan overdose may include:*
Disorientation, drowsiness, involuntary movements

Brand name:

RELAFEN

Pronounced: REL-ah-fen
Generic name: Nabumetone

Why is this drug prescribed?
Relafen, a nonsteroidal anti-inflammatory drug, is used to relieve the inflammation, swelling, stiffness, and joint pain associated with rheumatoid arthritis and osteoarthritis (the most common form of arthritis).

Most important fact about this drug
You should have frequent checkups with your doctor if you take Relafen regularly. Ulcers or internal bleeding can occur with or without warning.

How should you take this medication?
Relafen can be taken with or without food. Take it exactly as prescribed.

■ *If you miss a dose...*
Take the forgotten dose as soon as you remember. If it is almost time for your next dose, skip the one you missed and go back to your regular schedule. Never take a double dose.

■ *Storage instructions...*
Keep this medication in the container it came in, tightly closed, and away from moist places and direct light. It can be stored at room temperature.

What side effects may occur?
Side effects cannot be anticipated. If any develop or change in intensity, inform your doctor as soon as possible. Only your doctor can determine whether it is safe for you to continue taking Relafen.

■ *More common side effects may include:*
Abdominal pain, constipation, diarrhea, dizziness, fluid retention, gas, headache, indigestion, itching, nausea, rash, ringing in ears

■ *Less common side effects may include:*
Dry mouth, fatigue, inability to fall or stay asleep, increased sweating, inflammation of the mouth, inflammation of the stomach, nervousness, sleepiness, vomiting

■ *Rare side effects may include:*
Agitation, anxiety, confusion, dark, tarry, bloody stools, depression, difficult or labored breathing, difficulty swallowing, fluid retention, general feeling of illness, hives, increase or loss of appetite, large blisters, pins and needles, pneumonia or lung inflammation, sensitivity to light, severe allergic reactions, skin peeling, stomach and intestinal inflammation and/or bleeding, tremor, ulcers, vaginal bleeding, vertigo, vision changes, weakness, weight gain, yellow eyes and skin

Why should this drug not be prescribed?
Do not take this medication if you are sensitive to or have ever had an allergic reaction to Relafen, or if you have had asthma attacks, hives or other allergic reactions caused by Relafen, aspirin, or other nonsteroidal anti-inflammatory drugs.

Special warnings about this medication
Stomach and intestinal ulcers can occur without warning. Remember to get regular checkups.

Make sure the doctor knows if you have kidney or liver disease. Relafen should be used with caution.

This drug can cause fluid retention and swelling. It should be used with caution if you have congestive heart failure or high blood pressure.

Relafen can cause increased sensitivity to sunlight.

Possible food and drug interactions
when taking this medication
If Relafen is taken with certain other drugs, the effects of either could be increased, decreased, or altered. It is especially important to check with your doctor before combining Relafen with blood-thinning drugs such as Coumadin and aspirin.

Other drugs with which Relafen could possibly interact include:

Diuretics (HydroDIURIL, Lasix)
Lithium (Lithonate)
Methotrexate

Special information
if you are pregnant or breastfeeding
The effects of Relafen during pregnancy have not been adequately studied. If you are pregnant or plan to become pregnant, inform your doctor immediately. Relafen may appear in breast milk and could affect a nursing infant. If this medication is essential to your health, your doctor may advise you to discontinue breastfeeding until your treatment with Relafen is finished.

Recommended dosage

ADULTS

The usual starting dose is 1000 milligrams taken as a single dose. Dosage may be increased up to 2000 milligrams per day, taken once or twice a day.

CHILDREN

The safety and effectiveness of this drug in children have not been established.

Overdosage

Any medication taken in excess can have serious consequences. If you suspect an overdose, seek medical attention immediately.

Brand name:

REMERON

Pronounced: REM-ur-on
Generic name: Mirtazapine

Why is this drug prescribed?

Remeron is prescribed for the treatment of major depression—that is, a continuous depressed mood that interferes with everyday life. The symptoms of major depression often include changes in appetite and weight, difficulty sleeping, loss of interest in pleasurable activities, constant fidgeting or a slowdown in movement, fatigue, feelings of guilt or worthlessness, difficulty concentrating, slowed thinking, and suicidal thoughts.

Remeron is thought to work by adjusting the balance of the brain's natural chemical messengers, especially norepinephrine and serotonin.

Most important fact about this drug

Remeron makes some people drowsy or less alert, and may affect judgment and thinking. Don't drive or participate in any hazardous activity that requires full mental alertness until you know whether Remeron has this effect on you.

How should you take this medication?

Remeron may be taken with or without food. It is preferable to take it in the evening before you go to sleep. Even though you may begin to feel better in 1 to 4 weeks, continue taking this medication exactly as prescribed. Regular daily doses are needed for the drug to work properly.

■ *If you miss a dose...*
 Take the forgotten dose if you remember within a few hours. Otherwise, skip the dose. Never try to "catch up" by doubling the dose.

■ *Storage instructions...*
Store at room temperature in a tight, light-resistant container.

What side effects may occur?
Side effects cannot be anticipated. If any develop or change in intensity, tell your doctor as soon as possible. Only your doctor can determine if it is safe for you to continue taking Remeron.

■ *More common side effects may include:*
Abnormal dreams and thinking, constipation, dizziness, dry mouth, "flu-like" symptoms, increased appetite, sleepiness, weakness, weight gain

■ *Less common side effects may include...*
Back pain, confusion, difficult or labored breathing, fluid retention, frequent urination, muscle pain, nausea, swelling of ankles or hands, tremors

Why should this drug not be prescribed?
If you have ever had an allergic reaction to Remeron or similar drugs such as Ludiomil and Desyrel, you should not take this medication. Be sure to tell your doctor about any drug reactions you have experienced.

You should also avoid Remeron if you are taking the antidepressants Nardil or Parnate (see "Special warnings about this medication").

Special warnings about this medication
Serious, sometimes fatal reactions have been known to occur when drugs such as Remeron are taken in combination with other drugs known as MAO inhibitors, including the antidepressants Nardil and Parnate. Never take Remeron with one of these drugs or within 14 days of discontinuing therapy with one of them; and allow at least 14 days between stopping Remeron and starting an MAO inhibitor.

If you develop "flu-like" symptoms, a sore throat, chills or fever, mouth sores, or any other signs of infection, call your doctor; these symptoms may signal a serious underlying condition.

Remeron tends to raise cholesterol levels in some people. If you have a cholesterol problem, be sure to mention it to your doctor before starting therapy with Remeron.

Remeron should be used with caution if you have active liver or kidney disease, or heart or blood pressure problems. Also be sure to tell your doctor if you have a history of seizures, mania (extremely high spirits), hypomania (mild excitability), drug use, or any other physical or emotional problems.

While first taking this medication you may feel dizzy or light-headed, especially when getting up from a lying or sitting position. If getting up slowly doesn't help, or if this problem continues, notify your doctor.

Possible food and drug interactions
when taking this medication
Never combine Remeron with an MAO inhibitor; and do not drink alcohol while taking this medication. If Remeron is taken with certain other drugs, the effects of either could be increased, decreased, or altered. It is especially important to check with your doctor before combining Remeron with tranquilizers such as Valium, Xanax, and Ativan.

Special information
if you are pregnant or breastfeeding
The effects of Remeron during pregnancy have not been adequately studied. If you are pregnant or plan to become pregnant, tell your doctor immediately. It is not known whether Remeron appears in breast milk. However, because many drugs do make their way into breast milk, you should tell your doctor if you are breastfeeding or plan to breastfeed.

Recommended dosage

ADULTS

The usual starting dose is 15 milligrams taken daily before going to sleep. Depending upon your response, your dosage may be increased to as much as 45 milligrams a day.

CHILDREN

The safety and effectiveness of Remeron have not been established in children.

Overdosage
Any medication taken in excess can have serious consequences. If you suspect an overdose, seek medical attention immediately.

■ *Symptoms of Remeron overdose include:*
  Drowsiness, impaired memory, mental confusion, rapid heartbeat

Brand name:

RENOVA

See Retin-A and Renova, page 1114.

Generic name:

REPAGLINIDE

See Prandin, page 1022.

Brand name:

REQUIP

Pronounced: REE-kwip
Generic name: Ropinirole hydrochloride

Why is this drug prescribed?

Requip helps relieve the signs and symptoms of Parkinson's disease. Caused by a deficit of dopamine (one of the brain's chief chemical messengers), this disorder is marked by progressive muscle stiffness, tremor, and fatigue. Requip works by stimulating dopamine receptors in the brain, thus promoting better, easier movement.

Requip can be taken with or without levodopa (usually prescribed as Sinemet), another drug used to treat the symptoms of Parkinson's disease.

Most important fact about this drug

Requip is not a cure for Parkinson's disease. However, it does alleviate symptoms of the disease, and it can shorten the "off" periods of immobility that patients on long-term levodopa therapy often begin to experience.

How should you take this medication?

Take 3 doses a day, with or without food. If the drug upsets your stomach, combining it with food may relieve the problem. If you are also taking levodopa, its dosage may be gradually decreased when you start therapy with Requip.

- *If you miss a dose...*
  Take it as soon as you remember. If it is almost time for your next dose, skip the one you missed and go back to your regular schedule. Do not take 2 doses at once.

- *Storage instructions...*
  Store at room temperature away from light.

What side effects may occur?

Side effects cannot be anticipated. If any develop or change in intensity, inform your doctor as soon as possible. Only your doctor can determine if it is safe for you to continue taking Requip.

- *More common side effects may include:*
  Abdominal pain, abnormal dreaming, abnormal muscle movements, abnormal vision, amnesia, anxiety, arthritis, bronchitis, confusion, constipation, decreased muscle movements, diarrhea, difficulty breathing, dizziness, drowsiness, dry mouth, eye problems, fainting, falling, fatigue, hallucinations, headache, increased sweating, indigestion, joint pain, leg swelling, nausea, nervousness, pain, paralysis, respiratory tract infection, runny nose, sinus inflammation, skin tingling, sore throat, swelling, tremor, urinary tract infection, viral infections, vomiting, weakness

- *Less common side effects may include:*
  Back pain, blood in the urine, chills, cough, decreased heart rate, depression, difficulty swallowing, dry eyes, gas, gout, gum inflammation, high blood sugar, hot flashes, increased salivation, insomnia, leg cramps, low blood pressure, muscle aches, muscle spasms, muscle tone problems, nerve pain, rash, weight loss, worsening of Parkinson's disease symptoms

- *Rare side effects may include:*
  Abnormal coordination, acid indigestion, agitation, aggressive reaction, altered heart rate, asthma, boils, chest pain, conjunctivitis (pinkeye), convulsions, dandruff, decreased hearing, delirium, delusions, dementia, diabetes, disorders of the penis, earache, ear infection, eye inflammation, eye pain, enlarged abdomen, enlarged breasts, feeling of well-being, fever, flu-like symptoms, fungal infections, genital infections, hair loss, heart failure, hemorrhoids, herpes infections, hiccups, high cholesterol levels, hives, impaired concentration, increased or decreased sex drive, increased thirst, laryngitis, low blood sugar, loss of bowel control, loss of menstruation, loss of understanding, migraine, nose bleeds, osteoporosis, paranoid reaction, personality disorder, prostate disorder, psoriasis, purple skin patches, ringing in the ears, sensitivity to light, skin discoloration, skin itching, skin ulcers, stomach ulcers, thyroid problems, tongue swelling, toothache, twitching, urinary disorders, vaginal bleeding, varicose veins, vein inflammation, weight gain

Why should this drug not be prescribed?
If Requip gives you an allergic reaction, you will not be able to continue using it.

Special warnings about this medication
At the start of Requip therapy and whenever the dose is increased, you face a slightly increased risk of a fainting spell or other symptoms of low blood pressure such as dizziness, nausea, sweating, and light-headedness, particularly when you get up suddenly after sitting or reclining for a prolonged period. To avoid such symptoms, be careful to stand up slowly.

A few patients—especially older ones—also develop hallucinations. Let your doctor know if this occurs. You may have to stop Requip therapy.

There is also a slight chance of developing respiratory difficulties or problems with your eyesight. If you find it hard to breathe, have any swelling, or develop problems with your vision, alert your doctor at once.

If you are taking Sinemet with Requip, you may experience jerking muscle movements. Tell your doctor. He will need to decrease your dose of Sinemet.

With other Parkinson's medications, a sudden dose reduction has been known to cause high fever, muscle stiffness, and loss of consciousness. Although this has not happened with Requip, be alert for such problems and contact your doctor immediately if they occur.

Requip may cause drowsiness. Do not drive a car or operate machinery until you know how the drug affects you. Requip may also cause darkening of your skin and eye color. Tell your doctor if you notice any change.

Possible food and drug interactions
when taking this medication

If Requip is taken with certain other drugs, the effects of either can be increased, decreased, or altered. It is especially important to check with your doctor before combining Requip with the following:

Alcohol
Antidepressants such as Elavil, Pamelor, and Tofranil
Ciprofloxacin (Cipro)
Drugs that contain levodopa such as Dopar, Larodopa, and Sinemet
Estrogen medications such as ethinyl estradiol (Estinyl)
Major tranquilizers such as Haldol, Mellaril, Navane, Prolixin, and Thorazine
Metoclopramide (Reglan)
Tranquilizers such as the benzodiazepines Ativan, Librium, Valium, and Xanax

Special information
if you are pregnant or breastfeeding

Although the effects of Requip during pregnancy have not been adequately studied in humans, birth defects have occurred in animals. If you are pregnant or plan to become pregnant, inform your doctor immediately.

Requip may inhibit production of breast milk. There is also a possibility that it will appear in breast milk and affect the nursing infant. If this medication is essential to your health, your doctor may advise you to discontinue breastfeeding.

Recommended dosage

ADULTS

Requip is taken 3 times a day. During the first week of therapy, each dose is 0.25 milligram. During the second week, the amount rises to 0.5 milligram. In the third week, it increases to 0.75 milligram, and in the fourth week reaches 1 milligram (3 milligrams daily). If necessary, your doctor will gradually increase the dosage further, up to a maximum of 24 milligrams per day.

If you need to stop Requip therapy, the doctor will discontinue the drug gradually over a 7-day period, reducing the number of doses from 3 to 2 per day for the first 4 days, then to once a day for the remaining 3 days.

Overdosage

Any medication taken in excess can have serious consequences. If you suspect an overdose, seek medical treatment immediately.

■ *Symptoms of Requip overdose may include:*
Agitation, chest pain, confusion, drowsiness, facial muscle movements, grogginess, increased jerkiness of movement, symptoms of low blood pressure (dizziness, light-headedness) upon standing, nausea, vomiting

---

Generic name:

RESERPINE, HYDRALAZINE, AND HYDROCHLOROTHIAZIDE

See Ser-Ap-Es, page 1176.

Brand name:

RESTORIL

Pronounced: RES-tah-rill
Generic name: Temazepam

Why is this drug prescribed?

Restoril is used for the relief of insomnia (difficulty in falling asleep, waking up frequently at night, or waking up early in the morning). It belongs to a class of drugs known as benzodiazepines.

Most important fact about this drug

Sleep problems are usually temporary, requiring treatment for only a short time, usually 1 or 2 days and no more than 2 to 3 weeks. Insomnia that lasts longer than this may be a sign of another medical problem. If you find you need this medicine for more than 7 to 10 days, be sure to check with your doctor.

How should you take this medication?
Take this medication exactly as directed; never take more than the prescribed amount.

■ *If you miss a dose...*
Take only as needed.

■ *Storage instructions...*
Keep this medication in the container it came in, tightly closed, and out of the reach of children. Store it at room temperature.

What side effects may occur?
Side effects cannot be anticipated. If any develop or change in intensity, inform your doctor as soon as possible. Only your doctor can determine if it is safe for you to continue taking Restoril.

■ *More common side effects may include:*
Dizziness, drowsiness, fatigue, headache, nausea, nervousness, sluggishness

■ *Less common or rare side effects may include:*
Abdominal discomfort, abnormal sweating, agitation, anxiety, backache, blurred vision, burning eyes, confusion, constant, involuntary movement of the eyeball, depression, diarrhea, difficult or labored breathing, dry mouth, exaggerated feeling of well-being, fluttery or throbbing heartbeat, hallucinations, hangover, increased dreaming, lack of coordination, loss of appetite, loss of equilibrium, loss of memory, nightmares, overstimulation, restlessness, tremors, vertigo, vomiting, weakness

■ *Side effects due to rapid decrease in or abrupt withdrawal from Restoril:*
Abdominal and muscle cramps, convulsions, feeling of discomfort, inability to fall asleep or stay asleep, sweating, tremors, vomiting

Why should this drug not be prescribed?
If you are pregnant or plan to become pregnant, you should not take this medication. It poses a potential risk to the developing baby.

Special warnings about this medication

When you take Restoril every night for more than a few weeks, it loses its effectiveness to help you sleep. This is known as tolerance. You can also develop physical dependence on this drug, especially if you take it regularly for more than a few weeks, or take high doses.

When you first start taking Restoril, until you know whether the medication will have any "carry over" effect the next day, use extreme care while doing anything that requires complete alertness such as driving a car or operating machinery.

If you are severely depressed or have suffered from severe depression in the past, consult your doctor before taking this medication.

If you have kidney or liver problems or chronic lung disease, make sure your doctor is aware of it.

After you stop taking Restoril, you may have more trouble sleeping than you had before you started taking it. This is called "rebound insomnia" and should clear up after 1 or 2 nights.

Possible food and drug interactions
when taking this medication

Restoril may intensify the effects of alcohol. Do not drink alcohol while taking this medication.

If Restoril is taken with certain other drugs, the effects of either could be increased, decreased, or altered. It is especially important to check with your doctor before combining Restoril with the following:

Antidepressant drugs such as Elavil, Nardil, Parnate, and Tofranil
Antihistamines such as Benadryl
Barbiturates such as phenobarbital and Seconal
Major tranquilizers such as Mellaril and Thorazine
Narcotic pain relievers such as Percocet and Demerol
Oral contraceptives
Tranquilizers such as Valium and Xanax

Special information
if you are pregnant or breastfeeding

Do not take Restoril if you are pregnant or planning to become pregnant. There is an increased risk of birth defects. This drug may appear in breast milk and could affect a nursing infant. If this medication is essential to your health, your doctor may advise you to discontinue breastfeeding until your treatment with this medication is finished.

Recommended dosage

ADULTS

The usual recommended dose is 15 milligrams at bedtime; however, 7.5 milligrams may be all that is necessary, while some people may need 30 milligrams. Your doctor will tailor your dose to your needs.

CHILDREN

The safety and effectiveness of Restoril have not been established in children under 18 years of age.

OLDER ADULTS

The doctor will prescribe the smallest effective amount in order to avoid side effects such as oversedation, dizziness, confusion, and lack of muscle coordination. The usual starting dose is 7.5 milligrams.

Overdosage

Any medication taken in excess can cause symptoms of overdose. If you suspect an overdose, seek medical attention immediately.

- **The symptoms of Restoril overdose may include:**
  Coma, confusion, diminished reflexes, loss of coordination, low blood pressure, labored or difficult breathing, seizures, sleepiness, slurred speech

Brand names:

RETIN-A AND RENOVA

Pronounced: Ret-in-A, Re-NO-va
Generic name: Tretinoin
Other brand name: Avita

Why is this drug prescribed?

Retin-A, Avita, and Renova contain the skin medication tretinoin. Retin-A and Avita are used in the treatment of acne. Renova is prescribed to reduce fine wrinkles, discoloration, and roughness on facial skin (as part of a comprehensive program of skin care and sun avoidance).

Retin-A is available in liquid, cream, or gel form, and in a stronger gel called Retin-A Micro. Avita comes only as a gel. Renova is available in cream form only.

Most important fact about this drug

While using Retin-A, Avita, or Renova, keep exposure to sunlight, including sunlamps, to a minimum. If you have a sunburn, do not use the medication until you have fully recovered. Use of sunscreen products (at least SPF 15) and protective clothing over treated areas is recommended when exposure to the sun cannot be avoided. Weather extremes, such as wind and cold, may be irritating and should also be avoided while using these products.

How should you use this medication?

Retin-A and Avita should be applied once a day, at bedtime, to the skin where acne appears, using enough to lightly cover the affected area. The liquid form may be applied using a fingertip, gauze pad, or cotton swab. If you use gauze or cotton, avoid oversaturation, which might cause the liquid to run into areas where treatment is not intended.

Renova is also applied once daily at bedtime. Use only enough to lightly cover the affected area. Before you use Renova, wash your face with a mild soap, pat your skin dry, and wait 20 to 30 minutes. Then apply a dab of Renova cream the size of a pea and spread it lightly over your face, avoiding your eyes, ears, nostrils, mouth, and open wounds.

You may use cosmetics while being treated with these products; however, you should thoroughly cleanse the areas to be treated before applying the medication.

If your skin becomes too dry, you may want to use petroleum jelly or another emollient during the day.

If there is no immediate improvement, or new blemishes appear, don't get discouraged; it takes weeks for the medicine to take effect. Continue applying the prescribed amount. (Do not increase the dosage; it may irritate your skin.)

Do not stop treatment when improvement finally occurs. You must continue therapy to maintain the beneficial effect.

- *If you miss a dose...*
  Resume your regular schedule the next day.

- *Storage instructions...*
  Store at ordinary room temperature. Do not freeze Renova.

What side effects may occur?

If you have sensitive skin, the use of Avita or Retin-A may cause your skin to become excessively red, puffy, blistered, or crusted. If this happens, notify your doctor, who may recommend that you discontinue the medication until your skin returns to normal, or adjust the medication to a level that you can tolerate.

An unusual darkening of the skin or lack of color of the skin may occur temporarily with repeated application of Avita or Retin-A.

Side effects of Renova are generally not severe and may include burning, dry skin, itching, peeling, redness, and stinging.

Why should this drug not be prescribed?

If you are sensitive to or have ever had an allergic reaction to either of these products, avoid using them.

The safety and effectiveness of long-term use of Retin-A in the treatment of disorders other than acne have not been established.

The safety and effectiveness of Renova have not been established in children under age 18, adults over age 50, and people with heavily pigmented skin, nor in periods of greater than 48 weeks of daily use.

Special warnings about this medication

Be sure to keep these products away from the eyes, mouth, angles of the nose, and mucous membranes.

The medication may cause a brief feeling of warmth or slight stinging when applied. If it causes an abnormal irritation, redness, blistering, or peeling of the skin, notify your doctor. He may suggest that you use the medication less frequently, discontinue use temporarily, or discontinue use altogether. If a severe sensitivity reaction or chemical irritation occurs, you will probably need to stop using the drug.

If you have eczema (skin inflammation consisting of itching and small blisters that ooze and crust over) or other chronic skin conditions, use these products with extreme caution, as they may cause severe irritation.

During the early weeks of acne therapy, a worsening of the condition may occur due to the action of Avita or Retin-A on deep, previously unseen areas of inflammation. This is not a reason to discontinue therapy, but do notify your doctor if it occurs.

Retin-A gel and Avita are flammable and should be kept away from heat and flame.

Renova will not eliminate wrinkles, repair damage done by the sun, or reverse the aging process. After you stop using Renova, it is best to continue using a sunscreen and avoiding the sun.

Possible food and drug interactions
when taking this medication

If these medications are used with certain other drugs, the effects of either could be increased, decreased, or altered. It is especially important to check with your doctor before combining Avita or Retin-A with the following:

Preparations containing benzoyl peroxide, such as Benzac AC Wash 5, Benzshave, Desquam-E, PanOxyl

Preparations containing sulfur (ointments and other preparations used to treat skin disorders and infections)

Resorcinol (a drug, used in ointments to treat acne, that causes skin to peel)

Salicylic acid (a drug that kills bacteria and fungi and causes skin to peel)

"Resting" your skin is recommended between use of the above preparations and treatment with Avita or Retin-A.

Do not use Renova if you are taking other drugs that increase sensitivity to sunlight. These include:

Certain antibiotics, including Cipro, Noroxin, and tetracycline

Major tranquilizers such as Thorazine and Mellaril

Sulfa drugs such as Bactrim and Septra

Thiazide drugs (water pills) such as Diuril and HydroDIURIL

Caution should be exercised when using Avita, Retin-A, or Renova in combination with other topical medications, medicated or abrasive soaps and cleansers, soaps and cosmetics that have a strong drying effect, products with high concentrations of alcohol, astringents, spices, or lime (especially the peel), permanent wave solutions, electrolysis, hair depilatories or waxes, or other preparations that may dry or irritate the skin.

Special information
if you are pregnant or breastfeeding

If you are pregnant or plan to become pregnant, do not use these products. It is not known whether the drug appears in breast milk. Use with caution when breastfeeding.

Recommended dosage

RETIN-A AND AVITA

Apply once a day at bedtime.

You should begin to notice results after 2 to 3 weeks of treatment. More than 6 or 7 weeks of treatment are needed before consistent beneficial effects appear.

Once acne has responded satisfactorily, it may be possible to maintain the improvement with less frequent applications or other dosage forms. However, any change in formulation, drug concentration, or dose frequency should be closely monitored by your doctor to determine your tolerance and response.

RENOVA

Apply just enough to lightly cover the affected area once daily at bedtime. Do not apply more than the recommended amount; it will not improve results and may cause increased discomfort. You will see the most improvement during the first 24 weeks of therapy. After that, Renova will simply maintain the improvement. When therapy is stopped, the improvement will gradually diminish.

Overdosage

Applying Avita, Retin-A or Renova excessively will not produce faster or better results, and marked redness, peeling, or discomfort could occur.

Brand name:

RETROVIR

Pronounced: reh-troh-VEER
Generic name: Zidovudine

Why is this drug prescribed?

Retrovir is prescribed for adults infected with human immunodeficiency virus (HIV). HIV causes the immune system to break down so that it can no longer respond effectively to infection. This virus leads to the fatal disease known as acquired immune deficiency syndrome (AIDS). Retrovir slows down the progress of HIV. Combining Retrovir with other drugs such as Hivid can help slow the progression.

Retrovir is also prescribed for HIV-infected children over 3 months of age who have symptoms of HIV or who have no symptoms but, through testing, have shown evidence of impaired immunity.

Retrovir taken during pregnancy often prevents transmission of HIV from mother to child.

Signs and symptoms of HIV disease are significant weight loss, fever, diarrhea, infections, and problems with the nervous system.

Most important fact about this drug
The long-term effects of treatment with zidovudine are unknown. However, treatment with this drug may lead to blood diseases, including granulocytopenia (a severe blood disorder characterized by a sharp decrease of certain types of white blood cells called granulocytes) and severe anemia requiring blood transfusions. This is especially true in people with more advanced HIV and those who start treatment later in the course of their infection.

Also, because Retrovir is not a cure for HIV infections or AIDS, those who are infected may continue to develop complications, including opportunistic infections (exotic infections that develop when the immune system falters). Therefore, frequent blood counts by your doctor are strongly advised. Notify your doctor immediately of any changes in your general health.

How should you take this medication?
Take this medication exactly as prescribed by your doctor. Do not share this medication with anyone and do not exceed your recommended dosage. Take it at even intervals every 4 hours around the clock (children every 6 hours).

If you are pregnant, take the drug 5 times a day.

■ *If you miss a dose...*
Take it as soon as you remember. If it is almost time for your next dose, skip the one you missed and go back to your regular schedule. Do not take 2 doses at once.

■ *Storage instructions...*
Tablets and capsules should be stored at room temperature; keep capsules away from moisture. Syrup should be stored at room temperature, away from light.

What side effects may occur?
Side effects cannot be anticipated. If any develop or change in intensity, inform your doctor as soon as possible. Only your doctor can determine if it is safe for you to continue taking Retrovir.

The frequency and severity of side effects associated with the use of Retrovir are greater in people whose infection is more advanced when treatment is started. Sometimes it is difficult to distinguish side effects from the underlying signs of HIV disease or the infections caused by HIV.

■ *More common side effects may include:*
Change in sense of taste, constipation, diarrhea, difficult or labored breathing, dizziness, fever, general feeling of illness, inability to fall or stay

asleep, indigestion, loss of appetite, muscle pain, nausea, rash, severe headache, sleepiness, stomach and intestinal pain, sweating, tingling or pins and needles, vomiting, weakness

■ *Less common side effects may include:*
Acne, anxiety, back pain, belching, bleeding from the rectum, bleeding gums, body odor, changeable emotions, chest pain, chills, confusion, cough, decreased mental sharpness, depression, difficulty swallowing, dimness of vision, excess sensitivity to pain, fainting, fatigue, flu-like symptoms, frequent urination, gas, hearing loss, hives, hoarseness, increase in urine volume, inflammation of the sinuses or nose, itching, joint pain, light intolerance, mouth sores, muscle spasm, nervousness, nosebleed, painful or difficult urination, sore throat, swelling of the lip, swelling of the tongue, tremor, twitching, vertigo

Why should this drug not be prescribed?
If you have ever had a life-threatening allergic reaction to Retrovir or any of its ingredients, you should not take this drug.

Special warnings about this medication
This drug has been studied for only a limited period of time. Long-term safety and effectiveness are not known, especially for people who are in a less advanced stage of AIDS or AIDS-related complex (the condition that precedes AIDS), and for those using the drug over a prolonged period of time.

If you develop a blood disease, you may require a blood transfusion, and your doctor may reduce your dose or take you off the drug altogether. Make sure your doctor monitors your blood count on a regular basis.

The use of Retrovir has *not* been shown to reduce the risk of transmission of HIV to others through sexual contact or blood contamination or to nursing infants.

Retrovir should be used with extreme caution by people who have a bone marrow disease.

Some people taking Retrovir develop a sensitization reaction, often signaled by a rash. If you notice a rash developing, notify your doctor.

Because little data are available concerning the use of this drug in people with impaired kidney or liver function, check with your doctor before using Retrovir if you have either problem.

Possible food and drug interactions
when taking this medication

If Retrovir is taken with certain other drugs, the effects of either could be increased, decreased, or altered. It is especially important to check with your doctor before combining Retrovir with the following:

Acetaminophen (Tylenol)
Amphotericin B (Fungizone, a drug used to treat fungal infections)
Aspirin
Atovaquone (Mepron)
Dapsone (a drug used to treat leprosy)
Doxorubicin (Adriamycin, a cancer drug)
Fluconazole (Diflucan)
Flucytosine (Ancobon)
Indomethacin (Indocin)
Interferon (Intron A, Roferon-A)
Pentamidine (NebuPent, Pentam)
Phenytoin (Dilantin, a seizure medication)
Probenecid (Benemid, an antigout drug)
Ribavirin (Virazole)
Valproic acid (Depakene, a seizure medication)
Vinblastine (Velban, a cancer drug)
Vincristine (Oncovin, a cancer drug)

The combined use of phenytoin and Retrovir will be monitored by your doctor because of the possibility of seizures.

Special information
if you are pregnant or breastfeeding

The effects of Retrovir during pregnancy are under study. Use during pregnancy has been shown to protect the developing baby from contracting HIV. If you are pregnant or plan to become pregnant, inform your doctor immediately.

Since HIV can be passed on through breast milk to a nursing infant, do not breastfeed your baby.

Recommended dosage

ADULTS

All dosages of Retrovir must be very closely monitored by your physician. The following dosages are general; your physician will tailor the dose to your specific condition.

Tablets, Capsules, and Syrup
If you are also taking other HIV drugs, the usual total dose is 600 milligrams a day, divided into smaller doses. If you are taking Retrovir alone, the total daily dose is 500 milligrams (100 milligrams every 4 hours while awake) or 600 milligrams taken as several smaller doses.

If you are pregnant, the usual dosage is 100 milligrams in capsules, tablets, or syrup 5 times a day, beginning between 14 and 34 weeks of pregnancy, until you go into labor. You will then be given the drug intravenously until the baby is born. The baby will get Retrovir until it is 6 weeks old.

CHILDREN

The usual starting dose for children 3 months to 12 years of age is determined by body size. While the dose should not exceed 200 milligrams every 6 hours, it must still be individually determined. Safety and efficacy have not been determined for infants under 3 months of age.

Overdosage

Any medication taken in excess can have serious consequences. If you suspect an overdose, seek emergency medical treatment immediately.

■ *Symptoms of Retrovir overdose may include:*
 Nausea, vomiting

Brand name:

REVIA

Pronounced: reh-VEE-uh
Generic name: Naltrexone hydrochloride

Why is this drug prescribed?

ReVia is prescribed to treat alcohol dependence and narcotic addiction. ReVia is not a cure. You must be ready to make a change and be willing to undertake a comprehensive treatment program that includes professional counseling, support groups, and close medical supervision.

Most important fact about this drug

Before taking ReVia for narcotic addiction, you must be drug-free for at least 7 to 10 days. You must also be free of any drug withdrawal symptoms. If you think you are still in withdrawal, be sure to tell your doctor, since taking ReVia while narcotics are still in your system could cause serious physical problems. Your doctor will perform tests to confirm your drug-free condition.

How should you take this medication?

It is important to take ReVia on schedule as directed by your doctor, and to follow through with your counseling and support group therapy.

If you take small doses of heroin or other narcotic drugs while taking ReVia, they will have no effect. Large doses combined with ReVia can be fatal.

■ *If you miss a dose...*
Take the missed dose as soon as possible. If you do not remember until the next day, skip the missed dose and go back to your regular dosing schedule. Do not take 2 doses at once.

■ *Storage instructions...*
No special measures are needed.

What side effects may occur?

Side effects cannot be anticipated. If any side effects develop or change in intensity, tell your doctor immediately. Only your doctor can determine whether it is safe for you to continue taking ReVia.

■ *More common side effects of treatment for alcoholism may include:*
Dizziness, fatigue, headache, nausea, nervousness, sleeplessness, vomiting

■ *Less common side effects of treatment for alcoholism may include:*
Anxiety, sleepiness

■ *More common side effects of treatment for narcotic addiction may include:*
Abdominal pain/cramps, anxiety, difficulty sleeping, headache, joint and muscle pain, low energy, nausea and/or vomiting, nervousness

■ *Other side effects of treatment for narcotic addiction may include:*
Acne, athlete's foot, blurred vision and aching, burning, or swollen eyes, chills, clogged and aching ears, cold sores, cold feet, confusion, constipation, cough, decreased potency, delayed ejaculation, depression, diarrhea, disorientation, dizziness, dry mouth, fatigue, feeling down, fever, fluid retention, frequent urination, gas, hair loss, hallucinations, head "pounding," heavy breathing, hemorrhoids, hoarseness, "hot spells,"

increased appetite, increased blood pressure, increased energy, increased mucus, increased or decreased sexual interest, increased thirst, irregular or fast heartbeat, irritability, itching, light sensitivity, loss of appetite, nightmares, nosebleeds, oily skin, pain in shoulders, legs, or knees, pain in groin, painful urination, paranoia, restlessness, ringing in ears, runny nose, shortness of breath, side pains, sinus trouble, skin rash, sleepiness, sneezing, sore throat, stuffy nose, swollen glands, tremor, throbbing heartbeat, twitching, ulcer, weight loss or gain, yawning

Why should this drug not be prescribed?

If you are sensitive to or have ever had an allergic reaction to ReVia, you should not take it. If you have acute hepatitis (liver disease) or liver failure, do not start therapy with ReVia. Remember, too, that you must be narcotic-free before beginning ReVia therapy.

Special warnings about this medication

Since ReVia may cause liver damage when taken at high doses, if you develop symptoms that signal possible liver problems, you should stop taking ReVia immediately and see your doctor as soon as possible. These symptoms include abdominal pain lasting more than a few days, white bowel movements, dark urine, or yellowing of your eyes. Your doctor may periodically test your liver function while you are on ReVia therapy. Caution is also advisable if you have kidney problems.

If you are narcotic-dependent and accidentally take ReVia, you may experience severe withdrawal symptoms lasting up to 48 hours, including confusion, sleepiness, hallucinations, vomiting, and diarrhea. If this occurs, seek help immediately.

Do not attempt to use narcotics while taking ReVia. Small doses will have no effect, and large doses could lead to coma or even death.

Ask your doctor to give you a ReVia medication card to alert medical personnel that you are taking ReVia in case of an emergency. Carry this card with you at all times. If you do require medical treatment, be sure to tell the doctor that you are taking ReVia. You should also tell your dentist and pharmacist that you are taking ReVia.

The safety of ReVia in children under 18 years of age has not been established.

**Possible food and drug interactions
when taking this medication**
Since studies to evaluate the interaction of ReVia with drugs other than
narcotics have not been performed, do not take any medications, either over-
the-counter or prescription, without first notifying your doctor.

Do not use Antabuse while you are taking ReVia; both drugs can damage
your liver.

Do not take Mellaril (a drug used to treat depression and anxiety) while on
ReVia therapy, as the combination may make you feel very sleepy and
sluggish.

While taking ReVia avoid medicines that contain narcotics, including cough
and cold preparations, such as Actifed-C, Ryna-C, and Dimetane-DC;
antidiarrheal medications such as Lomotil; and narcotic painkillers such as
Percodan, Tylox, and Tylenol No. 3.

**Special information
if you are pregnant or breastfeeding**
The effects of ReVia during pregnancy have not been adequately studied. If
you are pregnant or are planning to become pregnant, tell your doctor
immediately. ReVia should be used during pregnancy only if clearly needed.
ReVia may appear in breast milk. If this medication is essential to your
health, your doctor may tell you to discontinue breastfeeding your baby until
your treatment with ReVia is finished.

Recommended dosage

ALCOHOLISM

The usual starting dose is 50 milligrams once a day.

NARCOTIC DEPENDENCE

The usual starting dose is 25 milligrams once a day. If no withdrawal
symptoms occur, the doctor may increase the dosage to 50 milligrams a day.

Overdosage
Any medication taken in excess can have serious consequences. If you
suspect an overdose of ReVia, seek medical attention immediately.

Brand name:

REZULIN

Pronounced: REZ-u-lin
Generic name: Troglitazone

Why is this drug prescribed?

Rezulin is used to hold down blood sugar levels in people with Type 2 diabetes. Sugar, one of the body's major energy sources, is usually transferred out of the bloodstream and into the cells with the help of a steady supply of insulin. In Type 2 diabetes, the body either fails to make enough insulin or can't use it properly, so that unused sugar builds up in the blood.

Rezulin brings down blood sugar levels in two ways: It cuts back the body's production of sugar; and it helps whatever insulin is available in the body to move sugar out of the blood and into muscle cells. It does not, however, improve the body's ability to produce insulin. Rezulin can be used alone or in conjunction with insulin injections or other oral diabetes medications. However, it should not be used as a substitute for other medications that successfully control your sugar levels.

Most important fact about this drug

Always remember that Rezulin is an aid to insulin, not a replacement for it. You need an adequate supply of insulin before Rezulin can do its job. Remember, too, that no diabetes medication can eliminate the need for good diet and exercise. Failure to stick with a good diet and exercise plan can lead to serious complications such as dangerously high or low blood sugar levels.

To make sure that your levels stay within the normal range, get regular tests of your blood sugar and glycosylated hemoglobin (a long-term measurement of blood sugar). Contact your doctor during periods of stress due to fever, infection, injury, surgery, and the like. Dosage of your diabetes medicines may need to be changed.

How should you take this medication?

Do not take any more or less of this medication than your doctor prescribes. Continue to take the same dose of insulin that you did before. Rezulin should be taken with a meal once a day, preferably at the same time each day.

- *If you miss a dose...*
  Take it at the next meal. If you completely miss a day, go back to your regular schedule on the following day. Never take 2 doses at the same time.

■ *Storage instructions...*
Store at room temperature away from moisture and humidity.

What side effects may occur?
Rezulin is unlikely to cause side effects. However, if any develop or change in intensity, tell your doctor as soon as possible. Only your doctor can determine if it is safe for you to continue taking Rezulin.

■ *Side effects may include:*
Anemia, back pain, diarrhea, dizziness, fainting, fever, flu-like symptoms, headache, heart failure, increased blood sugar, infections, nasal congestion, nausea, pain, sore throat, swelling, weakness, weight gain

Why should this drug not be prescribed?
Avoid Rezulin if it causes an allergic reaction.

Special warnings about this medication
Rezulin, by itself, will not cause excessively low blood sugar (hypoglycemia). However, when you combine it with insulin injections or other oral diabetes drugs, the chance of hypoglycemia increases. To avoid the problem, carefully follow your diet and exercise plan. If you begin to feel symptoms of hypoglycemia—shaking, sweating, agitation, clammy skin, or blurred vision—take some fast-acting sugar, such as 4 to 6 ounces of fruit juice. Let your doctor know about the incident; you may need a lower dose of insulin or oral medication.

Rezulin is not for Type 1 diabetics, who are unable to produce any insulin at all. Also, because there is a chance that Rezulin could aggravate congestive heart failure, it should be used in people with this condition only if urgently needed.

Although the chances are small, Rezulin has been known to damage the liver. If you have liver disease, you should not take this drug. Even if your liver is healthy, you should have monthly liver function tests for the first half year of therapy, tests every other month for the remainder of the year, and periodic tests thereafter. Notify your doctor immediately if you develop symptoms of liver damage such as nausea, vomiting, abdominal pain, fatigue, poor appetite, and dark urine.

Rezulin can affect the action of other diabetes medications. Ask your doctor whether a change of dosage will be needed for any of your other drugs.

Rezulin can increase your chances of pregnancy; and it cancels the effect of many birth control pills. To avoid an unwanted pregnancy, be sure to use some other form of contraception.

**Possible food and drug interactions
when taking this medication**

If Rezulin is taken with certain other drugs, the effects of either could be increased, decreased, or altered. It is especially important to check with your doctor before combining Rezulin with the following:

Astemizole (Hismanal)
Atorvastatin (Lipitor)
Calcium channel blockers such as Calan, Cardizem, Isoptin, and
    Procardia
Cerivastatin (Baycol)
Cholestyramine (Questran)
Cisapride (Propulsid)
Corticosteroids such as prednisone
Cyclosporine (Sandimmune, Neoral)
Fluvastatin (Lescol)
Lovastatin (Mevacor)
Oral contraceptives
Pravastatin (Pravachol)
Simvastatin (Zocor)
Tacrolimus (Prograf)
Terfenadine (Seldane)
Triazolam (Halcion)
Trimetrexate (Neutrexin)

**Special information
if you are pregnant or breastfeeding**

The effects of Rezulin during pregnancy have not been adequately studied, so your doctor will probably take you off the drug until the baby is born. Since it's important to maintain normal blood sugar levels during pregnancy, you should, however, continue to take insulin.

Researchers do not know whether Rezulin appears in breast milk. Use while breastfeeding is therefore not recommended.

Recommended dosage

ADULTS

Rezulin Alone

The usual starting dose is 400 or 600 milligrams once a day. If you start at the lower dose and your blood sugar doesn't respond after 6 to 8 weeks, the doctor may try the higher dose. If the 600-milligram dose fails to do the job, you'll need to switch to a different medication.

Rezulin with Insulin or Diabetes Pills
The usual starting dose is 200 milligrams once a day. Continue with your current dose of diabetes medication. Depending on your blood sugar response, your doctor may increase the dose of Rezulin after 2 to 4 weeks.

Long term, the usual dose is 400 milligrams once a day with a meal. The maximum daily dose is 600 milligrams.

As Rezulin begins working, your doctor may be able to lower your dosage of insulin or oral diabetes medication.

CHILDREN

Safety and effectiveness in children have not been established.

Overdosage
Although no specific information about Rezulin is available, any medication taken in excess can have serious consequences. If you suspect an overdose, seek medical attention immediately.

Generic name:

RHEUMATREX

See Methotrexate, page 776.

Brand name:

RHINOCORT

Pronounced: RYE-no-kort
Generic name: Budesonide

Why is this drug prescribed?
Rhinocort is an anti-inflammatory steroid medication. It is prescribed for relief of the symptoms of hay fever and other nasal inflammations.

Most important fact about this drug
Because steroids can suppress the immune system, people taking Rhinocort may become more susceptible to infections, and their infections could be more severe. Anyone taking Rhinocort or other corticosteroids who has not had infections such as chickenpox and measles should avoid exposure to them. If you are taking Rhinocort and are exposed, tell your doctor immediately.

How should you take this medication?

Rhinocort is prescribed as a nasal inhaler. Instructions for use are provided with the product. Do not use doses that are larger than recommended.

Relief of symptoms usually occurs 24 hours to a few days after starting Rhinocort. If symptoms do not improve within 3 weeks, or if nasal irritation worsens, contact your physician.

Shake the Rhinocort container well before using it. Do not use near an open flame.

Rhinocort is to be used within 6 months after opening it. If you have not used it for 8 weeks, spray into the air 4 times before you use it again.

■ *If you miss a dose...*
Take the forgotten dose as soon as you remember. If it is almost time for your next dose, skip the one you missed and go back to your regular schedule. Never take two doses at the same time.

■ *Storage instructions...*
Store at room temperature with the valve up.

Do not store near an open flame or heat above 120 degrees Fahrenheit. Do not store in areas of high humidity.

What side effects may occur?

Side effects cannot be anticipated. If any develop or change in intensity, inform your doctor as soon as possible. Only your doctor can determine if it is safe for you to continue taking Rhinocort.

■ *More common side effects may include:*
Increased coughing, irritation of the nasal passages, nosebleeds, sore throat

■ *Less common side effects may include:*
Bad taste in mouth, dry mouth, facial swelling, hoarseness, indigestion, inflammation of the skin, itching, muscle and joint pain, nasal sores or pain, nausea, nervousness, rash, reduced sense of smell, shortness of breath, yeast infection of the vagina or mouth, wheezing

Why should this drug not be prescribed?

If you develop an infection of your nose and throat, stop using Rhinocort and call your doctor. If you already have tuberculosis or any other kind of infection, be sure your doctor knows about it. Do not use Rhinocort if you have recently had nasal ulcers or nasal surgery; this drug would slow the healing process. You will also need to avoid Rhinocort if it gives you an allergic reaction.

Special warnings about this medication

If you have been taking a steroid in tablet form, such as prednisone, and are switched to Rhinocort, you may have symptoms of withdrawal, such as joint or muscle pain, lethargy, and depression. If you have been taking another steroid for a long time for asthma, your asthma may get worse if your medication is cut back too quickly. Using Rhinocort with another steroid drug can decrease the body's normal ability to make its own steroid chemicals.

Use Rhinocort with caution in children and teenagers. The drug can affect their rate of growth.

Possible food and drug interactions
when taking this medication

Talk to your doctor before using Rhinocort if you already take prednisone or any other steroid medication.

Special information
if you are pregnant or breastfeeding

The effects of Rhinocort during pregnancy have not been adequately studied. If you are pregnant or plan to become pregnant, inform your doctor immediately. Rhinocort should be used during pregnancy only if clearly needed. The effect of Rhinocort on nursing infants is also unknown, although we do know that similar drugs have been found in breast milk. Your doctor may have you stop breastfeeding while you are taking this drug.

Recommended dosage

The usual recommended starting dose for adults and children 6 years of age and older is 256 micrograms a day, either as two sprays in each nostril twice a day, morning and evening, or as four sprays in each nostril once a day in the morning. Your doctor may lower the dose once relief of symptoms occurs. Rhinocort is not recommended for use in children with nasal irritation not due to allergies.

Overdosage

Any medication taken in excess can have serious consequences. If you suspect an overdose, seek medical attention immediately.

Symptoms of Rhinocort overdose stem from a condition called hypercorticism, when the body produces an excess of its own steroid chemicals.

■ *Symptoms of overdose may include:*
Diabetes, excess hair growth, fatigue and weakness, fluid retention, impotence, lack of menstrual periods, skin discoloration

Brand name:

RIDAURA

Pronounced: ri-DOOR-ah
Generic name: Auranofin

Why is this drug prescribed?
Ridaura, a gold preparation, is given to help treat rheumatoid arthritis. Ridaura is taken by mouth, unlike other gold compounds, which are given by injection. It is recommended only for people who have not been helped sufficiently by nonsteroidal anti-inflammatory drugs (Anaprox, Dolobid, Indocin, Motrin, and others). Ridaura should be part of a comprehensive arthritis treatment program that includes non-drug forms of therapy.

You are most likely to benefit from Ridaura if you have active joint inflammation, especially in the early stages.

Most important fact about this drug
Unlike anti-inflammatory medications, Ridaura does not take effect immediately. In fact, you may have to wait for 3 to 6 months to get any benefit from Ridaura. Ridaura prevents or suppresses joint swelling, but does not cure rheumatoid arthritis.

How should you take this medication?
Read the patient information sheet provided with Ridaura, and take the medication exactly as prescribed.

You should observe good oral hygiene during therapy with Ridaura.

■ *If you miss a dose...*
If you take 1 dose a day, take the missed dose as soon as you remember. If you do not remember until the next day, skip the dose you missed and go back to your regular schedule.

If you take more than 1 dose a day, take the missed dose as soon as you remember. If it is almost time for your next dose, skip the one you missed and go back to your regular schedule.

Do not take 2 doses at once.

- *Storage instructions...*
  Store at room temperature in a tightly closed, light-resistant container.

What side effects may occur?
Side effects cannot be anticipated. If any side effects develop or change in intensity, tell your doctor immediately. Only your doctor can determine whether it is safe for you to continue taking Ridaura. Ridaura causes loose stools or diarrhea in about half of all people who take it; there may also be indigestion, abdominal pain and gas, loss of appetite, vomiting, or nausea.

- *Other commonly reported side effects include:*
  Blood-cell abnormalities which may result in bleeding, bronchitis, easy bruising, fever, gold dermatitis (inflammation of skin), itching, metallic taste, pinkeye, rash, sores in the mouth

- *Less common or rare side effects may include:*
  Altered sense of taste, anemia, black or bloody stools, blood in the urine, constipation, difficulty swallowing, fluid retention and swelling, hair loss, hives, inflammation of the tongue or gums, intestinal inflammation with ulcers, stomach or intestinal bleeding, yellowed eyes and skin

Why should this drug not be prescribed?
Do not take Ridaura if you have ever had any of the following reactions to a medication containing gold:

Anaphylaxis (life-threatening allergic reaction)
Blood or bone marrow abnormality
Fibrosis (scar tissue formation) in the lungs
Serious bowel inflammation
Skin peeling off in sheets

Special warnings about this medication
You should be monitored especially closely while taking Ridaura if you have any of the following:

History of a bone marrow abnormality
Inflammatory bowel disease
Kidney disease
Liver disease
Skin rash

Your doctor may order periodic blood and urine tests to check for unwanted effects.

Like other medications containing gold, Ridaura may cause serious blood abnormalities. If you start to bruise easily, or develop small red or purplish skin discolorations, see your doctor. He or she will have you stop taking Ridaura and will do some blood tests, including a platelet count.

Ridaura may cause protein or microscopic amounts of blood to spill into your urine. If a urine test shows that this is happening, your doctor will take you off of Ridaura immediately.

Gold compounds may cause your skin to become more sensitive to sunlight, so you may need to limit your exposure to the sun and wear a sunscreen.

Possible food and drug interactions
when taking this medication
If Ridaura is taken with certain other drugs, the effects of either could be increased, decreased, or altered. It is especially important to check with your doctor before combining Ridaura with the following:

Penicillamine (Cuprimine)
Phenytoin (Dilantin)

Special information
if you are pregnant or breastfeeding
If you are pregnant or plan to become pregnant, inform your doctor immediately. Because Ridaura may cause birth defects, it should not be taken during pregnancy.

Likewise, you should not take Ridaura while breastfeeding; although there are no data on Ridaura, injected gold appears in breast milk. If you are a new mother, you may have to choose between taking Ridaura and breastfeeding your baby.

Recommended dosage
The usual dosage of Ridaura is 6 milligrams daily in a single dose or divided into 2 smaller doses. After 6 months, your doctor may increase the dose to 9 milligrams, divided into 3 doses. Ridaura is prescribed only for adults.

Overdosage
Any medication taken in excess can have serious consequences. If you suspect an overdose of Ridaura, seek medical attention immediately.

Generic name:

RIFAMPIN, ISONIAZID, AND PYRAZINAMIDE

See Rifater, page 1135.

Brand Name:

RIFATER

Pronounced: RIF-a-tur
Generic ingredients: Rifampin, Isoniazid, Pyrazinamide

Why is this drug prescribed?

Rifater is a combination antibiotic used to treat the initial phase of tuberculosis. After a 2-month period, your doctor may prescribe another combination of antituberculosis drugs (Rifamate), which can be continued for longer periods.

Most important fact about this drug

Isoniazid, one of the components of Rifater, sometimes causes liver damage. Contact your doctor immediately if you develop yellowing of the eyes or skin, fatigue, weakness, loss of appetite, nausea, or vomiting.

How should you take this medication?

Take Rifater exactly as prescribed. Do not stop without consulting your doctor. It is important to take all of the drug prescribed for you, even if you feel better, and not to miss any doses.

Take Rifater on an empty stomach, either 1 hour before or 2 hours after a meal, with a full glass of water. Wait at least 1 hour before taking an antacid, as antacids may interfere with the drug.

If needed, your doctor may suggest taking vitamin B$_6$ while you are on Rifater therapy.

- *If you miss a dose...*
  Take it as soon as you remember. If it is almost time for the next dose, skip the one you missed and go back to your regular schedule. Never take 2 doses at once.

- *Storage instructions...*
  Store at room temperature. Protect from moisture.

What side effects may occur?

Side effects cannot be anticipated. If any develop or change in intensity, tell your doctor as soon as possible. Only your doctor can determine if it is safe for you to continue taking Rifater.

■ *More common side effects may include:*
Angina (crushing chest pain), anxiety, bone pain, chest pain, chest tightness, cough, coughing up blood, diabetic coma, diarrhea, difficult breathing, digestive pain, fast, fluttery heartbeat, headache, hepatitis, hives, itching, joint pain, nausea, numbness or tingling of the legs, rash, reddened skin, skin peeling or flaking, sleeplessness, sweating, swelling of the legs, vomiting, yellowing of skin and eyes

■ *Less common side effects may include:*
High or persistent fever, ringing in ears, vertigo

Why should this drug not be prescribed?

Do not take this medication if you have ever had an allergic reaction to or are sensitive to rifampin, isoniazid, or pyrazinamide. If you have serious liver disease or have ever had a severe side effect from isoniazid (such as fever, chills, and arthritis), do not take Rifater. Also, if you have a history of liver disease or have had acute and painful joint swelling (gout), avoid this drug.

Special warnings about this medication

Rifater may cause your urine, sputum, sweat, and tears to turn a red-orange color. This is to be expected and is not harmful. The drug may also permanently discolor contact lenses.

Since Rifater may cause eye problems, you should have a complete eye examination before starting therapy and periodically during Rifater treatment.

Limit the amount of alcohol you drink while on this medicine. Daily users of alcohol may be more prone to liver problems.

Use this medicine with caution if you have diabetes or kidney disease.

When rifampin, one of the drugs in Rifater, is taken at high doses (more than 600 milligrams) once or twice a week, it is likely that side effects may increase, including "flu-like" symptoms such as fever, chills, fatigue, weakness, upset stomach, and shortness of breath.

Possible food and drug interactions
when taking this medication

If Rifater is taken with certain other drugs, the effects could be increased, decreased, or altered. Consider another form of birth control if you are taking oral contraceptives, since Rifater lowers their effectiveness. Also check with your doctor before combining Rifater with the following:

Antacids such as Maalox or Tums
Anticonvulsants such as Dilantin, Depakene, Mysoline, Tegretol

Barbiturates such as phenobarbital and Nembutal
Blood pressure medicines such as Inderal, Tenormin, and Vasotec
Blood thinners such as Coumadin
Chloramphenicol (Chloromycetin)
Ciprofloxacin (Cipro)
Clofibrate (Atromid-S)
Cotrimoxazole (Bactrim, Septra)
Cycloserine (Seromycin)
Cyclosporine (Sandimmune)
Dapsone
Diabetes medications such as Diabinese and Orinase
Disulfiram (Antabuse)
Fluconazole (Diflucan)
Haloperidol (Haldol)
Heart medications such as Calan, Cardizem, Lanoxin, Mexitil, Norpace,
    Procardia, Quinidex, and Tonocard
Itraconazole (Sporanox)
Ketoconazole (Nizoral)
Levodopa (Sinemet)
Narcotic analgesics such as Darvon, Demerol, Percocet, Percodan
Nortriptyline (Pamelor)
Probenecid (Benemid)
Progestins such as Megace
Steroid drugs such as Deltasone and Prelone
Sulfasalazine (Azulfidine)
Theophylline (Theolair, Slo-Phyllin, Theo-Dur)
Tranquilizers such as Valium and Xanax

Foods such as cheese, fish, and red wine may cause reactions if you are
taking a medicine containing isoniazid. Call your doctor immediately if fast or
fluttery heartbeat, flushing, sweating, headache, or light-headedness occurs
while you are taking this medication.

Special information
if you are pregnant or breastfeeding
If you are pregnant or plan to become pregnant, tell your doctor immediately.
You may need to discontinue the drug. If needed for preventive treatment,
Rifater should be started after delivery. An ingredient in Rifater may cause
postnatal hemorrhaging in the mother and baby when given during the last
few weeks of pregnancy.

Rifater can pass into breast milk and may affect the nursing infant. Your
doctor may recommend that you stop breastfeeding until your treatment with
Rifater is finished.

Recommended dosage

ADULTS

Take once a day, as follows:

If you weigh 97 pounds or less: 4 tablets
If you weigh 98 to 120 pounds: 5 tablets
If you weigh 121 pounds or more: 6 tablets

CHILDREN

Safety and effectiveness in children under the age of 15 have not been established.

Overdosage

Any medication taken in excess can have serious consequences. An untreated overdose of Rifater can be fatal. If you suspect an overdose, seek medical attention immediately.

▪ *Symptoms of Rifater overdose may include:*
Blurred vision, coma, dizziness, hallucinations, increasing tiredness or sluggishness, liver enlargement or tenderness, nausea, seizures, shallow or difficult breathing, slurring of speech, stupor, vomiting, yellow eyes and skin

Brand name:

RISPERDAL

Pronounced: RIS-per-dal
Generic name: Risperidone

Why is this drug prescribed?

Risperdal is prescribed to treat severe mental illnesses such as schizophrenia.

Most important fact about this drug

Risperdal may cause tardive dyskinesia, a condition that causes involuntary muscle spasms and twitches in the face and body. This condition can become permanent and is most common among older people, especially women. Tell your doctor immediately if you begin to have any involuntary movement. You may need to discontinue Risperdal therapy.

How should you take this medication?
Do not take more or less of this medication than prescribed or use it for longer than the prescribed term of treatment as this may cause unwanted side effects.

Risperdal may be taken with or without food.

Risperdal oral solution comes with a calibrated pipette to use for measuring. The oral solution can be taken with water, coffee, orange juice, and low-fat milk, but *not* with cola drinks or tea.

- *If you miss a dose...*
  Take it as soon as you remember. If it is almost time for your next dose, skip the one you missed and go back to your regular schedule. Do not take 2 doses at once.

- *Storage instructions...*
  Store at room temperature. Protect tablets from light and moisture; protect oral solution from light and freezing.

What side effects may occur?
Side effects cannot be anticipated. If any develop or change in intensity, tell your doctor as soon as possible. Only your doctor can determine if it is safe for you to continue taking Risperdal.

- *More common side effects may include:*
  Abdominal pain, abnormal walk, agitation, aggression, anxiety, chest pain, constipation, coughing, decreased activity, diarrhea, difficulty with orgasm, diminished sexual desire, dizziness, dry skin, erection and ejaculation problems, excessive menstrual bleeding, fever, headache, inability to sleep, increased dreaming, increased duration of sleep, indigestion, involuntary movements, joint pain, lack of coordination, nasal inflammation, nausea, overactivity, rapid heartbeat, rash, reduced salivation, respiratory infection, sleepiness, sore throat, tremor, underactive reflexes, urination problems, vomiting, weight gain

- *Less common side effects may include:*
  Abnormal vision, back pain, dandruff, difficult or labored breathing, increased saliva, sinus inflammation, toothache

Why should this drug not be prescribed?
If you are sensitive to or have ever had an allergic reaction to Risperdal or other major tranquilizers, you should not take this medication.

Special warnings about this medication

You should use Risperdal cautiously if you have kidney, liver, or heart disease, seizures, breast cancer, thyroid disorders, or any other diseases that affect the metabolism (conversion of food into energy and tissue), or if you are exposed to extremes of temperature.

Be aware that Risperdal may mask signs and symptoms of drug overdose and of conditions such as intestinal obstruction, brain tumor, and Reye's syndrome (a dangerous neurological condition that may follow viral infections, usually occurring in children).

Risperdal may cause Neuroleptic Malignant Syndrome (NMS), a condition marked by muscle stiffness or rigidity, fast heartbeat or irregular pulse, increased sweating, high fever, and high or low blood pressure. Unchecked, this condition can prove fatal. Call your doctor immediately if you notice any of these symptoms. Risperdal therapy should be discontinued.

This drug may impair your ability to drive a car or operate potentially dangerous machinery. Do not participate in any activities that require full alertness if you are unsure of your ability.

Risperdal can cause orthostatic hypotension (low blood pressure when rising to a standing position), with dizziness, rapid heartbeat, and fainting, especially when you first start to take it. If you develop this problem, report it to your doctor. He can adjust your dose to reduce the symptoms.

Possible food and drug interactions
when taking this medication

If Risperdal is taken with certain other drugs, the effects of either can be increased, decreased, or altered. It is especially important to check with your doctor before combining Risperdal with the following:

Blood pressure medicines such as Aldomet, Procardia, and Vasotec
Bromocriptine mesylate (Parlodel)
Carbamazepine (Tegretol)
Clozapine (Clozaril)
Levodopa (Sinemet, Dopar)
Quinidine (Quinidex)

Risperdal tends to increase the effect of blood pressure medicines.

You may experience drowsiness and other potentially serious effects if Risperdal is combined with alcohol and other drugs that slow the central nervous system such as Valium, Percocet, Demerol, or Haldol.

Check with your doctor before taking any new medications.

Special information
if you are pregnant or breastfeeding

The safety and effectiveness of Risperdal during pregnancy have not been adequately studied. If you are pregnant or plan to become pregnant, tell your doctor immediately. It is not known whether Risperdal appears in breast milk. If this medication is essential to your health, your doctor may advise you to discontinue breastfeeding until your treatment with this medication is finished.

Recommended dosage

ADULTS

Doses of Risperdal can be taken once a day, or divided in half and taken twice daily. The usual dose on the first day is 2 milligrams or 2 milliliters of oral solution. On the second day, the dose increases to 4 milligrams or milliliters, and on the third day rises to 6 milligrams or milliliters. Further dosage adjustments can be made at intervals of 1 week. Over the long term, typical daily doses range from 4 to 8 milligrams or milliliters.

If you have a liver or kidney disease, your doctor will have you start with one-half of a 1-milligram tablet or 0.5 milliliter of oral solution twice daily and may then increase your dosage by one-half tablet or 0.5 milliliter per dose. Increases above the 1.5-milligram level are typically made at 1 week intervals.

CHILDREN

The safety and effectiveness of Risperdal in children have not been established.

OLDER ADULTS

Older adults generally take Risperdal at lower doses. The usual starting dose is one-half of a 1-milligram tablet or 0.5 milliliter of oral solution twice daily. Your doctor may increase the dose gradually and possibly switch you to a once-a-day dosing schedule after the first 2 to 3 days of drug therapy.

Overdosage

Any medication taken in excess can have serious consequences. If you suspect an overdose of Risperdal, seek medical attention immediately.

- *Symptoms of Risperdal overdose may include:*
  Drowsiness, low blood pressure, rapid heartbeat, sedation

Generic name:

RISPERIDONE

See Risperdal, page 1138.

Brand name:

RITALIN

Pronounced: RIT-ah-lin
Generic name: Methylphenidate hydrochloride

Why is this drug prescribed?

Ritalin is a mild central nervous system stimulant used in the treatment of attention deficit disorders in children. (This is a general term for several behavior problems previously known as minimal brain dysfunction in children; other names being used are hyperkinetic child syndrome, minimal brain damage, minimal cerebral dysfunction, and minor cerebral dysfunction.) Ritalin is also occasionally used in adults to treat narcolepsy (an uncontrollable desire to sleep).

This drug should be given as an integral part of a total treatment program that includes psychological, educational, and social measures. Symptoms of attention deficit disorder include continual problems with moderate to severe distractibility, short attention span, hyperactivity, emotional changeability, and impulsiveness.

Most important fact about this drug

Excessive doses of Ritalin over a long period of time can produce addiction. It is also possible to develop tolerance to the drug, so that larger doses are needed to produce the original effect. Because of these dangers, be sure to check with your doctor before making any change in dosage; and withdraw the drug only under your doctor's supervision.

How should you take this medication?

Follow your doctor's directions carefully.

Ritalin is available in standard and sustained-release tablets (Ritalin-SR). It is recommended that Ritalin be taken 30 to 45 minutes before meals. If the drug interferes with sleep, give the child the last dose before 6 p.m. Ritalin-SR tablets should be swallowed whole, never crushed or chewed.

- *If you miss a dose...*
  Give it to the child as soon as you remember. Give the remaining doses for the day at regularly spaced intervals. Do not give 2 doses at once.

- *Storage instructions...*
  Keep out of reach of children. Store below 86°F. in a tightly closed, light-resistant container. Protect Ritalin-SR from moisture.

What side effects may occur?
Side effects cannot be anticipated. If any develop or change in intensity, inform your doctor as soon as possible. Only your doctor can determine if it is safe for you to continue giving Ritalin.

- *More common side effects may include:*
  Inability to fall or stay asleep, nervousness

These side effects can usually be controlled by reducing the dosage and omitting the drug in the afternoon or evening.

In children, loss of appetite, abdominal pain, weight loss during long-term therapy, inability to fall or stay asleep, and abnormally fast heartbeat are more common side effects.

- *Less common or rare side effects may include:*
  Abdominal pain, abnormal heartbeat, abnormal muscular movements, blood pressure changes, chest pain, dizziness, drowsiness, fever, headache, hives, jerking, joint pain, loss of appetite, nausea, palpitations (fluttery or throbbing heartbeat), pulse changes, rapid heartbeat, reddish or purplish skin spots, skin reddening, skin inflammation with peeling, skin rash, Tourette's syndrome (severe twitching), weight loss during long-term treatment

Why should this drug not be prescribed?
This drug should not be prescribed for anyone experiencing anxiety, tension, and agitation, since the drug may aggravate these symptoms.

Anyone sensitive or allergic to this drug should not take it.

This medication should not be taken by anyone with the eye condition known as glaucoma, anyone who suffers from tics (repeated, involuntary twitches), or someone with a family history of Tourette's syndrome (severe and multiple tics).

Ritalin is not intended for use in children whose symptoms may be caused by stress or a psychiatric disorder.

Ritalin should not be used for the prevention or treatment of normal fatigue, nor should it be used for the treatment of severe depression.

Special warnings about this medication

Your doctor will do a complete history and evaluation before prescribing Ritalin. He or she will take into account the severity of the symptoms, as well as your child's age.

Ritalin should not be given to children under 6 years of age; safety and effectiveness in this age group have not been established.

There is no information regarding the safety and effectiveness of long-term Ritalin treatment in children. However, suppression of growth has been seen with the long-term use of stimulants, so your doctor will watch your child carefully while he or she is taking this drug.

Blood pressure should be monitored in anyone taking Ritalin, especially those with high blood pressure.

Some people have had visual disturbances such as blurred vision while being treated with Ritalin.

The use of Ritalin by anyone with a seizure disorder is not recommended. Be sure your doctor is aware of any problem in this area. Caution is also advisable for anyone with a history of emotional instability or substance abuse, due to the danger of addiction.

Possible food and drug interactions
when taking this medication

If Ritalin is taken with certain other drugs, the effects of either can be increased, decreased, or altered. It is especially important to check with your doctor before combining Ritalin with the following:

Antiseizure drugs such as phenobarbital, Dilantin and Mysoline
Antidepressant drugs such as Tofranil, Anafranil, Norpramin, and
    Effexor
Blood thinners such as Coumadin
Drugs that restore blood pressure, such as EpiPen
Guanethidine (Ismelin)
MAO inhibitors (drugs such as the antidepressants Nardil and Parnate)
Phenylbutazone

Special information
if you are pregnant or breastfeeding

The effects of Ritalin during pregnancy have not been adequately studied. If you are pregnant or plan to become pregnant, inform your doctor immediately. It is not known if Ritalin appears in breast milk. If this medication is essential to your health, your doctor may advise you to discontinue nursing your baby until your treatment with this medication is finished.

Recommended dosage

ADULTS

Tablets

The average dosage is 20 to 30 milligrams a day, divided into 2 or 3 doses, preferably taken 30 to 45 minutes before meals. Some people may need 40 to 60 milligrams daily, others only 10 to 15 milligrams. Your doctor will determine the best dose.

SR Tablets

Ritalin-SR tablets keep working for 8 hours. They may be used in place of Ritalin tablets if they deliver a comparable dose over an 8-hour period.

CHILDREN

Ritalin should not be given to children under 6 years of age.

Your doctor will start your child on small doses, then increase the dose gradually at weekly intervals. Your child should not take more than 60 milligrams in a day. If you do not see any improvement over a period of 1 month, check with your doctor. He or she may wish to discontinue the drug.

Tablets

The usual starting dose is 5 milligrams taken twice a day, before breakfast and lunch; your doctor will increase the dose by 5 to 10 milligrams a week.

SR Tablets

Ritalin-SR tablets continue working for 8 hours. Your doctor will decide if SR tablets should be used in place of Ritalin tablets.

Your doctor will periodically discontinue this drug in order to reassess your child's condition. Drug treatment should not, and need not, be indefinite and usually can be discontinued after puberty.

Overdosage

If you suspect an overdose, seek medical attention immediately.

■ *Symptoms of Ritalin overdose may include:*
Agitation, confusion, convulsions (may be followed by coma), delirium, dryness of mucous membranes, enlarging of the pupil of the eye, exaggerated feeling of elation, extremely elevated body temperature, flushing, hallucinations, headache, high blood pressure, irregular or rapid heartbeat, muscle twitching, sweating, tremors, vomiting

Generic name:

RITONAVIR

See Norvir, page 913.

Generic name:

RIZATRIPTAN

See Maxalt, page 755.

Brand name:

ROBAXIN

Pronounced: Ro-BAKS-in
Generic name: Methocarbamol

Why is this drug prescribed?
Robaxin is prescribed, along with rest, physical therapy, and other measures, for the relief of pain due to severe muscular injuries, sprains, and strains.

Most important fact about this drug
Robaxin is not a substitute for the rest or physical therapy needed for proper healing.

Although the drug may temporarily make an injury feel better, do not let that tempt you into pushing your recovery. Lifting or exercising too soon may further damage the muscle.

How should you take this medication?
Take Robaxin exactly as prescribed. Do not take a larger dose or use more often than directed.

■ *If you miss a dose...*
If only an hour or so has passed, take it as soon as you remember. If you do not remember until later, skip the dose and go back to your regular schedule. Do not take 2 doses at once.

■ *Storage instructions...*
Store at room temperature in a tightly closed container.

What side effects may occur?
Side effects cannot be anticipated. If any develop or change in intensity,

inform your doctor as soon as possible. Only your doctor can determine if it is safe for you to continue taking Robaxin.

■ *Side effects may include:*
Blurred vision, dizziness, drowsiness, fever, headache, hives, itching, light-headedness, nasal congestion, nausea, "pinkeye," rash

Why should this drug not be prescribed?
If you are sensitive to or have ever had an allergic reaction to Robaxin or other drugs of this type, you should not take this medication. Make sure your doctor is aware of any drug reactions you have experienced.

Special warnings about this medication
Robaxin causes drowsiness and blurred vision. Exercise extra caution while driving or performing tasks that require mental alertness.

Avoid or be careful using alcoholic beverages.

Robaxin may darken urine to brown, green, or black.

Possible food and drug interactions when taking this medication
If Robaxin is taken with certain other drugs, the effects of either can be increased, decreased, or altered. It is especially important to check with your doctor before combining Robaxin with drugs that slow the nervous system, including:

Narcotic pain relievers such as Percocet and Tylenol with Codeine
Sleep aids such as Halcion and Seconal
Tranquilizers such as Xanax and Valium

Special information if you are pregnant or breastfeeding
The effects of Robaxin during pregnancy have not been adequately studied. If you are pregnant or plan to become pregnant, inform your doctor immediately. It is not known if this drug appears in breast milk. If this medication is essential to your health, your doctor may advise you to discontinue breastfeeding your baby until your treatment is finished.

Recommended dosage
ADULTS

Robaxin
The usual starting dose is 3 tablets taken 4 times a day. The usual long-term dose is 2 tablets taken 4 times a day.

Robaxin-750
The usual starting dose is 2 tablets taken 4 times a day. The usual long-term dose is 1 tablet taken every 4 hours or 2 tablets taken 3 times a day.

CHILDREN

The safety and effectiveness of Robaxin have not been established in children under 12 years of age.

Overdosage

Any drug taken in excess can have dangerous consequences. If you suspect an overdose of Robaxin, seek emergency medical treatment immediately.

Brand name:

ROCALTROL

Pronounced: Ro-CAL-trol
Generic name: Calcitriol

Why is this drug prescribed?

Rocaltrol is a synthetic form of vitamin D used to treat people on dialysis who have hypocalcemia (abnormally low blood calcium levels) and resulting bone damage. Rocaltrol is also prescribed to treat low blood calcium levels in people who have hypoparathyroidism (decreased functioning of the parathyroid glands). When functioning correctly, these glands help control the level of calcium in the blood.

Rocaltrol is also prescribed for *hyper*parathyroidism (*increased* functioning of the parathyroid glands) and resulting bone disorders in people with kidney disease who are not yet on dialysis.

Most important fact about this drug

While you are taking Rocaltrol, your doctor may want you to follow a special diet or take calcium supplements. This is an important part of your therapy. On the other hand, too high a calcium level can be harmful. If you are already taking any medications containing calcium or calcium supplements, make sure your doctor knows about it.

How should you take this medication?

Be sure to get enough fluids and avoid dehydration while taking Rocaltrol.

■ *If you miss a dose...*
   If you take 1 dose every other day, and you remember before the next day, take the forgotten dose immediately, then go back to your regular

schedule. If you do not remember until the next day, take the dose immediately, skip a day, then go back to your regular schedule.

If you take 1 dose every day, take it as soon as you remember. Then go back to your regular schedule. If you do not remember until the next day, skip the dose you missed and go back to your regular schedule.

If you take Rocaltrol more than once a day, take the forgotten dose as soon as you remember. If it is almost time for your next dose, skip the one you missed and go back to your regular schedule.

Do not take 2 doses at once.

■ *Storage instructions...*
Keep capsules and oral solution away from heat and light.

What side effects may occur?
Side effects cannot be anticipated. If any develop or change in intensity, inform your doctor as soon as possible. Only your doctor can determine if it is safe for you to continue taking Rocaltrol.

■ *More common side effects occurring early may include:*
Bone pain, constipation, dry mouth, extreme sleepiness, headache, metallic taste, muscle pain, nausea, vomiting, weakness

■ *More common side effects occurring later may include:*
Abnormal thirst, decreased sex drive, elevated blood cholesterol levels, excessive urination, extremely high body temperature, high blood pressure, inflamed eyes, intolerance to light, irregular heartbeat, itchy skin, kidney problems, loss of appetite, nighttime urination, runny nose, weight loss, yellowish skin

■ *Rare side effects may include:*
Mental disturbances, red patches (irregular or circular shape) on arms and hands

Excessive amounts of Vitamin D may cause abnormally high calcium levels in the blood.

Why should this drug not be prescribed?
You should not use Rocaltrol if you have high blood levels of calcium, or if you have vitamin D poisoning.

Special warnings about this medication
You should not take additional doses of vitamin D while taking Rocaltrol.

People who are on dialysis should not take antacids containing magnesium (such as Maalox) while taking Rocaltrol.

Your doctor will monitor your calcium levels while you are taking Rocaltrol.

While taking Rocaltrol, you should have an adequate daily intake of calcium, either from foods (such as milk and dairy products) or from a calcium supplement. Your doctor will estimate your daily calcium intake before you take this drug to see if you will require more calcium.

Possible food and drug interactions when taking this medication

If Rocaltrol is taken with certain other drugs, the effects of either could be increased, decreased, or altered. It is especially important to check with your doctor before combining Rocaltrol with the following:

Antacids containing magnesium, such as Maalox
Calcium supplements
Cholestyramine (Questran)
Digitalis (Lanoxin)
Vitamin D pills

Special information if you are pregnant or breastfeeding

The effects of Rocaltrol during pregnancy have not been adequately studied. If you are pregnant or plan to become pregnant, inform your doctor immediately. Pregnant women should use Rocaltrol only if the possible benefit outweighs any possible risk to the unborn baby.

Rocaltrol may appear in breast milk. Because it may affect a nursing infant, you should not use Rocaltrol while you are breastfeeding.

Recommended dosage

ADULTS

For People on Dialysis
The suggested beginning dose is 0.25 microgram daily. Your doctor may increase the dose by 0.25 microgram daily at 4 to 8 week intervals if needed. Most people on dialysis require a dose of 0.5 to 1 microgram a day.

People with normal or only slightly low blood calcium levels may find it helpful to take 0.25 microgram every other day.

For Low Calcium Levels Due to Hypoparathyroidism
The suggested beginning dose is 0.25 microgram daily, taken in the morning. Your doctor may increase the dose at 2 to 4 week intervals.

For most adults, regular doses ranging from 0.5 to 2 micrograms daily are effective.

For People Not Yet on Dialysis
The recommended starting dose is 0.25 microgram a day, increased to 0.5 microgram if necessary.

CHILDREN

For Low Calcium Levels Due to Hypoparathyroidism
The starting dose is 0.25 microgram, taken in the morning.

For most children 6 years and older, doses ranging from 0.5 to 2 micrograms per day are effective.

Children from 1 to 5 years old are usually given 0.25 to 0.75 microgram a day. Doses have not been established for hypoparathyroidism in infants under 1 year, or for pseudohypoparathyroidism (a special form of the disorder) in children under 6.

For Children not yet on Dialysis
The recommended starting dose for children 3 years and older is 0.25 microgram a day, increased to 0.5 microgram if necessary.

For children less than 3 years old, the daily starting dose is 10 to 15 nanograms per 2.2 pounds of body weight.

Overdosage
Any medication taken in excess can have serious consequences. Severe overdosage of Rocaltrol may cause serious effects, such as extremely high blood levels of calcium. If you suspect an overdose, seek medical help immediately.

■ *Symptoms of Rocaltrol overdose may include:*
  Coma, confusion, extreme drowsiness

Brand name:

ROLAIDS

See Antacids, page 75.

Generic name:

ROPINIROLE

See Requip, page 1108.

Brand name:

ROWASA

Pronounced: ROH-ace-ah
Generic name: Mesalamine
Other brand names: Pentasa, Asacol

Why is this drug prescribed?
Rowasa Suspension Enema, Pentasa, and Asacol are used to treat mild to moderate ulcerative colitis (inflammation of the large intestine and rectum). Rowasa Suspension Enema is also prescribed for inflammation of the lower colon, and inflammation of the rectum.

Rowasa Suppositories are used to treat inflammation of the rectum.

Most important fact about this drug
Mesalamine, the active ingredient in these products, has been known to cause side effects such as:

Bloody diarrhea
Cramping
Fever
Rash
Severe headache
Sudden, severe stomach pain

If you develop any of these symptoms, stop taking this medication and consult your doctor.

How should you use this medication?

To Use Rowasa Suspension Enema:
1. Rowasa Suspension Enema comes in boxes of 7 bottles each. After the foil on the box has been unwrapped, all Rowasa Suspension Enemas should be used promptly, following your doctor's instructions. The Suspension Enema is normally off-white to tan in color, but may darken over time once its foil cover is unwrapped. You may still use the enema if it is slightly discolored, but do not use Rowasa Suspension Enema if it is dark brown. If you have any questions about using Rowasa Suspension Enema, contact your doctor.
2. Use Rowasa Suspension Enema at bedtime.
3. Shake the bottle thoroughly.
4. Uncover the applicator tip.
5. You may find it easier to use Rowasa Suspension Enema if you lie down

on your left side, extending your left leg and bending your right leg forward for a comfortable balance. An alternative position is to squat with your knees to your chest.
6. Pointing the applicator tip up, gently insert the tip into the rectum.
7. Squeeze the bottle steadily to discharge the contents.
8. The enema should be retained all night (8 hours) for best results.

To Use Rowasa Suppositories:
1. Rowasa Suppositories should be used twice a day.
2. You should handle the suppositories as little as possible, because they are designed to melt at body temperature.
3. Remove one suppository from the strip of suppositories.
4. While holding the suppository upright, carefully remove the foil wrapper.
5. Using gentle pressure, insert the suppository (with the pointed end first) completely into the rectum.
6. The suppository should be retained for 1 to 3 hours or longer for best results.

To take Pentasa or Asacol:
Swallow the capsule or tablet whole. Do not break, crush, or chew it before swallowing.

You may notice what looks like small beads in your stool. These are just empty shells that are left after the medication has been absorbed into your body. However, if this continues, check with your doctor.

■ *If you miss a dose...*
Take it as soon as you remember. If it is almost time for your next dose, skip the one you missed and go back to your regular schedule. Never take 2 doses at the same time.

■ *Storage instructions...*
Store these products at room temperature.

What side effects may occur?
Side effects cannot be anticipated. If any side effects develop or change in intensity, tell your doctor immediately. Only your doctor can determine whether it is safe to continue using this medication.

■ *More common side effects generally include:*
Diarrhea, dizziness, flu-like symptoms, gas, headache, nausea, stomach pain

■ *Other typical side effects may include:*
Abdominal pain, acne, back pain, belching, bloating, chest pain, chills, constipation, fever, hair loss, hemorrhoids, indigestion, insomnia, itching, joint pain, leg pain, menstrual problems, muscle pain, nasal inflammation, rash, rectal pain or bleeding, sore throat, stomach and intestinal bleeding, sweating, swelling of the arms and legs, tiredness, urinary burning, vomiting, weakness

Although quite rare, other problems are possible. If you notice any unusual symptoms, check with your doctor.

Why should this drug not be prescribed?
These products should not be used by anyone who is allergic or sensitive to mesalamine or their other ingredients.

Pentasa and Asacol should not be used if you are allergic or sensitive to salicylates (aspirin).

Special warnings about this medication
Your doctor should check your kidney function while you are taking mesalamine, especially if you have a history of kidney disease or you are using other anti-inflammatory drugs such as Dipentum.

You should use mesalamine cautiously if you are allergic to sulfasalazine (Azulfidine). If you develop a rash or fever, you should stop using the medication and notify your doctor.

Some people using mesalamine have developed flare-ups of their colitis.

Rare cases of pericarditis, in which the membrane surrounding the heart becomes inflamed, have been reported with products containing mesalamine. Symptoms may include chest, neck, and shoulder pain, and shortness of breath.

Rowasa Suspension Enema contains a sulfite that may cause allergic reactions in some people. These reactions may include shock and severe, possibly fatal asthma attacks. Most people aren't sensitive to sulfites. However, some people with asthma might be sensitive and should take any medication containing sulfites cautiously.

Rowasa Suspension Enema may stain clothes and fabrics.

Possible food and drug interactions
when taking this medication
If these products are taken with certain other drugs, the effects of either could be increased, decreased, or altered. It is especially important to check

with your doctor before combining Rowasa Suspension Enema or Rowasa Suppositories with sulfasalazine (Azulfidine).

Special information
if you are pregnant or breastfeeding

Pregnant women should use mesalamine only if clearly needed. Mesalamine has been found in breast milk. If this medication is essential to your health your doctor may advise you to discontinue breastfeeding until your treatment is finished.

Recommended dosage

ADULTS

Rowasa Suspension Enema

The usual dose is 1 rectal enema (60 milliliters) per day, preferably used at bedtime and retained for about 8 hours. Treatment time usually lasts from 3 to 6 weeks, although improvement may be seen within 3 to 21 days.

Rowasa Suppositories

The usual dose is one rectal suppository (500 milligrams) 2 times a day. To get the most benefit from a Rowasa Suppository, it should be retained for 1 to 3 hours or longer. Treatment time usually lasts from 3 to 6 weeks, although improvement may be seen within 3 to 21 days.

Pentasa Capsules

The usual dose is 4 capsules taken 4 times a day for a total of 16 capsules daily.

Asacol Tablets

The recommended dose for the treatment of ulcerative colitis is 2 tablets 3 times a day for 6 weeks.

To prevent a relapse, the usual dosage is 4 tablets a day, taken in 2 or more smaller doses, for 6 months.

CHILDREN

Safety and effectiveness in children have not been established.

Overdosage

There have been no proven reports of serious effects resulting from overdoses of Rowasa. An overdose of Pentasa or Asacol could cause any of the following symptoms:

Confusion, diarrhea, drowsiness, headache, hyperventilation, ringing in the ears, sweating, vomiting

Any medication taken in excess can have serious consequences. If you suspect an overdose, seek medical attention immediately.

Brand name:

ROXICET

See Percocet, page 979.

Brand name:

RU-TUSS TABLETS

Pronounced: ROO-tus
Generic ingredients: Phenylephrine hydrochloride,
  Phenylpropanolamine hydrochloride, Chlorpheniramine
  maleate, Hyoscyamine sulfate, Atropine sulfate,
  Scopolamine hydrobromide

Why is this drug prescribed?
Ru-Tuss is an antihistamine/decongestant that relieves the runny, stuffy nose, nasal drip, itching, watery eyes, and scratchy, itchy throat caused by allergies, colds, and other irritations of the sinus, nose, and upper respiratory tract. Chlorpheniramine, the antihistamine, relieves watery eyes, dries up post-nasal drip, and reduces sneezing. Phenylephrine and phenylpropanolamine combine to reduce congestion and make breathing easier. Hyoscyamine, atropine, and scopolamine, commonly called belladonna alkaloids, enhance the drying effects of Ru-Tuss.

Most important fact about this drug
Ru-Tuss tablets may cause drowsiness. Do not drive, operate machinery or participate in any hazardous activity that requires full mental alertness until you know how you react to this medication.

How should you take this medication?
Take this medication exactly as prescribed. The tablets act continuously for 10 to 12 hours. Tablets should be swallowed whole, not crushed or chewed.

If this medicine dries out your mouth, sucking on hard candy or chewing gum may help.

■ *If you miss a dose...*
Take it as soon as you remember. If it is almost time for your next dose, skip the one you missed and go back to your regular schedule. Never take 2 doses at the same time.

■ *Storage instructions...*
Store it at room temperature.

What side effects may occur?
Side effects cannot be anticipated. If any develop or change in intensity, inform your doctor as soon as possible. Only your doctor can determine if it is safe for you to continue taking Ru-Tuss.

■ *Side effects may include:*
Allergic reactions (rash, hives), blood disorders, blurred vision, constipation, diarrhea, difficulty sleeping (insomnia), dilated pupils, dizziness, drowsiness, dry mouth, dry nose and other mucous membranes, exhaustion, faintness, frequent urination, giddiness, headache, hyperirritability, increased chest congestion, itching, lack of coordination, loss of appetite, low blood pressure/high blood pressure, nausea, nervousness, painful or difficult urination, pounding heartbeat, rapid heartbeat, ringing in the ears, stomach upset, tightness in the chest, vision changes, vomiting

Why should this drug not be prescribed?
Ru-Tuss should be avoided if you are pregnant, if you are sensitive to or have ever had an allergic reaction to antihistamines or any of the ingredients in this medication, if you have glaucoma or bronchial asthma, or if you are taking antidepressant drugs known as MAO inhibitors (Nardil, for example). Ru-Tuss should not be given to children under 12 years of age.

Special warnings about this medication
This medication can make you feel drowsy. Be careful driving, operating machinery, or using appliances.

Ru-Tuss should be used with care if you have a bladder obstruction, high blood pressure, cardiovascular disease, or an overactive thyroid.

Possible food and drug interactions
when taking this medication
Ru-Tuss may increase the effects of alcohol. Do not drink alcohol while taking this medication.

Do not take Ru-Tuss while taking antidepressant drugs such as Nardil and Parnate.

If Ru-Tuss is taken with certain other drugs, the effects of either could be increased, decreased, or altered. It is especially important to check with your doctor before combining Ru-Tuss with the following:

Sleep medications such as Halcion and Dalmane
Tranquilizers such as Xanax and Valium

Special information
if you are pregnant or breastfeeding
Ru-Tuss is not recommended for use by pregnant women. If you are pregnant or plan to become pregnant, notify your doctor immediately.

Recommended dosage

ADULTS AND CHILDREN 12 YEARS OR OLDER

The usual dosage is 1 tablet in the morning and 1 tablet in the evening. This drug is not recommended for children under 12.

Overdosage
Any medication taken in excess can have serious consequences. Convulsions and death may occur from antihistamine overdose in children and infants. If you suspect an overdose, seek medical treatment immediately.

■ *Symptoms of Ru-Tuss overdose may include:*
Coma, delirium, fever, rapid breathing, respiratory failure, stupor

Brand name:

RYNATAN

Pronounced: RYE-nuh-tan
Generic ingredients: Phenylephrine tannate,
  Chlorpheniramine tannate, Pyrilamine tannate

Why is this drug prescribed?
Rynatan is an antihistamine/decongestant that relieves runny nose and nasal congestion caused by the common cold, inflamed sinuses, hay fever, and other upper respiratory conditions. Chlorpheniramine and pyrilamine, the antihistamines in the combination, reduce itching and swelling and dry up secretions from the eyes, nose, and throat. Phenylephrine, the decongestant, reduces congestion and makes breathing easier.

Most important fact about this drug
This medication can make you drowsy. You should not drive or operate dangerous machinery or participate in any hazardous activity that requires full mental alertness until you know how you react to Rynatan.

How should you take this medication?
Take this medication exactly as prescribed.

■ *If you miss a dose...*
Take it as soon as you remember. If it is almost time for the next dose, skip the one you missed and go back to your regular schedule. Do not take 2 doses at once.

■ *Storage instructions...*
Store at room temperature in a tightly closed container.

What side effects may occur?
Side effects cannot be anticipated. If any develop or change in intensity, inform your doctor as soon as possible. Only your doctor can determine if it is safe for you to continue taking Rynatan.

■ *Side effects may include:*
Drowsiness, dry nose, mouth, and throat, excessive calm (sedation), stomach and intestinal problems

Why should this drug not be prescribed?
Rynatan should not be given to newborn babies, or used by nursing mothers. It should also be avoided by people who have had an allergic reaction to any of its ingredients or to similar antihistamine and decongestant combinations.

Special warnings about this medication
Use Rynatan with care if you have high blood pressure, heart disease, circulatory problems, an overactive thyroid gland, diabetes, the eye condition known as narrow-angle glaucoma, or an enlarged prostate gland.

If you are taking a drug classified as an MAO inhibitor, such as the antidepressants Nardil and Parnate, or have taken one within the past two weeks, you should avoid taking Rynatan.

The antihistamines in Rynatan are more likely to cause dizziness, sedation, and low blood pressure in older adults. Antihistamines also can cause excitement, especially in children.

Possible food and drug interactions
when taking this medication

Rynatan may increase the effects of alcohol. Do not drink alcohol while taking this medication.

If Rynatan is taken with certain other drugs, the effects of either could be increased, decreased, or altered. It is especially important to check with your doctor before combining Rynatan with the following:

Drugs classified as MAO inhibitors, including the antidepressants Nardil and Parnate

Sleep aids such as Halcion and Dalmane

Tranquilizers such as Xanax and Valium

Special information
if you are pregnant or breastfeeding

The effects of Rynatan during pregnancy have not been adequately studied. If you are pregnant or plan to become pregnant, notify your doctor immediately. Rynatan should not be taken if you are breastfeeding.

Recommended dosage

RYNATAN TABLETS

Adults

The usual dosage is 1 or 2 tablets every 12 hours.

RYNATAN-S PEDIATRIC SUSPENSION

Children Over Age 6:

The usual dosage is 1 to 2 teaspoonfuls (5 to 10 milliliters) every 12 hours.

Children Aged 2 to 6:

The usual dosage is one-half to 1 teaspoonful (2.5 to 5 milliliters) every 12 hours.

Children Under Age 2:

Your doctor will determine the dose.

Overdosage

Any medication taken in excess can have serious consequences. Antihistamine overdose in young children can lead to convulsions and death. If you suspect an overdose, seek medical treatment immediately.

Symptoms of Rynatan overdose range from sedation to overstimulation (from restlessness to convulsions).

Brand name:

RYTHMOL

Pronounced: RITH-mol
Generic name: Propafenone

Why is this drug prescribed?
Rythmol is used to help correct certain life-threatening heartbeat irregularities (ventricular arrhythmias).

Most important fact about this drug
There is a possibility that Rythmol may cause new heartbeat irregularities or make the existing ones worse. Rythmol is therefore used only for serious problems, and should be accompanied by periodic electrocardiograms (EKGs) prior to and during treatment. Discuss this with your doctor.

How should you take this medication?
Rythmol may be taken with food or on an empty stomach.

Take Rythmol exactly as prescribed. It works best when there is a constant amount of the drug in the blood, so you should take it at evenly spaced intervals.

- *If you miss a dose...*
  Unless otherwise instructed by your doctor, take the forgotten dose as soon as possible. However, if it is almost time for your next dose or more than 4 hours have passed, skip the missed dose and go back to your regular schedule. Never take a double dose.

- *Storage instructions...*
  Keep this medication in the container it came in, tightly closed, away from direct light, at room temperature.

What side effects may occur?
Side effects cannot be anticipated. If any develop or change in intensity, inform your doctor as soon as possible. Only your doctor can determine if it is safe for you to continue taking Rythmol.

The most common side effects affect the digestive, cardiovascular, and nervous systems. The most serious are heartbeat abnormalities.

- *More common side effects may include:*
  Constipation, dizziness, heartbeat abnormalities, nausea, unusual taste in the mouth, vomiting

- *Other side effects may include:*
  Abdominal pain or cramps, anemia, angina (chest pain), anxiety, blood disorders, blurred vision, breathing difficulties, bruising, cardiac arrest, coma, confusion, congestive heart failure, depression, diarrhea, dreaming abnormalities, drowsiness, dry mouth, eye irritation, fainting or near fainting, fatigue, fever, flushing, gas, hair loss, headache, heart palpitations, heartbeat abnormalities (rapid, irregular, slow), hot flashes, impotence, increased blood sugar, indigestion, inflamed esophagus, stomach, or intestines, insomnia, itching, joint pain, kidney disease, kidney failure, lack of coordination, liver dysfunction, loss of appetite, loss of balance, low blood pressure, memory loss, muscle cramps, muscle weakness, numbness, pain, psychosis, rash, red or purple spots on the skin, ringing in the ears, seizures, speech abnormalities, sweating, swelling due to fluid retention, tingling or pins and needles, tremor, unusual smell sensations, vertigo, vision abnormalities, weakness

Why should this drug not be prescribed?
Do not take Rythmol if you have ever had an allergic reaction to or are sensitive to it. Your doctor will not prescribe Rythmol if you are suffering from any of the following conditions:

Abnormally slow heartbeat
Certain heartbeat irregularities, such as atrioventricular block or "sick sinus" syndrome, that have not been corrected by a pacemaker
Cardiogenic shock (shock due to a weak heart)
Chronic bronchitis or emphysema
Congestive heart failure that is not well controlled
Mineral (electrolyte) imbalance
Severe low blood pressure

Special warnings about this medication
If you have congestive heart failure, this condition must be brought under full medical control before you start taking Rythmol.

If you have a pacemaker, the pacemaker's settings must be monitored—and possibly reprogrammed—while you are taking Rythmol.

There is some risk that Rythmol may interfere with your body's normal ability to manufacture blood cells. Too few white blood cells may cause signs and symptoms that mimic infection. If you experience fever, chills, or sore throat while taking Rythmol—especially during the first 3 months of treatment—notify your doctor right away.

Rythmol may cause a lupus-like illness characterized by rashes and arthritic symptoms. If you have been taking Rythmol and testing shows that your

NORVIR

RITONAVIR
ABBOTT

100 MG

OGEN

ESTROPIPATE
PHARMACIA & UPJOHN

0.625 MG

1.25 MG

2.5 MG

OMNIPEN

AMPICILLIN
WYETH-AYERST

250 MG

500 MG

ORASONE

PREDNISONE
SOLVAY

1 MG

ORINASE

TOLBUTAMIDE
PHARMACIA & UPJOHN

250 MG

500 MG

ORUDIS

KETOPROFEN
WYETH-AYERST

25 MG

50 MG

75 MG

ORUVAIL

KETOPROFEN
WYETH-AYERST

100 MG

150 MG

200 MG

PAMELOR

NORTRIPTYLINE HCL
NOVARTIS

10 MG

25 MG

50 MG

75 MG

PANCREASE

PANCRELIPASE
ORTHO-MCNEIL

PARAFON FORTE DSC

CHLORZOXAZONE
ORTHO-MCNEIL

500 MG

PARLODEL

BROMOCRIPTINE MESYLATE
NOVARTIS

2.5 MG

5 MG

PAXIL

PAROXETINE HCL
SMITHKLINE BEECHAM

10 MG

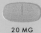
20 MG

30 MG

40 MG

PCE

ERYTHROMYCIN
ABBOTT

333 MG

500 MG

PENETREX

ENOXACIN
RHONE-POULENC RORER

200 MG

400 MG

PENTASA

MESALAMINE
HOECHST MARION ROUSSEL

250 MG

PEN-VEE K

PENICILLIN V POTASSIUM
WYETH-AYERST

250 MG

500 MG

PEPCID

FAMOTIDINE
MERCK

20 MG

40 MG

PERCOCET

**OXYCODONE HCL/
ACETAMINOPHEN**
ENDO

5 MG / 325 MG

PERIACTIN

CYPROHEPTADINE HCL
MERCK

4 MG

PERSANTINE

DIPYRIDAMOLE
BOEHRINGER INGELHEIM

25 MG   50 MG

75 MG

PHENAPHEN W/CODEINE NO. 3

ACETAMINOPHEN / CODEINE PHOSPHATE
A. H. ROBINS

325 MG / 30 MG

PHENERGAN

PROMETHAZINE HCL
WYETH-AYERST

12.5 MG

25 MG

50 MG

PLAQUENIL

HYDROXYCHLOROQUINE SULFATE
SANOFI

200 MG

PLENDIL

FELODIPINE
ASTRA

2.5 MG   5 MG

10 MG

POLY-VI-FLOR

**SODIUM FLUORIDE/
MULTIVITAMINS**
MEAD JOHNSON

0.5 MG

1 MG

PONSTEL KAPSEALS

MEFENAMIC ACID
PARKE-DAVIS

250 MG

PRANDIN

REPAGLINIDE
NOVO NORDISK

0.5 MG

1.0 MG

2.0 MG

PRAVACHOL

PRAVASTATIN SODIUM
BRISTOL-MYERS SQUIBB

10 MG

20 MG

40 MG

PRECOSE

ACARBOSE
BAYER

25 MG

50 MG

100 MG

PREMARIN

CONJUGATED ESTROGENS
WYETH-AYERST

0.3 MG

0.625 MG

0.9 MG

1.25 MG

2.5 MG

PREMPRO

**CONJUGATED ESTROGENS /
MEDROXYPROGESTERONE
ACETATE**
WYETH-AYERST

2.5 MG

PREMPHASE

**CONJUGATED ESTROGENS /
MEDROXYPROGESTERONE
ACETATE**
WYETH-AYERST

0.625 MG

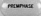

5 MG

PREVACID

LANSOPRAZOLE
TAP

15 MG

30 MG
DELAYED-RELEASE

PRILOSEC

OMEPRAZOLE
ASTRA

10 MG

20 MG

PRINCIPEN

AMPICILLIN
APOTHECON

250 MG

500 MG

PRINIVIL

LISINOPRIL
MERCK

2.5 MG   5 MG

10 MG   20 MG

40 MG

PRINZIDE

**LISINOPRIL/
HYDROCHLOROTHIAZIDE**
MERCK

10 MG / 12.5 MG

20 MG / 12.5 MG

20 MG / 25 MG

PROCANBID

PROCAINAMIDE HCL
PARKE-DAVIS

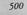
500

500 MG

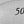
1000

1000 MG

PROCARDIA

NIFEDIPINE
PRATT

10 MG

20 MG

PRONESTYL

PROCAINAMIDE HCL
APOTHECON

250 MG

500 MG

PROPULSID

CISAPRIDE
JANSSEN

10 MG   20 MG

PROSCAR

FINASTERIDE
MERCK

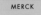

5 MG

PROSOM

ESTAZOLAM
ABBOTT

1 MG   2 MG

PROVENTIL

ALBUTEROL SULFATE
SCHERING

2 MG   4 MG

4 MG
REPETABS

PROVERA

MEDROXYPROGESTERONE ACETATE
PHARMACIA & UPJOHN

2.5 MG   5 MG

10 MG

PROZAC

FLUOXETINE HCL
DISTA

10 MG

20 MG

PYRIDIUM

PHENAZOPYRIDINE HCL
PARKE-DAVIS

100 MG

200 MG

QUINIDEX EXTENTABS

QUINIDINE SULFATE
A. H. ROBINS

300 MG

REGLAN

METOCLOPRAMIDE HCL
A. H. ROBINS

5 MG   10 MG

RELAFEN

NABUMETONE
SMITHKLINE BEECHAM

500 MG

750 MG

REMERON

MIRTAZAPINE
ORGANON

15 MG   30 MG

REQUIP

ROPINIROLE HCL
SMITHKLINE BEECHAM

0.25 MG

RESTORIL

TEMAZEPAM
NOVARTIS

7.5 MG

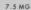

15 MG

30 MG

RETROVIR

ZIDOVUDINE
GLAXO WELLCOME

100 MG

REVIA

NALTREXONE HCL
DUPONT PHARMA

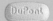

50 MG

REZULIN

TROGLITAZONE
PARKE-DAVIS

200
200 MG

400
400 MG

RIDAURA

AURANOFIN
CONNETICS

3 MG

RIFATER

ISONIAZID/ RIFAMPIN/ PYRAZINAMIDE
HOECHST MARION ROUSSEL

50 MG / 120 MG / 300 MG

RISPERDAL

RISPERIDONE
JANSSEN

R | 1
1 MG

R | 2
2 MG

R | 3
3 MG

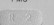
R | 4

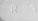

4 MG

RITALIN

METHYLPHENIDATE HCL
NOVARTIS

CIBA
5 MG

CIBA
10 MG

CIBA
20 MG

ROBAXIN

METHOCARBAMOL
A. H. ROBINS

ROBAXIN 2UB
500 MG

ROBAXIN 750
750 MG

ROCALTROL

CALCITRIOL
ROCHE

0.25 MCG

ROCA 0.5
0.5 MCG

RONDEC

CARBINOXAMINE MALEATE/ PSEUDOEPHEDRINE HCL
DURA

5126
4 MG / 60 MG

ROXICET

ACETAMINOPHEN/ OXYCODONE HCL
ROXANE

54 543
325 MG / 5 MG

RYTHMOL

PROPAFENONE HCL
KNOLL

150
150 MG

225
225 MG

300
300 MG

SECTRAL

ACEBUTOLOL HCL
WYETH-AYERST

WYETH 4177   SECTRAL 200
200 MG

WYETH 4176   SECTRAL 400
400 MG

SEMPREX D

**ACRIVASTINE/
PSEUDOEPHEDRINE HCL**
MEDEVA

8 MG / 60 MG

SEPTRA

**SULFAMETHOXAZOLE/
TRIMETHOPRIM**
GLAXO WELLCOME

400 MG / 80 MG

SERAX

OXAZEPAM
WYETH-AYERST

10 MG

15 MG

15 MG

30 MG

SEROQUEL

QUETIAPINE FUMARATE
ZENECA

25 MG   100 MG

200 MG

SERZONE

NEFAZODONE HCL
BRISTOL-MYERS SQUIBB

100 MG

150 MG

200 MG

250 MG

SINEMET

CARBIDOPA-LEVODOPA
DUPONT PHARMA

10 MG / 100 MG

25 MG / 100 MG

25 MG / 250 MG

SINEMET CR

CARBIDOPA-LEVODOPA
DUPONT PHARMA

25 MG / 100 MG
SUSTAINED RELEASE

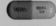

50 MG / 200 MG
SUSTAINED RELEASE

SINEQUAN

DOXEPIN HCL
ROERIG

10 MG

25 MG

50 MG

75 MG

100 MG

150 MG

SINGULAIR

MONTELUKAST SODIUM
MERCK

5 MG   10 MG
CHEWABLE

SLO-BID GYROCAPS

THEOPHYLLINE
RHONE-POULENC RORER

100 MG

200 MG

300 MG

SLO-PHYLLIN

THEOPHYLLINE
RHONE-POULENC RORER

100 MG   200 MG

SLOW-K

POTASSIUM CHLORIDE
NOVARTIS

8 MEQ

SOMA

CARISOPRODOL
WALLACE

350 MG

SORBITRATE

ISOSORBIDE DINITRATE
ZENECA

5 MG
SUBLINGUAL

5 MG
CHEWABLE

10 MG

SPORANOX

ITRACONAZOLE
JANSSEN

100 MG

STELAZINE

TRIFLUOPERAZINE HCL
SMITHKLINE BEECHAM

1 MG

2 MG

STUARTNATAL PLUS

VITAMINS, PRENATAL
WYETH-AYERST

SULAR

NISOLDIPINE
ZENECA

10 MG

20 MG

30 MG   40 MG

SUPRAX

CEFIXIME
LEDERLE

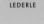
200 MG

400 MG

SURMONTIL

TRIMIPRAMINE MALEATE
WYETH-AYERST

25 MG

50 MG

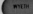
100 MG

SYNALGOS-DC

**DIHYDROCODEINE
BITARTRATE/ASPIRIN/
CAFFEINE**
WYETH-AYERST

16 MG / 356.4 MG / 30 MG

SYNTHROID

LEVOTHYROXINE SODIUM
KNOLL

0.025 MG   0.05 MG

0.075 MG   0.088 MG

0.1 MG   0.112 MG

0.125 MG   0.15 MG

0.175 MG   0.2 MG

0.3 MG

TAGAMET

CIMETIDINE
SMITHKLINE BEECHAM

200 MG

300 MG

400 MG

800 MG

TALWIN NX

PENTAZOCINE HCL
SANOFI

SCORED TABLET

TAMBOCOR

FLECAINIDE ACETATE
3M

50 MG

100 MG

150 MG

TARKA

**TRANDOLAPRIL/
VERAPAMIL HCL ER**
KNOLL

2 MG / 180 MG

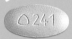

1 MG / 240 MG

2 MG / 240 MG

4 MG / 240 MG

TASMAR

TOLCAPONE
ROCHE

100 MG

200 MG

TAVIST

CLEMASTINE FUMARATE
NOVARTIS

2.68 MG

TEGRETOL

CARBAMAZEPINE
NOVARTIS

200 MG

100 MG
CHEWABLE

TENEX

GUANFACINE HCL
A. H. ROBINS

1 MG

2 MG

TENORETIC

**ATENOLOL /
CHLORTHALIDONE**
ZENECA

50 MG/25 MG

100 MG/25 MG

TENORMIN

ATENOLOL
ZENECA

25 MG   50 MG

100 MG

TENUATE

DIETHYLPROPION HCL
HOECHST MARION ROUSSEL

25 MG

75 MG

TESSALON PERLES

BENZONATATE
FOREST

100 MG

THEOCHRON

THEOPHYLLINE
FOREST

100 MG   200 MG

300 MG

THEO-DUR

THEOPHYLLINE
KEY

100 MG

200 MG

300 MG

450 MG

THEO-DUR

THEOPHYLLINE
KEY

50 MG

75 MG

125 MG

200 MG

THEOLAIR

THEOPHYLLINE
3M

125 MG

250 MG

THEOLAIR-SR

THEOPHYLLINE
3M

250 MG

300 MG

THORAZINE

CHLORPROMAZINE HCL
SMITHKLINE BEECHAM

25 MG

50 MG

75 MG

THYROLAR-1/2

LIOTRIX
FOREST

30 MG

THYROLAR-1

LIOTRIX
FOREST

60 MG

TIGAN

TRIMETHOBENZAMIDE HCL
ROBERTS

100 MG

250 MG

TOFRANIL

IMIPRAMINE HCL
NOVARTIS

10 MG   25 MG

50 MG

TOLECTIN

TOLMETIN SODIUM
ORTHO-MCNEIL

400 MG

600 MG

TONOCARD

TOCAINIDE HCL
MERCK

400 MG

600 MG

TORADOL

KETOROLAC TROMETHAMINE
ROCHE

10 MG

TRANDATE

LABETALOL HCL
GLAXO WELLCOME

100 MG   200 MG

300 MG

TRANXENE T-TAB

CLORAZEPATE DIPOTASSIUM
ABBOTT

3.75 MG

7.5 MG

15 MG

TRENTAL

PENTOXIFYLLINE
HOECHST MARION ROUSSEL

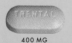

400 MG

TRIMOX

AMOXICILLIN
APOTHECON

250 MG

500 MG

TRINALIN REPETABS

AZATADINE MALEATE/ PSEUDOEPHEDRINE SULFATE
KEY

1 MG / 120 MG

TRITEC

RANITIDINE BISMUTH CITRATE
GLAXO WELLCOME

400 MG

TYLENOL W/CODEINE

ACETAMINOPHEN/ CODEINE PHOSPHATE
ORTHO-MCNEIL

300 MG / 30 MG

300 MG / 60 MG

TYLOX

OXYCODONE HCL/ ACETAMINOPHEN
ORTHO-MCNEIL

5 MG / 500 MG

ULTRAM

TRAMADOL HCL
ORTHO-MCNEIL

50 MG

UNIPHYL

THEOPHYLLINE
PURDUE FREDERICK

400 MG

UNIRETIC

MOEXIPRIL HCL / HYDROCHLOROTHIAZID
SCHWARZ PHARMA

7.5 MG / 12.5 MG

15 MG / 25 MG

UNIVASC

MOEXIPRIL HCL
SCHWARZ PHARMA

7.5 MG

15 MG

URISED	**VALTREX**	**VEETIDS**

URISED

**ATROPINE SULFATE/
BENZOIC ACID/
HYOSCYAMINE/
METHENAMINE/
METHYLENE BLUE/
PHENYL SALICYLATE**
POLYMEDICA

0.03 MG / 4.5 MG /
0.03 MG /40.8 MG /
5.4 MG / 18.1 MG

VALTREX

VALACYCLOVIR HCL
GLAXO WELLCOME

500 MG

1 G

VEETIDS

PENICILLIN V POTASSIUM
APOTHECON

250 MG

VENTOLIN

ALBUTEROL SULFATE
GLAXO WELLCOME

2 MG   4 MG

URISPAS

FLAVOXATE HCL
SMITHKLINE BEECHAM

100 MG

VASERETIC

**ENALAPRIL MALEATE/
HYDROCHLOROTHIAZIDE**
MERCK

5 MG /   10 MG /
12.5 MG   25 MG

VERELAN

VERAPAMIL HCL
LEDERLE

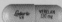

120 MG

180 MG

VALIUM

DIAZEPAM
ROCHE

2 MG

5 MG

10 MG

VASOTEC

ENALAPRIL MALEATE
MERCK

2.5 MG

5 MG

10 MG

20 MG

240 MG

VIBRAMYCIN

DOXYCYCLINE HYCLATE
PFIZER

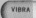

50 MG

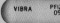

100 MG

VIBRA-TABS

DOXYCYCLINE HYCLATE
PFIZER

100 MG

VICODIN

HYDROCODONE BITARTRATE/ ACETAMINOPHEN
KNOLL

5 MG / 500 MG

VICOPROFEN

HYDROCODONE BITARTRATE / IBUPROFEN
KNOLL

7.5 MG / 200 MG

VIDEX

DIDANOSINE
BRISTOL MYERS
SQUIBB ONCOLOGY

100 MG

VIOKASE

PANCRELIPASE
A. H. ROBINS

VIRACEPT

NELFINAVIR MESYLATE
AGOURON

250 MG

VIRAMUNE

NEVIRAPINE
ROCHE

200 MG

VISKEN

PINDOLOL
NOVARTIS

5 MG

10 MG

VISTARIL

HYDROXYZINE PAMOATE
PFIZER

25 MG

50 MG

100 MG

VOLTAREN

DICLOFENAC SODIUM
NOVARTIS

25 MG   50 MG

75 MG

VOLTAREN-XR

DICLOFENAC SODIUM
NOVARTIS

100 MG

WELLBUTRIN

BUPROPION HCL
GLAXO WELLCOME

75 MG   100 MG

WYMOX

AMOXICILLIN
WYETH-AYERST

250 MG

500 MG

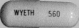

WYTENSIN

GUANABENZ ACETATE
WYETH-AYERST

4 MG   8 MG

XANAX

ALPRAZOLAM
PHARMACIA & UPJOHN

0.25 MG

0.5 MG

1 MG

2 MG

YOCON

YOHIMBINE HCL
GLENWOOD

5.4 MG

YOHIMEX

YOHIMBINE HCL
KRAMER

5.4 MG

ZANTAC

RANITIDINE HCL
GLAXO WELLCOME

150 MG

300 MG

ZAROXOLYN

METOLAZONE
MEDEVA

2.5 MG   5 MG

10 MG

ZERIT

STAVUDINE
BRISTOL MYERS
SQUIBB ONCOLOGY

15 MG

20 MG

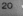

30 MG

40 MG

ZESTORETIC

**LISINOPRIL/
HYDROCHLOROTHIAZIDE**
ZENECA

10 MG / 12.5 MG

20 MG / 12.5 MG

20 MG / 25 MG

ZESTRIL

LISINOPRIL
ZENECA

5 MG   10 MG

20 MG   40 MG

ZITHROMAX

AZITHROMYCIN DIHYDRATE
PFIZER

250 MG

600 MG

ZOCOR

SIMVASTATIN
MERCK

 5 MG
 10 MG

 20 MG
 40 MG

ZOFRAN

ONDANSETRON HCL
GLAXO WELLCOME

 4 MG

 8 MG

ZOLOFT

SERTRALINE HCL
PFIZER

50 MG

100 MG

ZOMIG

ZOLMITRIPTAN
ZENECA

 2.5 MG

 5 MG

ZOVIRAX

ACYCLOVIR
GLAXO WELLCOME

 200 MG

400 MG

 800 MG

ZYBAN

BUPROPION HCL
GLAXO WELLCOME

 150 MG

ZYDONE

**HYDROCODONE
BITARTRATE/
ACETAMINOPHEN**
ENDO

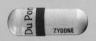 5 MG/500 MG

ZYFLO

ZILEUTON TABLETS
ABBOTT

 600 MG

ZYLOPRIM

ALLOPURINOL
GLAXO WELLCOME

 100 MG

 300 MG

ZYRTEC

CETIRIZINE HCL
PFIZER

 5 MG

 10 MG

blood contains ANA (antinuclear antibodies), your doctor may want to discontinue the medication.

Possible food and drug interactions
when taking this medication

If Rythmol is taken with certain other drugs, the effects of either could be increased, decreased, or altered. It is especially important to check with your doctor before combining Rythmol with the following:

Beta blockers such as Inderal and Lopressor
Cimetidine (Tagamet)
Cyclosporine (Neoral, Sandimmune)
Digoxin (Lanoxin)
Local anesthetics (such as Novocain used during dental work)
Quinidine (Cardioquin)
Rifampin (Rifadin)
Theophylline (Theo-Dur, Uni-Dur)
Warfarin (blood thinners such as Coumadin)

Special information
if you are pregnant or breastfeeding

If you are pregnant or plan to become pregnant, inform your doctor immediately. Because of a possible risk of birth defects, Rythmol is not recommended during pregnancy unless the benefit to the mother outweighs the potential risk to the unborn baby.

It is not known whether Rythmol appears in breast milk. You are advised not to take Rythmol if you are nursing a baby. If treatment with Rythmol is essential to your health, your doctor may advise you to stop breastfeeding until your treatment is finished.

Recommended dosage

ADULTS

In most cases, treatment with Rythmol begins in the hospital.

Your doctor will tailor your dosage according to your individual condition and the presence of other disorders.

The usual initial dose of Rythmol is 150 milligrams every 8 hours. Your doctor may increase the dosage depending on how you respond to the initial dosage. The maximum recommended daily dosage of Rythmol is 900 milligrams.

CHILDREN

Safety and effectiveness have not been established in children.

OLDER ADULTS

The doctor will increase the dosage more slowly at the beginning of treatment.

Overdosage

Any medication taken in excess can have serious consequences. If you suspect an overdose of Rythmol, seek medical attention immediately.

- *Symptoms of Rythmol overdose, which are usually most severe within the first 3 hours of taking the medication, may include:*
  Convulsions (rarely), heartbeat irregularities, low blood pressure, sleepiness

Generic name:

SALMETEROL

See Serevent, page 1183.

Generic name:

SALSALATE

See Disalcid, page 418.

Brand name:

SANDIMMUNE

Pronounced: SAN-dim-ewn
Generic name: Cyclosporine
Other brand name: Neoral

Why is this drug prescribed?

Sandimmune is given after organ transplant surgery to help prevent rejection of organs (kidney, heart, or liver) by holding down the body's immune system. It is also used to avoid long-term rejection in people previously treated with other immunosuppressant drugs, such as Imuran.

Neoral is a newer formulation of Sandimmune's active ingredient, cyclosporine. In addition to prevention of organ rejection, it is prescribed for certain severe cases of rheumatoid arthritis and psoriasis.

Some doctors also prescribe Sandimmune to treat alopecia areata (localized areas of hair loss), aplastic anemia (shortage of red and white blood cells and platelets), Crohn's disease (chronic inflammation of the digestive tract), and nephropathy (kidney disease). Sandimmune is sometimes used in the treatment of severe skin disorders, including psoriasis and dermatomyositis (inflammation of the skin and muscles causing weakness and rash). The drug is also used in procedures involving bone marrow, the pancreas, and the lungs.

Sandimmune is always given with prednisone or a similar steroid. It is available in capsules and liquid, or as an injection.

Most important fact about this drug

If you take Sandimmune orally over a period of time, your doctor will monitor your blood levels of cyclosporine to make sure your body is receiving the correct amount of Sandimmune. The reason for this repeated testing is that the absorption of this drug in the body is erratic. Constant monitoring is necessary to prevent toxicity due to overdosing or to prevent possible organ rejection due to underdosing. It is important to note that Sandimmune may need to be taken by mouth for an indefinite period following surgery.

How should you take this medication?

Take the Sandimmune capsule or oral liquid at the same time every day. You may take the medication either with a meal or between meals, but be consistent.

To make Sandimmune oral liquid more palatable, you may mix it with room-temperature milk, chocolate milk, or orange juice. Neoral oral solution may be mixed with room-temperature orange or pineapple juice. It does not taste good in milk. Use a container made of glass, not plastic. Never let the mixture stand; drink it as soon as you prepare it. To make sure you get your full dose, rinse the glass with a little more liquid and drink that too.

You should maintain good dental hygiene and see your dentist frequently for cleaning to prevent tenderness, bleeding, and gum enlargement.

After you use the dosage syringe to transfer the oral solution to a glass, dry the outside of the syringe with a clean towel and put it away. Do not rinse or wash it. If you do have to clean it, make sure it is thoroughly dry before you use it again.

You may notice an odor when you open the capsule container; this is nothing to worry about and will soon dissipate.

Neoral should start to work on rheumatoid arthritis in 4 to 8 weeks, and on psoriasis in 2 weeks. Psoriasis is usually controlled within 12 to 16 weeks; you should not take the drug for more than a year.

■ *If you miss a dose...*
If fewer than 12 hours have passed, take it as soon as you remember. If it is almost time for the next dose, skip the one you missed and go back to your regular schedule. Do not take 2 doses at once.

■ *Storage instructions...*
Store both the capsules and the oral solution below 86°F; do not store the liquid in the refrigerator. Keep the liquid from freezing. Sandimmune liquid, once opened, must be used within 2 months.

What side effects may occur?
Side effects cannot be anticipated. If any appear or change in intensity, inform your doctor immediately. Only your doctor can determine if it is safe for you to continue taking Sandimmune. The principal side effects of Sandimmune are high blood pressure, hirsutism (unusual growth of hair), kidney damage, excessive growth of the gums, and tremor.

■ *Other common side effects may include:*
Abdominal discomfort, acne, breathing difficulty, convulsions, coughing, cramps, diarrhea, flu-like symptoms, flushing, headache, liver damage, lymph system tumor, muscle, bone, or joint pain, nasal inflammation, nausea, numbness or tingling, sinus inflammation, vomiting, wheezing

■ *Less common side effects may include:*
Abdominal distention, allergic reactions, anemia, appetite loss or increase, bleeding gums, blood disorders, brittle fingernails, confusion, conjunctivitis (pinkeye), dizziness, fever, fluid retention, frequent urination, hearing loss, hiccups, high blood sugar, indigestion, infection, insomnia, nervousness, peptic ulcer, rash and other skin disorders, ringing in the ears, stomach inflammation, vertigo

■ *Rare side effects may include:*
Anxiety, blood in the urine, breast development in males, chest pain, constipation, depression, hair breaking, heart attack, itching, joint pain, lymph disorders, mouth sores, night sweats, sluggishness, stomach and upper intestinal bleeding, swallowing difficulty, tingling, visual disturbance, weakness, weight loss

Why should this drug not be prescribed?

Do not take these products if you have ever had an allergic reaction to them. Avoid Sandimmune by injection if you have ever had an allergic reaction to an injection of the drug or you are especially sensitive to castor oil.

Avoid taking Neoral for arthritis or psoriasis if you have a kidney condition, high blood pressure, or cancer. While taking the drug, you should avoid most other psoriasis treatment, including ultraviolet light, coal tar, methotrexate, and radiation.

Special warnings about this medication

When your immune system is suppressed by Sandimmune, you are at increased risk of infection and of certain malignancies, including skin cancer and lymph system cancer.

High-dose Sandimmune is toxic to the liver and kidneys and may cause serious kidney damage. Because this toxicity has symptoms similar to those of transplant rejection, you must be monitored closely. If your body is trying hard to reject a transplanted organ, your doctor will probably allow the rejection to occur rather than give you a very high dose of Sandimmune.

This drug can raise blood pressure, especially in older people. If high blood pressure develops while you are taking Neoral for transplant rejection, the doctor will prescribe blood pressure medication. If it develops while you are taking the drug for arthritis or psoriasis, the doctor may lower your dose.

Sandimmune and Neoral are not directly interchangeable. Your doctor may need to adjust the dosage if you switch.

If you take large doses of a prednisone-like drug called methylprednisolone (Medrol) along with Sandimmune, you may be at increased risk of convulsions.

Use a barrier method of contraception, such as diaphragms or condoms, during Sandimmune therapy. Do not use oral contraceptive pills without your doctor's approval.

Do not try to change dosage forms without consulting your doctor.

If you take Neoral for arthritis or psoriasis, the condition will eventually return when you stop taking the drug, generally within 1 or 2 months. Neoral treatments for psoriasis should be replaced with other types of therapy after 1 year.

**Possible food and drug interactions
when taking this medication**

Avoid getting vaccinations and immunizations while you are taking Sandimmune. The drug may make vaccinations less effective or increase your risk of contracting an illness from a live vaccine.

If taking Neoral for psoriasis, remember to avoid other psoriasis treatments.

Avoid grapefruit and grapefruit juice while taking this drug.

If Sandimmune is taken with certain other drugs, the effects of either could be increased, decreased, or altered. It is especially important to check with your doctor before combining Sandimmune with the following:

Allopurinol (Zyloprim)
Amphotericin B (Fungizone, Abelcet)
Bromocriptine (Parlodel)
Calcium-blocking heart and blood pressure medications such as Calan, Cardene, Procardia, and Cardizem
Carbamazepine (Tegretol)
Cimetidine (Tagamet)
Clarithromycin (Biaxin)
Danazol (Danocrine)
Diclofenac (Voltaren, Cataflam)
Digoxin (Lanoxin, Lanoxicaps)
Erythromycin (E.E.S., Erythrocin, others)
Fluconazole (Diflucan)
Gentamicin (Garamycin)
Indinavir (Crixivan)
Itraconazole (Sporanox)
Ketoconazole (Nizoral)
Lovastatin (Mevacor)
Melphalan (Alkeran)
Methotrexate
Methylprednisolone (Depo-Medrol, Medrol, Solu-Medrol)
Metoclopramide (Reglan)
Nafcillin (Unipen)
Nelfinavir
Nonsteroidal anti-inflammatory drugs such as Clinoril and Naprasyn
Octreotide (Sandostatin)
Phenobarbital
Phenytoin (Dilantin)
Potassium-sparing diuretics (Dyrenium, Midamor, Aldactone)
Prednisolone (Delta-Cortef, Prelone)

Ranitidine (Zantac)
Rifampin (Rifadin, Rifamate, Rimactane)
Ritonavir (Norvir)
Saquinavir (Fortovase)
Ticlopidine (Ticlid)
Tobramycin (Nebcin)
Trimethoprim/sulfamethoxazole (Bactrim, Septra)
Vancomycin (Vancocin)

Special information
if you are pregnant or breastfeeding

The effects of Sandimmune in pregnancy have not been adequately studied. If you are pregnant or plan to become pregnant, inform your doctor immediately. Sandimmune should be used during pregnancy only if the benefit justifies the potential risk to the unborn child. Since Sandimmune appears in breast milk, it should not be used during breastfeeding. If you are a new mother, you may need to choose between taking Sandimmune and breastfeeding your baby.

Recommended dosage

ADULTS

Transplant Rejection

Your doctor will tailor your dosage of Sandimmune in accordance with your body's response. Expect a single dose of 15 milligrams per 2.2 pounds of body weight 4 to 12 hours before a transplant and 1 dose daily for 1 to 2 weeks after the operation. After that, the doctor may keep you on a daily dose of 5 to 10 milligrams per 2.2 pounds of body weight.

The dosage of Neoral depends on the type of transplant and the other drugs you are taking. It is always taken twice a day.

Psoriasis or Rheumatoid Arthritis

The starting dosage is 2.5 milligrams of Neoral per 2.2 pounds of body weight divided into 2 doses per day. Your doctor may gradually increase the daily dose to a maximum of 4 milligrams per 2.2 pounds.

Overdosage

Although no specific information is available, an overdose of Sandimmune would be expected to cause liver and kidney problems. Any medication taken in excess can have serious consequences. If you suspect an overdose of Sandimmune, seek medical attention immediately.

Generic name:

SAQUINAVIR

See Fortovase, page 550.

Brand name:

SECTRAL

Pronounced: SEK-tral
Generic name: Acebutolol hydrochloride

Why is this drug prescribed?

Sectral, a type of medication known as a beta blocker, is used in the treatment of high blood pressure and abnormal heart rhythms. When used to treat high blood pressure, it is effective used alone or in combination with other high blood pressure medications, particularly with a thiazide-type diuretic. Beta blockers decrease the force and rate of heart contractions, thus reducing pressure within the circulatory system.

Most important fact about this drug

If you have high blood pressure, you must take Sectral regularly for it to be effective. Since blood pressure declines gradually, it may be several weeks before you get the full benefit of Sectral; and you must continue taking it even if you are feeling well. Sectral does not cure high blood pressure; it merely keeps it under control.

How should you take this medication?

Sectral can be taken with or without food. Take it exactly as prescribed, even if your symptoms have disappeared.

Try not to miss any doses. If this medication is not taken regularly, your condition may worsen.

■ *If you miss a dose...*
 Take the forgotten dose as soon as you remember. If it's within 4 hours of your next scheduled dose, skip the one you missed and go back to your regular schedule. Never take 2 doses at the same time.

■ *Storage instructions...*
 Store at room temperature. Keep the container tightly closed. Protect from light.

What side effects may occur?

Side effects cannot be anticipated. If any develop or change in intensity, inform your doctor as soon as possible. Only your doctor can determine if it is safe for you to continue taking Sectral.

■ *More common side effects may include:*
Abnormal vision, chest pain, constipation, cough, decreased sexual ability, depression, diarrhea, dizziness, fatigue, frequent urination, gas, headache, indigestion, joint pain, nasal inflammation, nausea, shortness of breath or difficulty breathing, strange dreams, swelling due to fluid retention, trouble sleeping, weakness

■ *Less common or rare side effects may include:*
Abdominal pain, anxiety, back pain, burning eyes, cold hands and feet, conjunctivitis, dark urine, excessive urination at night, eye pain, fever, heart failure, impotence, itching, loss of appetite, low blood pressure, muscle pain, nervousness, painful or difficult urination, rash, slow heartbeat, throat inflammation, vomiting, wheezing

Why should this drug not be prescribed?

If you have heart failure, inadequate blood supply to the circulatory system (cardiogenic shock), heart block (a type of irregular heartbeat), or a severely slow heartbeat, you should not take this medication.

Special warnings about this medication

If you have had severe congestive heart failure in the past, Sectral should be used with caution.

Sectral should not be stopped suddenly. This can cause increased chest pain and heart attack. Dosage should be gradually reduced.

If you suffer from asthma, seasonal allergies, other bronchial conditions, coronary artery disease, or kidney or liver disease, this medication should be used with caution.

Ask your doctor if you should check your pulse while taking Sectral. This medication can cause your heartbeat to become too slow.

This medication may mask the symptoms of low blood sugar or alter blood sugar levels. If you are diabetic, discuss this with your doctor.

Notify your doctor or dentist that you are taking Sectral if you have a medical emergency, or before you have any surgery.

Tell your doctor if you are taking over-the-counter cold medications and nasal drops. They may interact with Sectral.

If you experience difficulty breathing, or develop hives or large areas of swelling, seek medical attention immediately. You may be having a serious allergic reaction to the medicine. Sectral can also make other severe allergies worse.

Possible food and drug interactions
when taking this medication

If Sectral is taken with certain other drugs, the effects of either could be increased, decreased, or altered. It is especially important to check with your doctor before combining Sectral with the following:

Albuterol (the airway-opening drug Ventolin)
Certain blood pressure medicines such as reserpine (Diupres)
Certain over-the-counter cold remedies and nasal drops such as Afrin, Neo-Synephrine, and Sudafed
Nonsteroidal anti-inflammatory drugs such as Motrin and Voltaren
Oral diabetes drugs such as Micronase

Special information
if you are pregnant or breastfeeding

The effects of Sectral during pregnancy have not been adequately studied. If you are pregnant or plan to become pregnant, inform your doctor immediately. Sectral appears in breast milk and could affect a nursing infant. If this medication is essential to your health, your doctor may advise you to discontinue breastfeeding until your treatment with Sectral is finished.

Recommended dosage

ADULTS

Hypertension

The usual initial dose for mild to moderate high blood pressure is 400 milligrams per day. It may be taken in a single daily dose or in 2 doses of 200 milligrams each. The usual daily dosage ranges from 200 to 800 milligrams.

People with severe high blood pressure may take up to 1,200 milligrams per day divided into 2 doses. Sectral may be taken alone or in combination with another high blood pressure medication.

Irregular heartbeat

The usual starting dosage is 400 milligrams per day divided into 2 doses. Your doctor may gradually increase the dose to 600 to 1,200 milligrams per day. If your doctor wants you to stop taking this medication, he or she will have you taper off over a period of 2 weeks.

CHILDREN

The safety and effectiveness of Sectral have not been established in children.

OLDER ADULTS

Your doctor will determine the dosage based on your particular needs. Do not take more than 800 milligrams per day.

Overdosage

Any medication taken in excess can have serious consequences. If you suspect an overdose, seek medical attention immediately.

- *There is no specific information available on Sectral; however, overdose symptoms seen with other beta blockers include:*
  Difficulty breathing, extremely slow heartbeat, irregular heartbeat, low blood pressure, low blood sugar, seizures, severe congestive heart failure

Generic name:

SELEGILINE

See Eldepryl, page 464.

Brand name:

SEMPREX-D

Pronounced: SEM-precks-D
Generic ingredients: Acrivastine, Pseudoephedrine hydrochloride

Why is this drug prescribed?

Semprex-D is an antihistamine and decongestant drug that relieves sneezing, running nose, itching, watery eyes, and stuffy nose caused by seasonal allergies such as hay fever.

Most important fact about this drug

Semprex-D may cause drowsiness. Do not drive or operate dangerous machinery or participate in any hazardous activity that requires full mental alertness until you know how you react to this medication.

How should you take this medication?

Take Semprex-D exactly as prescribed by your doctor. Do not take more of this drug or use it more often than your doctor recommends.

- *If you miss a dose...*
  Take it as soon as you remember. If it is almost time for your next dose, skip the one you missed and go back to your regular schedule. Never take 2 doses at the same time.

- *Storage instructions...*
  Store at room temperature in a dry place; protect the drug from light.

What side effects may occur?
Side effects cannot be anticipated. If any develop or change in intensity, inform your doctor as soon as possible. Only your doctor can determine if it is safe for you to continue taking Semprex-D.

- *Side effects may include:*
  Cough, dizziness, drowsiness, dry mouth, headache, indigestion, menstrual problems, nausea, nervousness, skin eruptions, sleeplessness, sore throat, weakness, wheezing

Severe allergic reactions are rare. There have been isolated reports of swelling of the throat, lips, neck, face, hands, or feet. Pseudoephedrine, one of the ingredients of this drug, has also been known to cause rapid or fluttery heartbeat.

Why should this drug not be prescribed?
You should not take Semprex-D if you are sensitive to or have ever had an allergic reaction to acrivastine, pseudoephedrine, or similar drugs such as Actifed, Dimetane, Trinalin, or Seldane-D. Make sure your doctor is aware of any drug reactions you have experienced.

Avoid using Semprex-D if you have extremely high blood pressure or severe heart problems.

Do not take this drug within 14 days of taking any drug known as an MAO inhibitor, including the antidepressants Nardil and Parnate.

Special warnings about this medication
Use this drug with caution if you have high blood pressure, diabetes, heart problems, peptic ulcer or other stomach problems, or an enlarged prostate gland. Use Semprex-D with care, too, if you have increased eye pressure, an overactive thyroid gland, or kidney disease. Make sure the doctor has taken these conditions into account.

Antihistamines are more likely to cause dizziness, extreme calm (sedation), bladder obstruction, and low blood pressure in the elderly (over age 60). The elderly are also more likely to have more side effects from the decongestant (pseudoephedrine) in Semprex-D.

Possible food and drug interactions
when taking this medication

If Semprex-D is taken with certain other drugs, the effects of either could be increased, decreased, or altered. It is especially important to check with your doctor before combining this drug with the following:

Alcoholic beverages
Blood pressure medications such as Inderal and Lopressor
MAO inhibitors, including the antidepressants Nardil and Parnate
Other antihistamines such as Actifed, Seldane-D, and Entex
Other decongestants such as Quibron and Rynatan

Special information
if you are pregnant or breastfeeding

The effects of Semprex-D during pregnancy have not been adequately studied. If you are pregnant or plan to become pregnant, tell your doctor immediately.

It is not known whether acrivastine appears in breast milk, but pseudoephedrine does. If the drug is essential to your health, your doctor may tell you to stop nursing until your treatment is finished.

Recommended dosage

ADULTS

The usual dose for adults and children 12 years of age and older is 1 capsule, taken by mouth, every 4 to 6 hours, 4 times a day.

CHILDREN

The safety and effectiveness of Semprex-D in children less than 12 years old have not been established.

Overdosage

Although there have been few reports of overdosage with Semprex-D, overdosage with similar drugs has caused a variety of serious symptoms. If you suspect an overdose of Semprex-D, seek medical attention immediately.

■ *Symptoms of overdose may include:*
Anxiety, convulsions, difficult breathing, drowsiness, fear, hallucinations, heart failure with low blood pressure, irregular heartbeat, loss of consciousness, painful urination, paleness, restlessness, sleeplessness, tenseness, trembling, weakness

Brand name:

SEPTRA

See Bactrim, page 135.

Brand name:

SER-AP-ES

Pronounced: Sir-AP-ess
Generic ingredients: Serpasil (reserpine), Apresoline
(hydralazine hydrochloride), Esidrix (hydrochlorothiazide)

Why is this drug prescribed?
Ser-Ap-Es is a combination drug used in the treatment of high blood pressure. It combines two high blood pressure medications—Serpasil and Apresoline—with a thiazide diuretic, Esidrix. Serpasil and Apresoline improve blood flow throughout your body. Esidrix helps your body produce and eliminate more urine, which also helps lower blood pressure.

Most important fact about this drug
You must take Ser-Ap-Es regularly for it to be effective. Since blood pressure declines gradually, it may be several weeks before you get the full benefit of Ser-Ap-Es; and you must continue taking it even if you are feeling well. Ser-Ap-Es does not cure high blood pressure; it merely keeps it under control.

How should you take this medication?
Take Ser-Ap-Es exactly as prescribed by your doctor, even if your symptoms have disappeared.

Try not to miss any doses. If this medication is not taken regularly, your condition may worsen.

- *If you miss a dose...*
  Take the forgotten dose as soon as you remember. If it is almost time for the next dose, skip the one you missed and go back to your regular schedule. Never try to "catch up" by doubling the dose.

- *Storage instructions...*
  Ser-Ap-Es can be stored at room temperature. Use the container it came in.

What side effects may occur?
Side effects cannot be anticipated. If any develop or change in intensity, inform your doctor as soon as possible. Only your doctor can determine if it is safe for you to continue taking Ser-Ap-Es.

■ *Side effects may include:*
Anemia, anxiety, blockage in the intestines, blood disorders, blurred vision, breast development in males, breast engorgement, change in potassium levels (dry mouth, excessive thirst, weak or irregular heartbeat, muscle pain or cramps), chills, conjunctivitis, constipation, cramping (stomach and intestinal), crushing chest pain (angina), deafness, decreased sex drive, depression, diarrhea, difficult or labored breathing, difficult or painful urination, disorientation, dizziness, dizziness when standing up, drowsiness, dry mouth, enlarged spleen, eye disorders, fainting, fever, fluid in the lungs, fluid retention, flushing, glaucoma, headache, hepatitis, high blood sugar, hives, impotence, inflammation of the lungs, inflammation of the pancreas, inflammation of the salivary glands, irregular heartbeat, irritation of the stomach, itching, joint pain, loss of appetite, low blood pressure, muscle aches, muscle cramps, muscle spasm, nasal congestion, nausea, nervousness, nightmares, nosebleeds, numbness, parkinsonian syndrome (tremors, muscle weakness, shuffling walk, stooped posture, drooling), pounding heartbeat, rapid heartbeat, rash, red or purple skin discoloration, respiratory distress, restlessness, skin peeling, skin sensitivity to light, slow heartbeat, sugar in the urine, teary eyes, tingling or pins and needles, tremors, vertigo, vision changes, vomiting, weakness, weight gain, yellow eyes and skin

Why should this drug not be prescribed?
If you are being treated for depression you should avoid this medication.

Ser-Ap-Es should not be prescribed if you have an active peptic ulcer, ulcerative colitis (chronic inflammation of the large intestine and rectum), coronary artery disease, or rheumatic heart disease, or if you are unable to urinate, or are receiving electroshock therapy. Make sure your doctor is aware of all your medical problems.

If you are sensitive to or have ever had an allergic reaction to Ser-Ap-Es, any of its ingredients, or sulfa drugs, do not take this medication. Inform your doctor of any drug reactions you have experienced.

Special warnings about this medication
Diuretics can cause your body to lose too much potassium. Signs of an excessively low potassium level include muscle weakness and rapid or irregular heartbeat. To boost your potassium level, your doctor may

recommend eating potassium-rich foods such as bananas and orange juice, or may prescribe a potassium supplement.

Ser-Ap-Es can cause depression. It can last for several months after you have stopped taking the drug, and it can be severe. If you develop any signs of depression—despondency, waking early in the morning, loss of appetite, impotence, loss of self-esteem—contact your doctor immediately.

If you have a history of peptic ulcer, ulcerative colitis, or gallstones you should use this medication cautiously.

Some people have developed symptoms similar to those of lupus erythematosus, a disease characterized by rash, fever, and sometimes the symptoms of arthritis. These symptoms usually disappear when the Ser-Ap-Es is discontinued.

If you already have lupus erythematosus, Ser-Ap-Es may activate or worsen its symptoms.

If you have coronary artery, kidney, or liver disease, you should be carefully monitored while taking Ser-Ap-Es.

This medication may mask the symptoms of low blood sugar or alter blood sugar levels. If you are diabetic, discuss this with your doctor.

Allergic reactions are more likely to occur if you have a history of allergies or bronchial asthma.

In rare cases, abnormal amounts of uric acid in the blood may develop while taking this medication, leading to an attack of gout.

Notify your doctor or dentist that you are taking Ser-Ap-Es if you have a medical emergency, or before you have surgery or dental treatment.

Possible food and drug interactions
when taking this medication
If Ser-Ap-Es is taken with certain other drugs, the effects of either could be increased, decreased, or altered. It is especially important to check with your doctor before combining Ser-Ap-Es with the following:

ACTH (adrenal hormone)
Amphetamines such as Dexedrine
Antidepressant drugs such as Elavil and Norpramin
Cholestyramine (Questran)
Colestipol (Colestid)
Digitalis (Lanoxin)

Drugs that stimulate the central nervous system such as Cylert and Desoxyn

Drugs that stimulate the sympathetic nervous system such as epinephrine, ephedrine, isoproterenol, metaraminol, tyramine, and phenylephrine

Insulin

Lithium (Eskalith)

MAO inhibitors (antidepressant drugs such as Nardil and Parnate)

Nonsteroidal anti-inflammatory drugs (arthritis drugs and painkillers such as Motrin)

Norepinephrine (Levophed)

Other high blood pressure drugs such as Aldomet and Hyperstat

Quinidine (Quinidex)

Steroids such as Deltasone

Special information
if you are pregnant or breastfeeding

The effects of Ser-Ap-Es during pregnancy have not been adequately studied. If you are pregnant or plan to become pregnant, notify your doctor immediately. Ser-Ap-Es appears in breast milk and could seriously affect a nursing infant. If this medication is essential to your health, your doctor may advise you to discontinue breastfeeding until your treatment is finished.

Recommended dosage

ADULTS

Your doctor will determine the dosage according to your specific needs. You should not take more than 0.25 milligram of reserpine daily (the amount in 2½ tablets).

CHILDREN

The safety and effectiveness of this drug in children have not been established.

Overdosage

Any medication taken in excess can have serious consequences. If you suspect an overdose, seek medical attention immediately.

■ *Symptoms of Ser-Ap-Es overdose may include:*
Coma, confusion, constricted pupils, cramps of the calf muscles, decreased amounts of urine, diarrhea, dizziness, drowsiness, fatigue, flushing, headache, heart attack, inability to urinate, increased amounts of urine, increased

salivation, irregular heartbeat, low blood pressure, low body temperature, nausea, rapid heartbeat, severe loss of fluid, shock, slow heartbeat, slowed breathing, thirst, tingling or pins and needles, vomiting, weakness

Brand name:

SERAX

Pronounced: SER-aks
Generic name: Oxazepam

Why is this drug prescribed?
Serax is used in the treatment of anxiety disorders, including anxiety associated with depression.

This drug seems to be particularly effective for anxiety, tension, agitation, and irritability in older people. It is also prescribed to relieve symptoms of acute alcohol withdrawal.

Serax belongs to a class of drugs known as benzodiazepines.

Most important fact about this drug
Serax can be habit-forming or addicting and can lose its effectiveness over time, as you develop a tolerance for it. You may experience withdrawal symptoms if you stop using the drug abruptly. When discontinuing the drug, your doctor will reduce the dose gradually.

How should you take this medication?
Take Serax exactly as prescribed.

- *If you miss a dose...*
  If you remember within an hour or so, take the dose immediately. If you do not remember until later, skip the dose you missed and go back to your regular schedule. Do not take 2 doses at once.

- *Storage instructions...*
  Store at room temperature in a tightly closed container.

What side effects may occur?
Side effects cannot be anticipated. If any develop or change in intensity, inform your doctor as soon as possible. Only your doctor can determine if it is safe for you to continue taking Serax. Your doctor should periodically reassess the need for this drug.

- *More common side effects may include:*
  Drowsiness

- *Less common or rare side effects may include:*
  Blood disorders, change in sex drive, dizziness, excitement, fainting, headache, hives, liver problems, loss or lack of muscle control, nausea, skin rashes or eruptions, sluggishness or unresponsiveness, slurred speech, swelling due to fluid retention, tremors, vertigo, yellowed eyes and skin

- *Side effects due to rapid decrease or abrupt withdrawal from Serax:*
  Abdominal and muscle cramps, convulsions, depressed mood, inability to fall or stay asleep, sweating, tremors, vomiting

Why should this drug not be prescribed?

If you are sensitive to or have ever had an allergic reaction to Serax or other tranquilizers such as Valium, you should not take this medication. Make sure your doctor is aware of any drug reactions you have experienced.

Anxiety or tension related to everyday stress usually does not require treatment with Serax. Discuss your symptoms thoroughly with your doctor.

Serax should not be prescribed if you are being treated for mental disorders more serious than anxiety.

Special warnings about this medication

Serax may cause you to become drowsy or less alert; therefore, you should not drive or operate dangerous machinery or participate in any hazardous activity that requires full mental alertness until you know how this drug affects you.

This medication may cause your blood pressure to drop. If you have any heart problems, consult your doctor before taking this medication.

The 15-milligram tablet of this drug contains the coloring agent FD&C Yellow No. 5, which may cause an allergic reaction. If you are sensitive to aspirin or susceptible to allergies, consult your doctor before taking the tablet.

Possible food and drug interactions
when taking this medication

Serax may intensify the effects of alcohol. It may be best to avoid alcohol while taking this medication.

If Serax is taken with certain other drugs, the effects of either could be increased, decreased, or altered. It is especially important to check with your doctor before combining Serax with the following:

Antihistamines such as Benadryl
Narcotic painkillers such as Percocet and Demerol
Sedatives such as Seconal and Halcion
Tranquilizers such as Valium and Xanax

Special information
if you are pregnant or breastfeeding

Do not take Serax if you are pregnant or planning to become pregnant. There is an increased risk of birth defects. Serax may appear in breast milk and could affect a nursing infant. If this drug is essential to your health, your doctor may advise you to stop breastfeeding until your treatment with this medication is finished.

Recommended dosage

ADULTS

Mild to Moderate Anxiety with Tension, Irritability, Agitation
The usual dose is 10 to 15 milligrams 3 or 4 times per day.

Severe Anxiety, Depression with Anxiety, or Alcohol Withdrawal
The usual dose is 15 to 30 milligrams, 3 or 4 times per day.

CHILDREN

Safety and effectiveness have not been established for children under 6 years of age, nor have dosage guidelines been established for children 6 to 12 years. Your doctor will adjust the dosage to fit the child's needs.

OLDER ADULTS

The usual starting dose is 10 milligrams, 3 times a day. Your doctor may increase the dose to 15 milligrams 3 or 4 times a day, if needed.

Overdosage

An overdose of Serax can be fatal. If you suspect an overdose, seek medical attention immediately.

- *Symptoms of mild Serax overdose may include:*
  Confusion, drowsiness, lethargy

- *Symptoms of more serious overdose may include:*
  Coma, hypnotic state, lack of coordination, limp muscles, low blood
  pressure

Brand name:

SEREVENT

Pronounced: SER-ah-vent
Generic name: Salmeterol xinafoate
Other brand name: Serevent Diskus

Why is this drug prescribed?
Serevent relaxes the muscles in the walls of the bronchial tubes, allowing the passageways to expand and carry more air. Taken regularly (twice a day), the drug helps prevent wheezing and other symptoms of asthma, as well as exercise-induced asthma. A relatively long-acting medication, it is recommended for people who need shorter-acting bronchodilators such as Alupent and Ventolin on a frequent, regular basis.

Serevent is available in an aerosol inhaler and as Serevent Diskus inhalation powder. The aerosol inhaler is also used to treat the airway constriction that marks such chronic lung diseases as emphysema and chronic bronchitis. Both forms of Serevent can be used with or without inhaled or oral steroid therapy.

Most important fact about this drug
Serevent is intended only for long-term prevention of symptoms, and should not be used more than twice a day. Do not use it to treat acute asthma attacks, and do not attempt to relieve worsening asthma by increasing the frequency of your doses. (Your doctor will prescribe a short-acting bronchodilator to relieve acute attacks.)

Seriously worsening asthma is a dangerous—even life-threatening—condition that needs immediate medical attention. Alert your doctor if your short-acting bronchodilator is becoming less effective or you need more inhalations than usual. Also consider it a warning sign if you need 4 or more inhalations daily for 2 days or more in a row, or find that you are finishing a 200-dose canister in less than 8 weeks.

How should you take this medication?
Use no more than the prescribed dose and follow package directions closely.
Space your two daily doses approximately 12 hours apart, in the morning
and evening. To be effective, the drug must be used regularly every day.

Serevent aerosol inhaler must be shaken thoroughly before each use. Test-
spray the inhaler 4 times before the first use and whenever 4 weeks have
passed since the last use. Avoid spraying in the eyes.

Serevent Diskus should never be used with a spacer. Always activate the
Diskus device in a level, horizontal position. Never exhale into the Diskus
device, and always keep it dry. Do not wash the mouthpiece or any other
part of the device.

■ *If you miss a dose...*
Take it as soon as you remember. If it is almost time for your next dose,
skip the one you missed and go back to your regular schedule. Never
double your dose.

■ *Storage instructions...*
Store the Serevent aerosol inhaler and Serevent Diskus at room temperature away from direct sunlight and freezing temperatures. Leave the
aerosol inhaler canister with the nozzle end down. Throw away the Diskus
inhalation device after every blister has been used (when the dose
indicator reads "0") or 2 months after the blisters have been removed
from their foil pouch.

What side effects may occur?
Side effects cannot be anticipated. If any develop or change in intensity,
inform your doctor as soon as possible. Only your doctor can determine if it
is safe for you to continue using Serevent.

■ *More common side effects may include:*
Asthma, back pain, bronchitis, chest congestion, cough, diarrhea, headache, nasal, inflammation, pallor, respiratory tract infection, sinus headache, sinus infection, sinus problems, sore throat, stomachache, tremor

■ *Less common side effects may include:*
Abdominal pain, arm pain, chest discomfort, constipation, dental pain,
difficulty breathing, dry mouth, earache, eczema, fatigue, feeling of illness,
fever, heartburn, hives, indigestion, insomnia, joint pain, laryngitis, leg
cramps, mouth infection, mouth problems, muscle, aches or cramps, nasal
congestion, nausea, neck pain, nervousness, nosebleed, painful menstruation, pneumonia, rapid heartbeat, rash, shortness of breath, shoulder pain,

skin, tingling, sneezing, stomach pain, urinary tract infection, vomiting, wheezing

Why should this drug not be prescribed?
If Serevent gives you an allergic reaction, you cannot continue using it.

Special warnings about this medication
Serevent is not for the treatment of seriously worsening asthma, and should not be started if your asthma is deteriorating.

If you are taking inhaled or oral steroid medications for your asthma, continue using them along with Serevent. This drug does not replace them.

If you develop an allergic reaction (throat irritation, choking, hives, face and throat swelling, rash, and wheezing) after using Serevent, call your doctor immediately. Likewise, if symptoms of asthma or chronic lung disease get worse after inhaling Serevent, stop using it and check with your doctor at once.

Although such effects are rare, Serevent can cause an increase in blood pressure and heart rate. Use this medication carefully if you have high blood pressure, heart disease, or an irregular heartbeat. Caution is also advised if you have a seizure disorder or an overactive thyroid.

Serevent aerosol inhaler can be given to children 12 years of age and older. The Diskus inhalation powder can be given to children 4 and older.

Possible food and drug interactions
when taking this medication
If Serevent is taken with certain other drugs, the effects of either drug could be increased, decreased, or altered. It is especially important to check with your doctor before combining Serevent with the following:

Airway-opening medications such as Alupent, Proventil, and Ventolin
Blood pressure medications known as beta-blockers, including Inderal, Lopressor, and Tenormin
MAO inhibitors such as the antidepressants Marplan, Nardil, and Parnate
Tricyclic antidepressants such as Elavil and Tofranil
Water pills (diuretics) such as furosemide (Lasix) and hydrochlorothiazide (HydroDIURIL)

Special information
if you are pregnant or breastfeeding
Serevent has not been adequately tested in pregnant women. Check with your doctor immediately if you are pregnant or are planning a pregnancy.

Serevent's effects during breastfeeding are also unknown. You and your doctor should decide whether to discontinue nursing or give up Serevent.

Recommended dosage

SEREVENT AEROSOL INHALER

Asthma and chronic lung disease
The usual dose is 2 inhalations (42 micrograms) twice a day (morning and evening).

Prevention of exercise-induced asthma
Take 2 inhalations at least 30 to 60 minutes before exercise. Do not take another dose for 12 hours. (If you are on a twice daily dosage schedule, do NOT take additional Serevent before exercise.)

SEREVENT DISKUS INHALATION POWDER

Asthma
The usual dose is 1 inhalation (50 micrograms) twice a day (morning and evening).

Prevention of exercise-induced asthma
Take 1 inhalation at least 30 minutes before exercise. Do not take another dose for 12 hours. (If you are on a twice daily dosage schedule, do NOT take additional Serevent before exercise.)

Overdosage

Any medication taken in excess can have serious consequences. If you suspect an overdose, seek medical attention immediately.

■ *Symptoms of Serevent overdose may include:*
  Angina (chest pain), dizziness, dry mouth, fatigue, flu-like symptoms, headache, heart irregularities, high or low blood pressure, high blood sugar, insomnia, muscle cramps, nausea, nervousness, rapid heartbeat, seizures, tremor

Brand name:

SEROPHENE

See Clomiphene Citrate, page 262.

Brand name:

SEROQUEL

Pronounced: SER-oh-kwell
Generic name: Quetiapine fumarate

Why is this drug prescribed?

Seroquel combats the symptoms of schizophrenia, a mental disorder marked by delusions, hallucinations, disrupted thinking, and loss of contact with reality. It is the first in a new class of antipsychotic medications. Researchers believe that it works by diminishing the action of dopamine and serotonin, two of the brain's chief chemical messengers.

Most important fact about this drug

Seroquel may cause tardive dyskinesia—a condition characterized by uncontrollable muscle spasms and twitches in the face and body. This problem can be permanent, and appears to be most common among older adults, especially women.

How should you take this medication?

Your doctor will increase your dose gradually until the drug takes effect. If you stop Seroquel for more than 1 week, you'll need to build up to your ideal dosage once again.

- *If you miss a dose...*
  Take it as soon as you remember. If it is almost time for the next dose, skip the one you missed and go back to your regular schedule. Do not take 2 doses at once.

- *Storage instructions...*
  Store at room temperature.

What side effects may occur?

Side effects cannot be anticipated. If any develop or change in intensity, inform your doctor as soon as possible. Only your doctor can determine if it is safe for you to continue taking Seroquel.

- *More common side effects may include:*
  Abdominal pain, constipation, diminished movement, dizziness, drowsiness, dry mouth, excessive muscle tone, headache, indigestion, low blood pressure, nasal inflammation, neck rigidity, rapid heartbeat, rash, tremor, uncontrollable movements, weakness

- *Less common side effects may include:*
  Back pain, cough, difficulty breathing, difficulty speaking, ear pain, fever, flu, loss of appetite, palpitations, sore throat, sweating, swelling, weight gain

- *Rare side effects may include:*
  Abnormal dreams, abnormal ejaculation, abnormal vision, abnormal gait, abnormal thinking, acne, alcohol intolerance, amnesia, arthritis, asthma, bleeding gums, bone pain, bruising, chills, confusion, conjunctivitis (pinkeye), dehydration, delusions, diabetes, difficulty swallowing, dry eyes, ear ringing, eczema, eye pain, face swelling, fungal infection, gas, gum inflammation, hallucinations, heavy menstruation, hemorrhoids, impotence, increased appetite, increased sex drive, increased salivation, irregular pulse, itching, jerky or irregular movement, joint pain, lack of coordination, lack of emotion, leg cramps, loss of menstruation, low blood sugar, manic reaction, migraine, mouth sores, muscle weakness, neck pain, nosebleeds, painful menstruation, painful urination, paralysis, paranoia, pelvic pain, pneumonia, rash, rectal bleeding, seborrhea, sensitivity to light, skin inflammation or ulcer, slow heart rate, stomach and intestinal inflammation, stupor, swollen testicles, taste disturbances, teeth grinding, thirst, tongue swelling, twitching, uncontrollable bowel movements, underactive thyroid, urinary frequency or incontinence, urinary retention, urinary tract infection, vaginal bleeding, vaginal inflammation, vaginal yeast infection, vertigo, weight loss

Why should this drug not be prescribed?
If Seroquel gives you an allergic reaction, you will not be able to use it.

Special warnings about this medication
If you develop muscle stiffness, confusion, irregular or rapid heartbeat, excessive sweating, and high fever call your doctor immediately. These are signs of a serious—and potentially fatal—reaction to the drug. Be especially wary if you have a history of heart attack, heart disease, heart failure, circulation problems, or irregular heartbeat.

Particularly during the first few days of therapy, Seroquel can cause low blood pressure, with accompanying dizziness, fainting, and rapid heart beat. To minimize these effects, your doctor will increase your dose gradually. If you are prone to low blood pressure, take blood pressure medication, or become dehydrated, use Seroquel with caution.

Seroquel also tends to cause drowsiness, especially at the start of therapy, and can impair your judgment, thinking, and motor skills. Until you are certain of the drug's effect, use caution when operating machinery or driving a car.

If you are having problems with your vision, tell your doctor. There is a chance that Seroquel may cause cataracts, and you may be asked to see an eye doctor when you start Seroquel therapy, and every 6 months thereafter.

Seroquel poses a very slight risk of seizures, especially if you are over 65, or have epilepsy or Alzheimer's disease. The drug can also suppress an underactive thyroid, and generally causes a minor increase in cholesterol levels. There is also a remote chance that it will trigger a prolonged and painful erection.

Other antipsychotic medications have been known to interfere with the body's temperature-regulating mechanism, causing patients to overheat. Although this problem has not occurred with Seroquel, caution is still advisable. Avoid exposure to extreme heat, strenuous exercise, and dehydration.

Possible food and drug interactions
when taking this medication

Seroquel increases the effects of alcohol. Avoid alcoholic beverages while on Seroquel therapy.

If Seroquel is taken with certain other drugs, the effects of either could be increased, decreased, or altered. It is especially important to check with your doctor before combining Seroquel with the following:

Barbiturates such as phenobarbital
Carbamazepine (Tegretol)
Cimetidine (Tagamet)
Erythromycin (Eryc, Ery-Tab)
Fluconazole (Diflucan)
Itraconazole (Sporanox)
Ketoconazole (Nizoral)
Levodopa (Laradopa, Sinemet)
Lorazepam (Ativan)
Phenytoin (Dilantin)
Rifampin (Rifadin, Rimate, Rimactane)
Steroid medications such as hydrocortisone and prednisone
Thioridazine (Mellaril)

Special information
if you are pregnant or breastfeeding

The possibility of harm to a developing baby has not been ruled out. You should take Seroquel during pregnancy only if the benefits outweigh this potential risk. Notify your doctor as soon as you become pregnant or decide to become pregnant.

It is not known whether Seroquel appears in breast milk, and breastfeeding is not recommended.

Recommended dosage

ADULTS

On the first day of therapy, you'll take 2 doses of 25 milligrams each. On the second and third day, doses are usually increased by 25 to 50 milligrams apiece. Frequency may be increased to 3 times daily.

Long-term, the usual dosage is 300 to 400 milligrams a day, taken as 2 or 3 smaller doses. Doses as low as 150 milligrams a day sometimes prove effective, and daily dosage rarely exceeds 750 milligrams. Doses of 800 milligrams or more per day have not been tested for safety.

Dosage is increased more gradually—and is maintained at a lower level—for older adults, those with liver disease, those prone to low blood pressure reactions, and the debilitated.

Overdosage

Any medication taken in excess can have serious consequences. If you suspect an overdose, seek medical help immediately.

- *Symptoms of Seroquel overdose may include:*
  Dizziness, drowsiness, fainting, rapid heartbeat

Generic name:

SERTRALINE

See Zoloft, page 1470.

Brand name:

SERZONE

Pronounced: sur-ZONE
Generic name: Nefazodone hydrochloride

Why is this drug prescribed?
Serzone is prescribed for the treatment of depression severe enough to interfere with daily functioning. Possible symptoms include changes in appetite, sleep habits, and mind/body coordination, decreased sex drive, increased fatigue, feelings of guilt or worthlessness, difficulty concentrating, slowed thinking, and suicidal thoughts.

Most important fact about this drug
It may be several weeks before you feel the full antidepressant effect of
Serzone. Once you do begin to feel better, it is important to keep taking the
drug.

How should you take this medication?
Take Serzone exactly as prescribed by your doctor. It may be several weeks
before you begin to feel better; once you do, it is important to keep taking the
drug as prescribed. Your doctor should check your progress periodically.

- *If you miss a dose...*
  Take it as soon as you remember. If it is within 4 hours of your next dose,
  skip the one you missed and go back to your regular schedule. Do not take
  2 doses at once.

- *Storage instructions...*
  Store at room temperature in a tightly closed container.

What side effects may occur?
Side effects cannot be anticipated. If any develop or change in intensity, tell
your doctor as soon as possible. Only your doctor can determine if it is safe
for you to continue taking Serzone.

- *More common side effects may include:*
  Blurred or abnormal vision, confusion, constipation, dizziness, dry mouth,
  light-headedness, nausea, sleepiness, weakness

- *Less common side effects may include:*
  Abnormal dreams, cough, decreased concentration, diarrhea, dizziness on
  getting up, flu-like symptoms, headache, increased appetite, water retention

- *Rare side effects may include:*
  Breast pain, chills, decreased sex drive, difficulty urinating, fever, frequent
  urination, lack of coordination, ringing in ears, stiff neck, taste change,
  thirst, urinary tract infection, vaginal inflammation

Why should this drug not be prescribed?
If you are sensitive to or have ever had an allergic reaction to Serzone or
similar drugs, such as Desyrel, you should not take this medication.

Serious, sometimes fatal reactions have occurred when Serzone is used in
combination with drugs known as MAO inhibitors, including the antidepres-

sants Nardil and Parnate. Never take Serzone with one of these drugs; and do not begin therapy with Serzone within 14 days of discontinuing treatment with one of them. Also, allow at least 7 days between the last dose of Serzone and the first dose of an MAO inhibitor.

Serzone should also be avoided if you are taking Halcion, Hismanal, Propulsid, or Seldane.

You also should never combine Serzone with Seldane, Hismanal, or Propulsid. Heart problems could result.

Special warnings about this medication

Your doctor will prescribe Serzone with caution if you have a history of seizures or mania (extreme agitation or excitability) or heart or liver disease. Serzone should also be used with caution if you have had a heart attack or stroke, or suffer from dehydration. Be sure to discuss all of your medical problems with your doctor before taking Serzone.

Serzone may cause you to become drowsy or less alert and may affect your judgment. Do not drive or operate dangerous machinery or participate in any hazardous activity that requires full mental alertness until you know how the drug affects you.

Before having surgery, dental treatment, or any diagnostic procedure requiring anesthesia, tell the doctor or dentist you are taking Serzone. If you develop an allergic reaction such as a skin rash or hives while taking Serzone, notify your doctor. If you are male and experience a prolonged or inappropriate erection while taking Serzone, discontinue this drug and call your doctor.

If you have ever been addicted to drugs, tell your doctor before you start Serzone.

Possible food and drug interactions
when taking this medication

If Serzone is taken with certain other drugs, the effects of either could be increased, decreased, or altered. It is especially important to check with your doctor before combining Serzone with the following:

Alcohol
Astemizole (Hismanal)
Cisapride (Propulsid)
Digoxin (Lanoxin)
MAO inhibitors, including Nardil and Parnate
Sleep aids such as Halcion and Dalmane
Terfenadine (Seldane)
Tranquilizers such as Adapin and Xanax

**Special information
if you are pregnant or breastfeeding**

The effects of Serzone during pregnancy have not been adequately studied. If you are pregnant or are planning to become pregnant, tell your doctor immediately. Serzone should be used during pregnancy only if clearly needed. Serzone may appear in breast milk. If this medication is essential to your health, your doctor may tell you to discontinue breastfeeding until your treatment with Serzone is finished.

Recommended dosage

ADULTS

The usual starting dose for Serzone is 200 milligrams a day, divided into 2 doses. If needed, your doctor may increase your dose gradually to 300 to 600 milligrams a day.

CHILDREN

The safety and effectiveness of Serzone have not been established in children under 18 years of age.

OLDER ADULTS

The usual starting dose for older people and those in a weakened condition is 100 milligrams a day, taken in 2 doses. Your doctor will adjust the dose according to your response.

Overdosage

Any medication taken in excess can have serious consequences. If you suspect an overdose, seek medical attention immediately.

■ *Symptoms of Serzone overdose include:*
  Nausea, sleepiness, vomiting

Generic name:

SIBUTRAMINE

See Meridia, page 770.

Generic name:

SILDENAFIL CITRATE

See Viagra, page 1400.

Brand name:

SILVADENE CREAM 1%

Pronounced: SIL-vuh-deen
Generic name: Silver sulfadiazine

Why is this drug prescribed?

Silvadene Cream 1% is applied directly to the skin. The cream is used along with other medications to prevent and treat wound infections in people with second- and third-degree burns. It is effective against a variety of bacteria as well as yeast.

Most important fact about this drug

Silvadene is a sulfa derivative. If burn wounds cover extensive areas of the body, Silvadene may be absorbed into the bloodstream, and if you have ever had an allergic reaction to sulfa drugs, such as Bactrim or Septra, this could lead to a similar reaction. Make sure your doctor is aware of any drug reactions you have experienced.

How should you use this medication?

Silvadene cream is for external use only.

Bathe the burned area daily.

You should continue using Silvadene Cream until the area has healed or is ready for skin grafting.

Clean your skin and apply Silvadene with a sterile, gloved hand. Apply a thin layer (about one-sixteenth of an inch) to the affected area.

- *If you miss a dose...*
  Keep the burn areas covered with Silvadene at all times. Reapply the medicine if it is rubbed or washed off.

- *Storage instructions...*
  Silvadene can be stored at room temperature.

What side effects may occur?

Side effects cannot be anticipated. If any side effects develop or change in intensity, tell your doctor immediately. Only your doctor can determine whether it is safe for you to continue using Silvadene.

■ *Side effects may include:*
Areas of dead skin, burning sensation, red and raised rash on the body, skin discoloration

Why should this drug not be prescribed?
You should not use Silvadene if you are allergic to sulfa drugs such as Bactrim or Septra.

Do not use Silvadene at the end of pregnancy, on premature infants, or on newborn infants during the first 2 months of life.

Special warnings about this medication
Make sure your doctor knows about any kidney or liver problems you may have. If either organ becomes impaired, it may be necessary to stop using Silvadene.

There is a small chance of fungal infection when using Silvadene.

Possible food and drug interactions
when using this medication
If Silvadene is used with certain other drugs, the effects of either could be increased, decreased, or altered. It is especially important to check with your doctor before combining Silvadene with the following:

Topical enzyme preparations such as Panafil and Santyl that contain collagenase, papain, or sutilains

Special information
if you are pregnant or breastfeeding
If you are pregnant or plan to become pregnant, inform your doctor immediately.

The safety of Silvadene during pregnancy has not been fully studied, but you definitely should not take this drug at the end of your pregnancy, as it can lead to complications for the baby.

Although it is not known whether Silvadene appears in breast milk, other sulfa drugs are excreted in breast milk and can cause harm to a nursing infant. If this medication is essential to your health, your doctor may advise you to stop breastfeeding until your treatment is finished.

Recommended dosage
Apply Silvadene Cream 1% to the affected area once or twice daily to a thickness of one-sixteenth of an inch. Treatment with Silvadene should be continued until your doctor is satisfied that healing has occurred or determines that the burn site is ready for grafting.

Overdosage

Any medication taken in excess can have serious consequences. If you suspect an overdose, seek medical treatment immediately.

Generic name:

SILVER SULFADIAZINE

See Silvadene Cream 1%, page 1194.

Generic name:

SIMVASTATIN

See Zocor, page 1464.

Brand name:

SINEMET CR

Pronounced: SIN-uh-met see-are
Generic ingredients: Carbidopa, Levodopa

Why is this drug prescribed?

Sinemet CR is a controlled-release tablet that may be given to help relieve the muscle stiffness, tremor, and weakness caused by Parkinson's disease. It may also be given to relieve Parkinson-like symptoms caused by encephalitis (brain fever), carbon monoxide poisoning, or manganese poisoning.

Sinemet CR contains two drugs, carbidopa and levodopa. The drug that actually produces the anti-Parkinson's effect is levodopa. Carbidopa prevents vitamin B_6 from destroying levodopa, thus allowing levodopa to work more efficiently.

Parkinson's drugs such as Sinemet CR relieve the symptoms of the disease, but are not a permanent cure.

Most important fact about this drug

There is also a regular, non-controlled-release form of this medication, which is called Sinemet. Over a period of hours, Sinemet CR, the controlled-release form, gives a smoother release of the drug than regular Sinemet. If you have been taking regular Sinemet, be aware that you may need a somewhat higher dosage of Sinemet CR to get the same degree of relief. Your first morning dose of Sinemet CR may take as much as an hour longer to start working than your first morning dose of regular Sinemet.

How should you take this medication?
Take Sinemet CR after meals, rather than before or between meals. Swallow the tablets whole without chewing or crushing them.

Sinemet CR releases its ingredients slowly over a period of 4 to 6 hours. It is important to follow a careful schedule, taking your doses at the same time every day.

You should not change the prescribed dosage or add another product for Parkinson's disease without first consulting your doctor.

Sinemet CR works best when there is a constant amount in the blood. Try not to miss any doses, and take them at evenly spaced intervals day and night.

■ *If you miss a dose...*
If you forget to take a dose, take it as soon as you remember. If it is almost time for your next dose, skip the one you missed and go back to your regular schedule. Do not take 2 doses at once.

■ *Storage instructions...*
Store at room temperature in a tightly closed container.

What side effects may occur?
Side effects from Sinemet CR cannot be anticipated. If any develop or change in intensity, inform your doctor immediately.

Only your doctor can determine if it is safe for you to continue taking Sinemet CR.

■ *More common side effects may include:*
Confusion, hallucinations, nausea, uncontrollable twitching or jerking

■ *Less common or rare side effects may include:*
Abdominal or stomach pain, abnormal dreams, agitation, anemia, anxiety, back pain, bizarre breathing patterns, bleeding from stomach, blurred vision, burning sensation of tongue, chest pain, clumsiness in walking, common cold, constipation, convulsions, cough, dark sweat, dark urine, delusions, depression, diarrhea, disorientation, dizziness, dizziness upon rising from a sitting or lying position, dream abnormalities, drooling, drowsiness, dry mouth, euphoria, eyelid twitching, faintness, falling, fatigue, fever, flatulence, fluid retention, flushing, hair loss, headache, heart attack, heart palpitations, heartburn, hiccups, high or low blood pressure, hoarseness, hot flashes, increased tremor, insomnia or other sleep problems, irregular heartbeat, leg pain, locked jaw, loss of appetite,

malignant melanoma, memory problems, mental changes, muscle cramps, muscle twitching, nervousness, numbness, "on-off" phenomena, paralysis of certain muscles and unwanted movement of others, paranoia, persistent erection, phlebitis (swelling of a vein), rash, shortness of breath, shoulder pain, slowed physical movements, sore throat, speech impairment, stomach ulcer, suicidal tendencies, swallowing difficulties, sweating, taste changes, teeth-grinding, tingling or pins and needles, upper respiratory infection, upset stomach, urinary frequency, urinary incontinence, urinary retention, urinary tract infections, vomiting, weakness, weight loss or gain, writhing or flailing movements

Why should this drug not be prescribed?
Do not take Sinemet CR if you are sensitive to or have ever had an allergic reaction to its ingredients.

Sinemet CR should not be prescribed if you have a suspicious, undiagnosed mole or a history of melanoma.

Special warnings about this medication
Make sure your doctor knows if you have any of the following:

  Bronchial asthma
  Cardiovascular or lung disease (severe)
  Endocrine (glandular) disorder
  History of active peptic ulcer
  History of heart attack or heartbeat irregularity
  Kidney disorder
  Liver disorder
  Wide-angle glaucoma (pressure in the eye)

Your doctor will monitor your liver, blood, kidney and heart functions during extended therapy with Sinemet CR.

If you have been taking levodopa alone, you should stop taking levodopa for at least 12 hours before starting to take Sinemet CR.

The carbidopa contained in Sinemet CR cannot eliminate side effects caused by levodopa. Since carbidopa helps levodopa reach your brain, Sinemet CR may, in fact, produce some levodopa side effects—particularly twitching, jerking, or writhing—sooner and at a lower dosage than levodopa alone or even regular Sinemet. If such involuntary movements develop while you are taking Sinemet CR, you may need a dosage reduction.

Like levodopa, Sinemet CR may cause depression. Make sure your doctor knows if you have mental or emotional problems.

Muscle rigidity, high temperature, rapid heartbeat or breathing, sweating, blood pressure changes, and mental changes may occur when Sinemet CR is reduced suddenly or discontinued. If you stop taking this medication abruptly, your doctor should monitor your condition carefully.

You may see a red, brown, or black coloration in your saliva, urine, or sweat. This is not harmful, but may stain your clothes. Too much stomach acid can interfere with absorption of the medication.

Possible food and drug interactions
when taking this medication

If Sinemet CR is taken with certain other drugs, the effects of either could be increased, decreased, or altered. It is especially important to check with your doctor before combining Sinemet CR with the following:

Antacids such as Di-Gel, Maalox, and Mylanta
Antihypertensives such as Aldomet and Clonidine
Antiseizure drugs such as Dilantin
Antispasmodic drugs such as Artane and Cogentin
High-protein foods
Isoniazid (Nydrazid)
Major tranquilizers such as Haldol, Mellaril, and Thorazine
MAO inhibitors such as the antidepressants Nardil and Parnate
Methionine drugs such as Odor-Scrip and Pedameth
Metoclopramide (Reglan)
Papaverine (Pavabid)
Pyridoxine (Vitamin B$_6$)
Tranquilizers such as Dalmane, Valium, and Xanax
Tricyclic antidepressants such as Elavil and Tofranil

If you have been taking an MAO inhibitor such as Nardil or Parnate, you must discontinue it at least 2 weeks before starting to take Sinemet CR.

A high-protein diet may impair the effectiveness of Sinemet CR. Iron supplements can also reduce its effect.

Special information
if you are pregnant or breastfeeding

If you are pregnant or plan to become pregnant, inform your doctor immediately. Sinemet CR should be used during pregnancy only if the benefit outweighs the potential risk to the unborn child. It is not known whether Sinemet CR appears in breast milk. If this medication is essential to your health, your doctor may advise you to stop nursing your baby until your treatment with this drug is finished.

Recommended dosage
Your doctor will tailor your individual dosage carefully, depending on your response to previous therapy and symptoms.

ADULTS

For patients with mild to moderate symptoms, the initial recommended dose is 1 tablet of Sinemet CR taken 2 times a day.

Starting doses should be spaced out every 4 to 8 hours and then adjusted to each patient's individual response.

The usual long-term dose is 2 to 8 tablets per day, taken in divided doses every 4 to 8 hours during the waking day.

Higher doses (12 or more tablets per day) and shorter intervals (less than 4 hours) have been used, but are not usually recommended.

When doses of Sinemet CR are given at intervals of less than 4 hours, and/or if the divided doses are not equal, it is recommended that the smaller doses be given at the end of the day.

An interval of at least 3 days between dosage adjustments is recommended.

Dosage adjustment of Sinemet CR may be necessary if your doctor prescribes additional medications.

CHILDREN

Use of Sinemet CR in children under 18 is not recommended.

Overdosage
Too much Sinemet CR may cause muscle twitches, inability to open the eyes, or other symptoms of levodopa overdosage. Like other medications, Sinemet CR taken in excess can have serious consequences. If you suspect symptoms of a Sinemet CR overdose, seek medical attention immediately.

Brand name:

SINEQUAN

Pronounced: SIN-uh-kwan
Generic name: Doxepin hydrochloride

Why is this drug prescribed?
Sinequan is used in the treatment of depression and anxiety. It helps relieve tension, improve sleep, elevate mood, increase energy, and generally ease the feelings of fear, guilt, apprehension, and worry most

people experience. It is effective in treating people whose depression and/or anxiety is psychological, associated with alcoholism, or a result of another disease (cancer, for example) or psychotic depressive disorders (severe mental illness). It is in the family of drugs called tricyclic antidepressants.

Most important fact about this drug

Serious, sometimes fatal, reactions have occurred when Sinequan is used in combination with drugs known as MAO inhibitors, including the antidepressants Nardil and Parnate. Any drug of this type should be discontinued at least 2 weeks prior to starting treatment with Sinequan, and you should be carefully monitored by your doctor.

If you are taking any prescription or nonprescription drugs, consult your doctor before taking Sinequan.

How should you take this medication?

Take this medication exactly as prescribed. It may take several weeks for you to feel better.

■ *If you miss a dose...*
If you are taking several doses a day, take the missed dose as soon as you remember, then take any remaining doses for that day at evenly spaced intervals. If it is almost time for your next dose, skip the one you missed and go back to your regular schedule. Never take 2 doses at the same time.

If you are taking a single dose at bedtime and do not remember until the next morning, skip the dose. Do not take a double dose to make up for a missed one.

■ *Storage instructions...*
Store at room temperature.

What side effects may occur?

Side effects cannot be anticipated. If any develop or change in intensity, inform your doctor as soon as possible. Only your doctor can determine if it is safe for you to continue taking Sinequan.

The most common side effect is drowsiness.

■ *Less common or rare side effects may include:*
Blurred vision, breast development in males, bruises, buzzing or ringing in the ears, changes in sex drive, chills, confusion, constipation, diarrhea, difficulty urinating, disorientation, dizziness, dry mouth, en-

larged breasts, fatigue, fluid retention, flushing, fragmented or incomplete movements, hair loss, hallucinations, headache, high fever, high or low blood sugar, inappropriate breast milk secretion, indigestion, inflammation of the mouth, itching and skin rash, lack of muscle control, loss of appetite, loss of coordination, low blood pressure, nausea, nervousness, numbness, poor bladder control, rapid heartbeat, red or brownish spots on the skin, seizures, sensitivity to light, severe muscle stiffness, sore throat, sweating, swelling of the testicles, taste disturbances, tingling sensation, tremors, vomiting, weakness, weight gain, yellow eyes and skin

Why should this drug not be prescribed?
If you are sensitive to or have ever had an allergic reaction to Sinequan or similar antidepressants, you should not take this medication. Make sure that your doctor is aware of any drug reactions that you have experienced.

Unless you are directed to do so by your doctor, do not take this medication if you have the eye condition known as glaucoma or difficulty urinating.

Special warnings about this medication
Sinequan may cause you to become drowsy or less alert; driving or operating dangerous machinery or participating in any hazardous activity that requires full mental alertness is not recommended.

Notify your doctor or dentist that you are taking Sinequan if you have a medical emergency, and before you have surgery or dental treatment.

Possible food and drug interactions
when taking this medication
Alcohol increases the danger in a Sinequan overdose. Do not drink alcohol while taking this medication.

Never combine Sinequan with drugs known as MAO inhibitors. Medications in this category include the antidepressants Nardil and Parnate.

If you are switching from Prozac, wait at least 5 weeks after your last dose of Prozac before starting Sinequan.

If Sinequan is taken with certain other drugs, the effects of either could be increased, decreased, or altered. It is especially important to check with your doctor before combining Sinequan with the following:

Antidepressants that act on serotonin, such as Prozac, Zoloft, and Paxil
Other antidepressants such as Elavil and Serzone

Carbamazepine (Tegretol)
Cimetidine (Tagamet)
Clonidine (Catapres)
Flecainide (Tambocor)
Guanethidine (Ismelin)
Major tranquilizers such as Compazine, Mellaril, and Thorazine
Propafenone (Rythmol)
Quinidine (Quinidex)
Tolazamide (Tolinase)

Special information
if you are pregnant or breastfeeding

The effects of Sinequan during pregnancy have not been adequately studied. If you are pregnant or planning to become pregnant, inform your doctor immediately. Sinequan may appear in breast milk and could affect a nursing infant. If this medication is essential to your health, your doctor may advise you to discontinue breastfeeding your baby until your treatment is finished.

Recommended dosage

ADULTS

The starting dose for mild to moderate illness is usually 75 milligrams per day. This dose can be increased or decreased by your doctor according to individual need. The usual ideal dose ranges from 75 milligrams per day to 150 milligrams per day, although it can be as low as 25 to 50 milligrams per day. The total daily dose can be given once a day or divided into smaller doses. If you are taking this drug once a day, the recommended dose is 150 milligrams at bedtime.

The 150-milligram capsule strength is intended for long-term therapy only and is not recommended as a starting dose.

For more severe illness, gradually increased doses of up to 300 milligrams may be required as determined by your doctor.

CHILDREN

Safety and effectiveness have not been established for use in children under 12 years of age.

OLDER ADULTS

A once-a-day dosage should be carefully adjusted by your doctor, depending upon the severity of your illness.

Overdosage

■ *Symptoms of Sinequan overdose may include:*
Agitation, coma, confusion, convulsions, dilated pupils, disturbed concentration, drowsiness, hallucinations, high or low body temperature, irregular heartbeat, overactive reflexes, rigid muscles, severely low blood pressure, stupor, vomiting

If you experience any of these symptoms, seek medical attention immediately. An overdose of this drug can be fatal.

Brand name:

SINGULAIR

Pronounced: sing-you-LAIR
Generic name: Montelukast sodium

Why is this drug prescribed?
Singulair is used for long-term prevention of asthma. It reduces the swelling and inflammation that tend to close up the airways, and relaxes the walls of the bronchial tubes, expanding the airways and permitting more air to pass through.

Most important fact about this drug
Singulair alleviates the on-going symptoms of asthma, but it won't stop an acute asthma attack. For that you need a fast-acting, orally inhaled airway opener such as Alupent or Proventil.

How should you take this medication?
Take a Singulair tablet regularly every evening, whether or not you have any symptoms. The tablet can be taken with or without food.

■ *If you miss a dose...*
Take it as soon as you remember. If it is almost time for your next dose, skip the one you missed and go back to your regular schedule. Do not take 2 doses at once.

■ *Storage instructions...*
Store at room temperature, away from moisture and light.

What side effects may occur?
Side effects cannot be anticipated. If any develop or change in intensity, inform your doctor as soon as possible. Only your doctor can determine if it is safe for you to continue taking Singulair.

- *More common side effects may include:*
  Flu, headache

- *Less common side effects may include:*
  Abdominal pain, cough, dental pain, diarrhea, dizziness, ear infection, fatigue, fever, indigestion and other digestive problems, laryngitis, nasal congestion, nausea, rash, sinus inflammation, sore throat, viral infection, weakness

Why should this drug not be prescribed?
If Singulair gives you an allergic reaction, you cannot continue using the drug.

Special warnings about this medication
After you begin taking Singulair, your doctor may be able to slowly reduce the dosage of other asthma medications such as inhaled steroids. However, Singulair is not a complete replacement for such drugs, so you should not abruptly stop using them unless your doctor recommends it.

If your asthma gets worse after exercise, you'll need to continue using a short-acting inhaled airway opener to prevent the problem and relieve attacks.

If you are allergic to aspirin and other nonsteroidal anti-inflammatory drugs (NSAIDs), you should continue to avoid them. Singulair does not remedy this problem.

If you have difficulty breathing while taking Singulair, or find that you need your orally inhaled bronchodilator more often than usual (or require more puffs than prescribed), notify your doctor.

If you suffer from phenylketonuria, be aware that Singulair chewable tablets contain phenylalanine.

Possible food and drug interactions when taking this medication
If Singulair is taken with certain other drugs, the effects of either could be increased, decreased, or altered. It is especially important to check with your doctor before combining Singulair with the following:

Phenobarbital
Rifampin (Rifadin, Rifamate, Rimactane)

Special information if you are pregnant or breastfeeding
Singulair should be used during pregnancy only if clearly needed. If you are pregnant or plan to become pregnant, inform your doctor immediately.

It is not known whether Singulair appears in breast milk. Because many drugs do make their way into breast milk, use Singulair with caution if you are breastfeeding.

Recommended dosage

ADULTS AND CHILDREN 15 AND OVER

The usual dose is one 10-milligram tablet once a day in the evening.

CHILDREN 6 TO 14 YEARS OLD

The usual dose is one 5-milligram chewable tablet once a day in the evening.

Safety and effectiveness have not been studied in children younger than 6 years old.

Overdosage

Little is known about the effects of Singulair overdose. However, any medication taken in excess can have serious consequences. If you suspect an overdose, seek medical attention immediately.

Brand name:

SLO-BID

See Theo-Dur, page 1293.

Brand name:

SLOW-K

See Micro-K, page 791.

Generic name:

SODIUM FLUORIDE

See Luride, page 741.

Brand name:

SODIUM SULAMYD

Pronounced: SOH-dee-um SOO-lah-mid
Generic name: Sulfacetamide sodium
Other brand name: Bleph-10

Why is this drug prescribed?

Sodium Sulamyd is used in the treatment of eye inflammations, corneal ulcer, and other eye infections. It may be used along with an oral sulfa drug to treat a serious eye infection called trachoma.

Most important fact about this drug

Sodium Sulamyd is similar to oral sulfa drugs such as Bactrim, Gantanol, and Gantrisin. If you are allergic to any of these medications, you may also be allergic to Sodium Sulamyd. In addition, if you have taken one of these medications in the past, you may have developed a "hidden" allergy to sulfa drugs that might show up when you take Sodium Sulamyd. Be alert for a rash, itching, or other signs of allergy. If any of these symptoms develop, stop taking Sodium Sulamyd immediately and consult your doctor.

How should you use this medication?

Sodium Sulamyd is available in eyedrop and ointment form. Use it exactly as prescribed. Your doctor may tell you to use both the eyedrops and the ointment.

To apply Sodium Sulamyd, pull down your lower eyelid to form a pouch, then squeeze in the medication. To avoid contaminating the eyedrops or the ointment, do not touch your eye with the dropper bottle or the tip of the tube. Keep the dropper bottle or tube poised slightly above your eye as you instill the drops or squeeze out the ointment.

- *If you miss a dose...*
  Apply it as soon as you remember. If it is almost time for your next dose, skip the one you missed and go back to your regular schedule.

- *Storage instructions...*
  Store at room temperature. Protect the ointment from excessive heat.

What side effects may occur?

Side effects cannot be anticipated. If any develop or change in intensity, inform your doctor as soon as possible. Only your doctor can determine if it is safe for you to continue taking this medication.

Sodium Sulamyd may irritate your eye, causing stinging and burning. The irritation usually lasts only a short time. If it is very painful or lasts for a long time, you may have to stop using the medication.

In rare cases, people using Sodium Sulamyd have developed a severe blistering skin rash. Be alert for skin reactions. If a rash appears, stop using Sodium Sulamyd and call your doctor.

Why should this drug not be prescribed?
Do not use Sodium Sulamyd if you have ever had an allergic reaction to or are sensitive to this medication or any other sulfa drug.

Special warnings about this medication
Stay in close touch with your doctor while using Sodium Sulamyd. In some cases, an eye ointment may actually delay healing of the cornea. If you have a pus-producing eye infection, the pus may inactivate Sodium Sulamyd. Since sulfa drugs do not kill fungi, it is possible to develop a fungus infection in your eye while using Sodium Sulamyd.

Possible food and drug interactions
when taking this medication
Sodium Sulamyd should not be used with medications containing silver. Check with your doctor if you are unsure of any medications you are taking.

Special information
if you are pregnant or breastfeeding
If you are pregnant or plan to become pregnant, inform your doctor immediately. There is no information about the safety of Sodium Sulamyd during pregnancy.

It is not known whether Sodium Sulamyd appears in breast milk. If Sodium Sulamyd is essential to your health, it may be necessary to stop breastfeeding during treatment.

Recommended dosage
SODIUM SULAMYD OPHTHALMIC SOLUTION 30%

Inflamed Eyes or Corneal Ulcer
Place 1 drop inside the lower eyelid every 2 hours or less frequently; your doctor will determine the schedule according to the severity of the infection.

Trachoma (Contagious Inflammation)
Use 2 drops every 2 hours.

SODIUM SULAMYD OPHTHALMIC SOLUTION 10%

Place 1 or 2 drops inside the lower eyelid every 2 or 3 hours during the day, less often at night.

SODIUM SULAMYD OPHTHALMIC OINTMENT 10%

Apply a small amount of the ointment 4 times daily and at bedtime. The ointment may be used at the same time as either of the solutions.

Overdosage

Although no specific information is available on overdose with Sodium Sulamyd, any medication used in excess can have serious consequences. If you suspect you may have used too much Sodium Sulamyd, seek medical attention immediately.

Brand name:

SOF-LAX

See Colace, page 277.

Brand name:

SOMA

Pronounced: SOE-muh
Generic name: Carisoprodol

Why is this drug prescribed?

Soma is used, along with rest, physical therapy, and other measures, for the relief of acute, painful muscle strains and spasms.

Most important fact about this drug

Soma alone will not heal your muscles. You need to follow the program of physical therapy, rest, or exercise that your doctor prescribes. Do not attempt any more physical activity than your doctor recommends, even though Soma temporarily makes it seem feasible.

How should you take this medication?

Take Soma exactly as prescribed by your doctor.

- *If you miss a dose...*
  Take it as soon as you remember if only an hour or so has passed. If you do not remember until later, skip the dose you missed and go back to your regular schedule. Do not take 2 doses at once.

- *Storage instructions...*
  Store at room temperature in a tightly closed container.

What side effects may occur?

Side effects cannot be anticipated. If any develop or change in intensity, inform your doctor as soon as possible. Only your doctor can determine if it is safe for you to continue taking Soma.

- *Side effects may include:*
  Agitation, depression, dizziness, drowsiness, facial flushing, fainting, headache, hiccups, inability to fall or stay asleep, irritability, light-headedness upon standing up, loss of coordination, nausea, rapid heart rate, stomach upset, tremors, vertigo, vomiting

Allergic reactions usually seen between the first and fourth doses of Soma in patients who have never taken this drug before include: itching, red welts on the skin, and skin rash. A more severe allergic reaction may include symptoms such as asthmatic attacks, dizziness, fever, low blood pressure, shock, stinging of the eyes, swelling due to fluid retention, and weakness.

Why should this drug not be prescribed?
If you are sensitive to or have ever had an allergic reaction to Soma or drugs of this type, such as meprobamate (Miltown), you should not take this medication. Make sure your doctor is aware of any drug reactions you have experienced.

Unless you are directed to do so by your doctor, do not take this medication if you have porphyria (an inherited blood disorder).

Special warnings about this medication
In rare cases, the first dose of Soma may cause unusual symptoms that appear within minutes or hours of taking the medication. Symptoms reported include: agitation, confusion, disorientation, dizziness, double vision, enlargement of pupils, exaggerated feeling of well-being, extreme weakness, lack of coordination, speech problems, temporary loss of vision, and temporary paralysis of arms and legs. These symptoms usually subside within a few hours. If you experience any of them, contact your doctor immediately.

Soma may impair the mental or physical abilities you need to drive a car or operate dangerous machinery. Do not participate in hazardous activities until you know how this drug affects you.

If you have a history of drug dependence, make sure your doctor is aware of it before you start taking this medication.

Withdrawal symptoms, including abdominal cramps, chilliness, headache, insomnia, and nausea, have occurred in people who suddenly stop taking Soma.

Take this drug cautiously if you have any kidney or liver problems.

Possible food and drug interactions
when taking this medication

Soma may intensify the effects of alcohol. Be careful drinking alcoholic beverages while you are taking this medication.

If Soma is taken with certain other drugs, the effects of either could be increased, decreased, or altered. It is especially important to check with your doctor before combining Soma with the following:

Antidepressant drugs such as Elavil, Tofranil, and Nardil
Major tranquilizers such as Haldol, Stelazine, and Thorazine
Sedatives such as Nembutal and Halcion
Tranquilizers such as Librium, Valium, and Xanax

Special information
if you are pregnant or breastfeeding

The effects of Soma during pregnancy have not been adequately studied. If you are pregnant or plan to become pregnant, inform your doctor immediately. This drug appears in breast milk and could affect a nursing infant. If this medication is essential to your health, your doctor may advise you to discontinue breastfeeding until your treatment is finished.

Recommended dosage

ADULTS

The usual dosage of Soma is one 350-milligram tablet, taken 3 times daily and at bedtime.

CHILDREN

The safety and effectiveness of this drug have not been established in children under 12 years of age.

Overdosage

A severe overdose of Soma can be fatal. If you suspect an overdose, seek medical help immediately.

■ *Symptoms of Soma overdose may include:*
Breathing difficulty, coma, shock, stupor

Brand name:

SORBITRATE

See Isordil, page 649.

Brand name:

SPECTAZOLE CREAM

Pronounced: SPEK-tah-zole
Generic name: Econazole nitrate

Why is this drug prescribed?

Spectazole cream is prescribed for fungal skin diseases commonly called ringworm (tinea). It is used to treat athlete's foot (tinea pedis), "jock itch" (tinea cruris), a fungus infection of the entire body (tinea corporis), and a skin infection that causes yellow- or brown-colored skin eruptions (tinea versicolor). It is also prescribed for yeast infections of the skin caused by candida fungus (cutaneous candidiasis).

Most important fact about this drug

Do not use Spectazole in or near the eyes.

How should you use this medication?

Use Spectazole Cream exactly as prescribed by your doctor.

Continue using the medication for the full time prescribed even if your symptoms have been relieved.

When applied, the cream should completely cover the affected area.

- *If you miss a dose...*
  Apply it as soon as you remember. If it is almost time for your next dose, skip the one you missed and go back to your regular schedule.

- *Storage instructions...*
  Store at room temperature.

What side effects may occur?

Side effects cannot be anticipated. If any develop or change in intensity, inform your doctor as soon as possible. Only your doctor can determine whether it is safe for you to continue using Spectazole.

- *More common side effects may include:*
  Burning, itching, skin redness, stinging

- *Less common or rare side effects may include:*
  Itching rash

Why should this drug not be prescribed?

Spectazole Cream should not be used if you are sensitive to it or have ever had an allergic reaction to any of its ingredients.

Special warnings about this medication

If you develop an irritation or an allergic reaction to Spectazole, stop using the cream and inform your doctor.

Spectazole is only for external use.

Possible food and drug interactions when taking this medication

No interactions have been reported.

Special information if you are pregnant or breastfeeding

Spectazole should be used during the first trimester (3 months) of pregnancy only if it is essential to your health, and during the remainder of your pregnancy only if your doctor feels it is clearly needed. If you are pregnant or plan to become pregnant, inform your doctor immediately. Spectazole may appear in breast milk and could affect a nursing infant. If this medication is essential to your health, your doctor may advise you to stop breastfeeding until your treatment with Spectazole is finished.

Recommended dosage

ATHLETE'S FOOT, JOCK ITCH, TINEA CORPORIS, TINEA VERSICOLOR

Apply sufficient Spectazole Cream to completely cover the affected area once a day. Athlete's foot is treated for 1 month; jock itch and tinea corporis are treated for 2 weeks. Tinea versicolor is usually treated for 2 weeks.

CUTANEOUS CANDIDIASIS

Apply sufficient Spectazole Cream to completely cover the affected area 2 times a day, once in the morning and once in the evening. Cutaneous candidiasis is treated for 2 weeks.

Overdosage

Although no specific information is available on Spectazole Cream overdosage, any medication used in excess can have serious consequences. If you suspect an overdose, seek medical attention immediately.

Generic name:

SPIRONOLACTONE

See Aldactone, page 28.

Generic name:

SPIRONOLACTONE WITH HYDROCHLOROTHIAZIDE

See Aldactazide, page 25.

Brand name:

SPORANOX

Pronounced: SPORE-ah-nocks
Generic name: Itraconazole

Why is this drug prescribed?
Sporanox capsules are used to treat four types of serious fungal infection: blastomycosis, histoplasmosis, aspergillosis, and onychomycosis. Blastomycosis can affect the lungs, bones, and skin. Histoplasmosis can affect the lungs, heart, and blood. Aspergillosis can affect the lungs, kidneys, and other organs. Onychomycosis affects the nails. Sporanox is also used against fungal infections in people with weak immune systems, such as AIDS patients.

Sporanox oral solution is used to treat candidiasis (fungal infection) of the mouth, throat, and gullet (esophagus).

Most important fact about this drug
Be sure to take Sporanox for as long as your doctor prescribes. It will take 3 months or more to cure some infections completely. If you stop taking Sporanox too soon, the infection may return.

How should you take this medication?
Take Sporanox exactly as prescribed. To make sure the capsules are properly absorbed, you should take them with a full meal; the oral solution should be taken without food. A cola drink can help some people absorb the capsules better. Continue taking Sporanox until all the medication is gone. Do not take antacids at the same time as Sporanox.

Swish the oral solution, 10 milliliters at a time, in your mouth for a few seconds before swallowing it.

Mouth and throat candidiasis should clear up in several days.

The oral solution and capsules cannot be used interchangeably.

■ *If you miss a dose...*
Take the forgotten dose as soon as you remember. If it is almost time for the next dose, skip the one you missed and go back to your regular schedule. Never try to "catch up" by doubling the dose.

■ *Storage instructions...*
Store at room temperature. Protect the capsules from light and moisture. Do not freeze the oral solution.

What side effects may occur?
Side effects cannot be anticipated. If any develop or change in intensity, inform your doctor as soon as possible. Only your doctor can determine if it is safe for you to continue taking Sporanox.

■ *More common side effects may include:*
Anxiety, bursitis, diarrhea, fatigue, fever, gas, headache, high blood pressure, indigestion, injury, muscle pain, nasal and sinus inflammation, nausea, pain, rash, respiratory infection, swelling due to water retention, urinary infection, vomiting

■ *Less common side effects may include:*
Abdominal pain, abnormal dreams, decreased sexual drive, dizziness, extreme sleepiness, feeling of general discomfort, gum inflammation, hives, increased appetite, inflamed stomach and intestines, itching, loss of appetite, reproductive disorders such as male impotence, sleepiness, sore throat, tremor, weakness

■ *Rare side effects may include:*
Constipation, depression, hepatitis, male breast development, male breast pain, menstrual disorders, ringing in the ears, severe allergic reaction, skin peeling, sleeplessness

■ *Additional side effects that may be seen with the oral solution are:*
Back pain, blood in the urine, breast pain or development in males, breathing difficulty, chest pain, cough, dehydration, difficulty swallowing, hemorrhoids, hot flushes, insomnia, pneumonia, ringing in the ears, sweating, vision problems, weight loss

People being treated for onychomycosis may experience stomach and intestinal disorders or rash, or, less commonly, headache, light-headedness upon standing up, low blood pressure, muscle pain, a sick feeling, or vertigo.

Why should this drug not be prescribed?

If you are sensitive to or have ever had an allergic reaction to Sporanox or similar antifungal drugs such as Nizoral, you should not take this medication. Make sure that your doctor is aware of any drug reactions that you have experienced.

Serious heart problems, such as irregular heartbeats and even death, have occurred in people who have taken Sporanox at the same time as Seldane, Hismanal, or Propulsid. Never take these drugs with Sporanox, and avoid Halcion, Versed, Mevacor, and Zocor capsules as well.

During pregnancy, Sporanox should not be used for treatment of fungal nail infections.

Special warnings about this medication

If you have liver disease, or if you take Sporanox continuously for more than a month, your doctor should monitor your liver function periodically. If you develop such symptoms of liver disease as unusual fatigue, loss of appetite, nausea, vomiting, jaundice, dark urine, or pale stool, report them to your doctor so that the appropriate laboratory testing can be performed.

Possible food and drug interactions when taking this medication

If Sporanox is taken with certain other drugs, the effects of either could be increased, decreased, or altered. It is especially important to check with your doctor before combining Sporanox with any of the following:

Acid-blocking drugs such as Tagamet, Pepcid, and Zantac
Astemizole (Hismanal)
Blood-thinning drugs such as Coumadin
Calcium channel blockers such as Cardene and Norvasc
Carbamazepine (Tegretol)
Cisapride (Propulsid)
Cyclosporine (Sandimmune, Neoral)
Diazepam (Valium)
Digoxin (Lanoxin)
Indinavir (Crixivan)
Isoniazid
Lovastatin (Mevacor)

Methylprednisolone
Midazolam (Versed)
Oral diabetes medications such as DiaBeta, Diabinese, Glucotrol,
    Micronase, Orinase, and Tolinase
Phenobarbital
Phenytoin (Dilantin)
Quinidine (Quinidex)
Rifabutin (Mycobutin)
Rifampin (Rifadin, Rimactane)
Ritonavir (Norvir)
Simvastatin (Zocor)
Tacrolimus (Prograf)
Terfenadine (Seldane, Seldane-D)
Triazolam (Halcion)

**Special information
if you are pregnant or breastfeeding**
The effects of Sporanox during pregnancy have not been adequately studied.
If you are pregnant or plan to become pregnant, inform your doctor
immediately. You should not take Sporanox to treat onychomycosis if you are
or may become pregnant. In any event, Sporanox should not be used during
pregnancy if the problem is a nail infection. In other cases, check with your
doctor before you take Sporanox.

Sporanox appears in breast milk and could affect a nursing infant. If this
medication is essential to your health, your doctor may advise you to
discontinue breastfeeding until your treatment with Sporanox is finished.

Recommended dosage

ADULTS

Blastomycosis and Histoplasmosis
The usual dose is two 100-milligram capsules, taken after a full meal once a
day. If you feel no improvement, or if there is evidence that the fungal
disease has spread, your doctor will increase the dose 100 milligrams at a
time to a maximum of 400 milligrams a day. Daily dosages above 200
milligrams a day should be divided into 2 smaller doses.

Aspergillosis
The usual dose is 200 to 400 milligrams a day. Treatment usually continues
for a minimum of 3 months, until tests indicate that the fungal infection has
subsided.

Onychomycosis
The usual dose for a toenail infection, whether or not fingernails are also involved, is 200 milligrams once a day for 12 weeks.

If only fingernails are infected, treatment is given in two 7-day-long sessions during which you take 200 milligrams of Sporanox twice a day, with a 3-week rest period between sessions.

Candidiasis-mouth and throat
The usual dose is 20 milliliters of oral solution a day for 1 to 2 weeks. If the infection does not go away, your dose will be changed to 10 milliliters twice a day.

Candidiasis-esophagus
The usual dose is 10 milliliters of oral solution a day for at least 3 weeks. You should continue the treatment for 2 weeks after your symptoms clear up. If necessary, the doctor may increase the dose to 20 milliliters a day.

CHILDREN

The safety and effectiveness of Sporanox in children have not been established.

Overdosage
Any drug taken in excess can have dangerous consequences. If you suspect an overdose, seek emergency medical treatment immediately.

Generic name:

STAVUDINE

See Zerit, page 1450.

Brand name:

STELAZINE

Pronounced: STEL-ah-zeen
Generic name: Trifluoperazine hydrochloride

Why is this drug prescribed?
Stelazine is used to treat severe mental disturbances as well as anxiety that does not respond to ordinary tranquilizers.

Most important fact about this drug

Stelazine may cause tardive dyskinesia—a condition marked by involuntary muscle spasms and twitches in the face and body. This condition may be permanent and appears to be most common among the elderly, especially women. Ask your doctor for information about this possible risk.

How should you take this medication?

If taking Stelazine in a liquid concentrate form, you will need to dilute it with a liquid such as a carbonated beverage, coffee, fruit juice, milk, tea, tomato juice, or water. You can also use puddings, soups, and other semisolid foods. Stelazine should be diluted just before you take it.

You should not take Stelazine with alcohol.

■ *If you miss a dose...*

If you take 1 dose a day, take the dose you missed as soon as you remember. Then go back to your regular schedule. If you do not remember until the next day, skip the missed dose and go back to your regular schedule.

If you take more than 1 dose a day, take the dose you missed if it is within an hour or so of the scheduled time. If you do not remember until later, skip the missed dose and go back to your regular schedule. Do not take 2 doses at once.

■ *Storage instructions...*

Store at room temperature. Protect the concentrate from light.

What side effects may occur?

Side effects cannot be anticipated. If any develop or change in intensity, inform your doctor as soon as possible. Only your doctor can determine if it is safe for you to continue taking Stelazine.

■ *Side effects may include:*

Abnormal secretion of milk, abnormal sugar in urine, abnormalities in movement and posture, agitation, allergic reactions (sometimes severe), anemia, asthma, blood disorders, blurred vision, body rigidly arched backward, breast development in males, chewing movements, constipation, constricted pupils, difficulty swallowing, dilated pupils, dizziness, drooling, drowsiness, dry mouth, ejaculation problems, exaggerated or excessive reflexes, excessive or spontaneous flow of milk, eye problems causing a state of fixed gaze, eye spasms, fatigue, fever or high fever, flu-like symptoms, fluid accumulation and swelling (including the brain), fragmented movements, headache, heart attack, high or low blood sugar, hives, impotence, inability to urinate, increase in appetite and weight, infections, insomnia, intestinal blockage, involuntary movements of tongue, face, mouth, jaw, arms, and legs, irregular blood pressure, pulse, and heartbeat, irregular or no menstrual periods, jitteriness, light-headedness (especially when standing up), liver damage, lockjaw, loss of appetite, low blood pressure, mask-like face, muscle stiffness and rigidity, nasal congestion, nausea, persistent, painful erections, pill-rolling move-ment, protruding tongue, puckering of mouth, puffing of cheeks, purple or red spots on the skin, rapid heartbeat, restlessness, rigid arms, feet, head, and muscles, seizures, sensitivity to light, shuffling walk, skin inflamma-tion and peeling, skin itching, pigmentation, reddening, or rash, spasms in jaw, face, tongue, neck, hands, feet, back, and mouth, sweating, swelling of the throat, totally unresponsive state, tremors, twisted neck, weakness, yellowing of skin and whites of eyes

Why should this drug not be prescribed?

You should not be using Stelazine if you have liver damage, or if you are taking central nervous system depressants such as alcohol, barbiturates, or narcotic pain relievers. Stelazine should not be used if you have an abnormal bone marrow or blood condition.

Special warnings about this medication

You should use Stelazine cautiously if you have ever had a brain tumor, breast cancer, intestinal blockage, the eye condition called glaucoma, heart or liver disease, or seizures. Be cautious, too, if you are exposed to certain pesticides or extreme heat. Be aware that Stelazine may hide the signs of overdose of other drugs and may make it more difficult for your doctor to diagnose intestinal obstruction, brain tumor, and the dangerous neurological condition called Reye's syndrome.

Tell your doctor if you have ever had an allergic reaction to any major tranquilizer similar to Stelazine.

Dizziness, nausea, vomiting, and tremors can result if you suddenly stop taking Stelazine. Follow your doctor's instructions when discontinuing this drug.

Tell your doctor immediately if you experience symptoms such as a fever or sore throat, mouth, or gums. These signs of infection may signal the need to stop Stelazine treatment. Notify your doctor, too, if you develop flu-like symptoms with fever.

This drug may impair your ability to drive a car or operate potentially dangerous machinery, especially during the first few days of treatment. Do not participate in any activities that require full alertness if you are unsure about your ability.

If you have any trouble with your vision, tell your doctor.

Stelazine concentrate contains a sulfite that may cause allergic reactions in some people, especially in those with asthma.

Stelazine can cause a group of symptoms called Neuroleptic Malignant Syndrome. Signs are high body temperature, rigid muscles, irregular pulse or blood pressure, rapid or abnormal heartbeat, and excessive perspiration.

Possible food and drug interactions
when taking this medication

Extreme drowsiness and other potentially serious effects can result if Stelazine is combined with alcohol, tranquilizers such as Valium, narcotic painkillers such as Percocet, antihistamines such as Benadryl, and barbiturates such as phenobarbital.

If Stelazine is taken with certain other drugs, the effects of either could be increased, decreased, or altered. It is especially important to check with your doctor before combining Stelazine with the following:

Antiseizure drugs such as Dilantin
Atropine (Donnatal)
Blood thinners such as Coumadin
Guanethidine (Ismelin)
Lithium (Lithobid, Eskalith)
Propranolol (Inderal)
Thiazide diuretics such as Dyazide

Special information
if you are pregnant or breastfeeding

Pregnant women should use Stelazine only if clearly needed. The effects of Stelazine during pregnancy have not been adequately studied. If you are pregnant or plan to become pregnant, inform your doctor immediately. Stelazine appears in breast milk and may affect a nursing infant. If this medication is essential to your health, your doctor may have you discontinue breastfeeding while you are taking it.

Recommended dosage

ADULTS

Nonpsychotic Anxiety
Doses usually range from 2 to 4 milligrams daily. This amount should be divided into 2 equal doses and taken twice a day. Do not take more than 6 milligrams a day or take the medication for more than 12 weeks.

Psychotic Disorders
The usual starting dose is 4 to 10 milligrams a day, divided into 2 equal doses; doses range from 15 to 40 milligrams daily.

CHILDREN

Doses are based on the child's weight and the severity of his or her symptoms.

Psychotic Children 6 to 12 Years Old Who Are Closely Monitored or Hospitalized
The starting dose is 1 milligram a day, taken all at once or divided into 2 doses. Your doctor will increase the dosage gradually, up to 15 milligrams a day.

OLDER ADULTS

Older people usually take Stelazine at lower doses. Because you may develop low blood pressure while taking this drug, your doctor will watch you closely. Older people (especially older women) may be more susceptible to tardive dyskinesia—a possibly permanent condition characterized by involuntary muscle spasms and twitches in the face and body. Consult your doctor for information about these potential risks.

Overdosage
Any medication taken in excess can have serious consequences. If you suspect an overdose of Stelazine, seek medical help immediately.

- *Symptoms of Stelazine overdose may include:*
  Agitation, coma, convulsions, difficulty breathing, difficulty swallowing, dry mouth, extreme sleepiness, fever, intestinal blockage, irregular heart rate, low blood pressure, restlessness

Brand name:

STIMATE

See DDAVP, page 341.

Brand name:

STUARTNATAL PLUS

Pronounced: STU-art NAY-tal plus
Generic ingredients: Prenatal vitamins and minerals
Other brand names: Materna, Natalins Rx

Why is this drug prescribed?
Stuartnatal Plus contains vitamins and minerals including iron, calcium, zinc, and folic acid. The tablets are given during pregnancy and after childbirth to ensure an adequate supply of these critical nutrients. They may also be prescribed to improve a woman's nutritional status before she becomes pregnant.

Most important fact about this drug
Nutritional supplementation is especially important during pregnancy. Be sure to take Stuartnatal Plus regularly as prescribed.

How should you take this medication?
Take Stuartnatal Plus exactly as prescribed. The usual dosage is 1 tablet per day with or without food. (For Natalins Rx, 2 tablets.) Do not take more than the recommended dose.

- *If you miss a dose...*
  Take it as soon as you remember, then return to your regular schedule.

- *Storage instructions...*
  Store at room temperature in a tightly closed container, away from excessive heat.

Why should this drug not be prescribed?
Certain rare diseases allow copper or iron to accumulate in the body. If you've been diagnosed with such a disease, you should avoid vitamin and mineral supplements such as Stuartnatal Plus.

Special warnings about this medication
Your doctor will test you for pernicious anemia before you take this drug, since folic acid can cover up the symptoms.

If you have kidney stones, you need to limit your calcium intake. Your doctor should take this into account when prescribing a vitamin and mineral supplement.

Keep this product out of children's reach. An overdose could be fatal.

Special information
if you are pregnant or breastfeeding
Pregnancy and breastfeeding impose special nutritional demands on the mother. A vitamin and mineral supplement can help ensure that there are enough nutrients for both you and your baby.

Recommended dosage

ADULTS

Before, during, and after pregnancy, take 1 tablet daily, (2 tablets of Natalins Rx), or as directed by your doctor.

Overdosage
Although no specific overdose information is available, even a nutritional supplement can have serious consequences when taken in extremely large amounts. In children, an overdose of the iron in Stuartnatal Plus could be dangerous or even fatal. If you suspect an overdose, seek medical attention immediately.

Generic name:

SUCRALFATE

See Carafate, page 196.

Brand name:

SULAR

Pronounced: SOO-lar
Generic name: Nisoldipine

Why is this drug prescribed?
Sular controls high blood pressure. A long-acting tablet, Sular may be used alone or in combination with other blood pressure medications.

Sular is a type of medication called a calcium channel blocker. It inhibits the flow of calcium through the smooth muscles of the heart, delaying the passage of nerve impulses, slowing down the heart, and expanding the blood vessels. This eases the heart's workload and reduces your blood pressure.

Most important fact about this drug
You must take Sular regularly for it to be effective. Since blood pressure declines gradually, it may be several weeks before you get the full benefit of Sular, and you must continue taking it even if you are feeling well. Sular does not cure high blood pressure, it merely keeps it under control.

How should you take this medication?
Take Sular exactly as prescribed. Swallow the tablets whole. They should not be crushed, chewed, or divided. Avoid eating high-fat meals with Sular, as the medication will not work properly. Do not take grapefruit products before or after taking Sular.

■ *If you miss a dose...*
Take it as soon as you remember. If it is almost time for your next dose, skip the one you missed and go back to your regular schedule. Never take 2 doses at the same time.

■ *Storage instructions...*
Store at room temperature in a tight, light-resistant container. Protect from moisture.

What side effects may occur?
Side effects cannot be anticipated. If any develop or change in intensity, tell your doctor as soon as possible. Only your doctor can determine if it is safe for you to continue taking Sular.

■ *More common side effects may include:*
Dizziness, flushing, headache, heart palpitations, sinus inflammation, sore throat, swelling of the hands and feet

■ *Less common side effects may include:*
Chest pain, nausea, rash

Why should this drug not be prescribed?
Avoid Sular if you have ever had an allergic reaction to it, or to similar calcium channel blockers such as Plendil and Procardia.

Special warnings about this medication
If you have a heart condition or liver disease, be sure the doctor is aware of it. Sular should be used with caution.

Sular may cause an excessive drop in blood pressure, especially when you are first taking the medication or when the dosage is increased. Low blood pressure can also become a problem if you are taking other blood pressure medications. If you develop symptoms of low blood pressure such as dizziness or light-headedness, call your doctor.

If you have angina (chest pain) or clogged coronary arteries, there is a remote possibility that Sular will make the condition worse—or even trigger a heart attack—when you first start taking the drug or its dosage is increased. Your doctor should be especially cautious if you have angina, heart failure, or other heart problems, particularly if you are also taking a medication known as a beta blocker, such as Tenormin.

Possible food and drug interactions
when taking this medication

If Sular is taken with certain other drugs, the effects of either could be increased, decreased, or altered. It is especially important to check with your doctor before combining Sular with the following:

Atenolol (Tenormin)
Cimetidine (Tagamet)
Quinidine (Quinidex)

Special information
if you are pregnant or breastfeeding

The effects of Sular during pregnancy have not been adequately studied. If you are pregnant or plan to become pregnant, tell your doctor immediately. It is not known whether Sular makes its way into breast milk. Your doctor will advise whether to stop taking Sular or to forgo breastfeeding.

Recommended dosage

ADULTS

Your doctor will adjust the dosage to your individual needs. The usual starting dose is 20 milligrams once a day. At weekly intervals, the doctor may make 10-milligram increases in the dosage, depending on how your blood pressure responds. For the long term, the usual dosage ranges from 20 to 40 milligrams once daily. Doses above 60 milligrams are not recommended.

OLDER ADULTS

The usual starting dose is 10 milligrams. Dosage is adjusted upward according to your needs.

CHILDREN

Safety and effectiveness have not been established.

Overdosage

Any medication taken in excess can have serious consequences. Although no specific information is available, extremely low blood pressure is the most likely symptom of a Sular overdose. If you suspect an overdose, seek medical attention immediately.

Generic name:

SULFACETAMIDE

See Sodium Sulamyd, page 1206.

Generic name:

SULFASALAZINE

See Azulfidine, page 131.

Generic name:

SULFISOXAZOLE

See Gantrisin, page 556.

Generic name:

SULINDAC

See Clinoril, page 259.

Generic name:

SUMATRIPTAN

See Imitrex, page 619.

Brand name:

SUMYCIN

See Tetracycline, page 1289.

Brand name:

SUPRAX

Pronounced: SUE-praks
Generic name: Cefixime

Why is this drug prescribed?

Suprax, a cephalosporin antibiotic, is prescribed for bacterial infections of the chest, ears, urinary tract, and throat and for uncomplicated gonorrhea.

Most important fact about this drug

If you are allergic to either penicillin or cephalosporin antibiotics in any form, consult your doctor *before taking* Suprax. An allergy to either type of medication may signal an allergy to Suprax, and if a reaction occurs, it could be extremely severe. If you take the drug and feel signs of a reaction, seek medical attention immediately.

How should you take this medication?

Suprax can be taken with or without food. If the medication causes stomach upset, take it with meals. Food, however, will slow down the rate at which medication is absorbed into your bloodstream.

If you are taking a liquid form of Suprax, use the specially marked measuring spoon to measure each dose accurately. Shake well before using.

It is important that you finish taking all of this medication even if you are feeling better, in order to obtain the medicine's maximum benefit.

■ *If you miss a dose...*
If you are taking this medication once a day and you forget to take a dose, take it as soon as you remember. Wait at least 10 to 12 hours before taking your next dose. Then return to your regular schedule.

If you are taking this medication 2 times a day and you forget to take a dose, take it as soon as you remember and take your next dose 5 to 6 hours later. Then go back to your regular schedule.

If you are taking this medication 3 times a day and you forget to take a dose, take it as soon as you remember and take your next dose 2 to 4 hours later. Then return to your regular schedule.

■ *Storage instructions...*
Suprax liquid may be kept for 14 days, either at room temperature or in the refrigerator. Keep the bottle tightly closed. Do not store in damp places.

Keep out of reach of children and away from direct light and heat. Discard any unused portion after 14 days.

What side effects may occur?

Side effects cannot be anticipated. If any develop or change in intensity, inform your doctor as soon as possible. Only your doctor can determine if it is safe for you to continue taking Suprax.

- *More common side effects may include:*
  Abdominal pain, gas, indigestion, loose stools, mild diarrhea, nausea, vomiting

- *Less common side effects may include:*
  Colitis, dizziness, fever, headaches, hives, itching, skin rashes, vaginitis

- *Rare side effects may include:*
  Bleeding, decrease in urine output, seizures, severe abdominal or stomach cramps, severe diarrhea (sometimes accompanied by blood), shock, skin redness

Why should this drug not be prescribed?

If you are sensitive to or have ever had an allergic reaction to Suprax, other cephalosporin antibiotics, or any form of penicillin, you should not take this medication. Make sure that your doctor is aware of any drug reactions that you have experienced.

Special warnings about this medication

Notify your doctor if you have had allergic reactions to penicillins or other cephalosporin antibiotics.

If you have a history of stomach or intestinal disease such as colitis, check with your doctor before taking Suprax.

If your symptoms of infection do not improve within a few days, or if they get worse, notify your doctor immediately.

If you suffer nausea, vomiting, or severe diarrhea while taking Suprax, check with your doctor before taking a diarrhea medication. Some of these medications, such as Lomotil and Paregoric, may make your diarrhea worse or cause it to last longer.

If you are a diabetic, it is important to note that Suprax may cause false urine-sugar test results. Notify your doctor that you are taking this medication before being tested for sugar in the urine. Do not change diet or dosage of diabetes medication without first consulting with your doctor.

When prescribing Suprax, your doctor may perform laboratory tests to make certain it is effective against the bacteria causing the infection. Some bacteria do not respond to Suprax, so do not give it to other people or use it for other infections.

If you have a kidney disorder, check with your doctor before taking Suprax. You may need a reduced dose of this medication because of your medical condition.

Repeated use of Suprax may result in an overgrowth of bacteria that do not respond to the medication and can cause a secondary infection. Therefore, do not save this medication for use at another time. Take this medication only when directed to do so by your doctor.

**Possible food and drug interactions
when taking this medication**
When Suprax and the seizure medication Tegretol are used together, the amount of Tegretol in the bloodstream may show an increase. No other interactions are currently known.

**Special information
if you are pregnant or breastfeeding**
The effects of Suprax during pregnancy have not been adequately studied. If you are pregnant or plan to become pregnant, inform your doctor immediately. Suprax may appear in breast milk and could affect a nursing infant. If this medication is essential to your health, your doctor may advise you to discontinue breastfeeding your baby until your treatment with this medication is finished.

Recommended dosage

ADULTS

Infections Other Than Gonorrhea
The usual adult dose is 400 milligrams daily. This may be taken as a single 400-milligram tablet once a day or as a 200-milligram tablet every 12 hours. If you have kidney disease, the dose may be lower.

Uncomplicated Gonorrhea
A single 400-milligram oral dose is usually prescribed.

CHILDREN

The safety and effectiveness of Suprax in children less than 6 months old have not been established. The usual child's dose is 8 milligrams of liquid per

2.2 pounds of body weight per day. This may be given as a single dose or in 2 half doses every 12 hours. Children weighing more than 110 pounds or older than 12 years of age should be treated with an adult dose.

If your child has a middle ear infection (otitis media), your doctor will probably prescribe Suprax suspension. The tablet form is less effective against this type of infection.

OLDER ADULTS

Your doctor may start you on a low dosage because this drug is eliminated from your body by the kidneys and kidney function tends to decrease with age.

Overdosage

Any medication taken in excess can cause symptoms of overdose. If you suspect an overdose, seek medical attention immediately.

■ *Symptoms of Suprax overdose may include:*
Blood in the urine, diarrhea, nausea, upper abdominal pain, vomiting

Brand name:

SURMONTIL

Pronounced: SIR-mon-til
Generic name: Trimipramine maleate

Why is this drug prescribed?
Surmontil is used to treat depression. It is a member of the family of drugs known as tricyclic antidepressants.

Most important fact about this drug
Serious, sometimes fatal, reactions have been known to occur when drugs such as Surmontil are taken with another type of antidepressant called an MAO inhibitor. Drugs in this category include Nardil and Parnate. Do not take Surmontil within 2 weeks of taking one of these drugs. Make sure your doctor and pharmacist know of all the medications you are taking.

How should you take this medication?
Surmontil may be taken in 1 dose at bedtime. Alternatively, the total daily dosage may be divided into smaller amounts taken during the day. If you are on long-term therapy with Surmontil, the single bedtime dose is preferred.

It is important to take Surmontil exactly as prescribed, even if the drug seems to have no effect. It may take up to 4 weeks for its benefits to appear.

Surmontil can make your mouth dry. Sucking hard candy or chewing gum can help this problem.

■ *If you miss a dose...*
Take it as soon as you remember. If it is almost time for the next dose, skip the one you missed and go back to your regular schedule. Do not take 2 doses at once. If you take Surmontil once a day at bedtime and you miss a dose, do not take it in the morning. It could cause disturbing side effects during the day.

■ *Storage instructions...*
Store at room temperature in a tightly closed container. Capsules in blister strips should be protected from moisture.

What side effects may occur?
Side effects cannot be anticipated. If any develop or change in intensity, inform your doctor as soon as possible. Only your doctor can determine if it is safe for you to continue taking Surmontil.

■ *Side effects may include:*
Abdominal cramps, agitation, anxiety, black tongue, blocked intestine, blood disorders, blurred vision, breast development in men, confusion (especially in older adults), constipation, delusions, diarrhea, difficulty urinating, dilated pupils, disorientation, dizziness, drowsiness, dry mouth, excessive or spontaneous milk excretion, fatigue, fever, flushing, fluttery or throbbing heartbeat, frequent urination, hair loss, hallucinations, headache, heart attack, high blood pressure, high blood sugar, hives, impotence, increased or decreased sex drive, inflammation of the mouth, insomnia, irregular heart rate, lack of coordination, loss of appetite, low blood pressure, low blood sugar, nausea, nightmares, numbness, peculiar taste in mouth, purple or reddish-brown spots on skin, rapid heartbeat, restlessness, ringing in the ears, seizures, sensitivity to light, skin itching, skin rash, sore throat, stomach upset, stroke, sweating, swelling of breasts, swelling of face and tongue, swelling of testicles, swollen glands, tingling, pins and needles, tremors, visual problems, vomiting, weakness, weight gain or loss, yellowing of the skin and whites of the eyes

Why should this drug not be prescribed?
Surmontil should not be used if you are recovering from a recent heart attack.

You should not take Surmontil if you are sensitive to it or have ever had an allergic reaction to it or to similar drugs such as Tofranil.

Special warnings about this medication

Use Surmontil cautiously if you have a seizure disorder, the eye condition known as glaucoma, heart disease, or a liver disorder. Also use caution if you have thyroid disease or are taking thyroid medication. People who have had problems urinating should also be careful about taking Surmontil.

Nausea, headache, and a general feeling of illness may result if you suddenly stop taking Surmontil. This does not mean you are addicted, but you should follow your doctor's instructions closely when discontinuing the drug.

This drug may impair your ability to drive a car or operate potentially dangerous machinery. Do not participate in any activities that require full alertness if you are unsure of the drug's effect on you.

Possible food and drug interactions
when taking this medication

People who are taking antidepressants known as MAO inhibitors (Parnate and Nardil) should not take Surmontil. Wait 2 weeks after stopping an MAO inhibitor before you begin taking Surmontil.

If Surmontil is taken with certain other drugs, the effects of either could be increased, decreased, or altered. It is especially important to check with your doctor before combining Surmontil with the following:

Antidepressants such as Desyrel and Wellbutrin
Antidepressants that act on serotonin, such as Prozac, Paxil, and
  Zoloft
Antispasmodic drugs such as Donnatal and Cogentin
Cimetidine (Tagamet)
Drugs for heart irregularities, such as Rythmol and Tambocor
Guanethidine (Ismelin)
Local anesthetics containing epinephrine
Local decongestants such as Dristan Nasal Spray
Major tranquilizers such as Thorazine and Mellaril
Quinidine (Quinidex, Quinaglute)
Stimulants such as Proventil, Sudafed, and EpiPen
Thyroid medications such as Synthroid

Extreme drowsiness and other potentially serious effects may result if you drink alcoholic beverages while you are taking Surmontil.

Special information
if you are pregnant or breastfeeding

The effects of Surmontil in pregnancy have not been adequately studied. Pregnant women should use Surmontil only when the potential benefits clearly outweigh the potential risks.

Recommended dosage

ADULTS

The usual starting dose is 75 milligrams per day, divided into equal smaller doses. Your doctor may gradually increase your dose to 150 milligrams per day, divided into smaller doses. Doses over 200 milligrams a day are not recommended. Doses in long-term therapy may range from 50 to 150 milligrams daily. You can take this total daily dosage at bedtime or spread it throughout the day.

CHILDREN

Safety and effectiveness of Surmontil in children have not been established.

OLDER ADULTS AND ADOLESCENTS

Dosages usually start at 50 milligrams per day. Your doctor may increase the dose to 100 milligrams a day, if needed.

Overdosage

Any medication taken in excess can have serious consequences. An overdose of Surmontil can be fatal. If you suspect an overdose, seek medical help immediately.

■ *Symptoms of Surmontil overdose may include:*
Agitation, coma, confusion, convulsions, dilated pupils, disturbed concentration, drowsiness, hallucinations, high fever, irregular heart rate, low body temperature, muscle rigidity, overactive reflexes, severely low blood pressure, stupor, vomiting

You may also have any of the symptoms listed under "What side effects may occur?"

Brand name:

SYNALGOS-DC

Pronounced: SIN-al-gose dee-cee
Generic ingredients: Dihydrocodeine bitartrate, Aspirin,
   Caffeine

Why is this drug prescribed?
Synalgos-DC is a narcotic analgesic prescribed for the relief of moderate to moderately severe pain.

Most important fact about this drug
Narcotics such as Synalgos-DC can be habit-forming or addicting if they are taken over long periods of time.

How should you take this medication?
Take Synalgos-DC exactly as prescribed. Do not increase the amount you take without your doctor's approval.

Avoid or reduce use of alcohol while taking Synalgos-DC.

■ *If you miss a dose...*
If you take this drug on a regular schedule, take the forgotten dose as soon as you remember. If it is almost time for your next dose, skip the one you missed and go back to your regular schedule. Do not take 2 doses at once.

■ *Storage instructions...*
Store at room temperature in a tightly closed container.

What side effects may occur?
Side effects cannot be anticipated. If any develop or change in intensity, inform your doctor as soon as possible. Only your doctor can determine if it is safe for you to continue taking Synalgos-DC.

■ *Side effects may include:*
Constipation, dizziness, drowsiness, itching, light-headedness, nausea, sedation, skin reactions, vomiting

Why should this drug not be prescribed?
If you are sensitive to or have ever had an allergic reaction to Synalgos-DC, other narcotic pain relievers, or aspirin, you should not take this medication.

Make sure your doctor is aware of any drug reactions you have experienced.

Special warnings about this medication
Synalgos-DC may cause you to become drowsy or less alert; therefore, you should not drive or operate dangerous machinery or participate in any hazardous activity that requires full mental alertness until you know how this drug affects you.

If you have ever been dependent on or addicted to drugs, consult your doctor before taking Synalgos-DC.

If you are being treated for a stomach ulcer or blood-clotting disorder, consult your doctor before taking this medication.

Possible food and drug interactions
when taking this medication

Synalgos-DC slows brain activity and intensifies the effects of alcohol. Therefore, you should reduce your intake of alcoholic beverages or avoid them altogether.

If Synalgos-DC is taken with certain other drugs, the effects of either could be increased, decreased, or altered. It is especially important to check with your doctor before combining Synalgos-DC with the following:

Narcotic pain relievers such as Percocet and Demerol
Sedatives such as Halcion and Seconal
Tranquilizers such as Valium and Xanax

Taking blood thinners such as Coumadin in combination with Synalgos-DC may cause internal bleeding.

The use of Synalgos-DC in combination with antigout medications such as Benemid may alter its effects.

Special information
if you are pregnant or breastfeeding

The effects of Synalgos-DC during pregnancy have not been adequately studied. If you are pregnant or plan to become pregnant, inform your doctor immediately. This drug may appear in breast milk and could affect a nursing infant. If this medication is essential to your health, your doctor may advise you to discontinue breastfeeding until your treatment is finished.

Recommended dosage

ADULTS

Your doctor will prescribe a dosage based on the severity of your pain and how you respond to this medication. The usual dose of Synalgos-DC is 2 capsules taken every 4 hours as needed.

CHILDREN

The safety and effectiveness of this medication have not been established in children 12 years of age and under.

OLDER ADULTS

Synalgos-DC should be taken with caution by older adults or anyone in a weakened or run-down condition. Therefore, your doctor will adjust the dosage accordingly.

Overdosage

Although no specific information is available, any medication taken in excess can have serious consequences. If you suspect an overdose of Synalgos-DC, seek medical attention immediately.

Brand name:

SYNTHROID

Pronounced: SIN-throid
Generic name: Levothyroxine
Other brand names: Levothroid, Levoxyl

Why is this drug prescribed?

Synthroid, a synthetic thyroid hormone available in tablet or injectable form, may be given in any of the following cases:

If your own thyroid gland is not making enough hormone;

If you have an enlarged thyroid (a goiter) or are at risk for developing a goiter;

If you need a "suppression test" to determine whether your thyroid gland is making too much hormone;

If you have certain cancers of the thyroid;

If your thyroid production is low due to surgery, radiation, certain drugs, or disease of the pituitary gland or hypothalamus in the brain.

Most important fact about this drug

If you are taking Synthroid to make up for a lack of natural hormone, it is important to take it regularly at the same time every day. You will probably need to take it for the rest of your life.

How should you take this medication?

Take Synthroid exactly as directed. Take no more or less than the prescribed amount and take it no more or less often than prescribed. Take your dose at the same time every day for consistent effect. Do not use it for any other condition or let anyone else use it for whatever reason.

If a child cannot swallow whole tablets, you may crush a Synthroid tablet and mix it into a spoonful of liquid or sprinkle it over a small amount of food such as cooked cereal or applesauce. Give this mixture while it is very fresh; never store it for future use.

While taking Synthroid, your doctor will perform periodic blood tests to determine whether you are getting the right amount.

■ *If you miss a dose...*
Take it as soon as you remember. If it is almost time for your next dose, skip the one you missed and go back to your regular schedule. Never take 2 doses at the same time. If you miss 2 or more doses in a row, consult your doctor.

■ *Storage instructions...*
Keep this medication in a tightly closed container. Store it at room temperature, away from heat, light, and moisture.

What side effects may occur?
Side effects from Synthroid, other than overdose symptoms, are rare. People who are treated with Synthroid may initially lose some hair, but this effect is usually temporary. You may have an allergic reaction such as a rash or hives. Children may have an increase in pressure within the skull. Excessive dosage or a too rapid increase in dosage may lead to overstimulation of the thyroid gland. Notify your doctor immediately if you develop any if the following symptoms.

■ *Symptoms of overstimulation:*
Abdominal cramps, changes in appetite, change in menstrual periods, chest pain, diarrhea, fever, headache, heat intolerance, increased heart rate, irregular heartbeat, irritability, leg cramps, nausea, nervousness, palpitations, shortness of breath, sleeplessness, sweating, tremors, vomiting, weight loss

Why should this drug not be prescribed?
You should not be treated with Synthroid if you have ever had an allergic reaction to it; your thyroid gland is making too much thyroid hormone; you have had a recent heart attack; or your adrenal glands are not making enough corticosteroid hormone. If you are sensitive to dyes, you can take the Synthroid 50-microgram tablet, which is made without color additives.

Although Synthroid will speed up your metabolism, it is not effective as a weight-loss drug and should not be used as such. An overdose may cause life-threatening side effects, especially if you take Synthroid with an appetite-suppressant medication.

Special warnings about this medication
Synthroid has profound effects on the body. Make sure your doctor is aware of all your medical problems, especially conditions related to the heart and

disorders of the adrenal or pituitary glands. The doctor will also need to know about any allergies you may have to food or medicine, and will ask for the names of any medications you take, whether prescription or over-the-counter.

You should receive low doses of Synthroid, under very close supervision, if you are an older person, or if you suffer from high blood pressure, angina (chest pain caused by a heart condition), or other types of heart disease. You may have to stop taking the drug if you develop chest pain or additional circulatory problems.

If you have diabetes, or if your body makes insufficient adrenal corticosteroid hormone, Synthroid will tend to make your symptoms worse. If you take medication for any of these disorders, the dosage will probably have to be adjusted once you begin taking Synthroid. If diabetes is the problem, you should immediately report to your doctor any change in your glucose readings.

Synthroid may cause seizures at the beginning of treatment, although this is rare. You may also notice some hair loss at first, but this is temporary.

It may take a few weeks for Synthroid to begin working, and you may not see any change in your symptoms until then.

Tell your doctor or dentist you are taking Synthroid before you have surgery of any kind.

Tell your doctor if you become pregnant while you are taking Synthroid. Your dose may need to be increased.

Do not switch to another brand of levothyroxine without consulting your doctor.

Excessive doses of Synthroid in infants may cause the top of the skull to close too early.

Possible food and drug interactions
when taking this medication
Synthroid can interact with a wide variety of medications. It's advisable to check with your doctor before taking *any* other drug, but you should be especially wary of the following:

Androgens (male hormones)
Antacids containing aluminum hydroxide
Antidepressants such as Elavil, Nardil, and Prozac
Blood-thinning drugs such as Coumadin
Diabetes medicines such as insulin and Micronase
Diet drugs, including amphetamines

Digitalis-type drugs such as Lanoxin
Epinephrine injections such as EpiPen
Iron supplements
Soy-containing supplements
Sucralfate (Carafate)
The cholesterol-lowering drugs Colestid and Questran

Special information
if you are pregnant or breastfeeding
If you need to take Synthroid because of a thyroid hormone deficiency, you can continue to take the medication during pregnancy. In fact, your doctor will test you regularly and may increase your dose. Once your baby is born, you may breastfeed while continuing to take carefully regulated doses of Synthroid.

Recommended dosage
Your doctor will tailor the dosage to meet your individual requirements, taking into consideration the status of your thyroid gland and other medical conditions you may have. He or she will monitor your thyroid hormone level with periodic blood tests.

Overdosage
If you suspect a Synthroid overdose, seek emergency medical attention immediately. Taken in excess, the drug may have serious consequences.

- *Symptoms of Synthroid overdose may include:*
  Abdominal cramps, chest pain, diarrhea, excessive sweating, fever, headache, heat intolerance, increased appetite, increased pulse and blood pressure, insomnia, irregular heartbeat, menstrual irregularities, nervousness, palpitations, tremors, weight loss

Generic name:

TACRINE

See Cognex, page 274.

Brand name:

TAGAMET

Pronounced: TAG-ah-met
Generic name: Cimetidine
Other brand name: Tagamet HB

Why is this drug prescribed?

Tagamet is prescribed for the treatment of certain kinds of stomach and intestinal ulcers and related conditions. These include: active duodenal (upper intestinal) ulcers; active benign stomach ulcers; erosive gastroesophageal reflux disease (backflow of acid stomach contents); prevention of upper abdominal bleeding in those who are critically ill; and excess-acid conditions such as Zollinger-Ellison syndrome (a form of peptic ulcer with too much acid). It is also used for maintenance therapy of duodenal ulcer following the healing of active ulcers. Tagamet is known as a histamine blocker.

Some doctors also use Tagamet to treat acne and to prevent stress-induced ulcers. It may also be used to treat chronic hives, herpesvirus infections (including shingles), abnormal hair growth in women, and overactivity of the parathyroid gland.

Tagamet HB is an over-the-counter version of the drug used to relieve heartburn, acid indigestion, and sour stomach.

Most important fact about this drug

Short-term treatment with Tagamet can result in complete healing of a duodenal ulcer. However, there can be a recurrence of the ulcer after Tagamet has been discontinued. The rate of ulcer recurrence may be slightly higher in people healed with Tagamet rather than other forms of therapy. However, Tagamet is usually prescribed for more severe cases.

How should you take this medication?

You can take Tagamet with or between meals. Do not take antacids within 1 to 2 hours of a dose of Tagamet. Avoid excessive amounts of caffeine while taking this drug.

It may take several days for Tagamet to begin relieving stomach pain. Be sure to continue taking the drug exactly as prescribed even if it seems to have no effect.

Do not take the maximum daily dose of Tagamet HB for more than 2 weeks continuously without consulting your doctor.

■ *If you miss a dose...*
   Take it as soon as you remember. If it is almost time for your next dose, skip the one you missed and go back to your regular schedule. Do not take 2 doses at once.

■ *Storage instructions...*
Store at room temperature in a tightly closed container, away from light.

What side effects may occur?
Side effects cannot be anticipated. If any develop or change in intensity, inform your doctor as soon as possible. Only your doctor can determine if it is safe for you to continue taking Tagamet.

■ *More common side effects may include:*
Breast development in men, headache

■ *Less common side effects may include:*
Agitation, anxiety, confusion, depression, disorientation, and hallucinations may appear in severely ill individuals who have been treated for 1 month or longer. However, these reactions are not permanent and have cleared up within 3 to 4 days of discontinuation of the drug.

■ *Rare side effects may include:*
Allergic reactions, anemia, blood disorders, diarrhea, dizziness, fever, hair loss, impotence, inability to urinate, joint pain, kidney disorders, liver disorders, mild rash, muscle pain, pancreas inflammation, rapid heartbeat, skin inflammation or peeling, sleepiness, slow heart beat

Why should this drug not be prescribed?
If you have ever had an allergic reaction to Tagamet; do not take this medication.

Special warnings about this medication
Ulcers may be more difficult to heal if you smoke cigarettes.

If you are being treated for a liver or kidney disorder, make sure the doctor is aware of it.

If you are over 50 years old, have liver or kidney disease, or are severely ill, you may experience temporary mental confusion while taking Tagamet. Notify your doctor.

If you have trouble swallowing or persistent abdominal pain, do not take Tagamet HB; instead, check with your doctor. You may have a serious condition that requires different treatment.

**Possible food and drug interactions
when taking this medication**

If Tagamet is taken with certain other drugs, the effects of either can be increased, decreased, or altered. It is especially important that you check with your doctor before combining Tagamet with the following:

Antidiabetic drugs such as Micronase and Glucotrol
Antifungal drugs such as Diflucan and Nizoral
Aspirin
Augmentin
Benzodiazepine tranquilizers such as Valium and Librium
Beta-blocking blood pressure drugs such as Inderal and Lopressor
Calcium-blocking blood pressure drugs such as Cardizem, Calan, and
    Procardia
Chlorpromazine (Thorazine)
Cisapride (Propulsid)
Cyclosporine (Sandimmune)
Digoxin (Lanoxin)
Medications for irregular heartbeat, such as Cordarone, Tonocard,
    Quinidex, and Procan
Metoclopramide (Reglan)
Metronidazole (Flagyl)
Narcotic pain relievers such as Demerol and Morphine
Nicotine (Nicoderm, Nicorette)
Paroxetine (Paxil)
Pentoxifylline (Trental)
Phenytoin (Dilantin)
Quinine
Sucralfate (Carafate)
Theophylline (Theo-Dur, others)
Warfarin (Coumadin)

Avoid alcoholic beverages while taking Tagamet. This medication increases the effects of alcohol.

Antacids can reduce the effect of Tagamet when taken at the same time. If you take an antacid to relieve the pain of an ulcer, the doses should be separated by 1 to 2 hours.

If you need to take an antifungal drug such as Nizoral, you should take it at least 2 hours before you take Tagamet.

Special information
if you are pregnant or breastfeeding

The effects of Tagamet during pregnancy have not been adequately studied. If you are pregnant or plan to become pregnant, notify your doctor immediately. Tagamet appears in breast milk and could affect a nursing infant. If this medication is essential to your health, your doctor may advise you to discontinue breastfeeding until treatment with this drug is finished.

Recommended dosage

TAGAMET (ADULTS)

Active Duodenal Ulcer

The usual dose is 800 milligrams once daily at bedtime. However, other doses shown to be effective are:

300 milligrams 4 times a day with meals and at bedtime

400 milligrams twice a day, in the morning and at bedtime

Most people heal in 4 weeks.

If you require maintenance therapy, the usual dose is 400 milligrams at bedtime.

Active Benign Gastric Ulcer

The usual dose is 800 milligrams once a day at bedtime or 300 milligrams taken 4 times a day with meals and at bedtime.

Erosive Gastroesophageal Reflux Disease

The usual dosage is a total of 1,600 milligrams daily divided into doses of 800 milligrams twice a day or 400 milligrams 4 times a day for 12 weeks. The beneficial use of Tagamet beyond 12 weeks has not been firmly established.

Pathological Hypersecretory Condition

The usual dosage is 300 milligrams 4 times a day with meals and at bedtime. Your doctor may adjust your dosage based on your needs, but you should take no more than 2,400 milligrams per day.

TAGAMET (CHILDREN)

Safety and effectiveness have not been established in children under 16 years old. However, your doctor may decide that the potential benefits of Tagamet use outweigh the potential risks. Doses of 20 to 40 milligrams per 2.2 pounds of body weight have been used.

TAGAMET HB

Heartburn, Acid Indigestion, Sour Stomach
The usual dosage is 2 tablets, taken with water, once or up to twice a day. Do not take more than 4 tablets in 24 hours.

Do not give Tagamet HB to children under 12 years unless your doctor tells you to.

Overdosage
Information concerning overdosage is limited. However, respiratory failure, an increased heartbeat, exaggerated side effect symptoms or reactions such as unresponsiveness may be signs of Tagamet overdose. If you experience any of these symptoms, notify your doctor immediately.

Brand name:

TALWIN COMPOUND

Pronounced: TAL-win
Generic ingredients: Pentazocine hydrochloride, Aspirin

Why is this drug prescribed?
Talwin Compound combines the strong analgesic properties of pentazocine and the analgesic, anti-inflammatory, and fever-reducing properties of aspirin. It is used for the relief of moderate pain.

Most important fact about this drug
Talwin Compound can cause physical and psychological dependence. Do not share Talwin Compound with other people.

How should you take this medication?
Take Talwin Compound exactly as prescribed by your doctor. Do not increase the amount you take without your doctor's approval.

- *If you miss a dose...*
  And you take this medication on a regular schedule, take the forgotten dose as soon as you remember. If it is almost time for your next dose, skip the one you missed and go back to your regular schedule. Do not take 2 doses at once.

■ *Storage instructions...*
Store at room temperature. Protect from heat.

What side effects may occur?
Side effects cannot be anticipated. If any develop or change in intensity, inform your doctor as soon as possible. Only your doctor can determine if it is safe for you to continue taking Talwin.

■ *More common side effects may include:*
Confusion, disorientation, dizziness, feelings of elation, hallucinations, headache, light-headedness, nausea, sedation, sweating, vomiting

If any of these side effects occur, it may help if you lie down after taking the medication.

■ *Less common side effects may include:*
Blurred vision, constipation, depression, difficulty in focusing, disturbed dreams, fainting, flushing, inability to fall or stay asleep, lowered blood pressure, rapid heart rate, rash, weakness

■ *Rare side effects may include:*
Abdominal distress, chills, diarrhea, excitement, facial swelling, fluid retention, hives, inability to urinate, irritability, lack or loss of appetite, ringing in the ears, skin peeling, tingling sensation, tremors, troubled or slowed breathing

Why should this drug not be prescribed?
If you are sensitive to or have ever had an allergic reaction to pentazocine or salicylates (anti-inflammatory drugs such as aspirin), or other drugs of this type, you should not take this medication. Make sure your doctor is aware of any drug reactions you have experienced.

Because there is a possible association between aspirin and the dangerous neurological condition called Reye's syndrome, Talwin should not be given to children and teenagers who have chickenpox or flu, which predispose them to development of the condition.

Special warnings about this medication
Drug dependence and withdrawal symptoms—if you stop taking the drug abruptly—can occur with the use of pentazocine. If you have a history of drug dependence, Talwin should be used only under the close supervision of your doctor.

Talwin Compound may cause you to become drowsy, dizzy, or less alert; therefore, you should not drive or operate dangerous machinery or participate in any hazardous activity that requires full mental alertness until you know how this drug affects you.

Talwin Compound contains aspirin. If you have a stomach ulcer, consult your doctor before taking this medication. Aspirin may irritate the stomach lining and may cause bleeding.

If you have a kidney or liver disorder, or if you are prone to seizures, consult your doctor before taking Talwin.

Talwin Compound may cause breathing difficulties. If you have severe bronchial asthma or other respiratory problems, check with your doctor before taking this medication.

Talwin should be used with caution if you have had a heart attack or if you are nauseated or are vomiting.

Talwin Compound should be used with extreme caution in patients being treated by a doctor for a head injury. This medication may cause troubled breathing and pressure on the skull from increased brain and spinal fluid—which can be exaggerated by a head injury. This drug may also mask or hide the pain from head injury, making it difficult for your doctor to treat.

Use Talwin Compound only to relieve pain, not in anticipation of pain.

Possible food and drug interactions
when taking this medication

Talwin Compound slows brain activity and intensifies the effects of alcohol. Limit your intake of alcohol while taking this medication.

If Talwin Compound is taken with certain other drugs, the effects of either could be increased, decreased, or altered. It is especially important to check with your doctor before combining Talwin Compound with the following:

Benzodiazepines (tranquilizers such as Valium and Xanax)
MAO inhibitors (such as the antidepressants Nardil and Parnate)
Other analgesics (pain relievers such as Demerol)
Sleep aids such as Dalmane and Halcion

The use of these drugs with Talwin Compound increases their sedative or calming effects and may lead to overdose symptoms.

The use of blood thinners such as Coumadin in combination with Talwin Compound may cause bleeding. If you are taking a blood thinner, consult your doctor before taking this drug.

The use of narcotics, including methadone (prescribed for the daily treatment of drug dependence), with Talwin Compound may produce withdrawal symptoms.

Special information
if you are pregnant or breastfeeding

The effects of Talwin Compound during pregnancy have not been adequately studied. Consult your physician before taking Talwin Compound when pregnant. It is not known whether Talwin Compound appears in breast milk. If this medication is essential to your health, your doctor may advise you to discontinue breastfeeding until your treatment is finished.

Recommended dosage

ADULTS

The usual dose of Talwin Compound is 2 caplets, 3 or 4 times per day.

CHILDREN

The safety and effectiveness of Talwin Compound have not been established in children under 12 years of age.

Overdosage

Any medication taken in excess can have dangerous consequences. If you suspect an overdose, seek medical attention immediately.

- *Symptoms of an overdose of Talwin Compound, because of its aspirin content, may include:*
  Coma, confusion, convulsions, diarrhea, dizziness, gasping, headache, heavy perspiration, nausea, rapid breathing, rapid heart rate, ringing in the ears, thirst, vomiting

An inability to breathe may lead to death.

Brand name:

TAMBOCOR

Pronounced: TAM-ba-kore
Generic name: Flecainide acetate

Why is this drug prescribed?

Tambocor is prescribed to treat certain heart rhythm disturbances, including paroxysmal atrial fibrillation (a sudden attack or worsening of irregular heartbeat in which the upper chamber of the heart beats irregularly and very rapidly) and paroxysmal supraventricular tachycardia (a sudden attack or worsening of an abnormally fast but regular heart rate that occurs in intermittent episodes).

Most important fact about this drug

Tambocor may sometimes cause or worsen heartbeat irregularities and certain heart conditions, such as heart failure (the inability of the heart to sustain its workload of pumping blood). Before prescribing Tambocor, your doctor will weigh the drug's risks and benefits. Your condition will be monitored throughout your treatment.

How should you take this medication?

In almost every case, your doctor will initiate Tambocor therapy in the hospital.

Take Tambocor exactly as prescribed by your doctor. Serious heartbeat disturbances may result if you do not follow your doctor's instructions, if you miss any regular doses, or if you increase or decrease the dosage without consulting your doctor.

Your doctor may order regular blood tests to monitor your therapy.

- *If you miss a dose...*
  Take it as soon as you remember if it is within 6 hours of your scheduled time. If you do not remember until later, skip the dose you missed and go back to your regular schedule. Do not take 2 doses at once.

- *Storage instructions...*
  Store at room temperature in a tightly closed container, away from light.

What side effects may occur?

Tambocor has a wide variety of possible effects on the heart, including new or worsened heartbeat abnormalities, heart attack, congestive heart failure, and heart block—an interference with the heart's contraction. If any develop, inform your doctor immediately. Only your doctor can determine whether it is safe for you to continue taking Tambocor.

- *Other side effects may include:*
  Abdominal pain, angina pectoris (crushing chest pain), anxiety, apathy, appetite loss, chest pain, confusion, constipation, convulsions, decreased sex drive, depression, diarrhea, difficult or labored breathing, dizziness (light-headedness, faintness, near fainting, unsteadiness), dry mouth, edema (accumulation of fluid in the tissues), exaggerated feeling of well-being, excessive urine, eye pain or irritation, fainting, fatigue, fever, flushing, gas, hair loss, headache, heart palpitations (fluttery heartbeat),

high or low blood pressure, hives, impotence, inability to urinate, indigestion, insomnia, intolerance of light, involuntary eye movements, itching, joint pain, lack of coordination, loss of sense of identity, lung inflammation or other conditions, malaise (feeling unwell or ill), memory loss, morbid dreams, muscle pain, nausea, numbness or tingling, paralysis, rash, reduced sensitivity to touch, ringing in the ears, skin inflammation and peeling, sleepiness, speech problems, stupor, sweating, swollen lips, tongue, and mouth, taste changes, tremor, twitching, vertigo, vision problems (blurred vision, difficulty in focusing, double vision, spots before the eyes), vomiting, weakness, wheezing

Why should this drug not be prescribed?
Your doctor should not prescribe Tambocor if you have ever had an allergic reaction to it or you are sensitive to it, if you have heart block (without a pacemaker), or if your heart cannot supply enough blood to the body.

Special warnings about this medication
If you have a pacemaker, you should be monitored very closely while taking Tambocor—your pacemaker may need to be adjusted.

If you have liver disease, Tambocor could build up in your system. Your doctor will prescribe the drug only if the benefits outweigh the risks. In addition, you should have frequent blood tests to make sure your dosage is not too high.

If you have a history of congestive heart failure or a weak heart, you may be at increased risk for dangerous cardiac side effects from Tambocor.

If you have very alkaline urine, perhaps caused by a kidney condition or by a strict vegetarian diet, your body will tend to process and eliminate Tambocor rather slowly and you may need a lower-than-average dosage.

If the potassium levels in your blood are too high or too low, your doctor will want to correct the condition before allowing you to take Tambocor.

If you have kidney failure, your doctor will want to watch you closely.

Possible food and drug interactions
when taking this medication
If Tambocor is taken with certain other drugs, the effects of either could be increased, decreased, or altered. It is especially important to check with your doctor before combining Tambocor with the following:

Amiodarone (Cordarone)
Beta blockers (blood pressure drugs such as Inderal, Tenormin, and Sectral)
Carbamazepine (Tegretol)

Cimetidine (Tagamet)
Diltiazem (Cardizem)
Disopyramide (Norpace)
Nifedipine (Procardia)
Phenobarbital
Phenytoin (Dilantin)
Quinidine (Quinidex)
Verapamil (Calan, Isoptin)

Special information
if you are pregnant or breastfeeding

The effects of Tambocor during pregnancy have not been adequately studied. If you are pregnant or plan to become pregnant, inform your doctor immediately. Tambocor should be used during pregnancy only if the benefit justifies the potential risk to the unborn child. Tambocor appears in breast milk. Check with your doctor before breastfeeding your baby.

Recommended dosage

ADULTS

Treatment with Tambocor almost always begins in the hospital.

The usual starting dose is 50 to 100 milligrams every 12 hours, depending on the condition under treatment. Every 4 days, your doctor may increase your dose by 50 milligrams every 12 hours until your condition is under control.

CHILDREN

Children's dosage is based on body surface area and is always supervised by a cardiac physician.

Overdosage

An overdose of Tambocor is likely to cause slowed or rapid heartbeat, other cardiac problems, fainting, low blood pressure, nausea, vomiting, convulsions, and heart failure. Taken even in moderate excess, Tambocor may have serious consequences and can be fatal. If you suspect an overdose, seek medical attention immediately.

Generic name:

TAMOXIFEN

See Nolvadex, page 890.

Generic name:

TAMSULOSIN

See Flomax, page 535.

Brand name:

TARKA

Pronounced: TAR-kah
Generic ingredients: Trandolapril, Verapamil hydrochloride

Why is this drug prescribed?
Tarka is used to treat high blood pressure. It combines two blood pressure drugs: an ACE inhibitor and a calcium channel blocker. The ACE inhibitor (trandolapril) lowers blood pressure by preventing a chemical in your blood called angiotensin I from converting to a more potent form that narrows the blood vessels and increases salt and water retention. The calcium channel blocker (verapamil hydrochloride) also works to keep the blood vessels open, and eases the heart's workload by reducing the force and rate of your heartbeat.

Most important fact about this drug
Doctors usually prescribe Tarka for patients who have been taking one of its components—trandolapril (Mavik) or sustained-release verapamil (Calan SR, Isoptin SR)—without showing improvement. Like other blood pressure medications, Tarka must be taken regularly for it to be effective. Since blood pressure declines gradually, it may take a few weeks before you get the full benefit of Tarka; and you must continue taking it even if you are feeling well. Tarka does not cure high blood pressure; it merely keeps it under control.

How should you take this medication?
Take each dose with food, exactly as prescribed.

■ *If you miss a dose...*
Take it as soon as you remember. If it is almost time for your next dose, skip the one you missed and go back to your regular schedule. Never take 2 doses at the same time.

■ *Storage instructions...*
Keep the container tightly closed. Store at room temperature.

What side effects may occur?
Side effects cannot be anticipated. If any develop or change in intensity, inform your doctor as soon as possible. Only your doctor can determine if it is safe for you to continue taking Tarka.

■ *More common side effects may include:*
Constipation, cough, dizziness, headache, heartbeat irregularities, upper respiratory tract infection

■ *Less common side effects may include:*
Back pain, bronchitis, chest pain, diarrhea, difficulty breathing, fatigue, joint pain, nausea, pain in arms and legs, slow heartbeat, swelling, upper respiratory tract congestion

■ *Rare side effects may include:*
Anxiety, drowsiness, dry mouth, fast heartbeat, flushing, general feeling of illness, impotence, indigestion, muscle aches, rash, weakness

Why should this drug not be prescribed?
Avoid Tarka if you have ever had an allergic reaction to it, or to verapamil or any of the ACE inhibitors, including Capoten, Vasotec, and Zestril.

You should also avoid Tarka if you have low blood pressure or certain types of heart disease or irregular heartbeat. Make sure your doctor is aware of any cardiac problems you may have.

In addition, Tarka is not for you if you have ever developed a swollen throat and difficulty swallowing (angioedema) while taking an ACE inhibitor. Make sure your doctor is aware of the incident.

Special warnings about this medication
Call your doctor immediately if you begin to suffer angioedema while taking Tarka. Warning signs include swelling of the face, lips, tongue, or throat; swelling of the arms and legs; and difficulty swallowing or breathing.

Bee or wasp venom given to prevent an allergic reaction to stings may cause a severe allergic reaction to Tarka. Kidney dialysis can also prompt an allergic reaction to the drug.

Tarka sometimes causes a severe drop in blood pressure. The danger is especially great if you have been taking water pills (diuretics), or if you have heart disease, kidney disease, or a potassium or salt imbalance. Excessive sweating, severe diarrhea, and vomiting are also a threat. They can rob the body of water, causing a dangerous drop in blood pressure. If you feel light-headed or faint, you should lie down and contact your doctor immediately.

Because another of the ACE inhibitors, Capoten, has been known to cause serious blood disorders, your doctor will check your blood regularly while you are taking Tarka. If you develop signs of infection such as a sore throat or a fever, you should contact your doctor at once—an infection could be a signal of blood abnormalities.

Tarka may also affect the liver, so your doctor will perform liver function tests periodically. Report these symptoms of liver problems to your doctor immediately: a generally run-down feeling, fever, pain in the upper right abdomen, or yellowing of the skin or the whites of your eyes.

If you have a heart condition, heart failure, cardiac irregularities, kidney disease, liver disease, diabetes, or Duchenne's dystrophy (the most common type of muscular dystrophy), make certain that your doctor knows about it. Tarka should be used with caution under these circumstances.

Possible food and drug interactions when taking this medication

If Tarka is taken with certain other drugs, the effects of either could be increased, decreased, or altered. It is especially important to check with your doctor before combining Tarka with the following:

Drugs classified as "beta blockers," such as Inderal, Lopressor, and Tenormin
Carbamazepine (Tegretol)
Cimetidine (Tagamet)
Cyclosporine (Sandimmune, Neoral)
Digoxin (Lanoxin)
Disopyramide (Norpace)
Diuretics such as Lasix and HydroDIURIL
Flecainide (Tambocor)
Lithium (Lithonate, Lithobid)
Phenobarbital
Potassium-sparing diuretics such as Aldactone, Midamor, Dyrenium
Potassium supplements such as K-Lyte, K-Tabs, and Slow-K
Quinidine (Quinidex)
Rifampin (Rifadin)
Theophylline (Theo-Dur)

Because Tarka can increase the potassium level in your blood, you should avoid salt substitutes that contain potassium unless your doctor approves.

Special information if you are pregnant or breastfeeding

Because of its ACE-inhibitor component (trandolapril), Tarka should not be used during pregnancy. When taken during the last 6 months of pregnancy, ACE inhibitors can cause birth defects, premature birth, and death of the developing or newborn baby. If you become pregnant, inform your doctor immediately.

The verapamil component of Tarka does appear in breast milk and could affect a nursing infant. Do not breastfeed while taking Tarka.

Recommended dosage

ADULTS

Tarka comes in four strengths of trandolapril and sustained-release verapamil. Your doctor will prescribe a dose of Tarka that is comparable to the doses you were taking separately. Doses range from 1 to 4 milligrams of trandolapril and 180 to 240 milligrams of verapamil. Tarka is taken once a day with food.

If you have impaired liver or kidney function, your doctor will adjust your dosage accordingly.

CHILDREN

The safety and effectiveness of Tarka in children under 18 have not been established.

OLDER ADULTS

If you are over 65 years old, you may be more sensitive to Tarka. Your doctor will monitor your blood pressure more closely and adjust your medication dose accordingly.

Overdosage

An overdose of Tarka can cause dangerously low blood pressure and life-threatening heart problems. If you suspect an overdose, seek medical treatment immediately.

Brand name:

TASMAR

Pronounced: TAZ-mahr
Generic name: Tolcapone

Why is this drug prescribed?

Tasmar helps to relieve the muscle stiffness, tremor, and weakness caused by Parkinson's disease. When taken with Sinemet (levodopa/carbidopa), it sustains the blood levels of dopamine needed for normal muscle function.

Like all Parkinson's medications, Tasmar can provide long-term relief of symptoms, but won't cure the underlying disease.

Most important fact about this drug
During the first few weeks of Tasmar treatment, be prepared for certain side effects that appear most frequently at the start of therapy. Among the possibilities: attacks of dizziness or fainting when you first stand up, hallucinations, nausea, and increased stiffness. These problems tend to diminish with the passage of time or a reduction in your Sinemet dosage. However, they have forced a few people to discontinue Tasmar therapy.

How should you take this medication?
Tasmar works by boosting the efficacy of Sinemet, and will not work without it. It can be taken with either the immediate-release or controlled-release form of the drug (Sinemet or Sinemet CR). You may take it with or without food.

This drug is taken 3 times a day. Always take the first dose of Tasmar with your first dose of Sinemet. Take your second and third doses of Tasmar 6 and 12 hours later. (Your doctor will probably decrease your dose of Sinemet when you start taking Tasmar.)

■ *If you miss a dose...*
Take it as soon as you remember. If it is almost time for your next dose, skip the one you missed and go back to your regular schedule. Do not take 2 doses at once.

■ *Storage instructions...*
Store at room temperature in a tightly sealed container.

What side effects may occur?
Side effects cannot be anticipated. If any develop or change in intensity, inform your doctor as soon as possible. Only your doctor can determine if it is safe for you to continue taking Tasmar.

■ *More common side effects may include:*
Abdominal pain, abnormal muscle movements, acid indigestion, breathing difficulty, chest pain, confusion, constipation, decreased muscle movement, diarrhea, dizziness, drowsiness, dry mouth, excessive dreaming, falling, fatigue, fainting, flu, gas, hallucination, headache, increased muscle movement, loss of appetite, loss of balance, muscle cramps,

muscle stiffness, nausea, skin tingling, sleep disturbances, sweating, tiredness, upper respiratory tract infection, urinary tract infection, urine discoloration, vomiting

■ *Less common side effects may include:*
Agitation, arthritis, bronchitis, burning, cataract, chest discomfort, depression, excessive emotional reactions, eye inflammation, feeling of well-being, fever, hair loss, hyperactivity, impaired mental function, impotence, increased heart rate, increased muscle tone, infection, irritability, lack of sensibility, low blood pressure, lower back pain, muscle ache, neck pain, panic reaction, rash, ringing in the ears, salivation, sinus congestion, skin bleeding, skin tumor, speech disorder, stiffness, throat inflammation, tooth disorder, tremor, uneasy feeling, urinary frequency or incontinence, urination problems, uterine tumor, weight loss

■ *Rare side effects may include:*
Abnormal thinking, allergic reaction, amnesia, apathy, asthma, bloody nose, chills, cough, decreased heart rate, dehydration, delusions, diabetes, difficulty swallowing, ear infection, ear pain, eczema, eye problems, facial swelling, heart disorders, hiccups, high blood pressure, hostility, increased or decreased sex drive, irregular or rapid heartbeat, itching, joint problems, laryngitis, manic reaction, migraine headache, mouth ulcers, nervousness, nosebleeds, paranoia, prostate problems, salivation, skin disorders, stomach or intestinal bleeding or inflammation, thirst, tongue disorders, twitching, vaginal inflammation

Why should this drug not be prescribed?
If Tasmar gives you an allergic reaction, you will not be able to continue using it.

Special warnings about this medication
Especially at the start of therapy, Tasmar can cause severe low blood pressure, marked by nausea, sweating, dizziness, or fainting. To avoid these symptoms, get up very slowly from a seated or reclining position.

Hallucinations are most likely to occur within the first 2 weeks of therapy, and are most common in people over 75. If this problem surfaces, report it to your doctor immediately.

Diarrhea, occasionally severe, is also a possibility, typically after 6 to 12 weeks of therapy. If this becomes a problem, let your doctor know. Also be quick to inform your doctor if you develop a high fever, muscle rigidity, or altered consciousness.

Because Tasmar has been known to cause drowsiness and affect mental and motor skills, you should avoid operating machinery or driving until you know how the drug affects you.

Possible food and drug interactions when taking this medication

If Tasmar is taken with certain other drugs, the effects of either could be increased, decreased, or altered. It is especially important to check with your doctor before combining Tasmar with the following:

Apomorphine
Desipramine (Norpramin)
Isoproterenol (Isuprel)
MAO inhibitors such as the antidepressants Marplan, Nardil, and Parnate
Methyldopa (Aldomet)
Nervous system depressants such as alcohol and the sedatives Phenobarbital and Seconal
Warfarin (Coumadin)

Special information if you are pregnant or breastfeeding

The safety of Tasmar during pregnancy has not been confirmed. If you are pregnant or plan to become pregnant, inform your doctor immediately. You should continue taking the drug only if the benefits clearly outweigh the risk.

It is not known whether Tasmar appears in breast milk. Notify your doctor if you plan to breastfeed.

Recommended dosage

ADULTS

The usual dose is 100 to 200 milligrams 3 times daily. Take no more than a total of 600 milligrams a day.

Dosing for Liver Disease:

If you have cirrhosis of the liver, your doctor will prescribe a lower dose.

Overdosage

Any medication taken in excess can have serious consequences. If you suspect an overdose, seek medical attention immediately.

■ *Symptoms of Tasmar overdose may include:*
Dizziness, nausea, vomiting

Brand name:

TAVIST

Pronounced: TAV-ist
Generic name: Clemastine fumarate

Why is this drug prescribed?

Tavist is an antihistamine. Both Tavist and Tavist-1 are used in treatment of the sneezing, runny nose, itching, and watery eyes caused by hay fever. Tavist Tablets also relieve mild allergic skin reactions such as hives and swelling. Antihistamines reduce itching and swelling and dry up secretions from the eyes, nose, and throat.

Most important fact about this drug

Tavist may cause drowsiness. Be especially careful driving or operating dangerous machinery or participating in any hazardous activity that requires full mental alertness until you know how you react to this medication.

How should you take this medication?

Tavist should be taken exactly as prescribed.

Tavist may make your mouth dry. Sucking hard candy, chewing gum, or melting bits of ice in your mouth can provide relief.

- *If you miss a dose...*
  If you are taking this medication on a regular schedule, take the forgotten dose as soon as you remember. If it is almost time for your next dose, skip the one you missed and go back to your regular schedule. Do not take 2 doses at once.

- *Storage instructions...*
  Store at room temperature in a dry, cool place, away from direct sunlight. Keep container tightly closed.

What side effects may occur?

Side effects cannot be anticipated. If any develop or change in intensity, inform your doctor as soon as possible. Only your doctor can determine if it is safe for you to continue taking Tavist.

- *More common side effects may include:*
  Disturbed coordination, dizziness, drowsiness, extreme calm (sedation), increased chest congestion, sleepiness, upset stomach

■ *Less common or rare side effects may include:*
Acute inflammation of the inner ear, anemia, blurred vision, chills, confusion, constipation, convulsions, diarrhea, difficulty sleeping, difficulty urinating, double vision, dry mouth, nose, and throat, early menstruation, exaggerated sense of well-being, excessive perspiration, excitement, fatigue, frequent urination, headache, hives, hysteria, inability to urinate, irregular heartbeat, irritability, loss of appetite, low blood pressure, nausea, nerve inflammation, nervousness, palpitations, rapid heartbeat, rash, restlessness, ringing in the ears, sensitivity to light, severe allergic reaction (anaphylactic shock), stuffy nose, tightness of chest, tingling or pins and needles, tremor, vertigo, vomiting, weakness, wheezing

Why should this drug not be prescribed?
Do not take Tavist if you are breastfeeding. Also avoid this drug if you are sensitive to or have ever had an allergic reaction to clemastine fumarate or similar antihistamines.

Special warnings about this medication
Use antihistamines very cautiously if you have the eye condition known as narrow-angle glaucoma, a peptic ulcer, intestinal blockage, a bladder obstruction, or an enlarged prostate. Antihistamines can make these problems worse.

Antihistamines are more likely to cause dizziness, sedation, and low blood pressure in the elderly (over age 60).

Use Tavist with care if you have a history of bronchial asthma, heart disease, circulatory problems, an overactive thyroid, or high blood pressure.

Possible food and drug interactions
when taking this medication
Tavist may increase the effects of alcohol. Do not drink alcohol—or at least limit your use—while taking this medication.

If Tavist is taken with certain other drugs, the effects of either could be increased, decreased, or altered. It is especially important to check with your doctor before combining Tavist with the following:

Drugs known as MAO inhibitors, such as the antidepressants Nardil and Parnate
Sleeping pills such as Nembutal and Seconal
Tranquilizers such as Xanax and Valium

Special information
if you are pregnant or breastfeeding

The effects of Tavist during pregnancy have not been adequately studied. If you are pregnant or plan to become pregnant, inform your doctor immediately. Tavist should not be used if you are breastfeeding.

Recommended dosage

TAVIST-1 TABLETS

The recommended starting dose is 1 tablet twice daily. Your doctor may increase the dose to a maximum of 6 tablets daily.

TAVIST TABLETS

The maximum recommended dosage is 1 tablet 3 times daily. Many people do well on a single dose. You should take no more than 3 tablets daily.

TAVIST SYRUP

ADULTS AND CHILDREN 12 YEARS AND OVER

For Symptoms of Hay Fever

The starting dose of Tavist Syrup is 2 teaspoonfuls (1 milligram) 2 times a day. Your doctor may increase the dosage, but it should not be more than 12 teaspoonfuls (6 milligrams) daily.

For Hives and Swelling

The starting dose of Tavist Syrup is 4 teaspoonfuls (2 milligrams) twice a day; you should not take more than 12 teaspoonfuls (6 milligrams) daily.

CHILDREN 6 THROUGH 11

For Symptoms of Hay Fever

The starting dose of Tavist Syrup is 1 teaspoonful (0.5 milligram) 2 times per day. Your doctor may increase the dosage to a maximum of 6 teaspoonfuls (3 milligrams) daily.

For Hives and Swelling

The starting dose of Tavist Syrup is 2 teaspoonfuls (1 milligram) twice a day, not to exceed 6 teaspoonfuls (3 milligrams) daily.

Overdosage

An overdose of Tavist can be fatal, especially in children. If you suspect an overdose, seek medical treatment immediately.

- *Symptoms of Tavist overdose may include:*
  Coma, drowsiness, severe heart problems

- *Symptoms of Tavist overdose in children may include:*
  Bluish color to the skin, coma, convulsions, dry mouth, excitement, fever, fixed, dilated pupils, flushing, hallucinations, high body temperature, severe heart problems, slow twisting movements of hand and arms, tremors, twitching, uncoordinated movements

Generic name:

TAZAROTENE

See Tazorac, below.

Brand name:

TAZORAC

Pronounced: TAZZ-o-rack
Generic name: Tazarotene

Why is this drug prescribed?

Tazorac gel comes in two strengths, 0.05% and 0.1%. Both strengths are used to treat the type of psoriasis that causes large plaques on the skin. The 0.1% strength is also used to treat mild to moderate facial acne. The drug is chemically related to vitamin A.

Most important fact about this drug

Tazorac may cause severe birth defects. If you are a woman in your child-bearing years, do not use Tazorac if there is any chance that you are pregnant. Your doctor should give you a pregnancy test within 2 weeks of starting Tazorac therapy, and you should take reliable birth control measures as long as you use the drug. If you accidentally become pregnant, stop using Tazorac and call your doctor immediately.

How should you take this medication?

For psoriasis, apply a thin film of Tazorac to the affected areas each evening. Make sure your skin is dry before you begin. Keep the gel away from normal skin.

To treat acne, first wash your face and dry it thoroughly. Then apply a thin film of Tazorac to the acne eruptions. Repeat each evening.

■ *If you miss a dose...*
Apply it as soon as you remember. If it is almost time for the next dose, skip the one you missed and go back to your regular schedule.

■ *Storage instructions...*
Store at room temperature.

What side effects may occur?
Side effects cannot be anticipated. If any develop or change in intensity, inform your doctor as soon as possible. Only your doctor can determine if it is safe for you to continue using Tazorac.

■ *More common side effects may include:*
Burning, dry skin, irritation, itching, skin pain, skin peeling, skin reddening, stinging, worsening of psoriasis

■ *Less common side effects may include:*
Discoloration, rash, skin bleeding, skin cracking, skin inflammation, skin reddening due to sun-exposure, swelling

Why should this drug not be prescribed?
If Tazorac gives you an allergic reaction, you cannot continue using it.

Special warnings about this medication
Use Tazorac only on affected areas of the skin. Be careful to avoid your eyes and mouth. Tazorac is for external use only.

Avoid prolonged exposure to the sun or sunlamps while using Tazorac. Apply sunscreen (at least SPF 15) and wear protective clothing when you go into the sunlight. If you are normally sensitive to sunlight, be especially cautious. If you have a sunburn, wait until it heals before using Tazorac.

Tazorac may cause a temporary feeling of burning or stinging. If this irritation is excessive, or you develop extreme itching, burning, peeling, or reddening, stop using Tazorac and call your doctor. Do not restart therapy until your skin returns to normal. Never use Tazorac while your skin is inflamed.

While on Tazorac therapy, remember that extreme wind or cold may cause skin irritation.

The safety and effectiveness of this drug have not been tested in children under 12.

Possible food and drug interactions when taking this medication. Check with your doctor before combining Tazorac with other skin medications and cosmetics. Skin products that have a drying effect should not be used with

Tazorac. If you've been using such products, wait for their effects to disappear before using Tazorac.

Possible food and drug interactions
when taking this medication

Certain drugs can increase your sensitivity to sunlight. Check with your doctor before taking any other medication while using Tazorac, and be especially cautious when using the following:

Major tranquilizers such as Compazine, Stelazine, and Thorazine
Quinolone antibiotics such as Cipro, Floxin, and Noroxin
Sulfa drugs such as Bactrim and Septra
Tetracycline antibiotics such as Achromycin V, Minocin, and Vibramycin
Thiazide-type water pills such as Dyazide and HydroDIURIL

Special information
if you are pregnant or breastfeeding

Remember that Tazorac may cause birth defects and must never be used during pregnancy. Tazorac may appear in breast milk; use it with caution, if at all, while breastfeeding.

Recommended dosage

ADULTS

Apply the prescribed gel to affected areas once a day in the evening.

Overdosage

Excessive external use of Tazorac can cause redness, peeling, and skin discomfort. An oral overdose produces the same symptoms as an overdose of Vitamin A.

■ *Symptoms of ORAL Tazorac include:*
Abdominal pain, dizziness, dry or cracked lips, facial flushing, headache, lack of coordination and clumsiness, vomiting

Brand name:

TEGRETOL

Pronounced: TEG-re-tawl
Generic name: Carbamazepine
Other brand names: Atretol, Epitol, Tegretol-XR

Why is this drug prescribed?

Tegretol is used in the treatment of seizure disorders, including certain types of epilepsy. It is also prescribed for trigeminal neuralgia (severe pain in the jaws) and pain in the tongue and throat.

In addition, some doctors use Tegretol to treat alcohol withdrawal, cocaine addiction, and emotional disorders such as depression and abnormally aggressive behavior. The drug is also used to treat migraine headache and "restless legs."

Most important fact about this drug

There are potentially dangerous side effects associated with the use of Tegretol. If you experience symptoms such as fever, sore throat, rash, ulcers in the mouth, easy bruising, or reddish or purplish spots on the skin, you should notify your doctor immediately. These symptoms could be signs of a blood disorder brought on by the drug.

How should you take this medication?

This medication should only be taken with meals, never on an empty stomach.

Shake the suspension well before using.

Tegretol-XR (extended-release) tablets must be swallowed whole; do not crush or chew them and do not take tablets that have been damaged.

■ *If you miss a dose...*
Take it as soon as you remember. If it is almost time for your next dose, skip the one you missed and go back to your regular schedule. Do not take 2 doses at once. If you miss more than 1 dose in a day, check with your doctor.

■ *Storage instructions...*
Store Tegretol at room temperature. Keep the container tightly closed. Protect the tablets from light and moisture. Keep the liquid suspension away from light.

What side effects may occur?

Side effects cannot be anticipated. If any develop or change in intensity, inform your doctor as soon as possible. Only your doctor can determine if it is safe for you to continue taking Tegretol.

■ *More common side effects, especially at the start of treatment, may include:*
Dizziness, drowsiness, nausea, unsteadiness, vomiting

■ *Other side effects may include:*
Abdominal pain, abnormal heartbeat and rhythm, abnormal involuntary movements, abnormal sensitivity to sound, aching joints and muscles, agitation, anemia, blood clots, blurred vision, chills, confusion, congestive heart failure, constipation, depression, diarrhea, double vision, dry mouth and throat, fainting and collapse, fatigue, fever, fluid retention, frequent urination, hair loss, hallucinations, headache, hepatitis, hives, impotence, inability to urinate, inflammation of the mouth and tongue, inflamed eyes, involuntary movements of the eyeball, itching, kidney failure, labored breathing, leg cramps, liver disorders, loss of appetite, loss of coordination, low blood pressure, pancreatitis (inflammation of the pancreas), pneumonia, reddened skin, reddish or purplish spots on the skin, reduced urine volume, ringing in the ears, sensitivity to light, skin inflammation and scaling, skin peeling, skin rashes, skin pigmentation changes, speech difficulties, stomach problems, sweating, talkativeness, tingling sensation, worsening of high blood pressure, yellow eyes and skin

Why should this drug not be prescribed?
You should not use Tegretol if you have a history of bone marrow depression (reduced function), a sensitivity to Tegretol, or a sensitivity to tricyclic antidepressant drugs such as amitriptyline (Elavil). You should also not be taking Tegretol if you are on an MAO inhibitor antidepressant such as Nardil or Parnate, or if you have taken such a drug within the past 14 days.

Tegretol is not a simple pain reliever and should not be used for the relief of minor aches and pains.

Special warnings about this medication
If you have a history of heart, liver, or kidney damage, an adverse blood reaction to any drug, glaucoma, or serious reactions to other drugs, you should discuss this history thoroughly with your doctor before taking this medication.

Anticonvulsant drugs such as Tegretol should not be stopped abruptly if you are taking the medication to prevent major seizures. There exists the strong possibility of continuous epileptic attacks without return to consciousness, leading to possible severe brain damage and death. Only your doctor should determine if and when you should stop taking this medication.

Since dizziness and drowsiness may occur while taking Tegretol, you should refrain from operating machinery or driving an automobile or participating in any high-risk activity that requires full mental alertness until you know how this drug affects you.

Older adults, especially, can become confused or agitated when taking Tegretol.

In very rare cases, some people have had severe, even fatal, skin reactions to Tegretol. Contact your doctor at the first sign of a skin problem.

The coating of the Tegretol-XR tablet is not absorbed and passes through your body intact. If you notice it in your stool, it is not a cause for alarm.

Possible food and drug interactions
when taking this medication
The use of the antiseizure medications phenobarbital, phenytoin (Dilantin), or primidone (Mysoline) may reduce the effectiveness of Tegretol. Take other anticonvulsants along with Tegretol only if your doctor advises it. The use of Tegretol with other anticonvulsants may change thyroid gland function.

The following drugs may also reduce the effectiveness of Tegretol: cisplatin (Platinol), doxorubicin HCl (Adriamycin), felbamate (Felbatol), rifampin (Rifadin), and theophylline (Theo-Dur).

The effectiveness of acetaminophen (Tylenol), alprazolam (Xanax), clonazepam (Klonopin), clozapine (Clozaril), dicumarol, doxycycline (Doryx), ethosuximide (Zarontin), haloperidol (Haldol), methsuximide (Celontin), oral contraceptives, phensuximide (Milontin), phenytoin (Dilantin), theophylline (Theo-Dur), valproic acid (Depakene), and warfarin (Coumadin) may be reduced when these drugs are taken with Tegretol.

Tegretol may increase the effectiveness of clomipramine HCl (Anafranil), phenytoin, or primidone if the drugs are taken together.

All of the following drugs may raise the amount of Tegretol in the blood to harmful levels: cimetidine (Tagamet), clarithromycin (Biaxin), danazol (Danocrine), diltiazem (Cardizem), erythromycin (E-Mycin), fluoxetine (Prozac), isoniazid (Nydrazid), itraconazole (Sporanox), ketoconazole (Nizoral), loratadine (Claritin), niacinamide (Mega-B), nicotinamide (ILX B$_{12}$), propoxyphene (Darvon), terfenadine (Seldane), troleandomycin (Tao), valproate (Depakene), and calcium channel blockers such as Calan.

Lithium (Lithonate) used with Tegretol may cause harmful nervous system side effects.

If you are taking an oral contraceptive and Tegretol, you may experience blood spotting and your contraceptive may not be completely reliable.

Do not combine Tegretol suspension with other liquid medications such as Thorazine solution or Mellaril liquid. The mixture may congeal internally.

Special information
if you are pregnant or breastfeeding

There are no adequate safety studies regarding the use of Tegretol in pregnant women. However, there have been reports of birth defects in infants. Therefore, this medication should be used during pregnancy only if the potential benefits justify the potential risk to the fetus. If you are pregnant or plan on becoming pregnant, you should discuss this with your doctor.

Tegretol appears in breast milk. If you are breastfeeding, your doctor may advise you to discontinue doing so if taking Tegretol is essential to your health.

Recommended dosage

ADULTS

Seizures

The usual dose for adults and children over 12 years of age is 200 milligrams (1 tablet or 2 chewable or extended-release tablets) taken twice daily or 1 teaspoon 4 times a day. Your doctor may increase the dose at weekly intervals by adding 200-milligram doses twice a day for Tegretol-XR or 3 or 4 times per day for the other forms. Dosage should generally not exceed 1,000 milligrams daily in children 12 to 15 years old and 1,200 milligrams daily for adults and children over 15. The usual daily maintenance dosage range is 800 to 1,200 milligrams.

Trigeminal Neuralgia

The usual dose is 100 milligrams (1 chewable or extended-release tablet) twice or one-half teaspoon 4 times on the first day. Your doctor may increase this dose using increments of 100 milligrams every 12 hours or one-half teaspoonful 4 times daily only as needed to achieve freedom from pain. Doses should not exceed 1,200 milligrams daily and are usually in the range of 400 to 800 milligrams a day for maintenance.

CHILDREN

Seizures

The usual dose for children 6 to 12 years old is 100 milligrams twice daily or one-half teaspoon 4 times a day. Your doctor may increase the dose at weekly intervals by adding 100 milligrams twice a day for Tegretol-XR, 3 or

4 times a day for the other forms. Total daily dosage should generally not exceed 1,000 milligrams. The usual daily dosage range for maintenance is 400 to 800 milligrams.

The usual daily starting dose for children under 6 years of age is 10 to 20 milligrams per 2.2 pounds of body weight. The total daily dose is divided into smaller doses taken 2 or 3 times a day for tablets or 4 times a day for suspension. Daily dosage should not exceed 35 milligrams per 2.2 pounds.

OLDER ADULTS

To help determine the ideal dosage, your doctor may decide to periodically check the level of Tegretol in your blood.

Overdosage

Any medication taken in excess can have serious consequences. If you suspect an overdose, seek medical attention immediately. The first signs and symptoms of an overdose of Tegretol appear after 1 to 3 hours.

■ *The most prominent signs of a Tegretol overdose include:*
Coma, convulsions, dizziness, drowsiness, inability to urinate, involuntary rapid eye movements, irregular or reduced breathing, lack or absence of urine, lack of coordination, low or high blood pressure, muscular twitching, nausea, pupil dilation, rapid heartbeat, restlessness, severe muscle spasm, shock, tremors, unconsciousness, vomiting, writhing movements

Generic name:

TEMAZEPAM

See Restoril, page 1111.

Brand name:

TEMOVATE

Pronounced: TIM-oh-vate
Generic name: Clobetasol propionate
Other brand name: Cormax

Why is this drug prescribed?

Temovate and Cormax relieve the itching and inflammation of moderate to severe skin conditions. The scalp application is used for short-term treatment of scalp conditions; the cream, ointment, emollient cream, and gel are used for short-term treatment of skin conditions on the body. The products contain a steroid medication for external use only.

Most important fact about this drug

When you use Temovate, you inevitably absorb some of the medication through your skin and into the bloodstream. Too much absorption can lead to unwanted side effects elsewhere in the body. To keep this problem to a minimum, avoid using large amounts of Temovate over large areas, and do not cover it with airtight dressings such as plastic wrap or adhesive bandages unless specifically told to by your doctor.

How should you use this medication?

Use Temovate exactly as directed. Do not use it more often or for a longer time than ordered. Remember to avoid covering or bandaging the affected area.

Temovate is for use only on the skin. Be careful to keep it out of your eyes. If the scalp application gets into your eyes, flush your eyes with a lot of water.

A thin layer of cream, ointment, or gel should be gently rubbed into the affected area.

Do not use the scalp application near an open flame.

- **If you miss a dose...**
  Apply it as soon as you remember. If it is almost time for the next dose, skip the one you missed and go back to your regular schedule.

- **Storage instructions...**
  Store at room temperature. Do not refrigerate the creams, gel, or scalp application.

What side effects may occur?

Side effects cannot be anticipated. If any develop or change in intensity, inform your doctor as soon as possible. Only your doctor can determine if it is safe for you to continue using Temovate. This medication is generally well tolerated when used for 2 weeks. However, some side effects have been reported at the affected area.

CREAMS, OINTMENT, GEL

- **Side effects are infrequent but may include:**
  Burning, cracking/fissuring, irritation, itching, numbness of fingers, patches, reddened skin, shrinking of the skin, stinging

SCALP APPLICATION

- *More frequent side effects may include:*
  Burning, stinging

- *Less frequent side effects may include:*
  Eye irritation, hair loss, headache, inflammation, itching, tenderness and/or tightness of the scalp

These additional side effects have been known to result from use of topical steroids and may be particularly apt to occur with airtight dressings or higher strength steroids: Acne, allergic skin inflammation, dryness, excessive hair growth, infection, inflammation around the mouth, loss of skin color, prickly heat, skin softening, streaking.

Why should this drug not be prescribed?
All forms of Temovate should be avoided if you are sensitive to or have ever had an allergic reaction to clobetasol propionate, other corticosteroids such as Valisone and Topicort, or any of their ingredients. Do not use the scalp application if you have a scalp infection.

Special warnings about this medication
Temovate is a strong corticosteroid that can be absorbed into the bloodstream. It has caused Cushing's syndrome (a disorder characterized by a moon-shaped face, emotional disturbances, high blood pressure, weight gain, and, in women, abnormal growth of facial and body hair) and changes in blood sugar.

This medication should not be used for any condition other than the one for which it was prescribed.

If your skin becomes irritated, stop using the medication and call your doctor.

Temovate should not be used by children under 12 years of age.

Treatment should not last for more than 2 weeks.

Possible food and drug interactions
when using this medication
No interactions have been reported.

Special information
if you are pregnant or breastfeeding
Although Temovate is applied to the skin, there is no way of knowing how much medication is absorbed into the bloodstream. Strong corticosteroids have caused birth defects in animals. Temovate, a strong corticosteroid,

should be used only if the potential benefits outweigh the potential risks to the unborn baby; limit use to small amounts, on a limited area, for a short period of time. It is not known whether topical steroids are absorbed in sufficient amounts to appear in breast milk. If Temovate is essential to your health, your doctor may advise you to stop breastfeeding until your treatment with the medication is finished.

Recommended dosage

ADULTS AND CHILDREN 12 YEARS AND OLDER

Apply the medication to the affected area 2 times a day, once in the morning and once at night. Treatment should not last for more than 2 consecutive weeks, and the affected area should not be covered with a bandage. No more than 50 grams or 50 milliliters per week (approximately one large tube or bottle) should be used.

Overdosage

When absorbed into the bloodstream over a prolonged period, Temovate can cause disorders such as Cushing's syndrome. If you suspect an overdose of Temovate, seek medical attention immediately.

Brand name:

TENEX

Pronounced: TEN-ex
Generic name: Guanfacine hydrochloride

Why is this drug prescribed?

Tenex is given to help control high blood pressure. This medication reduces nerve impulses to the heart and arteries; this slows the heartbeat, relaxes the blood vessels, and thus reduces blood pressure. Tenex may be given alone or in combination with other high blood pressure medications, especially thiazide diuretics, such as Diuril, Esidrix, or Naturetin.

Most important fact about this drug

You must take Tenex regularly for it to be effective. Since blood pressure declines gradually, it may be several weeks before you get the full benefit of Tenex; and you must continue taking it even if you are feeling well. Tenex does not cure high blood pressure; it merely keeps it under control.

How should you take this medication?

Take Tenex exactly as prescribed by your doctor—usually 1 dose per day. Tenex should be taken at bedtime, since it will probably cause drowsiness.

After 3 or 4 weeks, if your blood pressure is still too high, your doctor may raise the dosage of Tenex. In some cases, you may take 2 evenly spaced doses per day rather than a single dose at bedtime.

■ *If you miss a dose...*
Take the forgotten dose as soon as you remember. This will help to keep the proper amount of medicine in your body. However, if it is almost time for the next dose, skip the one you missed and go back to your regular schedule. Never try to "catch up" by doubling the dose. If you miss taking Tenex for 2 or more days in a row, check with your doctor.

■ *Storage instructions...*
Store Tenex at room temperature. Use the container it came in.

What side effects may occur?
Side effects cannot be anticipated. If any develop or change in intensity, inform your doctor as soon as possible. Only your doctor can determine whether it is safe for you to continue taking Tenex. This medication will probably make you drowsy, especially when you first begin to take it.

■ *More common side effects may include:*
Constipation, dizziness, dry mouth, fatigue, headache, impotence, sleepiness, weakness

■ *Less common or rare side effects may include:*
Abdominal pain, amnesia, breathing difficulties, chest pain, confusion, conjunctivitis (red, puffy eyes), decreased sex drive, depression, diarrhea, difficulty swallowing, fainting, heart palpitations, indigestion, insomnia, itching, leg cramps, malaise (vague feeling of being sick), nausea, numbness or tingling of the skin, purplish spots on the skin, rash and peeling, ringing in the ears, "runny" nose, skin inflammation, slow heartbeat, stuffy nose, sweating, taste alterations, upset stomach, urinary incontinence, vision disturbance

Some of these side effects may lessen or disappear as your body gets used to Tenex.

Why should this drug not be prescribed?
Do not take Tenex if you are sensitive to it or have ever had an allergic reaction to it.

Tenex is not recommended for controlling the severe high blood pressure that accompanies toxemia of pregnancy (a disorder of pregnant women characterized by a rise in blood pressure, swelling, and leakage of protein into urine).

Special warnings about this medication

While taking Tenex, you should be monitored very closely by your doctor if you have any of the following medical conditions:

Chronic kidney or liver failure
Heart disease
History of stroke
Recent heart attack

Since Tenex causes drowsiness and may also make you dizzy, do not drive, climb, or perform hazardous tasks until you find out exactly how the medication affects you.

While taking Tenex, use alcoholic beverages with care; you may feel intoxicated after drinking only a small amount of alcohol.

If you have kidney damage and also take the antiseizure drug phenytoin (Dilantin), your body may process and eliminate Tenex rather quickly; in that case, you may need fairly frequent doses of Tenex to lower your blood pressure adequately.

If you have been taking Tenex for a while, do not stop taking it without consulting your doctor. Discontinuing abruptly may result in nervousness, rapid pulse, anxiety, heartbeat irregularities, and so-called rebound high blood pressure (higher than before you started taking Tenex). If you do have rebound high blood pressure, it will probably develop 2 to 4 days after your last dose of Tenex. Rebound high blood pressure, if it occurs, will usually diminish and then disappear over a period of 2 to 4 days.

Possible food and drug interactions
when taking this medication

If Tenex is taken with certain other drugs, the effects of either could be increased, decreased, or altered. It is especially important to check with your doctor before combining Tenex with the following:

Barbiturates such as Amytal, Seconal, Tuinal, and others
Benzodiazepines such as Tranxene, Valium, Xanax, and others
Phenothiazines such as Mellaril, Stelazine, Thorazine, and others
Phenytoin (Dilantin)

Special information
if you are pregnant or breastfeeding

If you are pregnant or plan to become pregnant, notify your doctor immediately. Tenex should be taken during pregnancy only if clearly needed.

It is not known whether Tenex appears in breast milk. Check with your doctor if you plan to breastfeed.

Recommended dosage

ADULTS

The usual recommended dose of Tenex is 1 milligram daily, taken at bedtime. If necessary, after 3 to 4 weeks your doctor may increase the daily dosage to 2 milligrams.

CHILDREN

The safety and effectiveness of Tenex have not been established in children under 12 years of age.

Overdosage

Any medication taken in excess can have serious consequences. If you suspect an overdose of Tenex, seek medical attention immediately.

- *Symptoms of Tenex overdose may include:*
  Drowsiness, lethargy, slowed heartbeat, very low blood pressure

Brand name:

TENORETIC

Pronounced: Ten-or-ET-ic
Generic ingredients: Atenolol, Chlorthalidone

Why is this drug prescribed?

Tenoretic is used in the treatment of high blood pressure. It combines a beta-blocker drug and a diuretic. Tenoretic can be used alone or in combination with other high blood pressure medications. Atenolol, the beta blocker, decreases the force and rate of heart contractions. Chlorthalidone, the diuretic, helps your body produce and eliminate more urine, which helps in lowering blood pressure.

Most important fact about this drug

You must take Tenoretic regularly for it to be effective. Since blood pressure declines gradually, it may be several weeks before you get the full benefit of Tenoretic; and you must continue taking it even if you are feeling well. Tenoretic does not cure high blood pressure; it merely keeps it under control.

How should you take this medication?

Tenoretic can be taken with or without food.

Take this medication exactly as prescribed by your doctor, even if your symptoms have disappeared.

Try not to miss any doses. If this medication is not taken regularly, your condition may worsen.

- *If you miss a dose...*
  Take the forgotten dose as soon as you remember. If it's within 8 hours of your next scheduled dose, skip the one you missed and go back to your regular schedule. Never take two doses at the same time.

- *Storage instructions...*
  Store Tenoretic at room temperature in the container it came in.

What side effects may occur?

Side effects cannot be anticipated. If any develop or change in intensity, inform your doctor as soon as possible. Only your doctor can determine if it is safe for you to continue taking Tenoretic.

- *More common side effects may include:*
  Dizziness, fatigue, nausea, slow heartbeat

- *Less common or rare side effects may include:*
  Blood disorders, constipation, cramping, decreased sexual ability, depression, diarrhea, difficult or labored breathing, dizziness when getting up, drowsiness, excessive thirst, hair loss, headache, high blood sugar, hives, impotence, light-headedness, loss of appetite, low potassium leading to symptoms like dry mouth, muscle pain or cramps, muscle spasm, Peyronie's disease (deformity of the penis), psoriasis-like rash, rash, reddish or purplish spots on skin, restlessness, skin sensitivity to light, sluggishness or unresponsiveness, stomach irritation, sugar in the urine, tingling or pins and needles, tiredness, vertigo, visual disturbances, vomiting, weak or irregular heartbeat, weakness, worsening of psoriasis, yellow eyes and skin

Why should this drug not be prescribed?

If you have a slow heartbeat; a history of serious heart block (conduction disorder); inadequate blood supply to the circulatory system (cardiogenic shock); heart failure; or inability to urinate; or if you are sensitive to or have ever had an allergic reaction to Tenoretic, its ingredients or similar drugs, or to other sulfonamide-derived drugs, you should not take this medication.

Special warnings about this medication

If you have a history of congestive heart failure or certain other heart problems, Tenoretic should be used with caution.

Tenoretic should not be stopped suddenly. It can cause increased chest pain and heart attack. When stopping the drug, your physician will gradually reduce your dosage.

When taking Tenoretic, if you suffer from asthma, seasonal allergies or other bronchial conditions, or liver or kidney disease, your doctor should monitor you more carefully.

Ask your doctor if you should check your pulse while taking Tenoretic. This medication can cause your heartbeat to become too slow.

This medication may mask the symptoms of low blood sugar or alter blood sugar levels. If you are diabetic, discuss this with your doctor.

Tenoretic can cause you to become drowsy or less alert; therefore, activity that requires full mental alertness is not recommended until you know how you respond to the drug.

Make sure the doctor knows that you are taking Tenoretic if you have a medical emergency, or plan to have surgery.

Possible food and drug interactions
when taking this medication

If Tenoretic is taken with certain other drugs, the effects of either could be increased, decreased, or altered. It is especially important to check with your doctor before combining Tenoretic with the following:

Blood pressure medicines containing reserpine
Other blood pressure drugs
Clonidine (Catapres)
Diltiazem (Cardizem)
Epinephrine (EpiPen)
Insulin
Lithium (Eskalith)
Nasal decongestants
Verapamil (Calan)

Special information
if you are pregnant or breastfeeding

When taken during pregnancy, Tenoretic may cause harm to the developing baby. If you are pregnant, or plan to become pregnant, inform your doctor immediately. Tenoretic appears in breast milk and could affect a nursing infant. If this medication is essential to your health, your doctor may advise you to discontinue breastfeeding until your treatment with this medication is finished.

Recommended dosage

ADULTS

Dosage is always individualized.

The usual starting dosage is 1 Tenoretic 50 tablet taken once a day. Your doctor may increase the dosage to 1 Tenoretic 100 tablet taken once a day. Your doctor may gradually add other high blood pressure medications.

Your doctor will adjust your dosage if your kidney function is impaired.

CHILDREN

The safety and effectiveness of Tenoretic have not been established in children.

Overdosage

Any medication taken in excess can have serious consequences. If you suspect an overdose, seek medical attention immediately.

■ *No specific information on Tenoretic is available, but common symptoms of overdose with the drug's atenolol component are:*

Congestive heart failure, constricted airways, low blood pressure, low blood sugar, slow heartbeat, sluggishness, wheezing

■ *Symptoms of overdose with the chlorthalidone component include:*
Dizziness, nausea, weakness

Brand name:

TENORMIN

Pronounced: Ten-OR-min
Generic name: Atenolol

Why is this drug prescribed?

Tenormin, a type of medication known as a beta blocker, is used in the treatment of high blood pressure, angina pectoris (chest pain, usually caused by lack of oxygen in the heart muscle due to clogged arteries), and heart attack. When used for high blood pressure it is effective alone or combined with other high blood pressure medications, particularly with a thiazide-type water pill (diuretic). Beta blockers decrease the force and rate of heart contractions.

Occasionally doctors prescribe Tenormin for treatment of alcohol withdrawal, prevention of migraine headache, and bouts of anxiety.

Most important fact about this drug

If you have high blood pressure, you must take Tenormin regularly for it to be effective. Since blood pressure declines gradually, it may be several weeks before you get the full benefit of Tenormin; and you must continue taking it even if you are feeling well. Tenormin does not cure high blood pressure; it merely keeps it under control.

How should you take this medication?

Tenormin can be taken with or without food. Take it exactly as prescribed, even if your symptoms have disappeared.

Try not to miss any doses, especially if you are taking Tenormin once a day. If this medication is not taken regularly, your condition may worsen.

■ *If you miss a dose...*
Take the forgotten dose as soon as you remember. If it's within 8 hours of your next scheduled dose, skip the one you missed and go back to your regular schedule. Never take 2 doses at the same time.

■ *Storage instructions...*
Store Tenormin at room temperature; protect from light.

What side effects may occur?

Side effects cannot be anticipated. If any develop or change in intensity, inform your doctor as soon as possible. Only your doctor can determine if it is safe for you to continue taking Tenormin.

■ *More common side effects may include:*
Dizziness, fatigue, nausea, slow heartbeat

■ *Less common or rare side effects may include:*
Depression, diarrhea, difficult or labored breathing, dizziness upon standing up, drowsiness, headache, heart failure, impotence, light-headedness, low blood pressure, penile deformity, psoriasis-like rash, red or purple spots on

the skin, rapid heartbeat, slow heartbeat, sluggishness, temporary hair loss, tiredness, vertigo, wheezing, worsening of psoriasis

Why should this drug not be prescribed?
If you have heart failure, inadequate blood supply to the circulatory system (cardiogenic shock), heart block (conduction disorder), or a severely slow heartbeat, you should not take this medication.

Special warnings about this medication
If you have a history of severe congestive heart failure, Tenormin should be used with caution.

Tenormin should not be stopped suddenly. It can cause increased chest pain and heart attack. Dosage should be gradually reduced.

If you suffer from asthma, seasonal allergies, or other bronchial conditions, coronary artery disease or kidney disease, this medication should be used with caution.

Ask your doctor if you should check your pulse while taking Tenormin. This medication can cause your heartbeat to become too slow.

This medication may mask the symptoms of low blood sugar or alter blood sugar levels. If you are diabetic, discuss this with your doctor.

Notify your doctor or dentist that you are taking Tenormin if you have a medical emergency, and before you have surgery or dental surgery.

Tenormin may cause harm to a developing baby when taken during pregnancy. If you are pregnant or become pregnant while taking this medication, inform your doctor immediately.

Possible food and drug interactions
when taking this medication
If Tenormin is taken with certain other drugs, the effects of either could be increased, decreased, or altered. It is especially important to check with your doctor before combining Tenormin with the following:

Ampicillin (Omnipen, others)
Calcium-blocking blood pressure drugs such as Calan and Cardizem
Calcium-containing antacids such as Tums
Certain other blood pressure drugs such as reserpine (Diupres)
Clonidine (Catapres)
Epinephrine (EpiPen)
Insulin
Oral diabetes drugs such as Micronase
Quinidine (Quinidex)

Special information
if you are pregnant or breastfeeding

The use of Tenormin during pregnancy may cause harm to a developing baby. If you are pregnant, become pregnant, or plan to become pregnant, inform your doctor immediately. Tenormin appears in breast milk and could affect a nursing infant. If this medication is essential to your health, your doctor may advise you to discontinue breastfeeding until your treatment is finished.

Recommended dosage

ADULTS

Hypertension

The usual starting dose is 50 milligrams a day in 1 dose, alone or with a diuretic. Full effects should be seen in 1 to 2 weeks. Dosage may be increased to a maximum of 100 milligrams per day in one dose. Your doctor can and may use this medication with other high blood pressure medications.

Angina Pectoris

The usual starting dose is 50 milligrams in 1 dose a day. Full effects should be seen in 1 week. Dosage may be increased to a maximum of 100 milligrams per day. In some cases, a single dose of 200 milligrams per day may be given. Dosage will be individualized by your doctor.

Heart Attack

This medication may be used in the acute treatment of heart attack in both injectable and tablet form. Your doctor will determine the proper dosage.

CHILDREN

The safety and effectiveness of Tenormin have not been established in children.

OLDER ADULTS

The doctor will determine the dosage for an older individual, according to his or her needs, especially in the case of reduced kidney function.

Overdosage

Any medication taken in excess can have serious consequences. If you suspect an overdose, seek medical attention immediately.

■ *Symptoms of Tenormin overdose may include:*
   Congestive heart failure, constricted airways, low blood pressure, low blood sugar, slow heartbeat, sluggishness, wheezing

Brand name:

TENUATE

Pronounced: TEN-you-ate
Generic name: Diethylpropion hydrochloride

Why is this drug prescribed?
Tenuate, an appetite suppressant, is prescribed for short-term use (a few weeks) as part of an overall diet plan for weight reduction. It is available in two forms: immediate-release tablets (Tenuate) and controlled-release tablets (Tenuate Dospan). Tenuate should be used with a behavior modification program.

Most important fact about this drug
Tenuate will lose its effectiveness within a few weeks. When this begins to happen, you should discontinue the medicine rather than increase the dosage.

How should you take this medication?
Take this medication exactly as prescribed. Tenuate may be habit-forming and can be addicting.

If you are taking Tenuate Dospan (the controlled release formulation), do not crush or chew the tablets. Swallow the medication whole.

- *If you miss a dose...*
  If you are taking the immediate-release form of Tenuate, go back to your regular schedule at the next meal.

  If you are taking Tenuate Dospan, take the missed dose as soon as you remember. If you do not remember until the next day, skip the dose. Never take 2 doses at once.

- *Storage instructions...*
  Store at room temperature in a tightly closed container. Protect from excessive heat.

What side effects may occur?
Side effects cannot be anticipated. If any develop or change in intensity, inform your doctor as soon as possible. Only your doctor can determine if it is safe for you to continue using Tenuate.

- *Side effects may include:*
  Abdominal discomfort, abnormal redness of the skin, anxiety, blood pressure elevation, blurred vision, breast development in males, bruising,

changes in sex drive, chest pain, constipation, depression, diarrhea, difficulty with voluntary movements, dizziness, drowsiness, dryness of the mouth, feelings of discomfort, feelings of elation, feeling of illness, hair loss, headache, hives, impotence, inability to fall or stay asleep, increased heart rate, increased seizures in epileptics, increased sweating, increased volume of diluted urine, irregular heartbeat, jitteriness, menstrual upset, muscle pain, nausea, nervousness, overstimulation, painful urination, palpitations, pupil dilation, rash, restlessness, shortness of breath or labored breathing, stomach and intestinal disturbances, tremors, unpleasant taste, vomiting

Why should this drug not be prescribed?
If you are sensitive to or have ever had an allergic reaction to Tenuate or other appetite suppressants, you should not take this medication. Make sure your doctor is aware of any drug reactions you have experienced.

Do not take this drug if you have severe hardening of the arteries, an overactive thyroid, glaucoma, or severe high blood pressure, or if you are agitated, have a history of drug abuse or are taking an MAO inhibitor (antidepressant drug such as Nardil) or have taken one within the last 14 days.

Special warnings about this medication
Tenuate or Tenuate Dospan may impair your ability to engage in potentially hazardous activities. Therefore, make sure you know how you react to this medication before you drive, operate dangerous machinery, or do anything else that requires alertness or concentration.

If you have heart disease or high blood pressure, use caution when taking this medication.

This drug may increase convulsions in some epileptics. Your doctor should monitor you carefully if you have epilepsy.

Psychological dependence has occurred while taking this drug. Talk with your doctor if you find you are relying on this drug to maintain a state of well-being.

The abrupt withdrawal of this medication following prolonged use at high doses may result in extreme fatigue, mental depression, and sleep disturbances.

Possible food and drug interactions
when taking this medication
Tenuate or Tenuate Dospan may interact with alcohol unfavorably. Do not drink alcohol while taking this medication.

If Tenuate or Tenuate Dospan is taken with certain other drugs, the effects of either could be increased, decreased, or altered. It is especially important that you consult your doctor before combining Tenuate with the following:

Blood pressure medications such as Ismelin
Insulin
Phenothiazine drugs such as the major tranquilizer Thorazine

Special information
if you are pregnant or breastfeeding
The effects of Tenuate or Tenuate Dospan during pregnancy have not been adequately studied. If you are pregnant or plan to become pregnant, inform your doctor immediately. This drug appears in breast milk. If the medication is essential to your health, your doctor may advise you to discontinue breastfeeding until your treatment is finished.

Recommended dosage

ADULTS

Tenuate Immediate-Release
The usual dosage is one 25-milligram tablet taken 3 times a day, 1 hour before meals; you may take 1 tablet in the middle of the evening, if you want, to overcome night hunger.

Tenuate Dospan Controlled-Release
The usual dosage is one 75-milligram tablet taken once daily, swallowed whole, in midmorning.

CHILDREN

Safety and effectiveness have not been established in children below 12 years of age.

Overdosage
Any medication taken in excess can have serious consequences. If you suspect an overdose, seek emergency medical treatment immediately.

■ *Symptoms of Tenuate overdose may include:*
Abdominal cramps, assaultiveness, confusion, depression, diarrhea, elevated blood pressure, fatigue, hallucinations, irregular heartbeat, lowered blood pressure, nausea, overreactive reflexes, panic state, rapid breathing, restlessness, tremors, vomiting

Brand name:

TERAZOL

Pronounced: TER-uh-zawl
Generic name: Terconazole

Why is this drug prescribed?

Terazol is prescribed to treat candidiasis (a yeast-like fungal infection) of the vulva and vagina.

Most important fact about this drug

Keep using Terazol for the full time of treatment, even if the infection seems to have disappeared. If you stop too soon, the infection could return. You should continue using this medicine during your menstrual period.

How should you use this medication?

Follow these steps to apply Terazol:

1. Load the applicator to the fill line with cream, or unwrap a suppository, wet it with warm water, and place it in the applicator as shown in the instructions you received with the product.
2. Lie on your back with knees drawn up.
3. Gently insert the applicator high into the vagina and push the plunger.
4. Withdraw the applicator and wash it with soap and water.

To protect your clothing, wear a sanitary napkin. Do not use tampons because they will absorb the medicine. Wear cotton underwear—avoid synthetic fabrics such as rayon or nylon. Do not douche unless your doctor tells you to do so.

Dry the genital area thoroughly after a shower, bath, or swim. Change out of a wet bathing suit or damp workout clothes as soon as possible. Moisture encourages the growth of yeast.

Try not to scratch. It can cause more irritation and can spread the infection.

■ *If you miss a dose...*
Apply it as soon as you remember. If it is almost time for your next dose, skip the one you missed and go back to your regular schedule.

■ *Storage instructions...*
Store at room temperature.

What side effects may occur?

Side effects cannot be anticipated. If any develop or change in intensity,

inform your doctor as soon as possible. Only your doctor can determine if it is safe for you to continue using Terazol.

■ *More common side effects may include:*
Abdominal pain, body pain, burning, genital pain or irritation, headache, menstrual pain

■ *Less common side effects may include:*
Chills, fever, itching

Why should this drug not be prescribed?
If you have ever had an allergic reaction to or are sensitive to terconazole or any other ingredients of Terazol, you should not use this medication. Make sure your doctor is aware of any drug reactions you have experienced.

Special warnings about this medication
If irritation, an allergic reaction, fever, chills, or flu-like symptoms develop while using this medication, notify your doctor.

To avoid re-infection while using Terazol, either avoid sexual intercourse or make sure your partner uses a non-latex condom.

Terazol 3 suppositories can interact with latex products such as diaphragms and certain types of condoms. Use some other method of birth control while you are using Terazol.

Possible food and drug interactions when taking this medication
No interactions have been reported.

Special information if you are pregnant or breastfeeding
Since Terazol is absorbed from the vagina, it should not be used during the first trimester (first 3 months) of pregnancy unless your doctor considers it essential to your health. It is not known whether this drug appears in breast milk. Your doctor may advise you to discontinue breastfeeding your baby while using this medication.

Recommended dosage

ADULTS

Terazol 3 and Terazol 7 Vaginal Cream
The recommended dose is 1 full applicator (5 grams) of cream inserted into the vagina once daily at bedtime. Apply Terazol 3 for 3 consecutive days; apply Terazol 7 for 7.

Terazol 3 Vaginal Suppositories
The recommended dose is 1 suppository inserted into the vagina once daily
at bedtime for 3 consecutive days.

CHILDREN

Safety and effectiveness have not been established in children.

Overdosage

There has been no reported overdose of this medication. Any medication
used in excess, however, can have serious consequences. If you suspect an
overdose of Terazol, seek medical attention immediately.

Generic name:

TERAZOSIN

See Hytrin, page 609.

Generic name:

TERBUTALINE

See Brethine, page 169.

Generic name:

TERCONAZOLE

See Terazol, page 1285.

Brand name:

TESSALON

Pronounced: TESS-ah-lon
Generic name: Benzonatate

Why is this drug prescribed?

Tessalon is taken for relief of a cough.

Most important fact about this drug

Tessalon should be swallowed whole, not chewed.

How should you take this medication?

Tessalon perles (soft capsule form) should be swallowed whole. If chewed, they can produce a temporary numbness of the mouth and throat that could cause choking or a severe allergic reaction.

■ *If you miss a dose...*
Take the forgotten dose as soon as you remember. If it is almost time for your next dose, skip the one you missed and go back to your regular schedule. Never double the dose.

■ *Storage instructions...*
Store Tessalon at room temperature.

What side effects may occur?

Side effects cannot be anticipated. If any occur or change in intensity, inform your doctor as soon as possible. Only your doctor can determine if it is safe to continue taking Tessalon.

■ *Side effects may include:*
Allergic reactions, burning sensation in the eyes, constipation, dizziness, extreme calm (sedation), headache, itching, mental confusion, nausea, numbness in chest, skin eruptions, stuffy nose, upset stomach, vague "chilly" feeling, visual hallucinations

Why should this drug not be prescribed?

Tessalon should not be used if you are sensitive to or have ever had an allergic reaction to benzonatate or similar drugs (such as local anesthetics).

Special warnings about this medication

Remember to swallow Tessalon perles whole.

Possible food and drug interactions
when taking this medication

There have been rare occurrences of bizarre behavior, including confusion and visual hallucinations, when Tessalon is taken with other prescribed drugs. Check with your doctor before taking Tessalon with other medications.

Special information
if you are pregnant or breastfeeding

The effects of Tessalon during pregnancy have not been studied adequately. Tessalon should be used during pregnancy only if clearly needed. If you are pregnant or plan to become pregnant, notify your doctor immediately. It is unknown if Tessalon appears in breast milk and could affect a nursing infant. If this medication is essential to your health, your doctor may advise you to stop breastfeeding until your treatment with Tessalon ends.

Recommended dosage

CHILDREN OVER AGE 10 AND ADULTS

The usual dose is a 100-milligram perle 3 times per day, as needed. The maximum dose is 600 milligrams, or 6 perles, a day.

Overdosage

If capsules are chewed or allowed to dissolve in the mouth, numbness of the mouth and throat will develop rapidly. Symptoms of restlessness and tremors may be followed by convulsions.

If you suspect a Tessalon overdose, seek medical attention immediately.

Generic name:

TETRACYCLINE

Pronounced: TET-ra-SY-clin
Brand name: Achromycin V, Sumycin

Why is this drug prescribed?

Tetracycline, a "broad-spectrum" antibiotic, is used to treat bacterial infections such as Rocky Mountain spotted fever, typhus fever, and tick fevers; upper respiratory infections; pneumonia; gonorrhea; amoebic infections; and urinary tract infections. It is also used to help treat severe acne and to treat trachoma (a chronic eye infection) and conjunctivitis (pinkeye). Tetracycline is often an alternative drug for people who are allergic to penicillin.

Most important fact about this drug

Tetracycline should not be used during the last half of pregnancy or in children under the age of 8. It may damage developing teeth and cause permanent discoloration.

How should you take this medication?

Tetracycline should be taken exactly as prescribed by your doctor. Be sure to use the entire prescription. If you are taking a liquid form of the drug, shake well before using.

Do not use outdated tetracycline. Outdated tetracycline is highly toxic to the kidneys.

Do not take antacids containing aluminum, calcium, or magnesium (e.g., Mylanta, Maalox) while taking this medication. They will affect the absorption of the drug.

Take tetracycline 1 hour before or 2 hours after meals. Foods, milk, and some other dairy products affect absorption of the drug.

Tetracycline should be continued for at least 24 to 48 hours after your symptoms have subsided.

■ *If you miss a dose...*
Take it as soon as you remember. If it is almost time for your next dose and you take tetracycline once a day (e.g., for acne), take the dose you missed, and then take the next one 10 to 12 hours later; if you take it twice a day, take the dose you missed, and then take the next one 5 to 6 hours later; if you take 3 or more doses a day, take the one you missed, and then take the next one 2 to 4 hours later. Then go back to your regular schedule.

■ *Storage instructions...*
Store capsules at room temperature. Keep the liquid form of tetracycline in the refrigerator, but do not allow it to freeze.

What side effects may occur?
Side effects cannot be anticipated. If any occur or change in intensity, inform your doctor as soon as possible. Only your doctor can determine if it is safe for you to continue taking tetracycline.

■ *More common side effects may include:*
Anemia, blood disorders, blurred vision and headache (in adults), bulging soft spot on the head (in infants), diarrhea, difficult or painful swallowing, dizziness, extreme allergic reactions, genital or anal sores or rash, hives, inflammation of large bowel, inflammation of the tongue, inflammation of the upper digestive tract, increased sensitivity to light, loss of appetite, nausea, rash, ringing in the ears, swelling due to fluid accumulation, vision disturbance, vomiting

■ *Less common or rare side effects may include:*
Inflamed skin, inflammation of the penis, liver poisoning, muscle weakness, peeling, skin eruptions, throat sores and inflammation

Why should this drug not be prescribed?
Do not take this medication if you are sensitive to or have ever had an allergic reaction to any tetracycline medication.

Special warnings about this medication
If you have kidney disease, make sure the doctor knows about it. A lower than usual dose of tetracycline may be needed.

Tetracycline drugs can make you more prone to sunburn when you are in sunlight or ultraviolet light. Take appropriate precautions.

Some adults may develop a headache and blurred vision while taking tetracycline, and infants may develop a bulging soft spot on the head. Contact your doctor if you experience or notice these symptoms. They usually disappear soon after the medication is stopped.

As with other antibiotics, use of this medication may cause other infections to develop. Contact your doctor if this occurs.

If you are taking tetracycline over an extended period of time, your doctor will perform blood, kidney, and liver tests periodically.

Possible food and drug interactions
when taking this medication
If tetracycline is taken with certain other drugs, the effects of either could be increased, decreased, or altered. It is especially important to check with your doctor before combining tetracycline with the following:

> Antacids containing aluminum, calcium, or magnesium, such as Mylanta and Maalox
> Blood thinners such as Coumadin
> Oral contraceptives
> Penicillin (Amoxil, Pen-Vee K, others)

Special information
if you are pregnant or breastfeeding
Tetracycline is not recommended for use during pregnancy. It can affect the development of the unborn child's bones and teeth. If you are pregnant or plan to become pregnant, inform your doctor immediately. Tetracycline appears in breast milk and may affect a nursing infant. If this medicine is essential to your health, your doctor may recommend that breastfeeding until your treatment is finished.

Recommended dosage

Your doctor will adjust your dose on the basis of the condition to be treated, your age, and risk factors such as kidney problems.

You should use this drug for at least 24 to 48 hours after symptoms and fever have subsided. For a streptococcal infection, doses should be taken for at least 10 days.

ADULTS

For most infections, the usual daily dose is 1 to 2 grams divided into 2 or 4 equal doses, depending on severity.

For Treatment of Brucellosis

The usual dose is 500 milligrams 4 times daily for 3 weeks; the drug should be accompanied by streptomycin.

For Treatment of Syphilis

You should take a total of 30 to 40 grams, divided into equal doses over a period of 10 to 15 days.

Gonorrhea patients sensitive to penicillin can take tetracycline, starting with 1.5 grams, followed by 0.5 gram every 6 hours for 4 days, to a total dosage of 9 grams.

For Urethral, Endocervical, or Rectal Infections in Adults Caused by Chlamydia Trachomatis

The usual dose is 500 milligrams, 4 times a day, for at least 7 days.

CHILDREN 8 YEARS OF AGE AND ABOVE

The usual daily dose is 10 to 20 milligrams per pound of body weight divided into 2 or 4 equal doses.

Overdosage

Any medication taken in excess can have serious consequences. Seek medical attention immediately if you suspect an overdose of tetracycline.

Brand name:

THALITONE

See Hygroton, page 605.

Brand name:

THEOCHRON

See Theo-Dur, below.

Brand name:

THEO-DUR

Pronounced: THEE-a-door
Generic name: Theophylline
Other brand names: Quibron-T/SR, Slo-bid, T-Phyl,
*   Theochron, Uni-Dur, Uniphyl*

Why is this drug prescribed?

Theo-Dur, an oral bronchodilator medication, is given to treat symptoms of asthma, chronic bronchitis, and emphysema. The active ingredient of Theo-Dur, theophylline, is a chemical cousin of caffeine. It opens the airways by relaxing the smooth muscle that circles the tubes and blood vessels in the lungs.

Most important fact about this drug

Theo-Dur is a controlled-release medication. For an acute attack you should take an immediate-release medication instead of more Theo-Dur. If you develop *status asthmaticus* (a severe breathing difficulty that does not clear up with your usual medications), do not take extra Theo-Dur; instead, seek medical treatment immediately. Since even a little extra Theo-Dur may constitute an overdose, you should be treated in a place where close monitoring is possible.

Individual doses are determined by a person's response (a decrease in symptoms of asthma). In order to avoid overdosing or underdosing, your doctor will perform regular tests to determine the amount of Theo-Dur in your bloodstream.

You should not change from Theo-Dur to another brand without first consulting your doctor or pharmacist. Products manufactured by different companies may not be equally effective.

How should you take this medication?

Take Theo-Dur exactly as prescribed. Do not change the dose, the time you take it, or how often you take it without consulting your doctor.

This drug is available in two forms. The extended-release tablets should be swallowed whole, not crushed or chewed. The tablets of some brands, including Theo-Dur, are scored; if the doctor prescribes a partial dosage, these tablets should be broken only at the score. You may take the tablets with or without food. If you are taking them on a once-a-day basis, do not take the dose at night.

The other form, Theo-Dur Sprinkle sustained-action capsules, must be taken either 1 hour before or 2 hours after a meal. You may take the capsule whole or open it and empty the contents onto a spoonful of food that is soft but not hot. Without chewing, immediately swallow the spoonful of food and follow it with a glass of cool water or juice. Always take the complete contents of the capsule.

When taking Theo-Dur, you should avoid large amounts of caffeine-containing beverages, such as tea or coffee.

■ *If you miss a dose...*
Take the next dose at the regular time. Do not try to make up the dose you missed.

■ *Storage instructions...*
Store at room temperature. Keep the container tightly closed. Protect from excessive heat, light, and moisture. Make sure this medicine is kept out of reach of children.

What side effects may occur?
Side effects from Theo-Dur cannot be anticipated. Nausea and restlessness may occur when you first start to take Theo-Dur, but will probably disappear as your body becomes used to the drug. If side effects persist, see your doctor; the dosage may be too high.

■ *Other side effects may include:*
Convulsions, diarrhea, disturbances of heart rhythm, excitability, frequent urination, hair loss, headache, heart palpitations, insomnia, irritability, muscle twitching, rash, severe seizures, tremors, vomiting

Why should this drug not be prescribed?
Do not take Theo-Dur if you have ever had an allergic reaction to it or similar drugs.

Do not take Theo-Dur if you have an active peptic ulcer or a seizure disorder such as epilepsy.

Special warnings about this medication
If you are a smoker, your body will tend to process and get rid of Theo-Dur rather quickly; thus, you may need to take more frequent doses than a

nonsmoker. Tell your doctor if you start or stop smoking. Even if you quit, the quick-clearance effect may linger for 6 months to 2 years.

You should take Theo-Dur cautiously and under close medical supervision if you are over age 60.

You should also take Theo-Dur cautiously and under close supervision if you have had a sustained high fever, or if you have heart disease, liver disease, heartbeat irregularities, fluid in the lungs, an underactive thyroid gland, the flu or another viral illness, or the symptoms of shock.

Call your doctor immediately if you develop nausea, vomiting, a lasting headache, insomnia, restlessness, or a too-rapid heartbeat; if you develop a new illness, especially with a fever; or if an illness you already have gets worse.

Possible food and drug interactions
when taking this medication

Theo-Dur interacts with a wide variety of drugs. Consult your doctor before combining any other medication with Theo-Dur. Let your doctor know whenever another doctor starts you on a new medication or stops an old one. Let every doctor you deal with know you are taking Theo-Dur.

Special information
if you are pregnant or breastfeeding

If you are pregnant or plan to become pregnant, inform your doctor immediately. Theo-Dur should not be taken during pregnancy unless it is clearly needed, and unless the benefits to the mother outweigh the potential risk to the developing child.

Theo-Dur does find its way into breast milk; it may make a nursing baby irritable or harm the baby in other ways. If you are a new mother, you will probably need to choose between breastfeeding and taking Theo-Dur.

Recommended dosage

ADULTS

Theo-Dur Extended Release Tablets

The usual initial dose is 1 Theo-Dur 150-milligram tablet every 12 hours. If this is not effective, your doctor will gradually increase the dose until you respond, up to a maximum of 600 milligrams per day. Once you have adjusted to the medication, your doctor may be able to put you on a once-a-day dose schedule.

Theo-Dur Sprinkle
The usual initial dose is no more than 200 milligrams every 12 hours. If this is not effective, your doctor will gradually increase the dose until you respond, up to a maximum of 900 milligrams per day. If a dose every 12 hours is inconvenient, your doctor may divide the daily total into 3 small doses taken every 8 hours.

CHILDREN AGED 6 to 16

Theo-Dur Extended Release Tablets
Maximum regular daily dosages are calculated by body weight as follows:

Less than 99 pounds—20 milligrams per 2.2 pounds up to a maximum of 600 milligrams
99 pounds or more—600 milligrams

Theo-Dur Sprinkle
For children under 55 pounds, a liquid preparation is recommended to establish proper dosage before switching to Theo-Dur Sprinkle. Maximum regular daily dosages are calculated by body weight as follows:

Children 6 through 8—24 milligrams per 2.2 pounds
Children 9 through 11—20 milligrams per 2.2 pounds
Children 12 through 15—18 milligrams per 2.2 pounds

OLDER ADULTS

Older adults are more likely than younger people to be seriously affected by Theo-Dur. Anyone over age 60 should not take more than 400 milligrams a day except in special circumstances.

Overdosage
Most of the symptoms listed in the "side effects" section are actually caused by slight overdosage.

Be aware that a flu shot, influenza itself, or another viral infection may make your usual dose of Theo-Dur act like an overdose. Consult your doctor if you anticipate getting a flu shot, or if you think you have the flu; you may need a temporary dosage reduction.

A mild overdose of Theo-Dur may cause nausea and restlessness. Taking too much over a long period of time may cause serious heartbeat irregularities, convulsions, or even death. If at any time you suspect symptoms of an overdose of Theo-Dur, seek medical attention immediately.

Generic name:

THEOPHYLLINE

See Theo-Dur, page 1293.

Brand name:

THERAGRAN

See Multivitamins, page 838.

Generic name:

THIORIDAZINE

See Mellaril, page 766.

Generic name:

THIOTHIXENE

See Navane, page 858.

Brand name:

THORAZINE

Pronounced: THOR-ah-zeen
Generic name: Chlorpromazine

Why is this drug prescribed?
Thorazine is used for the reduction of symptoms of psychotic disorders such as schizophrenia; for the short-term treatment of severe behavioral disorders in children, including explosive hyperactivity and combativeness; and for the hyperenergetic phase of manic-depressive illness (severely exaggerated moods).

Thorazine is also used to control nausea and vomiting, and to relieve restlessness and apprehension before surgery. It is used as an aid in the treatment of tetanus, and is prescribed for uncontrollable hiccups and acute intermittent porphyria (attacks of severe abdominal pain sometimes accompanied by psychiatric disturbances, cramps in the arms and legs, and muscle weakness).

Most important fact about this drug

Thorazine may cause tardive dyskinesia—a condition marked by involuntary muscle spasms and twitches in the face and body. This condition may be permanent, and appears to be most common among the elderly, especially women. Ask your doctor for information about this possible risk.

How should you take this medication?

If taking Thorazine in a liquid concentrate form, you will need to dilute it with a liquid such as a carbonated beverage, coffee, fruit juice, milk, tea, tomato juice, or water. Puddings, soups, and other semisolid foods may also be used. Thorazine will taste best if it is diluted immediately prior to use. You should not take Thorazine with alcohol.

Do not take antacids such as Gelusil at the same time as Thorazine. Leave at least 1 to 2 hours between doses of the two drugs.

■ *If you miss a dose...*
If you take Thorazine once a day, take the dose you missed as soon as you remember. If you do not remember until the next day, skip the dose, then go back to your regular schedule.

If you take more than 1 dose a day, take the one you missed as soon as you remember if it is within an hour or so of the scheduled time. If you do not remember until later, skip the dose, then go back to your regular schedule.

Never take 2 doses at once.

■ *Storage instructions...*
Store away from heat, light, and moisture. Do not freeze the liquid. Since the liquid concentrate form of Thorazine is light-sensitive, it should be stored in a dark place, but it does not need to be refrigerated.

What side effects may occur?

Side effects cannot be anticipated. If any develop or change in intensity, inform your doctor as soon as possible. Only your doctor can determine if it is safe for you to continue taking Thorazine.

■ *Side effects may include:*
Abnormal secretion of milk, abnormalities in movement and posture, agitation, anemia, asthma, blood disorders, breast development in males,

chewing movements, constipation, difficulty breathing, difficulty swallowing, dizziness, drooling, drowsiness, dry mouth, ejaculation problems, eye problems causing fixed gaze, fainting, fever, flu-like symptoms, fluid accumulation and swelling, headache, heart attack, high or low blood sugar, hives, impotence, inability to move or talk, inability to urinate, increase of appetite, infections, insomnia, intestinal blockage, involuntary movements of arms and legs, tongue, face, mouth, or jaw, irregular blood pressure, pulse, and heartbeat, irregular or no menstrual periods, jitteriness, light-headedness (on standing up), lockjaw, mask-like face, muscle stiffness and rigidity, narrow or dilated pupils, nasal congestion, nausea, pain and stiffness in the neck, persistent, painful erections, pill-rolling motion, protruding tongue, puckering of the mouth, puffing of the cheeks, rapid heartbeat, red or purple spots on the skin, rigid arms, feet, head, and muscles (including the back), seizures, sensitivity to light, severe allergic reactions, shuffling walk, skin inflammation and peeling, sore throat, spasms in jaw, face, tongue, neck, mouth, and feet, sweating, swelling of breasts in women, swelling of the throat, tremors, twitching in the body, neck, shoulders and face, twisted neck, visual problems, weight gain, yellowed skin and whites of eyes

Why should this drug not be prescribed?
You should not be using Thorazine if you are taking substances that slow down mental function such as alcohol, barbiturates, or narcotics.

You should not take Thorazine if you have ever had an allergic reaction to any major tranquilizer containing phenothiazine.

Special warnings about this medication
You should use Thorazine cautiously if you have ever had: asthma; a brain tumor; breast cancer; intestinal blockage; emphysema; the eye condition known as glaucoma; heart, kidney, or liver disease; respiratory infections; seizures; or an abnormal bone marrow or blood condition; or if you are exposed to pesticides or extreme heat. Be aware that Thorazine can mask symptoms of brain tumor, intestinal blockage, and the neurological condition called Reye's syndrome.

Stomach inflammation, dizziness, nausea, vomiting, and tremors may result if you suddenly stop taking Thorazine. Follow your doctor's instructions closely when discontinuing Thorazine.

Thorazine can suppress the cough reflex; you may have trouble vomiting.

This drug may impair your ability to drive a car or operate potentially dangerous machinery. Do not participate in any activities that require full alertness if you are unsure about your ability.

This drug can increase your sensitivity to light. Avoid being out in the sun too long.

Thorazine can cause a group of symptoms called Neuroleptic Malignant Syndrome, which can be fatal. Some symptoms are extremely high body temperature, rigid muscles, mental changes, irregular pulse or blood pressure, rapid heartbeat, sweating, and changes in heart rhythm.

If you are on Thorazine for prolonged therapy, you should see your doctor for regular evaluations, since side effects can get worse over time.

Possible food and drug interactions
when taking this medication

If Thorazine is taken with certain other drugs, the effects of either could be increased, decreased, or altered. It is especially important to check with your doctor before combining Thorazine with the following:

Anesthetics
Antacids such as Gelusil
Antiseizure drugs such as Dilantin
Antispasmodic drugs such as Cogentin
Atropine (Donnatal)
Barbiturates such as phenobarbital
Blood-thinning drugs such as Coumadin
Captopril (Capoten)
Cimetidine (Tagamet)
Diuretics such as Dyazide
Epinephrine (EpiPen)
Guanethidine (Ismelin)
Lithium (Lithobid, Eskalith)
MAO inhibitors (antidepressants such as Nardil and Parnate)
Narcotics such as Percocet
Propranolol (Inderal)

Extreme drowsiness and other potentially serious effects can result if Thorazine is combined with alcohol and other mental depressants such as narcotic painkillers like Demerol.

Because Thorazine prevents vomiting, it can hide the signs and symptoms of overdose of other drugs.

Special information
if you are pregnant or breastfeeding

The effects of Thorazine during pregnancy have not been adequately studied. If you are pregnant or plan to become pregnant, notify your doctor.

Pregnant women should use Thorazine only if clearly needed. Thorazine appears in breast milk and may affect a nursing infant. If this medication is essential to your health, your doctor may advise you not to breastfeed until your treatment is finished.

Recommended dosage

ADULTS

Psychotic Disorders
Your doctor will gradually increase the dosage until symptoms are controlled. You may not see full improvement for weeks or even months.

Initial dosages may range from 30 to 75 milligrams daily. The amount is divided into equal doses and taken 3 or 4 times a day. If needed, your doctor may increase the dosage by 20 to 50 milligrams at semiweekly intervals.

Nausea and Vomiting
The usual tablet dosage is 10 to 25 milligrams, taken every 4 or 6 hours, as needed.

One 100-milligram suppository can be used every 6 to 8 hours.

Uncontrollable Hiccups
Dosages may range from 75 to 200 milligrams daily, divided into 3 or 4 equal doses.

Acute Intermittent Porphyria
Dosages may range from 75 to 200 milligrams daily, divided into 3 or 4 equal doses.

CHILDREN

Thorazine is generally not prescribed for children younger than 6 months.

Severe Behavior Problems, Nausea, and Vomiting
Dosages are based on the child's weight.

Oral: The daily dose is one-quarter milligram for each pound of the child's weight, taken every 4 to 6 hours, as needed.

Rectal: the usual dose is one-half milligram per pound of body weight, taken every 6 to 8 hours, as necessary.

OLDER ADULTS

In general, older people take lower dosages of Thorazine, and any increase in dosage will be gradual. Because of a greater risk of low blood pressure, your doctor will watch you closely while you are taking Thorazine. Older people (especially older women) may be more susceptible to tardive dyskinesia—a possibly permanent condition characterized by involuntary muscle spasms and twitches in the face and body. Consult your doctor for information about these potential risks.

Overdosage

Any medication taken in excess can have serious consequences. An overdose of Thorazine can be fatal. If you suspect an overdose, seek medical help immediately.

- ■ *Symptoms of Thorazine overdose may include:*
  Agitation, coma, convulsions, difficulty breathing, difficulty swallowing, dry mouth, extreme sleepiness, fever, intestinal blockage, irregular heart rate, low blood pressure, restlessness

Generic name:

THYROID HORMONES

See Armour Thyroid, page 88.

Brand name:

TIAZAC

See Cardizem, page 205.

Brand name:

TIGAN

Pronounced: TIE-gan
Generic name: Trimethobenzamide hydrochloride

Why is this drug prescribed?
Tigan is prescribed to control nausea and vomiting.

Most important fact about this drug

Antiemetics (drugs that prevent or lessen nausea and vomiting) are not recommended for the treatment of simple vomiting in children. Use of Tigan in children should be limited to prolonged vomiting caused by a known disease.

Caution should always be exercised when using this drug in children, since there may be a link between the use of antiemetic drugs to treat symptoms of viral illnesses such as chickenpox and the development of Reye's syndrome, which is a potentially fatal childhood disease of the brain.

How should you take this medication?

Take this medication exactly as prescribed.

If you are using the suppository form of Tigan and find it is too soft to insert, you can firm it up by chilling it in the refrigerator for about 30 minutes or running cold water over it before removing the wrapper.

To insert a suppository, first remove the wrapper and moisten the suppository with cold water. Then lie down on your side and use a finger to push the suppository well up into the rectum.

■ *If you miss a dose...*
Take it as soon as you remember. If it is almost time for your next dose, skip the one you missed and go back to your regular schedule. Do not take 2 doses at once.

■ *Storage instructions...*
Store away from heat, light, and moisture.

What side effects may occur?

Side effects cannot be anticipated. If any develop or change in intensity, inform your doctor as soon as possible. Only your doctor can determine if it is safe for you to continue taking Tigan.

■ *Side effects may include:*
Allergic-type skin reactions, blurred vision, coma, convulsions, depression, diarrhea, disorientation, dizziness, drowsiness, headache, muscle cramps, severe muscle spasm, tremors, yellowed eyes and skin

Why should this drug not be prescribed?

If you are sensitive to or have ever had an allergic reaction to Tigan do not take this medication. Do not use the suppositories if you are allergic to benzocaine or other local anesthetics. Make sure your doctor is aware of any drug reactions you have experienced.

Unless you are directed to do so by your doctor, do not use suppositories in premature or newborn infants.

Special warnings about this medication

Tigan may cause you to become drowsy or less alert. Do not drive or operate dangerous machinery or participate in any hazardous activity that requires full mental alertness until you know how you respond to this drug.

Reye's syndrome has been associated with the use of Tigan during viral illnesses in children. Reye's syndrome is characterized by severe, persistent vomiting, sluggishness, irrational behavior, and a progressive brain disorder leading to coma, convulsions, and death.

Caution should be exercised when taking Tigan—especially in children, the elderly, or those in a weakened or run-down condition—if you have a severe illness accompanied by high fever, inflammation of the brain (encephalitis), inflammation of the stomach and intestines (gastroenteritis), or dehydration.

Severe vomiting should not be treated with Tigan alone. Your doctor should emphasize restoration of body fluids, the relief of fever, and the relief of the disease causing the vomiting. However, the overconsumption of fluids may result in cerebral edema (excessive accumulation of fluid in the brain).

The antinausea effects of Tigan may make it difficult to diagnose such conditions as appendicitis and may mask signs of drug poisoning due to overdosage of other drugs.

Possible food and drug interactions
when taking this medication

The use of alcohol in combination with this drug may produce an unfavorable reaction.

Caution should be exercised when taking Tigan in combination with central nervous system drugs such as phenothiazines (tranquilizers and antiemetics), barbiturates such as phenobarbital, and drugs derived from belladonna, such as Donnatal, if you are dehydrated or have a severe disease with fever, inflammation of the stomach, intestines, or brain.

Special information
if you are pregnant or breastfeeding

The effects of Tigan during pregnancy or breastfeeding have not been adequately studied. If you are pregnant or plan to become pregnant, inform your doctor immediately. If you are breastfeeding your baby, consult your doctor before taking this medication.

Recommended dosage
Dosage will be adjusted by your doctor according to your illness, the severity of your symptoms, and how well you do on the drug.

ADULTS

Capsules
The usual dosage is one 250-milligram capsule taken 3 or 4 times per day, as determined by your doctor.

Suppositories
The recommended dosage is 1 suppository (200 milligrams) inserted into the rectum 3 or 4 times per day, as determined by your doctor.

CHILDREN

Capsules
The usual dosage for children weighing 30 to 90 pounds is one or two 100-milligram capsules taken 3 or 4 times per day, as determined by the doctor.

Suppositories
The usual dosage for children weighing under 30 pounds is half a suppository (100 milligrams), inserted into the rectum 3 or 4 times a day, as determined by the doctor.

The usual dosage for children weighing 30 to 90 pounds is one-half to one 200-milligram suppository rectally 3 or 4 times a day, as determined by the doctor.

Pediatric Suppositories
The usual dosage for children weighing under 30 pounds is 1 suppository (100 milligrams) rectally 3 or 4 times a day, as determined by the doctor.

The usual dosage for children weighing 30 to 90 pounds is 1 to 2 suppositories (100 milligrams to 200 milligrams) rectally 3 or 4 times a day, as determined by the doctor.

Overdosage
Although no specific information is available, any medication taken in excess can have serious consequences. If you suspect a Tigan overdose, seek medical attention immediately.

Brand name:

TILADE

Pronounced: TILE-aid
Generic name: Nedocromil sodium

Why is this drug prescribed?
Tilade is an anti-inflammatory medication prescribed for use on a regular basis to control symptoms in people with mild to moderate asthma.

Most important fact about this drug
Tilade must be used regularly to be effective, even if you have no symptoms. It improves your condition, but won't help during an acute attack.

How should you take this medication?
Proper inhalation of Tilade is essential for it to be effective. Make sure you understand how to use the medication correctly, and take exactly the amount prescribed. It may be a week or more before you feel the full effect.

Tilade Inhaler should not be used with other mouthpieces.

Avoid spraying the medication in your eyes.

- *If you miss a dose...*
  To work properly, Tilade must be inhaled every day at regular intervals. If you miss a dose, take it as soon as you remember. If it is almost time for your next dose, skip the one you missed and go back to your regular schedule. Do not take double doses.

- *Storage instructions...*
  Store Tilade Inhaler at room temperature. Because the contents are under pressure, do not puncture, incinerate, or place near heat.

What side effects may occur?
Side effects cannot be anticipated. If any develop or change in intensity, inform your doctor as soon as possible. Only your doctor can determine if it is safe for you to continue using Tilade.

- *More common side effects may include:*
  Chest pain, coughing, fever, headache, inflamed nose and sinuses, nausea, sore throat, unpleasant taste, upper respiratory tract infection, wheezing

■ *Less common side effects may include:*
Abdominal pain, bronchitis, conjunctivitis (pinkeye), diarrhea, difficult or labored breathing, dizziness, dry mouth, fatigue, increased sputum, indigestion, rash, viral infection, vomiting

Why should this drug not be prescribed?

Tilade Inhaler should not be used if you are sensitive to or have ever had an allergic reaction to nedocromil sodium or any of Tilade's other ingredients. Make sure your doctor is aware of any drug reactions you have experienced.

Special warnings about this medication

This medication will not stop an asthma attack. However, you should continue to take it during an attack, along with a bronchodilator (a medication that increases air flow to your lungs) to relieve the acute symptoms.

If your symptoms do not improve or get worse, call your doctor right away; don't try increasing the dose to make the medication work.

Medications that are inhaled can cause coughing and wheezing in some people. If you experience these symptoms, stop taking Tilade and notify your doctor immediately.

Possible food and drug interactions when taking this medication

No interactions have been reported.

Special information if you are pregnant or breastfeeding

The effects of Tilade during pregnancy have not been adequately studied. If you are pregnant or plan to become pregnant, notify your doctor immediately. Tilade may appear in breast milk and could affect a nursing infant. If this medication is essential to your health, your doctor may advise you to discontinue breastfeeding until your treatment is finished.

Recommended dosage

ADULTS AND CHILDREN 12 YEARS OF AGE AND OVER

The recommended dose is 2 inhalations 4 times a day at regular intervals. If you are doing well on that dosage, your doctor may try reducing the dose after a time.

CHILDREN

The safety and effectiveness of Tilade Inhaler have not been established in children under 6 years of age.

Overdosage

A dangerous reaction is unlikely. However, any medication taken in excess can have serious consequences. If you suspect an overdose, seek medical attention immediately.

Generic name:

TIMOLOL

See Timoptic, below.

Brand name:

TIMOPTIC

Pronounced: Tim-OP-tic
Generic name: Timolol
Other brand name: Betimol

Why is this drug prescribed?

Timoptic is a topical medication (applied directly in the eye) that effectively reduces internal pressure in the eye. Timoptic is used in the treatment of glaucoma to lower elevated eye pressure that could damage vision and, with other glaucoma medications, to further reduce pressure in the eye.

Most important fact about this drug

Although Timoptic eyedrops are applied only to the eye, the medication is absorbed and may have effects in other parts of the body. If you have diabetes, asthma, or other respiratory disease, or decreased heart function, make sure your doctor is aware of the problem.

How should you use this medication?

Timoptic should be used exactly as prescribed by your doctor.

If you are using Timoptic in Ocudose, use the medication as soon as you open the individual unit and throw out any leftover solution.

If you are using Timoptic-XE, invert the closed container and shake it once—and only once—before each use. Do not enlarge the hole in the dispenser tip; it is designed to provide just 1 drop. Do not wash the dispenser tip with water, soap, or any other cleaner.

If you need to use other eye medications along with Timoptic-XE, use them at least 10 minutes before you instill Timoptic-XE. Allow 5 minutes with Betimol.

If you wear contact lenses, remove them before using Timoptic and wait 15 minutes before reinserting them.

Handle the Timoptic solution carefully to avoid contamination. Do not let the tip of the dispenser actually touch the eye.

To administer Timoptic, follow these steps:
1. Wash your hands thoroughly.
2. Gently pull your lower eyelid down to form a pocket.
3. Brace the bottle against the bridge of your nose or your forehead.
4. Tilt your head back and squeeze the medication into your eye.
5. Close your eyes gently.
6. Keep your eyes closed for 1 to 2 minutes.

■ *If you miss a dose...*
   If you use Timoptic once a day, apply it as soon as you remember. If you do not remember until the next day, skip the dose you missed and go back to your regular schedule. Do not take 2 doses at once. If you use it more than once a day, apply it as soon as you remember. If it is almost time for your next dose, skip the one you missed and go back to your regular schedule. Do not take 2 doses at once.

■ *Storage instructions...*
   Store at room temperature, protected from light. Keep from freezing.

What side effects may occur?
Side effects cannot be anticipated. If any side effects develop or change in intensity, tell your doctor immediately. Only your doctor can determine whether it is safe to continue using this medication. If Timoptic is absorbed into the bloodstream, it can cause additional side effects.

The most common side effects are burning and stinging on instillation of the drug.

■ *Other side effects may include:*
Abnormal overflow of tears, allergic reactions, anxiety, behavioral changes, blurred or abnormal vision, cataracts, chest pain, cold hands and feet, common cold, confusion, conjunctivitis (pinkeye), cough, decreased sex drive, depression, diarrhea, difficult or labored breathing, disorientation, dizziness, double vision, drooping eyelid, dry mouth, eye discharge, eye dryness or irritation and inflammation, eye pain or itching and tearing, fainting, fatigue, fluid in the lungs, hair loss, hallucinations, headache, heart failure, high blood pressure, hives, impotence, inability to breathe, increase in signs/symptoms of myasthenia gravis (severe muscle weakness), indigestion, inflammation or swelling of the eyelid, intolerance of light, itching, irregular heartbeat, loss of appetite, low blood pressure, memory loss, nausea, nervousness, nightmares, pain, pain or swelling in arms and legs, psoriasis, Peyronie's disease (curved and painful erection), rash, ringing in the ears, sensation of a foreign body in the eye, sinus inflammation, skin tingling, sleepiness, slow heartbeat, stroke, stuffy nose, swelling, swelling of the face and neck, throbbing or fluttering heartbeat, tingling or pins and needles, upper respiratory infection, visual disturbances, weakness, wheezing, worsened angina pectoris (crushing chest pain)

Why should this drug not be prescribed?

Do not use Timoptic if you have bronchial asthma, a history of bronchial asthma, or other serious breathing disorders such as emphysema, slow heartbeat, heart block (conduction disorder), active heart failure, or inadequate blood supply to the circulatory system (cardiogenic shock), or if you have ever had an allergic reaction or are sensitive to Timoptic or any of its ingredients.

Special warnings about this medication

Use Timoptic cautiously if you have a history of heart failure or poor circulation to the brain.

Tell your doctor if you have any type of allergy. The frequency and severity of allergic reactions may increase while you are using Timoptic.

Timoptic may mask the symptoms of low blood sugar. If you are diabetic, discuss this possibility with your doctor.

Tell your doctor or dentist that you are using Timoptic if you have a medical emergency or before you have surgery or dental treatment.

Timoptic may mask symptoms of an overactive thyroid. If your doctor suspects you have excessive thyroid function, he or she will manage your case carefully to avoid such symptoms as rapid heartbeat, which can occur when the drug is withdrawn too abruptly.

Timoptic's antiglaucoma effects may decrease if you use the medication for a long time.

Some older individuals may be more sensitive to this product than younger people. If you develop an eye infection, suffer an eye injury, or have eye surgery, check with your doctor. You may need to stop using Timoptic.

Possible food and drug interactions
when using this medication

If Timoptic is used with certain other drugs, the effects of either could be increased, decreased, or altered. It is especially important to check with your doctor before combining Timoptic with the following:

Epinephrine (EpiPen)
Catecholamine-depleting drugs, such as blood pressure drugs that
    contain reserpine (Serpasil)
Calcium antagonists such as Cardizem and Isoptin
Digitalis (Lanoxin)
Quinidine (Quinaglute, Quinidex)

Timoptic should not be used with other topical beta blockers and should be used with caution if you are taking oral beta blockers such as Inderal and Tenormin.

Special information
if you are pregnant or breastfeeding

If you are pregnant or plan to become pregnant, inform your doctor immediately. No information is available about the safety of using Timoptic during pregnancy.

Timolol appears in breast milk and may harm a nursing infant. If using Timoptic is essential to your health, your doctor may advise you to stop breastfeeding until your treatment is finished.

Recommended dosage

ADULTS

Your doctor will tailor an individual Timoptic dosage depending on your medical condition and how you responded to any previous glaucoma treatment.

The usual recommended initial dose is to place 1 drop of 0.25 percent Timoptic in the affected eye(s) twice a day. If you do not respond satisfactorily to this dosage, your doctor may tell you to place 1 drop of 0.5 percent Timoptic in the affected eye(s) twice a day.

The usual dose of Timoptic-XE is 1 drop of either 0.25 percent or 0.5 percent in the affected eye(s) once a day. Invert the closed container and shake it once before you use it.

The usual dose of Betimol is 1 drop of either 0.25 percent or 0.5 percent in the affected eye(s) twice a day.

Overdosage
Seek medical treatment immediately if you think you might have used too much Timoptic. Call your local poison control center or your doctor for assistance.

■ *Symptoms of Timoptic overdose may include:*
Dizziness, headache, heart failure, shortness of breath, slow heartbeat, wheezing

Generic name:

TOBRAMYCIN

See Tobrex, below.

Brand name:

TOBREX

Pronounced: TOE-breks
Generic name: Tobramycin
Other brand name: Aktob

Why is this drug prescribed?
Tobrex is an antibiotic applied to the eye to treat bacterial infections.

Most important fact about this drug
In order to clear up your infection completely, keep using Tobrex for the full time of treatment, even if your symptoms have disappeared.

How should you use this medication?

To apply Tobrex eyedrops:
1. Wash your hands thoroughly.
2. Gently pull your lower eyelid down to form a pocket between your eye and eyelid.
3. Brace the bottle on the bridge of your nose or your forehead.
4. Do not let the applicator tip touch your eye or any other surface.
5. Tilt your head back and squeeze the medication into the eye.

6. Close your eyes gently.
7. Keep your eyes closed for 1 to 2 minutes.
8. Do not rinse the dropper.
9. If you are using another eyedrop wait 5 to 10 minutes before applying it.

To apply the ointment form of this medication:
1. Tilt your head back.
2. Place a finger on your cheek just under your eye and gently pull down until a "V" pocket is formed between your eyeball and your lower lid.
3. Place about half an inch of Tobrex in the "V" pocket. Do not let the tip of the tube touch the eye.
4. Look downward before closing your eye.

■ *If you miss a dose...*
Apply it as soon as you remember. If it is almost time for your next dose, skip the one you missed and go back to your regular schedule.

■ *Storage instructions...*
Store Tobrex at room temperature, away from heat, or in the refrigerator. Do not allow to freeze.

What side effects may occur?
Side effects cannot be anticipated. If any develop or change in intensity, inform your doctor as soon as possible. Only your doctor can determine if it is safe for you to continue to take Tobrex.

■ *Side effects may include:*
Abnormal redness of eye tissue, allergic reactions, lid itching, lid swelling

Why should this drug not be prescribed?
If you are sensitive to or have ever had an allergic reaction to Tobrex or any of its ingredients, you should not use this medication. Make sure your doctor is aware of any drug reactions you have experienced.

Special warnings about this medication
If you experience an allergic reaction to this medication, discontinue use and inform your doctor.

Continued or prolonged use of Tobrex may result in a growth of bacteria that do not respond to this medication and can cause a secondary infection.

Possible food and drug interactions
when taking this medication
If you are taking any other prescription antibiotics for your eyes, check with

your doctor before using Tobrex. Using this medication with certain other antibiotics in your system may cause an overdose.

Special information
if you are pregnant or breastfeeding

The effects of Tobrex during pregnancy have not been adequately studied. If you are pregnant or plan to become pregnant, inform your doctor immediately. Tobrex may appear in breast milk. Your doctor may advise you to discontinue breastfeeding until your treatment with this medication is finished.

Recommended dosage

ADULTS

Solution

If the infection is mild to moderate, place 1 or 2 drops into the affected eye(s) every 4 hours. In severe infections, place 2 drops into the eye(s) every hour until there is improvement. Then you will be instructed to use less medication before you stop using it altogether.

Ointment

If the infection is mild to moderate, apply a half-inch ribbon into the affected eye(s) 2 or 3 times per day. In severe infections, apply a half-inch ribbon into the affected eye(s) every 3 or 4 hours until there is improvement. Then use less medication before stopping altogether.

CHILDREN

Your doctor will tailor a dose for the child.

Overdosage

Any medication used in excess can have serious consequences. If you suspect an overdose, seek medical assistance immediately.

▪ *Symptoms of Tobrex overdose may be similar to side effects. They include:*
Corneal redness and inflammation, excessive eye tearing, lid itching and swelling

Generic name:

TOCAINIDE

See Tonocard, page 1322.

Brand name:

TOFRANIL

Pronounced: toe-FRAY-nil
Generic name: Imipramine hydrochloride

Why is this drug prescribed?

Tofranil is used to treat depression. It is a member of the family of drugs called tricyclic antidepressants.

Tofranil is also used on a short-term basis, along with behavioral therapies, to treat bed-wetting in children aged 6 and older. Its effectiveness may decrease with longer use.

Some doctors also prescribe Tofranil to treat bulimia, attention deficit disorder in children, obsessive-compulsive disorder, and panic disorder.

Most important fact about this drug

Serious, sometimes fatal, reactions have been known to occur when drugs such as Tofranil are taken with another type of antidepressant called an MAO inhibitor. Drugs in this category include Nardil and Parnate. Do not take Tofranil within 2 weeks of taking one of these drugs. Make sure your doctor and pharmacist know of all the medications you are taking.

How should you take this medication?

Tofranil may be taken with or without food.

You should not take Tofranil with alcohol.

Do not stop taking Tofranil if you feel no immediate effect. It can take from 1 to 3 weeks for improvement to begin.

Tofranil can cause dry mouth. Sucking hard candy or chewing gum can help this problem.

- *If you miss a dose...*
  If you take 1 dose a day at bedtime, contact your doctor. Do not take the dose in the morning because of possible side effects.

  If you take 2 or more doses a day, take the forgotten dose as soon as you remember. If it is almost time for your next dose, skip the one you missed and go back to your regular schedule. Do not take 2 doses at once.

- *Storage instructions...*
  Store at room temperature in a tightly closed container.

What side effects may occur?

Side effects cannot be anticipated. If any develop or change in intensity, inform your doctor as soon as possible. Only your doctor can determine if it is safe for you to continue taking Tofranil.

■ *Side effects may include:*

Abdominal cramps, agitation, anxiety, black tongue, bleeding sores, blood disorders, blurred vision, breast development in males, confusion, congestive heart failure, constipation or diarrhea, cough, delusions, dilated pupils, disorientation, dizziness, drowsiness, dry mouth, episodes of elation or irritability, excessive or spontaneous flow of milk, fatigue, fever, flushing, frequent urination or difficulty or delay in urinating, hair loss, hallucinations, headache, heart attack, heart failure, high blood pressure, high or low blood sugar, high pressure of fluid in the eyes, hives, impotence, increased or decreased sex drive, inflammation of the mouth, insomnia, intestinal blockage, irregular heartbeat, lack of coordination, lightheadedness (especially when rising from lying down), loss of appetite, nausea, nightmares, odd taste in mouth, palpitations, purple or reddish-brown spots on skin, rapid heartbeat, restlessness, ringing in the ears, seizures, sensitivity to light, skin itching and rash, stomach upset, stroke, sweating, swelling due to fluid retention (especially in face or tongue), swelling of breasts, swelling of testicles, swollen glands, tendency to fall, tingling, pins and needles, and numbness in hands and feet, tremors, visual problems, vomiting, weakness, weight gain or loss, yellowed skin and whites of eyes

■ *The most common side effects in children being treated for bed-wetting are:*

Nervousness, sleep disorders, stomach and intestinal problems, tiredness

■ *Other side effects in children are:*

Anxiety, collapse, constipation, convulsions, emotional instability, fainting

Why should this drug not be prescribed?

Tofranil should not be used if you are recovering from a recent heart attack.

People who take drugs known as MAO inhibitors, such as the antidepressants Nardil and Parnate, should not take Tofranil. You should not take Tofranil if you are sensitive or allergic to it.

Special warnings about this medication

You should use Tofranil cautiously if you have or have ever had: narrow-angle glaucoma (increased pressure in the eye); difficulty in urinating; heart, liver, kidney, or thyroid disease; or seizures. Also be cautious if you are taking thyroid medication.

General feelings of illness, headache, and nausea can result if you suddenly stop taking Tofranil. Follow your doctor's instructions closely when discontinuing Tofranil.

Tell your doctor if you develop a sore throat or fever while taking Tofranil.

This drug may impair your ability to drive a car or operate potentially dangerous machinery. Do not participate in any activities that require full alertness if you are unsure about your ability.

This drug can make you sensitive to light. Try to stay out of the sun as much as possible while you are taking it.

If you are going to have elective surgery, your doctor will take you off Tofranil.

Possible food and drug interactions
when taking this medication
Never combine Tofranil with an MAO inhibitor. If Tofranil is taken with certain other drugs, the effects of either could be increased, decreased, or altered. It is especially important to check with your doctor before combining Tofranil with the following:

Albuterol (Proventil, Ventolin)
Antidepressants that act on serotonin, including Prozac, Paxil, and
    Zoloft
Barbiturates such as Nembutal and Seconal
Blood pressure medications such as Ismelin, Catapres, and Wytensin
Carbamazepine (Tegretol)
Cimetidine (Tagamet)
Decongestants such as Sudafed
Drugs that control spasms, such as Cogentin
Epinephrine (EpiPen)
Flecainide (Tambocor)
Major tranquilizers such as Mellaril and Thorazine
Methylphenidate (Ritalin)
Norepinephrine
Other antidepressants such as Elavil and Pamelor
Phenytoin (Dilantin)
Propafenone (Rythmol)
Quinidine (Quinaglute)
Thyroid medications such as Synthroid
Tranquilizers and sleep aids such as Halcion, Xanax, and Valium

Extreme drowsiness and other potentially serious effects can result if Tofranil is combined with alcohol or other mental depressants, such as narcotic painkillers (Percocet), sleeping medications (Halcion), or tranquilizers (Valium).

If you are switching from Prozac, wait at least 5 weeks after your last dose of Prozac before starting Tofranil.

Special information
if you are pregnant or breastfeeding

The effects of Tofranil during pregnancy have not been adequately studied. Pregnant women should use Tofranil only when the potential benefits clearly outweigh the potential risks. If you are pregnant or plan to become pregnant, inform your doctor immediately. Tofranil may appear in breast milk and could affect a nursing infant. If this medication is essential to your health, your doctor may advise you to stop breastfeeding until your treatment is finished.

Recommended dosage

ADULTS

The usual starting dose is 75 milligrams a day. The doctor may increase this to 150 milligrams a day. The maximum daily dose is 200 milligrams.

CHILDREN

Tofranil is not to be used in children to treat any condition but bed-wetting, and its use will be limited to short-term therapy. Safety and effectiveness in children under the age of 6 have not been established.

Total daily dosages for children should not exceed 2.5 milligrams for each 2.2 pounds of the child's weight.

Doses usually begin at 25 milligrams per day. This amount should be taken an hour before bedtime. If needed, this dose may be increased after 1 week to 50 milligrams (ages 6 through 11) or 75 milligrams (ages 12 and up), taken in one dose at bedtime or divided into 2 doses, 1 taken at mid-afternoon and 1 at bedtime.

OLDER ADULTS AND ADOLESCENTS

People in these two age groups should take lower doses. Dosage starts out at 30 to 40 milligrams per day and can go up to no more than 100 milligrams a day.

Overdosage

Any medication taken in excess can have serious consequences. An overdose of Tofranil can cause death. It has been reported that children are more sensitive than adults to overdoses of Tofranil. If you suspect an overdose, seek medical help immediately.

- *Symptoms of Tofranil overdose may include:*
  Agitation, bluish skin, coma, convulsions, difficulty breathing, dilated pupils, drowsiness, heart failure, high fever, involuntary writhing or jerky movements, irregular or rapid heartbeat, lack of coordination, low blood pressure, overactive reflexes, restlessness, rigid muscles, shock, stupor, sweating, vomiting

Generic name:

TOLBUTAMIDE

See Orinase, page 931.

Generic name:

TOLCAPONE

See Tasmar, page 1255.

Brand name:

TOLECTIN

Pronounced: toe-LEK-tin
Generic name: Tolmetin sodium

Why is this drug prescribed?

Tolectin is a nonsteroidal anti-inflammatory drug used to relieve the inflammation, swelling, stiffness, and joint pain associated with rheumatoid arthritis and osteoarthritis (the most common form of arthritis). It is used for both acute episodes and long-term treatment. It is also used to treat juvenile rheumatoid arthritis.

Most important fact about this drug

You should have frequent checkups with your doctor if you take Tolectin regularly. Ulcers or internal bleeding can occur without warning.

How should you take this medication?

If Tolectin upsets your stomach, it may be taken with food or an antacid, and with a full glass of water. It may also help to prevent upset if you avoid lying down for 20 to 30 minutes after taking the drug.

Take this medication exactly as prescribed by your doctor.

■ *If you miss a dose...*
Take it as soon as you remember. If it is almost time for your next dose, skip the one you missed and go back to your regular schedule. Never take 2 doses at the same time.

■ *Storage instructions...*
Store at room temperature in a tightly closed container, away from light.

What side effects may occur?

Side effects cannot be anticipated. If any develop or change in intensity, inform your doctor as soon as possible. Only your doctor can determine if it is safe for you to continue taking Tolectin.

■ *More common side effects may include:*
Abdominal pain, change in weight, diarrhea, dizziness, gas, headache, heartburn, high blood pressure, indigestion, nausea, stomach and intestinal upset, swelling due to fluid retention, vomiting, weakness

■ *Less common or rare side effects may include:*
Anemia, blood in urine, chest pain, congestive heart failure, constipation, depression, drowsiness, fever, hepatitis, hives, inflammation of the mouth or tongue, kidney failure, painful urination, peptic ulcer, purple or reddish spots on skin, ringing in the ears, severe allergic reactions, skin irritation, stomach inflammation, stomach or intestinal bleeding, urinary tract infection, visual disturbances, yellow eyes or skin

Why should this drug not be prescribed?

If you are sensitive to or have ever had an allergic reaction to Tolectin, aspirin, or other nonsteroidal anti-inflammatory drugs, or if you have had asthma, hives, or nasal inflammation caused by aspirin or other nonsteroidal anti-inflammatory drugs, you should not take this medication. Make sure your doctor is aware of any drug reactions you have experienced.

Special warnings about this medication

Tolectin can cause kidney problems, especially if you are elderly, suffer from heart failure or liver disease, or take diuretics.

This drug can also affect the liver. If you develop symptoms such as yellow skin and eyes, notify your doctor. You should be taken off Tolectin.

Do not take aspirin or any other anti-inflammatory medications while taking Tolectin unless your doctor tells you to do so.

Tolectin can cause visual disturbances. If you experience a change in your vision, inform your doctor.

Tolectin prolongs bleeding time. If you are taking blood-thinning medication, this drug should be taken with caution.

This drug can increase water retention. Use with caution if you have heart disease or high blood pressure.

Tolectin causes some people to become drowsy or less alert. If it has this effect on you, driving or operating dangerous machinery or participating in any hazardous activity that requires full mental alertness is not recommended.

Possible food and drug interactions
when taking this medication
If Tolectin is taken with certain other drugs, the effects of either could be increased, decreased, or altered. It is especially important to check with your doctor before combining Tolectin with the following:

Aspirin
Blood thinners such as Coumadin
Carteolol (Cartrol)
Diuretics such as Lasix
Glyburide (Micronase)
Lithium (Lithonate)
Methotrexate

Special information
if you are pregnant or breastfeeding
The effects of Tolectin during pregnancy have not been adequately studied. If you are pregnant or plan to become pregnant, inform your doctor immediately. Tolectin appears in breast milk and could affect a nursing infant. If this medication is essential to your health, your doctor may advise you to discontinue breastfeeding until your treatment is finished.

Recommended dosage

ADULTS

Rheumatoid Arthritis or Osteoarthritis

The starting dosage is usually 1,200 milligrams a day divided into 3 doses of 400 milligrams each. Take 1 dose when you wake up and 1 at bedtime, and 1 sometime in between. Your doctor may adjust the dosage after 1 to 2 weeks. Most people will take a total daily dosage of 600 to 1,800 milligrams usually divided into 3 doses.

You should see the benefits of Tolectin in a few days to a week.

CHILDREN

The starting dose for children 2 years and older is usually a total of 20 milligrams per 2.2 pounds of body weight per day, divided into 3 or 4 smaller doses. Your doctor will advise you on use in children. The usual dose ranges from 15 to 30 milligrams per 2.2 pounds per day.

The safety and effectiveness of Tolectin have not been established in children under 2 years of age.

Overdosage

Although no specific information is available, any medication taken in excess can have serious consequences. If you suspect an overdose of Tolectin, seek medical attention immediately.

Generic name:

TOLMETIN

See Tolectin, page 1319.

Brand name:

TONOCARD

Pronounced: TAH-nuh-card
Generic name: Tocainide hydrochloride

Why is this drug prescribed?

Tonocard is used to treat severe irregular heartbeat (arrhythmias). Arrhythmias are generally divided into two main types: heartbeats that are faster than normal (tachycardia), or heartbeats that are slower than normal (bradycardia). Irregular heartbeats are often caused by drugs or disease but can occur in otherwise healthy people with no history of heart disease or other illness. Tonocard works differently from other antiarrhythmic drugs, such as quinidine (Quinidex), procainamide (Procan SR), and disopyramide (Norpace). It is similar to lidocaine (Xylocaine) and is effective in treating severe ventricular arrhythmias (irregular heartbeats that occur in the main chambers of the heart).

Most important fact about this drug

Tonocard can cause serious blood and lung disorders in some patients, especially in the first 3 months of treatment. Be sure to notify your doctor if any of the following occurs: painful or difficult breathing, wheezing, cough, easy bruising or bleeding, tremors, palpitations, rash, soreness or ulcers in the mouth, sore throat, fever, and chills.

How should you take this medication?

It is important to take Tonocard on a regular schedule, exactly as prescribed by your doctor. Try not to miss any doses. If this medication is not taken regularly, your condition can worsen.

■ *If you miss a dose...*
   If less than 2 hours have passed, take the forgotten dose as soon as you remember. If you are more than 2 hours late, skip the dose. Never try to "catch up" by taking a double dose.

■ *Storage instructions...*
   Keep the container tightly closed, and store it at room temperature. Protect from extreme heat.

What side effects may occur?

Side effects cannot be anticipated. If any develop or change in intensity, inform your doctor as soon as possible. Only your doctor can determine if it is safe for you to continue taking Tonocard.

■ *More common side effects may include:*
   Confusion/disorientation, diarrhea/loose stools, dizziness/vertigo, excessive sweating, hallucinations, increased irregular heartbeat, lack of coordination, loss of appetite, nausea, nervousness, rash/skin eruptions, tingling or pins and needles, tremor, vision disturbances, vomiting

■ *Less common side effects may include:*
   Anxiety, arthritis, chest pain, congestive heart failure, drowsiness, exhaustion, fatigue, headache, hearing loss, hot/cold feelings, involuntary

eyeball movement, joint pain, low blood pressure, muscle pain, pounding heartbeat, rapid heartbeat, ringing in ears, sleepiness, slow heartbeat, sluggishness, unsteadiness, walking disturbances

■ *Rare side effects may include:*
Abdominal pain/discomfort, agitation, allergic reactions, anemia, angina, blood clots in lungs, blood disorders, changes in blood counts, changes in heart function, chills, cinchonism (a sensitivity reaction with symptoms including ringing in the ears, loss of hearing, dizziness, light-headedness, headache, nausea, and/or disturbed vision), cold hands and feet, coma, constipation, decreased mental ability, decreased urination, depression, difficulty breathing, difficulty sleeping, difficulty speaking, difficulty swallowing, disturbed behavior, disturbed dreams, dizziness on standing, double vision, dry mouth, earache, enlarged heart, fainting, fever, fluid in lungs, fluid retention, flushing, general bodily discomfort, hair loss, heart attack, hepatitis, hiccups, high blood pressure, hives, increased stuttering, increased urination, lung disorders, memory loss, muscle cramps, muscle twitching/spasm, myasthenia gravis, neck pain or pain extending from the neck, pallor, pneumonia, seizures, skin peeling, slurred speech, smell disturbance, stomach upset, taste disturbance, thirst, weakness, yawning, yellow eyes and skin

Why should this drug not be prescribed?
If you have heart block (conduction disorder) and do not have a pacemaker, or if you are sensitive to or have ever had an allergic reaction to Tonocard or certain local anesthetics such as Xylocaine, do not take this medication.

Special warnings about this medication
Be alert for signs of the blood and lung disorders that can occur early in your treatment. (See "Most important fact about this drug.")

If you have congestive heart failure, make sure the doctor is aware of it. Tonocard could worsen this condition.

Also make certain that the doctor is aware of any kidney or liver problems that you have. You will need to be monitored more carefully.

Before any kind of surgery, including dental surgery and emergency treatment, make sure the surgeon knows that you are taking Tonocard.

Possible food and drug interactions
when taking this medication
If Tonocard is taken with certain other drugs, the effects of either could be increased, decreased, or altered. It is especially important to check with your doctor before combining Tonocard with any of the following:

The anesthetic Lidocaine (Xylocaine)
The blood pressure medicine Metoprolol (Lopressor)
Other antiarrhythmics such as Quinidex, Procan, Mexitil

**Special information
if you are pregnant or breastfeeding**

The effects of Tonocard during pregnancy have not been adequately studied. However, animal studies have shown an increase in stillbirths and spontaneous abortions. If you are pregnant or plan to become pregnant, inform your doctor immediately. Tonocard may appear in breast milk and could affect a nursing infant. If this medication is essential to your health, your doctor may advise you to discontinue breastfeeding until your treatment is finished.

Recommended dosage

ADULTS

Dosages of Tonocard must be adjusted according to its effects on each individual. Your doctor should monitor you carefully to determine if the dosage you are taking is working properly. He may divide your doses further or make other changes, such as shortening the time between doses, if side effects occur.

The usual starting dose is 400 milligrams every 8 hours.

The usual dose range is between 1,200 and 1,800 milligrams total per day divided into 3 doses. This medication can be taken in 2 doses a day with careful monitoring by your doctor.

Doses beyond 2,400 milligrams per day are rarely used.

Some people, particularly those with reduced kidney or liver function, may be treated successfully with less than 1,200 milligrams per day.

CHILDREN

The safety and effectiveness of this drug in children have not been established.

Overdosage

Any medication taken in excess can have serious consequences. If you suspect an overdose, seek medical attention immediately.

There are no specific reports of Tonocard overdose. However, the first and most important signs of overdose would be expected to appear in the central nervous system. Disorders of the stomach and intestines might follow. Convulsions and heart and lung slowing or stopping might occur.

Brand name:

TOPICORT

Pronounced: TOP-i-court
Generic name: Desoximetasone

Why is this drug prescribed?
Topicort is a synthetic steroid medication in cream, gel, or ointment form that relieves the inflammation and itching caused by a variety of skin conditions.

Most important fact about this drug
When you use Topicort, you may absorb some of the medication through your skin and into the bloodstream. Too much absorption can lead to unwanted side effects elsewhere in the body. To keep this problem to a minimum, avoid using large amounts of Topicort over large areas, do not use it for extended periods of time, and do not cover it with airtight dressings such as plastic wrap or adhesive bandages unless specifically told to by your doctor.

Children may absorb more medication than adults do.

How should you use this medication?
Topicort is for use only on the skin. Be careful to keep it out of your eyes.

Apply a thin coating of Topicort to the affected area. Rub in gently.

The treated area should not be covered unless your doctor has told you to do so.

If Topicort is being used for an infant or toddler with a genital rash, make sure the diapers or plastic pants are not too tight, so that air can circulate.

■ *If you miss a dose...*
Use Topicort only as needed, in the smallest amount required for relief.

■ *Storage instructions...*
Store Topicort at room temperature.

What side effects may occur?
Side effects cannot be anticipated. If any develop or change in intensity, inform your doctor as soon as possible. Only your doctor can determine if it is safe for you to continue using Topicort. The side effects listed below occur

infrequently, but may occur more often if the treated area is covered with a bandage.

■ *Side effects may include:*
Acne-like pimples, blackheads, blistering, burning of the skin, dryness, excessive growth of hair, infection, inflammation of the hair follicles, irritation, itching, loss of skin pigmentation, prickly heat, rash, redness, skin inflammation around the mouth, stretch marks on the skin, thinning of the skin

Why should this drug not be prescribed?
Do not use Topicort if you are sensitive to it or have ever had an allergic reaction to any of its ingredients.

Special warnings about this medication
Remember to avoid getting Topicort in your eyes. Do not use Topicort to treat any condition other than the one for which it was prescribed.

Long-term use of steroids such as Topicort may interfere with the growth and development of children. They may also develop headaches, or bulging at the top of the head.

Avoid covering a treated area with tight waterproof diapers or plastic pants. They can increase unwanted absorption of Topicort.

If your skin becomes irritated or infected, stop using Topicort and call your doctor.

Possible food and drug interactions
when using this medication
No interactions have been reported.

Special information
if you are pregnant or breastfeeding
Topicort should not be used over large areas, in large amounts, or for long periods of time during pregnancy unless the benefit outweighs any potential risk to the unborn child. If you are pregnant or plan to become pregnant, inform your doctor immediately.

It is not known whether topical steroids are absorbed in sufficient amounts to appear in breast milk. If your doctor considers Topicort essential to your health, he or she may advise you to stop breastfeeding until your treatment with the medication is finished.

Recommended dosage

ADULTS

Apply a thin film of Topicort cream, gel, or ointment to the affected area 2 times a day. Rub in gently.

CHILDREN

Use the least amount of Topicort necessary to relieve symptoms. Ask your doctor for specific instructions.

Overdosage

Large doses of steroids such as Topicort applied over a large area or for a long time, especially when the treated area is covered, can cause increases in blood sugar and Cushing's syndrome, a condition characterized by a moon-shaped face, emotional disturbances, high blood pressure, weight gain, and, in women, baldness or growth of body and facial hair. Cushing's syndrome may also trigger the development of diabetes. If left uncorrected, Cushing's syndrome may become serious. If you suspect your use of Topicort has led to this problem, seek medical attention immediately.

Brand name:

TORADOL

Pronounced: TOH-rah-dol
Generic name: Ketorolac tromethamine

Why is this drug prescribed?

Toradol, a nonsteroidal anti-inflammatory drug, is used to relieve moderately severe, acute pain. It is prescribed for a limited amount of time (no more than 5 days), not for long-term therapy.

Most important fact about this drug

Toradol can cause serious side effects, including ulcers and internal bleeding. Never take it for more than 5 days.

How should you take this medication?

Toradol works fastest when taken on an empty stomach, but an antacid can be taken if it causes upset. Take this medication exactly as prescribed.

Take Toradol with a full glass of water. Also, do not lie down for about 20 minutes after taking it. This will help to prevent irritation of your upper digestive tract.

- *If you miss a dose...*
  If you take Toradol on a regular schedule, take it as soon as you remember. If it is almost time for your next dose, skip the one you missed and go back to your regular schedule. Never take 2 doses at the same time.

- *Storage instructions...*
  Store at room temperature, away from light.

What side effects may occur?

Side effects cannot be anticipated. If any develop or change in intensity, inform your doctor as soon as possible. Only your doctor can determine if it is safe for you to continue using Toradol.

- *More common side effects may include:*
  Diarrhea, dizziness, drowsiness, headache, indigestion, nausea, stomach and intestinal pain, swelling due to fluid retention

- *Less common side effects may include:*
  Abdominal fullness, constipation, gas, high blood pressure, inflammation of the mouth, itching, rash, red or purple spots on the skin, sweating, vomiting

- *Rare side effects may include:*
  Abnormal dreams, allergic reactions, anemia, asthma, belching, black stools, blood in the urine, convulsions, difficult or labored breathing, exaggerated feeling of well-being, fainting, fever, fluid in the lungs, flushing, gastritis (inflammation of the lining of the stomach), hallucinations, hearing problems, hives, increased appetite, kidney failure, kidney inflammation, loss of appetite, low blood pressure, nosebleeds, pallor, peptic ulcer, rapid heartbeat, skin inflammation and flaking, skin peeling, stomach and intestinal bleeding, swelling of the throat or tongue, thirst and dry mouth, tremors, urinary problems, vertigo, vision problems, weight gain, yellow skin and eyes

Why should this drug not be prescribed?

Do not take Toradol if it has ever given you an allergic reaction. Also avoid this medication if you have ever had an allergic reaction—such as nasal polyps (tumors), swelling of the face, limbs, and throat, hives, wheezing, light-headedness—to aspirin or other nonsteroidal anti-inflammatory drugs (NSAIDs) such as Motrin.

Do not take Toradol if you have ever had a peptic ulcer or stomach or intestinal bleeding. Avoid it if you have severe kidney disease or bleeding problems.

Never combine this drug with aspirin, NSAIDs, or probenecid. Make sure your doctor is aware of any drug reactions you have experienced.

Special warnings about this medication

Remember that Toradol has been known to cause peptic ulcers and bleeding. Contact your doctor immediately if you suspect a problem.

This drug should be used with caution if you have kidney or liver disease. It may cause liver inflammation or kidney problems in some people.

Toradol is not recommended for long-term use, since side effects increase over time. This medication should be taken for no more than 5 days.

If you are an older adult, use this drug cautiously.

Toradol can increase water retention. If you have heart disease or high blood pressure, use this drug with care.

This medication can prolong bleeding time. If you are taking blood-thinning medication, take Toradol with caution.

Possible food and drug interactions
when using this medication

If Toradol is taken with certain other drugs, the effects of either could be increased, decreased, or altered. It is especially important to check with your doctor before combining Toradol with the following:

ACE inhibitor drugs such as the blood pressure medications Vasotec and
    Capoten
Antidepressants such as Prozac
Antiepileptic drugs (Dilantin, Tegretol)
Aspirin and other nonsteroidal anti-inflammatory drugs such as Motrin
Blood thinners such as Coumadin
Lithium (Lithonate)
Major tranquilizers such as Navane
Methotrexate (Rheumatrex)
Probenecid (Benemid)
Tranquilizers such as Xanax
Water pills such as Lasix and Dyazide

Special information
if you are pregnant or breastfeeding

The effects of Toradol during pregnancy have not been adequately studied. If you are pregnant or plan to become pregnant, inform your doctor immediately. Toradol appears in breast milk and could affect a nursing infant. This medication should not be used while you are breastfeeding.

Recommended dosage

ADULTS

Your doctor will give you Toradol intravenously or intramuscularly to start, then have you switch to the tablets. You will take 2 tablets for the first dose (20 milligrams) and then 1 tablet (10 milligrams) every 4 to 6 hours. You should not take more than 40 milligrams per day and should not take Toradol for more than 5 days in all.

CHILDREN

The safety and effectiveness of Toradol in children under age 16 have not been established.

OLDER ADULTS

Doses are usually lower for people over 65, those with kidney problems, and those who weigh less than 110 pounds. Your doctor will tailor the best dosage for you.

Overdosage

Although no specific information is available, any medication taken in excess can have serious consequences. If you suspect an overdose, seek medical attention immediately.

■ *Symptoms of Toradol overdose may include:*
   Abdominal pain, peptic ulcer

Brand name:

TOTACILLIN

See Omnipen, page 922.

Brand name:

T-PHYL

See Theo-Dur, page 1293.

Generic name:

TRAMADOL

See Ultram, page 1369.

Brand name:

TRANDATE

See Normodyne, page 896.

Generic name:

TRANDOLAPRIL

See Mavik, page 751.

Generic name:

TRANDOLAPRIL WITH VERAPAMIL

See Tarka, page 1252.

Brand name:

TRANSDERM-NITRO

See Nitroglycerin, page 882.

Brand name:

TRANXENE

Pronounced: TRAN-zeen
Generic name: Clorazepate dipotassium
Other brand names: Tranxene-SD, Tranxene-SD Half
*   Strength*

Why is this drug prescribed?
Tranxene belongs to a class of drugs known as benzodiazepines. It is used in the treatment of anxiety disorders and for short-term relief of the symptoms of anxiety.

It is also used to relieve the symptoms of acute alcohol withdrawal and to help in treating certain convulsive disorders such as epilepsy.

Most important fact about this drug
Tranxene can be habit-forming if taken regularly over a long period. You may experience withdrawal symptoms if you stop using this drug abruptly. Consult your doctor before discontinuing Tranxene or making any change in your dose.

How should you take this medication?
Tranxene should be taken exactly as prescribed by your doctor.

■ *If you miss a dose...*
Take it as soon as you remember if it is within an hour or so of your scheduled time. If you do not remember until later, skip the dose you missed and go back to your regular schedule. Do not take 2 doses at once.

■ *Storage instructions...*
Store at room temperature. Protect from excessive heat.

What side effects may occur?
Side effects cannot be anticipated. If any develop or change in intensity, inform your doctor as soon as possible. Only your doctor can determine if it is safe for you to continue taking Tranxene.

■ *More common side effects may include:*
Drowsiness

■ *Less common or rare side effects may include:*
Blurred vision, depression, difficulty in sleeping or falling asleep, dizziness, dry mouth, double vision, fatigue, genital and urinary tract disorders, headache, irritability, lack of muscle coordination, mental confusion, nervousness, skin rashes, slurred speech, stomach and intestinal disorders, tremors

■ *Side effects due to rapid decrease or abrupt withdrawal from Tranxene may include:*
Abdominal cramps, convulsions, diarrhea, difficulty in sleeping or falling asleep, hallucinations, impaired memory, irritability, muscle aches, nervousness, tremors, vomiting

Why should this drug not be prescribed?
If you are sensitive to or have ever had an allergic reaction to Tranxene, you should not take this medication. Make sure your doctor is aware of any drug reactions you have experienced.

Do not take this medication if you have the eye condition known as acute narrow-angle glaucoma.

Anxiety or tension related to everyday stress usually does not require treatment with such a strong drug. Discuss your symptoms thoroughly with your doctor.

Tranxene is not recommended for use in more serious conditions such as depression or severe psychological disorders.

Special warnings about this medication

Tranxene may cause you to become drowsy or less alert; therefore, you should not drive or operate dangerous machinery or participate in any hazardous activity that requires full mental alertness until you know how this drug affects you.

If you are being treated for anxiety associated with depression, your doctor will have you take a low dose of this medication. Do not increase your dose without consulting your doctor.

The elderly and people in a weakened condition are more apt to become unsteady or oversedated when taking Tranxene.

Possible food and drug interactions
when taking this medication

Tranxene slows down the central nervous system and may intensify the effects of alcohol. Do not drink alcohol while taking this medication.

If Tranxene is taken with certain other drugs, the effects of either could be increased, decreased, or altered. It is especially important to check with your doctor before combining Tranxene with the following:

  Antidepressant drugs known as MAO inhibitors (Nardil, Parnate) and
    other antidepressants such as Elavil and Prozac
  Barbiturates such as Nembutal and Seconal
  Narcotic pain relievers such as Demerol and Percodan
  Major tranquilizers such as Mellaril and Thorazine

Special information
if you are pregnant or breastfeeding

The effects of Tranxene during pregnancy have not been adequately studied. However, because there is an increased risk of birth defects associated with this class of drug, its use during pregnancy should be avoided. Tranxene may appear in breast milk and could affect a nursing infant. If this medication is essential to your health, your doctor may advise you to discontinue breastfeeding until your treatment with this medication is finished.

Recommended dosage

ANXIETY

Adults

The usual daily dosage is 30 milligrams divided into several smaller doses. A normal daily dose can be as little as 15 milligrams. Your doctor may increase the dosage gradually to as much as 60 milligrams, according to your individual needs.

Tranxene can also be taken in a single bedtime dose. The initial dose is 15 milligrams, but your doctor will adjust the dosage to suit your individual needs.

Tranxene-SD, a 22.5-milligram tablet, and Tranxene-SD Half Strength, an 11.25-milligram tablet, can be taken once every 24 hours. Your doctor may switch you to this form of the drug after you have been taking Tranxene for several weeks.

Older Adults

The usual starting dose is 7.5 to 15 milligrams per day.

ACUTE ALCOHOL WITHDRAWAL

Tranxene can be used in a multi-day program for relief of the symptoms of acute alcohol withdrawal. Dosages are usually increased in the first 2 days from 30 to 90 milligrams and then reduced over the next 2 days to lower levels. After that, your doctor will gradually lower the dose still further, and will take you off the drug when you are ready.

WHEN USED WITH ANTIEPILEPTIC DRUGS

Tranxene can be used in conjunction with antiepileptic drugs. Follow the recommended dosages carefully to avoid drowsiness.

Adults and Children over 12 Years Old

The starting dose is 7.5 milligrams 3 times a day. Your doctor may increase the dosage by 7.5 milligrams per week to a maximum of 90 milligrams a day.

Children 9 to 12 Years Old

The starting dose is 7.5 milligrams twice a day. Your doctor may increase the dosage by 7.5 milligrams a week to a maximum of 60 milligrams a day.

Safety and effectiveness in children under 9 years of age have not been established.

Overdosage
Any medication taken in excess can have serious consequences. If you suspect an overdose, seek medical treatment immediately.

- *Symptoms of Tranxene overdose may include:*
  Coma, low blood pressure, sedation

Generic name:

TRAZODONE

See Desyrel, page 376.

Brand name:

TRENTAL

Pronounced: TREN-tall
Generic name: Pentoxifylline

Why is this drug prescribed?
Trental is a medication that reduces the viscosity or "stickiness" of your blood, allowing it to flow more freely. It helps relieve the painful leg cramps caused by "intermittent claudication," a condition that results when hardening of the arteries reduces the leg muscles' blood supply.

Some doctors also prescribe Trental for dementia, strokes, circulatory and nerve problems caused by diabetes, and Raynaud's syndrome (a disorder of the blood vessels in which exposure to cold causes the fingers and toes to turn white). The drug is also used to treat impotence and to increase sperm motility in infertile men.

Most important fact about this drug
Trental can ease the pain in your legs and make walking easier but should not replace other treatments such as physical therapy or surgery.

How should you take this medication?
Trental comes in controlled-release tablets. Do not break, crush, or chew the tablets; swallow them whole. Take Trental exactly as prescribed.

- *If you miss a dose...*
  Take it as soon as you remember. If it is almost time for your next dose, skip the one you missed and go back to your regular schedule. Never take 2 doses at the same time.

■ *Storage instructions...*
Keep this medication in the container it came in, tightly closed and away from light. Store it at room temperature.

What side effects may occur?
Side effects cannot be anticipated. If any develop or change in intensity, inform your doctor as soon as possible. Only your doctor can determine if it is safe for you to continue taking Trental.

Trental's side effects are fairly uncommon.

■ *Side effects may include:*
Allergic reaction (symptoms include: swelling of face, lips, tongue, throat, arms, or legs, sore throat, fever and chills, difficulty swallowing, chest pain), anxiety, bad taste in the mouth, blind spot in vision, blurred vision, brittle fingernails, chest pain (sometimes crushing), confusion, conjunctivitis (pinkeye), constipation, depression, difficult or labored breathing, dizziness, dry mouth/thirst, earache, excessive salivation, flu-like symptoms, fluid retention, general body discomfort, headache, hives, indigestion, inflammation of the gallbladder, itching, laryngitis, loss of appetite, low blood pressure, nosebleeds, rash, seizures, sore throat/swollen neck glands, stuffy nose, tremor, vomiting, weight change

Why should this drug not be prescribed?
Do not take Trental if you have recently had a stroke or bleeding in the retina of your eye.

If you are sensitive to or have ever had an allergic reaction to Trental, caffeine, theophylline (medication for asthma or other breathing disorders), or theobromine, do not take this medication. Make sure that your doctor is aware of any drug reactions that you have experienced.

Special warnings about this medication
If you are taking a blood thinner, or have recently had surgery, peptic ulcers, or other disorders that involve bleeding, the doctor should test your blood periodically.

Most people tolerate Trental well, but there have been occasional cases of crushing chest pain, low blood pressure, and irregular heartbeat in people with heart disease and brain disorders.

Possible food and drug interactions
when taking this medication

If Trental is taken with certain other drugs, the effects of either could be increased, decreased, or altered. It is especially important to check with your doctor before combining Trental with the following:

Blood pressure medications such as Vasotec and Cardizem SR
Blood-thinning drugs such as Coumadin
Clot inhibitors such as Persantine
Theophylline (Theo-Dur)
Ulcer medicines such as Tagamet

Special information
if you are pregnant or breastfeeding

The effects of Trental during pregnancy have not been adequately studied. If you are pregnant or plan to become pregnant, inform your doctor immediately. Trental appears in breast milk and could affect a nursing infant. If this medication is essential to your health, your doctor may advise you to discontinue breastfeeding until your treatment with this medication is finished.

Recommended dosage

ADULTS

The usual dosage of Trental in controlled-release tablets is one 400-milligram tablet 3 times a day with meals.

While the effect of Trental may be seen within 2 to 4 weeks, it is recommended that treatment be continued for at least 8 weeks.

Any stomach or central nervous system (affecting the brain and spinal cord) side effects are related to the dose. If any of these side effects occur, the dosage should be lowered to 1 tablet, 2 times a day, for a total of 800 milligrams a day. If side effects persist at this lower dosage, your doctor may consider stopping this drug.

CHILDREN

The safety and effectiveness of this drug in children have not been established.

Overdosage

Any medication taken in excess can have serious consequences. If you suspect symptoms of a Trental overdose, seek medical attention immediately. Symptoms appear within 4 to 5 hours and may last for 12 hours.

■ *Symptoms of Trental overdose may include:*
Agitation, convulsions, fever, flushing, loss of consciousness, low blood
pressure, sleepiness

Generic name:

TRETINOIN

See Retin-A and Renova, page 1114.

Generic name:

TRIAMCINOLONE

See Azmacort, page 126.

Brand name:

TRIAVIL

Pronounced: TRY-uh-vill
Generic ingredients: Amitriptyline hydrochloride,
Perphenazine

Why is this drug prescribed?
Triavil is used to treat anxiety, agitation, and depression. Triavil is a
combination of a tricyclic antidepressant (amitriptyline) and a tranquilizer
(perphenazine).

Triavil can also help people with schizophrenia (distorted sense of reality)
who are depressed and people with insomnia, fatigue, loss of interest, loss
of appetite, or a slowing of physical and mental reactions.

Most important fact about this drug
Triavil may cause tardive dyskinesia—a condition marked by involuntary
muscle spasms and twitches in the face and body. This condition may be
permanent and appears to be most common among the elderly, especially
women. Ask your doctor for information about this possible risk.

How should you take this medication?
Triavil may be taken with or without food. You should not take it with
alcohol.

■ *If you miss a dose...*
Take it as soon as you remember. If it is within 2 hours of your next dose, skip the one you missed and go back to your regular schedule. Do not take 2 doses at once.

■ *Storage instructions...*
Store at room temperature in a tightly closed container. Protect Triavil 2-10 tablets from light.

What side effects may occur?
Side effects cannot be anticipated. If any develop or change in intensity, inform your doctor as soon as possible. Only your doctor can determine if it is safe for you to continue taking Triavil.

■ *Side effects may include:*
Abnormal secretion of milk, abnormalities of movements and posture, anxiety, asthma, black tongue, blood disorders, blurred vision, body rigidly arched backward, breast development in males, change in pulse rate, chewing movements, coma, confusion, constipation, convulsions, delusions, diarrhea, difficulty breathing, difficulty concentrating, difficulty swallowing, dilated pupils, disorientation, dizziness, drowsiness, dry mouth, eating abnormal amounts of food, ejaculation failure, episodes of elation or irritability, excessive or spontaneous flow of milk, excitement, exhaustion, eye problems, eye spasms, eyes in a fixed position, fatigue, fever, fluid accumulation and swelling (including throat and brain, face and tongue, arms and legs), frequent urination, hair loss, hallucinations, headache, heart attacks, hepatitis, high blood pressure, high fever, high or low blood sugar, hives, impotence, inability to stop moving, inability to urinate, increased or decreased sex drive, inflammation of the mouth, insomnia, intestinal blockage, intolerance to light, involuntary jerky movements of tongue, face, mouth, lips, jaw, body, or arms and legs, irregular blood pressure, pulse, and heartbeat, irregular menstrual periods, lack of coordination, light-headedness upon standing up, liver problems, lockjaw, loss or increase of appetite, low blood pressure, muscle stiffness, nasal congestion, nausea, nightmares, odd taste in the mouth, overactive reflexes, pain and stiffness around neck, palpitations, protruding tongue, puckering of the mouth, puffing of the cheeks, purple-reddish-brown spots on skin, rapid heartbeat, restlessness, rigid arms, feet, head, and muscles, ringing in the ears, salivation, sedation, seizures, sensitivity to light, severe allergic reactions, skin rash or inflammation, scaling, spasms in the hands and feet, speech problems, stomach upset, stroke, sweating, swelling of breasts, swelling of testicles, swollen glands, tingling, pins and needles, and numbness in hands and feet, tremors, twisted neck, twitching in the body, neck, shoulders, and face, uncontrollable and

involuntary urination, urinary problems, visual problems, vomiting, weakness, weight gain or loss, writhing motions, yellowed skin and whites of eyes

Why should this drug not be prescribed?

You should not be using Triavil if you are taking drugs that slow down the central nervous system, including alcohol, barbiturates, analgesics, antihistamines, or narcotics.

Triavil should not be used if you are recovering from a recent heart attack, or if you have an abnormal bone marrow condition. Avoid Triavil if you have ever had an allergic reaction to phenothiazines or amitriptyline.

People who are taking antidepressant drugs known as MAO inhibitors (including Nardil and Parnate) should not take Triavil.

Special warnings about this medication

Before using Triavil, tell your doctor if you have ever had: the eye condition known as glaucoma; difficulty urinating; breast cancer; seizures; heart, liver, or thyroid disease; or if you are exposed to extreme heat or pesticides. Be aware that Triavil may mask signs of brain tumor, intestinal blockage, and overdose of other drugs.

Nausea, headache, and a general ill feeling can result if you suddenly stop taking Triavil. Follow your doctor's instructions closely when discontinuing Triavil. If your dose is gradually reduced, you may experience irritability, restlessness, and dream and sleep disturbances, but these effects will not last.

This drug may impair your ability to drive a car or operate potentially dangerous machinery. Do not participate in any activities that require full alertness if you are unsure about your ability.

If you develop a fever that has no other cause, stop taking Triavil and call your doctor.

Possible food and drug interactions
when taking this medication

If Triavil is taken with certain other drugs, the effects of either could be increased, decreased, or altered. It is especially important to check with your doctor before combining Triavil with the following:

Airway-opening drugs such as Proventil
Antidepressant drugs classified as MAO inhibitors, including Nardil and Parnate
Antihistamines such as Benadryl

Antispasmodic drugs such as Bentyl
Antiseizure drugs such as Dilantin
Atropine (Donnatal)
Barbiturates such as phenobarbital
Blood-thinning drugs such as Coumadin
Cimetidine (Tagamet)
Disulfiram (Antabuse)
Epinephrine (EpiPen)
Ethchlorvynol (Placidyl)
Fluoxetine (Prozac)
Furazolidone (Furoxone)
Guanethidine (Ismelin)
Major tranquilizers such as Haldol
Narcotic analgesics such as Percocet
Thyroid medications such as Synthroid

Extreme drowsiness and other potentially serious effects can result if Triavil is combined with alcohol or other central nervous system depressants such as narcotics, painkillers, and sleep medications.

Special information
if you are pregnant or breastfeeding
Triavil may cause false-positive results on pregnancy tests. Triavil should not be used by pregnant women or mothers who are breastfeeding.

Recommended dosage
Your doctor will individualize your dose.

You should not take more than 4 tablets of Triavil 4-50 or 8 tablets of any other strength in one day. It may be a few days to a few weeks before you notice any improvement.

ADULTS

For Non-Psychotic Anxiety and Depression
The usual dose is 1 tablet of Triavil 2-25 or 4-25 taken 3 or 4 times a day, or 1 tablet of Triavil 4-50 taken twice a day.

For Anxiety in People with Schizophrenia
The usual dose is 2 tablets of Triavil 4-25 taken 3 times a day. Your doctor may tell you to take another tablet of Triavil 4-25 at bedtime, if needed.

If you need to keep taking Triavil, your doctor will probably have you take 1 tablet of Triavil 2-25 or 4-25 from 2 to 4 times a day or 1 tablet of Triavil 4-50 twice a day.

CHILDREN

Children should not use Triavil.

OLDER ADULTS AND ADOLESCENTS

For Anxiety

The usual dose is 1 tablet of Triavil 4-10, taken 3 or 4 times a day. People in these age groups usually take Triavil at lower doses.

Overdosage

Any medication taken in excess can have serious consequences. An overdose of Triavil can be fatal. If you suspect an overdose, seek medical help immediately.

- **Symptoms of Triavil overdose may include:**
  Abnormalities of posture and movements, agitation, coma, convulsions, dilated pupils, drowsiness, extreme low body temperature, eye movement problems, heart failure, high fever, overactive reflexes, rapid or irregular heartbeat, rigid muscles, stupor, very low blood pressure, vomiting

Brand name:

TRIAZ

See Desquam-E, page 375.

Generic name:

TRIAZOLAM

See Halcion, page 579.

Brand name:

TRIDESILON

Pronounced: tri-DESS-ill-on
Generic name: Desonide
Other brand name: DesOwen

Why is this drug prescribed?

Tridesilon is a steroid preparation that relieves the itching and inflammation of a variety of skin problems. It is applied directly to the skin.

Most important fact about this drug
When you use Tridesilon, you inevitably absorb some of the medication through your skin and into the bloodstream. Too much absorption can lead to unwanted side effects elsewhere in the body. To keep this problem to a minimum, avoid using large amounts of Tridesilon over large areas, and do not cover it with airtight dressings such as plastic wrap or adhesive bandages unless specifically told to by your doctor.

How should you use this medication?
Use Tridesilon exactly as directed by your doctor. Shake lotion well before using.

Tridesilon is for use only on the skin. Be careful to keep it out of your eyes.

Remember to avoid wrapping the treated area with bandages or other coverings unless your doctor has told you to do so.

■ *If you miss a dose...*
Apply it as soon as you remember. If it is almost time for the next dose, skip the one you missed and go back to your regular schedule.

■ *Storage instructions...*
Store at room temperature.

What side effects may occur?
Side effects cannot be anticipated. If any develop or change in intensity, notify your doctor as soon as possible. Only your doctor can determine if it is safe for you to continue using Tridesilon. Many of the side effects listed below are rare, but may occur more often if the affected area is covered with a bandage or treated for a long time.

■ *Side effects may include:*
Acne, additional infections, allergic reactions of the skin, burning and stinging, dryness, excessive hair growth, irritation, itching, loss of skin color, prickly heat, rash, scaly skin, skin inflammation around the mouth, skin loss, skin peeling or redness, skin softening, stretch marks, worsening of the condition

■ *Side effects that may occur in children include:*
Delayed weight gain, headaches, slowed growth

Why should this drug not be prescribed?
You should not take this medication if you are sensitive or allergic to any of its ingredients.

Because steroid medications may interfere with their growth and development, children should be given the lowest strength that provides effective therapy. Safety and effectiveness of DesOwen in children have not been established.

Special warnings about this medication
If an irritation develops, or if your skin condition does not heal within 2 weeks, inform your doctor.

Avoid covering a treated area with waterproof diapers or plastic pants. They can increase unwanted absorption of Tridesilon.

Large doses of steroids applied over a large area, and long-term use of these preparations, especially when the treated areas are covered, can cause increases in blood sugar or sugar in the urine, Cushing's syndrome (a condition characterized by a moon-shaped face, emotional disturbances, high blood pressure, weight gain, and, in women, growth of body hair), and effects on the adrenal gland, pituitary, and hypothalamus.

Possible food and drug interactions
when using this medication
No interactions have been reported.

Special information
if you are pregnant or breastfeeding
Although Tridesilon is applied to the skin, there is no way of knowing how much medication is absorbed into the bloodstream. The more powerful steroids have caused birth defects in animals. In general, these preparations should not be used extensively, in large amounts, or for prolonged periods of time by pregnant women. They should be used only if the potential benefits outweigh the potential risks to the unborn baby. If you are pregnant or plan to become pregnant, inform your doctor immediately. It is not known whether steroid creams and ointments are absorbed in sufficient amounts to appear in breast milk. If your doctor considers Tridesilon essential to your health, he or she may advise you to stop breastfeeding until your treatment with the medication is finished.

Recommended dosage

ADULTS AND CHILDREN

Tridesilon should be applied to the affected area as a thin film, from 2 to 4 times a day, depending on the severity of the condition. Apply DesOwen 2 or 3 times daily.

A bandage or other covering may be prescribed by your doctor to apply over the affected area for psoriasis or conditions that are not responding as well as expected.

Overdosage

Any medication taken in excess can have serious consequences. With overuse or misuse of Tridesilon, too much medicine can enter the body, causing increases in blood sugar and Cushing's syndrome, with symptoms such as a moon-shaped face, emotional disturbances, high blood pressure, weight gain, and, in women, growth of body and facial hair.

Generic name:

TRIFLUOPERAZINE

See Stelazine, page 1218.

Generic name:

TRIHEXYPHENIDYL

See Artane, page 91.

Brand name:

TRILISATE

Pronounced: TRILL-ih-sate
Generic name: Choline magnesium trisalicylate

Why is this drug prescribed?

Trilisate, a nonsteroidal, anti-inflammatory medication, is prescribed for the relief of the signs and symptoms of rheumatoid arthritis (chronic joint inflammation disease), osteoarthritis (degenerative joint disease), and other forms of arthritis. This drug is used in the long-term management of these diseases and especially for flare-ups of severe rheumatoid arthritis.

Trilisate may also be prescribed for the treatment of acute painful shoulder, for mild to moderate pain in general, and for fever.

In children, this medication is prescribed for severe conditions—such as juvenile rheumatoid arthritis—that require relief of pain and inflammation.

Most important fact about this drug
Because there is a possible association between the development of the rare but serious nerve disorder known as Reye's syndrome and the use of medicines containing salicylates or aspirin during bouts of chickenpox or flu, Trilisate should not be used by children or teenagers during these illnesses unless otherwise advised by their doctor.

How should you take this medication?
Trilisate is available in tablet or liquid form. Take Trilisate exactly as prescribed by your doctor.

■ *If you miss a dose...*
If you take Trilisate on a regular schedule, take the forgotten dose as soon as you remember. If it is almost time for your next dose, skip the one you missed and go back to your regular schedule. Do not take 2 doses at once.

■ *Storage instructions...*
Store at room temperature.

What side effects may occur?
Side effects cannot be anticipated. If any develop or change in intensity, inform your doctor as soon as possible. Only your doctor can determine if it is safe for you to continue taking Trilisate.

■ *More common side effects may include:*
Constipation, diarrhea, heartburn, indigestion, nausea, ringing in the ears, stomach pain and upset, vomiting

■ *Less common side effects may include:*
Dizziness, drowsiness, headache, hearing impairment, light-headedness, sluggishness

■ *Rare side effects may include:*
Asthma, blood in the stool, bruising, confusion, distorted sense of taste, hallucinations, hearing loss, hepatitis, hives, inflammation of the upper gastric tract, itching, loss of appetite, nosebleed, rash, skin eruptions or discoloration, stomach or intestinal ulcers, swelling due to fluid accumulation, weight gain

Why should this drug not be prescribed?

If you are sensitive to or have ever had an allergic reaction to Trilisate or drugs of this type, such as aspirin, you should not take this medication. Make sure your doctor is aware of any drug reactions you have experienced.

Special warnings about this medication

Use Trilisate with caution if you have severe or recurring kidney or liver disorder, gastritis (inflammation of the stomach lining), or a stomach or intestinal ulcer. Consult your doctor regarding any medical problems you may have.

If you are an asthmatic allergic to aspirin, tell your doctor before taking Trilisate.

It may be 2 to 3 weeks before you feel the effect of this medication.

If you are an older adult, you are more likely to suffer side effects from Trilisate.

Possible food and drug interactions
when taking this medication

If Trilisate is taken with certain other drugs, the effects of either could be increased, decreased, or altered. It is especially important to check with your doctor before combining Trilisate with the following:

Antacids such as Gaviscon and Maalox

Antigout medications

Blood-thinners such as Coumadin

Carbonic anhydrase inhibitors such as acetazolamide (Diamox) used to
    treat heart failure, the eye condition called glaucoma, and certain
    convulsive disorders

Diabetes medications such as insulin, Micronase, and Tolinase

Methotrexate, an anticancer drug

Other salicylates used to reduce fever, inflammation, and pain, such as
    aspirin

Phenytoin (the seizure medication Dilantin)

Steroids such as prednisone

Valproic acid (the seizure medication Depakene)

Special information
if you are pregnant or breastfeeding

The effects of Trilisate during pregnancy have not been adequately studied. If you are pregnant or plan to become pregnant, inform your doctor immediately. This drug does appear in breast milk and could affect a nursing infant. If this medication is essential to your health, your doctor may advise you not to breastfeed until your treatment is finished.

Recommended dosage

ADULTS

In rheumatoid arthritis, osteoarthritis, more severe arthritis, and acute painful shoulder, the recommended starting dose is 1,500 milligrams taken 2 times a day or 3,000 milligrams taken once a day. Your doctor will adjust the dosage based on your response to this medication.

If you have a kidney disorder, your doctor will monitor you and adjust your dose accordingly.

For mild to moderate pain or to reduce a high fever, the usual dosage is 2,000 to 3,000 milligrams per day divided into 2 equal doses as recommended by your doctor.

CHILDREN

For reduction of inflammation or pain, the recommended dose for children is determined by weight. The usual dose for children who weigh 81 pounds or less is 50 milligrams per 2.2 pounds of body weight, taken twice a day. For heavier children, the usual dose is 2,250 milligrams per day, divided into 2 doses.

Trilisate liquid can be taken by younger children and by adults who are unable to swallow a tablet.

OLDER ADULTS

The usual dosage is 2,250 milligrams divided into 3 doses of 750 milligrams each.

Overdosage

Any medication taken in excess can have serious consequences. If you suspect an overdose, seek medical treatment immediately. An overdose of Trilisate can be fatal.

■ *Symptoms of Trilisate overdose may include:*
  Confusion, diarrhea, dizziness, drowsiness, headache, hearing impairment, rapid breathing, ringing in the ears, sweating, vomiting

Generic name:

TRIMETHOBENZAMIDE

See Tigan, page 1302.

Generic name:

TRIMETHOPRIM WITH SULFAMETHOXAZOLE

See Bactrim, page 135.

Generic name:

TRIMIPRAMINE

See Surmontil, page 1231.

Brand name:

TRIMOX

See Amoxil, page 58.

Brand name:

TRINALIN REPETABS

Pronounced: TRIN-uh-lin
Generic ingredients: Azatadine maleate, Pseudoephedrine sulfate

Why is this drug prescribed?

Trinalin Repetabs is a long-acting antihistamine/decongestant that relieves nasal stuffiness and middle ear congestion caused by hay fever and ongoing nasal inflammation. It can be used alone or with antibiotics and analgesics such as aspirin or acetaminophen. Azatadine, the antihistamine in this product, reduces itching and swelling and dries up secretions from the nose, eyes, and throat. Pseudoephedrine, the decongestant, reduces nasal congestion and makes breathing easier.

Most important fact about this drug

Trinalin Repetabs may cause drowsiness. You should not drive or operate dangerous machinery or participate in any hazardous activity that requires full mental alertness until you know how you react to this medication.

How should you take this medication?
Take this medication as indicated; do not take more than your doctor has prescribed.

■ *If you miss a dose...*
If you take Trinalin on a regular schedule, take the forgotten dose as soon as you remember. If it is almost time for your next dose, skip the one you missed and go back to your regular schedule. Do not take 2 doses at once.

■ *Storage instructions...*
Store at room temperature in a cool place.

What side effects may occur?
Side effects cannot be anticipated. If any develop or change in intensity, inform your doctor as soon as possible. Only your doctor can determine if it is safe for you to continue taking Trinalin.

■ *Side effects may include:*
Abdominal cramps, acute inflammation of the inner ear, anemia, anxiety, blood disorders, blurred vision, chest pain, chills, confusion, constipation, convulsions, diarrhea, difficulty breathing, dilated pupils, disturbed coordination, dizziness, dry mouth, nose, and throat, early menstruation, exaggerated feeling of well-being, excessive perspiration, excitement, extreme calm (sedation), fatigue, fear, fluttery heartbeat, frequent urination, hallucinations, headache, high blood pressure, hives, hysteria, increased chest congestion, increased sensitivity to light, insomnia, irregular heartbeat, irritability, loss of appetite, low blood pressure, nausea, nervousness, painful or difficult urination, pale skin, rapid heartbeat, rash, restlessness, ringing in the ears, severe allergic reaction, sleepiness, stuffy nose, tension, tightness in chest, tingling or pins and needles, tremor, upset stomach, urinary retention, vertigo, vomiting, weakness, wheezing

Why should this drug not be prescribed?
Trinalin should be avoided if you have narrow-angle glaucoma or difficulty urinating, if you are taking one of the antidepressant drugs known as MAO inhibitors or have taken one within the past two weeks, if you have severe high blood pressure, severe heart disease, or an overactive thyroid, or if you are sensitive to or have ever had an allergic reaction to any of its ingredients.

This drug should not be used to treat asthma and other lower respiratory tract diseases.

Special warnings about this medication
Trinalin should be used with care if you have a peptic ulcer or other upper intestinal obstruction, bladder obstruction due to an enlarged prostate or other bladder problems, a history of bronchial asthma, heart disease, high blood pressure, increased eye pressure, or diabetes.

Pseudoephedrine can be habit-forming at high doses. Remember that this medication can make you feel drowsy. Be careful driving, operating machinery, or using appliances.

Trinalin may cause dizziness, extreme calm (sedation), and low blood pressure in people aged 60 and over. It is also more likely to cause such side effects as confusion, convulsions, hallucinations, and death in this age group.

**Possible food and drug interactions
when taking this medication**
Alcohol may increase the effects of Trinalin. Do not drink alcohol while taking this medication.

If Trinalin is taken with certain other drugs, the effects of either could be increased, decreased, or altered. It is especially important to check with your doctor before combining Trinalin with the following:

Antacids such as Maalox
Barbiturates such as phenobarbital
Beta-blocking blood pressure drugs such as Tenormin and Inderal
Blood thinners such as Coumadin
Digitalis (Lanoxin)
Drugs for depression such as Prozac and Elavil
High blood pressure drugs such as Aldomet and Inversine
Kaolin (Kaopectate)
MAO inhibitor drugs such as the antidepressants Nardil and Parnate
Sedatives such as Nembutal and Seconal
Tranquilizers such as Xanax and Valium

**Special information
if you are pregnant or breastfeeding**
Although the effects of Trinalin during pregnancy have not been adequately studied, antihistamines have caused severe reactions in premature and newborn babies when used in the last 3 months of pregnancy. If you are pregnant or plan to become pregnant, notify your doctor immediately. Trinalin may appear in breast milk and could affect a nursing infant. If this medication is essential to your health, your doctor may advise you to discontinue breastfeeding until your treatment with Trinalin is finished.

Recommended dosage

ADULTS AND CHILDREN AGED 12 AND OVER

The usual dosage is 1 tablet twice a day.

Children under age 12 should not take Trinalin.

Overdosage

Any medication taken in excess can have serious consequences. An overdose of Trinalin can be fatal. If you suspect an overdose, seek medical attention immediately.

- *Symptoms of Trinalin overdose may include:*
  Anxiety, bluish color caused by lack of oxygen, blurred vision, chest pain, coma, convulsions, decreased mental alertness, delusions, difficulty sleeping, difficulty urinating, dizziness, excitement, extreme calm (sedation), exaggerated sense of well-being, fluttery heartbeat, giddiness, hallucinations, headache, high blood pressure/low blood pressure, irregular heartbeat, lack of muscle coordination, muscle tenseness, muscle weakness, nausea, perspiration, rapid heartbeat, restlessness, ringing in the ears, temporary interruption of breathing, thirst, tremors, vomiting

- *Overdose symptoms more common in children may include:*
  Dry mouth, fixed, dilated pupils, flushing, overstimulation, stomach and intestinal problems, very high body temperature

Brand name:

TRIPHASIL

See Oral Contraceptives, page 926.

Brand name:

TRITEC

Pronounced: TRIGH-tek
Generic name: Ranitidine bismuth citrate

Why is this drug prescribed?

Scientists have discovered that a germ called H. pylori is frequently the cause of ulcers that form in the duodenum (the part of the digestive system just past the stomach). Tritec, taken in combination with the antibiotic Biaxin, helps to cure H. pylori infection and improves your chances of staying ulcer-free.

Most important fact about this drug
Tritec alone will not cure the infection. You must also take Biaxin for the treatment to work.

How should you take this medication?
Take Tritec exactly as prescribed. For the first 2 weeks, you should take Biaxin along with Tritec. You should then continue taking Tritec alone for an additional 2 weeks. Tritec can be taken with or without food.

- *If you miss a dose...*
  Take it as soon as you remember. If it is almost time for the next dose, skip the one you missed and go back to your regular schedule. Do not take 2 doses at the same time.

- *Storage instructions...*
  Store at room temperature in a tightly closed container away from moisture and light.

What side effects may occur?
Side effects cannot be anticipated. If any develop or change in intensity, inform your doctor as soon as possible. Only your doctor can determine if it is safe for you to continue taking Tritec.

- *Side effects may include:*
  Abdominal discomfort, changes in taste, constipation, diarrhea, dizziness, female reproductive problems, gas, headache, itching, nausea, severe allergic reaction, skin rash, sleep disturbances, stomach pain, vomiting

Why should this drug not be prescribed?
If you have ever had an allergic reaction to Tritec or any of its ingredients, you should not take this drug.

Special warnings about this medication
Tritec/Biaxin treatment is not for people with severe kidney disease or the inherited condition called porphyria. If you have kidney problems, make sure the doctor is aware of them.

Tritec may cause darkening of the tongue and the stool. This reaction is harmless and temporary.

Possible food and drug interactions
when taking this medication

If Tritec is taken with certain other drugs, the effects of either can be increased, decreased, or altered. It is especially important to check with your doctor before combining Tritec with the following:

Alcohol
Antacids such as Maalox and Mylanta
Blood-thinning drugs such as Coumadin
Diazepam (Valium)
Diltiazem (Cardizem)
Enoxacin (Penetrex)
Glipizide (Glucotrol)
Glyburide (Diabeta, Micronase)
Itraconazole (Sporanox)
Ketoconazole (Nizoral)
Metformin (Glucophage)
Nifedipine (Procardia)
Phenytoin (Dilantin)
Procainamide (Procan SR)
Sucralfate (Carafate)
Theophylline (Theo-Dur)

Special information
if you are pregnant or breastfeeding

The effects of Tritec in pregnancy have not been adequately studied. If you are pregnant or plan to become pregnant, inform your doctor immediately. It is not known whether Tritec appears in breast milk. However, your doctor will probably want you to avoid nursing while taking the drug.

Recommended dosage

ADULTS

The recommended dose is 400 milligrams twice a day for 4 weeks (in combination with 500 milligrams of Biaxin 2 or 3 times a day for the first 2 weeks).

CHILDREN

The safety and effectiveness of Tritec have not been established in children.

Overdosage

Although doctors have had little experience with Tritec overdose, it's known that an overdose of bismuth, one of the ingredients, can damage the kidneys and the nerves. If you suspect an overdose of Tritec, seek medical attention immediately.

Generic name:

TROGLITAZONE

See Rezulin, page 1126.

Brand name:

T-STAT

See Erythromycin, Topical, page 487.

Brand name:

TUMS

See Antacids, page 75.

Brand name:

TUSSIONEX

Pronounced: TUSS-ee-uh-nex
Generic ingredients: Hydrocodone polistirex,
  Chlorpheniramine polistirex

Why is this drug prescribed?
Tussionex Extended-Release Suspension is a cough-suppressant/antihistamine combination used to relieve coughs and the upper respiratory symptoms of colds and allergies. Hydrocodone, a mild narcotic similar to codeine, is believed to work directly on the cough center. Chlorpheniramine, an antihistamine, reduces itching and swelling and dries up secretions from the eyes, nose, and throat.

Most important fact about this drug
This medication can cause considerable drowsiness and make you less alert. You should not drive or operate machinery or participate in any activity that requires full mental alertness until you know how you react to Tussionex.

How should you take this medication?
Tussionex should be taken exactly as prescribed.

It should not be diluted with other liquids or mixed with other drugs. Shake well before using.

■ *If you miss a dose...*
If you take Tussionex on a regular schedule, take the forgotten dose as soon as you remember. If it is almost time for your next dose, skip the one you missed and go back to your regular schedule. Do not take 2 doses at once.

■ *Storage instructions...*
Store at room temperature in a tightly closed container.

What side effects may occur?
Side effects cannot be anticipated. If any develop or change in intensity, inform your doctor as soon as possible. Only your doctor can determine if it is safe for you to continue taking Tussionex.

■ *Side effects may include:*
Anxiety, constipation, decreased mental and physical performance, difficulty breathing, difficulty urinating, dizziness, drowsiness, dry throat, emotional dependence, exaggerated feeling of depression, extreme calm (sedation), exaggerated sense of well-being, fear, itching, mental clouding, mood changes, nausea, rash, restlessness, sluggishness, tightness in chest, vomiting

Why should this drug not be prescribed?
Do not take Tussionex if you are sensitive to or have ever had an allergic reaction to hydrocodone or chlorpheniramine. Make sure your doctor is aware of any drug reactions you have experienced.

Special warnings about this medication
Tussionex contains a mild narcotic that can cause dependence and tolerance when the drug is used for several weeks. However, it is unlikely that dependence will develop when Tussionex is used for the short-term treatment of a cough.

Like all narcotics, Tussionex may produce slowed or irregular breathing. If you have lung disease or a breathing disorder, use this medication cautiously.

Use Tussionex with care if you have the eye condition known as narrow-angle glaucoma, asthma, an enlarged prostate gland, urinary difficulties, an intestinal disorder, liver or kidney disease, an underactive thyroid gland, or Addison's disease (a disorder of the adrenal glands), or if you have recently suffered a head injury.

Extra caution should be used when giving Tussionex to the elderly and those in a weakened condition.

Remember that Tussionex can cause drowsiness.

Narcotics can cause intestinal blockage or mask a severe abdominal condition.

Possible food and drug interactions
when taking this medication

Tussionex may increase the effects of alcohol. Do not drink alcohol while taking this medication.

If Tussionex is taken with certain other drugs, the effects of either could be increased, decreased, or altered. It is especially important to check with your doctor before combining Tussionex with the following:

Antispasmodic medications such as Bentyl and Cogentin
Major tranquilizers such as Thorazine and Compazine
MAO inhibitor drugs (antidepressant drugs such as Nardil and Parnate)
Medications for anxiety such as Xanax and Valium
Medications for depression such as Elavil and Prozac
Other antihistamines such as Benadryl
Other narcotics such as Percocet and Demerol

Special information
if you are pregnant or breastfeeding

The safety of Tussionex during pregnancy has not been adequately studied. However, babies born to mothers who have been taking narcotics regularly before delivery will be born addicted. If you are pregnant or plan to become pregnant, inform your doctor immediately. Tussionex may appear in breast milk and could affect a nursing infant. If this medication is essential to your health, your doctor may recommend that you stop breastfeeding until your treatment with Tussionex is finished.

Recommended dosage

ADULTS

The usual dose is 1 teaspoonful (5 milliliters) every 12 hours. Do not take more than 2 teaspoonfuls in 24 hours.

CHILDREN AGED 6 TO 12

The usual dose is one-half teaspoonful every 12 hours. Do not take more than 1 teaspoonful in 24 hours.

Tussionex is not recommended for children under 6 years old.

Overdosage

Any medication taken in excess can have serious consequences. A narcotic overdose can be fatal. If you suspect an overdose, seek medical treatment immediately.

■ *Symptoms of Tussionex overdose may include:*
Blue skin color due to lack of oxygen, cardiac arrest, cold and clammy skin, decreased or difficult breathing, extreme sleepiness leading to stupor or coma, low blood pressure, muscle flabbiness, slow heartbeat, temporary cessation of breathing

Brand name:

TUSSI-ORGANIDIN NR

Pronounced: TUSS-ee or-GAN-i-din
Generic ingredients: Guaifenesin, Codeine phosphate
Other brand name: Brontex

Why is this drug prescribed?

Tussi-Organidin NR is used to relieve coughs and chest congestion in adults and children. It contains guaifenesin, which helps thin and loosen mucus in the lungs, making it easier to cough up. It also contains a cough suppressant, the narcotic codeine.

Most important fact about this drug

Tussi-Organidin NR may cause you to become drowsy or less alert. Alcohol will intensify this effect. Driving, operating dangerous machinery, or participating in any hazardous activity that requires your full mental alertness is not recommended until you know how you react to this medication.

How should you take this medication?

Take Tussi-Organidin NR exactly as described. When giving the liquid to a child, use a calibrated dropper to measure the dose.

■ *If you miss a dose...*
Take the missed dose as soon as you remember. If it is almost time for your next dose, skip the one you missed and go back to your regular schedule. Never take 2 doses at once.

■ *Storage instructions...*
Store at room temperature in a tightly closed container, away from light.

What side effects may occur?
Side effects cannot be anticipated. If any side effects develop or change in intensity, tell your doctor as soon as possible. Only your doctor can determine whether it is safe to continue taking Tussi-Organidin NR.

■ *More common side effects may include:*
Constipation, nausea, pinpoint pupils of the eye, vomiting

■ *Less common side effects may include:*
Dizziness, headache, rash

At higher doses, this medication may also cause light-headedness, drowsiness, slowed breathing, and an exaggerated sense of well-being.

Why should this drug not be prescribed?
Do not take Tussi-Organidin NR if you are allergic to codeine or guaifenesin.

Special warnings about this medication
Because it contains codeine, Tussi-Organidin NR may cause drug dependence and tolerance with continued use.

Do not use this product in children under 2 years of age. Be cautious if the child has an allergy.

Do not take Tussi-Organidin NR for the constant cough brought on by smoking, asthma, chronic bronchitis, or emphysema unless your doctor recommends it. If your cough lasts for more than 1 week, tends to come back, or is accompanied by fever, rash, or persistent headache, check with your doctor.

Be sure to tell the doctor if you have any breathing problems, a severe abdominal condition, kidney or liver problems, an underactive thyroid gland, or an enlarged prostate. Also alert the doctor if you suffer from seizures, have had a head injury, or have recently had stomach, intestinal, or urinary tract surgery.

**Possible food and drug interactions
when taking this medication**
If Tussi-Organidin NR is taken with certain other drugs, the effects of either could be increased, decreased, or altered. It is especially important to check with your doctor before combining Tussi-Organidin NR with the following:

Alcohol

Antihistamines such as Actifed or Benadryl

Drugs used to treat anxiety or depression, such as Librium and Prozac

Sedatives such as Dalmane

Special information
if you are pregnant or breastfeeding

If you are pregnant or plan to become pregnant, inform your doctor immediately. The safety of Tussi-Organidin NR during pregnancy has not been established. Tussi-Organidin NR should not be taken if you are breastfeeding.

Recommended dosage

ADULTS AND CHILDREN 12 YEARS AND OLDER

Tussi-Organidin NR

The usual dosage is 2 teaspoonfuls every 4 hours, not to exceed 12 teaspoonfuls in 24 hours.

Brontex

The usual dosage is 1 tablet or 4 teaspoonfuls every 4 hours. Do not take more than 6 tablets in a 24-hour period.

CHILDREN 6 TO 12 YEARS OF AGE

Tussi-Organidin NR

The usual dosage is 1 teaspoonful every 4 hours, not to exceed 6 teaspoonfuls in 24 hours.

Brontex

The usual dosage is 2 teaspoonfuls every 4 hours. Do not give tablets.

CHILDREN 2 TO 6 YEARS OF AGE

Tussi-Organidin NR

Your doctor will determine the dosage according to weight. The recommended total daily dosage is 1 milligram per 2.2 pounds of body weight, divided into 4 small doses.

Overdosage

Any medication taken in excess can have serious consequences. If you suspect an overdose, seek medical treatment immediately.

- *Symptoms of Tussi-Organidin NR overdose may include:*
  Alternate periods of not breathing and rapid, deep breathing, bluish skin coloration, cold and clammy skin, constriction of the pupils of the eye, delirium, delusions, double vision, excitement, extreme sleepiness progressing to stupor or coma, flaccid muscles, hallucinations, low blood pressure, restlessness, slow, shallow, or labored breathing, slow heartbeat, speech disturbances, vertigo

Brand name:

TYLENOL

Pronounced: TIE-len-all
Generic name: Acetaminophen
Other brand names: Panadol, Aspirin Free Anacin

Why is this drug prescribed?

Tylenol is a fever- and pain-reducing medication that is widely used to relieve simple headaches and muscle aches; the minor aches and pains associated with the common cold; backache; toothache; minor pain of arthritis; and menstrual cramps.

Children's Tylenol is used to relieve fever, pain and discomfort due to colds, flu, teething, immunizations, and tonsillectomy.

Most important fact about this drug

Do not use Tylenol to relieve pain for more than 10 days, or to reduce fever for more than 3 days unless your doctor has specifically told you to do so.

How should you take this medication?

Follow the dosing instructions on the label. Do not take more Tylenol than is recommended.

- *If you miss a dose...*
  Take this medication only as needed.

- *Storage instructions...*
  Store at room temperature. Keep the liquid form from freezing.

What side effects may occur?

Tylenol is relatively free of side effects. Rarely, an allergic reaction may occur. If you develop any allergic symptoms such as rash, hives, swelling, or difficulty breathing, stop taking Tylenol immediately and notify your doctor.

Special warnings about this medication

Remember that Tylenol should not be used for more than 10 days for pain, or 3 days for fever. Children's Tylenol should not be used for more than 5 days for pain, or 3 days for fever. If pain or fever persists or gets worse, if new symptoms develop, or if there is any redness or swelling, contact your doctor. These symptoms could indicate a more serious illness.

If you generally drink 3 or more alcoholic beverages per day, check with your doctor about using Tylenol and other acetaminophen-containing products, and never take more than the recommended dosage. There is a possibility of damage to the liver when large amounts of alcohol and acetaminophen are combined.

**Possible food and drug interactions
when taking this medication**

If Tylenol is taken with certain other drugs the effects of either could be increased, decreased, or altered. It is especially important to check with your doctor before combining Tylenol with the following:

Alcohol
Cholestyramine (Questran)
Isoniazid (Nydrazid)
Nonsteroidal anti-inflammatory drugs such as Dolobid and Motrin
Oral Contraceptives
Phenytoin (Dilantin)
Warfarin (Coumadin)
Zidovudine (Retrovir)

Tylenol should not be used with other products containing acetaminophen.

**Special information
if you are pregnant or breastfeeding**

As with all medications, ask your doctor or health care professional whether it is safe for you to use Tylenol while you are pregnant or breastfeeding.

Recommended dosage

ADULTS AND CHILDREN 12 YEARS AND OLDER

Tylenol Regular Strength
The usual dose is 2 caplets or tablets every 4 to 6 hours. Do not take more than 12 caplets or tablets in 24 hours.

Tylenol Extended Relief
The usual dose is 2 caplets every 8 hours, not to exceed 6 caplets in any 24-hour period. Swallow each caplet whole. Do not crush, chew, or dissolve the caplets.

CHILDREN 6 TO 12 YEARS OLD

Tylenol Regular Strength
One-half to 1 caplet or tablet every 4 to 6 hours. Children in this age group should not be given more than 5 doses in 24 hours.

Children's Tylenol
All doses of Children's Tylenol may be repeated every 4 hours, but not more than 5 times daily. Chewable tablets: The usual dose for children 6 to 8 years of age is 4 tablets; 9 to 10 years, 5 tablets; 11 to 12 years, 6 tablets. Elixir and suspension liquid (a special cup for measuring dosage is provided): The usual dose for children 6 to 8 years of age is 2 teaspoons; 9 to 10 years, 2½ teaspoons; 11 to 12 years, 3 teaspoons.

CHILDREN UNDER 6 YEARS OLD

Regular Strength Tylenol
Consult your physician or health care professional.

Children's Tylenol
All doses of Children's Tylenol may be repeated every 4 hours, but not more than 5 times daily. Children under 2 years old should be given Children's Tylenol only on the advice of a physician. Chewable tablets: The usual dose for children 2 to 3 years of age is 2 tablets; 4 to 5 years, 3 tablets. Elixir and suspension liquid (a special cup for measuring dosage is provided): The usual dose for children 4 to 11 months of age is ½ teaspoon; 12 to 23 months, ¾ teaspoon; 2 to 3 years, 1 teaspoon; 4 to 5 years, 1½ teaspoons.

Infants' Tylenol Drops and Suspension Drops
The usual dose for children 0 to 3 months of age is 0.4 milliliter; 4 to 11 months, 0.8 milliliter; 12 to 23 months, 1.2 milliliters; 2 to 3 years, 1.6 milliliters; 4 to 5 years, 2.4 milliliters.

Overdosage
Any medication taken in excess can have serious consequences. If you suspect an overdose, seek medical attention immediately. Massive doses of Tylenol may cause liver damage.

■ *Symptoms of Tylenol overdose may include:*
  Excessive perspiration, exhaustion, general discomfort, nausea, vomiting

Brand name:

TYLENOL WITH CODEINE

Pronounced: TIE-len-awl with CO-deen
Generic ingredients: Acetaminophen, Codeine phosphate
Other brand name: Phenaphen with Codeine

Why is this drug prescribed?
Tylenol with Codeine, a narcotic analgesic, is used to treat mild to moderately severe pain. It contains two drugs—acetaminophen and codeine. Acetaminophen, an antipyretic (fever-reducing) analgesic, is used to reduce pain and fever. Codeine, a narcotic analgesic, is used to treat pain that is moderate to severe.

People who are allergic to aspirin can take Tylenol with Codeine.

Most important fact about this drug
Tylenol with Codeine contains a narcotic (codeine) and, even if taken in prescribed amounts, can cause physical and psychological addiction if taken for a long enough time.

Addiction may be more of a risk for a person who has been addicted to alcohol or drugs. Be sure to follow your doctor's instructions carefully when taking Tylenol with Codeine (or any other drugs that contain a narcotic).

How should you take this medication?
Tylenol with Codeine may be taken with meals or with milk (but not with alcohol).

■ *If you miss a dose...*
  If you take this medication on a regular schedule, take the forgotten dose as soon as you remember. If it is almost time for your next dose, skip the one you missed and go back to your regular schedule. Do not take 2 doses at once.

■ *Storage instructions...*
  Store away from heat, light, and moisture. Keep the liquid from freezing.

What side effects may occur?
Side effects cannot be anticipated. If any develop or change in intensity, inform your doctor as soon as possible. Only your doctor can determine if it is safe for you to continue taking Tylenol with Codeine.

- *More common side effects may include:*
  Dizziness, light-headedness, nausea, sedation, shortness of breath, vomiting

- *Less common side effects may include:*
  Abdominal pain, allergic reactions, constipation, depressed feeling, exaggerated feeling of well-being, itchy skin

- *Rare side effects may include:*
  Decreased breathing (when Tylenol with Codeine is taken at higher doses)

Why should this drug not be prescribed?
You should not use Tylenol with Codeine if you are sensitive to either acetaminophen (Tylenol) or codeine.

Special warnings about this medication
You should take Tylenol with Codeine cautiously and only according to your doctor's instructions, as you would take any medication containing a narcotic. Make sure your doctor is aware of any problems you have had with drug or alcohol addiction.

Tylenol with Codeine tablets contain a sulfite that may cause allergic reactions in some people. These reactions may include shock and severe, possibly life-threatening, asthma attacks. People with asthma are more likely to be sensitive to sulfites.

If you have experienced a head injury, consult your doctor before taking Tylenol with Codeine.

If you have stomach problems, such as an ulcer, check with your doctor before taking Tylenol with Codeine. Tylenol with Codeine may obscure the symptoms of stomach problems, making them difficult to diagnose and treat.

If you have ever had liver, kidney, thyroid, or adrenal disease, difficulty urinating, or an enlarged prostate, consult your doctor before taking Tylenol with Codeine.

If you generally drink 3 or more alcoholic beverages per day, check with your doctor before using Tylenol with Codeine and other acetaminophen-containing products, and never take more than the recommended dosage.

There is a possibility of damage to the liver when large amounts of alcohol and acetaminophen are combined.

This drug may cause drowsiness and impair your ability to drive a car or operate potentially dangerous machinery. Do not participate in any activities that require full attention when using this drug until you are sure of its effect on you.

Possible food and drug interactions
when taking this medication
Alcohol may increase the sedative effects of Tylenol with Codeine. Therefore, do not drink alcohol while you are taking this medication.

If Tylenol with Codeine is taken with certain other drugs, the effects of either could be increased, decreased, or altered. It is especially important to check with your doctor before combining Tylenol with Codeine with the following:

Antidepressants such as Elavil, Nardil, Parnate, and Tofranil
Drugs that control spasms, such as Cogentin
Major tranquilizers such as Clozaril and Thorazine
Other narcotic painkillers such as Darvon
Tranquilizers such as Xanax and Valium

Special information
if you are pregnant or breastfeeding
It is not known if Tylenol with Codeine could injure a baby, or if it could affect a woman's reproductive capacity. Using any medication that contains a narcotic during pregnancy may cause babies to be born with a physical addiction to the narcotic. If you are pregnant or plan to become pregnant, you should not take Tylenol with Codeine unless the potential benefits clearly outweigh the possible dangers. As with other narcotic painkillers, taking Tylenol with Codeine shortly before delivery (especially at higher dosages) may cause some degree of breathing difficulty in the mother and newborn.

Some studies (but not all) have reported that codeine appears in breast milk and may affect a nursing infant. Therefore, nursing mothers should use Tylenol with Codeine only if the potential gains are greater than the potential hazards.

Recommended dosage

ADULTS

Dosage will depend on how severe your pain is and how you respond to the drug.

To Relieve Pain

A single dose may contain from 15 milligrams to 60 milligrams of codeine phosphate and from 300 to 1,000 milligrams of acetaminophen. The maximum dose in a 24-hour period should be 360 milligrams of codeine phosphate and 4,000 milligrams of acetaminophen. Your doctor will determine the amounts of codeine phosphate and acetaminophen taken in each dose. Doses may be repeated up to every 4 hours.

Single doses above 60 milligrams of codeine do not give enough pain relief to balance the increased number of side effects.

Adults may also take Tylenol with Codeine elixir (liquid). Tylenol with Codeine elixir contains 120 milligrams of acetaminophen and 12 milligrams of codeine phosphate per teaspoonful.

The usual adult dose is 1 tablespoonful every 4 hours as needed.

CHILDREN

The safety of Tylenol with Codeine elixir has not been established in children under 3 years old.

Children 3 to 6 years old may take 1 teaspoonful 3 or 4 times daily.

Children 7 to 12 years old may take 2 teaspoonsfuls 3 or 4 times daily.

OLDER ADULTS

Older people and anyone in a weakened or run-down condition should use Tylenol with Codeine cautiously.

Overdosage

Any medication taken in excess can cause symptoms of overdose. Severe overdosage of Tylenol with Codeine can cause death. If you suspect an overdose, seek medical attention immediately.

■ *Symptoms of Tylenol with Codeine overdose may include:*
Bluish skin, cold and clammy skin, coma due to low blood sugar, decreased, irregular, or stopped breathing, extreme sleepiness progressing to stupor or coma, general bodily discomfort, heart attack, kidney failure, liver failure, low blood pressure, muscle weakness, nausea, slow heartbeat, sweating, vomiting

Brand name:

TYLOX

See Percocet, page 979.

Brand name:

ULTRAM

Pronounced: UL-tram
Generic name: Tramadol hydrochloride

Why is this drug prescribed?
Ultram is prescribed to relieve moderate to moderately severe pain.

Most important fact about this drug
You should not drive a car, operate machinery, or perform any other potentially hazardous activities until you know how this drug affects you.

How should you take this medication?
It's important to take Ultram exactly as prescribed. Do not increase the dosage or length of time you take this drug without your doctor's approval.

- *If you miss a dose...*
  Take it as soon as you remember. However, if it is almost time for your next dose, skip the one you missed and go back to your regular schedule. Never take 2 doses at once.

- *Storage instructions...*
  Store in a tightly closed container at room temperature.

What side effects may occur?
Side effects cannot be anticipated. If any develop or change in intensity, tell your doctor as soon as possible. Only your doctor can determine if it is safe for you to continue taking Ultram.

- *More common side effects may include:*
  Agitation, anxiety, bloating and gas, constipation, convulsive movements, diarrhea, dizziness, drowsiness, dry mouth, feeling of elation, hallucinations, headache, indigestion, itching, nausea, nervousness, sweating, tremor, vomiting, weakness

■ *Less common side effects may include:*
Abdominal pain, confusion, coordination problems, feeling of illness, flushing, frequent urination, inability to urinate, loss of appetite, menopausal symptoms, rash, sleeping problems, visual problems

■ *Rare side effects may include:*
Accidental injury, allergic reaction, altered taste, amnesia, difficult or labored breathing, difficulty concentrating, dizziness or light-headedness upon standing, fainting, feeling of "pins and needles," hives, menstrual problems, mental sluggishness or clouding, painful urination, rapid heartbeat, seizures, suicidal tendencies, weight loss

Why should this drug not be prescribed?
Avoid Ultram if it has ever given you an allergic reaction. Also avoid Ultram after taking large doses of sleeping pills such as Halcion, Dalmane, and Restoril; narcotic pain relievers such as Demerol, morphine, Darvon, and Percocet; or psychotherapeutic drugs such as antidepressants and tranquilizers. And do not take Ultram after drinking excessive amounts of alcohol.

Special warnings about this medication
If you have stomach problems such as an ulcer, make sure your doctor is aware of them. Ultram may hide the symptoms, making them difficult to diagnose and treat.

If you have become dependent on such drugs as Percocet, Demerol, or morphine, you may experience withdrawal symptoms when you switch to Ultram.

You can also experience withdrawal symptoms if you stop taking Ultram abruptly. Such symptoms include anxiety, sweating, insomnia, pain, nausea, tremor, diarrhea, and respiratory problems. A gradual decrease in dosage will help prevent these symptoms.

Do not take more than the recommended dose of Ultram, since larger doses have been known to cause seizures, especially if you have epilepsy or are taking medications that also increase the risk of seizures. Among the medications with this effect are almost all antidepressant drugs, plus narcotics and major tranquilizers such as Loxitane and Stelazine.

If you have liver or kidney disease, be sure your doctor knows about it. Your dosage may have to be reduced.

Before you have any kind of surgery, make sure the doctor knows you are taking Ultram.

If you have experienced a head injury, consult your doctor before taking Ultram. The medication's effects may be stronger and could hide warning signs of serious trouble.

Possible food and drug interactions when taking this medication

Ultram may increase the drowsiness caused by alcohol. Do not drink alcohol while taking this medication.

If Ultram is taken with certain other drugs, the effects of either could be increased, decreased, or altered. It is especially important to check with your doctor before combining Ultram with the following:

Carbamazepine (Tegretol)
Cyclobenzaprine (Flexeril)
Drugs known as MAO inhibitors, including the antidepressants Nardil
  and Parnate
Serotonin-boosting antidepressants such as Paxil, Prozac, and Zoloft
"Tricyclic" antidepressants such as Elavil, Norpramin, and Tofranil
Major tranquilizers such as Thorazine and Stelazine
Narcotic pain relievers (Demerol, morphine, Darvon, Percocet)
Promethazine (Mepergan, Phenergan)
Quinidine (Quinidex)
Sleeping pills (Halcion, Dalmane, Restoril)
Tranquilizers (Valium, Xanax)

Special information if you are pregnant or breastfeeding

The effects of Ultram during pregnancy have not been adequately studied. If you are pregnant or plan to become pregnant, tell your doctor immediately. Ultram appears in breast milk and may affect a nursing infant. If this medication is essential to your health, your doctor may advise you to discontinue breastfeeding until your treatment is finished.

Recommended dosage

ADULTS

The usual starting dose of Ultram is 50 to 100 milligrams every 4 to 6 hours, depending on the severity of pain. The most you should take is 400 milligrams a day (300 milligrams for those over age 75).

For people with kidney problems, the usual starting dose is 50 to 100 milligrams every 12 hours; and the maximum per day is 200 milligrams. For those with cirrhosis, the usual dose is 50 milligrams every 12 hours.

People taking the anti-seizure medication Tegretol in regular doses of up to 800 milligrams a day may need double the usual dosage of Ultram.

CHILDREN

Safety and effectiveness in children under 16 years of age have not been established.

Overdosage

An overdose of Ultram can be fatal. If you suspect an overdose, seek emergency medical treatment immediately.

- *Symptoms of Ultram overdose include:*
  Difficult or slowed breathing, seizures

Brand name:

ULTRASE

See Pancrease, page 947.

Brand name:

UNI-DUR

See Theo-Dur, page 1293.

Brand name:

UNIPHYL

See Theo-Dur, page 1293.

Brand name:

UNIRETIC

Pronounced: you-nih-RET-ick
Generic ingredients: Moexipril hydrochloride,
*   Hydrochlorothiazide*

Why is this drug prescribed?

Uniretic combines two types of blood pressure medication. The first, moexipril hydrochloride, is an ACE (angiotensin-converting enzyme) inhibitor.

It works by preventing a chemical in your blood called angiotensin I from converting into a more potent form (angiotensin II) that increases salt and water retention in the body and causes the blood vessels to constrict—two actions that tend to increase blood pressure.

To aid in clearing excess water from the body, Uniretic also contains hydrochlorothiazide, a diuretic that promotes production of urine. Diuretics often wash too much potassium out of the body along with the water. However, the ACE inhibitor part of Uniretic tends to keep potassium in the body, thereby canceling this unwanted effect.

Uniretic is not used for the initial treatment of high blood pressure. It is saved for later use, when a single blood pressure medication is not sufficient for the job.

Most important fact about this drug
You must take Uniretic regularly for it to be effective, and you must continue taking it even if you are feeling well. Like other blood pressure medications, Uniretic does not cure high blood pressure; it merely keeps it under control.

How should you take this medication?
Take Uniretic once a day, 1 hour before a meal. Try not to miss any doses. Stopping Uniretic suddenly could cause a rise in blood pressure.

■ *If you miss a dose...*
Take it as soon as you remember. If it is almost time for your next dose, skip the one you missed and go back to your regular schedule. Never take 2 doses at the same time.

■ *Storage instructions...*
Store at room temperature, away from moisture, in a tightly closed container.

What side effects may occur?
Side effects cannot be anticipated. If any develop or change in intensity, inform your doctor as soon as possible. Only your doctor can determine if it is safe for you to continue taking Uniretic.

■ *Common side effects may include:*
Abdominal pain, back pain, bronchitis, chest pain, cough, diarrhea, dizziness, fatigue, fever, flu symptoms, headache, impotence, increased blood sugar, indigestion, infection, inflammation of the nasal passages,

pain, rash, sinus inflammation, sore throat, swelling, tension, upper respiratory tract infection, urinary tract infection, vertigo

■ *Rare side effects may include:*
Constipation, difficulty breathing, dizziness upon standing, drowsiness, eczema, fainting, flushing, gynecological problems, inflammation of the digestive tract, insomnia, itching, loss of strength, low blood counts, muscle aches, nosebleed, pinkeye, pneumonia, rapid heartbeat, sweating, urinary problems

Why should this drug not be prescribed?
Do not take Uniretic if you've had a severe reaction called angioedema (swelling of the face, arms, legs, and throat) to any other ACE inhibitor (for example, Capoten, Prinivil, or Zestril). Avoid this drug, too, if you've had an allergic reaction to either of its ingredients, or to any sulfa drug. (Allergic reactions to Uniretic are more likely if you have a history of allergy or bronchial asthma.)

If you have problems with urination, do not take this drug.

Special warnings about this medication
Contact your doctor immediately if you develop swelling around your lips, tongue, or throat, or in your arms and legs, or if you begin to have difficulty breathing or swallowing. You may need emergency room treatment.

If you have poor kidneys, use Uniretic with caution. For people with severe kidney disease, Uniretic is not recommended at all. Your doctor should test your kidney function at the start of treatment, and continue to monitor it as long as you take the drug.

Uniretic can cause light-headedness, especially during the first few days of treatment. If you faint, stop taking the medication and call your doctor immediately.

Uniretic can cause a severe drop in blood pressure if you lose too much liquid through excessive sweating, severe diarrhea, or vomiting. Contact your doctor immediately if you develop one of these problems.

Low blood pressure is especially dangerous if you have congestive heart failure or other heart conditions. Your doctor should monitor your pressure with extra care if that's the case.

This drug should be used with caution if you are on dialysis. There have been reports of extreme allergic reactions during dialysis in people taking ACE inhibitors such as the one in Uniretic. A severe reaction is also more likely if you've ever had desensitization treatments with bee or wasp venom.

If you have liver disease or a disease of connective tissue called lupus erythematosus, Uniretic should be used with caution. Tell your doctor immediately if you notice a yellowish color to your skin or the whites of your eyes.

While taking Uniretic, do not use potassium supplements, salt substitutes that contain potassium, or diuretics that leave potassium levels high (such as Dyrenium and Moduretic) unless your doctor recommends it.

Diuretics such as the one in Uniretic sometimes leave the body with too little sodium, chloride, or potassium, leading to symptoms such as dry mouth, thirst, weakness, sluggishness, drowsiness, restlessness, muscle pain or cramps, muscular fatigue, low urine output, rapid heartbeat, nausea, and vomiting. If you develop any of these symptoms, alert your doctor.

Uniretic can aggravate diabetes or high cholesterol. If you have one of these conditions, your doctor should closely monitor your blood sugar or cholesterol levels.

If you develop unusual or increased coughing, tell your doctor. Contact your doctor immediately if you develop a sore throat or fever; they could be signs of a more serious illness.

If you are having a surgical procedure that requires anesthesia, make sure the doctor knows that you are taking Uniretic.

Possible food and drug interactions
when taking this medication
If Uniretic is taken with certain other drugs, the effects of either could be increased, decreased, or altered. It is especially important to check with your doctor before combining Uniretic with the following:

ACTH
Alcohol
Barbiturates such as phenobarbital or Seconal
Cholestyramine (Questran)
Colestipol (Colestid)
Diabetes medications such as glyburide and insulin
Guanabenz (Wytensin)
Lithium (Lithobid, Lithonate)
Narcotics such as Percocet
Nonsteroidal anti-inflammatory painkillers such as Motrin and Naprosyn
Potassium-sparing diuretics such as Dyrenium or Moduretic

Potassium supplements such as Slow-K
Propantheline (Pro-Banthine)
Salt substitutes containing potassium
Steroid medications such as prednisone (Deltasone)

Special information
if you are pregnant or breastfeeding
ACE inhibitors such as Uniretic have been shown to cause injury and even
death of the developing baby when used during the second and third
trimesters of pregnancy. If you are pregnant, contact your doctor immediately
for instructions on how to safely discontinue Uniretic. If you plan to become
pregnant, discuss the situation with your doctor as soon as possible.

Researchers do not know whether Uniretic appears in breast milk. If Uniretic
is essential to your health, your doctor may advise you to stop breastfeeding
while you are taking the drug.

Recommended dosage

ADULTS

Dosages of this drug are always tailored to the individual's response. The
doctor will probably start with a relatively low dosage, then after 2 or 3
weeks adjust it upward if necessary. In general, the daily dose of moexipril
should not exceed 30 milligrams. For hydrochlorothiazide, the maximum is 50
milligrams a day.

Your doctor may prescribe other blood pressure medications along with
Uniretic.

CHILDREN

The safety and effectiveness of Uniretic have not been established in
children.

Overdosage
Any medication taken in excess can have serious consequences. If you
suspect an overdose, seek medical attention immediately.

■ *Symptoms of Uniretic overdose are likely to include:*
Low blood pressure, dehydration (loss of body fluids), low levels of
sodium, potassium, and chloride

Brand name:

UNIVASC

Pronounced: YOO-ni-vask
Generic name: Moexipril Hydrochloride

Why is this drug prescribed?

Univasc is used in the treatment of high blood pressure. It is effective when used alone or with thiazide diuretics that help rid the body of excess water. Univasc belongs to a family of drugs called angiotensin-converting enzyme (ACE) inhibitors. It works by preventing the transformation of a hormone in your blood called angiotensin I into a more potent substance that increases salt and water retention in your body. Univasc also enhances blood flow throughout your blood vessels.

Most important fact about this drug

You must take Univasc regularly for it to be effective. Since blood pressure declines gradually, it may be several weeks before you get the full benefit of Univasc; and you must continue taking it even if you are feeling well. Univasc does not cure high blood pressure; it merely keeps it under control.

How should you take this medication?

Univasc should be taken 1 hour before a meal. Try to get in the habit of taking your medication at the same time each day, such as 1 hour before breakfast, so that it is easier to remember. Always take Univasc exactly as prescribed.

- *If you miss a dose...*
  Take the forgotten dose as soon as you remember. If it is almost time for the next dose, skip the one you missed and go back to your regular schedule. Never try to "catch up" by doubling the dose.

- *Storage instructions...*
  Store at room temperature in a tightly closed container, away from moisture.

What side effects may occur?

Side effects cannot be anticipated. If any develop or change in intensity, tell your doctor as soon as possible. Only your doctor can determine if it is safe for you to continue taking Univasc.

■ *More common side effects may include:*
Cough, diarrhea, dizziness, "flu-like" symptoms

If you develop swelling of your face, around the lips, tongue, or throat; swelling of arms and legs; sore throat, fever, and chills; or difficulty breathing or swallowing, stop taking the drug and contact your doctor immediately. You may need emergency treatment.

■ *Less common side effects may include:*
Fatigue, flushing, muscle pain, rash, sore throat

■ *Rare side effects may include:*
Abdominal pain, anemia, anxiety, changes in appetite and weight, changes in taste, chest pain, constipation, difficult or labored breathing, difficulty sleeping, drowsiness, dry mouth, fainting, feeling of illness, fluid retention, heart attack, hives, irregular heart rhythm, itching, joint pain, kidney problems, light-headedness on standing up, liver disease, low blood pressure, mood changes, nervousness, rash or skin disease, reduced amount of urine, ringing in ears, sensitivity to light, stroke, sweating, swelling of the arms, face, legs, throbbing, fluttery heartbeat, vomiting, wheezing

Why should this drug not be prescribed?
If you have ever had an allergic reaction to Univasc or other ACE inhibitors such as Capoten, Vasotec, and Zestril, you should not take this medication.

Special warnings about this medication
Your doctor will check your kidney function when you start taking Univasc and watch it carefully for the first few weeks.

Univasc can cause low blood pressure, especially if you are taking high doses of diuretics. You may feel light-headed or faint, especially during the first few days of therapy. If these symptoms occur, contact your doctor. Your dosage may need to be adjusted or discontinued. If you actually faint, stop taking the drug and contact your doctor immediately.

If you have congestive heart failure or other heart or circulatory disorders, use this drug with caution. Be cautious, too, if you have kidney disease, diabetes, or a collagen-vascular disease such as lupus erythematosus or scleroderma.

Excessive sweating, severe diarrhea, or vomiting could make you lose too much water, causing your blood pressure to become too low. Call your doctor if you have any of those conditions.

If you notice a yellow coloring to your skin or the whites of your eyes, stop taking the drug and notify your doctor immediately. You could be developing liver problems.

If you are using bee or wasp venom to prevent severe reactions to stings, you may have an allergic reaction to Univasc.

Some people on dialysis have had an allergic reaction to this type of drug (ACE inhibitor).

If you develop a persistent, dry cough, tell your doctor. It may be due to the medication and, if so, will disappear if you stop taking Univasc. If you develop a sore throat or fever, you should contact your doctor immediately. It could indicate a more serious illness.

Do not take potassium supplements or salt substitutes containing potassium without talking to your doctor first. In a medical emergency and before you have surgery, notify your doctor or dentist that you are taking Univasc.

Possible food and drug interactions when taking this medication

If Univasc is taken with certain other drugs, the effects of either could be increased, decreased, or altered. It is especially important to check with your doctor before combining Univasc with the following:

Diuretics (Diuril, HydroDIURIL, Lasix)
Lithium (Eskalith, Lithobid)
Potassium-sparing diuretics (Aldactone, Moduretic, Maxzide)
Potassium supplements (Slow-K)

Special information if you are pregnant or breastfeeding

Univasc can cause injury or death to developing and newborn babies if taken during the second and third trimesters of pregnancy. If you are pregnant and are taking Univasc, contact your doctor immediately. It is not known whether Univasc appears in human breast milk. Therefore, Univasc should be used with caution if you are breastfeeding.

Recommended dosage

ADULTS

For people not taking a diuretic drug, the usual starting dose is 7.5 milligrams taken once a day, an hour before a meal. The dosage after that can range from 7.5 to 30 milligrams per day, taken in either a single dose or divided into 2 equal doses daily. The maximum dose is 60 milligrams per day.

Your doctor will closely monitor the effect of this drug and adjust it according to your individual needs.

People already taking a diuretic should stop taking it, if possible, 2 to 3 days before starting Univasc. This reduces the possibility of fainting or light-headedness. If the diuretic cannot be discontinued, the starting dosage of Univasc should be 3.75 milligrams. If Univasc alone does not control your blood pressure, your doctor will have you start taking a diuretic again.

For people with kidney problems, the usual starting dose is 3.75 milligrams a day; your doctor may gradually raise the dose to a maximum of 15 milligrams a day.

CHILDREN

The safety and effectiveness of Univasc have not been established in children.

Overdosage

Although there is no specific information available, a sudden drop in blood pressure would be the most likely symptom of Univasc overdose.

If you suspect an overdose, seek medical attention immediately.

Brand name:

URISED

Pronounced: YOUR-i-said
*Generic ingredients: Methenamine, Methylene blue, Phenyl
    salicylate, Benzoic acid, Atropine sulfate, Hyoscyamine*

Why is this drug prescribed?

Urised relieves lower urinary tract discomfort caused by inflammation or diagnostic procedures. It is used to treat urinary tract infections including cystitis (inflammation of the bladder and ureters), urethritis (inflammation of the urethra), and trigonitis (inflammation of the mucous membrane of the bladder). Methenamine, the major component of this drug, acts as a mild antiseptic by changing into formaldehyde in the urinary tract when it comes in contact with acidic urine.

Most important fact about this drug

Urised may give a blue to blue-green color to urine and discolor stools as well.

How should you take this medication?
If dry mouth occurs, hard candy or gum, saliva substitute, or crushed ice may provide temporary relief.

Take this medication exactly as prescribed; do not take more than the recommended dose.

Drinking plenty of fluids will help the medication work better and relieve discomfort.

■ *If you miss a dose...*
Take it as soon as you remember. If it is almost time for your next dose, skip the one you missed and go back to your regular schedule. Never take 2 doses at the same time.

■ *Storage instructions...*
Store Urised at room temperature, in a dry place.

What side effects may occur?
Side effects cannot be anticipated. If any develop or change in intensity, inform your doctor as soon as possible. Only your doctor can determine if it is safe for you to continue taking Urised.

■ *Side effects with long-term use may include:*
Acute urinary retention (in men with an enlarged prostate), blurry vision, difficulty urinating, dizziness, dry mouth, flushing, rapid pulse, skin rash

Why should this drug not be prescribed?
Urised should be avoided if you have glaucoma, a bladder blockage, cardiospasm, or a disorder that obstructs the passage of food through the stomach. Also avoid Urised if you are sensitive to or have ever had an allergic reaction to any of its ingredients.

Special warnings about this medication
Urised should be used cautiously if you have heart disease or have ever had a reaction to medications that are chemically similar to atropine.

Your doctor may ask you to check your urine with phenaphthazine paper to see if it is acidic. Urine acidifiers, such as vitamin C, may be recommended if the urine is not acidic enough.

Possible food and drug interactions
when taking this medication

If Urised is taken with certain other drugs, the effects of either could be increased, decreased, or altered. It is especially important to check with your doctor before combining Urised with the following:

Acetazolamide (Diamox)
Potassium supplements such as Slow-K
Sodium bicarbonate antacids such as Alka-Seltzer
Sulfa drugs such as Gantrisin, Gantanol, Bactrim, and Septra

Drugs and foods that produce alkaline urine (such as sodium bicarbonate, antacids, and orange juice) should be limited.

Special information
if you are pregnant or breastfeeding

The effects of Urised during pregnancy have not been adequately studied. If you are pregnant or plan to become pregnant, inform your doctor immediately. Urised may appear in breast milk and could affect a nursing infant. If this medication is essential to your health, your doctor may advise you to stop breastfeeding until your treatment with Urised ends.

Recommended dosage

ADULTS

The usual dose is 2 tablets, 4 times a day.

CHILDREN 6 YEARS AND OLDER

The dosage must be determined by your doctor.

CHILDREN UNDER 6 YEARS

Use is not recommended in children under 6 years old.

Overdosage

Any medication taken in excess can have serious consequences. If you suspect an overdose, seek medical treatment immediately.

■ *Symptoms of Urised overdose may include:*
Abdominal pain, bladder and abdominal irritation, bloody diarrhea, bloody urine, burning pain in throat and mouth, circulatory collapse, coma, dilated pupils (large pupils), dizziness, dry nose, mouth, and throat, elevated blood pressure, extremely high body temperature, headache, hot, dry, flushed skin, painful and frequent urination, pallor (paleness), pounding heartbeat

(pounding sensation against the chest), rapid heartbeat (increased pulse rate), respiratory failure, ringing in ears, sweating, vomiting, weakness, white sores in mouth

Brand name:

URISPAS

Pronounced: YOUR-eh-spaz
Generic name: Flavoxate hydrochloride

Why is this drug prescribed?

Urispas prevents spasms in the urinary tract and relieves the painful or difficult urination, urinary urgency, excessive nighttime urination, pubic area pain, frequency of urination, and inability to hold urine caused by urinary tract infections. Urispas is taken in combination with antibiotics to treat the infection.

Most important fact about this drug

Urispas can cause blurred vision and drowsiness. Be careful driving, operating machinery, or performing any activity that requires complete mental alertness until you know how you will react to this medication.

How should you take this medication?

Take this medication exactly as prescribed. Urispas may make your mouth dry. Sucking on a hard candy, chewing gum, or melting bits of ice in your mouth can provide relief.

- *If you miss a dose...*
  Take it as soon as you remember. If it is almost time for your next dose, skip the one you missed and go back to your regular schedule. Do not take 2 doses at once.

- *Storage instructions...*
  Store away from heat, light, and moisture.

What side effects may occur?

Side effects cannot be anticipated. If any develop or change in intensity, notify your doctor as soon as possible. Only your doctor can determine whether it is safe for you to continue taking Urispas.

- *Side effects may include:*
  Allergic skin reactions, including hives, blurred vision and vision changes, drowsiness, dry mouth, fluttery heartbeat, headache, high body tempera-

ture, mental confusion (especially in the elderly), nausea, nervousness, painful or difficult urination, rapid heartbeat, vertigo, vomiting

Why should this drug not be prescribed?

You should not take Urispas if you have stomach or intestinal blockage, muscle relaxation problems (especially the sphincter muscle), abdominal bleeding, or urinary tract blockage.

Special warnings about this medication

Use Urispas cautiously if you have the eye condition known as glaucoma.

Possible food and drug interactions
when taking this medication

No interactions involving Urispas have been noted.

Special information
if you are pregnant or breastfeeding

The effects of Urispas during pregnancy have not been adequately studied. If you are pregnant or plan to become pregnant, inform your doctor immediately. Urispas may appear in breast milk and could affect a nursing infant. If this medication is essential to your health, your doctor may advise you to stop breastfeeding until your treatment is finished.

Recommended dosage

ADULTS AND CHILDREN OVER AGE 12

The usual dose of Urispas is one or two 100-milligram tablets 3 or 4 times a day.

When your symptoms have improved, your doctor may reduce the dosage.

CHILDREN

Safety and effectiveness of Urispas in children under 12 years of age have not been established.

Overdosage

Any medication taken in excess can have serious consequences. If you suspect an overdose of Urispas, seek medical attention immediately.

■ *Symptoms of Urispas overdose may include:*
  Convulsions, decreased ability to sweat (warm, red skin, dry mouth, and increased body temperature), hallucinations, increased heart rate and blood pressure, mental confusion

Generic name:

URSODIOL

See Actigall, page 14.

Generic name:

VALACYCLOVIR

See Valtrex, page 1389.

Brand name:

VALIUM

Pronounced: VAL-ee-um
Generic name: Diazepam

Why is this drug prescribed?
Valium is used in the treatment of anxiety disorders and for short-term relief of the symptoms of anxiety. It belongs to a class of drugs known as benzodiazepines.

It is also used to relieve the symptoms of acute alcohol withdrawal, to relax muscles, to relieve the uncontrolled muscle movements caused by cerebral palsy and paralysis of the lower body and limbs, to control involuntary movement of the hands (athetosis), to relax tight, aching muscles, and, along with other medications, to treat convulsive disorders such as epilepsy.

Most important fact about this drug
Valium can be habit-forming or addictive. You may experience withdrawal symptoms if you stop using this drug abruptly. Discontinue or change your dose only on your doctor's advice.

How should you take this medication?
Take this medication exactly as prescribed. If you are taking Valium for epilepsy, make sure you take it every day at the same time.

■ *If you miss a dose...*
   Take it as soon as you remember if it is within an hour or so of the scheduled time. If you do not remember until later, skip the dose you missed and go back to your regular schedule. Never take 2 doses at the same time.

■ *Storage instructions...*
Store away from heat, light, and moisture.

What side effects may occur?
Side effects cannot be anticipated. If any develop or change in intensity, inform your doctor as soon as possible. Only your doctor can determine if it is safe for you to continue taking Valium.

■ *More common side effects may include:*
Drowsiness, fatigue, light-headedness, loss of muscle coordination

■ *Less common or rare side effects may include:*
Anxiety, blurred vision, changes in salivation, changes in sex drive, confusion, constipation, depression, difficulty urinating, dizziness, double vision, hallucinations, headache, inability to hold urine, low blood pressure, nausea, overstimulation, rage, seizures (mild changes in brain wave patterns), skin rash, sleep disturbances, slow heartbeat, slurred speech and other speech problems, stimulation, tremors, vertigo, yellowing of eyes and skin

■ *Side effects due to rapid decrease in dose or abrupt withdrawal from Valium:*
Abdominal and muscle cramps, convulsions, sweating, tremors, vomiting

Why should this drug not be prescribed?
If you are sensitive to or have ever had an allergic reaction to Valium, you should not take this medication.

Do not take this medication if you have the eye condition known as acute narrow-angle glaucoma.

Anxiety or tension related to everyday stress usually does not require treatment with such a powerful drug as Valium. Discuss your symptoms thoroughly with your doctor.

Valium should not be prescribed if you are being treated for mental disorders more serious than anxiety.

Special warnings about this medication
Valium may cause you to become drowsy or less alert; therefore, you should not drive or operate dangerous machinery or participate in any hazardous activity that requires full mental alertness until you know how this drug affects you.

If you have liver or kidney problems, use this medication cautiously.

Possible food and drug interactions
when taking this medication

Valium slows down the central nervous system and may intensify the effects of alcohol. Do not drink alcohol while taking this medication.

If Valium is taken with certain other drugs, the effects of either could be increased, decreased, or altered. It is especially important to check with your doctor before combining Valium with any of the following:

Antidepressant drugs such as Elavil and Prozac
Antiseizure drugs such as Dilantin
Barbiturates such as phenobarbital
Cimetidine (Tagamet)
Digoxin (Lanoxin)
Disulfiram (Antabuse)
Fluoxetine (Prozac)
Isoniazid (Rifamate)
Levodopa (Larodopa, Sinemet)
Major tranquilizers such as Mellaril and Thorazine
MAO inhibitors (antidepressant drugs such as Nardil)
Narcotics such as Percocet
Omeprazole (Prilosec)
Oral contraceptives
Propoxyphene (Darvon)
Ranitidine (Zantac)
Rifampin (Rifadin)

Special information
if you are pregnant or breastfeeding

Do not take Valium if you are pregnant or planning to become pregnant. There is an increased risk of birth defects.

If this medication is essential to your health, your doctor may advise you to discontinue breastfeeding until your treatment is finished.

Recommended dosage

ADULTS

Treatment of Anxiety Disorders and Short-Term Relief of the Symptoms of Anxiety
The usual dose, depending upon severity of symptoms, is 2 milligrams to 10 milligrams 2 to 4 times daily.

Acute Alcohol Withdrawal
The usual dose is 10 milligrams 3 or 4 times during the first 24 hours, then 5 milligrams 3 or 4 times daily as needed.

Relief of Muscle Spasm
The usual dose is 2 milligrams to 10 milligrams 3 or 4 times daily.

Convulsive Disorders
The usual dose is 2 milligrams to 10 milligrams 2 to 4 times daily.

CHILDREN

Valium should not be given to children under 6 months of age.

The usual starting dose for children over 6 months is 1 to 2.5 milligrams 3 or 4 times a day. Your doctor may increase the dosage gradually if needed.

OLDER ADULTS

The usual dosage is 2 milligrams to 2.5 milligrams once or twice a day, which your doctor will increase as needed. Your doctor will limit the dosage to the smallest effective amount because older people are more apt to become oversedated or uncoordinated.

Overdosage
Any medication taken in excess can have serious consequences. If you suspect an overdose, seek medical attention immediately.

■ *Symptoms of Valium overdose may include:*
Coma, confusion, diminished reflexes, sleepiness

Generic name:

VALPROIC ACID

See Depakene, page 367.

Generic name:

VALSARTAN

See Diovan, page 410.

Brand name:

VALTREX

Pronounced: VAL-trex
Generic name: Valacyclovir hydrochloride

Why is this drug prescribed?
Valtrex is used to treat herpes zoster (the painful rash known as shingles). It is also prescribed to relieve the sores caused by genital herpes.

Most important fact about this drug
Valtrex should not be used by anyone with a weak immune system, such as those with HIV infection or those who have undergone a bone marrow or kidney transplant. Valtrex can cause serious side effects, including death, in such people.

How should you use this medication?
If you are taking Valtrex for shingles, you should start using it as soon as possible after your doctor has made a diagnosis. It's best to see a doctor and start the drug within 48 hours of first noticing the rash. If you wait more than 72 hours after you first get a herpes zoster rash, the medication may not be effective.

If you are using Valtrex for genital herpes, begin taking it at the first sign of an attack. The medication may not be effective if you wait longer than 72 hours after the first attack or 24 hours after a later attack. You may take Valtrex with or without food.

- *If you miss a dose...*
  Take it as soon as you remember. If it is almost time for your next dose, skip the one you missed and go back to your regular schedule. Do not take 2 doses at the same time.

- *Storage instructions...*
  Store at room temperature.

What side effects may occur?
Side effects cannot be anticipated. If any develop or change in intensity, inform your doctor as soon as possible. Only your doctor can determine if it is safe for you to continue using Valtrex.

■ *Side effects may include:*
Abdominal pain, aggressive behavior, agitation, allergic reactions, confusion, depression, diarrhea, dizziness, facial swelling, hallucinations, headache, high blood pressure, joint pain, mania, menstrual problems, nausea, rapid heartbeat, rash, vomiting

Why should this drug not be prescribed?
Avoid Valtrex if you are sensitive to it or the similar drug acyclovir (Zovirax).

Special warnings about this medication
High doses of Valtrex have proved dangerous in people whose immune system is compromised because of HIV infection, bone marrow transplant, or kidney transplant.

If your kidneys are not functioning properly, or you are taking drugs that may damage the kidneys such as Neomycin or Streptomycin, Valtrex can make your condition worse or affect your central nervous system (brain and spinal cord).

Valtrex relieves the symptoms of genital herpes, but it is not a cure. There's also no evidence that it will prevent transmission of the disease. To avoid spreading the infection, don't have sexual intercourse during a flare-up.

Valtrex is not intended for use in children.

Possible food and drug interactions
when taking this medication
If you are taking Valtrex with certain other drugs, the effect of either drug could be increased, decreased, or altered. Check with your doctor before combining Valtrex with cimetidine (Tagamet) and/or probenecid (Benemid).

Special information
if you are pregnant or breastfeeding
The effects of Valtrex during pregnancy and breastfeeding have not been adequately studied. If you are pregnant or plan to become pregnant, notify your doctor immediately. If you are nursing and need to use Valtrex, your doctor may advise you to discontinue breastfeeding while using the medication.

Recommended dosage

SHINGLES
The usual dose is 1 gram 3 times a day for 7 days.

GENITAL HERPES

The usual dose for the first attack is 1 gram twice a day for 10 days. For later attacks, the dose is 500 milligrams twice a day for 5 days. To keep the condition from returning, the dose is 1 gram once a day.

If your kidneys are not functioning well, your doctor may reduce the dosage.

Overdosage
When taken by people with kidney disorders excessive doses of Valtrex have been known to cause psychological problems and kidney failure. If you suspect an overdose, check with your doctor immediately.

Brand name:

VANCENASE

See Beclomethasone, page 143.

Brand name:

VANCERIL

See Beclomethasone, page 143.

Brand name:

VASERETIC

Pronounced: Vaz-err-ET-ik
Generic ingredients: Enalapril maleate,
Hydrochlorothiazide

Why is this drug prescribed?
Vaseretic is used in the treatment of high blood pressure. It combines an ACE inhibitor with a thiazide diuretic. Enalapril, the ACE inhibitor, works by preventing a chemical in your blood called angiotensin I from converting into a more potent form that increases salt and water retention in your body. Enalapril also enhances blood flow throughout your blood vessels. Hydrochlorothiazide, a diuretic, prompts your body to produce and eliminate more urine, which helps in lowering blood pressure.

Most important fact about this drug
You must take Vaseretic regularly for it to be effective. Since blood pressure declines gradually, it may be several weeks before you get the full benefit of

Vaseretic; and you must continue taking it even if you are feeling well. Vaseretic does not cure high blood pressure; it merely keeps it under control.

How should you take this medication?
Take this medication exactly as prescribed by your doctor.

■ *If you miss a dose...*
Take it as soon as you remember. If it is almost time for your next dose, skip the one you missed and go back to your regular schedule. Never take 2 doses at the same time.

■ *Storage instructions...*
Keep container tightly closed. Store at room temperature and protect from moisture. Keep out of reach of children.

What side effects may occur?
Side effects cannot be anticipated. If any develop or change in intensity, inform your doctor as soon as possible. Only your doctor can determine if it is safe for you to continue taking Vaseretic.

■ *More common side effects may include:*
Cough, diarrhea, dizziness, drop in blood pressure upon standing up, fatigue, headache, impotence, low potassium levels (leading to symptoms such as dry mouth, excessive thirst, weak or irregular heartbeat, muscle pain or cramps), muscle cramps, nausea, rash, tingling or pins and needles, weakness

■ *Less common or rare side effects may include:*
Abdominal pain, abnormal dreams, abnormal skin sensations such as numbness, prickling, or burning, allergic reactions, arthritis, back pain, black stools, blisters, blood clots in lungs, blurred vision, bronchitis, chest pain, confusion, conjunctivitis, constipation, decrease in sex drive, depression, disturbances in heart rhythm, dry eyes, dry mouth, excessive sweating, fainting, fluid in lungs, flushing, gas, gout, heart attack, hepatitis, hives, hoarseness, inability to sleep, indigestion, inflammation of mouth and tongue, inflammation of the pancreas, itching, joint pain, kidney failure, liver failure, loss of appetite, loss of coordination, loss of hair, low blood pressure, muscle cramps, nervousness, rapid heartbeat, rash, Raynaud's phenomenon (in which the fingers periodically turn pale, then blue), restlessness, ringing in ears, runny nose, sensitivity to light, shortness of breath, sleepiness, sore throat, stroke, tearing, urinary tract infection, vomiting, yellow eyes and skin

Why should this drug not be prescribed?

If you are sensitive to or have ever had an allergic reaction to enalapril, hydrochlorothiazide, or similar drugs, or if you are sensitive to other sulfa drugs, you should not take this medication.

If you have a history of angioedema (swelling of face, extremities, and throat) or inability to urinate, you should not take this medication. Tell your doctor of all allergic reactions you have experienced.

Special warnings about this medication

If you develop swelling of your face, eyes, lips, tongue, or throat; swelling of your arms and legs; or difficulty swallowing, you should contact your doctor immediately. You may need emergency treatment.

If you are taking bee or wasp venom to prevent an allergic reaction to stings, you may have a severe allergic reaction to Vaseretic.

If you develop chest pain, a sore throat, or fever you should contact your doctor immediately. It could indicate a more serious illness.

If you are taking Vaseretic, a complete assessment of your kidney function should be done. Kidney function should continue to be monitored. Some people on dialysis have had a severe allergic reaction to Vaseretic.

If you have liver disease or lupus erythematosus (a form of rheumatism), Vaseretic should be used with caution.

If your skin or the whites of your eyes turn yellow, stop taking Vaseretic and notify your doctor at once.

If you have severe congestive heart failure, you should be carefully watched for low blood pressure.

Excessive sweating, dehydration, severe diarrhea, or vomiting could cause you to lose too much water and cause your blood pressure to become too low. Be careful when exercising and in hot weather.

Vaseretic can cause some people to become drowsy or less alert. If it has this effect on you, driving or operating dangerous machinery or participating in any hazardous activity that requires full mental alertness is not recommended.

If you are diabetic, blood sugar levels should be monitored.

Vaseretic may increase your sensitivity to sunlight. Be careful to avoid overexposure.

Possible food and drug interactions
when taking this medication

Vaseretic may intensify the effects of alcohol. Do not drink alcohol while taking this medication.

If Vaseretic is taken with certain other drugs, the effects of either could be increased, decreased, or altered. It is especially important to check with your doctor before combining Vaseretic with the following:

Alcohol
Barbiturates such as phenobarbital
Certain other antihypertensives
Corticosteroids such as prednisone
Digitalis (Lanoxin)
Insulin
Lithium (Eskalith, Lithonate)
Narcotics (Percocet)
Nonsteroidal anti-inflammatory drugs such as Naprosyn, Advil, and
   Motrin
Norepinephrine
Oral antidiabetic drugs such as Micronase
Potassium supplements (K-Lyte, K-Tab, others)
Potassium-containing salt substitutes
Potassium-sparing diuretics such as Midamor

Special information
if you are pregnant or breastfeeding

Vaseretic can cause birth defects, prematurity, and death to the newborn baby. If you are pregnant or plan to become pregnant and are taking Vaseretic, contact your doctor immediately to discuss the potential hazard to your unborn child. Vaseretic appears in breast milk and could affect a nursing infant. If this medication is essential to your health, your doctor may advise you to discontinue breastfeeding until your treatment is finished.

Recommended dosage

ADULTS

The doctor will adjust your dosage until your blood pressure is in the desired range. If you are taking the 5 milligrams enalapril/12.5 milligrams hydrochlorothiazide combination, the maximum daily dosage is 4 tablets. For the 10/25 combination, the maximum is 2 tablets.

CHILDREN

The safety and effectiveness of Vaseretic in children have not been established.

OLDER ADULTS

Your doctor will prescribe Vaseretic cautiously, starting with small doses.

Overdosage

Any medication taken in excess can cause symptoms of overdose. If you suspect an overdose, seek medical attention immediately.

■ *Symptoms of a Vaseretic overdose may include:*
Dehydration, low blood pressure

Brand name:

VASOTEC

Pronounced: VAZ-oh-tek
Generic name: Enalapril maleate

Why is this drug prescribed?

Vasotec is a high blood pressure medication known as an ACE inhibitor. It works by preventing a chemical in your blood called angiotensin I from converting into a more potent form that increases salt and water retention in your body. It is effective when used alone or in combination with other medications, especially thiazide-type diuretics. It is also used in the treatment of congestive heart failure, usually in combination with diuretics and digitalis, and is prescribed as a preventive measure in certain conditions that could lead to heart failure.

Most important fact about this drug

If you have high blood pressure, you must take Vasotec regularly for it to be effective. Since blood pressure declines gradually, it may be several weeks before you get the full benefit of Vasotec; and you must continue taking it even if you are feeling well. Vasotec does not cure high blood pressure; it merely keeps it under control.

How should you take this medication?

Vasotec can be taken with or without food.

Do not use salt substitutes containing potassium without first consulting your doctor.

Take this medication exactly as prescribed by your doctor.

■ *If you miss a dose...*
Take it as soon as you remember. If it is almost time for your next dose, skip the one you missed and go back to your regular schedule. Never take two doses at the same time.

■ *Storage instructions...*
Keep container tightly closed. Store at room temperature and protect from moisture.

What side effects may occur?
Side effects cannot be anticipated. If any develop or change in intensity, inform your doctor as soon as possible. Only your doctor can determine if it is safe for you to continue taking Vasotec.

■ *Side effects may include:*
Abdominal pain, abnormal dreams, abnormal skin sensations such as numbness or prickling, anaphylactoid reactions (severe allergic reactions), angina pectoris (chest pain, often accompanied by a feeling of choking or impending death), angioedema (swelling of face, lips, tongue, throat, arms and legs, difficulty swallowing), asthma, blisters, blood abnormalities, blood clots or foreign material in the lungs, blurred vision, breast enlargement in males, bronchitis, confusion, constipation, cough, dark, tarry stool containing blood, decreased urination, depression, diarrhea, difficulty breathing, difficulty sleeping, digestive difficulty and stomach discomfort, dizziness, dizziness upon standing, dry eyes, dry mouth, excessive perspiration, fainting, fatigue, flank pain, fluid in lungs, flushing, hair loss, headache, heart palpitations, heart rhythm disturbances, hepatitis, herpes zoster, hives, impotence, inflammation of the mouth, inflammation of the tongue, itching, lack of muscle coordination, liver failure, loss of appetite, loss of sense of smell, low blood pressure, low blood pressure upon standing, muscle cramps, nausea, nervousness, pinkeye (conjunctivitis), pneumonia, pounding heartbeat, rapid or slow heartbeat, rash, Raynaud's phenomenon (in which the fingers periodically turn pale, then blue), red skin (like sunburn), ringing in ears, runny nose, sensitivity to light, sleepiness, sore throat and hoarseness, stroke, taste alteration, tearing, tingling or pins and needles or burning sensation, upper respiratory infection, upset stomach, urinary tract infection, vertigo, vomiting, weakness, wheezing

Why should this drug not be prescribed?
If you are sensitive or have ever had an allergic reaction to Vasotec or similar drugs, or if you have a history of angioedema (swollen throat and difficulty swallowing) related to previous treatment with ACE inhibitors, you should not take this medication. Make sure that your doctor is aware of any drug reactions that you have experienced.

Special warnings about this medication
Vasotec has been known to cause a serious allergic reaction called angioedema. The symptoms are swelling of the face, lips, tongue, or throat; swelling of arms and legs; and difficulty swallowing or breathing. If you notice any of these symptoms, call your doctor immediately.

If you are taking bee or wasp venom to prevent an allergic reaction to stings, you may have a severe allergic reaction to Vasotec.

If you are taking high doses of diuretics and Vasotec, you may develop excessively low blood pressure. You are at special risk if you have heart disease, kidney disease, or a potassium or salt imbalance. Some people on kidney dialysis have had a severe allergic reaction to Vasotec.

There have been cases of serious blood disorders reported with the use of captopril, another ACE inhibitor drug. Your doctor should check your blood regularly while you are taking Vasotec.

ACE inhibitors can cause fetal abnormalities and fetal and newborn deaths when used in pregnancy during the second and third trimesters.

When pregnancy is detected, Vasotec should be discontinued as soon as possible.

If you develop a sore throat or fever, you should contact your doctor immediately. It could indicate a more serious illness. Also, if your skin and the whites of your eyes turn yellow, contact your doctor at once.

Excessive sweating, dehydration, severe diarrhea, or vomiting could prompt you to lose too much water, causing your blood pressure to drop dangerously. Be careful when exercising or when exposed to excessive heat.

Possible food and drug interactions
when taking this medication
If Vasotec is taken with certain other drugs, the effects of either could be increased, decreased, or altered. It is especially important to check with your doctor before combining Vasotec with the following:

  Diuretics such as Lasix and HydroDIURIL
  Lithium (Eskalith, Lithobid)

Potassium-containing salt substitutes
Potassium-sparing diuretics such as Aldactazide and Moduretic
Potassium supplements such as K-Lyte and K-Tab

Special information
if you are pregnant or breastfeeding

Vasotec can cause birth defects, prematurity, and death to the developing or newborn baby. If you are pregnant or plan to become pregnant, inform your doctor immediately. Vasotec appears in breast milk and could affect a nursing infant. If this medication is essential to your health, your doctor may advise you to stop breastfeeding until your treatment with Vasotec is finished.

Recommended dosage

ADULTS

Hypertension

The usual starting dose for people not using diuretics is 5 milligrams, taken once a day. The usual dose is 10 to 40 milligrams per day, taken as a single dose or divided into 2 smaller doses.

If you are taking a diuretic, your physician may ask you to stop for 2 to 3 days before using Vasotec. Otherwise, he or she may give an initial dose of 2.5 milligrams of Vasotec under medical supervision before any further medication is prescribed.

If you have a kidney disorder, your dosage will be adjusted according to its severity.

To Treat Heart Failure

This medication can be used in conjunction with digitalis and diuretics in people with heart disease. The usual starting dose is 2.5 milligrams twice a day.

The usual regular dose is 2.5 to 20 milligrams each day, taken in 2 separate doses. The maximum daily dose is 40 milligrams, in 2 separate doses.

To Prevent Heart Failure

The usual starting dose is 2.5 milligrams twice a day, to be gradually increased to 20 milligrams a day divided into smaller doses.

CHILDREN

The safety and effectiveness of Vasotec in children have not been established.

Overdosage

Any medication taken in excess can have serious consequences. If you suspect symptoms of a Vasotec overdose, seek medical attention immediately.

A sudden drop in blood pressure is the primary effect of a Vasotec overdose.

Brand name:

V-CILLIN K

See Penicillin V Potassium, page 971.

Brand name:

VEETIDS

See Penicillin V Potassium, page 971.

Brand name:

VELOSULIN

See Insulin, page 639.

Generic name:

VENLAFAXINE

See Effexor, page 453.

Brand name:

VENTOLIN

See Proventil, page 1073.

Generic name:

VERAPAMIL

See Calan, page 181.

Brand name:

VERELAN

See Calan, page 181.

Brand name:

VIAGRA

Pronounced: vye-AG-ruh
Generic name: Sildenafil citrate

Why is this drug prescribed?
Viagra is the first oral drug for male impotence. It works by dilating blood vessels in the penis, allowing the inflow of blood needed for an erection.

Most important fact about this drug
Viagra causes erections only during sexual excitement. It does not work in the absence of arousal.

How should you take this medication?
Taking Viagra approximately 1 hour before sexual activity works best for most men. Depending on how and when the drug works for you, an interval of one-half hour to as much as 4 hours may prove ideal.

- *If you miss a dose...*
  Viagra is *not* for regular use. Take it only before sexual activity.

- *Storage instructions...*
  Store at room temperature.

What side effects may occur?
Side effects cannot be anticipated. If any develop or change in intensity, inform your doctor as soon as possible. Only your doctor can determine if it is safe for you to continue taking Viagra.

- *More common side effects may include:*
  Abnormal vision (color tinge, blurring, sensitivity to light), acid indigestion, diarrhea, flushing, headache, nasal congestion, urinary tract infection

- *Less common to rare side effects may include:*
  Abdominal pain, abnormal dreams, abnormal ejaculation, allergic reactions, anxiety, asthma, bloodshot eyes, bone pain, breast enlargement, cataracts, chest pain, chills, coordination problems, cough, depression, difficulty breathing, difficulty swallowing, dilated pupils, dizziness, drowsiness, dry eyes, dry mouth, emotional or mental disturbances, eye inflammation or pain, other eye disorders, fainting, falling, genital problems, gout, gum inflammation, heart problems, increased night-time urination, increased pressure in the eyes, insomnia, itchy skin, joint

disease, light sensitivity, loss of bladder control (urinary incontinence), low blood pressure, migraine headache, muscle ache, numbness, oral inflammation, pain, painful erection, prolonged erection, raised skin patches, rapid or throbbing heartbeat, rectal bleeding, respiratory inflammation, ringing in the ears, seizure, sinus and throat inflammation, skin rash, skin ulcer, slow reflexes, stomach or intestinal inflammation, sweating, swelling, thirst, tremor, vomiting, weakness

Heart attack, stroke, heart irregularities, dangerous surges in blood pressure, and sudden death have all been reported after use of Viagra, usually in men with existing cardiac risk factors, and typically during or shortly after sex.

Why should this drug not be prescribed?
Do not take Viagra if you are taking any nitrate-based drug, including nitroglycerin patches (Nitro-Dur, Transderm-Nitro), nitroglycerin ointment (Nitro-Bid, Nitrol), nitroglycerin pills (Nitro-Bid, Nitrostat), and isosorbide pills (Dilatrate-SR, Isordil, Sorbitrate). Combining Viagra with these drugs can cause a severe drop in blood pressure.

If Viagra gives you an allergic reaction, do not use it again.

Special warnings about this medication
If you have heart problems severe enough to make sexual activity a danger, you should avoid using Viagra. Use it cautiously—if at all—if you've had a heart attack, stroke, or life-threatening heart irregularities within the past 6 months. Be equally cautious if you have severe high or low blood pressure, heart failure, or unstable angina (crushing heart pain that occurs at any time).

If you take Viagra and develop cardiac symptoms (for example, dizziness, nausea, and chest pain) during sexual activity, do not continue. Alert your doctor to the problem as soon as possible.

If you have a condition that might result in long-lasting erections, such as sickle cell anemia, multiple myeloma (a disease of the bone marrow), or leukemia, use Viagra with caution. Also use cautiously if you have a genital problem or deformity such as Peyronie's disease. If an erection lasts more than 4 hours, seek treatment immediately. Permanent damage and impotence could result.

If you have a bleeding disorder, a stomach ulcer, or the inherited eye condition known as retinitis pigmentosa, use this medication with caution. Its safety under these circumstances has not yet been studied.

Remember that Viagra offers no protection from transmission of sexually transmitted diseases, such as HIV, the virus that causes AIDS.

This drug is not for use by women. Its effects during pregnancy have not been studied.

Possible food and drug interactions when using this medication

If Viagra is taken with certain other drugs, the effects of either could be increased, decreased, or altered. It is especially important to check with your doctor before combining Viagra with the following:

Other impotence remedies including Caverject and Muse
Amlodipine (Norvasc)
Cimetidine (Tagamet)
Erythromycin (E-Mycin, Ery-Tab, PCE)
Itraconazole (Sporanox)
Ketoconazole (Nizoral)
Nitrates such as Isordil, Nitro-Bid, and Nitro-Dur
Rifampin (Rifadin, Rimactane)

Recommended dosage

Doses range from 25 milligrams to 100 milligrams, depending on the drug's effect. The usual dose is 50 milligrams. If you are over 65, have liver or kidney problems, or are taking erythromycin, ketoconazole, or itraconazole, a dose of 25 milligrams may be sufficient. Your doctor will adjust the dosage if the drug is not working properly for you.

Take Viagra only before sexual activity. The manufacturer recommends a maximum of 1 dose per day.

Overdosage

No overdose of Viagra has been reported. However, any medication taken in excess can have serious consequences. If you suspect an overdose, seek medical attention immediately.

Brand name:

VIBRAMYCIN

See Doryx, page 437.

Brand name:

VIBRA-TABS

See Doryx, page 437.

Brand name:

VICODIN

Pronounced; VY-koe-din
Generic ingredients: Hydrocodone bitartrate,
  Acetaminophen
Other brand names: Anexsia, Co-Gesic, Hydrocet, Lorcet,
  Lortab, Zydone

Why is this drug prescribed?
Vicodin combines a narcotic analgesic (painkiller) and cough reliever with a nonnarcotic analgesic for the relief of moderate to moderately severe pain.

Most important fact about this drug
Vicodin can be habit-forming. If you take this drug over a long period of time, you can become mentally and physically dependent on it, and you may find the drug no longer works for you at the prescribed dosage.

How should you take this medication?
Take Vicodin exactly as prescribed. Do not increase the amount you take or the frequency without your doctor's approval. Do not take this drug for any reason other than the one prescribed.

Do not give this drug to others who may have similar symptoms.

- *If you miss a dose...*
  If you take Vicodin regularly, take the forgotten dose as soon as you remember. If it is almost time for your next dose, skip the one you missed and go back to your regular schedule. Do not take 2 doses at once.

- *Storage instructions...*
  Store at room temperature in a tightly closed container, away from light.

What side effects may occur?
Side effects cannot be anticipated. If any develop or change in intensity, inform your doctor as soon as possible. Only your doctor can determine if it is safe for you to continue taking Vicodin.

- *More common side effects may include:*
  Dizziness, light-headedness, nausea, sedation, vomiting

If these side effects occur, it may help if you lie down after taking the medication.

■ *Less common or rare side effects may include:*
Allergic reactions, anxiety, blood disorders, constipation, decreased mental and physical capability, difficulty urinating, drowsiness, fear, itching, mental clouding, mood changes, restlessness, skin rash, slowed breathing, sluggishness

Why should this drug not be prescribed?

If you are sensitive to or have ever had an allergic reaction to hydrocodone or acetaminophen (Tylenol), you should not take this medication. Make sure your doctor is aware of any drug reactions you have experienced.

Special warnings about this medication

Vicodin may make you drowsy, less alert, or unable to function well physically. Do not drive a car, operate machinery, or perform any other potentially dangerous activities until you know how this drug affects you.

Use caution in taking Vicodin if you have a head injury. Narcotics tend to increase the pressure of the fluid within the skull, and this effect may be exaggerated by head injuries. Side effects of narcotics can interfere in the treatment of people with head injuries.

Use Vicodin with caution if you have a severe liver or kidney disorder, an underactive thyroid gland, Addison's disease (a disease of the adrenal glands), an enlarged prostate, or urethral stricture (narrowing of the tube carrying urine from the bladder).

Older adults and those in a weakened condition should be careful using this drug, since it contains a narcotic.

Narcotics such as Vicodin may interfere with the diagnosis and treatment of people with abdominal conditions.

Hydrocodone suppresses the cough reflex; therefore, be careful using Vicodin after an operation or if you have a lung disease.

High doses of hydrocodone may produce slowed breathing; if you are sensitive to this drug, you are more likely to experience this effect.

Possible food and drug interactions
when taking this medication

Hydrocodone slows the nervous system. Alcohol can intensify this effect.

If hydrocodone is taken with certain other drugs, the effects of either may be increased, decreased, or altered. It is especially important to check with your doctor before combining Vicodin with the following:

Antianxiety drugs such as Valium and Librium
Antidepressants such as Elavil, Nardil, and Tofranil

Antihistamines such as Tavist
Major tranquilizers such as Thorazine and Haldol
Other central nervous system depressants such as Halcion and Restoril
Other narcotic analgesics such as Demerol

Special information
if you are pregnant or breastfeeding

The effects of Vicodin in pregnancy have not been adequately studied. Do not take this drug if you are pregnant or plan to become pregnant unless you are directed to do so by your doctor. Drug dependence occurs in newborns when the mother has taken this drug regularly prior to delivery. If you take it shortly before delivery, the baby's breathing may be slowed. Acetaminophen does, and hydrocodone may, appear in breast milk and could affect a nursing infant. If this medication is essential to your health, your doctor may advise you to discontinue breastfeeding your baby until your treatment is finished.

Recommended dosage

ADULTS

Your doctor will adjust the dosage according to the severity of the pain and the way the medication affects you.

The dosages given below are for Vicodin and Vicodin ES only. If your doctor prescribes other brands, your daily dose may vary.

The usual dose is 1 or 2 tablets every 4 to 6 hours as needed for pain. Take no more than 8 tablets of Vicodin per day. For Vicodin ES, the maximum is 5 tablets per day.

CHILDREN

The safety and effectiveness of Vicodin have not been established in children.

Overdosage

Any medication taken in excess can have serious consequences. A severe overdose of Vicodin can be fatal. If you suspect an overdose, seek emergency medical treatment immediately.

- *Symptoms of a Vicodin overdose include:*
  Blood disorders, bluish tinge to skin, cold and clammy skin, extreme sleepiness progressing to a state of unresponsiveness or coma, general feeling of bodily discomfort, heart problems, heavy perspiration, kidney problems, limp muscles, liver failure, low blood pressure, nausea, slow heartbeat, troubled or slowed breathing, vomiting

Brand name:

VICOPROFEN

Pronounced: VY-koe-pro-fen
Generic ingredients: Hydrocodone bitartrate, Ibuprofen

Why is this drug prescribed?

Vicoprofen is a chemical cousin of the well-known painkiller Vicodin. Both products contain the prescription pain medication hydrocodone. However, while Vicodin also includes acetaminophen (the active ingredient in Tylenol), Vicoprofen replaces it with ibuprofen (the active ingredient in Advil).

Vicoprofen relieves acute pain. It is generally prescribed for less than 10 days, and cannot be used in the long-term treatment of osteoarthritis or rheumatoid arthritis.

Most important fact about this drug

Vicoprofen can be habit-forming. If you take this drug over a long period of time, you can become both mentally and physically dependent on it, and you may find that it no longer works for you at the prescribed dose.

How should you take this medication?

Take Vicoprofen exactly as prescribed. Do not increase the amount you take or the number of doses per day without your doctor's approval. Vicoprofen should be used only for pain—and only as needed.

■ *If you miss a dose...*
   Take it as soon as you remember. If it is almost time for your next dose, skip the one you missed and go back to your regular schedule. Never take 2 doses at the same time.

■ *Storage information...*
   Store at room temperature in a tightly sealed, light-resistant container.

What side effects may occur?

Side effects cannot be anticipated. If any develop or change in intensity, inform your doctor as soon as possible. Only your doctor can determine if it is safe for you to continue taking Vicoprofen.

■ *More common side effects may include:*
   Abdominal pain, anxiety, constipation, diarrhea, dizziness, drowsiness, dry mouth, gas, headache, indigestion, infection, insomnia, itching, loss of strength, nausea, nervousness, sweating, swelling, vomiting

- *Less common side effects may include:*
  Confusion, dark tarry stool, difficulty breathing, fever, flu symptoms, frequent urination, hiccups, inflammation of the throat and nasal passages, loss of appetite, mouth ulcers, pain, ringing in the ears, skin tingling, stomach inflammation, tension, thinking abnormalities, thirst, throbbing heartbeat

- *Rare side effects may include:*
  Abnormal dreams, agitation, allergic reaction, altered vision, asthma, bad taste, bronchitis, chalky stool, decreased sex drive, depression, difficulty swallowing, dry eyes, elevated mood, hives, hoarseness, impotence, increased cough, inflamed sinuses, inflammation of the tongue or intestines, joint pain, low blood pressure, lung congestion, mood changes, muscle ache, pneumonia, rapid or irregular heartbeat, rash, shallow breathing, skin swelling, slurred speech, teeth clenching, tremor, urinary problems, vertigo, weight loss

Why should this drug not be prescribed?

If ibuprofen, aspirin, or brands such as Advil, Aleve, and Naprosyn have ever given you asthma, hives, or any other type of allergic attack, do not take this medication. You should also avoid Vicoprofen if you've ever had an allergic reaction to hydrocodone or other narcotic painkillers.

Special warnings about this medication

Vicoprofen can make you drowsy and slow. Do not drive a car, operate machinery, or perform any other potentially dangerous activities until you know how this drug affects you. Alcohol, sedatives, tranquilizers, and other narcotic painkillers can increase drowsiness. Do not combine them with Vicoprofen.

High doses of hydrocodone may produce troubled, irregular, or slowed breathing; if you are sensitive to this drug, or have a head injury, such problems are more likely. Narcotics tend to increase the pressure of the fluid inside the skull, and this effect can be exaggerated by a head injury. Avoid Vicoprofen if possible.

Use Vicoprofen with caution if you have a severe liver or kidney disorder, heart failure, lupus, underactive thyroid or adrenal glands, an enlarged prostate, or any narrowing of the duct that drains the bladder. Caution is also called for in those who are weak, elderly, or dehydrated.

Hydrocodone suppresses the cough reflex; use it cautiously if you have a lung condition or have just had surgery.

The ibuprofen in Vicoprofen has been known to cause ulcers, and stomach bleeding can start without warning. If you've had such problems in the past, make sure the doctor is aware of it. Smoking, drinking, old age, and poor health make stomach problems more likely.

Vicoprofen can prolong bleeding time and cause a decrease in blood cell count. If you are taking a blood-thinning medication, use Vicoprofen with caution. This drug can also cause water retention. Be cautious if you have high blood pressure or poor heart function.

Contact your doctor if you notice any signs of stomach or intestinal bleeding, suffer blurred vision or other eye problems, get a skin rash, or notice any weight gain or swelling. If you have a severe allergic reaction, stop taking the drug and seek medical help immediately.

Possible food and drug interactions
when taking this medication
If Vicoprofen is taken with certain other drugs, the effects of either can be increased, decreased, or altered. It is especially important to check with your doctor before combining Vicoprofen with the following:

ACE-inhibitor-type blood pressure and heart drugs such as Capoten and
  Vasotec
Alcohol
Antidepressants such as Elavil, Norpramin, and Pamelor
Antihistamines such as Benadryl, chlorpheniramine, and Tavist
Aspirin
Blood-thinning drugs such as Coumadin
Drugs that control muscle spasms such as Artane and Cogentin
Lithium (Lithobid, Lithonate)
Major tranquilizers such as Haldol and Thorazine
Methotrexate (Rheumatrex)
Other narcotic painkillers such as Demerol, morphine, and Percocet
Sleeping pills such as Halcion and Restoril
Tranquilizers such as Ativan, Valium, and Xanax
Water pills (diuretics) such as Lasix and HydroDIURIL

Special information
if you are pregnant or breastfeeding
Do not take this drug during pregnancy unless directed by your doctor. Drug dependence occurs in newborns when mothers take narcotics regularly prior to delivery.

Vicoprofen may appear in breast milk and could affect a nursing infant. If this medication is essential to your health, your doctor may advise you to discontinue breastfeeding until your treatment is finished.

Recommended dosage

ADULTS

Your doctor will adjust the dosage according to the severity of the pain and the way the medication affects you. The usual dose is 1 tablet every 4 to 6 hours as needed. Do not take more than 5 tablets a day.

CHILDREN

The safety and effectiveness of Vicoprofen have not been established in children below 16 years of age.

OLDER ADULTS

A reduced dosage is recommended.

Overdosage

A massive overdose of Vicoprofen can be fatal. If you suspect an overdose, seek medical attention immediately.

■ *Symptoms of Vicoprofen overdose may include:*
Slowed breathing, extreme drowsiness, muscle weakness, cold and clammy skin, low blood pressure, slowed heart rate, stomach and intestinal irritation, headache, dizziness, ringing in the ears, confusion, blurred vision, eye problems, inflammation of the skin in the mouth, skin rash, swelling, difficulty breathing, heart attack, coma

Brand name:

VI-DAYLIN

See Multivitamins, page 838.

Brand name:

VIDEX

Pronounced: VIE-decks
Generic name: Didanosine

Why is this drug prescribed?

Videx is one of the drugs used to fight the human immunodeficiency virus (HIV)—the deadly cause of AIDS. Over a period of years, HIV slowly destroys the immune system, leaving the body defenseless against infection.

Videx disrupts reproduction of HIV, thereby staving off the immune system's collapse.

Signs and symptoms of advanced HIV infection include diarrhea, fever, headache, infections, problems with the nervous system, rash, sore throat, and significant weight loss.

Most important fact about this drug
Although Videx can slow the progress of HIV, it is not a cure. You may continue to develop complications, including frequent infections. Even if you feel better, regular physical exams and blood counts by your doctor are highly advisable. And notify your doctor immediately if you experience any changes in your general health.

How should you take this medication?
Videx should be taken every 12 hours, exactly as prescribed. It is important to keep levels of the drug in your body as constant as possible, so be sure to take every scheduled dose. Videx should be taken on an empty stomach, at least 30 minutes before or 2 hours after a meal. Never take more than the prescribed dose; nerve disorders could result.

Videx Tablets
There should be 2 tablets in each dose. Do NOT swallow the tablets whole. Instead, take them in one of these three ways:

1. Chew the tablets thoroughly before swallowing.
2. Crush the tablets before you take them.
3. Dissolve the tablets in at least 1 ounce of water, stirring until the particles are evenly dispersed. Swallow the mixture immediately. If desired, you can add 1 ounce of apple juice to the water/Videx mixture. This combination should be taken within 1 hour of preparation. Be sure to stir it immediately before drinking.

Buffered Powder for Oral Solution
Open the packet and pour the contents into 4 ounces of water. Stir for 2 to 3 minutes, until the powder is completely dissolved. Drink the entire solution immediately. Do not mix with fruit juice.

Videx Pediatric Oral Solution
The pediatric version of Videx comes premixed from the pharmacy. Shake well before using.

- *If you miss a dose...*
  Take it as soon as you remember. If it is almost time for your next dose, skip the one you missed and go back to your regular schedule. Do not take 2 doses at once.

- *Storage instructions...*
  Videx tablets and powder can be stored at room temperature. The pediatric oral solution should be stored in a refrigerator and used within 30 days.

What side effects may occur?
The higher your dosage, the greater your chance of side effects. However, it's often hard to tell a side effect from a symptom of the disease. If you think the drug is causing problems, keep taking it until you've checked with your doctor. Only your doctor can determine whether the drug is at fault and adjust your dosage accordingly.

- *More common side effects may include:*
  Abdominal pain, chills, diarrhea, fever, headache, itching, nausea, pain, rash, tingling, burning, numbness, or pain in the feet and hands, vomiting, weakness

- *Less common side effects may include:*
  Allergic reactions, changes in blood sugar levels, dry mouth, dry eyes, gas, indigestion, joint pain, loss of appetite, muscle disorders, swollen glands, vision problems

Why should this drug not be prescribed?
If Videx gives you an allergic reaction, you should not take the drug.

Special warnings about this medication
It's important to remember that Videx will not prevent the spread of HIV through sexual relations or contact with infected blood.

Videx can cause serious side effects such as pancreatitis (a potentially dangerous inflammation of the pancreas), vision changes, nerve disorders, and liver failure. Notify your physician if you experience abdominal pain, nausea and vomiting, changes in your eyesight, or a feeling of tingling, numbness, or pain in your hands or feet. Make sure your doctor is aware of any liver, kidney, or pancreas problems you may have.

If you are on a sodium-restricted diet, you should be aware that Videx powder contains 1,380 milligrams of sodium per packet. Those with the hereditary disease phenylketonuria should remember that Videx tablets contain phenylalanine.

Possible food and drug interactions when taking this medication

Alcohol increases your risk of developing serious side effects such as pancreatitis.

If Videx is taken with certain other medications, the effect of either may be increased, decreased, or altered. It is especially important to check with your doctor before taking any of the following:

Antacids containing magnesium or aluminum, including Maalox and Mylanta
Allopurinol (Zyloprim)
IV pentamidine (Pentam)
Tetracycline

If you are taking Dapsone, Nizoral or Sporanox, you should allow at least 2 hours to pass before taking Videx. When taking antibiotics known as quinolones, including Cipro, Floxin, and Noroxin, you should take Videx at least 6 hours before the antibiotic, or wait for 2 hours after it.

Special information if you are pregnant or breastfeeding

The effects of Videx during pregnancy have not been adequately studied. If you are pregnant or plan to become pregnant, inform your doctor immediately.

HIV can be passed to a baby through breast milk, so you should not plan on breastfeeding.

Recommended dosage

Videx should be taken every 12 hours, at least 30 minutes before eating. If you have a kidney or liver problem, your dosage may be reduced.

ADULTS

Tablets

For adults weighing 132 pounds or more, the recommended dose is 200 milligrams every 12 hours. Those weighing less than 132 pounds usually take 125 milligrams every 12 hours.

Buffered Powder for Oral Solution
For adults weighing 132 pounds or more, the recommended dose is 250 milligrams every 12 hours. Those weighing less than 132 pounds usually take 167 milligrams every 12 hours.

CHILDREN

The recommended dose varies according to the child's size.

Overdosage

■ *Symptoms of Videx overdose may include:*
  Abdominal pain, diarrhea, pain, numbness, burning, and tingling in the hands and feet

If you suspect an overdose, seek medical attention immediately.

Brand name:

VIOKASE

See Pancrease, page 947.

Brand name:

VIRACEPT

Pronounced: VYE-ruh-sept
Generic name: Nelfinavir mesylate

Why is this drug prescribed?

Viracept is one of the drugs prescribed to fight HIV, the human immunodeficiency virus that causes AIDS (acquired immune deficiency syndrome). Once inside the body, HIV spreads through certain key cells in the immune system, weakening the body's ability to fight off other infections. Viracept works by interfering with an important step in the virus's reproductive cycle. This slows the spread of the virus and prolongs the strength of the immune system.

Viracept belongs to the new class of drugs that has successfully reversed the course of HIV infection in many people. Called protease inhibitors, these drugs work better when used in combination with other HIV medications called nucleoside analogues (Retrovir, Hivid, and others) which act against the virus in other ways.

Most important fact about this drug
Although Viracept can keep HIV at bay, it is not a complete cure. If you stop taking the drug, the infection will re-emerge and progress to AIDS, leaving you vulnerable to a host of opportunistic infections (rare infections that develop only when the immune system falters, such as certain types of pneumonia, tuberculosis, and fungal infections). It's imperative, therefore, that you continue to see your doctor regularly and keep all your follow-up appointments.

How should you take this medication?
Take Viracept every day, exactly as prescribed. Do not stop taking it or change the dose without first consulting your doctor.

To achieve higher blood levels of the drug, always take Viracept with a meal or light snack.

If your child is taking Viracept oral powder, mix it with a small amount of water, milk, formula, soy formula, soy milk, or a liquid nutritional product such as Ensure, Sustacal, or Advera, then use within 6 hours. Make sure the child drinks the entire dose. Do not mix the powder with apple juice, applesauce, or orange juice; these combinations will taste bitter.

■ *If you miss a dose...*
Take it as soon as possible. If it is almost time for the next dose, skip the one you missed and go back to your regular schedule. Never double the dose.

■ *Storage instructions...*
Both tablets and powder may be stored at room temperature.

What side effects may occur?
Side effects cannot be anticipated. If any develop or change in intensity, tell your doctor as soon as possible. Only your doctor can determine if it is safe for you to continue taking Viracept.

The most frequent side effect associated with Viracept is diarrhea. If it develops, it can be controlled with over-the-counter medications such as Imodium A-D.

■ *More common side effects may include:*
Abdominal pain, gas, loss of strength, nausea, skin rash

■ *Less common side effects may include:*
Allergic reaction, anxiety, arthritis, back pain, blood disorders, dehydration, depression, difficulty breathing, dizziness, drowsiness, emotional

problems, eye problems, fever, flu-like symptoms, headache, hepatitis, hives, increased or decreased blood sugar, indigestion, itching, joint pain, kidney problems, loss of appetite, migraine, mouth ulcers, muscle pain or cramps, muscle weakness or disorders, nasal and sinus congestion, overactivity, pain, seizures, sexual dysfunction, skin rash, skin tingling or numbness, sleep problems, sore throat, stomach and intestinal bleeding, stomach pain, suicidal thoughts, sweating, vomiting

Why should this drug not be prescribed?
If you have ever had an allergic reaction to Viracept or any of its ingredients, do not take this drug.

Special warnings about this medication
Although Viracept reduces the amount of HIV in the blood, its long-term effect on survival is still unknown. We do know, however, that the drug does NOT reduce the risk of passing HIV to others through sexual contact or blood contamination. You will need to continue avoiding practices that spread the virus.

If you have been using oral contraceptives, you'll need to take other measures. Viracept dramatically reduces the effectiveness of the Pill.

Viracept may trigger diabetes or make existing diabetes worse. If this occurs, you may have to start taking insulin or oral diabetes medication, or have your present dosage adjusted.

People with hemophilia type A and B may experience increased bleeding. If this happens, alert your doctor immediately. Make sure, too, that your doctor is aware of any liver problems you may have.

Viracept oral powder contains phenylalanine. If your child has the hereditary disease known as phenylketonuria, do not give the powder form.

Possible food and drug interactions
when taking this medication
Do not take Viracept with any of the following medications. The combination could cause serious or even life-threatening problems.

Amiodarone (Cordarone)
Astemizole (Hismanal)
Cisapride (Propulsid)
Ergot derivatives such as Cafergot, Ercaf, and Ergostat
Midazolam (Versed)
Quinidine (Cardioquin, Quinaglute, Quinidex)
Rifampin (Rifadin, Rimactane)

Terfenadine (Seldane)
Triazolam (Halcion)

Viracept may also interact with certain other drugs, and the effects of either could be increased, decreased, or altered. It is especially important to check with your doctor before combining Viracept with the following:

Calcium channel blockers such as Cardene, Norvasc, Procardia, and Sular
Carbamazepine (Tegretol)
Indinavir (Crixivan)
Oral contraceptives such as Ovcon-35
Phenobarbital
Phenytoin (Dilantin)
Rifabutin (Mycobutin)
Ritonavir (Norvir)
Saquinavir (Fortovase)

Special information
if you are pregnant or breastfeeding

The effects of Viracept during pregnancy have not been adequately studied. If you are pregnant or plan to become pregnant, tell your doctor immediately.

Do not breastfeed your baby. HIV appears in breast milk and can infect a nursing infant.

Recommended dosage

ADULTS

The recommended dose is 750 milligrams (three 250-milligram tablets) 3 times a day with a meal or snack.

CHILDREN

Viracept oral powder is available for children who are unable to take tablets. The recommended dose for children 2 to 13 years of age is 20 to 30 milligrams per 2.2 pounds of body weight, 3 times a day with a meal or snack. The oral powder can be measured out with the provided scooper or a teaspoon—your doctor will tell you how much—and mixed with a small amount of water or any other fluid listed under "How should you take this medication?"

The safety and effectiveness of Viracept in children below age 2 have not been established.

Overdosage

Information on acute overdose with Viracept is limited. However, any medication taken in excess can have serious consequences. If you suspect an overdose, seek emergency medical treatment immediately.

Brand name:

VIRAMUNE

Pronounced: VIE-ruh-mewn
Generic name: Nevirapine

Why is this drug prescribed?

Viramune is prescribed for advanced cases of HIV. HIV—the human immunodeficiency virus that causes AIDS—undermines the immune system over a period of years, eventually leaving the body defenseless against infection. Viramune is generally prescribed only after the immune system has declined and infections have begun to appear. It is always taken with at least one other HIV medication such as Retrovir or Videx. If taken alone, it can cause the virus to become resistant. Even if used properly, it may be effective for only a limited time.

Like other drugs for HIV, Viramune works by impairing the virus's ability to multiply.

Most important fact about this drug

Though Viramune can slow the progress of HIV, it is not a cure. HIV-related infections remain a danger, so frequent check-ups and tests are still advisable.

How should you take this medication?

Be sure to take this medication every day, exactly as prescribed. Increase the dosage only when directed. To avoid development of resistance, be careful to take your other HIV drugs as well.

If you are using the oral suspension, shake it gently before each dose. Give it to the child with an oral dosing syringe or dosing cup. After each dose, rinse the cup with water and give the rinse to the child as well.

■ *If you miss a dose...*
Take it as soon as you remember. If it is almost time for the next dose, skip the one you missed and go back to your regular schedule. Do not double the dose.

■ *Storage instructions...*
Store tablets and oral suspension at room temperature in a tightly closed bottle.

What side effects may occur?
Side effects cannot be anticipated. If any develop or change in intensity, inform your doctor as soon as possible. Only your doctor can determine if it is safe for you to continue using Viramune.

■ *More common side effects may include:*
Fever, headache, nausea, rash

■ *Less common side effects may include:*
Abdominal pain, diarrhea, liver problems, mouth sores, muscle pain, tingling sensation

Why should this drug not be prescribed?
If Viramune gives you an allergic reaction, you cannot use this drug.

Special warnings about this medication
The most important side effect of Viramune is a rash which occasionally becomes so serious as to be life-threatening. The rash strikes approximately one in three patients, and becomes severe in over 7 percent. It usually appears during the first 6 weeks of therapy. If you notice any signs of a rash, inform your doctor immediately. If it becomes severe or is accompanied by fever, blisters, mouth sores, red eyes, swelling, muscle or joint aches, or general fatigue, stop taking the drug and call your doctor.

If you have any kidney or liver problems, you should not take Viramune. When you begin taking the drug, your doctor will check your liver function through blood tests for at least the first 6 months. If a liver condition develops while you are on the drug, therapy will be stopped temporarily.

Remember that Viramune does not completely eliminate HIV from the body. The virus can still be passed to others during sex or through blood contamination.

Possible food and drug interactions
when taking this medication
Viramune should NOT be taken with the protease-inhibitor drugs Crixivan, Fortovase, Invirase, and Norvir. These drugs are part of the highly successful drug "cocktails" now being used against HIV, but unlike some other HIV drugs, Viramune can reduce their effectiveness.

You should also check with your doctor before combining Viramune with the following:

Cimetidine (Tagamet)
Hormonal contraceptives (implants and pills)
Ketoconazole (Nizoral)
Macrolide antibiotics such as Biaxin, Dynabac, Ery-Tab, Eryc, Tao, and Zithromax
Rifabutin (Mycobutin)
Rifampin (Rifadin, Rimactane)

Special information
if you are pregnant or breastfeeding
The effects of Viramune during pregnancy have not been adequately studied. If you are pregnant or plan to become pregnant, notify your doctor immediately.

Avoid breastfeeding. HIV can be passed to a nursing infant through breast milk.

Recommended dosage

ADULTS

For the first 14 days, the dose is 1 tablet a day. If no serious rash appears, the dose is then increased to 1 tablet twice a day. If you miss your doses for more than 7 days, the doctor will have to restart you at the lower initial dose.

CHILDREN

2 months to 8 years of age
For the first 14 days, the dose of oral suspension is 4 milligrams per 2.2 pounds of body weight once a day. If no serious rash appears, the dose is then increased to 7 milligrams per 2.2 pounds twice a day.

8 years and older
For the first 14 days, the dose of oral suspension is 4 milligrams per 2.2 pounds of body weight once a day. If no serious rash appears, the dose is then increased to 4 milligrams per 2.2 pounds twice a day.

For both adults and children, total daily dosage should never exceed 400 milligrams (2 tablets).

Overdosage

Any medication taken in excess can have serious consequences. If you suspect an overdose, seek medical attention immediately.

- *Symptoms of Viramune overdose may include:*
  Dizziness, fatigue, fever, headache, insomnia, nausea, rash, reddened bumps on the skin, respiratory problems, swelling, vomiting, weight loss

Brand name:

VISKEN

Pronounced: VIS-kin
Generic name: Pindolol

Why is this drug prescribed?

Visken, a type of medication known as a beta blocker, is used in the treatment of high blood pressure. It is effective alone or combined with other high blood pressure medications, particularly with a thiazide-type diuretic. Beta blockers decrease the force and rate of heart contractions.

Most important fact about this drug

You must take Visken regularly for it to be effective. Since blood pressure declines gradually, it may be several weeks before you get the full benefit of Visken; and you must continue taking it even if you are feeling well. Visken does not cure high blood pressure; it merely keeps it under control.

How should you take this medication?

Visken can be taken with or without food.

Take this medication exactly as prescribed, even if your symptoms have disappeared. Try not to miss any doses. If this medication is not taken regularly, your condition may worsen.

- *If you miss a dose...*
  Take it as soon as you remember. If it's within 4 hours of your next scheduled dose, skip the one you missed and go back to your regular schedule. Never take 2 doses at the same time.

- *Storage instructions...*
  Store Visken at room temperature in a tightly closed, light-resistant container.

What side effects may occur?
Side effects cannot be anticipated. If any develop or change in intensity, inform your doctor as soon as possible. Only your doctor can determine if it is safe for you to continue taking Visken.

■ *More common side effects may include:*
Abdominal discomfort, chest pain, difficult or labored breathing, dizziness, fatigue, joint pain, muscle pain or cramps, nausea, nervousness, strange dreams, swelling due to fluid retention, tingling or pins and needles, trouble sleeping, weakness

■ *Less common or rare side effects may include:*
Hallucinations, heart failure, itching, palpitations, rapid heartbeat, rash

Why should this drug not be prescribed?
If you have bronchial asthma; severe congestive heart failure; inadequate blood supply to the circulatory system (cardiogenic shock); heart block (a heart irregularity); or a severely slow heartbeat, you should not take this medication.

Special warnings about this medication
If you have had severe congestive heart failure in the past, Visken should be used with caution.

Visken should not be stopped suddenly. It can cause increased chest pain and heart attack. Dosage should be gradually reduced.

If you suffer from asthma, chronic bronchitis, emphysema, seasonal allergies or other bronchial conditions, coronary artery disease, or kidney or liver disease, this medication should be used with caution.

Ask your doctor if you should check your pulse while taking Visken. This medication can cause your heartbeat to become too slow.

This medication may mask the symptoms of low blood sugar in diabetics or alter blood sugar levels. If you are diabetic, discuss this with your doctor.

Visken may cause you to become disoriented. If it has this effect on you, driving or operating dangerous machinery or participating in any hazardous activity that requires full mental alertness is not recommended.

If you have a history of severe allergic reactions, inform your doctor before taking Visken.

Notify your doctor or dentist that you are taking Visken if you have a medical emergency and before you have surgery or dental treatment.

Possible food and drug interactions
when taking this medication

If Visken is taken with certain other drugs, the effects of either could be increased, decreased, or altered. It is especially important to check with your doctor before combining Visken with the following:

Airway-opening drugs such as Proventil and Ventolin
Blood pressure drugs such as reserpine
Digoxin (Lanoxin)
Epinephrine (EpiPen)
Hydrochlorothiazide (HydroDIURIL)
Insulin or oral antidiabetic agents such as Micronase
Nonsteroidal anti-inflammatory drugs such as Motrin
Ritodrine (Yutopar)
Theophylline (Theo-Dur, others)
Thioridazine (Mellaril)
Verapamil (Calan, Verelan)

Special information
if you are pregnant or breastfeeding

The effects of Visken during pregnancy have not been adequately studied. If you are pregnant or plan to become pregnant, inform your doctor immediately. Visken appears in breast milk and could affect a nursing infant. If this medication is essential to your health, your doctor may advise you to discontinue breastfeeding until your treatment with this medication is finished.

Recommended dosage

ADULTS

Your doctor will determine the dosage according to your specific needs.

The usual starting dose is 5 milligrams, 2 times per day, alone or with other high blood pressure medication. Your blood pressure should be lower in 1 to 2 weeks. If blood pressure is not reduced sufficiently within 3 to 4 weeks, your doctor may increase your total daily dosage by 10 milligrams at a time, at 3- to 4-week intervals, up to a maximum of 60 milligrams a day.

CHILDREN

The safety and effectiveness of Visken have not been established in children.

ELDERLY

The doctor will determine dosage for an elderly individual based on his or her particular needs.

Overdosage
Any medication taken in excess can have serious consequences. If you suspect an overdose, seek medical attention immediately.

- *Symptoms of Visken overdose may include:*
  Bronchospasm (spasm of the air passages), excessively slow heartbeat, heart failure, low blood pressure

Brand name:

VISTARIL

See Atarax, page 104.

Generic name:

VITAMINS WITH FLUORIDE

See Poly-Vi-Flor, page 1017.

Brand name:

VIVELLE

See Estraderm, page 490.

Brand name:

VOLMAX

See Proventil, page 1073.

Brand name:

VOLTAREN

Pronounced: vol-TAR-en
Generic name: Diclofenac sodium
Other brand name: Cataflam (Diclofenac potassium)

Why is this drug prescribed?
Voltaren and Cataflam are nonsteroidal anti-inflammatory drugs used to relieve the inflammation, swelling, stiffness, and joint pain associated with rheumatoid arthritis, osteoarthritis (the most common form of arthritis), and ankylosing spondylitis (arthritis and stiffness of the spine). Voltaren-XR, the extended-release form of Voltaren, is used only for long-term treatment.

Cataflam is also prescribed for immediate relief of pain and menstrual discomfort.

Most important fact about this drug
You should have frequent checkups with your doctor if you take Voltaren regularly. Ulcers or internal bleeding can occur without warning.

How should you take this medication?
To minimize stomach upset and related side effects, your doctor may recommend taking this medicine with food, milk, or an antacid. However, this may delay onset of relief.

Take this drug with a full glass of water. Also, do not lie down for about 20 minutes after taking it. This will help to prevent irritation in your upper digestive tract.

Take this medication exactly as prescribed.

■ *If you miss a dose...*
  If you take this medicine on a regular schedule, take it as soon as you remember. If it is almost time for your next dose, skip the one you missed and go back to your regular schedule. Do not take 2 doses at once.

■ *Storage instructions...*
  Store at room temperature. Keep the container tightly closed and protect from moisture.

What side effects may occur?
Side effects cannot be anticipated. If any develop or change in intensity, inform your doctor as soon as possible. Only your doctor can determine if it is safe for you to continue taking Voltaren.

■ *More common side effects may include:*
  Abdominal pain or cramps, constipation, diarrhea, dizziness, headache, indigestion, nausea

■ *Less common side effects may include:*
  Abdominal bleeding, abdominal swelling, fluid retention, gas, itching, peptic ulcers, rash, ringing in the ears

■ *Rare side effects may include:*
  Anaphylaxis (severe allergic reaction), anemia, anxiety, appetite change, asthma, black stools, blood disorders, bloody diarrhea, blurred vision, changes in taste, colitis, congestive heart failure, convulsions, decrease in

white blood cells, decreased urine production, depression, double vision, drowsiness, dry mouth, hair loss, hearing loss, hepatitis, high blood pressure, hives, inability to sleep, inflammation of mouth, irritability, kidney failure, low blood pressure, nosebleed, red or purple skin discoloration and itching, sensitivity to light, skin eruptions and inflammation, scaling, or peeling, sores in the gullet, Stevens-Johnson syndrome (a severe form of skin eruption), swelling of eyelids, lips, and tongue, swelling of the throat due to fluid retention, vague feeling of illness, vision changes, vomiting, yellow eyes and skin

Why should this drug not be prescribed?

If you have an allergic reaction to Voltaren or Cataflam, or if you have had asthma attacks, hives, or other allergic reactions caused by aspirin or other nonsteroidal anti-inflammatory drugs, you should not take this medication. Make sure your doctor is aware of any drug reactions you have experienced.

Special warnings about this medication

Remember that this medication has been known to cause peptic ulcers and bleeding. Contact your doctor immediately if you suspect a problem.

Use this drug cautiously if you have kidney problems, heart disease, or high blood pressure. It can cause fluid retention.

This medication can also cause liver problems. If you develop signs of liver disease such as nausea, fatigue, lethargy, itching, yellowish eyes and skin, tenderness in the upper right area of your abdomen, or flu-like symptoms, notify your doctor at once.

Rare cases of meningitis (inflammation of the membrane enclosing the brain) have been linked to this medication. If symptoms such as fever and coma develop, alert the doctor immediately.

In rare instances, this drug may also affect your vision. If you notice any problems, stop taking the drug and check with your doctor.

Possible food and drug interactions
when taking this medication

If Voltaren or Cataflam is taken with certain other drugs, the effects of either could be increased, decreased, or altered. It is especially important to check with your doctor before combining Voltaren with the following:

Aspirin
Blood thinners such as Coumadin
Cyclosporine (Sandimmune)

Digitalis drugs such as Lanoxin
Diuretics such as Dyazide, Midamor, and Lasix
Insulin or oral antidiabetes medications such as Micronase
Lithium (Lithonate)
Methotrexate
Phenobarbital

Special information
if you are pregnant or breastfeeding
Do not take this drug late in your pregnancy; it could harm the baby. Check with your doctor before taking the drug early in pregnancy; it should be used only if necessary. The drug does appear in breast milk and could affect a nursing infant. If this medication is essential to your health, your doctor may advise you to discontinue breastfeeding until your treatment with Voltaren is finished.

Recommended dosage

ADULTS

Osteoarthritis
The usual dose is 100 to 150 milligrams a day, divided into smaller doses of 50 milligrams 2 or 3 times a day (for Voltaren or Cataflam) or 75 milligrams twice a day (for Voltaren). The usual dose of Voltaren-XR (extended-release) is 100 milligrams taken once a day.

Rheumatoid Arthritis
The usual dose is 100 to 200 milligrams a day, divided into smaller doses of 50 milligrams 2 to 4 times a day (for Voltaren or Cataflam), 75 milligrams twice a day (for Voltaren), or 100 milligrams once or twice a day (for Voltaren-XR).

People with rheumatoid arthritis should not take more than 225 milligrams a day.

Ankylosing Spondylitis
The usual dose is 100 to 125 milligrams of Voltaren a day, divided into smaller doses of 25 milligrams 4 times a day, with another 25 milligrams at bedtime if necessary.

Pain and menstrual discomfort
The usual starting dose of Cataflam is 50 milligrams 3 times a day, although for the first day doctors sometimes prescribe a starting dose of 100 milligrams followed by two 50-milligram doses. After the first day, you should not take more than 150 milligrams in a day.

CHILDREN

The safety and effectiveness of Voltaren have not been established in children.

Overdosage

Any medication taken in excess can have serious consequences. If you suspect an overdose, seek medical attention immediately.

- *The symptoms of Voltaren overdose may include:*
  Acute kidney failure, drowsiness, loss of consciousness, lung inflammation, vomiting

Generic name:

WARFARIN

See Coumadin, page 303.

Brand name:

WELLBUTRIN

Pronounced: Well-BEW-trin
Generic name: Bupropion hydrochloride
Other brand name: Wellbutrin SR

Why is this drug prescribed?

Wellbutrin, a relatively new antidepressant medication, is given to help relieve certain kinds of major depression.

Major depression involves a severely depressed mood (for 2 weeks or more) and loss of interest or pleasure in usual activities accompanied by sleep and appetite disturbances, agitation or lack of energy, feelings of guilt or worthlessness, decreased sex drive, inability to concentrate, and perhaps thoughts of suicide.

Unlike the more familiar tricyclic antidepressants, such as Elavil, Tofranil, and others, Wellbutrin tends to have a somewhat stimulating effect.

The drug is available in regular and sustained-release formulations (Wellbutrin SR).

Most important fact about this drug

Although Wellbutrin occasionally causes weight gain, a more common effect is weight loss: Some 28 percent of people who take this medication lose 5 pounds or more. If depression has already caused you to lose weight, and if further weight loss would be detrimental to your health, Wellbutrin may not be the best antidepressant for you.

How should you take this medication?
Take Wellbutrin exactly as prescribed by your doctor. The usual dosing regimen is 3 equal doses spaced evenly throughout the day. Allow at least 6 hours between doses. Your doctor will probably start you at a low dosage and gradually increase it; this helps minimize side effects.

You should take Wellbutrin SR, the sustained-release form, in 2 doses, at least 8 hours apart. Swallow Wellbutrin SR tablets whole; do not chew, divide, or crush them.

If Wellbutrin works for you, your doctor will probably have you continue taking it for at least several months.

- *If you miss a dose...*
  Take it as soon as you remember. If it is within 4 hours of your next dose, skip the one you missed and go back to your regular schedule. Never take 2 doses at the same time.

- *Storage instructions...*
  Store at room temperature. Protect from light and moisture.

What side effects may occur?
Side effects cannot be anticipated. If any develop or change in intensity, inform your doctor as soon as possible. Only your doctor can determine if it is safe for you to continue taking Wellbutrin.

Seizures are perhaps the most worrisome side effect.

- *More common side effects may include:*
  Abdominal pain (Wellbutrin SR), agitation, anxiety (Wellbutrin SR), constipation, dizziness, dry mouth, excessive sweating, headache, loss of appetite (Wellbutrin SR), nausea, palpitations (Wellbutrin SR), vomiting, skin rash, sleep disturbances, sore throat (Wellbutrin SR), tremor

- *Other side effects may include:*
  Acne, allergic reactions (severe), bed-wetting, blisters in the mouth and eyes (Stevens-Johnson syndrome), blurred vision, breathing difficulty, chest pain, chills, complete or almost complete loss of movement, confusion, dry skin, episodes of over-activity, elation, or irritability, extreme calmness, fatigue, fever, fluid retention, flu-like symptoms, gum irritation and inflammation, hair color changes, hair loss, hives, impotence, incoordination and clumsiness, indigestion, itching, increased libido,

menstrual complaints, mood instability, muscle rigidity, painful ejaculation, painful erection, retarded ejaculation, ringing in the ears, sexual dysfunction, suicidal ideation, thirst disturbances, toothache, urinary disturbances, weight gain or loss

Why should this drug not be prescribed?

Do not take Wellbutrin if you are sensitive to or have ever had an allergic reaction to it.

Since Wellbutrin causes seizures in some people, do not take it if you have any type of seizure disorder or if you are taking another medication containing bupropion, such as Zyban, the quit smoking aid.

If you have had any kind of heart trouble or liver or kidney disease, be sure your doctor knows about it before you start taking this drug.

You should not take Wellbutrin if you currently have, or formerly had, an eating disorder. For some reason, people with a history of anorexia nervosa or bulimia seem to be more likely to experience Wellbutrin-related seizures.

Do not take Wellbutrin if, within the past 14 days, you have taken a monoamine oxidase inhibitor (MAO inhibitor) drug, such as the antidepressants Nardil or Parnate. This particular drug combination could cause you to experience a sudden, dangerous rise in blood pressure.

Special warnings about this medication

If you take Wellbutrin, you may be vulnerable to seizures if your dosage is too high or if you ever suffered brain damage or experienced seizures in the past.

The danger of seizures is greater in people addicted to narcotics, cocaine, or stimulants, and in those using over-the-counter stimulants or diet pills. Alcohol abue or withdrawal also increases the risk, as does the use of other antidepressants or major tranquilizers. The risk is higher, too, if you are taking insulin or oral diabetes medication.

Because seizures are possible, if you have been taking Valium or a similar tranquilizer but are ready to stop, taper off gradually rather than quitting abruptly.

Since Wellbutrin may impair your coordination or judgment, do not drive or operate dangerous machinery until you find out how the medication affects you.

Possible food and drug interactions
when taking this medication

Do not drink alcohol while you are taking Wellbutrin; an interaction between alcohol and Wellbutrin could increase the possibility of a seizure.

If Wellbutrin is taken with certain other drugs, the effects of either could be increased, decreased, or altered. It is especially important to check with your doctor before combining Wellbutrin with the following:

Cyclophosphamide (Cytoxan)
Dilantin
Levodopa (Larodopa)
Major tranquilizers such as Thorazine and Mellaril
MAO inhibitors (such as the antidepressants Parnate and Nardil)
Orphenadrine (Norgesic)
Other antidepressants such as Elavil and Tofranil
Phenobarbital (Luminal)
Steroid medications such as Prednisone
Tagamet
Tegretol
Theophylline (Theo-Dur)

Special information
if you are pregnant or breastfeeding

If you are pregnant or plan to become pregnant, notify your doctor immediately. Wellbutrin should be taken during pregnancy only if clearly needed.

Wellbutrin does pass into breast milk and may cause serious reactions in a nursing baby; therefore, if you are a new mother, you may need to discontinue breastfeeding while you are taking this medication.

Recommended dosage

No single dose of Wellbutrin should exceed 150 milligrams.

ADULTS

Wellbutrin

At the beginning, your dose will probably be 200 milligrams per day, taken as 100 milligrams 2 times a day. After at least 3 days at this dose, your doctor may increase the dosage to 300 milligrams per day, taken as 100 milligrams 3 times a day, with at least 6 hours between doses. This is the usual adult dose. The maximum recommended dosage is 450 milligrams per day taken in doses of no more than 150 milligrams each.

Wellbutrin SR

The usual starting dose is 150 milligrams in the morning. After 3 days, if you do well, your doctor will have you take another 150 milligrams at least 8 hours after the first dose. It may be 4 weeks before you feel the benefit and you will take the drug for several months. The maximum recommended dose is 400 milligrams a day, taken in doses of 200 milligrams each.

CHILDREN

The safety and effectiveness in children under 18 years old have not been established.

OLDER ADULTS

Although they are more sensitive to antidepressant drugs, older people have responded no differently to Wellbutrin than younger people.

Overdosage

Any medication taken in excess can have serious consequences. If you suspect an overdose of Wellbutrin, seek medical attention immediately.

- *Symptoms of Wellbutrin overdose may include:*
  Hallucinations, heart failure, loss of consciousness, rapid heartbeat, seizures

- *Symptoms of Wellbutrin SR overdose may include:*
  Blurred vision, confusion, jitteriness, lethargy, lightheadedness, nausea, seizures, vomiting

- *An overdose that involves other drugs in combination with Wellbutrin may also cause these symptoms:*
  Breathing difficulties, coma, fever, rigid muscles, stupor

Brand name:

WYMOX

See Amoxil, page 58.

Brand name:

WYTENSIN

Pronounced: why-TEN-sin
Generic name: Guanabenz acetate

Why is this drug prescribed?

Wytensin is used in the treatment of high blood pressure. It is effective used alone or in combination with a thiazide type of diuretic. Wytensin begins to lower blood pressure within 60 minutes after taking a single dose and may slow your pulse rate slightly.

Most important fact about this drug

You must take Wytensin regularly for it to be effective. Since blood pressure declines gradually, it may be several weeks before you get the full benefit of Wytensin; and you must continue taking it even if you are feeling well. Wytensin does not cure high blood pressure; it merely keeps it under control.

How should you take this medication?

Wytensin may be taken with or without food. Take it exactly as prescribed.

■ *If you miss a dose...*
Take it as soon as you remember. If it is almost time for the next dose, skip the one you missed and go back to your regular schedule. Do not take 2 doses at the same time. If you forget the medication 2 or more times in a row, contact your doctor.

■ *Storage instructions...*
Store at room temperature, in a tightly closed container, away from light.

What side effects may occur?

Side effects cannot be anticipated. If any develop or change in intensity, inform your doctor as soon as possible. Only your doctor can determine if it is safe for you to continue taking Wytensin.

■ *More common side effects may include:*
Dizziness, drowsiness, dry mouth, headache, weakness

■ *Less common side effects may include:*
Abdominal discomfort, aches in arms and legs, anxiety, blurred vision, breast development in males, changes in taste, chest pain, constipation, decreased sex drive, depression, diarrhea, fluid retention, frequent urination, impotence, irregular heartbeat, itching, lack of muscle coordination, muscle aches, nausea, pounding heartbeat, rash, shortness of breath, sleep disturbances, stomach pain, stuffy nose, vomiting

■ *Rare side effects may include:*
Heartbeat irregularities

Why should this drug not be prescribed?

Do not take Wytensin if you are sensitive to it or have ever had an allergic reaction to it.

Special warnings about this medication

Wytensin can make you drowsy or less alert. Driving or operating dangerous machinery or participating in any hazardous activity that requires full mental alertness is not recommended until you know how this drug affects you.

If you have severe heart disease, stroke or related disorders, or severe liver or kidney failure, or if you have recently had a heart attack, this drug should be used with caution.

Your doctor will monitor your blood pressure if you have disorders of the kidney or liver.

Possible food and drug interactions
when taking this medication

Wytensin may intensify the effects of alcohol. Use of alcohol should be avoided.

If Wytensin is taken with certain other drugs, the effects of either could be increased, decreased, or altered. It is especially important to check with your doctor before combining Wytensin with the following:

Antihistamines such as Benadryl, Clor-Trimeton, and Tavist
Drugs that depress the central nervous system such as Halcion, Valium,
and phenobarbital

Special information
if you are pregnant or breastfeeding

The effects of Wytensin during pregnancy have not been adequately studied, but it may affect the fetus. If you are pregnant or plan to become pregnant, inform your doctor immediately. Wytensin may appear in breast milk and could affect a nursing infant. If this medication is essential to your health, your doctor may advise you to discontinue breastfeeding until your treatment is finished.

Recommended dosage

ADULTS

Your doctor will adjust the dosage of this medication to meet your individual needs.

The usual starting dose is 4 milligrams 2 times per day, whether Wytensin is used alone or with a thiazide type of diuretic.

Your doctor may increase the dosage in increments of 4 to 8 milligrams per day every 1 to 2 weeks, depending on your response.

The maximum reported dose has been 32 milligrams twice daily, but doses as high as this are rarely needed.

CHILDREN

The safety and effectiveness of this drug have not been established in children under 12 years of age.

OLDER ADULTS

Older adults should use this drug with caution.

Overdosage

Any medication taken in excess can have serious consequences. If you suspect an overdose, seek medical attention immediately.

■ *Symptoms of Wytensin overdose may include:*
Excessive contraction of the pupils, irritability, low blood pressure, sleepiness, slow heartbeat, sluggishness

Brand name:

XALATAN

Pronounced: ZAL-a-tan
Generic name: Latanoprost

Why is this drug prescribed?

Xalatan is used to relieve high pressure within the eye (a hallmark of the condition known as open-angle glaucoma). Xalatan usually is prescribed when other medications have failed to do the job or have caused other problems.

Most important fact about this drug

Be careful not to let the tip of the Xalatan bottle touch your eye or anything else. Otherwise, the contents could become contaminated. A contaminated solution can cause an eye infection and lead to serious damage, including loss of vision.

How should you use this medication?

Use Xalatan exactly as prescribed. It should be applied only once a day; more frequent administration may reduce its effectiveness. Apply one drop to the eye in the evening. If you are using other eyedrops to lower pressure, allow at least 5 minutes between applications of the two medications. Contact lenses should be removed before the drug is applied. Wait 15 minutes before reinserting them.

■ *If you miss a dose...*
Apply it as soon as possible. If you don't remember until the next day, skip the dose and go back to your regular schedule. Never double the dose.

■ *Storage instructions...*
Store unopened bottles in the refrigerator. Once opened, the bottles may be stored at room temperature for up to 6 weeks. Protect from light.

What side effects may occur?
Side effects cannot be anticipated. If any develop or change in intensity, inform your doctor as soon as possible. Be especially quick to report pinkeye or any effects on the eyelids. Only your doctor can determine if it is safe for you to continue using Xalatan.

■ *More common side effects may include...*
Bloodshot eyes, blurred vision, burning, foreign body sensation, increased pigmentation of the iris, inflammatory disease of the cornea, itching, stinging, upper respiratory infection

■ *Less common side effects may include...*
Allergic reactions, back pain, chest pain, dry eye, excessive tearing, eye pain, eyelid crusting or reddening, eyelid swelling or pain, intolerance to light, joint and muscle pain, rash

■ *Rare side effects may include...*
Double vision, eye discharge, pinkeye

Why should this drug not be prescribed?
Do not use Xalatan if you are sensitive or allergic to any of its ingredients.

Special warnings about this medication
Xalatan may gradually turn the eye's iris brown. This change may not be noticed for months or years. Its long-term effects are unknown, but it may be permanent. Ask your doctor about the possibility of mismatched eye color if you will be treating only one eye with Xalatan.

If your eye sustains an injury or becomes infected, or you have eye surgery, you may need to start a new bottle of Xalatan. Be sure to check with your doctor.

Xalatan may cause blurred vision. Make certain it does not have this effect on you before you attempt to drive.

Possible food and drug interactions
when using this medication
Mixing Xalatan with eyedrops containing thiomersal can cause the formation of solid substances in the eye. To avoid this problem, administer the drops at least 5 minutes apart.

Special information
if you are pregnant or breastfeeding
The effects of Xalatan during pregnancy and breastfeeding have not been adequately studied. If you are pregnant or plan to become pregnant, notify your doctor immediately. It is not known whether Xalatan makes its way into breast milk. If you are nursing and need to use Xalatan, your doctor may advise you to discontinue breastfeeding while using the medication.

Recommended dosage
The usual dose is 1 drop in the affected eye once every evening.

Overdosage
Any medication taken in excess can have serious consequences. If you suspect an overdose, seek medical attention immediately.

■ *Symptoms of Xalatan overdose may include:*
  Bloodshot eyes, eye irritation

Brand name:

XANAX

Pronounced: ZAN-ax
Generic name: Alprazolam

Why is this drug prescribed?
Xanax is a tranquilizer used in the short-term relief of symptoms of anxiety or the treatment of anxiety disorders. Anxiety disorder is marked by unrealistic worry or excessive fears and concerns.

Xanax is also used in the treatment of panic disorder, which appears as unexpected panic attacks and may be accompanied by a fear of open spaces called agoraphobia. Only your doctor can diagnose panic disorder and best advise you about treatment. Anxiety associated with depression is also responsive to Xanax.

Some doctors prescribe Xanax to treat alcohol withdrawal, fear of open spaces and strangers, depression, irritable bowel syndrome, and premenstrual syndrome.

Most important fact about this drug
Tolerance and dependence can occur with the use of Xanax. You may experience withdrawal symptoms if you stop using the drug abruptly. Only your doctor should advise you to discontinue or change your dose.

How should you take this medication?
Xanax may be taken with or without food. Take it exactly as prescribed.

■ *If you miss a dose...*
If you are less than 1 hour late, take it as soon as you remember. Otherwise skip the dose and go back to your regular schedule. Never take 2 doses at the same time.

■ *Storage instructions...*
Store Xanax at room temperature.

What side effects may occur?
Side effects cannot be anticipated. If any develop or change in intensity, inform your doctor as soon as possible. Only your doctor can determine if it is safe for you to continue taking Xanax. Your doctor should periodically reassess the need for this drug.

Side effects of Xanax are usually seen at the beginning of treatment and disappear with continued medication. However, if dosage is increased, side effects will be more likely.

■ *More common side effects may include:*
Abdominal discomfort, abnormal involuntary movement, agitation, allergies, anxiety, blurred vision, chest pain, confusion, constipation, decreased or increased sex drive, depression, diarrhea, difficult urination, dream abnormalities, drowsiness, dry mouth, fainting, fatigue, fluid retention, headache, hyperventilation (too frequent or too deep breathing), impaired memory, inability to fall asleep, increase or decrease in appetite, increased or decreased salivation, irritability, lack of coordination, light-headedness, low blood pressure, menstrual problems, muscular twitching, nausea and vomiting, nervousness, palpitations, rapid heartbeat, rash, restlessness,

ringing in the ears, sexual dysfunction, skin inflammation, speech difficulties, stiffness, stuffy nose, sweating, tiredness/sleepiness, tremors, upper respiratory infections, weakness, weight gain or loss

■ *Less common or rare side effects may include:*
Abnormal muscle tone, concentration difficulties, decreased coordination, dizziness, double vision, fear, hallucinations, inability to control urination or bowel movements, infection, itching, loss of appetite, muscle cramps, muscle spasticity, rage, sedation, seizures, sleep disturbances, slurred speech, stimulation, talkativeness, taste alterations, temporary memory loss, tingling or pins and needles, uninhibited behavior, urine retention, warm feeling, weakness in muscle and bone, weight gain or loss, yellow eyes and skin

■ *Side effects due to decrease or withdrawal from Xanax:*
Blurred vision, decreased concentration, decreased mental clarity, diarrhea, heightened awareness of noise or bright lights, impaired sense of smell, loss of appetite, loss of weight, muscle cramps, seizures, tingling sensation, twitching

Why should this drug not be prescribed?
If you are sensitive to or have ever had an allergic reaction to Xanax or other tranquilizers, you should not take this medication. Also avoid Xanax while taking the antifungal drugs Sporanox or Nizoral. Make sure that your doctor is aware of any drug reactions that you have experienced.

Do not take this medication if you have been diagnosed with the eye condition called narrow-angle glaucoma.

Anxiety or tension related to everyday stress usually does not require treatment with Xanax. Discuss your symptoms thoroughly with your doctor.

Special warnings about this medication
Xanax may cause you to become drowsy or less alert; therefore, driving or operating dangerous machinery or participating in any hazardous activity that requires full mental alertness is not recommended.

If you are being treated for panic disorder, you may need to take a higher dose of Xanax than for anxiety alone. High doses—more than 4 milligrams a day—of this medication taken for long intervals may cause emotional and physical dependence. It is important that your doctor supervise you carefully when you are using this medication.

Remember that withdrawal symptoms can occur when Xanax is stopped suddenly.

Possible food and drug interactions
when taking this medication

Xanax may intensify the effect of alcohol. Do not drink alcohol while taking this medication.

Never combine Xanax with Sporanox or Nizoral. These drugs cause a build-up of Xanax in the body.

If Xanax is taken with certain other drugs, the effects of either could be increased, decreased, or altered. It is important to check with your doctor before combining Xanax with the following:

Amiodarone (Cordarone)
Antihistamines such as Benadryl and Tavist
Carbamazepine (Tegretol)
Certain antibiotics such as Biaxin and erythromycin
Certain antidepressant drugs, including Elavil, Norpramin, and Tofranil
Cimetidine (Tagamet)
Cyclosporine (Neoral, Sandimmune)
Digoxin (Lanoxin)
Diltiazem (Cardizem)
Disulfiram (Antabuse)
Ergotamine
Fluoxetine (Prozac)
Fluvoxamine (Luvox)
Grapefruit juice
Isoniazid (Rifamate)
Major tranquilizers such as Mellaril and Thorazine
Nefazodone (Serzone)
Nicardipine (Cardene)
Nifedipine (Adalat, Procardia)
Oral contraceptives
Other central nervous system depressants such as Valium and Demerol
Paroxetine (Paxil)
Propoxyphene (Darvon)
Sertraline (Zoloft)

Special information
if you are pregnant or breastfeeding

Do not take this medication if you are pregnant or planning to become pregnant. There is an increased risk of respiratory problems and muscular weakness in your baby. Infants may also experience withdrawal symptoms. Xanax may appear in breast milk and could affect a nursing infant. If this medication is essential to your health, your doctor may advise you to stop breastfeeding until your treatment with this medication is finished.

Recommended dosage

ADULTS

Anxiety disorder
The usual starting dose of Xanax is 0.25 to 0.5 milligram taken 3 times a day. The dose may be increased every 3 to 4 days to a maximum daily dose of 4 milligrams, divided into smaller doses.

Panic disorder
You may be given a dose from 1 up to a total of 10 milligrams, according to your needs. The typical dose is 5 to 6 milligrams a day.

The usual starting dose is 0.5 milligram 3 times a day. This dose can be increased by 1 milligram a day every 3 or 4 days.

Your doctor will reassess your treatment periodically to be sure you're getting the right amount of medication.

CHILDREN

Safety and effectiveness have not been established in children under 18 years of age.

OLDER ADULTS

The usual starting dose for an anxiety disorder is 0.25 milligram, 2 or 3 times daily. This dose may be gradually increased if needed and tolerated.

Overdosage
Any medication taken in excess can have serious consequences. If you suspect an overdose, seek medical attention immediately.

■ *Symptoms of Xanax overdose may include:*
Coma, confusion, impaired coordination, sleepiness, slowed reaction time

An overdose of Xanax, alone or after combining it with alcohol, can be fatal.

Brand name:

YOCON

Pronounced: YOE-kon
Generic name: Yohimbine hydrochloride
Other brand name: Yohimex

Why is this drug prescribed?

Yocon is used in the treatment of male impotence. The drug is thought to work by stimulating the release of norepinephrine, one of the body's natural chemical regulators. This results in increased blood flow to the penis.

Most important fact about this drug

Yocon does not work for all men. Your doctor will determine if Yocon can be prescribed for you.

How should you take this medication?

Take this medication exactly as prescribed.

■ *If you miss a dose...*

Take it as soon as you remember. If it is almost time for your next dose, skip the one you missed and go back to your regular schedule. Never take 2 doses at the same time.

■ *Storage instructions...*

Keep this medication in the container it came in, tightly closed, and out of the reach of children. Store it at room temperature, away from moist places and direct light.

What side effects may occur?

Side effects cannot be anticipated. If any develop or change in intensity, inform your doctor as soon as possible. Only your doctor can determine if it is safe for you to continue taking Yocon.

■ *Side effects may include:*

Decreased urination, dizziness, flushing, headache, increase in blood pressure, increased heart rate, increased motor activity, irritability, nausea, nervousness, tremor

Why should this drug not be prescribed?

Yocon should not be used if you have kidney disease, or if you are sensitive to or have ever had an allergic reaction to yohimbine. Make sure your doctor is aware of any drug reactions you have experienced.

Special warnings about this medication

Yocon is generally not recommended for use by children, the elderly, or men with heart and kidney disease who also have a history of stomach or duodenal ulcer. The drug is also not recommended for men being treated for a psychiatric disorder.

Possible food and drug interactions
when taking this medication
It is important that you consult with your doctor before taking Yocon with drugs for depression such as Elavil or other drugs that change mood.

Special information
if you are pregnant or breastfeeding
Yocon is not recommended for use in women generally and certainly must not be used during pregnancy.

Recommended dosage

ADULTS

Dosages of this drug are based on experimental research in the treatment of male impotence.

This dosage is one 5.4-milligram tablet, 3 times a day.

If you experience nausea, dizziness, or nervousness, your doctor will reduce the dose to one-half tablet 3 times a day, and then increase it gradually back up to 1 tablet 3 times a day.

CHILDREN

This drug is not for use in children.

OLDER ADULTS

This drug should not be used by older men.

Overdosage
Any medication taken in excess can cause symptoms of overdose. If you suspect an overdose, seek medical attention immediately. No specific symptoms of Yocon overdose have been reported.

Generic name:

YOHIMBINE

See Yocon, page 1440.

Brand name:

YOHIMEX

See Yocon, page 1440.

Generic name:

ZAFIRLUKAST

See Accolate, page 1.

Generic name:

ZALCITABINE

See Hivid, page 593.

Brand name:

ZANTAC

Pronounced: ZAN-tac
Generic name: Ranitidine hydrochloride

Why is this drug prescribed?
Zantac is prescribed for the short-term treatment (4 to 8 weeks) of active duodenal ulcer and active benign gastric ulcer, and as maintenance therapy for gastric or duodenal ulcer, at a reduced dosage, after the ulcer has healed. It is also used for the treatment of conditions in which the stomach produces too much acid, such as Zollinger-Ellison syndrome and systemic mastocytosis, for gastroesophageal reflux disease (backflow of acid stomach contents) and for healing—and maintaining healing of—erosive esophagitis (severe inflammation of the esophagus).

Some doctors prescribe Zantac to prevent damage to the stomach and duodenum from long-term use of nonsteroidal anti-inflammatory drugs such as Indocin and Motrin, and to treat bleeding of the stomach and intestine. Zantac is also sometimes prescribed for stress-induced ulcers.

Most important fact about this drug
Zantac helps to prevent the recurrence of gastric or duodenal ulcers and aids the healing of ulcers that do occur.

How should you take this medication?
Take this medication exactly as prescribed by your doctor. Make sure you follow the diet your doctor recommends.

Dissolve "Efferdose" tablets and granules in 6 to 8 ounces of water before taking them.

You can take an antacid for pain while you are taking Zantac.

- *If you miss a dose...*
  Take it as soon as you remember. If it is almost time for your next dose, skip the one you missed and go back to your regular schedule. Never take 2 doses at the same time.

- *Storage instructions...*
  Store this medication at room temperature in the container it came in, tightly closed and away from moist places and direct light. Keep Zantac Syrup from freezing.

What side effects may occur?
Side effects cannot be anticipated. If any develop or change in intensity, inform your doctor as soon as possible. Only your doctor can determine if it is safe for you to continue taking Zantac.

- *More common side effects may include:*
  Headache, sometimes severe

- *Less common or rare side effects may include:*
  Abdominal discomfort and pain, agitation, changes in blood count (anemia), changes in liver function, constipation, depression, diarrhea, difficulty sleeping, dizziness, hair loss, hallucinations, heart block, hepatitis, hypersensitivity reactions, inflammation of the pancreas, involuntary movements, irregular heartbeat, jaundice (yellowing of eyes and skin), joint pain, muscle pain, nausea and vomiting, rapid heartbeat, rash, reduced white blood cells, reversible mental confusion, sleepiness, slow heartbeat, vague feeling of bodily discomfort, vertigo, yellow eyes and skin

Why should this drug not be prescribed?
If you are sensitive to or have ever had an allergic reaction to Zantac or similar drugs such as Tagamet, you should not take this medication. Make sure that your doctor is aware of any drug reactions that you have experienced.

Special warnings about this medication
A stomach malignancy could be present, even if your symptoms have been relieved by Zantac.

If you have kidney or liver disease, this drug should be used with caution.

If you have phenylketonuria, you should be aware that the "Efferdose" tablets and granules contain phenylalanine.

Possible food and drug interactions
when taking this medication

If Zantac is taken with certain other drugs, the effects of either could be increased, decreased, or altered. It is especially important to check with your doctor before combining Zantac with the following:

Alcohol
Blood-thinning drugs such as Coumadin
Diazepam (Valium)
Diltiazem (Cardizem)
Enoxacin (Penetrex)
Glipizide (Glucotrol)
Glyburide (DiaBeta, Micronase)
Itraconazole (Sporanox)
Ketoconazole (Nizoral)
Metformin (Glucophage)
Nifedipine (Procardia)
Phenytoin (Dilantin)
Procainamide (Procan SR)
Sucralfate (Carafate)
Theophylline (Theo-Dur)
Triazolam (Halcion)

Special information
if you are pregnant or breastfeeding

The effects of Zantac in pregnancy have not been adequately studied. If you are pregnant or plan to become pregnant, inform your doctor immediately. Zantac appears in breast milk and could affect a nursing infant. If this medication is essential to your health, your doctor may advise you to discontinue breastfeeding until your treatment with this medication is finished.

Recommended dosage

ADULTS

Active Duodenal Ulcer

The usual starting dose is 150 milligrams 2 times a day or 10 milliliters (2 teaspoonfuls) 2 times a day. Your doctor also might prescribe 300 milligrams or 20 milliliters (4 teaspoonfuls) once a day, after the evening meal or at bedtime, if necessary for your convenience. The dose should be the lowest effective dose. Long-term use should be reduced to a daily total of 150 milligrams or 10 milliliters (2 teaspoonfuls), taken at bedtime.

Other Excess Acid Conditions (such as Zollinger-Ellison Syndrome)
The usual dose is 150 milligrams or 10 milliliters (2 teaspoonfuls) 2 times a day. This dose can be adjusted upwards by your doctor.

Benign Gastric Ulcer and Gastroesophageal Reflux Disease (GERD)
The usual dose is 150 milligrams or 10 milliliters (2 teaspoonfuls) 2 times a day. Once an ulcer has cleared up, a single bedtime dose is prescribed to maintain healing. Symptoms of GERD generally improve within 24 hours after the start of therapy.

Erosive Esophagitis
The usual dose is 150 milligrams or 10 milliliters (2 teaspoonfuls) 4 times a day. Maintenance dosage is 150 milligrams or 10 milliliters (2 teaspoonfuls) twice a day.

CHILDREN

The safety and effectiveness of Zantac have not been established in children.

Overdosage

Any medication taken in excess can have serious consequences. If you suspect an overdose, seek medical attention immediately.

Information concerning Zantac overdosage is limited. However, an abnormal manner of walking, low blood pressure, and exaggerated side effect symptoms may be signs of an overdose.

If you experience any of these symptoms, notify your doctor immediately.

Brand name:

ZAROXOLYN

Pronounced: Zar-OX-uh-lin
Generic name: Metolazone
Other brand name: Mykrox

Why is this drug prescribed?

Zaroxolyn is a diuretic used in the treatment of high blood pressure and other conditions that require the elimination of excess fluid from the body. These conditions include congestive heart failure and kidney disease. When used for high blood pressure, Zaroxolyn can be used alone or with other high blood pressure medications. Diuretics prompt your body to produce and eliminate more urine, which helps lower blood pressure.

Zaroxolyn is also occasionally prescribed for kidney stones.

Most important fact about this drug
If you have high blood pressure, you must take Zaroxolyn regularly for it to be effective. Since blood pressure declines gradually, it may be several weeks before you get the full benefit of Zaroxolyn; and you must continue taking it even if you are feeling well. Zaroxolyn does not cure high blood pressure; it merely keeps it under control.

How should you take this medication?
Take Zaroxolyn exactly as prescribed. Stopping Zaroxolyn suddenly could cause your condition to worsen.

■ *If you miss a dose...*
Take it as soon as you remember. If it is almost time for the next dose, skip the one you missed and go back to your regular schedule. Do not take 2 doses at the same time.

■ *Storage instructions...*
Store at room temperature in a tightly closed, light-resistant container.

What side effects may occur?
Side effects cannot be anticipated. If any develop or change in intensity, inform your doctor as soon as possible. Only your doctor can determine if it is safe for you to continue taking Zaroxolyn.

■ *Side effects may include:*
Anemia, bloating of the abdomen, blood clots, blurred vision, chest pain, chills, constipation, depression, diarrhea, dizziness on standing up, dizziness or light-headedness, drowsiness, fainting, fatigue, gout, head-ache, hepatitis, high blood sugar, hives, impotence, inflammation of the pancreas, inflammation of the skin, joint pain, loss of appetite, low potassium levels (leading to dry mouth, excessive thirst, weak or irregular heartbeat, or muscle pain or cramps), muscle spasms or cramps, nausea, rapid, pounding heartbeat, rash, reddish or purplish spots on the skin, restlessness, sensitivity to light, sugar in the urine, tingling or pins and needles, upset stomach, vertigo, vomiting, weakness, yellow eyes and skin

Why should this drug not be prescribed?
If you are unable to urinate or have severe liver disease, you should not take this medication.

If you are sensitive to or have ever had an allergic reaction to Zaroxolyn or other diuretics such as HydroDIURIL, you should not take this medication.

Special warnings about this medication
Diuretics can cause your body to lose too much potassium. Signs of an excessively low potassium level include muscle weakness and rapid or irregular heartbeat. To boost your potassium level, your doctor may recommend eating potassium-rich foods or taking a potassium supplement.

If you are taking Zaroxolyn, your doctor will do a complete assessment of your kidney function and continue to monitor it.

Do not interchange Zaroxolyn and other formulations of metolazone such as Mykrox. The brands vary in potency of action.

If you have liver disease, diabetes, gout, or lupus erythematosus (a disease of the immune system), Zaroxolyn should be used with caution.

If you have had an allergic reaction to sulfa drugs, thiazides, or quinethazone, you may be at greater risk for an allergic reaction to this medication. You can have an allergic reaction to Zaroxolyn even if you have never had allergies or asthma.

Dehydration, excessive sweating, severe diarrhea, or vomiting could deplete your fluids and cause your blood pressure to become too low. Be careful when exercising and in hot weather.

Notify your doctor or dentist that you are taking Zaroxolyn if you have a medical emergency and before you have surgery or dental treatment.

Possible food and drug interactions
when taking this medication
Zaroxolyn may intensify the effects of alcohol. Avoid drinking alcohol while taking this medication.

If Zaroxolyn is taken with certain other drugs, the effects of either could be increased, decreased, or altered. It is especially important to check with your doctor before combining Zaroxolyn with the following:

ACTH
Antidiabetic drugs such as Micronase
Barbiturates such as phenobarbital
Corticosteroids such as prednisone (Deltasone)

Digitalis glycosides such as Lanoxin
Insulin
Lithium (Lithonate)
Loop diuretics such as furosemide (Lasix)
Methenamine (Mandelamine)
Narcotics such as Percocet
Nonsteroidal anti-inflammatory agents such as Advil, Motrin, and
    Naprosyn
Norepinephrine (Levophed)
Other high blood pressure medications such as Aldomet
Tubocurarine

Special information
if you are pregnant or breastfeeding

The effects of Zaroxolyn during pregnancy have not been adequately studied.
If you are pregnant or plan to become pregnant, inform your doctor
immediately. Zaroxolyn appears in breast milk and could affect a nursing
infant. If this medication is essential to your health, your doctor may advise
you to discontinue breastfeeding until your treatment is finished.

Recommended dosage

ADULTS

Your doctor will adjust the dosage of this medication to your individual needs
and will use the lowest possible dose with the maximum effect. The time it
takes for this medication to become effective varies from person to person,
depending on the diagnosis.

Most starting doses of this medication will be given once a day.

Edema Due to Heart or Kidney Disorders
The usual dosage is 5 milligrams to 20 milligrams once a day.

Mild to Moderate High Blood Pressure
The usual dosage is 2.5 milligrams to 5 milligrams once a day.

CHILDREN

The safety and effectiveness of Zaroxolyn in children have not been
established.

Overdosage

Any medication taken in excess can have serious consequences. If you
suspect an overdose, seek medical attention immediately.

■ *Symptoms of Zaroxolyn overdose may include:*
Difficulty breathing, dizziness, dizziness on standing up, drowsiness, fainting, irritation of the stomach and intestines, lethargy leading to coma

Brand name:

ZERIT

Pronounced: ZAIR-it
Generic name: Stavudine

Why is this drug prescribed?
Zerit is one of the drugs used to fight the human immunodeficiency virus (HIV)—the deadly cause of AIDS. It is usually prescribed for people who have already been taking the HIV drug Retrovir for an extended period. HIV attacks the immune system, slowly destroying the body's ability to fight off infection. Zerit helps stave off the attack by disrupting the virus's ability to reproduce.

Signs and symptoms of HIV infection include diarrhea, fever, headache, infections, problems with the nervous system, rash, sore throat, and significant weight loss.

Most important fact about this drug
Although Zerit can slow the progress of HIV infection, it is not a cure. Because of the continuing danger of complications and infections, you should get frequent physical exams and blood counts. Be sure, too, to notify your doctor immediately if you experience any changes in your general health.

How should you take this medication?
Take Zerit every 12 hours, exactly as prescribed. It's important to keep a constant level of the drug in the body, so be sure to take each dose on schedule. Do not take more than the prescribed amount; nerve disorders could result.

Shake the oral solution vigorously before measuring the dose.

You can take Zerit with or without food.

■ *If you miss a dose...*
Take it as soon as you remember. If it is almost time for your next dose, skip the one you missed and go back to your regular schedule. Do not take 2 doses at once.

■ *Storage instructions...*
Keep the Zerit container tightly closed. Store the capsules at room temperature. Store Zerit oral solution in the refrigerator; throw out any unused medication after 30 days.

What side effects may occur?
The higher your dosage, the greater your chance of side effects. However, it's often hard to tell a side effect from a symptom of the disease. If you think the drug is causing problems, keep taking it until you've checked with your doctor. Only your doctor can determine whether the drug is at fault, and adjust your dosage accordingly.

■ *Side effects may include:*
Abdominal pain, allergic reaction, chills, diarrhea, fever, headache, loss of appetite, muscle pain, nausea and vomiting, nervous system abnormalities, pain or numbness and tingling in the hands and feet, rash, sleeplessness

Why should this drug not be prescribed?
If Zerit gives you an allergic reaction, you should not take the drug.

Special warnings about this medication
Remember that Zerit does not prevent the spread of HIV through sexual contact or contact with infected blood.

If you have ever had kidney or liver problems, or if you tend to abuse alcohol, make sure the doctor is aware of it. Your dosage may need adjustment.

One of the more common and dangerous side effects of Zerit is a problem called peripheral neuropathy, a serious condition in which certain nerves are damaged. If you notice numbness, tingling, or pain in your hands or feet, notify your physician immediately.

The benefit you get from Zerit may not last long. If your symptoms begin to get worse, tell your doctor immediately.

Possible food and drug interactions
when taking this medication
Combining Zerit with any of the following drugs may make peripheral neuropathy worse.

Chloramphenicol (Chloromycetin)
Cisplatin (Platinol)

Dapsone
Didanosine (Videx)
Ethambutol (Myambutol)
Hydralazine (Apresoline)
Lithium (Lithonate)
Metronidazole (Flagyl)
Nitrofurantoin (Macrodantin)
Phenytoin (Dilantin)
Vincristine (Oncovin)
Zalcitabine (Hivid)

Special information
if you are pregnant or breastfeeding

The use of Zerit during pregnancy has not been adequately studied. If you are pregnant or plan to become pregnant, inform your doctor immediately. Do not breastfeed; HIV can be passed to a newborn infant through breast milk.

Recommended dosage

ADULTS

For adults weighing 132 pounds or more, the usual dose is 40 milligrams every 12 hours. For those under 132 pounds, the dose is 30 milligrams every 12 hours.

CHILDREN

The usual starting dose for children weighing less than 66 pounds is 1 milligram per 2.2 pounds of body weight every 12 hours. Children weighing 66 pounds or more should take the adult dose.

Overdosage

Numbness, pain, and tingling of the hands and feet can be signs of an overdose. If you suspect an overdose, seek medical attention immediately.

Brand name:

ZESTORETIC

Pronounced: zest-or-ET-ik
Generic ingredients: Lisinopril, Hydrochlorothiazide
Other brand name: Prinzide

Why is this drug prescribed?

Zestoretic is used in the treatment of high blood pressure. It combines an ACE inhibitor drug with a diuretic. Lisinopril, the ACE inhibitor, works by limiting production of a substance that promotes salt and water retention in your body. Hydrochlorothiazide, a diuretic, prompts your body to produce and eliminate more urine, which helps in lowering blood pressure. Combination products such as Zestoretic are usually not prescribed until therapy is already under way.

Most important fact about this drug
You must take Zestoretic regularly for it to be effective. Since blood pressure declines gradually, it may be several weeks before you get the full benefit of Zestoretic; and you must continue taking it even if you are feeling well. Zestoretic does not cure high blood pressure; it merely keeps it under control.

How should you take this medication?
Zestoretic can be taken with or without food once a day. Take it exactly as prescribed.

■ *If you miss a dose...*
   Take the forgotten dose as soon as you remember. If it is almost time for your next dose, skip the one you missed and go back to your regular schedule. Never take a double dose.

■ *Storage instructions...*
   Zestoretic should be stored at room temperature. Keep the container tightly closed.

What side effects may occur?
Side effects cannot be anticipated. If any develop or change in intensity, inform your doctor as soon as possible. Only your doctor can determine if it is safe for you to continue taking Zestoretic.

■ *More common side effects may include:*
   Cough, dizziness, dizziness when standing up, fatigue, headache

■ *Less common side effects may include:*
   Asthma, diarrhea, hair loss, impotence, indigestion, low blood pressure, muscle cramps, nausea, rash, tingling or pins and needles, upper respiratory infection, vomiting, weakness

■ *Rare side effects may include:*
   Abdominal pain, anemia, arthritis, back pain, back strain, blurred vision, bronchitis, bruising, chest discomfort or pain, common cold, confusion, constipation, decreased sex drive, depression, difficulty breathing, difficul-

ty falling or staying asleep, dry mouth, earache, excessive perspiration, fainting, fever, flu, flushing, foot pain, gas, general feeling of illness, gout, hay fever, heart attack, heartburn, heart rhythm disturbances, hepatitis, hives, itching, joint pain, knee pain, loss of appetite, lung congestion, muscle pain, muscle spasm, nervousness, palpitations, rapid heartbeat, red or purple areas on the skin, reduced urine output, restlessness, ringing in ears, sensitivity to light, shortness of breath, severe allergic reaction, shoulder pain, sinus inflammation, skin inflammation, sleepiness, sore throat, stomach and intestinal cramps, stroke, stuffy nose, swelling of the face, lips, tongue, throat, or arms and legs, trauma, urinary tract infection, vertigo, virus infection, vision abnormality in which objects have a yellowish hue, yellow eyes and skin

Why should this drug not be prescribed?

If you are sensitive to or have ever had an allergic reaction to lisinopril or hydrochlorothiazide or if you are sensitive to other ACE inhibitor drugs such as Capoten or sulfa drugs such as Gantrisin, you should not take this medication. If you suffered angioedema (swelling of face, lips, tongue, throat, arms, or legs) during previous treatment with an ACE inhibitor, you should not take this medication; if you have ever developed angioedema for any reason, you run a higher risk of developing it while you are taking this kind of drug. You should also avoid Zestoretic if you are unable to urinate. Tell your doctor of all allergic reactions you have experienced.

Special warnings about this medication

If you develop swelling of your face, lips, tongue, or throat, or of your arms and legs, or have difficulty swallowing or breathing, you should stop taking the drug and contact your doctor immediately. You may need emergency treatment.

Zestoretic may cause your blood pressure to become too low. If you feel light-headed, especially during the first few days of treatment, inform your doctor. If you actually faint, stop taking Zestoretic until you have consulted your doctor.

Do not use salt substitutes containing potassium without first consulting your doctor.

Excessive sweating, dehydration, severe diarrhea, or vomiting could cause you to lose too much water and cause your blood pressure to drop dangerously.

If you develop chest pain, a sore throat, or fever and chills, contact your doctor immediately. It could indicate a more serious illness.

Make sure the doctor knows if you have congestive heart failure, diabetes, liver disease, a history of allergy or bronchial asthma, or lupus erythematosus (an arthritis-like disease sometimes accompanied by rashes). Zestoretic should be used cautiously. If you have kidney disease, your doctor should monitor your kidney function regularly.

If you are undergoing desensitization to bee or wasp venom, Zestoretic may cause a severe allergic reaction.

This medication is not recommended for people on dialysis; severe allergic reactions have occurred.

If you notice a yellowish cast to your skin or eyes, stop taking Zestoretic and contact your doctor immediately.

If you are diabetic, your doctor will want to keep an eye on your blood sugar levels.

Before any surgery, make sure your doctor or dentist knows you are taking Zestoretic.

Possible food and drug interactions
when taking this medication
Zestoretic may intensify the effects of alcohol. Do not drink alcohol while taking this medication.

If Zestoretic is taken with certain other drugs, the effects of either could be increased, decreased, or altered. It is especially important to check with your doctor before combining Zestoretic with the following:

Barbiturates such as Nembutal and Seconal
Cholestyramine (Questran)
Colestipol (Colestid)
Corticosteroids such as prednisone
High blood pressure drugs such as Procardia XL and Aldomet
Indomethacin (Indocin)
Insulin
Lithium (Lithonate)
Narcotics such as Darvon and Dilaudid
Nonsteroidal anti-inflammatory drugs such as Naprosyn
Oral antidiabetic drugs such as Micronase
Potassium supplements such as K-Dur and Slow-K
Potassium-containing salt substitutes
Potassium-sparing diuretics such as Midamor

Special information
if you are pregnant or breastfeeding

During the second and third trimesters, lisinopril can cause birth defects, prematurity, and death in the fetus and newborn. If you are pregnant or plan to become pregnant, contact your doctor immediately to discuss the potential hazard to your unborn child. Zestoretic may appear in breast milk and could affect a nursing infant. If this medication is essential to your health, your doctor may advise you to discontinue breastfeeding until your treatment with this medication is finished.

Recommended dosage

ADULTS

Zestoretic is designed to replace higher doses of either component. Dosages of the lisinopril component range from 10 to 80 milligrams a day; dosages of hydrochlorothiazide typically fall between 6.25 and 50 milligrams daily. If either component, when prescribed alone, fails to control your blood pressure, your doctor may try the Zestoretic combination, starting with either 10 or 20 milligrams of lisinopril and 12.5 milligrams of hydrochlorothiazide, and gradually increasing the dosage as needed.

If you are age 65 or older, or have kidney problems, your doctor will adjust your dosage with caution. This drug is not prescribed for people with severe kidney damage.

CHILDREN

Safety and effectiveness in children have not been established.

Overdosage

Any medication taken in excess can have serious consequences. If you suspect an overdose, seek medical treatment immediately.

- *Symptoms of Zestoretic overdose may include:*
  Dehydration, low blood pressure

Brand name:

ZESTRIL

Pronounced: ZEST-rill
Generic name: Lisinopril
Other brand name: Prinivil

Why is this drug prescribed?

Lisinopril is used in the treatment of high blood pressure. It is effective when used alone or when combined with other high blood pressure medications. It may also be used with other medications in the treatment of heart failure, and may be given within 24 hours of a heart attack to improve chances of survival.

Lisinopril is a type of drug called an ACE inhibitor. It works by reducing production of a substance that increases salt and water retention in your body.

Most important fact about this drug

If you have high blood pressure, you must take lisinopril regularly for it to be effective. Since blood pressure declines gradually, it may be several weeks before you get the full benefit of lisinopril; and you must continue taking it even if you are feeling well. Lisinopril does not cure high blood pressure; it merely keeps it under control.

How should you take this medication?

Lisinopril can be taken with or without food. Take it exactly as prescribed. Stopping lisinopril suddenly could cause your blood pressure to rise.

- *If you miss a dose...*
  Take the forgotten dose as soon as you remember. If it is almost time for your next dose, skip the one you missed and go back to your regular schedule. Never take 2 doses at the same time.

- *Storage instructions...*
  Store at room temperature, with the container sealed and dry. Avoid excessive heat or freezing cold.

What side effects may occur?

Side effects cannot be anticipated. If any develop or change in intensity, inform your doctor as soon as possible. Only your doctor can determine if it is safe for you to continue taking lisinopril.

- *More common side effects may include:*
  Chest pain, cough, diarrhea, dizziness, headache, low blood pressure

- *Less common or rare side effects may include:*
  Abdominal pain, anemia, arm pain, arthritis, asthma, back pain, blood clot in lungs, blurred vision, breast pain, bronchitis, changes in sense of taste, chills, common cold, confusion, constipation, coughing up blood, cramps in stomach/intestines, decreased sex drive, dehydration, diabetes, dizziness on standing, double vision, dry mouth, fainting, fatigue, feeling of illness, fever, flu, fluid retention, flushing, gas, gout, hair loss, heart attack, heartburn, hepatitis, hip pain, hives, impotence, inability to sleep or sleeping too much, incoordination, indigestion, inflamed stomach, intolerance to light, irregular heartbeat, irritability, joint pain, kidney trouble or failure, knee pain, laryngitis, leg pain, little or no urine, lung cancer, memory impairment, muscle pain or cramps, nasal congestion or inflammation, nausea, neck pain, nervousness, nosebleed, numbness or tingling, painful breathing, painful urination, pelvic pain, pneumonia, prickling or burning sensation, rapid or fluttery heartbeat, rash, reddening of skin, respiratory infection, ringing in ears, runny nose, sensitivity to light, skin infections or eruptions, shoulder pain, sinus inflammation, sleepiness, sore throat, spasm, stroke, sweating, swelling of face or arms and legs, thigh pain, tremor, urinary tract infection, vertigo, virus infection, vision changes, vomiting, weakness, weight loss or gain, wheezing, yellow eyes and skin

Why should this drug not be prescribed?
If you are sensitive to or have ever had an allergic reaction to lisinopril or other ACE inhibitors, you should not take this medication. Make sure your doctor is aware of any drug reactions you have experienced.

Special warnings about this medication
If you develop swelling of your face, lips, tongue, or throat, or of your arms and legs, or have difficulty swallowing or breathing, you should contact your doctor immediately. You may need emergency treatment.

If you are being given bee or wasp venom to guard against future reactions, you may have a severe reaction to lisinopril.

If you have a kidney disorder or connective tissue disease such as lupus, your doctor may perform periodic blood tests while you are taking this medication.

If you are taking lisinopril, a complete assessment of your kidney function should be done and kidney function should continue to be monitored. Lisinopril is used with great caution after a heart attack if the patient also has kidney problems.

This drug also should be used with caution if you are on dialysis. There have been reports of extreme allergic reactions during dialysis in people taking ACE inhibitor medications such as lisinopril.

If you are taking high doses of a diuretic (water pill) and lisinopril, you may develop excessively low blood pressure.

Lisinopril may cause some people to become dizzy, light-headed, or faint, especially if they are taking a water pill at the same time. Do not drive, operate dangerous machinery, or participate in any hazardous activity that requires full mental alertness until you are certain lisinopril does not have this effect on you.

If you develop chest pain, sore throat, fever, and chills, contact your doctor for medical attention.

If your skin and the whites of your eyes turn yellow, stop taking the medication and contact your doctor.

Avoid salt substitutes that contain potassium. Limit your consumption of potassium-rich foods such as bananas, prunes, raisins, orange juice, and whole and skim milk. Ask your doctor for advice on how much of these foods to consume.

Excessive sweating, dehydration, severe diarrhea, or vomiting could cause you to lose too much water and cause your blood pressure to drop dangerously.

Possible food and drug interactions
when taking this medication
If lisinopril is taken with certain other drugs, the effects of either could be increased, decreased, or altered. It is especially important to check with your doctor before combining lisinopril with any of the following:

Indomethacin (Indocin)
Lithium (Lithonate, Eskalith)
Potassium preparations such as K-Phos and Micro-K
Water pills such as HydroDIURIL and Lasix, and others that leave
    potassium in the body, such as Aldactone and Midamor

Special information
if you are pregnant or breastfeeding

If it is taken during the final 6 months of pregnancy, lisinopril can cause birth defects, prematurity, and death in the fetus and newborn. If you are pregnant or plan to become pregnant and are taking lisinopril, contact your doctor immediately to discuss the potential hazard to your unborn child. Lisinopril may appear in breast milk and could affect a nursing infant. If this medication is essential to your health, your doctor may advise you to discontinue breastfeeding until your treatment with this medication is finished.

Recommended dosage

ADULTS

High Blood Pressure

For people not on water pills (diuretics), the initial starting dose is usually 10 milligrams, taken 1 time a day. After blood pressure is adjusted, dosage is usually 20 to 40 milligrams a day, taken in a single dose.

Diuretic use should, if possible, be stopped before using lisinopril. If not, your physician may give an initial dose of 5 milligrams under supervision before any further medication is prescribed.

People with kidney disorders must be carefully monitored, and dosages will be adjusted to the individual's needs, depending on kidney function.

Heart Failure

The recommended dose is 5 milligrams, once a day, along with diuretics and digitalis. This starting dose should be taken under your doctor's supervision. The usual dosage range is 5 to 20 milligrams taken once a day.

Heart Attack

The usual dose is 5 milligrams within the first 24 hours after a heart attack, then 5 milligrams 24 hours later, 10 milligrams 48 hours later, and, finally, 10 milligrams once a day for 6 weeks. If low blood pressure is a problem, the doctor may recommend a lower dosage.

CHILDREN

The safety and effectiveness of lisinopril in children have not been established.

OLDER ADULTS

The physician will adjust the dosage carefully, according to the individual's needs.

Overdosage

Any medication taken in excess can cause symptoms of overdose. If you suspect an overdose, seek medical attention immediately.

A severe drop in blood pressure is the primary sign of a lisinopril overdose.

Generic name:

ZIDOVUDINE

See Retrovir, page 1118.

Generic name:

ZILEUTON

See Zyflo, page 1485.

Brand name:

ZITHROMAX

Pronounced: ZITH-roh-macks
Generic name: Azithromycin

Why is this drug prescribed?

Zithromax is an antibiotic related to erythromycin. It is prescribed for adults to treat certain mild to moderate skin infections; upper and lower respiratory tract infections, including pharyngitis (strep throat), tonsillitis, and pneumonia; sexually transmitted infections of the cervix or urinary tract; and genital ulcer disease in men. In children, Zithromax is used to treat middle ear infection, pneumonia, tonsillitis, and strep throat.

Most important fact about this drug

There is a possibility of rare but very serious reactions to Zithromax, including angioedema (swelling of the face, lips, and neck that impedes speaking, swallowing, and breathing), anaphylaxis (a violent, even fatal allergic reaction), and serious skin diseases. If you develop these symptoms, stop taking Zithromax and call your doctor immediately.

How should you take this medication?

Take Zithromax capsules or oral suspension at least 1 hour before or 2 hours after a meal. Zithromax tablets can be taken with or without food. Do not take any form with an antacid that contains aluminum or magnesium, such as Di-Gel, Gelusil, Maalox, and others.

If you are using single-dose packets of Zithromax powder for oral suspension, mix the entire contents of each packet with 2 ounces of water, drink immediately, then add an additional 2 ounces of water, mix again, and drink to make sure you've taken the entire dose. When giving the pediatric suspension, shake the bottle thoroughly before each use and measure the dose with the supplied calibrated dropper. Use the pediatric suspension within 10 days and throw out any that remains.

Be sure to take all the drug prescribed. If you stop taking Zithromax too soon, some germs may survive and the illness may return.

■ *If you miss a dose...*
Take the forgotten dose as soon as you remember. If you don't remember until the next day, skip the dose and go back to your regular schedule. Never try to "catch up" by doubling the dose.

■ *Storage instructions...*
Zithromax should be stored at room temperature.

What side effects may occur?

Side effects cannot be anticipated. If any develop or change in intensity, inform your doctor as soon as possible. Only your doctor can determine if it is safe for you to continue taking Zithromax.

■ *More common side effects may include:*
Abdominal pain, diarrhea or loose stools, nausea or vomiting

■ *Less common side effects may include:*
Blood in the stools, chest pain, dizziness, drowsiness, fatigue, gas, headache, heart palpitations, indigestion, jaundice (yellowing of the skin and the whites of the eyes), kidney infection, light sensitivity, rash, severe allergic reaction including swelling (as in hives), vaginal inflammation, vertigo, yeast infection

■ *Other uncommon side effects sometimes seen in children include:*
Agitation, constipation, feeling of illness, fever, insomnia, loss of appetite, nervousness, overactivity, pinkeye, stomach inflammation

The single large dose of Zithromax that is prescribed to treat sexually transmitted infection of the cervix or urinary tract is more likely to cause stomach and bowel side effects than the smaller doses prescribed for a skin or respiratory tract infection.

Why should this drug not be prescribed?
Do not take Zithromax if you have ever had an allergic reaction to it or to similar antibiotics such as erythromycin (E.E.S., PCE, and others).

Special warnings about this medication
Like certain other antibiotics, Zithromax may cause a potentially life-threatening form of diarrhea called pseudomembranous colitis. Pseudomembranous colitis may clear up spontaneously when the drug is stopped; if it doesn't, hospital treatment may be required. If you develop diarrhea, check with your doctor immediately.

If you have a liver problem, your doctor should monitor you very carefully while you are taking Zithromax.

Possible food and drug interactions
when taking this medication
If Zithromax is taken with certain other drugs, the effects of either could be increased, decreased, or altered. It is especially important to check with your doctor before combining Zithromax with antacids containing aluminum or magnesium, such as Maalox and Mylanta.

The following interactions can occur with erythromycin, a similar drug.

Carbamazepine (Tegretol)
Certain antihistamines such as Hismanal and Seldane
Cyclosporine (Neoral and Sandimmune)
Digoxin (Lanoxin, Lanoxicaps)
Ergot-containing drugs such as Cafergot and D.H.E.
Hexobarbital
Lovastatin (Mevacor)
Phenytoin (Dilantin)
Theophylline drugs such as Bronkodyl, Slo-Phyllin, Theo-Dur, and others
Triazolam (Halcion)
Warfarin (Coumadin)

Special information
if you are pregnant or breastfeeding
If you are pregnant or plan to become pregnant, inform your doctor immediately. You should take Zithromax during pregnancy only if it is clearly

needed. It is not known whether Zithromax can make its way into breast milk. If the drug is essential to your health, your doctor may advise you to stop breastfeeding until your treatment is finished.

Recommended dosage

ADULTS

Respiratory Diseases, Tonsillitis, Strep Throat, and Skin Infections
The usual dose of Zithromax is 500 milligrams in a single dose the first day. This is followed by 250 milligrams once daily for the next 4 days.

Genital Ulcer Disease
The usual dose is a single gram (1,000 milligrams) one time only.

Sexually Transmitted Diseases
The usual dose is a single 2-gram (2,000 milligrams) dose.

CHILDREN

Middle Ear Infection and Pneumonia
For children aged 6 months and up, the usual dose is 10 milligrams of Zithromax suspension per 2.2 pounds of body weight in a single dose the first day, followed by 5 milligrams per 2.2 pounds for the next 4 days.

Strep Throat and Tonsillitis
For children aged 2 years and up, the usual dose is 12 milligrams per 2.2 pounds of body weight once daily for 5 days.

Overdosage
Although no specific information on Zithromax overdose is available, any medication taken in excess can have serious consequences. If you suspect an overdose, seek medical attention immediately.

Brand name:

ZOCOR

Pronounced: ZOH-core
Generic name: Simvastatin

Why is this drug prescribed?

Zocor is a cholesterol-lowering drug. Your doctor may prescribe Zocor in addition to a cholesterol-lowering diet if your blood cholesterol level is too high, and if you have been unable to lower it by diet alone.

In people with high cholesterol and heart disease, Zocor reduces the risk of heart attack, stroke and "mini-stroke" (transient ischemic attack) and can stave off the need for bypass surgery or angioplasty to clear clogged arteries.

Most important fact about this drug

Zocor is usually prescribed only if diet, exercise, and weight-loss fail to bring your cholesterol level under control. It's important to remember that Zocor is a supplement to—not a substitute for—those other measures. To get the full benefit of the medication, you need to stick to the diet and exercise program prescribed by your doctor. All these efforts to keep your cholesterol levels normal are important because together they may lower your risk of heart disease.

How should you take this medication?

Take Zocor exactly as prescribed.

■ *If you miss a dose...*
Take it as soon as you remember. If it is almost time for your next dose, skip the one you missed and go back to your regular schedule. Do not take 2 doses at once.

■ *Storage instructions...*
Store at room temperature.

What side effects may occur?

Side effects cannot be anticipated. If any develop or change in intensity, inform your doctor as soon as possible. Only your doctor can determine whether it is safe for you to continue taking Zocor.

■ *More common side effects may include:*
Abdominal pain, headache

■ *Less common side effects may include:*
Constipation, diarrhea, gas, nausea, upper respiratory infection, upset stomach, weakness

Why should this drug not be prescribed?

Do not take Zocor if you have ever had an allergic reaction to it or are sensitive to it.

Do not take Zocor if you have active liver disease.

Do not take Zocor if you are pregnant or plan to become pregnant.

Avoid combining Zocor with the heart medication Posicor.

Special warnings about this medication

Because Zocor may damage the liver, your doctor may order a blood test to check your liver enzyme levels before you start taking the drug. Blood tests will probably be done before your treatment is started and at periodic intervals for a year after your final dosage increase. If your liver enzyme levels rise too high, your doctor may tell you to stop taking Zocor.

Since Zocor may cause damage to muscle tissue, be sure to tell your doctor of any unexplained muscle tenderness, weakness, or pain right away, especially if you also have a fever or feel sick. Your doctor may want to do a blood test to check for signs of muscle damage.

If you are scheduled for major surgery, your doctor will have you stop taking Zocor a few days before the operation.

Possible food and drug interactions
when taking this medication

If you take Zocor with certain other drugs, the effects of either could be increased, decreased, or altered. It is especially important to check with your doctor before combining Zocor with any of the following:

Blood-thinning drugs such as Coumadin and Dicumarol
Cimetidine (Tagamet)
Clarithromycin (Biaxin)
Clofibrate (Atromid-S)
Cyclosporine (Sandimmune, Neoral)
Digoxin (Lanoxin, Lanoxicaps)
Erythromycin (PCE and others)
Gemfibrozil (Lopid)
Itraconazole (Sporanox)
Ketoconazole (Nizoral)
Mibefradil (Posicor)
Nefazodone (Serzone)
Nicotinic acid
Spironolactone (Aldactone, Aldactazide)

Special information
if you are pregnant or breastfeeding

You must not become pregnant while taking Zocor. This drug lowers cholesterol, and cholesterol is needed for a baby to develop properly. If you do become pregnant while taking Zocor, notify your doctor right away. Based on studies of other cholesterol-lowering drugs, it is assumed that Zocor could appear in breast milk and could cause severe adverse effects in a nursing baby. Do not take Zocor while breastfeeding your baby.

Recommended dosage
You will have to follow a standard cholesterol-lowering diet before starting treatment with Zocor and continue this diet while using Zocor.

All doses should be adjusted to your individual needs.

ADULTS

The usual starting dose is 5 to 10 milligrams per day, taken as a single dose in the evening. The maximum recommended dose is 40 milligrams per day. Dosage adjustments may be made every 4 weeks, and dose levels should be reduced as cholesterol levels come down.

People with high cholesterol and heart disease may start with 20 milligrams daily taken as a single dose in the evening.

Those who have severe kidney disease should use Zocor with caution. The recommended dose is 5 milligrams per day.

Zocor may be used with other drugs. Your doctor will determine the proper dose based on your individual needs.

OLDER ADULTS

Doses of 20 milligrams per day or less may be sufficient.

Overdosage
Although no specific information about Zocor overdose is available, any medication taken in excess can have serious consequences. If you suspect an overdose of Zocor, seek medical attention immediately.

Brand name:

ZOFRAN

Pronounced: ZOH-fran
Generic name: Ondansetron hydrochloride

Why is this drug prescribed?
Zofran is used for the prevention of nausea and vomiting caused by radiation therapy and chemotherapy for cancer, and, in some cases, to prevent these problems following surgery.

Most important fact about this drug
To ensure the maximum effect, it is important to take all doses of Zofran exactly as prescribed by your doctor.

How should you take this medication?
Your doctor will tell you how much drug to take and how often, depending on the type of therapy you will be having.

■ *If you miss a dose...*
Take the forgotten dose as soon as you remember.

■ *Storage instructions...*
Store Zofran at room temperature. Protect from light. Keep the drug in the carton it came in. Store oral solution bottles upright.

What side effects may occur?
Side effects cannot be anticipated. If any develop or change in intensity, inform your doctor as soon as possible. Only your doctor can determine if it is safe for you to continue taking Zofran.

■ *More common side effects may include:*
Abdominal pain, constipation, diarrhea, dizziness, fatigue, headache

■ *Less common or rare side effects may include:*
Anaphylaxis (severe allergic reaction), dry mouth, rash, weakness, wheezing

When Zofran is used to prevent nausea and vomiting after surgery, the following side effects may occur:
Anxiety, difficulty breathing, difficulty urinating, dizziness, drowsiness, female reproductive disorders, fever, headache, itching, low blood pressure, shivers, slow heartbeat

Why should this drug not be prescribed?
If you are sensitive to or have ever had an allergic reaction to ondansetron hydrochloride, you should not take this medication. Make sure that your doctor is aware of any drug reactions that you have experienced.

Special warnings about this medication
If drugs similar to Zofran (for instance, Kytril) have given you a reaction, Zofran may cause one too.

**Possible food and drug interactions
when taking this medication**
No interactions with Zofran have been reported.

**Special information
if you are pregnant or breastfeeding**
The effects of Zofran during pregnancy have not been adequately studied. If you are pregnant or plan to become pregnant, inform your doctor immediately. Zofran may appear in breast milk and could affect a nursing infant. If this medication is essential to your health, your doctor may advise you to discontinue breastfeeding until your treatment with this medication is finished.

Recommended dosage

PREVENTION OF NAUSEA AND VOMITING DUE TO CHEMOTHERAPY

Adults and Children 12 Years of Age and Older
The recommended dose of Zofran is one 8-milligram tablet or 2 teaspoonfuls of oral solution taken twice a day. The first dose should be taken 30 minutes before the start of treatment. The other dose should be taken 8 hours after the first dose. One 8-milligram tablet or 2 teaspoonfuls should be taken twice a day (every 12 hours) for 1 to 2 days after completing chemotherapy.

Children 4 through 11 Years of Age
The recommended dose of Zofran is one 4-milligram tablet or 1 teaspoonful of oral solution taken 3 times a day. The first dose should be taken 30 minutes before the start of chemotherapy. The other 2 doses should be taken 4 and 8 hours after the first dose. One 4-milligram tablet or 1 teaspoonful should be taken 3 times a day (every 8 hours) for 1 to 2 days after completing chemotherapy.

PREVENTION OF NAUSEA AND VOMITING DUE TO RADIATION THERAPY

Adults
The usual dosage is one 8-milligram tablet or 2 teaspoonfuls of oral solution taken 3 times a day. You will take the first dose 1 to 2 hours before therapy; the other intervals will depend on the type of radiation therapy you are receiving.

Children
Zofran has not been used for this purpose in children.

PREVENTION OF NAUSEA AND VOMITING AFTER SURGERY

Adults
The usual dose is two 8-milligram tablets or 4 teaspoonfuls of oral solution taken 1 hour before undergoing anesthesia.

Children
Zofran has not been used for this purpose in children.

Overdosage
There are no specific symptoms of Zofran overdose to report. However, any medication taken in excess can have serious consequences. If you suspect an overdose, seek medical attention immediately.

Generic name:

ZOLMITRIPTAN

See Zomig, page 1474.

Brand name:

ZOLOFT

Pronounced: ZOE-loft
Generic name: Sertraline

Why is this drug prescribed?
Zoloft is prescribed for major depression—a persistently low mood that interferes with everyday living. Symptoms may include loss of interest in your usual activities, disturbed sleep, change in appetite, constant fidgeting or lethargic movement, fatigue, feelings of worthlessness or guilt, difficulty thinking or concentrating, and recurrent thoughts of suicide.

Zoloft is also used in the treatment of obsessive-compulsive disorder—symptoms of which include unwanted thoughts that won't go away and an irresistible urge to keep repeating certain actions, such as hand-washing or counting—and for the treatment of panic disorder (unexpected attacks of overwhelming anxiety, accompanied by fear of their return).

Zoloft is thought to work by boosting the amount of serotonin in the brain. Serotonin is one of the brain's natural chemical messengers.

Most important fact about this drug
Do not take Zoloft within 2 weeks of taking any drug classified as an MAO inhibitor. Drugs in this category include the antidepressants Marplan, Nardil, and Parnate. When serotonin boosters such as Zoloft are combined with MAO inhibitors, serious and sometimes fatal reactions can occur.

How should you take this medication?
Take Zoloft exactly as prescribed: once a day, in either the morning or the evening.

Improvement with Zoloft may not be seen for several days to a few weeks. You should expect to keep taking it for at least several months.

Zoloft may make your mouth dry. For temporary relief suck a hard candy, chew gum, or melt bits of ice in your mouth.

- *If you miss a dose...*
  Take the forgotten dose as soon as you remember. If several hours have passed, skip the dose. Never try to "catch up" by doubling the dose.

- *Storage instructions...*
  Store at room temperature.

What side effects may occur?
Side effects cannot be anticipated. If any develop or change in intensity, inform your doctor as soon as possible. Only your doctor can determine if it is safe for you to continue taking Zoloft.

- *More common side effects may include:*
  Agitation, anxiety, constipation, decreased sex drive, diarrhea or loose stools, difficulty with ejaculation, dizziness, dry mouth, fatigue, gas, headache, decreased appetite, increased sweating, indigestion, insomnia, nausea, nervousness, rash, sleepiness, tingling or pins and needles, tremor, vision problems, vomiting

- *Less common or rare side effects may include:*
  Acne, allergic reaction, altered taste, back pain, breast development in males, breast pain or enlargement, bruise-like marks on the skin, changeable emotions, chest pain, cold, clammy skin, conjunctivitis (pinkeye), coughing, difficulty breathing, difficulty swallowing, double vision, dry eyes, eye pain, fainting, feeling faint upon arising from a sitting

or lying position, feeling of illness, female and male sexual problems, fever, fluid retention, flushing, frequent urination, hair loss, heart attack, hemorrhoids, hiccups, high blood pressure, high pressure within the eye (glaucoma), hearing problems, hot flushes, impotence, increased appetite, increased salivation, increased sex drive, inflamed nasal passages, inflammation of the penis, intolerance to light, itching, joint pains, lack of coordination, lack of sensation, leg cramps, menstrual problems, low blood pressure, migraine, movement problems, muscle cramps, pain or weakness, need to urinate during the night, nosebleed, pain upon urination, persistent, painful erection, purplish spots on the skin, racing heartbeat, rectal hemorrhage, respiratory infection/lung problems, ringing in the ears, sensitivity to light, sinus inflammation, skin eruptions or inflammation, sleepwalking, sores on tongue, speech problems, stomach and intestinal inflammation, swelling of the face, swollen wrists and ankles, thirst, throbbing heartbeat, twitching, vaginal inflammation, hemorrhage or discharge, yawning

- *Zoloft may also cause mental or emotional symptoms such as:*
  Abnormal dreams or thoughts, aggressiveness, exaggerated feeling of well-being, depersonalization ("unreal" feeling), hallucinations, impaired concentration, memory loss, paranoia, rapid mood shifts, suicidal thoughts, tooth-grinding, worsened depression

Many people lose a pound or two of body weight while taking Zoloft. This usually poses no problem but may be a concern if your depression has already caused you to lose a great deal of weight.

In a few people, Zoloft may trigger the grandiose, inappropriate, out-of-control behavior called mania or the similar, but less dramatic, "hyper" state called hypomania.

Why should this drug not be prescribed?
Do not use this drug while taking an MAO inhibitor (see "Most important fact about this drug").

Special warnings about this medication
If you have a kidney or liver disorder, or are subject to seizures, take Zoloft cautiously and under close medical supervision.

Possible food and drug interactions when taking this medication
You should not drink alcoholic beverages while taking Zoloft.

If Zoloft is taken with certain other drugs, the effects of either could be increased, decreased, or altered. It is especially important to check with your doctor before combining Zoloft with the following:

Cimetidine (Tagamet)
Diazepam (Valium, Valrelease)
Digitoxin (Crystodigin)
Flecainide (Tambocor)
Lithium (Lithonate)
MAO inhibitor drugs such as the antidepressants Nardil and Parnate
Other serotonin-boosting drugs such as Paxil and Prozac
Other antidepressants such as Elavil and Serzone
Over-the-counter drugs such as cold remedies
Propafenone (Rythmol)
Tolbutamide (Orinase)
Warfarin (Coumadin)

Special information
if you are pregnant or breastfeeding

The effects of Zoloft during pregnancy have not been adequately studied. If you are pregnant or plan to become pregnant, inform your doctor immediately. Zoloft should be taken during pregnancy only if it is clearly needed. It is not known whether Zoloft appears in breast milk. Caution is advised when using Zoloft during breastfeeding.

Recommended dosage

ADULTS

Depression or Obsessive Compulsive Disorder
The usual starting dose is 50 milligrams once a day, taken either in the morning or in the evening.

Your doctor may increase your dose depending upon your response. The maximum dose is 200 milligrams in a day.

Panic Disorder
During the first week, the usual dose is 25 milligrams once a day. After that, the dose increases to 50 milligrams once a day.

CHILDREN

Obsessive-Compulsive Disorder
The starting dose for children aged 6 to 12 is 25 milligrams and for adolescents aged 13 to 17, 50 milligrams.

Your doctor will adjust the dose as necessary.

Safety and effectiveness have not been established for children under 6.

Overdosage

Any medication taken in excess can have serious consequences. If you suspect an overdose, seek medical attention immediately.

▪ *Symptoms of Zoloft overdose may include:*
Anxiety, dilated pupils, nausea, rapid heartbeat, sleepiness, vomiting

Generic name:

ZOLPIDEM

See Ambien, page 50.

Brand name:

ZOMIG

Pronounced: ZOE-mig
Generic name: Zolmitriptan

Why is this drug prescribed?

Zomig relieves migraine headaches. It's effective whether or not the headache is preceded by an aura (visual disturbances such as halos and flickering lights). For most people Zomig provides relief within 2 hours, but it will not abort an attack or reduce the number of headaches you experience.

Migraines are thought to be caused by expansion and inflammation of blood vessels in the head. Zomig ends a migraine attack by constricting these blood vessels and reducing inflammation.

Most important fact about this drug

Zomig is for use only on common and classic migraine headaches. It should not be used for other types of headache, including certain unusual types of migraine. It has not been tested for cluster headaches, a type of severe headache more common among men.

How should you take this medication?

Take Zomig as soon as your first symptoms appear. If the headache comes back after your first dose, you may take a second one 2 hours later. However, if the first dose has no effect at all, do not take a second one unless your doctor advises it, and never take more than 10 milligrams in a day. Throw away any unused tablets already removed from the blister packaging.

■ *If you miss a dose...*
Zomig is not for regular use. Take it only when you are having a migraine attack.

■ *Storage instructions...*
Store Zomig at room temperature, away from heat, light, and moisture. Throw away any remaining tablets after the expiration date printed on the package. Also discard any leftover medicine if your doctor decides to stop treatment with Zomig.

What side effects may occur?
Side effects cannot be anticipated. If any develop or change in intensity, inform your doctor as soon as possible. Only your doctor can determine if it is safe for you to continue taking Zomig.

■ *More common side effects may include:*
Chest pain or tightness, cold sensation, dizziness, drowsiness, dry mouth, feeling of heaviness in the chest or elsewhere, indigestion, jaw pain or tightness, nausea, neck pain or tightness, pain, skin tingling, sweating, throat pain or tightness, warm sensation, weakness

■ *Less common side effects may include:*
Difficulty swallowing, lack of sensation, muscle pain, muscle weakness, throbbing heartbeat

Why should this drug not be prescribed?
You should not take Zomig if you have certain types of heart disease, including angina (chest pain), a history of heart attack, and certain heart irregularities. Also avoid the drug if you have uncontrolled high blood pressure.

Do not use Zomig within 24 hours of taking an ergotamine-based migraine medication such as Cafergot, Ergostat, or Sansert, or a drug in the same class as Zomig, such as Imitrex.

Avoid using Zomig within 2 weeks of taking a drug classified as an MAO inhibitor, such as the antidepressants Nardil and Parnate.

If Zomig gives you an allergic reaction, do not take it again.

Special warnings about this medication
If the first dose of Zomig does not relieve your symptoms, ask your doctor to reevaluate you; migraine may not be the problem.

Although the danger is very remote, this type of medication has been known to trigger serious heart problems in people with heart disease. If you have risk factors for heart disease, your doctor may ask you to take your first dose of Zomig in the office, and may want to monitor you carefully thereafter. Risk factors that signal the need for caution include high blood pressure, high cholesterol, smoking, excess weight, diabetes, and a strong family history of heart disease or hardening of the arteries. Heart disease is also more likely in postmenopausal women and men over 40.

Use Zomig with caution if you have liver or kidney disease. These conditions could alter the effect of the drug. If you have a history of seizures, make sure the doctor is aware of it. Also, if you develop any trouble with your eyes, alert your doctor. There is a possibility the problem could be related to Zomig.

If you experience pain or tightness in your chest or throat when using Zomig, tell your doctor. If the chest pain is severe or does not go away, seek medical attention immediately. These pains could be symptoms of a previously undetected heart condition.

If you develop shortness of breath, wheezing, a throbbing heartbeat, swelling of the eyelids, face, or lips, or a skin rash, skin lumps, or hives after taking Zomig, call your doctor immediately, and do not take any more of the drug without your doctor's approval.

If a headache feels different from your usual migraine, check with your doctor before using Zomig.

Possible food and drug interactions
when taking this medication

Remember that Zomig should *never* be combined with the following drugs (see "Why should this drug not be prescribed?"):

MAO inhibitors such as the antidepressant drugs Nardil and Parnate
Ergotamine-type drugs such as Cafergot, D.H.E. 45 Injection, Ergostat, and Sansert
Sumatriptan (Imitrex)

If Zomig is taken with certain other drugs, the effects of either may be increased, decreased, or altered. It is especially important to check with your doctor before combining Zomig with the following:

Acetaminophen (Tylenol)
Cimetidine (Tagamet)
Fluoxetine (Prozac)
Fluvoxamine (Luvox)

Oral contraceptives
Paroxetine (Paxil)
Propranolol (Inderal)
Sertraline (Zoloft)

Special information
if you are pregnant or breastfeeding
The effects of Zomig during pregnancy have not been adequately studied. If you are pregnant or plan to become pregnant, inform your doctor immediately. Although researchers have not confirmed it, Zomig may appear in breast milk and could affect a nursing infant. Check with your doctor before using Zomig while breastfeeding.

Recommended dosage

ADULTS

The recommended starting dose is no more than 2.5 milligrams. Higher doses have little additional effect, but tend to cause more side effects. If the headache returns, the dose may be repeated after 2 hours. Do not exceed 10 milligrams in a day.

If you have liver disease, your doctor will prescribe a lower dose and closely monitor your blood pressure.

CHILDREN AND OLDER ADULTS

The safety and effectiveness of Zomig have not been established in children and adults over 65.

Overdosage
The only known symptom of Zomig overdose is drowsiness. However, any medication taken in excess can have serious consequences. If you suspect an overdose, seek medical attention immediately.

Brand name:

ZOVIRAX

Pronounced: zoh-VIGH-racks
Generic name: Acyclovir

Why is this drug prescribed?
Zovirax liquid, capsules, and tablets, are used in the treatment of certain infections with herpes viruses. These include genital herpes, shingles, and chickenpox. This drug may not be appropriate for everyone, and its use

should be thoroughly discussed with your doctor. Zovirax ointment is used to treat initial episodes of genital herpes and certain herpes simplex infections of the skin and mucous membranes.

Some doctors use Zovirax, along with other drugs, in the treatment of AIDS, and for unusual herpes infections such as those following kidney and bone marrow transplants.

Most important fact about this drug

Zovirax does not cure herpes. However, it does reduce pain and may help the sores caused by herpes to heal faster. Genital herpes is a sexually transmitted disease. To reduce the chance of infecting your partner, forgo intercourse and other sexual contact while you have sores or any other symptom.

How should you take this medication?

Your medication should not be shared with others, and the prescribed dose should not be exceeded. Zovirax ointment should not be used in or near the eyes.

To reduce the risk of spreading the infection, use a rubber glove to apply the ointment.

You can take Zovirax with or without food.

■ *If you miss a dose...*
Take it as soon as you remember. If it is almost time for your next dose, skip the one you missed and go back to your regular schedule. Never take 2 doses at the same time.

If you are using the ointment, apply it as soon as you remember and continue your regular schedule.

■ *Storage instructions...*
Store Zovirax at room temperature in a dry place.

What side effects may occur?

Side effects cannot be anticipated. If any develop or change in intensity, inform your doctor as soon as possible. Only your doctor can determine if it is safe for you to continue taking Zovirax.

■ *More common side effects may include:*
Diarrhea, general feeling of bodily discomfort, nausea, vomiting

- *Less common or rare side effects may include:*
  Headache

- *Common side effects of Zovirax ointment may include:*
  Burning, itching, mild pain, skin rash, stinging, vaginal inflammation

Why should this drug not be prescribed?

If you are sensitive to or have ever had an allergic reaction to Zovirax or similar drugs, you should not take this medication. Make sure that your doctor is aware of any drug reactions that you have experienced.

Special warnings about this medication

If you are being treated for a kidney disorder, consult your doctor before taking Zovirax.

Possible food and drug interactions
when taking this medication

If Zovirax is taken with certain other drugs, the effects of either could be increased, decreased, or altered. It is especially important to check with your doctor before combining Zovirax with the following:

Cyclosporine (Sandimmune, Neoral)
Interferon (Roferon-A)
Probenecid (Benemid)
Zidovudine (Retrovir)

Special information
if you are pregnant or breastfeeding

The effects of Zovirax during pregnancy have not been adequately studied. If you are pregnant or plan to become pregnant, inform your doctor immediately. Zovirax appears in breast milk and could affect a nursing infant. If this medication is essential to your health, your doctor may advise you to discontinue breastfeeding your baby until your treatment with Zovirax is finished.

Recommended dosage

ADULTS

For Genital Herpes

The usual dose is one 200-milligram capsule or 1 teaspoonful of liquid every 4 hours, 5 times daily for 10 days. If the herpes is recurrent, the usual adult dose is 400 milligrams (two 200-milligram capsules, one 400-milligram tablet or 2 teaspoonfuls) 2 times daily for up to 12 months.

If genital herpes is intermittent, the usual adult dose is one 200-milligram capsule or 1 teaspoon of liquid every 4 hours, 5 times a day for 5 days. Therapy should be started at the earliest sign or symptom.

Ointment: Apply ointment to affected area every 3 hours, 6 times per day, for 7 days. Use enough ointment (approximately one-half inch ribbon of ointment per 4 square inches of surface area) to cover the affected area.

For Herpes Zoster (Shingles)
The usual adult dose is 800 milligrams (one 800-milligram tablet or 4 teaspoonfuls of liquid) every 4 hours, 5 times daily for 7 to 10 days.

For Chickenpox:
The usual adult dose is 800 milligrams 4 times a day for 5 days.

If you have a kidney disorder, the dose will need to be adjusted by your doctor.

CHILDREN

The usual dose for chickenpox in children 2 years of age and older is 20 milligrams per 2.2 pounds of body weight taken orally 4 times daily, for a total of 80 milligrams per 2.2 pounds, for 5 days. A child weighing more than 88 pounds should take the adult dose.

The safety and effectiveness of oral Zovirax have not been established in children under 2 years of age. However, your doctor may decide that the benefits of this medication outweigh the potential risks. The safety and effectiveness of Zovirax ointment in children have not been established.

OLDER ADULTS

Your doctor will start you at the low end of the dosage range, since older adults are more apt to have kidney problems or other disease, or to be taking other medications.

Overdosage
Zovirax is generally safe; however, there have been cases of kidney disorder in people taking Zovirax orally. Any medication taken in excess can have serious consequences. If you suspect an overdose, seek medical attention immediately.

Brand name:

ZYBAN

Pronounced: ZIGH-ban
Generic name: Bupropion hydrochloride

Why is this drug prescribed?
Zyban is a new type of quit-smoking aid: It contains no nicotine. Instead, Zyban has the same active ingredient as the antidepressant medication Wellbutrin. It works by boosting the levels of several chemical messengers in the brain. With more of these chemicals at work, you experience a reduction in nicotine withdrawal symptoms and a weakening of the urge to smoke. More than a third of the people who take Zyban while participating in a support program are able to quit smoking for at least 1 month.

Most important fact about this drug
About 1 person in 1,000 suffers a seizure while taking Zyban. For this reason, people with epilepsy and certain other disorders should never take the drug. Don't share Zyban with friends. Only a doctor can decide whether it's safe for a particular individual.

How should you take this medication?
Treatment with this drug begins while you are still smoking. Zyban needs about a week to reach an effective level in your body; so to improve your chance of success, you should not attempt to quit until the second week of treatment. Set a firm date for quitting. If you are still smoking after that date, your odds of breaking the habit will be worse. You should keep taking Zyban for 7 to 12 weeks.

You can use nicotine patches along with Zyban. However, combining the two treatments can raise your blood pressure, so it's important to tell your doctor if you plan to use both. Do not smoke while using a patch, because too much nicotine can cause serious side effects.

Participating in a counseling or support program will make success more likely. Your doctor can recommend a local program for you.

Swallow Zyban tablets whole. Do not chew, divide, or crush them. Take them exactly as prescribed.

■ *If you miss a dose...*
   Do not take an extra tablet to "catch up" for the missed dose. Skip the dose and take your next tablet at the regularly scheduled time.

■ *Storage instructions...*
Store at room temperature in a tightly closed container. Keep out of direct sunlight.

What side effects may occur?
Side effects cannot be anticipated. If any develop or change in intensity, inform your doctor as soon as possible. Only your doctor can determine if it is safe for you to continue taking Zyban.

■ *The most common side effects are:*
Dry mouth and sleeplessness

These are generally mild and usually disappear after a few weeks. If you have difficulty sleeping, avoid taking Zyban close to bedtime and ask your doctor about reducing your dosage.

■ *More common side effects may include:*
Abdominal pain, abnormal dreams, anxiety, constipation, diarrhea, disturbed concentration, dizziness, increased cough, itching, joint pain, nasal inflammation, nausea, nervousness, rash, sore throat

■ *Less common side effects may include:*
Abnormal thinking, allergic reaction, bronchitis, changes in taste, difficulty breathing, dry skin, hives, hot flashes, increased appetite or loss of appetite, increased blood pressure, mouth ulcers, muscle pain, neck pain, nosebleed, ringing in the ears, shakiness, sinus inflammation, sleepiness, throbbing heartbeat

■ *Rare side effects may include:*
Chest pain, feeling of unhappiness, thirst, swelling of the face

Why should this drug not be prescribed?
Because Zyban has been known to trigger convulsions, no one with a seizure disorder should take this drug. Also avoid Zyban if you are taking Wellbutrin or any other drug that contains bupropion, Zyban's active ingredient. The more bupropion you take, the more likely you are to have a seizure.

Zyban's seizure-triggering potential is greater in people with an eating disorder such as bulimia or anorexia. If you suffer from one of these problems, never take Zyban. Avoid it, too, if you are taking a drug classified as an MAO inhibitor, such as the antidepressants Nardil and Parnate. Allow at least 14 days to pass between taking one of these drugs and starting your Zyban therapy.

If bupropion or any other ingredient in Zyban has ever given you an allergic reaction, the drug is not for you.

Special warnings about this medication

Because the chance of a seizure from Zyban rises with the amount in your system, never take more than one 150-milligram tablet at a time, and limit your total daily intake to 2 doses (300 milligrams).

A variety of conditions can predispose you to seizures, including:

Prior head injuries
Prior seizures
Central nervous system tumors
Too much alcohol
Abrupt withdrawal from alcohol, tranquilizers, or sedatives
Addiction to narcotics or cocaine
Use of over-the-counter stimulants or diet pills
Use of diabetes medications
Use of antidepressants, major tranquilizers, steroids, or theophylline

If any of these apply to you, use Zyban with care.

Stop taking Zyban and call your doctor immediately if you have difficulty breathing or swallowing; notice swelling in your face, lips, tongue, or throat; develop swollen arms and legs; or break out with itchy eruptions. These are warning signs of a potentially severe allergic reaction.

If you have a liver or kidney condition, make sure the doctor is aware of it. Your dosage may need to be reduced. Also make certain the doctor knows about any heart condition you may have.

Zyban can interfere with your driving ability. Don't drive or operate dangerous machinery until you are certain of the drug's effect on you.

**Possible food and drug interactions
when taking this medication**

If Zyban is used with certain other drugs, the effects of either could be increased, decreased, or altered. It is especially important to check with your doctor before combining Zyban with the following:

Alcohol
Carbamazepine (Tegretol)
Cimetidine (Tagamet)
Levodopa (Dopar, Larodopa, Sinemet)
Major tranquilizers such as Haldol and Thorazine
MAO inhibitors such as the antidepressants Nardil and Parnate
Orphenadrine (Norflex)
Phenobarbital

Phenytoin (Dilantin)
Theophylline (Theo-Dur, Theolair)

Special information
if you are pregnant or breastfeeding

Zyban has not been tested in pregnant women. If you are pregnant or plan to become pregnant, do your best to quit smoking with the aid of counseling and support before turning to drug therapy. For the sake of the baby, you should avoid smoking or taking nicotine in any other form while pregnant.

Zyban appears in breast milk and could affect a nursing infant. Ask your doctor whether it will be better to discontinue the medication or to stop breastfeeding.

Recommended dosage

ADULTS

The usual starting dose is one 150-milligram tablet in the morning for the first 3 days. After that, take one 150-milligram tablet in the morning and another in the early evening. Keep doses at least 8 hours apart. The maximum recommended dose is 300 milligrams daily.

Continue taking Zyban for 7 to 12 weeks.

Kidney and Liver Disease
Your doctor will start you at a lower dose to avoid high blood levels of Zyban.

CHILDREN

The safety and efficacy of Zyban have not been established in children under 18.

Overdosage

Information on Zyban overdose is limited. However, any medication taken in excess can have serious consequences. If you suspect an overdose, seek medical attention immediately.

■ *Symptoms of Zyban overdose may include:*
Blurred vision, confusion, grogginess, jitteriness, lightheadedness, nausea, seizure, sluggishness, visual hallucinations

Brand name:

ZYDONE

See Vicodin, page 1403.

Brand name:

ZYFLO

Pronounced: ZIGH-flow
Generic name: Zileuton

Why is this drug prescribed?
Zyflo tablets prevent and relieve the symptoms of chronic asthma. The drug works by relaxing the muscles in the walls of your airways, allowing them to open wider, and by reducing inflammation, swelling, and mucus secretion in the lungs.

Most important fact about this drug
While taking Zyflo, you should continue taking all other asthma medications your doctor has prescribed, unless directed otherwise. Do not decrease the dose or stop taking any of these drugs.

How should you take this medication?
Zyflo should be taken 4 times a day. Although you can take it with or without meals, it may be easier to remember if you take it with meals and at bedtime. Take Zyflo exactly as prescribed, even when symptoms subside.

- *If you miss a dose...*
  Take the forgotten dose as soon as you remember. If it is almost time for your next dose, skip the one you missed and go back to your regular schedule. Never take 2 doses at the same time.

- *Storage instructions...*
  Store at room temperature, away from light.

What side effects may occur?
Side effects cannot be anticipated. If any develop or change in intensity, inform your doctor as soon as possible. Only your doctor can determine if it is safe for you to continue taking Zyflo.

- *More common side effects may include:*
  Abdominal pain, headache, indigestion, loss of strength, muscle aches, nausea, pain

- *Less common side effects may include:*
  Chest pain, constipation, dizziness, drowsiness, fever, gas, general discomfort, inflamed eyes (conjunctivitis), inflammation of the vagina,

insomnia, itching, joint pain, muscle tension, neck pain or rigidity, nervousness, urinary tract infection, vomiting

Why should this drug not be prescribed?

If you have liver disease, you should not take this medication. You should also avoid Zyflo if you have ever had an allergic reaction to it or its ingredients.

Special warnings about this medication

Zyflo will not help an acute asthma attack in which immediate opening of the airways is needed.

If you find that you have to use your other asthma medications—such as an inhaler—more often, report this to your doctor.

Because Zyflo can affect the liver, make sure your doctor is aware of any problems you've had in the past. Warn the doctor, too, if you're a heavy drinker. Your liver function will be tested before you start Zyflo, and regularly thereafter. Be sure to go in for these tests. If they reveal liver damage, you'll have to stop taking Zyflo. Also be sure to tell your doctor immediately if you develop any symptoms of liver disease. These include pain in the upper right abdomen, nausea, fatigue, lethargy, itching, general discomfort, and jaundice (yellowing of the skin and eyes).

Possible food and drug interactions
when taking this medication

If Zyflo is taken with certain other drugs, the effects of either could be increased, decreased, or altered. You should check with your doctor before stopping or starting any prescription or nonprescription medicine. This is especially important with the following:

Astemizole (Hismanal)
"Beta blocker" drugs such as propranolol (Inderal) and others in this group
"Calcium channel blockers" such as Cardene, DynaCirc, Nimotop, Norvasc, Plendil, Procardia, Sular
Cisapride (Propulsid)
Cyclosporine (Sandimmune, Neoral)
Terfenadine (Seldane)
Theophylline (Theo-Dur)
Warfarin (Coumadin)

While you are taking Zyflo, your theophylline dosage may need to be lowered, and your theophylline levels will have to be carefully watched. Dosages of propranolol may also need reduction, and warfarin dosages may need adjustment as well.

Special information
if you are pregnant or breastfeeding
The effects of Zyflo in pregnancy have not been adequately studied. If you are pregnant or plan to become pregnant, ask your doctor whether you should continue taking Zyflo. It is not certain that the drug appears in breast milk, but taking Zyflo while nursing is not recommended. Discuss with your doctor whether it's best to stop taking the drug or to give up breastfeeding.

Recommended dosage

ADULTS

The recommended dosage is one 600-milligram tablet 4 times a day.

CHILDREN

The safety and effectiveness of this drug in children under 12 years of age have not been established.

Overdosage
Because Zyflo is a relatively new drug, little is known about overdosage. However, any medication taken in excess can have serious consequences. If you suspect an overdose, seek medical treatment immediately.

Brand name:

ZYLOPRIM

Pronounced: ZYE-loe-prim
Generic name: Allopurinol

Why is this drug prescribed?
Zyloprim is used in the treatment of many symptoms of gout, including acute attacks, tophi (collection of uric acid crystals in the tissues, especially around joints), joint destruction, and uric acid stones. Gout is a form of arthritis characterized by increased blood levels of uric acid. Zyloprim works by reducing uric acid production in the body, thus preventing crystals from forming.

Zyloprim is also used to manage the increased uric acid levels in the blood of people with certain cancers, such as leukemia. It is also prescribed to manage some types of kidney stones.

Most important fact about this drug

Zyloprim will not stop a gout attack that is already underway. However, when taken over a period of several months, this drug will begin to reduce your symptoms. It's important to keep taking it regularly, even if it seems to have no immediate effect.

How should you take this medication?

Take Zyloprim exactly as prescribed. Your doctor will probably start you on a low dosage, increasing it gradually each week until you reach the dosage that is best for you.

A typical starting dose is one 100-milligram tablet per day. You may want to take Zyloprim immediately after a meal to minimize the risk of stomach irritation.

You should avoid taking large doses of vitamin C because of the increased possibility of kidney stone formation.

While taking Zyloprim you should drink plenty of liquids—10 to 12 glasses (8 ounces each) per day—unless otherwise prescribed by your doctor.

To help prevent attacks of gout, you should also avoid beer, wine, and purine-rich foods such as anchovies, sardines, liver, kidneys, lentils, and sweetbreads.

If you have been taking colchicine and/or an anti-inflammatory drug, such as Anaprox, Indocin, and others, to relieve your gout, your doctor will probably want you to continue taking this medication while your Zyloprim dosage is being adjusted. Later, when you have had no attacks of gout for several months, you may be able to stop taking these other medications.

If you have been taking a drug that promotes the excretion of uric acid in the urine, such as probenecid (Benemid) or sulfinpyrazone (Anturane), to try to prevent attacks of gout, your doctor will probably want to reduce or stop your dosage of this drug while increasing your dosage of Zyloprim.

■ *If you miss a dose...*
   Take it as soon as you remember. If it is almost time for your next dose, skip the one you missed and go back to your regular schedule. Do not take 2 doses at once.

■ *Storage instructions...*
   Store at room temperature in a cool, dry place, away from light.

What side effects may occur?
Side effects cannot be anticipated. If any develop or change in intensity, inform your doctor as soon as possible. Only your doctor can determine if it is safe for you to continue taking Zyloprim.

Because a skin reaction, the most common side effect of Zyloprim, may occasionally become severe or even fatal, you should stop taking Zyloprim if you notice even the beginnings of a rash. Such a rash may be itchy or scaly or may make your skin peel off in sheets; it may be accompanied by chills and fever, aching joints, or jaundice.

■ *More common side effects may include:*
Acute attack of gout, diarrhea, nausea, rash

■ *Less common or rare side effects may include:*
Abdominal pain, bruising, chills, fever, hair loss, headache, hepatitis, hives, indigestion, itching, joint pain, kidney failure, loosening of nails, muscle disease, nosebleed, rare skin condition characterized by severe blisters and bleeding on the lips, eyes, or nose, reddish-brown or purplish spots on skin, skin inflammation or peeling, sleepiness, stomach inflammation, taste loss or change, tingling or pins and needles, unusual bleeding, vomiting, yellowing of skin and eyes

Why should this drug not be prescribed?
Do not take Zyloprim if you have ever had a severe reaction to it in the past.

Special warnings about this medication
If you notice a rash or other signs of an allergic reaction, stop taking Zyloprim immediately and consult your doctor. In some people, a Zyloprim-induced rash may lead to a serious skin disease, generalized inflammation of a blood or lymph vessel, irreversible liver damage, or even death.

You may experience acute attacks of gout more often in the early stages of Zyloprim therapy, even when normal uric acid levels have been attained. These attacks will become shorter and less severe after several months of therapy.

A kidney problem may turn a normal dose of Zyloprim into an overdose. If you have a kidney disease, or a condition such as diabetes or high blood pressure that may affect your kidneys, your doctor should prescribe Zyloprim cautiously and order periodic blood and urine tests to assess your kidney function.

Because Zyloprim may make you drowsy, do not drive or perform hazardous tasks until you know how the medication affects you.

It may be 2 to 6 weeks before you see any results from this medication.

Possible food and drug interactions
when taking this medication

If Zyloprim is taken with certain other drugs, the effects of either could be increased, decreased, or altered. It is especially important to check with your doctor before combining Zyloprim with the following:

Amoxicillin (Amoxil, Trimox, Wymox)
Ampicillin (Omnipen, Principen)
Azathioprine (Imuran)
Blood thinners such as Coumadin
Cyclosporine (Sandimmune, Neoral)
Drugs for diabetes, such as Diabinese and Orinase
Mercaptopurine (Purinethol)
Probenecid (Benemid, ColBENEMID)
Sulfinpyrazone (Anturane)
Theophylline (Theo-Dur, Slo-Phyllin, and others)
Thiazide diuretics such as HydroDIURIL, Diuril, and others
Vitamin C

Special information
if you are pregnant or breastfeeding

The effects of Zyloprim during pregnancy have not been adequately studied. If you are pregnant or plan to become pregnant, notify your doctor immediately. Zyloprim should be taken during pregnancy only if it is clearly needed.

Zyloprim appears in breast milk; what effect it may have on a nursing baby is unknown. Caution is advised when Zyloprim is taken during breastfeeding.

Recommended dosage

ADULTS

Your doctor will tailor the dosage of Zyloprim individually to control the severity of symptoms and to bring the uric acid levels to normal or near normal.

Gout
The usual starting dose is 100 milligrams once daily. Your doctor may increase your dose by 100 milligrams per day at 1-week intervals until desired results are attained. The average dose is 200 to 300 milligrams per day for mild gout and 400 to 600 milligrams daily for moderate to severe gout. The most you should take in a day is 800 milligrams.

Recurrent Kidney Stones
The usual dose is 200 to 300 milligrams daily, divided into smaller doses or taken as one dose.

Management of Uric Acid Levels in Certain Cancers
The usual dose is 600 to 800 milligrams daily for 2 to 3 days, together with a high fluid intake.

CHILDREN

The usual recommended dose for children 6 to 10 years of age is 300 milligrams daily for the management of uric acid levels in certain types of cancer. Children under 6 years of age are generally given 150 milligrams daily.

Overdosage
Although no specific information is available regarding Zyloprim overdosage, any medication taken in excess can have serious consequences. If you suspect an overdose of Zyloprim, seek medical attention immediately.

Brand name:

ZYPREXA

Pronounced: Zye-PRECKS-ah
Generic name: Olanzapine

Why is this drug prescribed?
Zyprexa helps manage symptoms of schizophrenia and other psychotic disorders. It is thought to work by opposing the action of serotonin and dopamine, two of the brain's major chemical messengers.

Most important fact about this drug
At the start of Zyprexa therapy, the drug can cause extreme low blood pressure, increased heart rate, dizziness, and, in rare cases, a tendency to faint when first standing up. These problems are more likely if you are

dehydrated, have heart disease, or take blood pressure medicine. To avoid such problems, your doctor may start with a low dose of Zyprexa and increase the dosage gradually.

How should you take this medication?

Zyprexa should be taken once a day with or without food.

■ *If you miss a dose...*
Take it as soon as you remember. If it is almost time for your next dose, skip the one you missed and go back to your regular schedule. Do not take 2 doses at once.

■ *Storage instructions...*
Store at room temperature away from light and moisture.

What side effects may occur?

Side effects cannot be anticipated. If any develop or change in intensity, inform your doctor as soon as possible. Only your doctor can determine if it is safe for you to continue taking Zyprexa.

■ *More common side effects may include:*
Abdominal pain, agitation, anxiety, back pain, behavior problems, blurred vision, chest pain, constipation, dizziness, drowsiness, dry mouth, extreme low blood pressure, fever, headache, hostility, increased cough, inflammation of the nasal passages and throat, insomnia, joint pain, movement disorders, muscle rigidity, nausea, nervousness, pain in arms and legs, rapid heartbeat, restlessness, tension, tremor, weakness, weight gain

■ *Less common side effects may include:*
Amnesia, difficulty breathing, eye problems, feeling of well-being, flu-like symptoms, increased appetite, increased salivation, involuntary movements, joint problems, low blood pressure, neck rigidity, rash, suicide attempt, stuttering, swelling of the arms and legs, thirst, twitching, urinary problems, vomiting, weight loss

■ *Rare side effects may include:*
Arthritis, asthma, blood problems, bone pain, chills, diabetes, digestive system problems, ear problems, face swelling, gynecological problems, light sensitivity, migraine, muscle ache, skin problems, stroke, taste disturbance

Why should this drug not be prescribed?
If Zyprexa gives you an allergic reaction, you cannot take the drug.

Special warnings about this drug
Zyprexa sometimes causes drowsiness and can impair your judgment, thinking, and motor skills. Use caution while driving and don't operate dangerous machinery until you know how the drug affects you.

Medicines such as Zyprexa can interfere with regulation of the body's temperature. Do not get overheated or become dehydrated while taking Zyprexa. Avoid extreme heat and drink plenty of fluids.

Use Zyprexa with caution if you have any of the following conditions: Alzheimer's disease, trouble swallowing, narrow angle glaucoma (high pressure in the eye), an enlarged prostate, heart irregularities, heart disease, heart failure, liver disease, or a history of heart attack, seizures, or intestinal blockage.

Drugs such as Zyprexa sometimes cause a condition called Neuroleptic Malignant Syndrome. Symptoms include high fever, muscle rigidity, irregular pulse or blood pressure, rapid heartbeat, excessive perspiration, and changes in heart rhythm. If these symptoms appear, your doctor will have you stop taking Zyprexa while the condition is under treatment.

There is also a risk of developing tardive dyskinesia, a condition marked by slow, rhythmical, involuntary movements. This problem is more likely to surface in older adults, especially elderly women. When it does, use of Zyprexa is usually stopped.

**Possible food and drug interactions
when taking this medication**
Avoid alcohol while taking Zyprexa. The combination can cause a sudden drop in blood pressure.

If Zyprexa is taken with certain other drugs, the effects of either can be increased, decreased, or altered. Ask your doctor before taking any prescription or over-the-counter drugs. It is especially important to check before combining Zyprexa with the following:

Blood pressure medications
Carbamazepine (Tegretol)
Diazepam (Valium)
Drugs that boost the effect of dopamine, such as the Parkinson's
    medications Mirapex, Parlodel, Permax, and Requip

Fluvoxamine (Luvox)
Levodopa (Dopar, Larodopa)
Omeprazole (Prilosec)
Rifampin (Rifadin, Rimactane)

Special information
if you are pregnant or breastfeeding

If you are pregnant or plan to become pregnant, inform your doctor immediately. Zyprexa should be used during pregnancy only if absolutely necessary. The drug may appear in breast milk; do not breastfeed while on Zyprexa therapy.

Recommended dosage

ADULTS

The usual starting dose is 5 to 10 milligrams once a day. If you start at the lower dose, after a few days the doctor will increase it to 10. After that, the dosage will be increased no more than once a week, 5 milligrams at a time, up to a maximum of 20 milligrams a day.

Those most likely to start at 5 milligrams are the debilitated, people prone to low blood pressure, and nonsmoking women over 65 (because they tend to have a slow metabolism).

Overdosage

An overdose of Zyprexa is usually not life-threatening. However, any medication taken in excess can have serious consequences. If you suspect an overdose, seek medical attention immediately.

■ *Symptoms of Zyprexa overdose may include:*
Drowsiness, slurred speech

Brand name:

ZYRTEC

Pronounced: ZEER-tek
Generic name: Cetirizine hydrochloride

Why is this drug prescribed?

Zyrtec is an antihistamine. It is prescribed to treat the sneezing; itchy, runny nose; and itchy, red, watery eyes caused by seasonal allergies such as hay fever. Zyrtec also relieves the symptoms of year-round allergies due to dust, mold, and animal dander. This medication is also used in the treatment of chronic itchy skin and hives.

Most important fact about this drug

Zyrtec may cause drowsiness. Be especially careful driving or operating dangerous machinery or participating in any hazardous activity that requires full mental alertness until you know how you react to this medication.

How should you take this medication?

Take Zyrtec once a day, exactly as prescribed. This medication can be taken with or without food.

Zyrtec may make your mouth dry. Sucking hard candy, chewing a stick of gum, or melting bits of ice in your mouth can provide relief.

■ *If you miss a dose...*
If you are taking this medication on a regular schedule, take the forgotten dose as soon as you remember. If it is almost time for your next dose, skip the one you missed and go back to your regular schedule. Do not take 2 doses at once.

■ *Storage instructions...*
Store tablets and syrup at room temperature.

What side effects may occur?

Side effects cannot be anticipated. If any develop or change in intensity, tell your doctor as soon as possible. Only your doctor can determine if it is safe for you to continue taking Zyrtec.

■ *More common side effects in adults may include:*
Drowsiness, dry mouth, fatigue

■ *Less common side effects in adults may include:*
Dizziness, sore throat

■ *More common side effects in children aged 6 to 11 may include:*
Abdominal pain, coughing, diarrhea, headache, nosebleed, sleepiness, sore throat, wheezing

■ *Less common side effects in children aged 6 to 11 may include:*
Nausea, vomiting

Why should this drug not be prescribed?

Avoid Zyrtec if it causes a reaction, or if you have ever had a reaction to the similar drug Atarax.

Special warnings about this medication

If you have kidney or liver disease, be sure to tell your doctor. Your dose of this medication may have to be reduced.

Possible food and drug interactions
when taking this medication

You should avoid drinking alcohol or taking sedatives, tranquilizers, sleeping pills, or muscle relaxants while using Zyrtec. They can lead to increased drowsiness and reduced mental alertness. Among the products to avoid are the following:

    Antidepressants such as Tofranil, Elavil, Ludiomil, and Anafranil
    Muscle relaxants such as Valium and Soma
    Pain-relieving narcotics such as codeine, Demerol, and Percocet
    Sedatives such as Nembutal, Seconal, and phenobarbital
    Sleeping pills such as Halcion, Restoril, and Ambien
    High doses of theophylline (Theo-Dur)

Special information
if you are pregnant or breastfeeding

The effects of Zyrtec during pregnancy have not been adequately studied. If you are pregnant or plan to become pregnant, tell your doctor immediately. Zyrtec appears in breast milk and should not be used if you are breastfeeding.

Recommended dosage

ADULTS AND CHILDREN 12 YEARS AND OLDER

The usual starting dose is 5 or 10 milligrams once a day, depending on the severity of your symptoms. If you have a kidney or liver condition, the doctor will probably prescribe 5 milligrams daily.

CHILDREN 6 TO 11 YEARS

The usual starting dose is 5 or 10 milligrams (1 or 2 teaspoonfuls of syrup) once a day. If your child has a kidney or liver condition, the doctor will probably prescribe the lower dose.

CHILDREN 2 TO 5 YEARS

The usual starting dose is 2.5 milligrams (half a teaspoonful) once a day. Dosage may be increased to a maximum of 5 milligrams (1 teaspoonful) once daily or 2.5 milligrams (half a teaspoonful) every 12 hours. If the child has a kidney or liver condition, Zyrtec should not be given.

Overdosage

Any medication taken in excess can have serious consequences. In adults, the primary symptom of a Zyrtec overdose is extreme sleepiness. In children, restlessness and irritability may precede drowsiness. If you suspect an overdose, seek medical treatment immediately.

APPENDIX 1

Safe Medication Use

Using medications safely is largely a matter of common sense and caution. The following are general guidelines to keep in mind:

You and your doctor

- Tell your doctor everything about your medical history, including reactions to medications you've used in the past.
- Tell the doctor about any medications you are using now, even if they are over-the-counter drugs.
- Keep track of your reactions to a medication and report them to your doctor.
- Ask your doctor what you can do when given a new drug. For example, are there any foods to avoid when taking the drug? Should you avoid alcohol?
- Never change your dose schedule unless your doctor tells you to do so.
- Ask about the addiction or dependence potential of any new drug.

You and your pharmacist

- See if there are any written instructions that you can take with you.
- Ask the pharmacist to explain clearly when and how to take the drug.
- Check the ingredients of over-the-counter drugs you may be taking to ensure that your prescription doesn't interact with them.
- If you are starting a new medication, ask your pharmacist to fill only half the prescription in case you have an adverse reaction and the drug is stopped.
- Ask how long the medication remains effective. Don't take it after its expiration date.
- If you are going on a vacation, make sure your drug can be used in different climates.

You and your medications

- Never take someone else's medication; and don't share your own medicines.
- Check the label each time you take a drug. Don't take a drug in the dark.

- Keep your medications in a dry, safe spot.
- Keep each medicine in the bottle from the drugstore. Don't mix medicines together in a single bottle.
- If you think you are pregnant, consult with your doctor before using any medication.
- Destroy any unused portions of a drug and throw out the bottle.
- If you need a certain medicine (for instance, insulin) in case of emergency, carry the information with you.

Your medicines and your children

- Keep all medications in a locked cabinet or in a spot well out of the reach of children.
- Ask for child-proof safety bottles.
- Be alert and awake when giving a child medication.
- Make sure that children know medications can be dangerous if misused.
- Keep antidotes such as Syrup of Ipecac on hand.
- Keep the numbers of your EMS (emergency medical service) and poison control centers handy.

APPENDIX 2
Poison Control Centers

Many of the centers listed below are certified by the American Association of Poison Control Centers. Certified centers are marked by an asterisk after the name. Each has to meet certain criteria. It must, for example, serve a large geographic area; it must be open 24 hours a day and provide direct-dial or toll-free access; it must be supervised by a medical director; and it must have registered pharmacists or nurses available to answer questions from the public.

The centers have a wide variety of toxicology resources, including a computerized database of some 750,000 substances maintained by MICROMEDEX, INC., an affiliate of *Red Book*. Staff members are trained to resolve toxic situations in the home of the caller, though hospital referrals are given in some instances. The centers also offer a range of educational services to both the public and healthcare professionals. In some states, these larger centers exist side by side with smaller centers offering a more limited range of services.

Within each state, centers are listed alphabetically by city. Telephone numbers designated "TTY" are teletype lines for the hearing-impaired. "TDD" numbers reach a telecommunication device for the deaf.

ALABAMA

BIRMINGHAM
Regional Poison Control Center,
The Children's Hospital
of Alabama (*)
1600 7th Ave. South
Birmingham, AL 35233-1711
Bus.:   205-939-9720
Emer.: 205-933-4050
            205-939-9201
            800-292-6678 (AL)
Fax: 205-939-9245

TUSCALOOSA
Alabama Poison Center,
Tuscaloosa (*)
2503 Phoenix Dr.
Tuscaloosa, AL 35405
Bus.:   205-345-0600
Emer.: 205-345-0600
            800-462-0800 (AL)
Fax: 205-759-7994

ALASKA

ANCHORAGE
Anchorage Poison Control Center,
Providence Hospital
P.O. Box 196604
3200 Providence Dr.
Anchorage, AK 99519-6604
Bus.:   907-562-2211
            ext. 3633
Emer.: 907-261-3193
            800-478-3193 (AK)
Fax: 907-261-3645

FAIRBANKS
Fairbanks Poison Control Center
1650 Cowles St.
Fairbanks, AK 99701
Bus.:   907-456-7182
Emer.: 907-456-7182
Fax: 907-458-5553

ARIZONA

PHOENIX
Samaritan Regional Poison Center (*)
Good Samaritan Regional
Medical Center
Ancillary-1
1111 East McDowell Rd.
Phoenix, AZ 85006
Bus.: 602-495-4884
Emer.: 602-253-3334
        800-362-0101 (AZ)
Fax: 602-256-7579

TUCSON
Arizona Poison & Drug
Information Center (*)
Arizona Health Sciences Center
1501 North Campbell Ave.
Rm. 1156
Tucson, AZ 85724
Emer.: 520-626-6016
        800-362-0101 (AZ)
Fax: 520-626-2720

ARKANSAS

LITTLE ROCK
Arkansas Poison and
Drug Information Center,
College of Pharmacy - UAMS
4301 West Markham St.,
Slot 522
Little Rock, AR 72205
Bus.:   501-661-6161
Emer.:   800-376-4766 (AR)
TDD/TTY: 800-641-3805

CALIFORNIA

FRESNO
Central Poison Control System-
Fresno/Madera (*)
Valley Children's Hospital
9300 Valley Children's Place
Madera, CA 93638-8762
Emer.: 800-876-4766 (CA)

SACRAMENTO
California Poison Control System-
Sacramento (*)
UCDMC-HSF Room 1024
2315 Stockton Blvd.
Sacramento, CA 95817
Bus.: 916-734-3415
Emer.: 800-876-4766 (CA)
Fax: 916-734-7796

SAN DIEGO
California Poison Control System-
San Diego (*)
UCSD Medical Center
200 West Arbor Dr.
San Diego, CA 92103-8925
Emer.: 800-876-4766 (CA)

SAN FRANCISCO
California Poison Control System-
San Francisco
San Francisco General Hospital
1001 Potrero Ave., Room E86
San Francisco, CA 94110
Emer.: 800-876-4766 (CA)

COLORADO

DENVER
Rocky Mountain Poison and Drug Center (*)
8802 East 9th Ave.
Denver, CO 80220-6800
Bus.:   303-739-1100
Emer.: 303-739-1123
        800-332-3073 (CO)
Fax: 303-739-1119

CONNECTICUT

FARMINGTON
Connecticut Regional Poison Control Center (*)
University of Connecticut Health Center
263 Farmington Ave.
Farmington, CT 06030-5365
Bus.:   860-679-3456
Emer.: 800-343-2722 (CT)
Fax: 860-679-1623

DELAWARE

(PHILADELPHIA, PA)
The Poison Control Center (*)
3535 Market St.
Suite 985
Philadelphia, PA 19104-3309
Emer.: 800-722-7112 (PA)
        215-386-2100

DISTRICT OF COLUMBIA

WASHINGTON, DC
National Capital Poison Center (*)
3201 New Mexico Ave., NW, Suite 310
Washington, DC 20016
Bus.:   202-362-3867
Emer.: 202-625-3333
TTY: 202-362-8563
Fax: 202-362-8377

FLORIDA

JACKSONVILLE
Florida Poison Information Center-Jacksonville (*)
University Medical Center
University of Florida Health Science Center-Jacksonville
655 W. 8th St.
Jacksonville, FL 32209
Emer.: 904-549-4480
        800-282-3171 (FL)
Fax: 904-549-4063

MIAMI
Florida Poison Information Center-Miami (*)
University of Miami,
School of Medicine
Department of Pediatrics
P.O. Box 016960 (R-131)
Miami, FL 33101
Emer.: 305-585-5253
        800-282-3171 (FL)
Fax: 305-242-9762

TAMPA
Florida Poison Information
Center-Tampa (*)
Tampa General Hospital
P.O. Box 1289
Tampa, FL 33601
Emer.: 813-253-4444 (Tampa)
   800-282-3171 (FL)
Fax: 813-253-4443

GEORGIA

ATLANTA
Georgia Poison Center (*)
Hughes Spalding Children's
Hospital, Grady Health System
80 Butler St. SE
P.O. Box 26066
Atlanta, GA 30335-3801
Emer.: 404-616-9000
   800-282-5846 (GA)
TDD: 404-616-9287
Fax: 404-616-6657

HAWAII

HONOLULU
Hawaii Poison Center
1319 Punahou St.
Honolulu, HI 96826
Emer.: 808-941-4411
Fax: 808-535-7922

IDAHO

(DENVER, CO)
Rocky Mountain Poison &
Drug Center (*)
8802 E. 9th Ave.
Denver, CO 80220-6800
Emer.: 800-860-0620 (ID)
   303-739-1123

ILLINOIS

CHICAGO
Illinois Poison Center (*)
222 South Riverside Plaza
Suite 1900
Chicago, IL 60606
Bus.: 312-906-6136
Emer.: 800-942-5969 (IL)
Fax: 312-803-5400

URBANA
ASPCA/National Animal Poison
Control Center (*)
1717 S. Philo Rd., Suite 36
Urbana, IL 61802
Bus.: 217-337-5030
Emer.: 888-426-4435
Fax: 217-337-0599

INDIANA

INDIANAPOLIS
Indiana Poison Center (*)
Methodist Hospital of Indiana
I-65 at 21st St.
Indianapolis, IN 46206-1367
Emer.: 317-929-2323
   800-382-9097 (IN)
Fax: 317-929-2337

IOWA

IOWA CITY
Poison Control Center,
The University of Iowa
Hospitals and Clinics
Dept. of Pharmaceutical Care,
CC101 GH
200 Hawkins Dr.
Iowa City, IA 52242
Emer.: 800-272-6477 (IA)

SIOUX CITY
Iowa Poison Center
2720 Stone Park Blvd.
Sioux City, IA 51104
Bus.: 712-277-2222
Emer.: 800-352-2222 (IA)
Fax: 712-279-7852

KANSAS

KANSAS CITY
Mid-America Poison Control Center,
University of Kansas Medical Center
3901 Rainbow Blvd., Room B-400
Kansas City, KS 66160-7231
Business &
Emer.: 913-588-6633
        800-332-6633 (KS)
TDD: 913-588-6639
Fax: 913-588-2350

TOPEKA
Stormont-Vail Regional Medical
Center Emergency Department
1500 S.W. 10th
Topeka, KS 66604-1353
Bus.: 785-354-6000
Emer.: 785-354-6100
Fax: 785-354-5004

KENTUCKY

LOUISVILLE
Kentucky Regional Poison Center
Medical Towers South, Suite 572
234 E. Gray St.
Louisville, KY 40202
Bus.: 502-629-7264
Emer.: 502-589-8222
Fax: 502-629-7277

LOUISIANA

MONROE
Louisiana Drug and Poison
Information Center (*)
Northeast Louisiana University
School of Pharmacy
Sugar Hall
Monroe, LA 71209-6430
Bus.: 318-342-1710
Emer.: 800-256-9822 (LA)
Fax: 318-342-1744

MAINE

PORTLAND
Maine Poison Control Center,
Maine Medical Center
22 Bramhall St.
Portland, ME 04102
Bus.: 207-871-2950
Emer.: 800-442-6305 (ME)
Fax: 207-871-6226

MARYLAND

BALTIMORE
Maryland Poison Center (*)
University of Maryland at
Baltimore
School of Pharmacy
20 North Pine St., PH 230
Baltimore, MD 21201
Bus.: 410-706-7604
Emer.: 410-706-7701
        800-492-2414 (MD)
TDD: 410-706-1858
Fax: 410-706-7184

MASSACHUSETTS

BOSTON
Massachusetts Poison Control
System (*)
300 Longwood Ave.
Boston, MA 02115
Emer.: 617-232-2120
      800-682-9211 (MA)
Fax: 617-738-0032

MICHIGAN

DETROIT
Poison Control Center (*)
Children's Hospital of Michigan
4160 John R. Harper Prof.
Office Bldg.
Suite 616
Detroit, MI 48201
Bus.:   313-745-5335
Emer.:   313-745-5711
          800-764-7661 (MI)
TDD/TTY: 800-356-3232
Fax: 313-745-5493

GRAND RAPIDS
Spectrum Health Regional Poison
Center (*)
1840 Wealthy SE
Grand Rapids, MI 49506-2968
Bus.:   616-774-5329
Emer.:   800-764-7661 (MI)
TDD/TTY: 800-356-3232
Fax: 616-774-7204

MINNESOTA

MINNEAPOLIS
Hennepin Regional Poison Center (*)
Hennepin County Medical Center
701 Park Ave.
Minneapolis, MN 55415
Bus.:   612-347-3144
Emer.: 800-764-7661 (MN, SD)
       612-347-3141
TTY: 612-904-4691
Fax: 612-904-4289

MISSISSIPPI

HATTIESBURG
Poison Center,
Forrest General Hospital
P.O. Box 16389
400 South 28th Ave.
Hattiesburg, MS 39404
Emer.: 601-288-2100
       601-288-2197
       601-288-2199
Fax: 601-288-2125

JACKSON
Mississippi Regional Poison
Control Center, University of
Mississippi Medical Center
2500 North State St.
Jackson, MS 39216
Bus.:   601-984-1675
Emer.: 601-354-7660
Fax: 601-984-1676

MISSOURI

KANSAS CITY
Poison Control Center,
Children's Mercy Hospital
2401 Gillham Rd.
Kansas City, MO 64108-4619
Bus.: 816-234-3053
Emer.: 816-234-3430
Fax: 816-234-3421

ST. LOUIS
Cardinal Glennon Children's Hospital
Regional Poison Center (*)
1465 South Grand Blvd.
St. Louis, MO 63104
Emer.: 800-366-8888 (MO)
314-772-5200
Fax: 314-577-5355

MONTANA

(DENVER, CO)
Rocky Mountain Poison and Drug
Center (*)
8802 E. 9th Ave.
Denver, CO 80220-6800
Emer.: 800-525-5042 (MT)
303-739-1123
Fax: 303-739-1119

NEBRASKA

OMAHA
The Poison Center (*)
Children's Hospital
8301 Dodge St.
Omaha, NE 68114
Emer.: 402-354-5555 (Omaha)
800-955-9119 (NE & WY)

NEVADA

(DENVER, CO)
Rocky Mountain Poison and Drug
Center (*)
8802 E. 9th Ave.
Denver, CO 80220-6800
Emer.: 800-446-6179 (NV)
303-739-1123
Fax: 303-739-1119

NEW HAMPSHIRE

LEBANON
New Hampshire Poison
Information Center, Dartmouth-
Hitchcock Medical Center
1 Medical Center Dr.
Lebanon, NH 03756
Emer.: 603-650-8000
(ask for Poison Center)
800-562-8236 (NH)
Fax: 603-650-8986

NEW JERSEY

NEWARK
New Jersey Poison Information
and Education System (*)
201 Lyons Ave.
Newark, NJ 07112
Bus.: 973-926-7443
Emer.: 800-764-7661 (NJ)
Fax: 973-705-8098

NEW MEXICO

ALBUQUERQUE
**New Mexico Poison and
Drug Information Center** (*)
University of New Mexico
Health Sciences Library, Rm. 125
Albuquerque, NM 87131-1076
Emer.: 505-272-2222
      800-432-6866 (NM)
Fax: 505-277-5892

NEW YORK

BUFFALO
**Western New York Regional
Poison Control Center** (*)
Children's Hospital of Buffalo
219 Bryant St.
Buffalo, NY 14222
Bus.: 716-878-7657
Emer.: 716-878-7654
      800-888-7655
      (NY Western Regions Only)

MINEOLA
**Long Island Regional Poison
Control Center** (*)
Winthrop University Hospital
259 First St.
Mineola, NY 11501
Emer.: 516-542-2323
      516-663-2650
TDD: 516-747-3323 (Nassau)
      516-924-8811 (Suffolk)
Fax: 516-739-2070

NEW YORK CITY
**New York City Poison Control
Center** (*)
NYC Dept. of Health
455 First Ave., Room 123
Box 81
New York, NY 10016
Bus.: 212-447-8154
Emer.: 800-210-3985
      212-340-4494
      212-POISONS
      212-VENENOS (Spanish)
TDD: 212-689-9014
Fax: 212-447-8223

ROCHESTER
**Finger Lakes Regional Poison
and Drug Information Center** (*)
**University of Rochester Medical
Center**
601 Elmwood Ave.
Box 321
Rochester, NY 14642
Bus.: 716-273-4155
Emer.: 716-275-3232
      800-333-0542 (NY)
TTY: 716-273-3854
Fax: 716-244-1677

SLEEPY HOLLOW
**Hudson Valley Regional Poison
Center** (*)
Phelps Memorial Hospital Center
701 N. Broadway
Sleepy Hollow, NY 10591
Emer.: 914-366-3030
      800-336-6997 (NY)
Fax: 914-353-1050

SYRACUSE
**Central New York Poison
Control Center** (*)
SUNY Health Science Center
750 East Adams St.
Syracuse, NY 13210
Bus.: 315-464-7073
Emer.: 315-476-4766
      800-252-5655 (NY)
Fax: 315-464-7077

NORTH CAROLINA

CHARLOTTE
Carolinas Poison Center (*)
Carolinas Medical Center
5000 Airport Center Pkwy.
Suite B
P.O. Box 32861
Charlotte, NC 28208
Bus.: 704-355-3054
Emer.: 704-355-4000
      800-848-6946 (NC)

NORTH DAKOTA

FARGO
North Dakota Poison Information
Center, Meritcare Medical Center
720 North 4th St.
Fargo, ND 58122
Bus.: 701-234-6062
Emer.: 701-234-5575
      800-732-2200 (ND, MN, SD)
Fax: 701-234-5090

OHIO

CINCINNATI
Cincinnati Drug and Poison
Information Center and Regional
Poison Control System (*)
2368 Victory Pkwy.
Suite 300
Cincinnati, OH 45206
Emer.: 513-558-5111
      800-872-5111 (OH)
Fax: 513-558-5301

CLEVELAND
Greater Cleveland Poison Control
Center
11100 Euclid Ave.
Cleveland, OH 44106-6010
Emer.: 216-231-4455
      888-231-4455 (OH)
Fax: 216-844-3242

COLUMBUS
Central Ohio Poison Center (*)
700 Children's Dr.
Room L032
Columbus, OH 43205-2696
Bus.: 614-722-2635
Emer.: 614-228-1323
      800-682-7625 (OH)
      800-762-0727 (Dayton only)
TTY: 614-222-2272
Fax: 614-221-2672

TOLEDO
Poison Information Center of NW
Ohio, Medical College of Ohio
Hospital
3000 Arlington Ave.
Toledo, OH 43614
Bus.: 419-383-3897
Emer.: 419-383-3897
      800-589-3897 (OH)
Fax: 419-383-6066

OKLAHOMA

OKLAHOMA CITY
Oklahoma Poison Control Center,
University of Oklahoma and
Children's Hospital of Oklahoma
940 Northeast 13th St.
Room 3512
Oklahoma City, OK 73104
Bus.: 405-271-5454
Emer.: 800-764-7661 (OK)
TTD: 405-271-1122
Fax: 405-271-1816

OREGON

PORTLAND
Oregon Poison Center (*)
Oregon Health Sciences University
3181 S.W. Sam Jackson Park Rd.
Portland, OR 97201
Emer.: 503-494-8968
       800-452-7165 (OR)
Fax: 503-494-4980

PENNSYLVANIA

HERSHEY
Central Pennsylvania
Poison Center (*)
University Hospital
Milton S. Hershey Medical Center
MC H043, P.O. Box 850
500 University Dr.
Hershey, PA 17033-0850
Emer.: 800-521-6110 (PA)
       717-531-6111
Fax: 717-531-6932

PHILADELPHIA
The Poison Control Center (*)
3535 Market St., Suite 985
Philadelphia, PA 19104-3309
Bus.: 215-590-2003
Emer.: 215-386-2100
       800-722-7112 (PA)
Fax: 215-590-4419

PITTSBURGH
Pittsburgh Poison Center (*)
Children's Hospital of Pittsburgh
3705 Fifth Ave.
Pittsburgh, PA 15213
Bus.: 412-692-5600
Emer.: 412-681-6669
Fax: 412-692-7497

PUERTO RICO

SANTURCE
San Jorge Children's
Hospital Poison Center
258 San Jorge St.
Santurce, PR 00912
Emer.: 787-726-5674

RHODE ISLAND

PROVIDENCE
Lifespan Poison Center (*)
Rhode Island Hospital
593 Eddy St.
Providence, RI 02903
Emer.: 401-444-5727
Fax: 401-444-8062

SOUTH CAROLINA

COLUMBIA
Palmetto Poison Center,
College of Pharmacy,
University of South Carolina
Columbia, SC 29208
Bus.: 803-777-7909
Emer.: 803-777-1117
       800-922-1117 (SC)
Fax: 803-777-6127

SOUTH DAKOTA

(FARGO, ND)
North Dakota Poison
Information Center
Meritcare Medical Center
720 North 4th St.
Fargo, ND 58122
Bus.: 701-234-6062
Emer.: 701-234-5575
        800-732-2200 (SD, MN, ND)
Fax: 701-234-5090

(MINNEAPOLIS, MN)
Hennepin Regional Poison
Center (*) Hennepin County
Medical Center
701 Park Ave.
Minneapolis, MN 55415
Bus.: 612-347-3144
Emer.: 800-764-7661 (MN, SD)
        612-347-3141
TTY: 612-904-4691

TENNESSEE

MEMPHIS
Southern Poison Center
847 Monroe Ave., Suite 104
Memphis, TN 38163
Bus.: 901-448-6800
Emer.: 901-528-6048
        800-288-9999 (TN)
Fax: 901-448-5419

NASHVILLE
Middle Tennessee Poison Center (*)
The Center for Clinical Toxicology,
Vanderbilt University Medical Center
1161 21st Ave. South
501 Oxford House
Nashville, TN 37232-4632
Bus.: 615-936-0760
Emer.: 615-936-2034
        800-288-9999 (TN)
TDD: 615-936-2047
Fax: 615-936-2046

TEXAS

AMARILLO
Texas Panhandle Poison Center
Northwest Texas Hospital
1501 S. Coulter Dr.
Amarillo, TX 79106
Emer.: 806-354-1000
        800-764-7661 (TX)

DALLAS
North Texas Poison Center (*)
5201 Harry Hines Blvd.
P.O. Box 35926
Dallas, TX 75235
Bus.: 214-590-6625
Emer.: 800-764-7661 (TX)
Fax: 214-590-5008

EL PASO
West Texas Regional
Poison Center (*)
Thomason Hospital
4815 Alameda Ave.
El Paso, TX 79905
Emer.: 800-764-7661 (TX)

GALVESTON
Southeast Texas Poison Center (*)
The University of Texas
Medical Branch
301 University Ave.
Galveston, TX 77555-1175
Bus.: 409-766-4403
Emer.: 800-764-7661 (TX)
Fax: 409-772-3917

SAN ANTONIO
South Texas Poison Center (*)
The University of Texas
Health Sciences Center
7703 Floyd Curl Dr., MC 7849
San Antonio, TX 78229-3900
Emer.: 210-567-5762
800-764-7661 (TX)
Fax: 210-567-5718

TEMPLE
Central Texas Poison Center (*)
Scott & White Memorial Hospital
2401 South 31st St.
Temple, TX 76508
Bus.: 254-724-4636
Emer.: 800-764-7661 (TX)
254-724-7401
Fax: 254-724-1731

UTAH

SALT LAKE CITY
Utah Poison Control Center (*)
410 Chipeta Way, Suite 230
Salt Lake City, UT 84108
Emer.: 801-581-2151
800-456-7707 (UT)
Fax: 801-581-4199

VERMONT

BURLINGTON
Vermont Poison Center,
Fletcher Allen Health Care
111 Colchester Ave.
Burlington, VT 05401
Bus.: 802-656-2721
Emer.: 802-658-3456
877-658-3456 (toll-free)
Fax: 802-656-4802

VIRGINIA

CHARLOTTESVILLE
Blue Ridge Poison Center (*)
University of Virginia Health
System
Box 437
Charlottesville, VA 22908
Emer.: 804-924-5543
800-451-1428 (VA)
Fax: 804-971-8657

RICHMOND
Virginia Poison Center (*)
Virginia Commonwealth University
P.O. Box 980522
Richmond, VA 23298-0522
Emer.: 804-828-9123
800-552-6337 (VA)
Fax: 804-828-5291

WASHINGTON

SEATTLE
Washington Poison Center (*)
155 N.E. 100th St.
Suite 400
Seattle, WA 98125-8012
Bus.: 206-517-2351
Emer.: 206-526-2121
       800-732-6985 (WA)
TDD: 800-572-0638
      206-517-2394
Fax: 206-526-8490

WEST VIRGINIA

CHARLESTON
West Virginia Poison Center (*)
3110 MacCorkle Ave. S.E.
Charleston, WV 25304
Bus.: 304-347-1212
Emer.: 304-348-4211
       800-642-3625 (WV)
Fax: 304-348-9560

WISCONSIN

MADISON
Poison Control Center, University
of Wisconsin Hospital and Clinics
600 Highland Ave., F6-133
Madison, WI 53792
Bus.: 608-262-7537
Emer.: 608-262-3702
       800-815-8855 (WI)

MILWAUKEE
Children's Hospital Poison Center,
Children's Hospital of Wisconsin
9000 W. Wisconsin Ave.
P.O. Box 1997
Milwaukee, WI 53201
Bus.: 414-266-2000
Emer.: 414-266-2222
       800-815-8855 (WI)
Fax: 414-266-2820

WYOMING

(OMAHA, NE)
The Poison Center (*)
Children's Hospital
8301 Dodge St.
Omaha, NE 68114
Emer.: 402-354-5555 (Omaha)
       800-955-9119 (WY, NE)

WASHINGTON

SEATTLE
Washington Poison Center (*)
155 N.E. 100th St.
Suite 400
Seattle, WA 98125-8012
Bus.: 206-517-2351
Emer.: 206-526-2121
800-732-6985 (WA)
TDD: 800-572-0638
206-517-2394
Fax: 206-526-8490

WEST VIRGINIA

CHARLESTON
West Virginia Poison Center (*)
3110 MacCorkle Ave. SE
Charleston, WV 25304
Bus.: 304-347-1212
Emer.: 304-348-4211
800-642-3625 (WV)
Fax: 304-348-9560

WISCONSIN

MADISON
Poison Center, University
of Wisconsin Hospital and Clinics
600 Highland Ave., F6-133
Madison, WI 53792
Bus.: 608-262-6527
Emer.: 800-262-3702
800-815-8855 (WI)

MILWAUKEE
Children's Hospital Poison Center
Children's Hospital of Wisconsin
9000 W. Wisconsin Ave.
P.O. Box 1997
Milwaukee, WI 53201
Bus.: 414-266-2000
Emer.: 414-266-2222
800-815-8855 (WI)
Fax: 414-266-2820

WYOMING

(OMAHA, NE)
The Poison Center (*)
Children's Hospital
8301 Dodge St.
Omaha, NE 68114
Emer.: 402-354-5555 (Omaha)
800-955-9119 (WY, NE)

Disease and Disorder Index

U se this index to find out which drugs are available for a specific medical problem. Both brand and generic names are listed; the generic names are shown in italics. Only brands covered in the drug profiles are included.

ReVia, 1122
Valium, 1385

Allergies, severe
Cyproheptadine. See Periactin
Decadron Tablets, 345
Deltasone, 357
Dexamethasone. See Decadron
  Tablets
Medrol, 762
Methylprednisolone. See Medrol
Orasone. *See* Deltasone
Pediapred, 960
Periactin, 982
Prednisolone Sodium Phosphate.
  See Pediapred
Prednisone. See Deltasone

Allergies, symptomatic relief of
Acrivastine with Pseudoephedrine.
  See Semprex-D
Allegra, 36
Astemizole. See Hismanal
Atarax, 104
Azatadine with Pseudoephedrine.
  See Trinalin Repetabs
Benadryl, 149
Budesonide. See Rhinocort
Cetirizine Hydrochloride.
  See Zyrtec
Claritin-D, 254
Clemastine. See Tavist
Cyproheptadine. See Periactin
Decadron Turbinaire and
  Respihaler, 349
Dexacort. See Decadron Turbinaire
  and Respihaler
Dexamethasone Sodium Phosphate.
  See Decadron Turbinaire and
  Respihaler
Diphenhydramine. See Benadryl
Fexofenadine Hydrochloride. See
  Allegra
Flonase. See Fluticasone

Fluticasone, 542
Hismanal, 590
Hydroxyzine. See Atarax
Loratadine with Pseudoephedrine.
  See Claritin-D
Periactin, 982
Phenergan, 990
Promethazine. See Phenergan
Rhinocort, 1129
Semprex-D, 1173
Tavist, 1259
Trinalin Repetabs, 1350
Vistaril. See Atarax
Zyrtec, 1494

Alzheimer's disease
Aricept, 84
Cognex, 274
Donepezil. See Aricept
Tacrine. See Cognex

Angina
Adalat. See Procardia
Amlodipine. See Norvasc
Atenolol. See Tenormin
Calan, 181
Cardene, 198
Cardizem, 205
Corgard, 294
Covera-HS. See Calan
Dilacor XR. See Cardizem
Diltiazem. See Cardizem
Imdur, 615
Inderal, 627
Ismo. See Imdur
Isoptin. See Calan
Isordil, 649
Isosorbide Dinitrate. See Isordil
Isosorbide Mononitrate. See
  Imdur
Lopressor, 718
Metoprolol. See Lopressor
Monoket. See Imdur
Nadolol. See Corgard

Nicardipine. See Cardene
Nifedipine. See Procardia
Nitro-Bid. See Nitroglycerin
Nitro-Dur. See Nitroglycerin
Nitroglycerin, 882
Nitrolingual Spray. See
    Nitroglycerin
Nitrostat Tablets. See Nitroglycerin
Norvasc, 910
Procardia, 1055
Propranolol. See Inderal
Sorbitrate. See Isordil
Tenormin, 1278
Transderm-Nitro. See Nitroglycerin
Verapamil. See Calan
Verelan. See Calan

Anxiety disorders
Alprazolam. See Xanax
Atarax, 104
Ativan, 107
BuSpar, 175
Buspirone. See BuSpar
Chlordiazepoxide. See Librium
Clorazepate. See Tranxene
Compazine, 286
Diazepam. See Valium
Equanil. See Miltown
Hydroxyzine. See Atarax
Librium, 694
Lorazepam. See Ativan
Meprobamate. See Miltown
Miltown, 804
Oxazepam. See Serax
Prochlorperazine. See
    Compazine
Serax, 1180
Stelazine, 1218
Tranxene, 1332
Trifluoperazine. See Stelazine
Valium, 1385
Vistaril. See Atarax
Xanax, 1436

Arthritis
Actron. See Orudis
Advil. See Motrin
Anaprox, 66
Ansaid, 72
Arava, 81
Arthrotec, 94
Aspirin, 98
Auranofin. See Ridaura
Azulfidine, 131
Cataflam. See Voltaren
Celebrex, 238
Celecoxib. See Celebrex
Choline Magnesium Trisalicylate.
    See Trilisate
Clinoril, 259
Cyclosporine. See Neoral
Daypro, 338
Decadron Tablets, 345
Deltasone, 357
Dexamethasone. See Decadron
    Tablets
Diclofenac. See Voltaren
Diclofenac and misoprostol. See
    Arthrotec
Diflunisal. See Dolobid
Disalcid, 418
Dolobid, 427
EC-Naprosyn. See Naprosyn
Ecotrin. See Aspirin
Empirin. See Aspirin
Enbrel, 474
Etanercept. See Enbrel
Etodolac. See Lodine
Feldene, 512
Flurbiprofen. See Ansaid
Genuine Bayer. See Aspirin
Hydroxychloroquine. See Plaquenil
Ibuprofen. See Motrin
Indocin, 635
Indomethacin. See Indocin
Ketoprofen. See Orudis
Leflunomide. See Arava
Lodine, 708

Simvastatin. *See* Zocor
Zocor

Heart attack, treatment of
Atenolol. See Tenormin
Inderal, 627
Lisinopril. See Zestril
Lopressor, 718
Mavik, 751
Metoprolol. See Lopressor
Prinivil. *See* Zestril
Propranolol. See Inderal
Tenormin, 1278
Trandolapril. See Mavik
Zestril, 1457

**Heartburn and related stomach
  problems**
Cimetidine. See Tagamet
Cisapride. See Propulsid
Famotidine. See Pepcid
Lansoprazole. See Prevacid
Metoclopramide. See Reglan
Pepcid, 975
Pepcid AC. *See* Pepcid
Prevacid, 1044
Propulsid, 1064
Reglan, 1099
Tagamet, 1240
Tagamet HB. *See* Tagamet

Heart failure, congestive
See also Fluid retention
Accupril, 3
Acetazolamide. See Diamox
Altace, 39
*Amiloride with Hydrochlorothiazide.
  See* Moduretic
Bumetanide. See Bumex
Bumex, 172
Capoten, 187
Captopril. See Capoten
Carvedilol. See Coreg
Coreg, 291

Diamox, 389
Digoxin. See Lanoxin
Enalapril. See Vasotec
Esidrix. See HydroDIURIL
Furosemide. See Lasix
Hydrochlorothiazide. See
  HydroDIURIL
HydroDIURIL, 601
Lanoxin, 669
Lasix, 673
Moduretic, 817
Quinapril. See Accupril
Ramipril. See Altace
Vasotec, 1395

Heart rhythms, abnormal
Acebutolol. See Sectral
Calan, 181
Cardioquin, 202
Digoxin. See Lanoxin
Disopyramide. See Norpace
Flecainide. See Tambocor
Inderal, 627
Isoptin. See Calan
Lanoxin, 669
Mexiletine. See Mexitil
Mexitil, 785
Norpace, 903
Procainamide. See Procan SR
Procanbid. See Procan SR
Procan SR, 1051
Pronestyl-SR. See Procan-SR
Propafenone. See Rythmol
Propranolol. See Inderal
Quinidex Extentabs, 1095
Quinidine Polygalacturonate. See
  Cardioquin
Quinidine Sulfate. See Quinidex
  Extentabs
Rythmol, 1161
Sectral, 1170
Tambocor, 1248
Tocainide. See Tonocard
Tonocard, 1322

Hives
*See Skin inflammations, swelling,
and redness*

Homocysteine levels, high